PA Review for the PANCE

PA Review for the PANCE

5TH EDITION

Julie J. Kinzel, MEd, PA-C
Assistant Clinical Professor
Physician Assistant Program
Drexel University
Philadelphia, Pennsylvania

Patrick C. Auth, PhD, PA-C
Clinical Professor
Physician Assistant Program
Drexel University
Philadelphia, Pennsylvania

Audio narration by **John T.K. Scherch,** MM Voice/Pedagogy,
Announcer/Producer, WBJC, Maryland's Classical Music Station

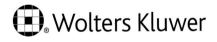

Philadelphia • Baltimore • New York • London
Buenos Aires • Hong Kong • Sydney • Tokyo

Acquisitions Editor: Matt Hauber
Development Editor: Andrea Vosburgh
Editorial Coordinator: Tim Rinehart
Marketing Manager: Phyllis Hitner
Production Project Manager: Barton Dudlick
Design Coordinator: Joan Wendt
Manufacturing Coordinator: Margie Orzech
Prepress Vendor: S4Carlisle Publishing Services

Fifth edition

Library of Congress Cataloging-in-Publication Data

Names: Kinzel, Julie J., editor. | Auth, Patrick C., editor.
Title: PA review for the PANCE / [edited by] Julie J. Kinzel, Patrick C. Auth.
Other titles: Physician assistant review
Description: Fifth edition. | Philadelphia, PA: Wolters Kluwer, [2020] |
    Preceded by: Physician assistant review / editor, Patrick C. Auth. 4th ed.
    c2013. | Includes bibliographical references and index.
Identifiers: LCCN 2019002887 | ISBN 9781496384188
Subjects: | MESH: Clinical Medicine | Physician Assistants | Examination
    Question | Outline
Classification: LCC R697.P45 | NLM WB 18.2 | DDC 610.76—dc23 LC record available at https://lccn.loc
    .gov/2019002887

shop.lww.com

PREFACE AND ACKNOWLEDGMENTS

This 5th edition of *PA Review for the PANCE* includes chapters written by a variety of experts in the PA field from across the United States and internationally. The content is aligned with the National Commission on Certification of Physician Assistants blueprint. The chapters have been revised to reflect current recommendations and practices. We included an expanded and updated online test bank and new end of chapter questions, all with rationales for the answers. The online question format allows readers to test their knowledge and focus on areas needing improvement.

The goal of this book is to prepare first-time PA board examination takers and recertifying examination takers to pass the examination on their first try. This book reviews primary care medical knowledge for physician assistants. It is organized into 21 chapters, which cover major body systems, disease etiology, pathology, epidemiology, signs and symptoms, physical examination findings, diagnostic studies, and management. The format is designed for easy reading using bullet points to highlight key concepts.

New with this edition is an accompanying audio component to the book. We designed a brief audio to permit the user to hear the most important content for each chapter. This allows for not only a test taker to hear the content in brief segments and return to the book for more detail at a later time, but also the busy practicing PA who will spend a short time listening to a quick topic review on a break or during a few minutes of free time.

This book has developed an excellent reputation over the years. The quality of this book is a result of the commitment of the contributors who are leaders in their field. I would like to thank each of the chapter contributors who devoted their time and talent to the PA profession and education of PAs. I especially would like to thank my coeditor, Dr. Patrick Auth, for his guidance and leadership. Without his drive and expertise, this book would not have been a reality. I am grateful to the team at Wolters Kluwer for their patience and editorial assistance throughout this process.

Julie J. Kinzel
Patrick C. Auth

CONTRIBUTORS

Adrian Andrews, DHSc, PA-C
Director
Physician Assistant Program
South University
Royal Palm Beach, Florida

Patrick C. Auth, PhD, PA-C
Clinical Professor
Physician Assistant Department
College of Nursing and Health Profession
Drexel University
Philadelphia, Pennsylvania

Matt Dane Baker, DHSc
Provost
Philadelphia University and Thomas Jefferson University
Philadelphia, Pennsylvania

Michael C. Barros, PharmD
Clinical Associate Professor
Department of Pharmacy Practice
Temple University School of Pharmacy
Philadelphia, Pennsylvania

Petar Breitinger, MPAS, PA-C, DFAAPA
Assistant Professor
School of Physician Assistant Studies
University of Florida
Gainesville, Florida

Lawrence P. Carey, PharmD
Associate Chair
Department of Pharmacy Practice
Temple University School of Pharmacy
Philadelphia, Pennsylvania

Daniela Cheles-Livingston, MD, PA-C
Assistant Clinical Professor
Physician Assistant Department
College of Nursing and Health Profession
Drexel University
Philadelphia, Pennsylva

Ryan J. Clancy, MSHS, PA-C
Clinical Instructor
Physician Assistant Department
College of Nursing and Health Profession
Drexel University
Philadelphia, Pennsylvania

Jesse Coale, MDiv, PA-C
Program Director
Associate Professor
Department of Physician Assistant Studies
Philadelphia University + Thomas Jefferson University
Philadelphia, Pennsylvania

Randi Beth Cooperman, DHSc, MCMSc, PA-C
Program Director
Physician Assistant Program
Barry University
Delray Beach, Florida

Rosalie G. Coppola, MHS, PA-C
Associate Clinical Professor
Physician Assistant Department
College of Nursing and Health Profession
Drexel University
Philadelphia, Pennsylvania

Eric Cucchi, MS, PA-C
Clinical Assistant Professor
Physician Assistant Studies
Bay Path University
Longmeadow, Massachusetts

Valerie Damon-Leduc, MA
Program Coordinator
Center for Learning and Academic Success Services
Drexel University
Philadelphia, Pennsylvania

Ellen D. Feld, MD
Clinical Professor Medical Director
PA Program
Drexel University College of Nursing and
    Health Professions
Philadelphia, Pennsylvania

Justine Filippelli, PA-C
Physician Assistant
Department of Surgery
Cleveland Clinic
Cleveland, Ohio

Ilaria Gadalla, MS, PA-C
Director of Clinical Education
South University
Royal Palm Beach, Florida

Juanita Gardner, MPH, PA-C
Assistant Clinical Professor
Physician Assistant Department
College of Nursing and Health Profession
Drexel University
Philadelphia, Pennsylvania

Abigail Gonnella, PA-C
Surgical Physician Assistant
Department of Surgery
Cleveland Clinic
Avon, Ohio

Michelle L. Heinan, EdD, PA-C
Program Director
Physician Assistant Studies
Concordia University
Mequon, Wisconsin

Janina Iwaszko, BSc, MSc, PhD, MBChB, MMed Ed
PA Course Director
Institute of Health and Society
University of Worcester
Worcester, United Kingdom

Jennifer Keat-Wysocki, PA-C
Physician Assistant
Trauma/Surgery
Capital Health Regional Medical Center
Asbury, New Jersey

Colleen M. Kennedy, MD, FACEP
Emergency Department
Chair and Medical Director
Lehigh Valley Hospital-Pocono
East Stroudsburg, Pennsylvania

Julie J. Kinzel, MEd, PA-C
Assistant Clinical Professor
Physician Assistant Program
Drexel University
Philadelphia, Pennsylvania

Tanya Konyesni, PA-C
Physician Assistant
Orthopedic Surgery
Cleveland Clinic
Medina, Ohio

Julie Le, PA-C
Physician Assistant
Trauma/Surgery
Capital Health Regional Medical Center
Philadelphia, Pennsylvania

Michael A. Mancano, PharmD
Clinical Professor
Temple University School of Pharmacy
Philadelphia, Pennsylvania

Lindsay Matias, MA
Assistant Director
Center for Learning and Academic Success Services
Drexel University
Philadelphia, Pennsylvania

Ann McDonugh Madden, MHS, PA-C
Clinical Assistant Professor
Physician Assistant Department
College of Nursing and Health Profession
Drexel University
Philadelphia, Pennsylvania

Nina Multak, PhD, MPAS, PA-C, DFAAPA
Clinical Associate Professor
Physician Assistant Department
College of Nursing and Health Profession
Drexel University
Philadelphia, Pennsylvania

Scott Naples, PA-C
Physician Assistant
Mid-Ohio Emergency Services
Columbus, Ohio

Catherine Nowak, MS, PA-C, DFAAPA
Clinical Associate Professor
Director of Clinical Education
Physician Assistant Department
College of Nursing and Health Profession
Drexel University
Philadelphia, Pennsylvania

Sonia V. Otte, MMS, PA-C
Director of Pre-Clinical Education
South University
Royal Palm Beach, Florida

Elizabeth Quinlan-Bohn, MS, PA-C
Clinical Assistant Professor
Physician Assistant Department
D'Youville University
Buffalo, New York

Theresa Riethle, MS, PA-C
Program Director
Physician Assistant
Bay Path University
East Longmeadow, Massachusetts

Robin Risling, MHS, PA-C
Assistant Professor
Physician Assistant Studies
University of South Alabama
Mobile, Alabama

Allison S. Rusgo, MPH, PA-C
Clinical Assistant Professor
Physician Assistant Department
College of Nursing and Health Profession
Drexel University
Philadelphia, Pennsylvania

Parmjeet S. Saini, DHsc, MPA, PA-C
Public Health Analyst
York College
Jamaica, New York

Megan Schneider, MMS, MSPH, PA-C
Clinical Instructor
Physician Assistant Department
College of Nursing and Health Profession
Drexel University
Philadelphia, Pennsylvania

William R. Short, MD, MPH
Associate Professor of Medicine
University of Pennsylvania
Philadelphia, Pennsylvania

Rebecca Signore, MA
Director
Center for Learning and Academic Success Services
Drexel University
Philadelphia, Pennsylvania

Diana Smith, MHS, PA-C
Assistant Clinical Professor
Physician Assistant Department
College of Nursing and Health Profession
Drexel University
Philadelphia, Pennsylvania

Charles Stream, MPH, PA-C
Clinical Assistant Professor
Physician Assistant Department
College of Nursing and Health Profession
Drexel University
Philadelphia, Pennsylvania

Jacqueline A. Theodorou, PharmD, BCPS
Clinical Assistant Professor
Temple University School of Pharmacy
Philadelphia, Pennsylvania

Michele Zawora, MD
Chair
Department of Physician Assistant Studies
Philadelphia University + Thomas Jefferson University
Philadelphia, Pennsylvania

QUESTION WRITERS

Victoria Coppola, MHS, PA-C
Nemours Children's Hospital
Wilmington, Delaware

Laura Jennings, MHS, PA-C
Stoltz and Hahn Medical Associates
Feasterville-Trevose, Pennsylvania

Claire Pisoni, MPAS, PA-C
Clinical Instructor
Physician Assistant Department
College of Nursing and Health Professions
Philadelphia, Pennsylvania

Estelle Whitney, MD, FACOG
Center for Advanced Gynecology and Minimally
    Invasive Surgery
Christiana Care Health Services
Newark, Delaware

Justin Allen Wolfe, MHS, PA-C
Clinical Instructor
Physician Assistant Program
College of Nursing and Health Professions
Drexel University
Philadelphia, Pennsylvania

CONTENTS

16 Infectious Diseases 396

William R. Short

17 Surgery Disorders 424

Abigail Gonnella • Randi Beth Cooperman • Justine Filippelli •
Jennifer Keat-Wysocki • Tanya Konyesni • Julie Le • Scott Naples

18 Preventive Medicine 461

Parmjeet S. Saini • Patrick C. Auth

19 Study and Test-Taking Strategies 478

Rebecca Signore • Lindsay Matias • Valerie Damon-Leduc

20 Pharmacology 481

Lawrence P. Carey • Michael C. Barros • Michael A. Mancano •
Jacqueline A. Theodorou

21 Pediatric Care and Common Disorders . . 510

Petar Breitinger

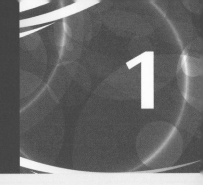

Renal and Urinary Tract Disorders

Eric Cucchi • Theresa Riethle

I. Urethritis

A. Etiology

- Urethral inflammation due to infectious or noninfectious causes.
- Most commonly associated with sexually transmitted infections.
- Urethritis is classified as gonococcal or nongonococcal.
- Nonsexually transmitted cases are most commonly seen in diabetics; organisms vary.
- Noninfectious causes include reactive arthritis as seen in Reiter syndrome.
- Posttraumatic urethritis can occur in patients practicing intermittent catheterization.

B. Pathology

- Acute inflammation of the urethra.
- Concurrent infection with several organisms is common.
- Most common.
  - Gonococcal urethritis.
    - Incubation period is between 2 and 7 days.
    - Coinfection *Chlamydia* is present in 30% to 40% of cases.
  - Nongonococcal urethritis.
    - Incubation period is 7 to 14 days.
    - *Chlamydia trachomatis* is present in 50% of cases.
  - Other common etiologic agents include *E. Coli, C. trachomatis, Ureaplasma urealyticum,* and *Trichomonas vaginalis.*

C. Clinical Features

1. Gonococcal Urethritis

- Men—Dysuria with discharge, discharge yellowish/green.
- Women—Dysuria, urinary frequency, and urgency less commonly with urethral discharge, possible dyspareunia. Symptoms can be worse with menses.
- Asymptomatic infection may occur in men and women.
- Fever, rash, tenosynovitis, conjunctivitis, and arthritis can be seen with disseminated disease.
- Complications—stricture, abscesses, fistula.

2. Nongonococcal Urethritis

- Men—Dysuria, associated with clear-to-white, scanty discharge.
- Women infected with *Chlamydia* may be asymptomatic or may have symptoms of cervicitis or pelvic inflammatory disease.
- Asymptomatic infection may occur in men and women.

D. Diagnostic Studies

- General.
  - Often clinical diagnosis.
  - Urinalysis.
  - Urine culture.
- Gonococcal urethritis.
  - Gram stain of discharge reveals intracellular gram-negative diplococci that may be seen in a smear or cultured from an infected site.
  - If Gram stain is inconclusive, culture on Thayer–Martin medium is recommended.
- Nongonococcal urethritis.
  - Gram stain shows no organisms.
  - Culture is reliable, but difficult and expensive.
  - Nucleic acid amplification of urine or cervical/urethral samples is recommended and diagnosis confirmed whenever possible.
  - Historically, diagnosis was often made clinically and by exclusion and presumptive treatment was administered.
  - Wet prep of discharge—may show *Trichomonas.*

E. Management

1. Gonococcal Urethritis

- In uncomplicated situations, ceftriaxone, 125 mg intramuscular, is the treatment of choice.
- Also treat for concurrent chlamydial infection with azithromycin 1 g orally as a single dose, or doxycycline (100 mg BID × 7 days).
- Treat partners.

2. Nongonococcal Urethritis

- Chlamydial infection and infection by *Ureaplasma* respond to azithromycin 1 g orally as a single dose, or doxycycline (100 mg BID × 7 days).
- If gonorrhea and chlamydia excluded, trimethoprim/sulfamethoxazole or fluoroquinolone may be used.

- Erythromycin, 500 mg four times a day for 7 days, is appropriate for pregnant women or patients allergic to tetracycline.
- Infection caused by *Trichomonas* responds to Flagyl (metronidazole)—2 g orally as a single dose or 250 mg TID × 7 days.
- In all cases, sexual partners also should be treated.
- Education of patients in prevention and safe sex practices is essential.

II. Cystitis
A. Etiology
- Typically ascending infection primarily due to coliform bacteria (especially *Escherichia coli*) and, occasionally, gram-positive bacteria (enterococci).
- Female predominance secondary to anatomy.
- Owing to the longer and protected urethra in men, cystitis in men may imply a pathologic process requiring further investigation.
- Risk factors include diabetes mellitus (DM), use of an indwelling catheter, obstruction, use of a diaphragm or spermicide, neurogenic bladder, pregnancy, immunocompromised state, and underlying anatomic abnormalities of the urinary tract.

B. Pathology
- In general, genitourinary (GU) tract infections occur as a result of ascension of the infecting agent up the urethra.
- Hematogenous spread is uncommon.

C. Clinical Features
- Dysuria, urinary frequency, urgency, burning, and sensation of incomplete bladder emptying are common.
- Hematuria or cloudy urine.
- Suprapubic discomfort.
- In women, symptoms may often appear after sexual intercourse.
- Physical examination is often unremarkable.
- Signs of systemic involvement (e.g., fever, nausea, or vomiting) are absent.

D. Diagnostic Studies
- Urinalysis discloses pyuria and bacteriuria with or without hematuria.
- Urine culture demonstrating bacteria >10^5 bacteria per mL confirms diagnosis.
- Additional or follow-up studies are warranted only with certain populations (children, men) recurrent infections, suspicion of anatomic abnormalities, or if pyelonephritis is suspected.

E. Management
1. Acute Uncomplicated Cystitis
- Antibiotics are appropriate to the causative agent.
  - A 3-day course of fluoroquinolones or nitrofurantoin is the recommended treatment.

- Trimethoprim/sulfamethoxazole (TMP/SMX) may be ineffective secondary to resistant organisms.
- Postcoital cystitis may require prompt voiding followed by a single dose of TMP/SMX or ciprofloxacin.
- Pregnant patients require 10- to 14-day treatment with pregnancy-safe antibiotic such as cephalexin or amoxicillin.
- Urinary analgesics (phenazopyridine, 200 mg orally three times daily), sitz baths, and fluids may provide symptomatic relief.
- Owing to the infrequent occurrence of uncomplicated cystitis in men, additional investigation is warranted and treatment is targeted to the underlying etiology.

2. Prevention for Women
- Increase fluids.
- Urinate after intercourse.
- Avoid use of spermicides.
- Postmenopausal women may need estrogen cream or suppositories.

III. Pyelonephritis
A. Etiology
- Ascending, infectious, inflammatory disease of the renal parenchyma and pelvis.
- Risk factors include underlying urinary tract abnormalities, nephrolithiasis, DM, immunocompromised conditions, elderly institutionalized women, and episode of acute pyelonephritis within the previous year.

B. Pathology
- Infection ascends from lower urinary tract, uncommonly from bacteria in bloodstream.
- Most common etiologic agents are gram-negative bacteria including *E. coli*, *Proteus*, *Klebsiella*, *Enterobacter*, and *Pseudomonas*.
- Gram-positive organisms are seen less commonly and include *Streptococcus faecalis* (enterococci) and *Staphylococcus aureus* (hematogenous route).

C. Clinical Features
- Patient presents with symptoms of fever, chills, flank, or back pain.
- Nausea, vomiting, and loose stool are also common.
- Irritative voiding symptoms are often present or were present before systemic symptoms.
- Physical examination may disclose costovertebral tenderness, fever, and tachycardia.

D. Diagnostic Studies
- Urinalysis discloses pyuria, bacteriuria with or without hematuria, and possibility of white blood cell (WBC) casts.
- Urine culture demonstrates specific offending agent.
- Complete blood count (CBC) typically shows a leukocytosis with a left shift.

- Blood cultures may be positive if sepsis suspected.
- Renal ultrasound (U/S) may reveal hydronephrosis or obstruction in complicated pyelonephritis.
- Computed tomography (CT) scanning is used if failure to respond to treatment or complicating factors are present.

E. Management
- Treat underlying organism.
- In the outpatient setting, fluoroquinolones or TMP/SMX may be initiated for 1 to 2 weeks.
- In patients in whom complicating factors or evidence of severe infection is present, hospital admission is required.
  - IV ampicillin and gentamycin or fluoroquinolones are administered until fever free for 24 hours.
  - Upon discharge, patients are converted to appropriate oral antibiotic therapy to complete a 2- to 3-week course.
- Follow-up urine cultures may be required after the completion of treatment.
- For repeat infections, further workup may be required.

IV. Nephrolithiasis
A. Etiology
- Calculi in the urinary tract.
- Major types of urinary stones.
  - Calcium oxalate/calcium phosphate—85% of stones.
  - Magnesium ammonium phosphate (or struvite)
  - Uric acid.
  - Cystine.
- Men are affected more frequently than women, in the ratio of 3:1.
- A medical history of gout uric acid, chronic urinary tract infections (UTIs), and chronic diarrhea or family history of renal calculi increases the risk of stone development.
- **Commonly used medications may increase the risk of stone formation:**
  - Antacids and carbonic anhydrase inhibitors may raise urinary pH, which facilitates calcium phosphate stone precipitation.
  - Calcium-containing antacids may increase the amount of calcium ingested and subsequently filtered by the kidney.
  - Loop diuretics may cause increased urinary calcium concentrations leading to an oversaturation state.
  - Large doses of vitamin C can result in hyperoxaluria in some patients because ascorbic acid is oxidized to oxalate.
- **Dietary factors have a significant effect on stone formation:**
  - Metabolic acidosis secondary to animal protein metabolism leads to an increased filtered load of calcium and a decrease in tubular calcium reabsorption and hypercalciuria.

- Meats and other purine-containing foods also augment uric acid excretion, increasing both calcium-based and uric acid stones.
- Thiazide diuretics and alcohol may increase the risk of uric acid stones.
- Oxalate-rich foods (green leafy vegetables, such as kale, spinach, mustard greens; nuts; tea; coffee) contribute to calcium oxalate nephrolithiasis.

B. Pathology
- Stones develop as the result of growth of crystalline components in a supersaturated urine.
- Hypercalciuria is present in 40% to 60% of calcium stone formers.
- **Secondary causes include:**
  - Hyperparathyroidism, hyperthyroidism, Cushing syndrome, granulomatous diseases (sarcoidosis, tuberculosis, disseminated candidiasis), immobilization, vitamin D intoxication, rapidly progressive bone disease.

C. Clinical Features
- Often asymptomatic when tiny.
- Patient may complain of sharp, colicky flank pain with radiation to the testicle or labia.
- Associated fever, chills, nausea, or vomiting may be present.
- Urinary symptoms include frequency and urgency, with or without dysuria.
- Hematuria.

D. Diagnostic Studies
1. **Acute Stone Disease**
   - Urinalysis may disclose microscopic or gross hematuria, pyuria, bacteriuria, crystals, and altered pH.
     - pH persistently <5.0 is correlated with uric acid or cystine stones.
     - pH persistently >7.2 is suggestive of struvite stones.
   - Noncontrast spiral CT is a test of choice and identifies radiopaque and radiolucent stones.
   - Other laboratory studies.
     - CBC demonstrates an elevated WBC if infection is present.
     - Electrolytes may show hypokalemia, hypercalcemia, and metabolic acidosis.
     - Uric acid may be elevated.
     - Creatinine may be elevated with bilateral obstruction or unilateral obstruction in a patient with one kidney.
   - Radiograph—kidney, ureter, and bladder.
     - Radiopaque stones are visible—calcium and struvite.
     - Radiolucent stones are not visible—uric acid and cystine.
   - Renal U/S can demonstrate the presence of stones and hydronephrosis secondary to obstruction.

Abdominal, transvaginal, or transrectal U/S can aid in identifying calculi in the ureterovesicular junction.
- Stone analysis should be performed on recovered stones.

2. Chronic Stone Disease
- Analysis of stones.
- Urinalysis to determine pH.
- Parathyroid hormone (PTH) level if calcium is elevated.
- Serum calcium, phosphate, and uric acid.
- Qualitative test for urinary cystine.
- Twenty-four-hour urine collection on a random diet to ascertain volume, urinary pH and calcium, uric acid, oxalate phosphate, and citrate excretion. A second collection on a restricted calcium and sodium diet is undertaken to subcategorize patients.

E. Management

1. Acute Stone Disease
- Initial management includes fluids and analgesia. Most stones <5 mm pass spontaneously.
- Stones of 5- to 10-mm size may need to be removed in the presence of intractable pain, severe obstruction, serious bleeding, or infection.
- Stones >10 mm may require inpatient treatment and removal.
- Extraction or stent placement via cystoscopy.
- Shock-wave lithotripsy or percutaneous nephrolithotomy.

2. Chronic Stone Disease
- Asymptomatic calculi need not be treated. They should be followed with serial abdominal radiographs or renal ultrasound. If stones become symptomatic or grow, treatment should be instituted.
- Treatment of any underlying disorder.
- Increased fluid intake is of great importance.

V. Ureteral Stones

A. Etiology
- See Nephrolithiasis.

B. Pathology
- Renal calculi may become lodged in the ureter, which interferes with the effect of peristalsis and leads to impediment of urine flow.
- Ureteral stones typically become lodged at three sites—(1) ureteropelvic junction, (2) crossing of the ureter over the iliac vessels, and (3) ureterovesical junction.
- Stones <5 mm in diameter frequently pass spontaneously.

C. Clinical Features
- See Nephrolithiasis.
- Fever in association with an upper urinary tract obstruction is a medical emergency.

D. Diagnostic Studies
- Urinalysis.
- Abdominal radiographs.
- Abdominal, transvaginal, or transrectal U/S.
- Noncontrast spiral CT.

E. Management
- Conservative observation with appropriate pain medication for up to 6 weeks. Indications for intervention earlier than 6 weeks include fever, persistent nausea and vomiting, severe pain, or unresponsiveness to medications.
- Distal ureteral stones respond to in situ extracorporeal shock-wave lithotripsy or ureteroscopic stone extraction.

VI. Urinary Incontinence

A. Etiology
- Multiple etiologies.
- Detrusor muscle hyperactivity = urge incontinence – most common.
- Outflow obstruction = overflow incontinence – least common.
- Urethral incompetence = stress incontinence.
- Cognitive impairment (physical or environmental barriers) = functional incontinence.
- May have mixed incontinence.
- Neurogenic bladder, loss of central nervous system (CNS) control.
- Risk factors include increasing age, female gender, multiparity, prostatic hypertrophy, dementia/spinal cord injury, multiple sclerosis, stroke, and diabetes.

B. Pathology
- Mechanical.
  - Pelvic muscle weakness.
  - Obstruction.
  - Spasm.
- Increased urine volume.
  - Involuntary loss of urine from the bladder.
  - The amount of urine lost can vary greatly.
- Typically comes to medical attention when it is perceived as a social and/or health problem by the patient or patient's family.

C. Clinical Features
- Depends on the type of incontinence.
- Involuntary loss of urine, urgency, dysuria, and perineal irritation.
- Physical examination may disclose distended bladder, and digital rectal examination may show prostatic hypertrophy.
- In addition, identifying neuropsychiatric disease, impaired mobility, or pharmaceutical issues is essential.
- In women, vaginal speculum examination and bimanual pelvic examination may disclose GU pathology.

D. Diagnostic Studies
- Urinalysis is typically normal, but may show glycosuria, proteinuria, WBCs, red blood cells (RBCs), or bacteria.
- Urodynamic testing.
  - Voiding cystogram may disclose bladder or urethral pathology.
  - Cystogram may disclose abnormal sphincter pressure or bladder physiology.
  - Postvoiding residual measurement may show increased residual urine.
    - If a postvoid residual is >150 mL in a male, a renal ultrasound is required to rule out hydronephrosis.

E. Management
- General measures.
  - Treat underlying etiology.
  - Modifying fluid intake.
- Specific.
  - Detrusor instability—bladder training and Kegel exercises.
    - Medications—oxybutynin or tolterodine (antimuscarinic agents).
  - Urethral incompetence—lifestyle modifications, Kegel exercises, and biofeedback.
    - Drug therapy is limited to trials with pseudoephedrine or duloxetine.
  - Bladder suspension surgery is a last resort but most effective.
  - Outflow obstruction—intermittent or indwelling catheterization.
    - Medication—bethanechol (Urecholine).
  - Overflow obstruction due to prostatic enlargement—intermittent or indwelling catheterization, electrical stimulation, and surgery.
    - Medications—prazosin (Minipress), terazosin, and finasteride (Proscar).
  - Cognitive impairment—direct treatment to underlying impairment.

VII. Cystic Diseases of the Kidney
A. Etiology
- Simple cysts or solitary cysts.
  - Account for up to 70% of all renal masses, must rule abscess, malignancy, or polycystic kidney disease.
- Medullary sponge kidney.
  - Autosomal dominant.
  - Common, benign disorder, present at birth, diagnosed in fourth or fifth decade.
  - Mutations in the *MCKD*1 or *MCKD*2 genes on chromosomes 1 and 16.
- Autosomal recessive polycystic kidney disease (ARPKD):
  - Rare. Occurs in 1 in 20,000 live births. Diagnosed in utero or in neonatal period.

- Autosomal dominant polycystic kidney disease (ADPKD):
  - ADPKD1—Defective gene on the short arm of chromosome 16 in 85% to 90% of cases.
  - ADPKD2—Defect on chromosome 4 in 10% to 15% of cases. Slower progression with longer life expectancy.
  - Age at onset is between 20 and 40 years.
  - Among the five leading causes of renal failure in adults, accounting for 10% of dialysis patients in the United States.

B. Pathology
- Renal cysts are epithelium-lined cavities filled with fluid or semisolid material that develop primarily from renal tubular elements.
- They are noted in isolated areas in the cortex, medulla, and interpapillary collecting ducts depending on the type of cystic kidney disease.
- One or more simple cysts are common in people >50 years of age.
- Generalized cystic diseases are associated with cysts scattered throughout the cortex and medulla of both the kidneys and can progress to end-stage renal disease (ESRD).

C. Clinical Features
- Simple or solitary cysts:
  - Usually asymptomatic, present on routine urographic examination.
- Medullary cystic disease:
  - Gross or microscopic hematuria, recurrent UTIs, or nephrolithiasis.
- ARPKD.
  - Presentation highly variable based on when disease is detected.
- ADPKD.
  - Abdominal or flank pain associated with hematuria and hypertension.
  - Extrarenal manifestations may include cerebral "berry" aneurysms, hepatic cysts, valvular heart disease, and colonic diverticula.
  - Positive family history may be obtained in the majority of patients.
  - Hypertension is present in <50% of the patients.
  - Palpable kidneys.

D. Diagnostic Studies
- Simple or solitary cysts
  - Concern is to differentiate from a malignant renal mass.
  - U/S and CT are recommended procedures for evaluation.
  - Both simple and complex cysts should be reevaluated periodically.
- Medullary sponge kidney.
  - Intravenous pyelogram (IVP)—which shows striations in the papillary portions, which represent the

accumulation of contrast in the dilated collecting ducts.
- ARPDK.
  - U/S reveals large echogenic kidneys.
- Polycystic kidneys.
  - Urinalysis may show hematuria and mild proteinuria.
  - Diagnosis is confirmed by U/S.
  - CT or MRI is recommended if sonogram is equivocal or to detect presymptomatic disease.

E. Management
- Simple cysts.
  - Benign cysts require observation and periodic reappraisal. If the cysts change, surgical exploration or percutaneous biopsy is recommended.
- Medullary sponge kidney.
  - No known treatment; provide supportive care, including adequate fluid intake and thiazide diuretics if hypercalciuria is present.
- ARPKD.
  - No specific therapy. Advances in neonatal management and kidney transplant have led to survival into adulthood.
- ADPDK.
  - Treatment is supportive including controlling hypertension, adequate fluid intake, dialysis, and transplantation if warranted.

VIII. Renovascular Hypertension

A. Etiology
- Renal artery stenosis is a common cause of secondary hypertension.
- May be due to atherosclerotic narrowing of one or both renal arteries.
- In Caucasian women younger than 50 years, may be due to fibromuscular hyperplasia (or fibrous dysplasia).

B. Pathology
- Excessive renin release due to reduction of renal blood flow and perfusion pressure.

C. Clinical Features
- May present in a manner similar to essential hypertension, but should be considered under the following circumstances:
  - Onset below age 20.
  - Hypertension is resistant to three or more drugs.
  - Stable hypertension that suddenly gets worse or is difficult to control.
  - Sudden-onset renal disease.
  - In the presence of renal artery or epigastric bruits.
  - If concomitant atherosclerosis is present.
  - Abrupt deterioration in renal function after the administration of angiotensin-converting enzyme (ACE) inhibitors.

D. Diagnostic Studies
- Renal arteriography is the definitive test and is suggested when suspicion is high.
  - Can be therapeutic for stent placement or angiography if needed.
- Noninvasive angiography through MRI/MRA or CT/CTA if moderate to low suspicion.
- Doppler sonography is playing an increasing role in detection and monitoring for progression; technician dependent.

E. Management
- Therapy is aimed at controlling the blood pressure (BP) and preserving the glomerular filtration rate (GFR).
- Medical therapy includes the use of ACE inhibitors, angiotension II receptor blockers (ARBs), and diuretics in most patients.
- Surgical management includes angioplasty with or without stent placement.
- In rare cases, renal bypass surgery is indicated in patients with severe, uncontrolled hypertension or in those with inevitable risk of losing a kidney due to ischemia.
- Close follow-up and monitoring is essential.

IX. Acute Kidney Injury

A. Etiology
- Prerenal.
  - Forty percent to 80% of acute renal injury (AKI) cases.
  - Failure of appropriate kidney perfusion.
- Intrinsic.
  - Up to 50% of AKI cases.
  - Acute tubular necrosis (ATN), acute interstitial nephritis (AIN), acute glomerulonephritis (AGN).
- Postrenal.
  - Five percent to 10% of ARI cases.
  - Obstruction.

B. Pathology
- An abrupt decrease in GFR, which results in the retention of nitrogenous wastes.

C. Clinical Features
- Typically, nonspecific.
- Symptoms and physical examination is variable based on the etiology and severity of AKI.
- Early.
  - Water retention, edema, decreased urine output.
- Late.
  - Fatigue, anorexia, nausea, pruritus.

D. Diagnostic Studies
- Serum blood chemistries for elevations of blood urea nitrogen (BUN), creatinine (although not specific for acute vs. chronic renal failure), hyperkalemia, hyperuricemia, hyperphosphatemia, and hypocalcemia.

- Urine analysis is a key initial test.
- **Prerenal.**
  - Increased specific gravity and hyaline casts. High osmolality and urea. Decreased urine sodium.
- **Intrinsic.**
  - AGN and vascular causes—proteinuria, hematuria, and RBC casts. In AIN: WBCs, eosinophils, and WBC casts. ATN: low urine specific gravity, high urine sodium, and "muddy brown casts."
  - Pigmented casts are seen in rhabdomyolysis and hemolysis.
- **Postrenal.**
  - Values can vary based on the duration of the obstruction.
- Special tests.
  - U/S is helpful to evaluate postrenal causes of ARI.
  - CT, MRI, and magnetic resonance angiography are useful adjuvant testing modalities to evaluate underlying causes of ARI.
  - Renal biopsy may be diagnostic for patients where the cause of intrinsic renal failure is not clear.

E. Management
- Prerenal.
  - Volume repletion with appropriate fluids ± blood products.
  - Occasional use of short-term dialysis until renal function restored.
- Intrinsic.
  - ATN—Diuresis, correct electrolyte disorders, nutritional support with low-protein diet.
  - AIN—Supportive measures with removal of inciting agent, corticosteroids, short-term dialysis.
  - AGN—high-dose corticosteroids, cytotoxic agents, and/or plasmapheresis.
- Postrenal.
  - Identify location of obstruction and treat definitively.
- All causes of ARI may need short-term dialysis treatment.

X. Chronic Kidney Disease

A. Etiology
- The result of renal pathology that interferes with renal excretory and regulatory function on a chronic basis.
- The major causes of chronic kidney disease (CKD) include glomerulopathies (diabetic nephropathy), tubulointerstitial nephritis (drug hypersensitivity), hereditary diseases (polycystic kidney disease), obstructive nephropathies (prostate disease), and vascular disease (hypertension).

B. Pathology
- Progressive and irreversible deterioration of renal function caused by a variety of diseases over a period of 3 months or longer.

- The underlying primary disease is often difficult to identify when advanced renal failure is diagnosed.
- The two most common causes of CKD include DM and systemic hypertension.
- Laboratory manifestations of CKD may not occur until ≥40% of renal function is lost, and clinical manifestations may not occur until ≥80% of renal function is lost.
- The following are the five stages of CKD:
  - Stage 1—slight kidney damage with normal or increased filtration, GFR >90.
  - Stage 2—mild decrease in kidney function, GFR 60 to 89.
  - Stage 3—moderate decrease in kidney function, GFR 30 to 59.
  - Stage 4—severe decrease in kidney function, GFR 15 to 29.
  - Stage 5—kidney failure, GFR <15 or dialysis.

C. Clinical Features
- Symptoms are nonspecific, but include:
  - Malaise, metallic taste, pruritis, easy bruising, edema, shortness of breath, dyspnea, orthopnea, nausea, vomiting, anorexia, restless legs, altered mental status, and irritability.
  - Physical examination may reveal hypertension, pallor or jaundice, cachexia, edema, asterixis, uremic fetor, and muscle wasting.

D. Diagnostic Studies
- Laboratory evaluation is divided into two categories:
  - Evaluate the etiology of CKD.
  - Monitor the progression of CKD.
- Evaluation includes serial measurements of serum creatinine, urinary protein excretion, estimations of GFR, urea, calcium, phosphate, bicarbonate, alkaline phosphatase, anemia, and lipids.
- Renal U/S—evaluates the presence of the two kidneys, obstruction, and renal size and symmetry. Bilateral small kidneys (<10 cm) supports the diagnosis of CKD.
- Renal biopsy—reserved when definitive diagnosis cannot be made.

E. Management
1. **Resolution of primary cause of CKD**
   - Lifestyle modifications including low-protein and low-potassium diet.
   - Strict diabetes and hypertension control.
   - Removal of obstructions.
   - Discontinuation or modification of medication that exacerbates CKD.
2. **Stabilization of CKD**
   - Medical therapy with ACE inhibitor or ARB.
   - Revascularization for renal artery stenosis.
   - Optimal control of comorbid conditions.
   - Minimize effects on other organ systems.

3. **Renal Replacement Therapy**
   - Dialysis.
   - Generally started when serum creatinine is >8 mg per dL or creatinine clearance is <10 mL per μm.
   - Hemodialysis or peritoneal dialysis.
   - Kidney transplantation.
     - Average wait for a deceased-donor transplant is 2 to 5 years depending on geographic location.
     - Requires chronic immunosuppressive therapy.

XI. Glomerulonephritis

A. Etiology
- Typically, glomerular diseases present as nephritic or nephrotic syndrome, or both.
- Accounts for 5% of all acute kidney injury (AKI).
- Glomerular diseases presenting as nephritic syndrome:
  - Postinfectious glomerulonephritis.
  - Immunoglobulin A (IgA) nephropathy (Buerger disease) and Henoch–Schönlein purpura.
  - Pauci-immune glomerulonephritis, which includes Wegener granulomatosis, microscopic polyangiitis, and Churg-Strauss disease.
  - Idiopathic crescentic glomerulonephritis.
  - Anti–glomerular basement membrane (GBM) or Goodpasture syndrome.
  - Essential (mixed) cryoglobulinemia.

B. Pathology
- Each underlying disease process utilizes different inflammatory pathways.
- An inflammatory process involving the glomerulus, although renal vasculature, interstitium, and tubular epithelium may be involved.
- Glomerular inflammation may result in damage to the GBM, mesangium, or capillary endothelium.
- The inflammatory process is often a result of formation and deposition of antigen–antibody complexes.

C. Clinical Features
- Gross hematuria may occur 1 to 2 days after an infection.
- Hematuria may occur in only a single episode; in some patients, recurrent episodes may occur over years.
- Postinfectious glomerulonephritis most commonly occurs 1 to 3 weeks after a group A (β-hemolytic) streptococci. It is characterized by the sudden onset of cola-colored urine (caused by red blood cell [RBC] cast proteinemia), edema, oliguria, and varying degrees of hypertension.
- IgA nephropathy (Buerger disease) is the most common form of glomerulonephritis in the world, mostly occurring in children and young adults.
  - It generally presents as an episode of macroscopic hematuria associated frequently with upper respiratory tract infection (50%), gastrointestinal (GI) symptoms, or flu-like illness.

- Approximately 50% of patients with IgA nephropathy develop progressive loss of renal function.
- Henoch–Schönlein purpura presents most commonly in male children and typically presents with palpable purpura secondary to leukocytoclastic vasculitis, arthralgias, and abdominal symptoms (e.g., nausea and colic melena).
  - Purpuric lesions are often located on lower extremities.
  - Patients rarely develop progressive renal disease and generally recover in several weeks.
- Pauci-immune glomerulonephritis is a small vessel antineutrophil cytoplasmic antibody (ANCA)–associated vasculitides.
  - Granulomatosis with polyangiitis generally presents with necrotizing vasculitis that can affect the pulmonary system as well as the renal system.
- Anti-GBM glomerulonephritis is generally associated with glomerulonephritis and pulmonary hemorrhage; however, one-third of patients do not have lung involvement.
  - More common in men than in women and usually occurs in the second and third decades of life and is usually preceded by an upper respiratory infection (URI).
- Cryoglobulin-associated glomerulonephritis occurs from the precipitation of cryoglobulins in the glomeruli and is associated with an underlying infection.
  - Skin necrosis in the dependent areas, arthralgias, fevers, and hepatosplenomegaly; associated with rapidly progressive glomerulonephritis.

D. Diagnostic Studies
- Initial evaluation in a patient suspected of having glomerulonephritis includes:
  - Urinalysis (UA) to determine hematuria, proteinuria, and cellular elements (i.e., RBCs, white blood cells [WBCs], and casts).
  - Twenty-four-hour urine for protein excretion.
  - Creatinine clearance.
  - Urine and serum protein electrophoresis to identify monoclonal or Bence Jones proteins suggestive of multiple myeloma or amyloidosis.
- Additional tests: depending on history and results in initial evaluation.
  - Complement levels CH50, C3, C4, antistreptolysin titer, cryoglobulins, ANCA, anti-GBM, serum IgA, serum eosinophils, antinuclear antibody (ANA), renal failure (RF), and hepatitis B and C serology.
  - Light and electron microscopy: for specific characteristics related to specific diseases.
  - Renal ultrasound (U/S) and biopsy (pathologic diagnosis is often definitive).

E. Management
- Treatment is directed toward correcting fluid overload, hypertension, uremia, and inflammatory injury to the kidney. Measures include sodium and water

restriction, diuretic therapy and dialysis, antihypertensive medications, and immunosuppressive therapy to reduce inflammatory injury.

- Postinfectious glomerulonephritis is usually self-limiting.
  - Supportive care, antibiotics for the underlying infection.
  - Most patients recover normal renal function within 2 months of onset.
  - No specific treatment other than antihypertensives, sodium restriction, and diuretics.
- IgA nephropathy.
  - Angiotensin-converting enzyme (ACE) inhibitors or angiotensin receptor blockers to decrease hypertension and proteinuria.
  - Corticosteroids.
  - Fish oil may have some benefit to improve proteinuria.
  - Patients with end-stage renal disease (ESRD) may need kidney transplant.
- Patients with Henoch–Schönlein purpura often recover renal function completely without long-term sequelae.
- Pauci-immune glomerulonephritis treatment includes corticosteroids and cytotoxic agents. Some patients may benefit from plasmapheresis.
- Anti-GBM glomerulonephritis is treated with plasmapheresis, corticosteroids, and cytotoxic agents.
- Cryoglobulin-associated glomerulonephritis is focused on treating the underlying disease. Some benefit may be seen with plasmapheresis, corticosteroids, cytotoxic agents and interferon alpha with ribavirin or direct acting antivirals in hepatitis C infection.

XII. Nephrotic Syndrome
A. Etiology
- May be a consequence of primary glomerulopathy or as a manifestation of one of a variety of systemic disorders.
- A majority of adult patients (50%–70%) who present with nephrotic syndrome have an associated systemic illness.
- Most common multisystem diseases associated with this syndrome are diabetic mellitus (DM), systemic lupus erythematosus (SLE), and other collagen vascular diseases and primary or secondary amyloidosis.
- Bacterial, viral, protozoan, and helminthic infections have been associated with nephrotic syndrome.
- Neoplasms including solid tumors, lymphomas, and leukemias are associated with nephrotic syndrome.
- Idiopathic nephrotic syndrome, in which no identifiable cause is present, or associated systemic disease occurs in 30% to 50% of adults with nephrotic syndrome.
- Idiopathic nephrotic syndrome is secondary to one of the four forms of glomerular disease:
  - Minimal change.
  - Focal glomerular sclerosis.
  - Membranous nephropathy.
  - Membranoproliferative glomerulonephritis.

B. Pathology
- Nephrotic syndrome is characterized by increased permeability of the glomerular capillary wall to circulating plasma proteins, primarily albumin.
- Albumin is the most abundant protein lost because it is the most abundant protein in plasma.
- Minimal change disease is usually associated with allergies, Hodgkin disease, and nonsteroidal anti-inflammatory drugs (NSAIDs). Seen with fusion of foot processes on electron microscopy.
- Focal segmental glomerulosclerosis is associated with heroin abuse, HIV, reflux nephropathy, and obesity. Seen with focal segmental sclerosis, IgM and C3 sclerotic lesions, and fusion of foot processes.
- Membranous nephropathy is associated with non–Hodgkin lymphoma, carcinoma, gold therapy, penicillamine, and SLE. Associated with thickened GBM, granular IgG and C3.
- Membranoproliferative glomerulonephropathy has two types:
  - Type 1 is associated with URIs. Seen with granular C3, C1q, C4, IgG, and IgM.
  - Type 2 is seen with C3 deposits only.

C. Clinical Features
- Most common sign of nephrotic syndrome is peripheral edema due to sodium retention as a result of renal dysfunction.
- As plasma albumin concentrations fall to <3 g per dL, ascites and anasarca develop.
- Hypercholesterolemia and hypertriglyceridemia are associated with increased hepatic production of proteins to compensate for the loss of albumin.
- Increased risk for a hypercoagulable state.
- If nephrotic syndrome is due to the presence of systemic disease, clinical manifestations pertinent to those diseases may be present.

D. Diagnostic Studies
- Quantification of urinary protein loss is necessary through 24-hour urine collection. Protein loss of >3.5 g per 24 hours is diagnostic.
- Urine dipstick analysis may be used as a screening test for proteinuria.
- On microscopic analysis, findings such as hematuria, cellular casts, or pyuria strongly suggest glomerular disease as the cause of nephrotic syndrome.
- Oval fat bodies, as a result of lipid deposition, are found in the urine, if there is hyperlipidemia present. They may present as "Maltese crosses" or "grape clusters" under polarized light.

- Blood chemistries associated with nephrotic syndrome include decreased serum albumin (<3 g per dL), decreased total serum protein (<6 g per dL), and elevated serum cholesterol (>200 mg per dL).
- Serum creatinine should be measured.
- Complement levels (C3, C4, CH150), fasting glucose serum and urine electrophoresis, ANA, and hepatitis B and C serology may also help determine the etiology of nephrotic syndrome.
- Renal biopsy may be used to obtain a histologic diagnosis.

E. Management
- Treatment issues common to all patients with nephrotic syndrome include:
  - Protein intake (0.6–0.8 g/kg/day with a glomerular filtration rate <25 mL per minute) may have some benefit.
  - Goal is generally to match protein loss with protein intake to avoid malnutrition.
  - Addition of an ACE inhibitor may reduce the amount of proteinuria.
- Peripheral edema and ascites respond to:
  - Dietary salt restriction.
- Diuretics:
  - Thiazide diuretics are appropriate for mild edema.
  - Loop diuretics are more appropriate for fluid retention associated with pleural effusions and ascites.
    - Metolazone or thiazide acting distal to the loop of Henle may potentiate the action of a loop diuretic if necessary.
- Hyperlipidemia:
  - Hypercholesterolemia and hypertriglyceridemia typically accompany nephrotic syndrome.
  - Low-fat diet with a weight control and exercise program is recommended.
  - Pharmacologic intervention should be instituted.
- Nephrotic proteinuria:
  - Increased loss of antithrombin III and other proteins involved in the clotting and fibrinolytic cascades, causing a relative hypercoagulable state.
  - If thrombosis is detected, heparin therapy followed by warfarin is necessary for at least 3 to 6 months.
- Minimal change disease:
  - Prednisone 1 mg/kg/day, adults often require a longer course, may take up to 16 weeks and should continue several weeks after remission. Frequent recurrences may require cyclophosphamide.
  - ESRD is rare.
- Membranous nephropathy:
  - Treatment depends on the risk of progression of disease. Management is based on the level of proteinuria.
    - Less than 3.5 g per day: low salt diet, blood pressure (BP) control, and ACE inhibitor.

- 3.5 to 8 g per day with normal renal function: can use corticosteroids and chlorambucil or cyclophosphamide × 6 months.
- More than 8 g per day: should receive a corticosteroid and cytotoxic agent.
- Focal segmental glomerular sclerosis:
  - Treatment includes supportive care and 1 to 1.5 mg/kg/day of corticosteroids for 2 to 3 months followed by a taper.
- Membranoproliferative glomerulonephropathy:
  - Treated with corticosteroids and antiplatelet therapy (because of increased platelet consumption). Fifty percent progress to ESRD in 10 years. Type 2 has a worse outcome than type 1. Both types will recur after transplant; however, it is more common in type 2.

XIII. Acute Tubulointerstitial Nephritis

A. Etiology
- Drug reactions to NSAIDs (which account for 70% of all causes), antibiotics (including penicillins, cephalosporins, sulfonamides, and rifampin), diuretics, proton pump inhibitors, and miscellaneous drugs such as allopurinol, cimetidine, and phenytoin.
- Systemic infections due to:
  - Bacteria: *Streptococcus*, *Corynebacterium diphtheriae*, *Legionella*.
  - Viruses: Epstein–Barr virus, cytomegalovirus.
  - Others: *Mycoplasma*, *Rickettsia rickettsii*, toxoplasmosis, leptospirosis, histoplasmosis.
- Systemic inflammatory diseases such as SLE, Sjögren, sarcoidosis, and cryoglobulinemia.
- Idiopathic diseases such as tubulointerstitial nephritis and uveitis (TINU).

B. Pathology
- Mostly caused by T lymphocytes, plasma cells, and macrophages, which appear to damage the interstitium by way of direct cytotoxicity.

C. Clinical Features
- Sudden decrease in renal function in a previously asymptomatic patient.
- Signs and symptoms are associated with allergic reactions:
  - Fever (seen in 80% of patients), transient maculopapular rash (seen in 25%–50% of patients), bilateral or unilateral flank pain secondary to renal capsule distension, RF failure evolves over days to weeks, and arthralgias.
- Hematuria.
- Peripheral eosinophilia.
- TINU:
  - Unknown etiology.
  - Characterized by anterior uveitis seen usually before or after acute tubulointerstitial nephritis.

- Associated with bone marrow granulomas, and chlamydia and mycoplasma infections.
- Usually seen in women.
- Associated with weight loss and anemia and with an elevated erythrocyte sedimentation rate.

D. Diagnostic Studies
- Peripheral eosinophils.
- UA may show pyuria, hematuria, proteinuria (<1 g per 24 hours), eosinophiluria, and WBC casts.
- Serum creatinine.
- U/S shows normal or enlarged kidneys with increased cortical echogenicity.
- Gallium scanning may show bilaterally nonspecific increased uptake of isotope.

E. Management
- Discontinue the offending drug.
- Dialysis may be necessary in up to one-third of patients.
- Some benefit may be seen with corticosteroids at high doses, which can be administered if drug discontinuation does not lead to return to baseline renal function within a few days.
- Most patients have complete recovery of renal function, although advanced age at onset and a prolonged period of acute RF are poor prognostic indicators.

XIV. Chronic Tubulointerstitial Nephritis

A. Etiology
- The most common cause is prolonged obstructive uropathy, vesicoureteral reflux, analgesics, and heavy metals.

B. Pathology
- Obstructive uropathy is the most common cause of chronic tubulointerstitial nephritis (CTIN).
  - It can be caused by prostatic hypertrophy, calculi, and carcinoma of the cervix, colon, bladder, and retroperitoneal space.
- Vesicoureteral reflex is usually seen in children and is the second most common cause.
  - Generally associated with retrograde flow of urine from the bladder back into the ureters to the kidneys during voiding because of an incompetent ureteral sphincter. The urine then causes inflammation in the interstitium, and this inflammation can cause fibrosis.
- Increased analgesic use.
  - Seen with the use of acetaminophen, aspirin, and NSAIDs.
- Environmental exposure to heavy metals such as lead and cadmium.
  - Chronic exposure to lead results in urinary concentrating defects by causing dysfunction in the proximal tubules, leading to decreased uric acid secretion.

C. Clinical Features
- Obstructive uropathy can result in urinary difficulty; additional symptoms are associated with the underlying pathology.
- Reflux nephropathy occurs before the age of 5, but focal renal deterioration continues. Focal glomerulosclerosis and hypertension are often sequelae, and the patient may progress to ESRD.
- Analgesic abuse can result in hematuria, mild proteinuria, polyuria, anemia (from GI bleed), and sterile pyuria, and may be present because of the necrosis caused by the analgesic medication(s).
- Chronic exposure of heavy metals can over years results in progressive azotemia, hyperuricemia, saturnine gout, and hypertension. Hypercalciuria can occur with cadmium exposure.

D. Diagnostic Studies
1. **General Characteristics**
   - Small, contracted kidneys.
   - Decreased urinary concentrating and diluting ability.
   - Hyperchloremic due to type 1 and 4 renal tubular acidosis.
   - Hyperkalemia due to the distal tubules becoming aldosterone resistant.
   - Proteinuria <2 g per day because of dysfunction to the proximal tubule, so that it cannot reabsorb protein well.
2. **General Studies**
   - UA in CTIN is essentially nonspecific and may show mild proteinuria, few cells, and broad granular casts.
   - Most characteristic finding is polyuria and sodium wasting out of proportion to the degree of renal impairment, and inability to acidify urine in association with hyperchloremic metabolic acidosis (renal tubular acidosis).
3. **Obstructive Uropathy**
   - Need to identify the presence of benign prostatic hyperplasia.
   - Renal U/S is useful for identifying hydronephrosis.
   - Antegrade or retrograde pyelography may be needed to confirm the diagnosis.
   - UA may show hematuria, pyuria, and bacteriuria.
   - May need further abdominal imaging to rule out carcinoma.
4. **Reflux Nephropathy**
   - May be diagnosed by proteinuria of >1 g per day and renal U/S or intravenous pyelogram (IVP) demonstrating renal scarring and potentially hydronephrosis.
5. **Analgesic-Associated Disease**
   - Associated with hematuria, proteinuria, and sterile pyuria or UA.
   - If gross hematuria occurs secondary to papillary necrosis, sloughed papillae may be noted in the urine.

- IVP demonstrates a "ring shadow" sign and the papillary tip in the case of papillary necrosis.
  6. **Heavy Metal Exposure**
     - May be diagnosed by performing an edetate disodium (EDTA) test to diagnose lead nephropathy.
     - Greater than 600 mg of lead in a 24-hour period after an IV infusion of 1 g of edetate indicates excessive lead exposure.

E. Management
- Treatment is directed toward the underlying cause.
- Recovery of renal function depends on the degree of interstitial fibrosis.
- Medical management of specific tubular dysfunction with dietary restriction of potassium, or sodium and bicarbonate supplements may be necessary if damage is irreversible.
- Treatment of analgesic nephropathy necessitates withdrawal of all analgesics and may result in stabilization or improvement in renal function if significant interstitial fibrosis has not already resulted.

XV. Hematuria
A. Etiology
- Can be gross hematuria or microscopic hematuria.
- Upper sources of bleeding are nephrolithiasis (40%), kidney disease (20%), renal cell carcinoma (10%), urothelial cell carcinoma (5%), trauma, medications, diabetes, and sickle cell trait disease.
- Lower sources of bleeding are infection, urothelial cell carcinoma (most common in the absences of infection), anticoagulation, trauma, and benign prostatic hypertrophy (most common form of microscopic hematuria in men).
- Hematuria associated with pyuria with or without symptoms of frequency, urgency, or dysuria suggests an infectious cause.
- Pseudohematuria may be caused by substances that impart a color to urine that may be mistaken for hematuria, such as porphyrins, myoglobin, and certain medications.

B. Pathology
- Pathology depends on underlying disease process.

C. Clinical Features
- May be asymptomatic, and hematuria may be incidentally found on routine dipstick UA.
- Patient may present with grossly, bloody urine with or without clots.
- Clots may result in bladder outlet obstruction, which can result in significant discomfort.
- Initial hematuria with presence of blood at the beginning of the urinary stream implies an anterior or penile urethral source.
- Terminal hematuria with presence of blood only at the end of the urinary stream is associated with bladder neck or prostatic urethral source.

- Total hematuria, presence of blood throughout the urinary stream, is associated with a bladder or upper tract source.
- Intermittent hematuria in patients younger than 40 years is less concerning for cancer. However, hematuria in patients older than 50 years should have a high concern for cancer.

D. Laboratory Diagnosis
- Hematuria is defined as >2 RBCs per high-power field (HPF) on at least two occasions. However, there is no lower limit that will definitively rule out underlying disease.
- Dipstick method can detect 1 to 2 RBCs per HPF; therefore, it is as sensitive as microscopic evaluation. However, they are not specific because they can have a high rate of false positives if there are myoglobins or oxidizing agents present.
- May see proteinuria and casts, which would suggest underlying renal disease.
- If it is unclear as to the source of hematuria, further evaluation of the underlying disease may be warranted.
  - CBC, an estimate of glomerular function (serum creatinine), sickle cell preparation, and 24-hour urine specimen to determine concentration of calcium and uric acid.
  - In patients suspected of having a bleeding disorder, a platelet count and partial prothrombin time/partial thromboplastin time should be obtained.
  - Computed tomography (CT) urography, magnetic resonance imaging (MRI), U/S, cystoscopy, and/or IVP.
  - Biopsy is not usually needed for isolated glomerular hematuria without proteinuria or renal insufficiency.
  - In older patients or those at risk for neoplasm, cytology should be performed and a urologist should be consulted.

E. Management
- Identifiable causes should be treated.
- Clots should be treated with continuous bladder irrigation.
- When neoplasm is suspected, a urologist should be consulted.
- When underlying renal disease is suspected, a nephrologist should be consulted.

XVI. Hyponatremia
A. Etiology
- Defined as a serum sodium concentration of <135 mEq per L; is the most common electrolyte abnormality observed in the general hospitalized population. No age or gender prevalence exists.
- There are three major types of hyponatremia based on serum osmolality.

- Isotonic hyponatremia.
- Hypertonic hyponatremia.
- Hypotonic hyponatremia, which is further divided depending on the patient's volume status:
  - Euvolemic hypotonic hyponatremia.
  - Hypervolemic hypotonic hyponatremia.
  - Hypovolemic hypotonic hyponatremia, which is further divided into:
    - Extrarenal losses.
    - Renal losses.

B. Pathology

1. **Isotonic Hyponatremia (Normal Serum Osmolality of 280–295 mOsm per kg)**
   - Any increase in plasma solids such as lipids and protein lowers the proportion of liquid in comparison with the number of solids.
   - Examples: Hyperlipidemia gives a milky-appearing serum as seen in familial hyperlipidemia or nephrotic syndrome. Hyperproteinemia such as in multiple myeloma or macroglobulinemia.
2. **Hypertonic Hyponatremia (High Serum Osmolality of >295 mOsm per kg)**
   - Introduction of osmotically active solutes (such as glucose and mannitol), which do not readily penetrate the cell membrane, will increase extracellular fluid osmolality.
   - Examples: Hyperglycemia and hypertonic therapy with mannitol.
3. **Hypotonic Hyponatremia (Low Serum Osmolality of <280 mOsm per kg)**
   - Euvolemic hypotonic hyponatremia.
     - No extracellular fluid expansion or depletion relative to the amount of sodium is present.
     - Examples: syndrome of inappropriate antidiuretic hormone (SIADH), psychogenic polydipsia, and beer potomania.
4. **Hypervolemic Hypotonic Hyponatremia**
   - Expansion of extracellular fluid relative to the amount of sodium present.
   - These patients have edema and other signs of intravascular volume overload.
   - Examples: congestive heart failure (CHF), nephrotic syndrome, and cirrhosis.
5. **Hypovolemic Hypotonic Hyponatremia**
   - Depletion of extracellular fluid relative to the amount of sodium due to extrarenal or renal volume/salt loss.
   - Extrarenal volume/salt loss (low urine sodium of <10 mEq per L in the setting of a low serum osmolality of <280 mOsm per kg).
     - Examples: dehydration, diarrhea, and vomiting.
   - Renal volume/salt loss (high urine sodium of >20 mEq per L in the setting of a low serum osmolality of <280 mOsm per kg):

- Examples: diuretics, ACE inhibitors, nephropathies, mineralocorticoid deficiency, and cerebral salt wasting.

C. Clinical Features
- Patients may be asymptomatic with a serum Na$^+$ in the range of 130 to 135 mEq per L.
- Symptoms are common with a serum Na$^+$ of <125 mEq per L.
- Uncommon for a serum Na$^+$ of <120 mEq per L to be acute.
- Symptoms include nausea, weakness, muscle cramps, and orthostatic hypotension.
- Neurologic symptoms and can be a change in mental status, lethargy, disorientation, obtundation, coma, and seizure.
- Slow progression of hyponatremia may be asymptomatic because the brain has time to shift idiogenic osmoles and change the intracellular tonicity to match the extracellular tonicity so that the brain does not become edematous. This can occur over days, weeks to months, and patients can then tolerate very low sodium levels.
- If hyponatremia occurs rapidly, over hours, the brain does not have time to shift the idiogenic osmoles and can result in varying levels of severity based on the rapidity and degree of hyponatremia.

D. Diagnostic Studies
- Sodium level.
- Blood urea nitrogen (BUN), creatinine to evaluate for renal dysfunction.
- Serum osmolality and urine sodium levels.
- Additional studies to help determine underlying cause:
  - Serum glucose, each 100 mg per dL rise in plasma glucose decreases serum sodium by approximately 1.5 mEq per L.
  - Urine dipstick for glucose and protein.
  - Serum albumin.
  - Serum cholesterol.
  - Serum electrophoresis when multiple myeloma is suspected.
  - Thyroid-stimulating hormone level to rule out hypothyroidism.
  - CT scan of the head if pituitary or central nervous system (CNS) disorder is considered.
  - Chest X-ray to rule out pulmonary pathology if SIADH.
  - Evaluate for other electrolyte abnormalities.

E. Management
- Inpatient management is needed if hyponatremia is symptomatic or acute, or if the patient is asymptomatic with a serum sodium <125 mEq per dL.
- Isotonic hyponatremia will require fluid restriction and treatment of the underlying condition.
- Treatment of hypertonic hyponatremia is to correct the underlying cause (i.e., correct hyperglycemia).

A loop diuretic may be added to enhance free water excretion.
- Euvolemic hypotonic hyponatremia can be treated with fluid restriction.
- Hypervolemic hypotonic hyponatremia can be treated with diuresis.
- Hypovolemic hypotonic hyponatremia treatment consists of volume replacement with isotonic crystalloid.
- Severe symptomatic hyponatremia may need to be repleted with hypertonic crystalloid (such as 3% saline), at the rate of 1 to 1.5 mL/kg/hour, and not to correct the serum sodium >8 mEq/L/day.
- Avoid a too-rapid correction, as the osmotic imbalance may cause water to preferentially enter brain cells leading to cerebral edema and potentially severe neurologic impairment (osmotic demyelination).
- Monitor electrolytes frequently, every 1 to 2 hours in the early treatment phase.
- Treat underlying and/or precipitating events (stop thiazide diuretics, thyroid hormone replacement therapy when indicated).

XVII. Hypernatremia

A. Etiology
- Defined as a serum sodium >145 mEq per L.
- Hypernatremia is always hyperosmolar and is usually hypovolemic because of excess water loss.
- Often accompanied by an impaired thirst mechanism.
- Occurs most commonly in hospitalized, elderly patients.
- Lactulose, mannitol osmotic therapy, and diabetes insipidus (DI), both central and nephrogenic, can cause hypernatremia.
- May occur with severe diarrhea, especially in at-risk populations such as the elderly, disabled, and infants.
- Occurs after the administration of hypertonic fluids.

B. Pathology
- Blunting of the thirst mechanism or limited access to water can result in decreased intake of water.
- Volume loss through mechanisms such as polyuria seen in diuresis and DI or severe diarrhea can result in hypernatremia.
- The brain attempts to shift idiogenic osmoles and change intracellular tonicity to match the extracellular tonicity so that the brain does not shrink.

C. Clinical Features
- Severity of symptoms correlates with the extent of hyperosmolality.
- Thirst may initially be present, but as the sodium levels continue to rise, the thirst mechanism may become dysfunctional.
- Dry mouth and mucous membranes, decreased tears, decreased salivation, oliguria, and orthostatic hypotension.
- Fever, hyperventilation, hyperthermia, delirium, and coma.
- Polydipsia, polyuria, and nocturia.
- Brain shrinkage may result in intracranial hemorrhages, permanent neurologic damage, or death.
- Osmotic demyelination syndrome is uncommon.

D. Diagnostic Studies
- Serum osmolality is always >290 mOsm per kg, which represents a hyperosmolar state.
- Urine osmolality >400 mOsm per kg indicates renal water-conserving ability is functioning, and therefore the free water loss is from extrarenal causes such as sweating, loss from the respiratory tract, and GI losses. Renal losses of free water are seen in severe hyperglycemia and osmotic diuresis.
- Urine osmolality <250 mOsm per kg with hypernatremia is characteristic of DI.
- Salt ingestion typically shows increased urine sodium and increased urine osmolality.
- Dehydration has decreased urine sodium and increased urine osmolality.

E. Management
- General measures include correcting the cause of the fluid loss, replacing water, and repletion of electrolytes as needed.
- Removal of salt from diet in the case of hypervolemic hypernatremia.
- Acute hypernatremia has a free water deficit similar to the amount of weight loss.
- Calculate free water deficit for chronic hypernatremia.
  - Volume (L) to be replaced = current body weight (kg) $\times$ ([serum sodium] − 140)/140.
- Fluid therapy should be administered over 48 hours with a goal of decreasing serum sodium to 1 mEq/L/hour. In response to increased plasma osmolality, brain cells synthesize solutes that increase osmotic flow of water back into the brain cells to regulate their volume. This process is initiated 4 to 6 hours after dehydration and takes several days to reach a steady state. A too-rapid correction of hypernatremia may cause water to preferentially enter brain cells, causing cerebral edema and severe neurologic impairment.
- Hypernatremia with hypovolemia that is causing hemodynamic instability should be treated with isotonic (0.9%) saline; otherwise, hypotonic crystalloids are adequate.
- In patients with hypernatremia with euvolemia, water drinking or 5% dextrose and IV water results in the excretion of excess sodium in the urine.
- In patients with hypervolemic hypernatremia, provide water as 5% dextrose in water to reduce hyperosmolality and loop diuretics (in severe renal insufficiency, hemodialysis may be required).

XVIII. Hypokalemia

A. Etiology

- Serum potassium <3.5 mEq per L is considered hypokalemia.
- Always associated with a total body potassium deficit.
- Deficits arise from poor intake or from excessive loss of body fluids.
- Nonrenal causes of hypokalemia:
  - Vomiting and nasogastric suctioning.
  - Metabolic alkalosis increases the magnitude of potassium loss by increasing renal potassium secretion.
  - Malabsorption of nutrients in patients with small bowel disorders or decreased intake.
  - Colonic losses due to diarrhea, laxatives, enemas, or colon preparation before lower endoscopy.
  - Villous adenoma and Zollinger–Ellison syndrome.
- Renal losses:
  - Diuretic treatment (most common cause in outpatients), digoxin intoxication.
  - Renal tubular acidosis I and II or parenchymal disease.
  - Adrenal hormones.
  - Primary hyperaldosteronism (second most common, generally occurs due to underlying heart or liver disease).
  - Secondary hyperaldosteronism (CHF, cirrhosis, nephrotic syndrome, rennin-producing tumors, and Bartter syndrome).
  - Excessive glucocorticoid (Cushing disease and exogenous glucocorticoid administration).
  - Genetic disorders.
  - Hypomagnesemia.

B. Pathology

- Hypokalemia can occur as a result of shift of potassium from outside to inside the cell.
- "Redistribution hypokalemia" is seen when potassium taken up by the cell is stimulated by insulin in the presence of glucose. It is also facilitated by β-adrenergic stimulation of the Na–K–ATPase pump, whereas α-adrenergic stimulation blocks it.
- Aldosterone regulates potassium uptake in the distal tubules.
- Magnesium is a cofactor for potassium uptake and for maintaining adequate intracellular potassium levels.

C. Clinical Features

- Any level of hypokalemia may potentially be dangerous.
- Skeletal muscle weakness and cramps.
- Smooth muscle involvement may result in constipation and ileus.
- Vasoconstriction with secondary distal tissue ischemia.
- When potassium level is <2.5 mEq per L, flaccid paralysis, hypercapnia, tetany, and rhabdomyolysis may be present.
- Cardiac involvement leads to ventricular dysrhythmias, hypotension, and cardiac arrest.
- Patients receiving digoxin are at increased risk of arrhythmias.
- Kidneys can lose H^+ ions, resulting in metabolic alkalosis.
- Renal involvement causes polyuria and nocturia due to impaired concentration ability.
- Hypertension may suggest aldosterone or mineralocorticoid excess.

D. Diagnostic Studies

- Serum potassium <3.5 mEq per L is diagnostic of hypokalemia.
- Urine potassium of <20 suggests extrarenal losses, and a urine potassium of >40 suggests renal losses.
- Electrocardiogram (ECG).
  - Findings include frequent premature ventricular contractions, decreased amplitude and broadening of T waves, prominent U waves, depressed ST segments, and, in severe deficits, atrioventricular block.
- Special tests:
  - Plasma renin and aldosterone levels to differentiate adrenal from nonadrenal causes.
  - A high urine chloride level in the absence of hypertension and acidosis suggests hypokalemia secondary to diuretics or Bartter syndrome.
  - A low urine chloride suggests GI losses by vomiting.

E. Management

- General measures include treatment of underlying cause.
- Mild-to-moderate deficiency may be treated with oral potassium phosphate in doses of 40 to 120 mEq/L/day.
- Potassium chloride (KCl) is suitable for all forms of hypokalemia, especially ones associated with hypochloremia.
- IV potassium replacement is indicated in patients with severe hypokalemia and those who cannot take oral supplements.
- If the serum potassium level is >2.5 mEq per L without ECG abnormalities, potassium can be given at the rate of 10 mEq/L/hour IV in concentrations not exceeding 40 mEq per L.
- In emergent situations (serum potassium <2.5 mEq per L), the rate of administration should not exceed 20 mEq/L/hour and maximum recommended concentration is 60 mEq per L. To replace potassium safely using higher concentrations, it should be administered through central venous access. These patients should have potassium levels checked every 4 to 6 hours.
- Continue to monitor ECGs and watch for signs of hyperkalemia.
- If hypomagnesemia is present, it must be repleted.

XIX. Hyperkalemia

A. Etiology
- May be due to increased potassium load, translocation of potassium between cellular compartments, or factitious.
- Most commonly associated with AKI.
- A common electrolyte disorder with plasma potassium concentration >5.0 mEq per L.
- Severe hyperkalemia (>6.5 mEq per L) could result in ventricular fibrillation and death.

B. Pathology
- Spurious causes of hyperkalemia can be associated with hemolysis, thrombocytosis/leukocytosis, repeated fist clenching during blood draw, and blood drawn from a line with potassium infusion.
- Decreased excretion can result in hyperkalemia from acute kidney disease or chronic kidney disease (CKD), renal secretory defects, decreased rennin/aldosterone, and medications that inhibit potassium secretion.
- Potassium can also shift from the intracellular to extracellular spaces causing hyperkalemia. This can occur from burns, rhabdomyolysis, hemolysis, severe infections, internal bleeding and extreme exercise, metabolic acidosis, hypertonicity, decreased levels of insulin, and medications.
- Excess intake of potassium can also result in hyperkalemia.

C. Clinical Features
- Half of all patients with serum potassium >6.5 mEq per L have no ECG findings.
- Effects of hyperkalemia constitute a medical emergency.
- Hyperkalemia can cause bradycardia, PR prolongation, and peaked T waves progressing to widened QRS complexes, sine waves, and asystole.
- Patients are initially hyperreflexic, but then progress to flaccid paralysis, because of decreased neuromuscular transmission.
- Hypotension secondary to vasodilation.

D. Diagnostic Studies
- Mild hyperkalemia is 5.5 to 5.9 mEq per L, moderate is 6 to 6.9 mEq per L, and severe is ≥7 mEq per L. A serum potassium >7.5 mEq per L will require immediate intervention.
- Special tests:
  - Cortisol and aldosterone levels to confirm suspected mineralocorticoid deficiency.

E. Management
- Evaluate for possible hemolysis resulting in spurious potassium levels.
- Discontinue potassium-sparing drugs or dietary potassium.
- Determine the underlying cause.
  - If hyperkalemia is severe (>6.5–7 mEq per L), treat it directly before determining underlying cause.
- Emergent treatment is indicated if cardiac toxicity or muscular paralysis is present.
- IV β-agonists, sodium bicarbonate, and insulin will temporarily shift potassium into the cell within a few minutes of administration.
- A source of dextrose should be given with insulin boluses to prevent hypoglycemia.
- Intravenous calcium gluconate will stabilize the cardiac membrane.
- Cation exchange resins, given orally or rectally, help with excretion of potassium in the GI tract within 1 to 2 hours of administration.
- Loop diuretics, or other non–potassium-sparing diuretics, can aid in the excretion of potassium from the kidneys if the kidneys are not in overt failure.
- In severe cases, dialysis can be used to excrete potassium and works immediately on initiation of treatment.

XX. Disorders of Calcium

A. Calcium
- Ninety-nine percent of calcium is stored in bone.
- The remaining 0.01% of calcium is stored in solution in body fluid.
- Fifty percent of calcium is bound to protein (mostly albumin), 10% is bound to other complexes, and the remaining 40% is "free" or ionized calcium.
- Ionized calcium is the physiologically active form.
- Normal serum total calcium level is 9 to 10 mg per dL.
- Normal serum ionized calcium level is 4.6 to 5.4 mg per dL.
- Serum ionized calcium is the most accurate measurement of serum calcium concentration.
- Functions of ionized calcium include neuromuscular function, smooth muscle contraction, plasma membrane stability, and permeability.
- Vitamin D is required for adequate absorption of calcium within intestines.

B. Hypocalcemia
1. Etiology
- Hypoalbuminemia is the most common cause of low calcium levels in the serum. When the albumin level is <4 g per dL, the serum calcium level decreases by 0.8 to 1 mg per dL for every drop in albumin of 1 g per dL.
- CKD is the most common cause of hypocalcemia because of decreased vitamin D_3 production and increased hyperphosphatemia.
- Sepsis, acute pancreatitis, and thyroid surgery.
- Hypoparathyroidism.
- Vitamin D deficiency.
- Alkalosis, blood transfusions, drugs (cimetidine, phenytoin), hyperphosphatemia, and calcitonin secretion with medullary carcinoma of the thyroid.

2. **Pathology**
   - Hypocalcemia is a result of decreased intestinal absorption (vitamin D deficiency due to RF or nutritional deficiencies), decreased calcium intake, decrease in parathyroid hormone (PTH) levels, and deposition of ionized calcium into soft tissues or bone.
   - Hypocalcemia causes a lowering of the excitation threshold of the neuromuscular and cardiovascular systems, thereby making these nerves more sensitive to stimulation and impulses.
   - Hypocalcemia causes a reduced contractile force in both vascular smooth muscle and cardiac muscle.

3. **Clinical Features**
   - General:
     - Generally, patients with hypocalcemia are asymptomatic.
     - Weakness/fatigue.
   - Neurologic:
     - Skeletal muscle cramps and tetany, hyperactive deep tendon reflexes, paresthesias of lips and fingertips, and laryngospasm with stridor that may lead to fatal asphyxia, seizures, and confusion.
     - Chvostek sign is defined as a contraction of the facial muscle in response to tapping facial nerve anterior to the ear.
     - Trousseau sign is defined as carpal spasm occurring after 3 minutes following inflation of BP cuff to proximal arm, just above systolic pressure.
   - GI: abdominal pain.
   - Cardiac: Arrhythmias, QT segment prolongation, heart block, ventricular fibrillation, hypotension, and heart failure.
   - Skeletal: Abnormal dentition, rickets, osteomalacia, and osteodystrophy.
   - Hypocalcemia from chronic hyperparathyroid.
   - Cataracts and calcification of basal ganglia.

4. **Diagnostic Studies**
   - Total serum Ca^{2+}.
     - Will need albumin level to calculate a corrected calcium.
       - Corrected calcium = $(0.8 \times$ [normal albumin − measure albumin]) + total serum calcium.
   - Ionized Ca^{2+}.
   - Commonly, hyperphosphatemia and hypomagnesemia are noted.
   - ECG demonstrates prolongation of QT interval.

5. **Management of Hypocalcemia**
   - If the patient is asymptomatic:
     - Oral calcium carbonate.
     - Vitamin D preparations such as ergocalciferol or calcifediol.
     - Magnesium replacement therapy, if low.
     - If total serum calcium is low and the ionized Ca^{2+} level is normal, then no calcium replacement is needed.

   - If the patient is symptomatic:
     - IV calcium gluconate 10% solution (92 mg of calcium per 10 mL).
     - IV calcium gluconate has a short duration and therefore continuous infusion is generally required.
     - IV calcium chloride 10% solution (272 mg of calcium per 10 mL) is more irritating to veins than the gluconate preparation.
     - Maintenance of serum Ca^{2+} level at 7 to 8 mg per dL.
     - Treat hypomagnesemia, if present.
     - Monitor serum calcium and other electrolytes.

C. **Hypercalcemia**
   1. **Etiology**
      - Increased calcium intake, milk-alkali syndrome, hyperparathyroid (most common), multiple myeloma, Paget disease, adrenal insufficiency, acromegaly, neoplasm, Zollinger–Ellison syndrome, excessive vitamin D or A intake, medications, and sarcoidosis.

   2. **Pathology**
      - Hypercalcemia causes an increase in the excitation threshold of the neuromuscular and cardiovascular systems, thereby requiring an increased level of stimulus or impulse to trigger a response.

   3. **Clinical Features**
      - General: malaise, weakness, polydipsia, and dehydration.
      - Neurologic: muscle weakness with hyporeflexia, hypotonia, tremor, lethargy, confusion, stupor, and coma.
      - Cardiovascular: arrhythmias.
      - Renal: polyuria, nocturia, renal calculi, and nephrogenic DI, which is caused by increased calcium in the collecting ducts resulting in decreased response to antidiuretic hormone (ADH).
      - GI: nausea, vomiting, abdominal pain, constipation, ileus, peptic ulcer disease, and pancreatitis.
      - Musculoskeletal: muscle weakness, bone pain, fractures, and deformities.

   4. **Diagnostic Studies**
      - Total serum calcium is >11 to 12 mg per dL.
      - Ionized serum calcium is >6 mg per dL or <2.7 mEq per L.
      - ECG demonstrates shortened QT interval.

   5. **Management**
      - Primary disease or cause identified and controlled.
      - Correct dehydration caused by increased Ca^{2+} levels interfering with ADH and ability of the kidney to concentrate urine.
      - Hydration with IV fluids forces urinary excretion of calcium.

- Patients with cardiac or renal disease may require adjustment of fluid replacement and/or peritoneal dialysis or hemodialysis.
- IV furosemide can also be used to enhance Ca^{2+} excretion and prevent volume overload.
- Thiazides may worsen hypercalcemia.
- Replacement of K^+ and Mg^{2+} is usually necessary.
- Additional treatment options for specific disease:
  - Metastatic bone disease:
    - Calcitonin (rapid, mild inhibition of bone resorption) and pamidronate (delayed onset, most potent inhibition of bone resorption).
  - Sarcoidosis, vitamin A or D intoxication, multiple myeloma, leukemia, or breast cancer:
    - Glucocorticoids that increase calcium urinary excretion, decrease GI absorption of calcium, and interfere with lymphoid neoplastic tissue growth.
  - Neoplasms producing PTH-like activity: consider irradiation or resection.
  - Surgical resection of the parathyroid glands in the setting of medically refractory hyperparathyroidism.

XXI. Disorders of Phosphorus
A. Phosphorous
- Mainly inorganic phosphates in the plasma.
- Intracellular phosphorus is 70% and intraskeletal phosphorus is 29%.
- Serum phosphorus is approximately <1% of total body phosphorus.
- Phosphorus levels are based on renal excretion and release from bone caused by PTH (major factor), intestinal absorption caused by 1,25-dihydroxy-vitamin D_3, and intercellular and extracellular shifts.
- Because PTH and vitamin D are involved in the metabolism of phosphorus and calcium, often if there is a disorder of phosphorus, there will be a disorder of calcium present as well.

B. Hypophosphatemia
1. Etiology
- Diminished supply or decreased intestinal absorption such as starvation, refeeding syndrome, decreased intake, and vitamin D deficiency.
- Increased loss from medications, hyperparathyroid, and hyperthyroid.
- Intracellular shift caused by increased glucose, anabolic steroids, hungry bone syndrome, respiratory alkalosis, diabetic ketoacidosis, postoperative phase, trauma, sepsis, and salicylate toxicity.
- Electrolyte abnormalities such as hypercalcemia and hypomagnesemia.
- Common in patients who abuse alcohol.

2. Pathology
- Pathology is based on the underlying disease process.
- Severe hypophosphatemia results in decreased affinity of hemoglobin for oxygen.
3. Clinical Features
- Severe hypophosphatemia (<1 mg per dL) can result in rhabdomyolysis, paresthesias, encephalopathy, irritability, confusion, dysarthria, seizures, and coma.
- Because serum phosphorus levels do not reflect the total amount of phosphorus, low levels of serum phosphorus may be asymptomatic.
- May see respiratory failure or failure to wean in ventilated patients because of diaphragmatic weakness.
4. Diagnostic Studies
- Serum phosphate levels <2.5 mg per dL.
- Urine phosphate >20 mg per dL suggests renal loss.
- PTH levels may be elevated.
- Bone biopsy may show osteomalacia in adults.
- If creatinine kinase levels are elevated, it may suggest rhabdomyolysis.
5. Management
- Phosphate repletion with oral replacement of sodium or potassium phosphate.
- IV phosphate repletion can result in hypocalcemia.
- Moderate or chronic hypophosphatemia (1–2.5 mg per dL) is generally asymptomatic and does not require repletion.
- Severe hypophosphatemia (<1 mg per dL) may require IV replacement and when able should be switched to an oral regimen.
- Monitor phosphate levels when repleting, as well as calcium, potassium, and magnesium levels, and correct any other electrolyte abnormality.
- Phosphate repletion in hypoparathyroidism, hypercalcemia, and CKD should be done with caution.

C. Hyperphosphatemia
1. Etiology
- Most commonly seen in CKD, but may also be seen in AKI, hypoparathyroidism, and acromegaly because of decreased excretion.
- Phosphate shifts into the extracellular space due to increased intake, increased levels of vitamin D, rhabdomyolysis, cellular lysis, and metabolic or respiratory acidosis.
- Multiple myeloma, hyperbilirubinemia, hypertriglyceridemia, and hemolysis can result in pseudohyperphosphatemia.
2. Pathology
- Pathology is determined by the underlying cause.

- Hypercalcemia seen with hyperphoshatemia suggests underlying malignancy.

3. Clinical Features
- Signs and symptoms are based on the underlying disease.

4. Diagnostic Studies
- Phosphate level is elevated.
- Tests ordered will be based on the underlying disease.

5. Management
- Treat the underlying disease.
- Oral phosphate binders such as calcium carbonate, calcium acetate, sevelamer carbonate, lanthanum carbonate, and aluminum hydroxide.
- Sevelamer, lanthanum, and aluminum hydroxide are used if there is hypercalcemia in addition to the hyperphosphatemia.
- Aluminum hydroxide can cause neurotoxicity if used for a prolonged period of time.
- Dialysis can be used in AKI and CKD.

XXII. Disorders of Magnesium
A. Magnesium
- Normal magnesium levels are 1.5 to 2.5 mEq per L.
- One percent of total body magnesium is within the extracellular fluid.
- One-third of serum magnesium is bound to protein.
- Two-thirds of serum magnesium is in the cation form.
- Excretion of magnesium is primarily from the kidneys.
- Hypomagnesemia and hypermagnesemia can decrease PTH production.
- Magnesium concentration disorders are usually associated with changes in calcium levels and can be associated with changes in potassium levels.

B. Hypomagnesemia
1. Etiology
- Hypomagnesemia caused by decrease absorption from chronic diarrhea, small bowel bypass, increased gastric suction, alcoholism, and malnutrition.
- Increased renal loss from diuretics, hyperaldosteronism, hyperparathyroid, hyperthyroid, hypercalcemia, hypervolemia, tubulointerstitial disease, medications, and kidney transplantation can all cause hypomagnesemia.
- Diabetes, hungry bone syndrome, respiratory alkalosis, and pregnancy are all other potential causes of hypomagnesemia.

2. Pathology
- Pathology is determined by the underlying cause.
- Severe hypomagnesemia can cause decreased resistance to PTH in end organs and results in hypocalcemia that is resistant to repletion until the magnesium level is normalized.

- Increased renal excretion of potassium can be secondary to hypomagnesemia, and therefore the hypokalemia may be resistant to repletion until the magnesium level is normalized.

3. Clinical Features
- Signs and symptoms are similar to those of hypokalemia and hypocalcemia.
- Weakness, hyperreflexia, cramps, hyperirritability, tremors, athetoid movements, jerking, nystagmus, a Babinski reflex, confusion, disorientation, hypertension, tachycardia, and ventricular arrhythmias.

4. Diagnostic Studies
- Magnesium level is <1.5 mEq per L.
- Urinary magnesium level of >10 to 30 mg per day or a fractional excretion of >2% suggests a renal loss of magnesium.
- Calcium and potassium levels may also be low.
- ECG may see a prolonged QT and prolonged ST.
- PTH levels may be low.

5. Management
- For chronic, mild, or asymptomatic hypomagnesemia, may treat with magnesium oxide orally.
- For severe or symptomatic hypomagnesemia, may treat with IV magnesium sulfate.
- Replete potassium and calcium levels.
- Monitor electrolyte levels and watch for hypermagnesemia.

C. Hypermagnesemia
1. Etiology
- Hypermagnesemia is usually associated with CKD or increased intake of magnesium.

2. Pathology
- Pathology is determined by the underlying cause.
- Severe hypermagnesemia (>5 mEq per L) can depress PTH and cause hypocalcemia. This can be seen in patients with preeclampsia receiving magnesium therapy.

3. Clinical Features
- Signs and symptoms can be muscle weakness, hyperreflexia, mental obtundation, flaccid paralysis, ileus, urinary retention, confusion, hypotension, cardiac arrest, or respiratory muscular paralysis.

4. Diagnostic Studies
- Magnesium level >2.5 mEq per L.
- If CKD is present, may also see a rise in BUN/Cr and other electrolyte abnormalities.
- ECG may show a prolonged PR, widened QRS, and peaked T waves.

5. Management
- Decrease the magnesium intake.
- Calcium will antagonize magnesium and should be given IV.
- Dialysis can be performed for patients with CKD.

XXIII. Acid–Base Disturbances

A. Normal Physiology

- Acid–base balance is dependent on the maintenance of the hydrogen (H^+) ion concentration in body fluids.
- Normal physiologic processes cause increased amounts of carbonic acid and noncarbonic acids.
  - $CO_2 + H_2O \Leftrightarrow H_2CO_3$ (carbonic acid) $\Leftrightarrow H^+ + HCO_3^-$.
- Reactions work to buffer the pH using internal, rapid changes that work within a fraction of a second to change strong acids and bases into weak ones.
- The lungs work to alter respirations to buffer the CO_2 side of the carbonic acid reaction.
  - Adjusting rate and depth of respiration can compensate for pH shifts. It takes approximately 1 to 3 minutes for an adjustment to occur.
    - Increasing the respiratory rate or increasing the volume of the breath (tidal volume) will decrease $PaCO_2$.
    - Slowing the respiratory rate or decreasing the tidal volume will increase $PaCO_2$.
- The kidneys work to excrete or retain HCO_3^- to buffer the HCO_3^- side of the carbonic acid reaction.
  - H^+ can then be secreted into the tubules and HCO_3^- into blood at the level of the proximal tubules. These changes in secretion can also be reversed. Can take hours or days to see changes.
- Total venous CO_2 is a better measurement of bicarbonate because it is almost in all the bicarbonate forms within the serum. Therefore, the CO_2 level is ± 3 mEq per L of the actual serum bicarbonate level.
- Pathology:
  - Normal pH is 7.35 to 7.45; even minor deviations can affect physiologic responses.
  - Acidosis is when pH is <7.35.
  - Alkalosis is when pH is >7.45.

B. Metabolic Acidosis

1. Etiology

- Characterized by decreased bicarbonate and decreased pH.
- Divided into two categories:
  - Without increased anion gap:
    - Hyperchloremia.
    - Loss of bicarbonate.
  - With increased anion gap.
- Increased presence of an acid other than carbonic acid resulting in an anion gap.
  - Anion gap is a measurement of the difference between anions, which are negatively charged, and cations, which are positively charged.
  - ([Measured serum Na^+] – [Measured serum HCO_3^- + Measured serum Cl^-]).
  - Normally 8 to 16 mEq per L.
- Metabolic acidosis with an increased or widened anion gap includes:
  - Lactic acidosis.
  - Ketoacidosis: diabetic, alcohol (ETOH) abuse, and starvation.
  - Intoxication overdose (salicylates, methanol, and ethylene glycol).
  - Uremia.
- Metabolic acidosis with normal anion gap includes:
  - Diarrhea.
  - Mild renal insufficiency.
  - Diuretic treatment.
  - Renal tubular acidosis types I (classic distal), II (proximal), and IV (hyporeninemic-hypoaldosteronemic).
  - Aggressive normal saline resuscitation.

2. Pathology

- Pathology of metabolic acidosis is due to underlying causes.

3. Clinical Features

- A pH above 7.2 is usually well tolerated.
- Symptoms depend on underlying cause.

4. Diagnostic Studies

- Arterial blood gases (ABGs) show $\downarrow HCO_3^-$ and $\downarrow$pH.
- Other studies as needed for underlying cause.

5. Management

- Treat underlying cause.
- Varying practices on administration of bicarbonate to correct academia.
  - Monitor for hypokalemia.
- Alkali administration for type I and II renal tubular acidosis (RTA). Type IV (RTA) may need potassium restriction.

C. Metabolic Alkalosis

1. Etiology

- Characterized by increased bicarbonate and increased pH.
- Happens in two ways: by adding bicarbonate or by the loss of H^+ ions.
- If lost H^+ through stomach, will always be associated with the accompanying loss of chloride.
- Mechanisms causing a primary metabolic alkalosis:
  - Vomiting/too aggressive suctioning of gastric contents.
  - Diuretics (depletion of K^+ leads to the stimulation of proximal tube secretion and H^+, causing the so-called contraction alkalosis).
  - Overcorrection of bicarbonate in cardiac arrest or respiratory acidosis.
  - Volume depletion (especially as the kidney tries to compensate for other problems, i.e., diuretics, chloride depletion).

- Adrenal cortical overactivity.
  - Posthypercapnia, a rapid decrease in $PaCO_2$, can result in the HCO_3^- remaining elevated.
2. **Pathology**
   - Pathology of the metabolic alkalosis is due to the underlying cause.
   - Patients may hypoventilate to increase $PaCO_2$, as a compensation mechanism.
3. **Clinical Features**
   - Weakness, irritability, hyporeflexia, and tetany.
   - Hypoventilation.
   - Orthostatic hypotension.
   - Rarely symptoms other than those of underlying illness.
4. **Diagnostic Studies**
   - ABGs show $\uparrow HCO_3^-$ and $\uparrow pH$.
   - Check for urine chloride levels.
   - Other studies as needed for underlying cause.
5. **Management**
   - Severe alkalosis (pH > 7.6) needs immediate treatment.
   - Treat underlying cause.
   - Acetazolamide will increase renal bicarbonate excretion; use with caution in hypercapnic patients as it may result in respiratory acidosis.
   - Fluids with sodium chloride (NaCl) as determined by underlying causes.
   - Administration of KCl as determined by underlying causes.

D. **Respiratory Acidosis**
1. **Etiology**
   - Hypoventilation leading to increased $PaCO_2$.
   - Disorders that result in hypoventilation may cause respiratory acidosis.
     - Paralysis of chest/respiratory muscles (i.e., trauma and neuromuscular disorders).
     - Narcotic or sedative-hypnotic overdose.
     - Morbid obesity.
     - Severe kyphoscoliosis.
   - Obstructive disorders of the airways:
     - Chronic obstructive pulmonary disease (COPD).
     - Severe asthma.
2. **Pathology**
   - May have an acute or chronic respiratory acidosis.
   - Renal compensation occurs with increased H^+ excretion and increased reabsorption of HCO_3^- at proximal renal tubules.
3. **Clinical Features**
   - Symptoms depend on underlying cause.
   - $PaCO_2$ regulates blood flow to brain and increases cerebrospinal fluid pressure; leads to generalized CNS depression.
   - Cardiac output decreases, leading to decreased blood flow to organs.
   - Asterixis and myoclonus.

4. **Diagnostic Studies**
   - ABGs show $\uparrow PaCO_2$ and $\downarrow pH$.
   - Studies determined by underlying cause.
5. **Management**
   - Treat underlying cause.
   - Hyperventilate to "blow off" excess CO_2 if an acute respiratory acidosis.

E. **Respiratory Alkalosis**
1. **Etiology**
   - Hyperventilation leading to decreased $PaCO_2$.
   - Disorders that result in hyperventilation may cause respiratory alkalosis.
   - Anxiety resulting in hyperventilation is the most common source of respiratory alkalosis.
   - Fever.
   - Cerebral injury.
   - Pulmonary disorders such as asthma, pneumonia, and fibrosis.
   - Acetylsalicylic acid (aspirin) in extremely high doses can increase respirations by directly affecting the respiratory center.
2. **Pathology**
   - Renal compensation occurs with decreased H^+ excretion and decreased HCO_3^- reabsorption in the proximal renal tubules.
3. **Clinical Features**
   - Carpal/pedal spasm.
   - Tetany, paresthesias, and perioral numbness.
   - Light-headedness.
   - Anxiety.
   - Cardiac output increases due to alkalemia, but can then decrease if the pH is >7.7.
   - Symptoms also depend on underlying cause.
4. **Diagnostic Studies**
   - ABGs show $\downarrow PaCO_2$ and $\uparrow pH$.
5. **Management**
   - Treat underlying cause.
   - Evaluate underlying cause, then may need to control ventilation to increase CO_2, although usually only in severe cases.

F. **Mixed Acid–Base Disturbances**
   Etiology/Pathology
   - The kidneys and the lungs work in combination to balance the following chemical reaction.
     - $CO_2 + H_2O \Leftrightarrow H_2CO_3$ (carbonic acid) $\Leftrightarrow H^+ + HCO_3^-$.
     - If the CO_2 rises due to hypoventilation, the kidneys will hold onto more HCO_3^- to maintain balance.
     - When this "balance mechanism" is ineffective, it can result in a second or third acid–base disturbance.
       - Example: HCO_3^- is low because of GI losses, but patient, rather than hyperventilating to lower the $PaCO_2$, has an elevated $PaCO_2$ due to underlying COPD resulting in a second acid–base disturbance.

- Patients can present with two to three concomitant acid–base disturbances.
- Three disturbances can occur only when there is a primary anion gap metabolic acidosis.
- The only combination that cannot coexist is respiratory alkalosis and respiratory acidosis because one is secondary to hypoventilation and the other to hyperventilation.

G. Steps to Determine Acid–Base Disturbance

1. **Look Whether the pH Is High, Low, or Normal**
   - A high pH means alkalosis.
   - A low pH means acidosis.
   - Normal does not necessarily mean there are no abnormalities.

2. **Look the $PaCO_2$ and the HCO_3 for the Primary Acid–Base Disorder (or the Reason the pH Is High or Low)**
   - High $PaCO_2$ (nl 35–45) means respiratory acidosis.
   - Low $PaCO_2$ (nl 35–45) means respiratory alkalosis.
   - High HCO_3 (nl 24–32) means metabolic alkalosis.
   - Low HCO_3 (nl 24–32) means metabolic acidosis.

3. **Is There an Appropriate Response?**
   - The lungs and the kidneys work in combination to balance the need to calculate the response (see Table 1–1).
   - The purpose of the response equations is to determine a second, if any, acid–base disorder or whether there is an appropriate response by the opposite molecule (HCO_3 or CO_2).

4. **Is There an Anion Gap?**
   - Needed to perform only if you find a primary metabolic acidosis.
   - $Na - (Cl + HCO_3^-)$.
   - Greater than 16 equals an anion gap.

5. **Is There a Third Disorder?**
   - When there is an anion gap metabolic acidosis, there is an extra anion present that is unaccounted for in the equation; $Na - (Cl + HCO_3)$.
   - This means there is an extra anion other than sodium (Na), chloride (Cl), and bicarbonate (HCO_3). Normally, the extra anion is organic protein such as albumin or globulin; a normal anion gap is 3 to 12.
     - A low anion gap should suggest the need for evaluation for hypoproteinemia or hypoglobulinemia.
   - If the anion gap is elevated, then there is perhaps an unknown anion present. These extra anions are the cause of the unexpected difference between anions and cations. What they do *not* account for is the change in HCO_3 (because they are extra).
   - The delta–delta gap accounts for the HCO_3^-.
     - Delta–delta is calculated by the equation change in the anion gap divided by the change in the bicarbonate level ($\Delta AG/\Delta HCO_3$).
     - If the delta–delta gap is <1, then that means there is a non–anion gap metabolic acidosis

TABLE 1–1.	Compensatory Changes in Simple Acid–Base Disorders
Metabolic Acidosis	
Primary change: HCO_3^- decreased Predicted compensation[a]: $PaCO_2 = (10.5 \times HCO_3^-) + 8 \pm 2$	
Metabolic Alkalosis	
Primary change: HCO_3^- increased Predicted compensation[b]: $PaCO_2 = (0.9 \times HCO_3^-) + 9$	
Respiratory Acidosis	
Primary change: $PaCO_2$ increased Predicted compensation Acute acidosis: HCO_3^- increases 1 mEq/L for every 10 mm Hg increase in $PaCO_2$ Chronic acidosis: HCO_3^- increases 3.5 mEq/L for every 10 mm Hg increase in $PaCO_2$	
Respiratory Alkalosis	
Primary change: $PaCO_2$ decreased Predicted compensation Acute alkalosis: HCO_3^- decreases 2 mEq/L for every 10 mm Hg decrease in $PaCO_2$ Chronic alkalosis: HCO_3^- decreases 5 mEq/L for every 10 mm Hg decrease in $PaCO_2$	

[a]Full compensation may require 12 hours.

[b]Actual compensation is erratic and only approximated by this formula.

From Fishman M, Hoffman A, Klausner R, et al. Fluids, electrolytes, and pH homeostasis. In: Fishman M, Hoffman A, Klausner R, et al, eds. *Medicine*. 3rd ed. Philadelphia, PA: JB Lippincott; 1991: chap 21:159–172, with permission.

superimposed on top of an anion gap metabolic acidosis.
- If the delta–delta gap is >1.5, then that means there is a metabolic alkalosis superimposed on the top of an anion gap metabolic acidosis.

REVIEW QUESTIONS

1. A 23-year-old 4-month pregnant woman presents to Emergency Department (ED) with difficulty concentrating and blurred vision. Vitals: blood pressure (BP) 122/84, body mass index (BMI) 32.2 (pre-pregnancy BMI 28), pulse 112. A blood glucose was performed at 47. What condition is this patient at greater risk of developing during her pregnancy?

a) Diabetes, type I
b) Cushing disease
c) Hemorrhoids
d) Eclampsia
e) Cystitis

2. A 42-year-old African American man presents to his primary care provider with hematospermia for 2 days without dysuria, hematuria, or previous urologic evaluation. He reports that his father had been evaluated by a urologist in the past and had surgery but unfortunately patient is unsure of his father's diagnosis, and patient's father died of myocardial infarction (MI) 2 years ago. What imaging study is preferred for complete evaluation of this patient?

a) Computed tomography (CT) pelvis
b) Ultrasound (U/S) scrotum
c) Magnetic resonance imaging (MRI) prostate
d) No diagnostic imaging is necessary

3. As you go to leave after seeing a patient for annual physical, he asks, "Is it common for men as they age to ... you know ... (patient blushes) ejaculate sooner than desired?" You explain that it appears that he may have premature ejaculation and you need to ask a complete sexual history. He states that he would prefer to keep his sexual life private. How should you best proceed?

a) Explain a complete sexual history is imperative to diagnose premature ejaculation.
b) Complete a short five-question sexual history and attempt to treat based on those answers.
c) Skip sexual history given patient's preference and empirically treat based on his report.
d) Refer to urology.

4. An 83-year-old woman with history of chronic obstructive pulmonary disease (COPD), hypertension (HTN), and hyperlipidemia (HLD) all well controlled on medications, presents with frequent urination, urgency, urge incontinence with nocturia × 4 for the past month and is very bothered by her symptoms and wants immediate relief. Urine culture was negative. What is the first-line treatment for this patient?

a) Trial of mirabegron prior to urology referral
b) Posterior tibial nerve stimulation
c) Oxybutynin
d) Intradetrusor onabotulinumtoxinA (100 U)
e) Cystotomy
f) None of the above

5. A new patient, Ms. Bailey, presents to the office for routine physical exam. The patient states that she recently moved to the United States about 6 months ago from Thailand as she was living there for "health reasons." When asked as to what health issues led her to live in Thailand, the patient explained that she was there to have gender affirmation surgery. Unfortunately, there has not been a known transgender person who has been evaluated at the office before Ms. Bailey. Which of the following is the best response to Ms. Bailey's request for care?

a) "I can't help you as we have never had a transgender person in this office. You must see someone else."
b) "I don't know much about transgender healthcare, but I will just treat you as I would any other female patient."

c) "I am not as knowledgeable about transgender healthcare as I should be, but let's meet today to complete a comprehensive history and physical and I will speak with some of my colleagues who are more knowledgeable than I am."
d) "I unfortunately cannot discuss your health today until I get your previous records, so we need to reschedule after I obtain your records from Thailand. This may take some time, so I will call you in a few weeks."

6. A 56-year-old man presents to ED with erection lasting more than 4 hours that was unrelieved by ejaculation. He reports a past medical history significant for insomnia and depression. He is unsure of his medication list, but he takes a medication at night which he was told can cause sexual side effects and/or drowsiness. What medication is this patient likely taking?

a) Zolpidem
b) Duloxetine
c) Amitriptyline
d) Alprazolam
e) Trazadone

7. A 16-year-old girl presents with acute left knee pain without trauma; however, she does report chills and a one-week history of multiple joint pain. Temperature 102.6, pulse 90, BP 122/70. After a complete sexual history, she reports multiple partners and prefers not to have her male partners use a condom as it "feels different." Upon examination, the left knee is with edema, erythematous, and tender to palpation. The left knee joint was aspirated and found to demonstrate gram-negative diplococcic. What is the most likely diagnosis?

a) Rheumatoid arthritis
b) Systemic lupus erythematosus
c) Viral hepatitis myositis
d) Reiter's syndrome
e) Gonoccocal arthritis

8. Which of the following terms refer to the retracted foreskin becoming trapped proximal to glans penis resulting in edema, inflammation, and pain?

a) Phimosis
b) Priapism
c) Paraphimosis
d) Fornier gangrene

9. A 55-year-old woman presents to the office with her husband with dyspareunia for 6 months. Of the following, which is the most appropriate question to ask?

a) When was her last menstrual cycle?
b) Does her partner experience premature ejaculation?
c) Does the patient experience an inability to orgasm?
d) Does this patient experience inhibited sexual desire?

10. In those with Klinefelter syndrome, the primary feature is which of the following:

a) Low-set ears, short stature
b) Sterility

c) Wide-set eyes

d) Small jaw

11. Which of the following is a risk factor for prostate cancer?

a) Caribbean descent

b) Cigarette smoking

c) Recurrent urinary tract infections

d) South American residency

e) In men who eat a primary fruit and vegetable diet

12. A 19-year-old woman presents with cough, sore throat, and overall malaise over the past 3 to 4 days, suspect viral upper respiratory. Bloodwork including urinalysis was obtained for thorough evaluation noting 10 to 30 red blood cells (RBCs) and proteinuria in urinalysis and creatinine of 1.8. What is the likely diagnosis?

a) IgA nephropathy (Buerger disease)

b) Henoch–Schonlein purpura

c) Pauci-immune glomerulonephritis

d) Anti-GBM glomerulonephritis

e) Cryoglobulin-associated glomerulonephritis

13. What is a necessary diagnostic study in nephrotic syndrome?

a) Microscopic urinalysis

b) Renal biopsy

c) 24-hour urine collection

d) Liver function tests

14. Which of the following would result in the greatest increase in glomerular filtration rate (GFR)?

a) Renal artery stenosis

b) Renal vein constriction

c) Afferent arteriolar constriction

d) Efferent arteriolar constriction

15. A 12-year-old boy presents with nausea and one episode of bloody diarrhea in the past 24 hours with initially erythematous macules noted on upper thighs, which has been developing to palpable purpura. What is the best treatment option for this patient?

a) Amoxicillin (or clindamycin) × 10 days

b) Angiotensin-converting-enzyme (ACE) inhibitors or angiotensin II receptor blockers (ARBs)

c) 5-day course of steroids

d) Supportive

16. Acute tubulointerstitial nephritis (ATIN) is related to a drug reaction to which common medication over 70% of the time?

a) Naproxen

b) Allopuriniol

c) Hydralazine

d) Amoxicillin

17. A 62-year-old woman with a history of HTN on diuretic therapy only presents after a cruise in which she developed gastrointestinal (GI) symptoms (i.e., nausea, vomiting). She developed muscle cramps and weakness with a 2-day course of constipation. Labwork was obtained. What is a likely finding?

a) Serum hemoglobin > 16.0

b) Serum sodium < 125 mEq per dL

c) >2 RBCs/high-power field (HPF) on urinalysis

d) Serum potassium < 3.5

18. Metabolic acidosis is characterized by the following on arterial blood gases (ABGs):

a) $\downarrow HCO_3^-$ and $\downarrow pH$

b) $\uparrow HCO_3^-$ and $\uparrow pH$

c) $\uparrow PaCO_2$ and $\downarrow pH$

d) $\downarrow PaCO_2$ and $\uparrow pH$

ANSWERS TO REVIEW QUESTIONS

1. **Answer: D**. Gestational hypoglycemia is common in women whose pre-pregnancy BMI <30 and age <25. Gestational hypoglycemia increases risk of preeclampsia and eclampsia. (Formulating Most Likely Diagnosis)

2. **Answer: C**. Hematospermia can be associated with prostate cancer. CT tends to have poor performance characteristics for assessing prostate nodule/metastasis. Transrectal ultrasound can be used as an alternative imaging study for older patients and/or patients who cannot obtain an MRI. Imaging is necessary for this patient. MRI is preferred imaging study for evaluation of prostate nodule, cyst, and/or metastasis. (Using Laboratory & Diagnostic Studies)

3. **Answer: A**. A complete sexual history is vital to diagnosing premature ejaculation; however, some patients may feel uncomfortable in disclosing this information. It is important to explain that a complete sexual history is necessary. Please offer a male provider to complete sexual history if possible. If the patient still does not want to disclose, a referral to urology can be made. However, a diagnosis cannot be made without a complete sexual history. (History Taking & Performing Physical Examinations)

4. **Answer: F**. The first-line treatment for the suspected diagnosis of overactive bladder is behavioral therapies, including bladder training, pelvic floor muscle training, fluid management, and bladder journaling. For older adults with multiple pharmacologic agents, the Beers Criteria for Potentially Inappropriate Medication Use in Older Adults needs to be considered, which is a concern for starting an antimuscarinic in this 83-year-old with multiple comorbidities. Mirabegron (antispasmodic) has anticholingeric-like effects and should be a considered late in evaluation given possible side effects. (Pharmaceutical Therapeutics)

5. **Answer: C**. It is important to be honest about your knowledge or lack thereof with transgender healthcare. However, a referral to a more knowledgeable provider is not always necessary. It is vital to perform an organ inventory to ensure that specific tests and physical exam is or is not necessary (i.e., prostate intact may need prostate cancer screening). Although previous records are very helpful, it is inappropriate to delay care or treatment to

obtain previous records. (History Taking & Performing Physical Examination)

6. **Answer: E.** A serious adverse reaction of trazadone is priapism. Priapism is an involuntary, prolonged erection unrelated to sexual stimulation and unrelieved by ejaculation. Zolpidem is a nonbenzodiazepine hypnotic that can cause headache, drowsiness, and back pain and, in serious cases, can cause depression exacerbation. Duloxetine is a serotonin and norepinephrine reuptake inhibitor (SNRI) that can cause nausea, headache, and, in severe cases, suicidal ideation, but not associated with priapism. Amitriptyline is a tricyclic antidepressants (TCA) that can cause drowsiness, blurred vision, and, in severe cases, orthostatic hypotension, but not associated with priapism. Alprazolam is a benzodiazepine that can cause sedation, depression, and, in severe cases, respiratory distress, but is not associated with priapism. (Clinical Intervention)

7. **Answer: E.** Gonoccocal arthritis is an infection of a joint caused by the bacteria Neisseria gonorrhoeae. This infection does affect women more often than men and is common in sexually active teen girls. (Formulating Most Likely Diagnosis)

8. **Answer: C.** Paraphimosis refers to the retracted foreskin becoming trapped proximal to glans penis, resulting in edema, inflammation, and pain. (Formulating Most Likely Diagnosis)

9. **Answer: A.** This patient's dyspareunia is most likely related to postmenopausal decrease in estrogen. For most postmenopausal women, inadequate lubrication is a result of low estrogen levels. A topical estrogen can be applied to the vagina as treatment. Hypoactive sexual desire (HSD) is experienced by 10% to 15% of women in which there is little desire for sexual activity. An inability to orgasm is common in female sexual arousal disorder (FSAD) where patients experience a lack of psychologic and/or physical response to sexual stimulation. (History Taking & Performing Physical Examination)

10. **Answer: B.** The primary feature of Klinefelter syndrome is sterility. Most males are diagnosed in adulthood during infertility evaluation and is one of the leading causes of male infertility, with approximately 3% of all infertile males. (History Taking & Performing Physical Examination)

11. **Answer: A.** Men of African American and Caribbean descent are seen to have a higher likelihood of having prostate cancer. Men who eat primarily fruit and vegetables and those of South American residency tend to have less risk for prostate cancer. Urinary tract infections (UTIs) and cigarette smoking are not known to be a risk factor for prostate cancer. (Formulating Most Likely Diagnosis)

12. **Answer: A.** IgA nephropathy is most likely. (Formulating Most Likely Diagnosis)

13. **Answer: C.** Renal biopsy can be used, but only in rare circumstances. A 24-hour urine collection is the necessary diagnostic study to determine if protein loss is >3.5 g per 24 hours. (Using Laboratory & Diagnostic Studies)

14. **Answer: D.** Efferent arteriolar constriction. (Applying Basic Science Concepts)

15. **Answer: D.** Henoch–Schönlein purpura typically is self-limiting, and renal function typically returns without any intervention. (Formulating Most Likely Diagnosis)

16. **Answer: A.** Nonsteroidal anti-inflammatory drugs (NSAIDs) account for approximately 70% of all cases of ATIN, although all other medications listed can cause ATIN. (Pharmaceutical Therapeutics)

17. **Answer: D.** Hypokalemia is typically a result of nasogastric suctioning or vomiting along with diuretic therapy. It is typically managed by treating underlying cause (i.e., vomiting) along with oral potassium supplementation in mild-to-moderate deficiency. (Formulating Most Likely Diagnosis)

18. **Answer: A.** $\downarrow HCO_3^-$ and $\downarrow pH$. (Using Laboratory & Diagnostic Studies)

Hematologic Disorders

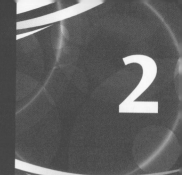

2

Elizabeth Quinlan-Bohn

I. Anemia
A. General Definition, Red Cell Morphology
- Anemia occurs when hemoglobin (Hgb) in blood is too low to fulfill oxygen (O_2) demands of the body.
- Can be measured by a decrease in the red blood cell (RBC) volume (hematocrit [HCT]) or decrease in the amount of Hgb.
- RBC: Adult normals.
  - Males: 4.4 to 5.9×10^6 per mm³.
  - Females: 3.8 to 5.2×10^6 per mm³.
- Hgb consists of a protein called globin composed of four polypeptide chains and four nonprotein pigments (heme) that contain iron to carry O_2—Hgb A ($\alpha_2\beta_2$), Hgb A_2 ($\alpha_2\delta_2$), and Hgb F ($\alpha_2\gamma_2$).
- HGB: Adult normals.
  - Males: 13.3 to 17.7 g per dL.
  - Females: 11.7 to 15.7 g per dL.
- Normal adult blood contains Hgb A (95%–98%), Hgb A_2 (1.5%–3.5%), and Hgb F (<2%).
- HCT: percentage of blood volume that is RBCs, usually approximately three times the Hgb concentration.
- Example: A patient with an Hgb of 12 g per dL would have an approximate HCT of 36%.
- HCT: Adult normals.
  - Males: 40% to 52%.
  - Females: 35% to 47%.
- Factors that may account for variations in normal values: increased HCT due to secondary erythrocytosis among tobacco smokers and people living at high altitudes; decreased HCT due to dilutional effect from plasma volume expansion of pregnancy.
  - HCT values may be artificially high or low in hypovolemia/hypervolemia.
  - Gold standard: RBC mass, a nuclear medicine test that measures milliliter RBCs per kilogram of body weight, generally obtained only in the evaluation of abnormally elevated values (polycythemia).
- Erythrocyte indices.
  - Erythrocyte indices classify RBCs by size and Hgb content.
  1. **Mean Cell Volume or Mean Corpuscular Volume**
     - Measure of average RBC size.
     - **Normocytic cells** have a mean corpuscular volume (MCV) of 80 to 100 fL.
     - **Microcytic cells** have an MCV of <80 fL.
     - **Macrocytic cells** have an MCV of >100 fL.
  2. **Mean Corpuscular Hgb Concentration**
     - Measure of average Hgb concentration per RBC.
     - Percentage of Hgb in RBC.
     - Measure of *color*.
     - **Normochromic cells** have a mean corpuscular Hgb concentration (MCHC) of 32 to 36 g per dL.
     - **Hypochromic cells** have an MCHC of <32 g per dL.
     - **Hyperchromic cells:** The MCHC cannot exceed 37 g per dL, because this is the maximum amount of Hgb that RBCs can contain. No real hyperchromic cells exist except the spherocyte secondary to decreased surface–volume ratio.
  3. **Mean Corpuscular Hgb**
     - Measure of the average amount of Hgb per RBC.
     - Measure of *weight*.
     - **NOTE:** mean corpuscular Hgb (MCH) does not take into account cell size—should be correlated with MCV.
     - **Normochromic cells** have an MCH of 26 to 34 pg.
     - **Hypochromic cells** have an MCH of <26 pg.
     - **Hyperchromic cells** have an MCH of >34 pg.
  4. **Reticulocyte**
     - Immature RBC with no nucleus and residual ribonucleic acid and mitochondria that lives in bone marrow 2 to 3 days; is then extruded into peripheral blood where it lives in this form for another day or two.
     - Laboratory normals: 0.5% to 1.5% of all RBCs.
     - Values higher than these indicate increased production of RBCs.
     - Elevated reticulocyte count indicates increased production of RBCs. Must take into account that an increased reticulocyte count does not always indicate a hyperproliferative bone marrow and also must determine the corrected reticulocyte count reticulocyte count (CRC):
       - CRC = (% reticulocytes) × (patient's HCT/ normal HCT).

B. Blood Loss (Acute and Chronic)
  1. **Acute Blood Loss**
     a. **Etiology**
        - Acute blood loss caused by hemorrhage from such disorder as trauma.
        - Massive gastrointestinal (GI) bleed.
        - Ruptured aneurysm.

b. **Pathology**
- Blood loss of >1,500 mL causes cardiovascular collapse.

c. **Clinical Features**
- Patient may complain of dizziness, lightheadedness, or both, or be stuporous or comatose.
- Physical examination may show tachycardia, hypotension, orthostatic change in pulse and blood pressure, melena, hematemesis, or signs of trauma.

d. **Diagnostic Studies**
- Laboratory values may be normal initially; then increased white blood cells (WBCs) with neutrophil predominance; decreased platelets following massive RBC transfusion; increased reticulocytes; heme-positive stool (if GI source of blood loss).
- Elevated blood urea nitrogen (BUN)-to-creatinine ratio >36:1 is suggestive of upper GI bleeding as cause.
- Upper endoscopy is the diagnostic test of choice for acute upper GI bleeding; once lesion is identified, endoscopy can achieve hemostasis and prevent recurrent bleeding in most cases.
- If an upper GI bleeding source has been excluded by upper endoscopy, the initial diagnostic test of choice for acute lower GI bleeding is colonoscopy; allows for localization of lesion, collection of pathologic specimens, and potential therapeutic intervention.

e. **Management**
- Maintain volume by placing two large-bore intravenous (IV) lines and transfuse with fluids and blood products, as clinically indicated.
- When site of blood loss is identified, treat underlying condition.

2. **Chronic Blood Loss**
- May be due to occult bleeding.
- Patients usually present with signs/symptoms of iron deficiency anemia.
- Perform appropriate diagnostic studies—for example, upper GI series, upper endoscopy, colonoscopy, flexible sigmoidoscopy, arteriogram, pelvic examination, ultrasound (U/S).
- Then correct underlying disorder.

C. **Microcytic Anemia**
1. **Iron Deficiency Anemia**
   a. **Etiology**
   - Caused by blood loss (e.g., menstruation, chronic GI blood loss, and genitourinary blood loss), inadequate dietary intake, physiologic states of increased utilization (e.g., pregnancy), malabsorption (e.g., postgastrectomy, celiac sprue, chronic achlorhydria, and atrophic gastritis).

   b. **Epidemiology**
   - Most common anemia worldwide.
   - Can occur at any age.
   - Common cause of iron deficiency in developing countries is hookworm infestation in areas where this parasite is endemic.

   c. **Pathology**
   - Iron is absorbed most efficiently in the duodenum.
   - Occurs gradually; initially, iron stores depleted and RBC count normal (iron deficiency without anemia).
   - No stored iron remains.
   - Total iron-binding capacity (TIBC) increases.
   - After all stores are depleted, RBC formation continues with low-serum iron values (<30 μg per dL), transferrin saturation falls to <15%.
   - MCV then decreases, with anisocytosis, poikilocytosis, hypochromia.

   d. **Clinical Features**
   - History: may be of multiple pregnancies, excess menstrual bleeding, alcoholism, poor diet, gastric surgery, celiac sprue, peptic ulcer disease.
   - Symptoms: depending on the degree of anemia, the patient may be asymptomatic or may have symptoms including fatigue, weakness, palpitations, dyspnea on exertion, dizziness, syncope, bleeding, bruising, melena, bright red blood per rectum, headache, confusion, depression, pica, muscle weakness, angina, and dysphagia due to pharyngeal web (Plummer–Vinson syndrome).
   - Physical examination: may show hypotension, tachycardia, pallor, ecchymoses, pale palpebral conjunctiva, glossitis, cheilosis, heme-positive stool, hemorrhoids, pelvic masses, and koilonychias.

   e. **Diagnostic Studies**
   - Decrease in RBCs, Hgb, HCT.
   - Serum iron <30 μg per dL.
   - Serum ferritin (SF) <20 μg per L. (Because SF is an *acute-phase reactant*, in the presence of microcytic MCV and anemia, SF may be higher than 20 μg per L and may still support a diagnosis of iron deficiency anemia, depending on underlying medical conditions.)
   - Increased TIBC.
   - Transferrin saturation of <15%.
   - Microcytosis (MCV < 80 fL).
   - Hypochromia (MCHC < 30 g per dL and MCH < 26 pg).
   - Anisocytosis, poikilocytosis on peripheral blood smear.
   - Platelet count may be increased.
   - "Gold standard": bone marrow biopsy with iron stain to assess bone marrow iron stores. However, bone marrow is not routinely required to diagnose iron deficiency and would

generally only be indicated if etiology of anemia was uncertain.

   f. **Management**

- Treat underlying disorder, if any.
- Administer oral iron (e.g., $FeSO_4$ 325 mg PO TID [three times a day], taken between meals) until iron levels are normal. If patient experiences GI side effects (e.g., nausea, constipation) while taking oral iron, it may be beneficial to start patient on $FeSO_4$ 325 mg PO once daily, and gradually increase dose as tolerated, until therapeutic dose of $FeSO_4$ 325 mg PO TID is achieved. **NOTE:** Enteric-coated forms of oral iron are not well absorbed and should generally be avoided.
- Monitor response to treatment by checking to determine whether reticulocyte count increases. Period of maximum reticulocytosis generally occurs approximately 1 week after starting oral iron therapy.
- Hgb should normalize in 6 to 10 weeks, but oral iron should be continued until iron stores replete (generally requires continuation of oral iron therapy for approximately 6 months following normalization of Hgb). It is important to follow the SF level during iron replacement therapy to document repletion of iron stores.
- Occasionally, owing to inability to take oral iron supplement or intestinal malabsorption, patients cannot receive oral iron therapy and must be given parenteral iron. Parenteral iron therapy in the form of low-molecular-weight iron dextran may be administered by intramuscular (IM) injection (using Z-track technique in the buttock) or IV infusion; dosage is calculated on the basis of the patient's body weight and Hgb. Parenteral iron therapy has significant potential systemic side effects including, but not limited to, fever, rash, arthralgias, lymphadenopathy, splenomegaly, and anaphylaxis. Patients must receive a test dose to assess for hypersensitivity, before a course of iron dextran treatment is started, because of the risk of anaphylaxis.

2. **Thalassemia**

   a. **Etiology**

- Hereditary disorder resulting from inherited defect in the synthesis of globin chains, resulting in decreased or absent α- or β-globin chain production.
- Most common among Southeast Asian, Mediterranean, and African American populations.

   b. **Pathology**

- Chromosomes 11 and 16 are responsible for globin chain synthesis. One gene on chromosome 11 is responsible for the synthesis of β chains, and two genes on chromosome 16 are responsible for the synthesis of α chains.
  - Owing to gene deletion or point mutations that cause decrease in synthesis or production of globin chains, either α or β chains, of Hgb.
  - Deficiency or total absence of α-globin chains results in the α-thalassemia disorders, and deficiency or total absence of β-globin chains results in the β-thalassemia disorders.

   c. **Clinical Features**

- Presentation varies widely depending on whether person has α- or β-thalassemia and whether they are homozygous or heterozygous.
- α-Thalassemia severity depends on the number of α-globin genes present (four α-globin genes are normally present).
- Three α-globin genes present: silent carrier state (also known as α-thalassemia minima); involves deletion of one of four alleles on chromosome 16; the patient is clinically normal.
- Two α-globin genes present: α-thalassemia trait (also known as α-thalassemia minor) with microcytic anemia; the patient is clinically normal.
- One α-globin gene present: Hgb H disease (also known as α-thalassemia intermedia). Only a small amount of Hgb A is formed, and the excess β-globin chains form tetramers; Hgb H (β_4). Clinical findings include microcytic chronic hemolytic anemia; pallor and splenomegaly may be present.
- Total absence of α-globin genes; excess γ-globin chains form tetramers; Hgb Barts (γ_4); resulting in no fetal or adult Hgb synthesis; generally incompatible with life; causes Hgb Barts hydrops fetalis syndrome, which is a frequent cause of stillbirth in Southeast Asia.
- β-Thalassemia minor found in heterozygotes with mild microcytic anemia, clinically normal.
- β-Thalassemia intermedia: mild homozygous form with microcytic hemolytic anemia, hepatosplenomegaly, bony deformities.
- β-Thalassemia major: severe homozygous form that develops within the first year of life; with severe anemia and hepatosplenomegaly, bony deformities, osteopenia, fractures.

   d. **Diagnostic Studies**

- Microcytic anemia that varies according to severity of disease; RBC number is typically normal or elevated in thalassemia and may help distinguish between thalassemia and iron deficiency anemia.
- On peripheral blood smear target cells, basophilic stippling, nucleated RBCs may be seen.
- Hgb electrophoresis testing is indicated for the diagnosis of β-thalassemia and more severe forms of α-thalassemia.

NOTE: In patients with α-thalassemia silent carrier state or α-thalassemia trait, Hgb electrophoresis will generally be normal; DNA mutation analysis is required to make the definitive diagnosis.

- Thalassemia should be suspected in patients with microcytosis, normal iron levels.
- **Complications**
  - Frequent transfusion requirements may result in iron overload causing cardiomyopathy, congestive heart failure, hepatomegaly, and death.
  - Misdiagnosis as iron deficiency anemia results in inappropriate iron therapy.
- e. **Management**
  - Mild disease generally requires no treatment.
  - Genetic counseling should be given.
  - Severe forms of thalassemia may require RBC transfusions with iron chelation therapy to prevent iron overload, folic acid, and vitamin C.
  - In select cases in patients with β-thalassemia major and transfusion-dependent anemia, allogeneic hematopoietic stem cell transplant (HSCT) is the only curative option.

3. **Acquired Sideroblastic Anemia of Lead Poisoning**
   a. **Etiology**
   - Lead poisoning (also known as *plumbism*) among children may be caused by ingestion of lead paint chips or soil or water contaminated with lead.
   - Adults may develop lead poisoning by eating food that leached lead from pottery dishware or through inhalation of lead from industrial processes.
   - Currently, in the United States, approximately 4 million children are living in households with high lead levels, and approximately 500,000 U.S. children aged 1 to 5 years have lead levels that exceed the reference range of 5 μg per dL.
   b. **Pathology**
   - Lead poisons enzymes, causing cell death.
   - Shortens life span of RBCs.
   - Lead poisoning inhibits multiple enzyme steps required in heme synthesis, causing abnormal heme synthesis and resulting in an acquired sideroblastic anemia.
   c. **Clinical Features**
   - Children with lead toxicity may complain of abdominal pain and fatigue. Chronic lead toxicity may cause learning disability or other neurologic or behavioral problems.
   - On examination, they may be pale, ataxic, with slurred speech, or may be seizing or comatose because of acute encephalopathy.
   - Adults may have symptoms of abdominal pain, headache, peripheral neuropathies, and be pale, ataxic, with loss of memory, and foot or wrist drop.

- A *lead line* may be present along the gum line (dark blue-gray line along gingival border); generally indicates severe and prolonged lead exposure.
   d. **Diagnostic Studies**
   - Peripheral blood smear: microcytic, hypochromic anemia with basophilic stippling of RBCs.
   - Iron deficiency may coexist with lead poisoning; patients with elevated blood lead levels (BLLs) should undergo screening for iron deficiency with CBC and SF.
   - X-rays of long bones may show lead lines (increased density of metaphyseal plates).
   - Children should be screened for lead levels according to currently accepted pediatric guidelines.
   - No "nontoxic" BLL exists; in the United States, reference BLL for children as 5 μg per dL has been adopted, corresponding to 97.5th percentile of BLLs among U.S. children.
   - In 2015, National Institute for Occupational Safety and Health designated the adult reference BLL as 5 μg per dL.
   e. **Management**
   - Remove source of lead.
   - Specific treatment recommendations for lead poisoning are dependent on multiple factors (e.g., BLL and clinical presentation of patient). The decision regarding whether chelation therapy is indicated should, therefore, be made in consultation with a medical toxicologist.

D. Macrocytic Anemia
1. **Megaloblastic Anemia: Vitamin B12 (Cobalamin) Deficiency**
   a. **Etiology**
   - Most common cause of vitamin B_{12} deficiency is not inadequate intake, but inability to absorb; most adults have enough vitamin B_{12} stores to last 3 years.
   - Those at risk for vitamin B_{12} deficiency due to inadequate intake are strict vegetarians (e.g., veganism).
   b. **Pathology**
   - Following ingestion of B_{12}-containing food, vitamin B_{12} is bound to intrinsic factor (IF), and the vitamin B_{12}–IF complex is transported through the intestine and then absorbed in the terminal ileum.
   - Vitamin B_{12} is required for the synthesis of homocysteine to methionine, a main reaction in DNA synthesis.
   - It is theorized that a low vitamin B_{12} level causes folate to be "trapped" and, therefore, to be unavailable for DNA synthesis.
   - Vitamin B_{12} is present in all animal products (e.g., milk, eggs, and meat).

- Vitamin B_{12} deficiency may lead to defective myelin synthesis in the central nervous system (CNS) and subsequent neurologic dysfunction.
- Vitamin B_{12} deficiency may be caused by pernicious anemia, poor diet, malabsorption (e.g., due to partial or total gastrectomy, ileal resection, tropical sprue, small bowel lymphoma, inflammatory bowel disease, and pancreatic insufficiency), nitrous oxide (N_2O) inhalation, small intestine parasite infestation (fish tapeworm), bacterial overgrowth of small intestine, drugs (e.g., metformin, cholestyramine, neomycin, and colchicine), and congenital disorders (e.g., transcobalamin II deficiency).

c. **Clinical Features**
- Patient may complain of symptoms of anemia or neurologic dysfunction (e.g., paresthesias, ataxia, weakness, and change in mental status), anorexia, and diarrhea.
- Gastric atrophy and achlorhydria are present in pernicious anemia.
- On examination, assess for pallor, decrease in position and vibratory sense, Romberg sign, Babinski sign, neuropathy, and glossitis.

d. **Diagnostic Studies**
- Anemia may not be present in 25% of patients with vitamin B_{12} deficiency.
- Neuropsychiatric symptoms due to vitamin B_{12} (cobalamin) deficiency may occur when anemia or macrocytosis is not yet present.
- If present, anemia is typically macrocytic with MCV of 110 to 140. **NOTE:** In the setting of combined deficiencies (e.g., concurrent iron deficiency and vitamin B_{12} deficiency), MCV may be normal.
- Hypersegmented neutrophils ($\geq$5 lobes), serum $B_{12} < 100\ \mu g$ per mL, anisocytosis, poikilocytosis, macroovalocytes, decreased WBCs, and decreased platelets.
- Bone marrow may show megaloblasts and erythroid hyperplasia.
- Increased serum lactate dehydrogenase (LDH) and increased indirect bilirubin may be present because of underlying hemolysis and increased cell turnover.
- Serum IF antibodies are present in majority of patients with pernicious anemia, and are highly specific for this diagnosis in patients with megaloblastic anemia and elevated levels of IF antibodies.
- Parietal cell antibodies are present in 90% of patients with pernicious anemia, and support a diagnosis of pernicious anemia, but are not specific for this condition.
- Elevated serum gastrin levels in pernicious anemia.

- Schilling test is a two-step test utilizing radiolabeled B_{12} and IF to determine whether underlying cause of B_{12} deficiency is pernicious anemia. This test is rarely used and has been largely replaced by parietal cell and IF antibody testing.
- If vitamin B_{12} levels are low-normal and vitamin B_{12} deficiency is suspected, check serum levels of methylmalonic acid (MMA) and homocysteine.
- Elevated serum levels of both MMA and homocysteine confirm the diagnosis of B_{12} deficiency.

e. **Management**
- Management of megaloblastic anemia due to vitamin B_{12} deficiency generally involves parenteral administration of vitamin B_{12}. However, the specific dosage regimen and duration of vitamin B_{12} supplementation depend on the underlying cause of vitamin B_{12} deficiency.
- Vitamin B_{12} is available for administration in oral, nasal, or parenteral forms of delivery. When treating megaloblastic anemia due to vitamin B_{12} deficiency, initial vitamin B_{12} supplementation is generally given by parenteral route of administration. When hematologic parameters have normalized, nasal and oral forms of vitamin B_{12} are available as alternatives to continued parenteral treatment, for maintaining normal vitamin B_{12} levels. Patients receiving oral or nasal forms of vitamin B_{12} must be followed up closely to ensure that normal vitamin B_{12} levels are being maintained.
- Parenteral vitamin B_{12} is typically administered by IM injection and also may be administered by subcutaneous injection.

NOTE: Upon instituting vitamin B_{12} (cobalamin) replacement therapy, the patient must be monitored closely. *Patients may develop severe life-threatening hypokalemia requiring potassium supplementation.* Therefore, serum potassium levels must be followed up closely during treatment.

NOTE: Folate administration in sufficient doses may treat the underlying anemia of vitamin B_{12} deficiency while allowing the vitamin B_{12} deficiency–related neurologic dysfunction to progress. Therefore, patients with megaloblastic anemia should be evaluated for vitamin B_{12} deficiency and folate deficiency, and empiric treatment with a trial of folate is not recommended.

2. **Pernicious Anemia**
a. **Etiology**
- Hereditary autoimmune disorder is commonly present among Northern European and African populations; occurs infrequently among Asian population.
- Occurrence is rare before age 35.
- Most common cause of cobalamin deficiency.
- If family history exists of pernicious anemia, risk increases 20-fold.

- Patients also may have other autoimmune diseases—for example, autoimmune immunoglobulin A (IgA) deficiency, polyglandular endocrine insufficiency (e.g., Graves disease, thyroiditis, vitiligo, and hypoparathyroidism), and type I diabetes mellitus (DM).

  b. **Pathology**
  - Pernicious anemia is an autoimmune disorder characterized by immune-mediated atrophy of the gastric parietal cells, resulting in absent gastric acid and IF secretion. Lack of IF made by gastric parietal cells causes inability to absorb vitamin B_{12} in the gut; therefore, it manifests itself as vitamin B_{12} deficiency anemia.
  - Atrophic gastritis leads to increased risk of gastric cancer among persons with pernicious anemia.

  c. **Clinical Features/Diagnostic Studies**
  - See section I. D. 1.

  d. **Management of Pernicious Anemia**
  - A typical replacement schedule for the treatment of pernicious anemia is as follows: initially, 1,000 μg vitamin B_{12} IM daily for the first week, followed by 1,000 μg vitamin B_{12} IM once weekly for 1 month, followed by 1,000 μg vitamin B_{12} IM once monthly thereafter. Patients with pernicious anemia require lifelong vitamin B_{12} treatment.
  - **Complications**
    - Spinal cord damage due to vitamin B_{12} deficiency is generally irreversible.
    - Other CNS abnormalities (e.g., dementia) also may be irreversible if present >6 months.

3. **Megaloblastic Anemia: Folate Deficiency**
  a. **Etiology**
  - Folate: abundant in citrus fruits and green leafy vegetables (also in meat, eggs, and liver).
  - Total body stores generally last 3 to 6 months.
  - Deficiency may be caused by inadequate dietary intake (e.g., patients on hemodialysis and elderly persons). Folate deficiency associated with alcoholism is likely multifactorial (e.g., dietary malabsorption, decreased intracellular folate metabolism, and decreased hepatic storage of folate).
  - Other causes of folate deficiency include folate-antagonist drugs that interfere with DNA synthesis (e.g., methotrexate, trimethoprim, and pyrimethamine), increased folate utilization (e.g., pregnancy, exfoliative skin disorders, hemolytic anemia, and malignancy), malabsorption (e.g., tropical sprue, celiac disease, inflammatory bowel disease, small bowel lymphoma, and significant small bowel resection), congenital disorders (e.g., 5-methyltetrahydrofolate transferase deficiency), and anticonvulsant medications.

  b. **Pathology**
  - Folate absorption occurs primarily in the jejunum.
  - Folate is required for important steps in DNA synthesis.
  - Folate deficiency results in slow nuclear development with large cytoplasm and decreased RBC life.

  c. **Clinical Features**
  - Similar to vitamin B_{12} deficiency, but without neurologic abnormalities.

  d. **Diagnostic Studies**
  - Macrocytic anemia.
  - Hypersegmented neutrophils ($\geq$5 lobes).
  - Decreased serum folate level.
  - Decreased RBC folate level.
  - Normal serum B_{12} level.

  NOTE: The serum folate level is sensitive to recent dietary intake of folate-containing foods. Therefore, a serum RBC folate level also should generally be checked.
  - **Complications:** Deficiency in pregnancy may lead to neural tube defects.

  e. **Management**
  - Folic acid: 1 mg per day orally.

E. **Normocytic Anemia**
  1. **Hemolytic Anemia: Glucose-6-Phosphate Dehydrogenase Deficiency**
    a. **Etiology**
    - Glucose-6-phosphate dehydrogenase (G6PD) deficiency is an X-linked recessive disorder.
    - Occurs in 10% to 15% of African American males in the United States (G6PD A-variant).
    - Also present among Mediterranean population (G6PD Mediterranean variant).
    - Clinical G6PD deficiency occurs almost exclusively in males. Female carriers are variably clinically affected.

    b. **Pathology**
    - G6PD deficiency results in oxidation of Hgb to methemoglobin that then forms precipitants known as Heinz bodies, which cause membrane damage, osmotic fragility, and rigid cells.
    - Damaged cells are removed by the spleen.
    - Infection or exposure to drugs causes hemolysis.
    - Some drugs known to cause this condition—dapsone, quinine, quinidine, nitrofurantoin, primaquine, sulfonamides, and aspirin.
    - Fava beans may also be implicated, causing a severe hemolytic episode among affected persons.

    c. **Clinical Features**
    - Patients may complain of jaundice, dark urine, and abdominal and low back pain.
    - Physical examination may be normal until crisis occurs.

d. **Diagnostic Studies**
- Laboratory studies may be normal in the time between acute hemolytic episodes.
- During an acute hemolytic episode, characteristic laboratory test results include an elevated reticulocyte count and an elevated unconjugated (indirect) bilirubin level.
- Peripheral blood smear may show bite cells. Heinz bodies (seen with special stain preparation known as *Heinz body preparation*) may be present.
- Perform enzyme assay for G6PD.

NOTE: Patients with the G6PD A-variant will have *normal* G6PD levels immediately following the hemolytic episode because the new cells are not yet G6PD deficient. Therefore, it is advisable to wait several weeks after the hemolytic episode before checking the G6PD level in these patients.

- **Complications:** Renal failure (rare).

e. **Management**
- Avoid offending drugs, food, or both.
- Usually self-limiting.

2. **Hemolytic Anemia: Sickle Cell Anemia**
   a. **Etiology**
   - Hgb S occurs when valine substitutes for glutamic acid on the β-chain.
   - Decreased solubility of Hgb S in hypoxic tissues leads to sickle-shaped cells.

   b. **Pathology**
   - Sickled cells have difficulty passing through small capillaries, leading to blockage and tissue necrosis.
   - Sickled cells are destroyed, resulting in hemolytic anemia.
   - Sickle cell trait does not result in clinical problems unless patients are subjected to severe hypoxia.
   - **Epidemiology**
     - Autosomal recessive disorder.
     - Eight percent of African American persons are heterozygous for Hgb S (known as sickle cell trait).
     - Only 0.15% of African American children in the United States are homozygous for Hgb S (sickle cell anemia).
     - Frequency is highest in Africa, particularly where *Plasmodium falciparum* is common, and is thought to be so because the Hgb S carrier state offers a protective advantage by conferring increased resistance to *P. falciparum* malaria infection.

   c. **Clinical Features**
   - Usually appears at about 6 months of age when fetal Hgb is replaced with Hgb S.
   - Early signs are delayed growth and development, fevers, and infection.
   - Infarctions may result in skin ulceration, painful crises, retinopathy, ischemic necrosis of bones, renal dysfunction, hyposplenism, hepatic dysfunction, and priapism.
   - Hemolytic anemia may result in jaundice, gallstones.
   - Decreased O_2 affinity of Hgb S results in pulmonary hypertension (HTN), congestive heart failure, and symptoms of fatigue and shortness of breath.

   d. **Diagnostic Studies**
   - Hgb electrophoresis shows Hgb S ($\alpha_2\beta^s_2$) of 85% to 98%, Hgb F ($\alpha_2\gamma_2$) of 2% to 20%, and Hgb A$_2$ ($\alpha_2\delta_2$) of 2% to 4% in sickle cell anemia.
   - Sickle cell trait has Hgb S ($\alpha_2\beta^s_2$) of 40% and Hgb A ($\alpha_2\beta_2$) of 60%.
   - Normocytic normochromic anemia.
   - Reticulocytosis.
   - Sickled cells, Howell–Jolly bodies, and target cells on peripheral smear.
   - Increased WBC count and thrombocytosis may be seen.
   - **Complications**
     - Chronic multisystem failure from end-organ damage.
     - Heart failure, stroke.
     - Acute chest syndrome.
     - Skin ulcers.
     - Recurrent infections.
     - Bilirubin gallstones.
     - Osteonecrosis (femoral or humeral head).
     - Aplastic crisis (from infection with parvovirus B19 or folate deficiency).
     - Median age of death is 35 if >3 crises per year and 50 if <3 crises per year.

   e. **Management**
   - Genetic counseling for heterozygous carriers.
   - Avoid dehydration, treat infections aggressively.
   - Analgesics and O_2 administration during painful crises.
   - Hydroxyurea is a cytotoxic drug that has been shown to be beneficial in reducing the frequency of acute pain crises; generally considered in the treatment of patients who are more severely affected with manifestations of sickle cell disease (e.g., frequent severe acute pain crises, increased risk of stroke, and history of acute chest syndrome).
   - Folic acid supplementation.
   - Children should be immunized for *Haemophilus influenzae* type B, pneumococcus, and meningococcus, and should receive prophylactic penicillin up to age 6.
   - Allogeneic stem cell transplantation is the only potentially curative treatment available for sickle cell disease; has significant associated

risks, and therefore patients must be carefully selected and have a human leukocyte antigen–matched donor.

- RBC transfusion therapy is clinically indicated in the management of sickle cell disease, in situations requiring increased O_2-carrying capacity of the blood, decreased amount of sickle Hgb present in the blood, and increased Hgb concentration (e.g., acute chest syndrome, splenic sequestration, and preoperative transfusion).

F. Anemia of Chronic Disease (Also Known as Anemia of Chronic Inflammation)

1. **Etiology**
   - Caused by underlying chronic inflammatory conditions such as chronic infection, inflammatory bowel disease, rheumatoid arthritis, and malignancy.
   - Most common anemia of hospitalized patients.
2. **Pathology**
   - Unclear, but may be attributed to decreased RBC life span; increased production of hepcidin protein in response to inflammation, which blocks the release of iron from macrophages; cytokine inhibition of erythropoietin (EPO).
3. **Clinical Features**
   - Consistent with underlying disease.
   - Usually asymptomatic.
4. **Diagnostic Studies**
   - Mild normochromic normocytic anemia is most common, although it may also present with hypochromic microcytic anemia. Hgb is usually 10 to 11 g per dL range.
   - Decreased serum iron; normal or decreased TIBC; normal or low-normal transferrin saturation; normal or elevated SF.
     - Transferrin saturation (%) = (serum iron [μg/dL]/TIBC [μg/dL]) × 100.
   - Bone marrow iron stores are normal or increased, with decreased or absent sideroblasts.
   - Clinically, anemia of chronic disease is a diagnosis of exclusion.
5. **Management**
   - Treat the underlying disease. The anemia often improves when the underlying inflammatory condition is treated successfully.
   - No role exists for iron therapy in the treatment of anemia of chronic disease.
   - The anemia is generally mild and typically does not require blood transfusion.

II. Malignant Diseases

A. Lymphoma

1. **Hodgkin Lymphoma**
   a. **Etiology/Pathology**
      - No consistent chromosomal abnormalities are identified.
      - Malignant disorder of the lymphoreticular system characterized by Reed–Sternberg cells (large cells with multiloculated or bilobed nucleus with a halo around prominent inclusion-like nucleoli) in the background of benign lymphocytes, plasma cells, or histiocytes.
      - The role of Epstein–Barr virus (EBV) in etiology is suggested by increased risk of Hodgkin lymphoma (HL) in young adults with a history of infectious mononucleosis; frequent coinfection with EBV among patients with human immunodeficiency virus (HIV)-related HL.
      - In contrast to non-Hodgkin lymphoma (NHL), HL tends to spread in an orderly, predictable manner to adjacent sites of lymph tissue.
      - **Epidemiology**
        - Bimodal age distribution with increased incidence after 10 years of age, and first peak occurring approximately in the 20s, and second peak occurring after 50 years.
        - Approximately 85% of children who have HL are boys.
        - There is a wide geographic range of incidence; those with higher social class or education, small family size, and early birth order are more at risk.
   b. **Clinical Features**
      - Patients may complain of painless lump in the neck, fever, drenching night sweats, weight loss, malaise, and generalized pruritus.
      - Alcohol ingestion may cause pain in lymph nodes (LNs).
      - Physical examination may disclose lymphadenopathy often starting initially in the cervical and supraclavicular regions, spreading contiguously to adjacent LN groups. Common extranodal sites of involvement include spleen, liver, lung, and bone marrow.
      - *Pel–Ebstein fever pattern* may be present (period of days or weeks during which fever is present, alternating with periods during which patient is afebrile).
   c. **Diagnostic Studies**
      - Chest X-ray (CXR) may show mediastinal adenopathy.
      - Laboratory tests may show anemia, elevated sedimentation rate, elevated serum LDH, decreased lymphocytes, eosinophilia, increased platelets with mild leukocytosis.
      - Workup should include HIV serology.
      - Positron emission tomography (PET)/computed tomography (CT) scan of the chest, abdomen, and pelvis.
      - Bilateral bone marrow biopsy is also often required for staging.

- Excisional LN biopsy is needed for diagnosis.
- Immunohistochemical studies distinguish classic HL from nodular lymphocyte-predominant Hodgkin lymphoma (NLPHL): classic HL ($CD15^+$, $CD20^-$, $CD30^+$, $CD45^-$) and NLPHL ($CD15^-$, $CD20^+$, $CD30^-$, $CH45^+$).
- The World Health Organization (WHO) has adopted a classification system including *classical HL* (nodular sclerosis, mixed cellularity, lymphocyte rich, and lymphocyte depleted) and NLPHL (Table 2–1).
- Routine staging laparotomy is no longer recommended for all patients with a diagnosis of HL. The indications for staging laparotomy vary depending on clinical stage of patient at the time of diagnosis and anticipated treatment plan.
- **Complications**
  - Spinal cord compression.
  - Late treatment–related complications include cardiac and pulmonary diseases (related to prior irradiation and/or chemotherapy side effects) and second malignancy (e.g., secondary acute leukemia, NHL, and solid tumors).
  - Hypothyroidism occurs in approximately 50% of patients who received neck irradiation and occurs within 1 to 20 years of radiation treatment.
  - Infertility (related to pelvic irradiation and certain chemotherapy regimens).
  - Diminished cell-mediated immunity.
- d. **Management**
  - Treatment of HL depends on the stage of disease according to the Ann Arbor Staging System, which classifies disease stage on the basis of anatomic location as well as the presence or absence of "B" symptoms.
    - Ann Arbor staging system
      - Stage I: involvement of single LN region or single extralymphatic organ or site (Stage IE).

- Stage II: involvement of two or more LN regions on the same side of the diaphragm; also can include localized involvement of an extralymphatic organ or site (Stage IIE).
- Stage III: involvement of LN regions on both sides of the diaphragm; also can include localized involvement of an extralymphatic organ or site (Stage IIIE), or involvement of the spleen (Stage IIIS), or both (Stage IIISE).
- Stage IV: diffuse or disseminated involvement of one or more extralymphatic organs, with or without associated LN involvement.
- "A": B symptoms not present.
- "B": patient with history of fever ($>38°$ C), drenching night sweats, weight loss $>10\%$ of body weight in previous 6 months.
- "X": bulky disease; mediastinal widening greater than one-third of the diameter of the chest or LN mass >10 cm in any dimension.
- "E": involvement of a single extranodal site contiguous or proximal to a known site.
- Treatment of classic HL
  - **Early-stage favorable HL:** early-stage HL (Stages I and II) in the *absence of adverse risk factors, including* B symptoms, bulky disease, extranodal disease, >3 sites of nodal involvement, or erythrocyte sedimentation rate (ESR) ≥50 mm per hour.
  - Treatment options include ABVD combination chemotherapy (doxorubicin, bleomycin, vinblastine, and dacarbazine); ABVD + involved-field radiation therapy (IF-XRT); XRT alone (in selected circumstances).
  - Patients with early-stage favorable HL have reported long-term, disease-free survival rates of approximately 80% to 90%.
  - **Early-stage unfavorable HL:** early-stage HL (Stages I and II) in the *presence of one or more adverse risk factors, including* B symptoms, bulky disease, extranodal disease, ≥3 sites of nodal involvement, or ESR ≥50 mm per hour.
  - Treatment options include ABVD combination chemotherapy + IF-XRT; BEACOPP combination chemotherapy (bleomycin, etoposide, doxorubicin, cyclophosphamide, vincristine, procarbazine, and prednisone) + IF-XRT.
  - More than 75% of patients can be cured with this treatment approach.
  - **Advanced-stage classic HL:** treatment approach for advanced-stage (Stages III and IV) HL includes ABVD combination chemotherapy. Approximately 60% to 70% of patients with

TABLE 2–1.	WHO Classification: Morphologic Subtypes of Hodgkin Lymphoma
Classical Hodgkin lymphoma	
• Nodular sclerosis	
• Mixed cellularity	
• Lymphocyte rich	
• Lymphocyte depleted	
Nodular lymphocyte-predominant Hodgkin lymphoma	

Adapted from Cashen, AF, Van Tine, BA, eds. *The Washington Manual: Hematology Oncology Subspecialty Consult.* New York, NY: Lippincott Williams & Wilkins; 2016.

advanced HL can be cured with combination chemotherapy.

- **Nodular lymphocyte-predominant HL:** this subtype of HL follows a more indolent course and is associated with a favorable prognosis.
  - Most patients are first seen with early-stage disease (Stages I and II), and the treatment approach typically includes IF-XRT only. Trials with single-agent rituximab (monoclonal antibody) also have promising results.
  - For the infrequent patient with NLPHL who has advanced disease (Stages III and IV), treatment involves combination chemotherapy, and chemotherapy + rituximab has favorable results.
  - Approximate 10-year overall survival rate is 80%, and among the 20% of patients with NLPHL relapse, the 10-year overall survival rate is approximately 70%.

2. **Non-Hodgkin Lymphoma**
   a. **Etiology/Pathology**
      - Malignancy of lymphoreticular system.
      - Classified functionally as B cell or T cell.
      - Morphologically defined as small-, intermediate-, or large cell.
      - Several classification systems currently exist for NHL:
        - Working Formulation (developed in 1982) classifies NHL as low, intermediate, or high grade. NHL may be further classified on the basis of clinical behavior and Working Formulation categories (Table 2–2).
        - In 1993, the Revised European American Lymphoma (REAL) classification was developed. The WHO accepted the REAL classification with some modifications (2001), and this was further updated in 2016.
        - Cytogenic abnormalities are common.
      - **Epidemiology**
        - Median age: 50.
        - Incidence increases with age.
        - Approximately 75,000 new cases of NHL are diagnosed annually in the United States.
        - Mature B-cell neoplasms account for majority of NHL (88%); most common type of NHL in adults.
        - Mature T-cell and natural killer (NK) cell neoplasms account for 12% of NHL.
        - Increased incidence of NHL has been noted among persons with HIV disease.
        - Over the past several decades, there has been an increased incidence of NHL associated with pesticides and organic solvents.
        - Bacterial association with *Helicobacter pylori* infection and gastric MALT lymphoma.

TABLE 2–2.   Classification of Non-Hodgkin Lymphoma Based on Clinical Behavior and Working Formulation

Indolent Non-Hodgkin Lymphoma

- Small lymphocytic (low grade)
- Follicular, small-cleaved cell (low grade)
- Follicular, mixed small-cleaved and large cell (low grade)
- Diffuse, small-cleaved cell (intermediate grade)

Aggressive Non-Hodgkin Lymphoma

- Follicular, large cell (intermediate grade)
- Diffuse, mixed small and large cell (intermediate grade)
- Diffuse, large cell (intermediate grade)
- Diffuse, large cell immunoblastic (high grade)
- Small, noncleaved cell (high grade)
- Lymphoblastic (high grade)
- Burkitt lymphoma (high grade)

Adapted from Mazza JJ, ed. *Manual of Clinical Hematology*. 3rd ed. New York, NY: Lippincott Williams & Wilkins; 2002; Pillot G, Chantler M, Magiera H, et al, eds. *The Washington Manual Subspecialty Consult Series: Hematology and Oncology Subspecialty Consult*. New York, NY: Lippincott Williams & Wilkins; 2004.

b. **Clinical Features**
   - Two-thirds of patients have persistent painless lymphadenopathy including retroperitoneum, mesentery, and pelvis.
   - One-third of sites are extranodal; symptoms vary according to the site.
   - Fever, night sweats, and weight loss are much less common than in HL.
   - Pruritus is rare.
   - Laboratory tests may show only anemia, elevated serum LDH, and elevated ESR.
   - Workup should include HIV serology.

c. **Diagnostic Studies**
   - LN biopsy is needed for diagnosis, and an excisional LN biopsy is preferable.
   - Staging uses Ann Arbor classification (see section II. A. 1).
   - CXR: CT scan of the chest, abdomen, and pelvis. Initial PET scan imaging is recommended for fluorodeoxyglucose (FDG)-avid NHL subtypes (e.g., follicular, Burkitt, mantle cell, and diffuse large B cell); contrast-enhanced CT scan remains standard for NHL subtypes that are not reliably FDG-avid (e.g., marginal zone, chronic lymphocytic/small lymphocytic, cutaneous B cell, and mycosis fungoides).
   - Bilateral bone marrow biopsies are often indicated for staging.
   - Lumbar puncture if CNS involvement.
   - Treatment and prognosis depend on staging and histologic subtype.

d. **Management**
- The Ann Arbor Staging System is used in the staging of NHL (see section II. A. 1).
- Limited disease (Stages I and II) indolent NHL: treatment options include involved IF-XRT; rituximab with or without combination chemotherapy; watchful waiting in selected cases.
- Advanced-stage (Stages III and IV) indolent NHL: for patients who are asymptomatic, treatment is not always indicated; close observation without initial therapy may be appropriate in certain situations. For patients with advanced-stage (Stages III and IV) indolent NHL who are symptomatic, single-agent or combination chemotherapy regimens, or use of monoclonal antibodies (e.g., rituximab, obinutuzumab) may be effective in inducing a remission. Advanced-stage indolent lymphomas are generally not curable with standard treatments. The disease may respond well to chemotherapy or radiation therapy and may achieve a partial or complete remission. However, recurrence of disease is common.
- Limited disease (Stages I and II) aggressive NHL: treatment generally requires treatment with combination chemotherapy for several cycles, followed by involved IF-XRT. For Stages III and IV aggressive NHL, combination chemotherapy is generally the treatment of choice. Depending on the pathologic subtype and extent of disease, prophylactic CNS treatment using intrathecal chemotherapy also may be indicated.
- There may be a role for consideration of autologous or allogeneic HSCT in cases of relapsed intermediate- or high-grade NHL.

3. **Multiple Myeloma (Plasma Cell Myeloma)**
a. **Etiology/Pathology**
- Malignant proliferation of plasma cells.
- In multiple myeloma, all five classes of immunoglobulin are produced, with a single immunoglobulin produced in excess; therefore, monoclonal gammopathy.
- **Epidemiology**
  - Usually presents in older adults; only 2% of patients are younger than 40 years at the time of diagnosis.
  - Estimated 30,000 new cases are diagnosed annually in the United States.
  - Incidence increases with age; average age of diagnosis is 60.
  - More men than women are affected, with increased incidence among African American population.
  - Exposure to radiation, benzene, herbicides, and insecticides may play a role.

b. **Clinical Features**
- Patients may complain of bone pain, often in the spine and ribs (70%), at the time of diagnosis, resulting from osteolytic bone lesions or pathologic fractures.
- Bone marrow infiltration results in a normocytic, normochromic anemia; thrombocytopenia; and leucopenia.
- Bone resorption causes osteopenia and hypercalcemia.
  - Primary amyloidosis may coexist with a diagnosis of multiple myeloma.
  - Clinical findings may include macroglossia, carpal tunnel syndrome, skin involvement (e.g., periorbital ecchymosis), congestive heart failure, and nephrotic syndrome, among others.
- Fatigue, weakness, nausea, vomiting, bleeding, bruising (secondary to platelet dysfunction), or infection also may be presenting symptoms depending on the extent of disease.

c. **Diagnostic Studies**
- Diagnosis is made by serum protein electrophoresis and urine protein electrophoresis, demonstrating a monoclonal protein (M-protein) spike, followed by immunofixation electrophoresis to further identify the specific heavy-chain class and light-chain type in the M-protein. Diagnosis is confirmed by bone marrow biopsy.
- Bence Jones protein (monoclonal immunoglobulin light chains) in urine.
- Normochromic, normocytic anemia is present in approximately two-thirds of patients at the time of diagnosis. *Rouleaux formation* of RBCs may be present on peripheral blood smear.
- ESR elevation is commonly present.
- Obtain complete baseline serum chemistry panel to evaluate calcium, total protein, albumin, LDH, BUN, creatinine, electrolytes, uric acid, and liver function tests (LFTs).
- Serum C-reactive protein (marker for interleukin 6 activity, which stimulates myeloma cell growth) and serum β_2 microglobulin (reflects tumor burden in multiple myeloma) levels should also be checked (Table 2–3).
- Hypercalcemia may be present. Need to calculate corrected serum calcium level if serum albumin is low: (Corrected Ca^{+2}) = (serum Ca^{+2}) + (0.8 × [4.0 − patient's serum albumin]).
  - Example: Albumin = 2.0 mg per dL; calcium = 12.0 mg per dL; corrected Ca^{+2} = 12.0 + 1.6 = **13.6 mg per dL**.
- Renal function tests may show renal insufficiency in approximately 50% of patients at the time of diagnosis.
- Plain films show lytic bone lesions.

TABLE 2–3.	International Staging System for Multiple Myeloma		
Stage	Serum β2-Microglobulin (mg/L)	Serum Albumin (g/dL)	Median Survival (mo)
I	<3.5	≥3.5	62
II	<3.5	<3.5	44
	OR		
	3.5–5.5	—	
III	>5.5	—	29

Note: (—) indicates that stage is determined based on serum β2-microglobulin level, regardless of serum albumin level.
Adapted from Cashen AF, Wildes TM, Henderson KE, et al, eds. *The Washington Manual Subspecialty Consult Series: Hematology and Oncology Subspecialty Consult.* 2nd ed. Philadelphia, PA: Lippincott Williams & Wilkins; 2008:143; Greipp PR, Miguel JS, Durie BGM, et al. International staging system for multiple myeloma. *J Clin Oncol.* 2005;23(15):3412–3420. http://jco.ascopubs.org/content/23/15/3412.full. Accessed February 22, 2012.

NOTE: Because the bone lesions of multiple myeloma are generally purely lytic, a bone scan is not a useful diagnostic test. It is preferable to obtain a skeletal survey (plain film radiographs of skull, vertebrae, ribs, pelvis, and long bones) to assess for the extent of bony involvement.

- Serum β_2 microglobulin level can be a useful prognostic indicator; elevated level tends to be associated with a less favorable prognosis.
- CT/magnetic resonance imaging (MRI) or PET scan imaging for high-risk patients or patients with bone pain not explained by skeletal survey results.
- Bone marrow with mature and immature plasma cells, diffuse or in sheets, >30%.
- In asymptomatic patients, multiple myeloma may be suspected if routine laboratory tests show hypercalcemia, increased serum protein, anemia; diagnosis should then be confirmed by further testing.
- **Complications**
  - Renal failure.
  - Recurrent infections with *Streptococcus pneumonia, Staphylococcus aureus, H. influenzae, Pseudomonas aeruginosa, Escherichia coli,* or *Klebsiella.*
  - Spinal cord compression.
  - Carpal tunnel syndrome.
  - Visual disturbances.
  - Pathologic bone fractures.
- d. **Management**
  - Treatment decisions are based on whether the patient is eligible or ineligible for autologous stem cell transplant (ASCT). Determining

factors include age, performance status, and presence of comorbid conditions.
- Transplant-eligible patients: use of alkylating agents should be avoided, because of toxicity to stem cells. High-dose chemotherapy + ASCT is the standard of care for transplant-eligible patients; bortezomib-based three-drug regimens have shown increased rates of complete remission.
- Transplant-ineligible patients: standard induction chemotherapy regimens may include use of an alkylating agent, such as melphalan and prednisone (MP), or melphalan/prednisone/thalidomide (MPT). Bortezomib-based chemotherapy regimens or Revlimid/dexamethasone may also be used in newly diagnosed patients.
- Radiation therapy is generally reserved for palliative treatment of localized lesions, lesions causing spinal cord compression, or prophylactic treatment of large lytic lesions in long bones at risk for pathologic fracture.
- Supportive measures, aggressive hydration to delay renal insufficiency, bisphosphonates, such as pamidronate (Aredia) or zoledronic acid (Zometa), have been shown to delay skeletal disease in patients with multiple myeloma, decrease bone pain, and improve quality of life.

B. Acute Lymphoblastic Leukemia (Also known as Acute Lymphocytic Leukemia)

1. **Etiology/Pathology**
   - Malignant proliferation of lymphoid stem cells in bone marrow that invade LNs, spleen, liver, other organs.
   - May be classified as B-cell or T-cell origin.
   - FAB (French–American–British) classification has three subtypes of acute lymphoblastic leukemia (ALL) (L1–L3) based on morphology, heterogeneity of lymphocytes.
   - Has propensity for CNS, gonads.
   - **Epidemiology**
     - The incidence of ALL peaks between ages 2 and 4, then decreases to fairly steady levels, with increasing incidence again after age 50. Approximately 75% of ALL cases occur among patients who are <15 years.
     - ALL accounts for 80% of childhood leukemias and 20% of adult leukemias.
     - Most common childhood malignancy.
     - Cause is generally unknown; however, several genetic syndromes are associated with an increased risk of developing ALL (e.g., Down syndrome and ataxia-telangiectasia syndrome).

2. **Clinical Features**
   - Patients may complain of fever, fatigue, weight loss, irritability, anorexia, bone pain, arthralgias, and bleeding.

- If CNS involvement is present at the time of diagnosis, patient also may complain of headache, stiff neck, visual disturbances, and vomiting.
- On physical examination, there may be pallor, fever, petechiae, bruises, hepatosplenomegaly, lymphadenopathy, stiff neck, papilledema, cranial nerve palsies, seizures, and change in mental status.
- Hepatosplenomegaly and lymphadenopathy can be seen.

3. **Diagnostic Studies**
   - WBC typically varies from 5,000 to 100,000 per mm^3; however, it may be <5,000 or >100,000 per mm^3 at the time of diagnosis.
   - Anemia, neutropenia, and thrombocytopenia are commonly present at the time of diagnosis.
   - Hypercellular bone marrow with >30% lymphoblasts.
   - WBC differential often shows blast cells in peripheral blood at the time of diagnosis.
   - Elevated serum uric acid may be present.
   - Elevated serum LDH level often may be present.
   - CXR: anterior mediastinal mass may be present and is suggestive of T-cell ALL.
   - Cerebrospinal fluid may show blast cells, with increased protein and decreased glucose.
   - Presence of Philadelphia chromosome (t[9;22] [q34;q11]) in ALL is a poor prognostic sign.
   - **Complications**
     - Chemotherapy causes immunosuppression and results in increased risk of infections.
     - *Pneumocystis jiroveci* pneumonia: trimethoprim/sulfamethoxazole (Bactrim) for prophylaxis during chemotherapy treatment.
     - Sterility (related to chemotherapy).
     - Metabolic complications arising during chemotherapy treatment, including *tumor lysis syndrome* (hyperuricemia, hyperkalemia, hypocalcemia, hyperphosphatemia) with associated increased risk of cardiac arrhythmias, and acute renal failure.

4. **Management**
   a. **Approach to Treatment of Children with ALL**
      - Approximately 98% of children with ALL achieve a complete remission within 4 weeks of starting induction chemotherapy, and current clinical trial results suggest approximately 70% of children diagnosed currently with ALL can expect to be cured; children with favorable prognostic indicators may have an even better prognosis.
      - Initial treatment is known as *induction chemotherapy*, and the goal of treatment is to induce a complete remission. Typical regimens include vincristine, glucocorticoid, and L-asparaginase.

- CNS prophylaxis must be included in the initial treatment, and typically involves intrathecal chemotherapy. Cranial irradiation may be indicated for certain high-risk patients.
- Following induction of remission, the patient receives *consolidation/intensification* chemotherapy.
- After completion of the consolidation/intensification treatment phase, the patient must receive *maintenance chemotherapy* for approximately 2 to 3 years.
- Allogeneic HSCT is generally reserved for the treatment of relapsed disease and typically is not recommended for children with standard-risk ALL during the first complete remission.

   b. **Approach to Treatment of Adults with ALL**
      - ALL in adulthood is associated with decreased long-term survival when compared with that of children with ALL. Approximately 60% to 80% of adults with ALL can expect to achieve a complete remission with induction chemotherapy treatment, although many of these patients suffer a relapse of their disease. The overall cure rate for adults with ALL is approximately 30% to 40%. Presence of poor prognostic factors (e.g., age > 60, Philadelphia chromosome–positive, long time to achieve first remission, and high WBC at the time of diagnosis) is generally associated with reduced survival.
      - As with treatment of childhood ALL, the goal of initial treatment is to induce a complete remission using *induction chemotherapy* using multiple chemotherapy drugs. Typical regimens include vincristine, glucocorticoid, and an anthracycline drug. L-Asparaginase may also be included in some treatment regimens. Remission rates exceeding 90% were achieved among patients with Philadelphia chromosome–positive ALL when standard induction chemotherapy regimens are combined with *BCR-ABL* tyrosine kinase inhibitors.
      - Following the remission induction, the patient receives *consolidation therapy* with additional chemotherapy. Consolidation treatment also generally includes CNS prophylaxis using intrathecal chemotherapy and/or cranial irradiation. For adults with ALL, the (induction + consolidation) treatment typically takes approximately 6 months following diagnosis; then followed by the *maintenance chemotherapy* phase. The optimal duration of maintenance treatment is under investigation, although it generally continues until approximately 2 to 3 years from the time of diagnosis.

- Allogeneic HSCT for select adult patients with ALL has been associated with improved long-term, disease-free survival rates.
- Relapse is common in adult ALL; patients may be considered for further reinduction chemotherapy, followed by allogeneic HSCT.

C. Chronic Lymphocytic Leukemia

1. **Etiology/Epidemiology**
   - Usually occurs in adults older than 50 years.
   - Men outnumber women, 2:1.
   - The disease is rare among Asian persons.
   - Cause of chronic lymphocytic leukemia (CLL) is unknown; however, evidence exists to suggest that hereditary and cytogenetic factors may have a role. CLL is associated with some common cytogenetic abnormalities (e.g., trisomy 12 and 13q deletion). There also have been familial clusters of patients identified, with relatives having 2- to 3-fold increased risk of CLL compared with that of the general population.
   - CLL is the most common form of adult leukemia in Western countries.
   - There have not yet been any proven environmental factors leading to increased CLL risk.

2. **Pathology**
   - Caused by proliferation of mature-appearing lymphocytes in peripheral blood that invade bone marrow, spleen, LNs.
   - Usually of B-lymphocyte origin (>90%), with monoclonal surface immunoglobulin expressed by >90% of patients.
   - WHO classification of lymphoid neoplasms recognizes CLL and small lymphocytic lymphoma (SLL) (a type of NHL) as being on the same clinical spectrum. CLL manifests as a "leukemic" lymphoid process, with more prominent involvement of the peripheral blood than is present in SLL.

3. **Clinical Features**
   - May have no signs or symptoms.
   - In 25% of patients, CLL is noted initially on routine complete blood count.
   - Patients may complain of weakness, fatigue, dyspnea on exertion, infections.
   - On physical examination, lymphadenopathy and hepatosplenomegaly often seen. Advanced disease also may be associated with weight loss, fever, or bruising.

4. **Diagnostic Studies**
   - Elevated WBC count of 15,000 to 100,000 per mm^3 in 70% to 95% of cases.
   - Absolute lymphocyte count >5,000 per mm^3 (required criteria to distinguish between CLL and SLL).
   - Peripheral blood smear: mature-appearing lymphocytes with characteristic *smudge cells* present.
   - Anemia may be present and may be multifactorial (e.g., splenic sequestration, autoimmune hemolytic anemia, and bone marrow infiltration).

- Thrombocytopenia may be present and may be multifactorial (e.g., splenic sequestration, autoimmune thrombocytopenia, and bone marrow infiltration).
- Bone marrow: >30% well-differentiated lymphocytes.
- Hypogammaglobulinemia is often present.
- CXR: to evaluate for pleural effusion, infiltrates, and adenopathy associated with the disease.
- Direct Coombs test (direct antiglobulin test) will be positive in the presence of autoimmune hemolytic anemia associated with CLL.

- **Complications**
  - Approximately 10% of patients may develop Coombs-positive warm antibody hemolytic anemia, and approximately 5% of patients may develop autoimmune thrombocytopenia during the course of their disease.
  - Hypogammaglobulinemia leads to impaired immunity and subsequent infection.
  - Approximately 5% of patients with CLL undergo transformation into a more aggressive lymphoma (*Richter syndrome*).
  - Pancytopenia is often associated with advanced disease and may result in life-threatening infections.

5. **Management**
   - Because CLL is often an indolent disease, no indication for treatment of an asymptomatic patient with stable disease generally exists. Decision whether to initiate treatment is based on several clinical indicators including disease stage, as well as presence or absence of systemic symptoms (fever, sweats, weight loss), evidence of advanced disease, whether lymphadenopathy is causing mechanical obstruction or significant physical discomfort, and if rapid doubling time for peripheral blood lymphocyte count exists.
   - Two staging systems are available for the staging of CLL: (1) the Binet staging system and (2) the modified Rai classification system.
   - **Binet staging system**
     - LN groups: cervical, axillary, inguinal, liver, spleen.
     - Stage A: lymphocytosis with <3 lymph node groups involved; no anemia or thrombocytopenia.
     - Stage B: lymphocytosis with >3 lymph node groups involved.
     - Stage C: anemia and/or thrombocytopenia regardless of number of LN groups.
   - **Modified Rai classification system**
     - Stage 0: lymphocytosis of peripheral blood and bone marrow (>40% lymphocytes in bone marrow; >5,000 per μL blood lymphocytes).
     - Stage I: Stage 0 + lymphadenopathy.

- Stage II: Stage 0 or I + splenomegaly and/or hepatomegaly.
- Stage III: Stage 0, I, or II + anemia (Hgb < 11 g per dL).
- Stage IV: Stage 0, I, II, or III + thrombocytopenia (platelet count < 100,000 per μL)
- Chemotherapy options include single-agent chemotherapy—purine analogs (e.g., fludarabine and cladribine); combination chemotherapy utilizing alkylating agents (e.g., cyclophosphamide), monoclonal antibodies (e.g., rituximab), and/or purine analogs.
- For treatment of autoimmune hemolytic anemia or autoimmune thrombocytopenia associated with CLL, glucocorticoid treatment is indicated (e.g., prednisone 1 mg/kg/day orally as starting dose, to be gradually tapered once blood counts have stabilized).
- Splenectomy may be indicated for patients with CLL and autoimmune hemolytic anemia or autoimmune thrombocytopenia who do not respond adequately to glucocorticoid therapy.
- Local radiation therapy may be indicated to relieve symptoms caused by lymphadenopathy or splenomegaly.
- Allogeneic HSCT currently being studied as treatment option for select cases, particularly among young patients with high-risk disease.

D. Acute Myelogenous Leukemia

1. **Etiology/Epidemiology**
   - Acute myelogenous leukemia (AML) accounts for approximately 80% of all new cases of adult acute leukemias. Primarily occurs in adults older than 50 years, but also may occur in young adults and children.
   - In most cases, the cause of AML is unknown. However, some risk factors have been identified including prior treatment with certain chemotherapy agents, exposure to ionizing radiation, benzene exposure, congenital disorders (e.g., Down syndrome).
   - Can be preceded by chronic myelogenous leukemia (CML), polycythemia vera (PV), idiopathic myelofibrosis, or myelodysplastic syndromes (MDSs).

2. **Pathology**
   - Caused by proliferation of abnormal myeloid cells (precursors of erythrocytes, granulocytes, monocytes, platelets) that do not mature.
   - Classified by FAB classification into eight subtypes (M_0 to M_7) depending on the degree of differentiation and maturation of predominant cells.

3. **Clinical Features**
   - Patient may complain of fever, fatigue, weakness, bleeding, bruising, and recurrent infection.
   - Bone pain, CNS occurrence rare.

- Hepatosplenomegaly and lymphadenopathy are less common than in acute lymphocytic leukemia.
- Gingival hypertrophy and skin infiltration by leukemia (*leukemia cutis*) may be present in patients with acute monocytic leukemia (M_5 variant).
- Retinal hemorrhages may be present (due to thrombocytopenia).
- Bleeding symptoms due to disseminated intravascular coagulation (DIC) may be present, particularly with acute promyelocytic leukemia (M_3 variant).
- Leukostasis may occur, especially if WBC >100,000 per mm^3, and may cause CNS manifestations (e.g., confusion, headache, and cranial nerve deficits) or severe respiratory distress (due to leukostasis in the pulmonary vasculature). Emergent leukapheresis is indicated.

4. **Diagnostic Studies**
   - Normocytic normochromic anemia is often present.
   - Peripheral blood smear: the presence of Auer rods in the blast cytoplasm is pathognomonic for AML.
   - Decreased neutrophils; absolute neutrophil count (ANC) is often low, and approximately 50% of patients have ANC <1,500 at the time of diagnosis.
   - WBCs may be low, normal, high.
   - Bone marrow hypercellular with >30% blasts.
   - Serum uric acid and serum LDH may be elevated (related to increased cell turnover).
   - Thrombocytopenia is often present.
   - If the WBC >100,000, additional laboratory findings may be present, including *pseudohypoxemia* (as a result of O_2 consumption by blast cells in vitro), *pseudohyperkalemia* (as a result of elevated WBC), and *pseudohypoglycemia* (as a result of glucose consumption by blast cells in vitro).
   - **Complications**
     - Chemotherapy causes immunosuppression, with resultant increased risk of infections.
     - Leukostasis may occur; typically associated with WBC >100,000 per mm^3.
     - Bleeding complications may occur because of thrombocytopenia, DIC.
     - *Tumor lysis syndrome* may occur during chemotherapy treatment (see Complications in section II. B. 3)

5. **Management**
   - The prognosis for AML varies significantly and is dependent on multiple factors including age at diagnosis, whether AML occurred de novo or is secondary to toxin exposure, or preceding MDS. In addition, the cytogenetic profile is also a useful prognostic factor. Poor prognostic factors include advanced age at the time of diagnosis, unfavorable cytogenetic profile, secondary AML due to toxin exposure (e.g., benzene, alkylating agent

chemotherapy, and ionizing radiation), poor performance status at the time of diagnosis, and AML preceded by myelodysplasia.

- As with ALL, initial phase of treatment is known as *induction chemotherapy*. Multiple effective induction chemotherapy regimens are available and generally include an anthracycline (e.g., daunorubicin and idarubicin) in combination with cytosine arabinoside (Ara-C). Complete remission may be obtained in 70% to 80% of patients 60 years and younger and in 50% of older patients.
- Induction chemotherapy is then followed by postinduction treatment, and options generally include additional chemotherapy with high-dose Ara-C, ASCT, and allogeneic HSCT. The decision regarding which treatment to offer depends largely on the prognostic category of the patient. Patients with poor prognostic factors are at significant risk for relapse and generally should be considered for HSCT after induction. Patients with good prognostic factors would typically be offered additional chemotherapy as the postinduction treatment, with a significant chance for cure with this approach. For patients who have intermediate prognostic factors, management must be considered on an individual basis.
  - CNS involvement with leukemia may be treated with intrathecal Ara-C or methotrexate.
  - In case of relapse, consider SCT.

E. Chronic Myelogenous Leukemia

1. **Etiology/Epidemiology**
   - Median age at presentation is 45 to 55.
   - CML accounts for approximately 15% of all cases of leukemia in adults.
   - Cause is unclear; however, increased incidence of CML has been noted among persons with a history of organic solvent exposure (such as benzene) and among persons with a history of exposure to high levels of ionizing radiation (e.g., Hiroshima and Nagasaki).

2. **Pathology**
   - CML is a myeloproliferative disorder caused by proliferation of myeloid cells that retain their capacity to differentiate.
   - Chronic phase is characterized by elevated WBCs >100,000 per mm^3 with <5% blasts in blood or bone marrow.
   - Accelerated phase (>5%, <30% blasts in blood or bone marrow) is often heralded by worsening anemia and refractory response to treatment.
   - Acute blast crisis phase (>30% blasts in blood or bone marrow) is an aggressive phase of the disease, because CML evolves into a secondary acute leukemia.

- Most patients who transform into an acute blast phase have disease poorly responsive to therapy and will die in this phase.
- Philadelphia chromosome–negative CML is associated with a poor prognosis.

3. **Clinical Features**
   - May be asymptomatic.
   - Patient may complain of left upper quadrant (LUQ) pain secondary to enlarged spleen, or weight loss, fever, arthralgias, and bleeding.
   - Physical examination may disclose marked splenomegaly, hepatomegaly, lymphadenopathy (rare), ecchymoses, and bone tenderness.

4. **Diagnostic Studies**
   - WBCs elevated >100,000 per mm^3 with increased numbers of granulocytes, especially neutrophils.
   - WBC differential also may show an increase in basophils and eosinophils.
   - Normocytic normochromic anemia may be present.
   - Chromosomal abnormality: presence of Philadelphia chromosome t(9;22). Approximately 90% of patients with CML are Philadelphia chromosome–positive.
   - Low leukocyte alkaline phosphatase score.
   - Elevated serum B_{12} level.
   - Thrombocytosis may be present at the time of diagnosis.
   - Peripheral blood smear: WBCs present at all stages of maturation.

5. **Management**
   - The majority of patients with CML are in *chronic phase* at the time of diagnosis. Treatment options for newly diagnosed patients with CML diagnosed in chronic phase include tyrosine kinase inhibitors (e.g., imatinib), chemotherapy followed by allogeneic SCT, interferon-alpha (IFN-α), or hydroxyurea.
   - Allogeneic SCT is the only potentially curative option for CML and should be considered early in disease for select patients; best chance for success if done in chronic phase.
   - Treatment options for acute blast phase of CML are limited.
   - **For patients who develop a secondary AML:**
     - Imatinib may be helpful in inducing a remission. If remission is achieved, consideration should be given to allogeneic SCT, if patient is eligible and a donor is available.
   - **For patients who develop a secondary ALL:**
     - Imatinib may be helpful in inducing a remission. If remission is achieved, consideration should be given to allogeneic SCT, if patient is eligible and a donor is available. If patient has a relapse following treatment with imatinib,

consideration may be given to treatment with an ALL chemotherapy regimen (e.g., vincristine/prednisone), which can occasionally be helpful in allowing patients to return to chronic phase for a period of time.

- With advances in treatment of CML, approximately 7% of patients diagnosed in chronic phase will progress to accelerated phase or blast crisis within 5 years; survival of patients in blast crisis who do not respond to treatment is approximately 2 to 4 months.

III. Platelet Disorders

A. Acquired Coagulopathy: Disseminated Intravascular Coagulation

1. **Etiology/Pathology**
   - DIC: consumption of coagulation factors resulting from intravascular activation of coagulation process with secondary activation of fibrinolysis, which may lead to either hemorrhage or thrombosis.
   - Most common causes: infection (usually gram-negative endotoxins), complications of pregnancy, massive tissue injury, malignancy, hypoxia, acidosis, snakebite, cancer, acute promyelocytic leukemia (M_3 variant of AML).
   - **Epidemiology**
     - DIC occurs in 1/1,000 hospitalized patients.
     - Twenty percent are asymptomatic.
     - Most often occurs in young or elderly patients.
2. **Clinical Features**
   - Acute: may present as sudden onset of bleeding, hemorrhage (80%–90%).
   - Chronic: bleeding symptoms may be mild or patient may be asymptomatic.
   - Thrombosis may occur and generally involves small or midsize vessels.
   - May see hematuria, GI bleed, epistaxis, petechiae, bleeding from surgical or venipuncture sites or uterus.
   - Thrombi may infarct the heart, kidney, brain, liver, pancreas, causing shock secondary to increased vascular permeability and hypotension.
3. **Diagnostic Studies**
   - Decreased platelets, decreased fibrinogen level, increased prothrombin time (PT)/partial thromboplastin time (PTT), elevated fibrin degradation products (FDPs), elevated D-dimer level, and elevated thrombin time.
   - Peripheral blood smear: schistocytes and low platelet count are generally present.
   - Low levels of clotting factors are present due to increased consumption.
   - **Complications**
     - Renal failure.
     - Exsanguination.
     - Mortality rates: 50% to 60%.

4. **Management**
   - Timely and appropriate treatment of the underlying disorder is of paramount importance when managing a patient with DIC.
   - Although there is a theoretical concern that giving a patient in DIC transfusion support may worsen the condition, current clinical recommendations seem to support the use of blood products for patients in DIC with documented factor deficiencies who are actively bleeding, or who require surgery or other invasive procedures, and are at high risk for bleeding. In this situation, transfusion support with appropriate blood products would generally be given (e.g., platelets, fresh frozen plasma [FFP], and cryoprecipitate).
   - If thrombosis is occurring, it may be appropriate to consider initiating anticoagulation with heparin. However, the decision regarding whether to use heparin anticoagulation for a patient with DIC must always be determined on an individual basis, and the associated potential risks and benefits must be considered carefully. In the absence of thrombosis, heparin anticoagulation as a treatment for acute DIC is rarely indicated.

B. Thrombotic Thrombocytopenic Purpura

1. **Etiology/Pathology**
   - Although the underlying mechanism for the development of thrombotic thrombocytopenic purpura (TTP) is not entirely understood, the etiology of TTP is thought to be due, in part, to a deficiency of a von Willebrand factor (vWF) cleaving proteolytic enzyme (ADAMTS13) responsible for cleaving high-molecular-weight vWF molecules into their usual length. Elevated levels of high-molecular-weight vWF molecules are believed to be associated with abnormal platelet aggregation. This enzyme deficiency may either be inherited or caused by the inhibition of the enzyme by an antibody.
   - TTP may be idiopathic or related to other underlying causes—for example, drug-induced (e.g., mitomycin C), pregnancy, HIV infection, connective tissue disease.
   - Thrombi form in capillaries and arterioles.
   - May be acute, chronic, relapsing.
   - **Epidemiology**
     - Peak incidence between ages 30 and 50; relatively uncommon before age 20.
     - Rare disorder with annual incidence of 2 to 6 per million population in the United States.
     - Affects women more than men at ages <50; approximately equal male-to-female ratio at ages >60.
2. **Clinical Features**
   - Patients may complain of headache, confusion, seizures, jaundice, visual defects, abdominal pain, bleeding, and fever.

- The classic *pentad of clinical findings* characterizes this condition: microangiopathic hemolytic anemia, thrombocytopenia, CNS abnormalities, fever, and renal dysfunction. Not all findings must be present to confirm the diagnosis.
- Patients may appear pale with purpura, petechiae, jaundice, and abdominal tenderness; and neurologic examination may show abnormal findings (e.g., confusion and seizures).

3. Diagnostic Studies

- Thrombocytopenia.
- Anemia.
- Peripheral blood smear: evidence of microangiopathic hemolysis including schistocytes, helmet cells, nucleated RBCs, and polychromasia.
- Increased reticulocytes.
- Elevated BUN and creatinine.
- Elevated serum LDH.
- Elevated serum indirect bilirubin.
- Decreased level of ADAMTS13 activity (typically <10%).
- Leukocytosis with a neutrophil predominance may be present.
- Coagulation tests—PT/international normalized ratio (INR), PTT—results are normal, which differentiates it from DIC.
- Direct Coombs test result is negative.
- Hemoglobinuria may be present.
- **Complications**
  - Without treatment, mortality rate is >90% because of multiorgan failure. With treatment, the mortality rate is <30%.
  - Chronic renal failure.
  - In some patients, the disease follows a chronic, relapsing course.

4. Management

- Prompt initiation of plasma exchange (plasmapheresis) is the mainstay of therapy and is generally done on a daily basis, until the platelet count normalizes, the neurologic abnormalities resolve, and serum LDH level returns to near normal. The frequency of plasmapheresis is then generally tapered gradually over the following 1 to 2 weeks; however, it may take longer for some patients to achieve a disease remission.
- Splenectomy may have a role in the treatment of patients who have a suboptimal response to plasmapheresis or continue to require plasmapheresis after 4 to 6 weeks.
- Corticosteroids also have a role in the treatment of patients with TTP and are sometimes given in addition to plasmapheresis.
- It is unclear whether the use of antiplatelet agents (e.g., aspirin and dipyridamole) confers any additional benefit in the treatment of TTP.
- Chronic renal insufficiency may occur in 25% of patients; dialysis-dependent renal failure occurs in 3% to 8% of patients.

C. Idiopathic (Immune) Thrombocytopenic Purpura

1. Etiology/Pathology

- Idiopathic thrombocytopenic purpura (ITP) is an acquired autoimmune disorder characterized by isolated thrombocytopenia, without other apparent causes or underlying conditions contributing to the thrombocytopenia. An autoantibody that binds to platelets is produced. The antibody-coated platelets are then bound to splenic macrophages and destroyed in the spleen. The thrombocytopenia occurs as a result of splenic sequestration and accelerated platelet destruction.
- May be classified as *acute* (<3 months), *persistent* (3–12 months), or *chronic* (>12 months) course.
- Childhood ITP usually occurs acutely, 1 to 3 weeks after viral illness, and is often self-limited.
- Viral antigen–antibody immune complexes thought to bind to platelet receptors.
- Adults usually have a more chronic form with no predisposing cause.
- In adult ITP, an autoantibody forms against platelet membrane antigen, thereby destroying platelets.
- **Epidemiology**
  - Most common cause of isolated thrombocytopenia.
  - Occurs predominately in young children and young women (usually younger than 40 years).
  - Peak incidence for childhood ITP is from 2 to 4 years; resolves spontaneously in 90% of cases.
  - May be associated with HIV infection.

2. Clinical Features

- Bruising, petechiae, and purpura are seen commonly at the time of diagnosis.
- Purpuric lesions in ITP are not palpable and do not blanch with pressure.
- Mucocutaneous bleeding is commonly present (e.g., epistaxis and gingival bleeding).
- Presence of extensive purpura or hemorrhagic bullae in mucosal areas (known as *wet purpura*) may be a predictor of life-threatening bleeding and must be treated accordingly.
- Adult women may experience menorrhagia.
- No fever or hepatosplenomegaly. **NOTE:** If splenomegaly is present, need to question the diagnosis of ITP, because presence of enlarged spleen suggests other underlying diagnosis.
- Intracranial hemorrhage is an infrequent occurrence; however, it is the most common cause of death among adult patients with ITP.

3. Diagnostic Studies

- Hallmark: thrombocytopenia (<20,000 per mm^3 in acute form, 30,000–80,000 per mm^3 in chronic form).

- Peripheral blood smear: platelets may be normal in size or may appear enlarged. **NOTE:** It is important to evaluate the peripheral smear to rule out platelet clumping as the cause of *pseudothrombocytopenia.*
- WBC and Hgb are generally normal.
- Coagulation studies (PT/INR, PTT) are normal.
- Bone marrow may show increased number of megakaryocytes.
- Serum platelet autoantibodies may be present in chronic cases.
- HIV test may be indicated in patients with risk factors.

4. **Management**
   - Avoidance of trauma and medications that can cause bleeding (e.g., aspirin and other nonsteroidal anti-inflammatory drugs [NSAIDs]) should be advised.
   - **Treatment of childhood ITP**
     - Childhood ITP is often a self-limited disease, and specific treatment is not always recommended, particularly if the symptoms are mild.
     - For children receiving treatment, management options for childhood ITP include intravenous immunoglobulin (IVIG), short course of corticosteroids, or IV Rh(D) immune globulin (RhIG); child must be nonsplenectomized, Rh$^+$, and not have history of autoimmune hemolytic anemia to receive RhIG.
     - Because of the considerable risks of serious infection following splenectomy, consideration of splenectomy for the treatment of childhood ITP is generally reserved for selected patients with demonstrated severe thrombocytopenia and associated bleeding concerns.
   - **Treatment of adult ITP**
     - For patients who are clinically stable, treatment is generally initiated with prednisone (1 mg/kg/day); the platelet count typically begins to increase within 1 week. After the platelet count has normalized, the prednisone dose can be tapered down gradually to the lowest effective dose that will allow the platelet count to remain in an acceptable range. Other treatment options include IVIG and RhIG; RhIG may only be used in Rh+ patients who have not undergone removal of spleen and do not have history of autoimmune hemolytic anemia.
   - Given the more chronic course typical of adult ITP, patients may need further treatment. For a patient who has not responded to a trial of steroid treatment, or who continues to require high steroid doses to maintain an acceptable platelet count, splenectomy may be a consideration. If a patient does not respond to steroid trial or splenectomy, some favorable responses have been observed using other agents (e.g., danazol, azathioprine, and cyclophosphamide).
   - Thrombopoietin analogs are also available for the treatment of chronic refractory adult ITP (e.g., romiplostim and eltrombopag).
   - Rituximab (monoclonal antibody) may be an effective treatment option for patients who are refractory to corticosteroids and IVIG.
   - In the case of life-threatening bleeding when a more rapid increase in the platelet count is needed, the patient is typically treated with IVIG and parenteral glucocorticoid therapy (e.g., methylprednisolone). Although there is generally no role for platelet transfusion in the treatment of ITP (because the transfused platelets will have limited survival given the presence of antiplatelet antibody), in the setting of life-threatening hemorrhage, consideration may be given to the administration of platelet transfusion in an attempt to achieve hemostasis.

IV. Factor Deficiencies
A. Hemophilia A and B
1. **Hemophilia A (Classic Hemophilia)**
   a. **Etiology/Pathology**
      - X-linked recessive disorder affecting only males (with rare exceptions); results in deficiency of coagulation factor VIII.
      - Mild form if level of coagulation factor VIII activity is 6% to 30%; severe form if level of coagulation factor VIII activity is <1%.
      - First episode of bleeding usually occurs when patient is <18 months old.
      - **Epidemiology**
        - After von Willebrand disease (vWD), the most common congenital bleeding disorder.
        - Occurs in 1/5,000 male births in the United States; occurs in all ethnic groups.
        - Eighty percent of all patients with hemophilia have hemophilia A.
   b. **Clinical Features**
      - Patients may complain of pain in weight-bearing joints.
      - Bleeding into joints occurs (hemarthroses). Commonly affected joints include knees, ankles, and elbows.
      - Patients can also bleed into muscles, the GI tract, or base of the tongue.
      - Severe disease is associated with spontaneous bleeding; mild disease is typically associated with bleeding due to trauma or surgery, and spontaneous bleeding is rare.
      - Hemophilia A and hemophilia B are clinically indistinguishable.
   c. **Diagnostic Studies**
      - Decreased levels of factor VIII. Specific assay for factor VIII activity is necessary for diagnosis.

- Increased PTT, normal PT, normal bleeding time, and normal fibrinogen.
- Level of vWf is normal.
- Mixing study: mixing plasma of normal patients with that of plasma from a patient with hemophilia A will result in normal PTT.
- **Complications**
  - Hemarthroses may lead to joint deformities.
  - Some patients transfused with factor VIII develop inhibitors to it and need to be identified and managed differently.
  - Lack of normalization of the PTT mixing study is a diagnostic of factor VIII anticoagulant activity (inhibitor).
  - d. **Management**
    - Infusion of factor VIII concentrate to levels of 25% to 100%. Optimal level for factor VIII replacement is dependent on the underlying situation (e.g., patient with only mild bleeding may require only 25% factor VIII level for control of bleeding).
    - Desmopressin acetate (DDAVP) may cause transient rise in factor VIII levels for several hours. **NOTE:** With repeated doses of DDAVP, tachyphylaxis occurs.
    - Primary prophylaxis with factor VIII concentrate may be indicated.
    - Avoid trauma.
    - Avoid medications that may cause bleeding (e.g., aspirin and other NSAIDs).
    - Avoid IM injections.
    - Genetic counseling for carriers.
  2. **Hemophilia B (Christmas Disease)**
    - a. **Etiology**
      - Occurs in 1/30,000 male births.
    - b. **Etiology/Pathology**
      - X-linked recessive disorder affecting only males (with rare exceptions); results in deficiency of coagulation factor IX.
    - c. **Clinical Features**
      - See section IV. A. 1.
    - d. **Diagnostic Studies**
      - Decreased levels of factor IX. Specific assay for factor IX activity is necessary for diagnosis.
      - Increased PTT, normal PT, normal bleeding time, normal fibrinogen.
      - Mixing study: mixing plasma of normal patients with that of plasma from a patient with hemophilia B will result in normal PTT.
      - **Complications**
        - Risk of thrombosis secondary to proteins (activated coagulation factors) is related to the use of some preparations of factor IX concentrate; risk has been significantly diminished

with the availability of higher purity factor IX concentrates.
- Lack of normalization of the PTT mixing study is diagnostic of factor IX anticoagulant activity (inhibitor).
- e. **Management**
  - Infusion of factor IX concentrate.
  - Primary prophylaxis with factor IX concentrate may be indicated.
  - Avoid medications that may cause bleeding (e.g., aspirin and other NSAIDs).
  - Avoid IM injections.
  - Genetic counseling for carriers.

B. **von Willebrand Disease**
1. **Etiology/Pathology**
   - Autosomal dominant disorder that results from deficient or defective vWF and causes *ineffective platelet adhesion.*
   - Platelet aggregation is normal.
   - vWF is produced in megakaryocytes and endothelial cells; it also functions to bind factor VIII and protects it from breaking down; therefore, decreased vWF also may cause reduced levels of factor VIII.
   - **Epidemiology**
     - Most common inherited bleeding disorder; affects approximately 1% of population.
     - Affects both men and women.
2. **Clinical Features**
   - Patients may commonly have mucosal bleeding (e.g., epistaxis and gingival bleeding) or increased menstrual bleeding.
   - Spontaneous hemarthroses do not generally occur.
   - GI bleeding is less common.
   - Bleeding is worsened by aspirin.
3. **Diagnostic Studies**
   - Prolonged bleeding time (usually, but wide fluctuations can occur); worse after taking aspirin.
   - Mild increase in PTT may be present.
   - In type I vWD, levels of vWF are reduced.
   - Low ristocetin cofactor activity.
   - Normal number and morphology of platelets.
4. **Management**
   - Avoid aspirin.
   - In type I, treatment with DDAVP may be helpful.
   - Infusion of plasma factor VIII concentrate containing vWF (e.g., Humate-P), or cryoprecipitate.
   - Check bleeding time immediately before elective procedures.

C. **Coagulopathy of Liver Disease**
1. **Etiology**
   - Damage to the liver may be caused by cancer, alcoholism, drugs, hemochromatosis, abscess, obstruction, viral hepatitis, and ischemia.

2. Pathology
   - **Reasons that liver dysfunction results in coagulopathy:**
     - The liver produces all coagulation factors except vWF.
     - Impaired hepatic synthetic function results in deficiencies of most clotting factors.
     - Liver macrophages remove activated factors (e.g., fibrin split products [FSPs] and fibrinolytic enzymes).
     - Liver produces antithrombin III, factors C and S.
     - Liver disease causes malabsorption of vitamin K.
     - Portal HTN can lead to splenomegaly, mild thrombocytopenia, varices, peptic ulcer disease, and bleeding.
3. Clinical Features
   - Bleeding: classic finding.
   - Assess for clinical signs of alcoholism (i.e., cardiomegaly, caput medusa, hepatomegaly, jaundice, scleral injection, and ecchymoses).
4. Diagnostic Studies
   - Prolonged PT > PTT.
   - Early liver disease is generally associated with prolonged PT only. Advanced liver disease may be associated with a prolonged PT and PTT.
     - Elevated factor VIII level is often present in chronic liver disease; extrahepatic synthesis of factor VIII also occurs.
   - Mixing study (50:50 mix of normal plasma and patient plasma) corrects PT/PTT elevation completely.
   - No response to vitamin K.
   - Low fibrinogen level; decreased platelets may be present, due to portal HTN and splenic sequestration.
   - Peripheral blood smear: target cells, macrocytes may be present.
5. Management
   - FFP may be given to replace deficient clotting factors if patient is bleeding or needs to undergo an invasive procedure.
   - Cryoprecipitate contains concentrated form of fibrinogen and may be given to replace fibrinogen in a patient with severe hypofibrinogenemia if patient is bleeding or needs to undergo an invasive procedure.
   - Vitamin K may be given in the setting of vitamin K deficiency; however, it does not typically correct the coagulopathy because patients with chronic liver disease often have significant impairment in hepatic synthetic function as well.
   - Avoid alcohol consumption.
   - Correct underlying disorder.

D. Vitamin K Deficiency

1. Etiology
   - Vitamin K deficiency can be caused by poor diet, malabsorption, antibiotics, warfarin, and biliary obstruction.
   - Dietary sources of vitamin K present in leafy vegetables.
   - Vitamin K is synthesized by intestinal bacteria.
   - Body stores are small and may be depleted in <1 week.
2. Pathology
   - Vitamin K is necessary for γ carboxylation of the vitamin K–dependent clotting factors (II, VII, IX, X) in the liver.
   - These clotting factors, along with calcium and platelets, activate factors X and II in coagulation cascade.
3. Clinical Features
   - Bleeding.
4. Diagnostic Studies
   - Prolonged PT > PTT.
   - Early vitamin K deficiency is associated with elevated PT only; severe vitamin K deficiency is generally associated with prolonged PT and PTT.
   - Normal fibrinogen level, platelets.
   - Mixing study (50:50 mix of normal plasma and patient plasma) completely corrects PT/PTT abnormalities.
5. Management
   - Diet including consumption of green leafy vegetables.
   - Depending on the etiology of vitamin K deficiency and goal of treatment, management may differ. Depending on the clinical situation, patients with warfarin-induced vitamin K deficiency and an excessive elevation of PT/INR, who are not actively bleeding and will continue to require anticoagulation for treatment of an underlying hypercoagulable disorder, may not require complete correction of PT/INR, and smaller doses of vitamin K may be sufficient. Each case must be carefully evaluated on an individual basis.
   - Vitamin K replacement is typically given by oral or subcutaneous route, with subsequent correction of PT/PTT abnormalities generally within 12 to 24 hours. **NOTE:** Absorption of subcutaneous vitamin K may be less predictable in patients who are edematous.
   - For the treatment of vitamin K deficiency in the setting of active bleeding, or if the patient requires an invasive procedure, administration of FFP may be indicated.

V. Hypercoagulability
A. Antithrombin III Deficiency

1. Etiology
   - May be inherited as an autosomal dominant trait, or acquired (e.g., liver disease, nephrotic syndrome, in DIC, or from certain chemotherapy drugs).
2. Pathology
   - Antithrombin III inactivates surplus thrombin.
   - Its activity is potentiated by heparin.

- Deficiency of antithrombin III (25%–60%) results in venous thrombosis.

3. **Clinical Features**
   - Patients may have a family history of thromboembolism or have recurrent deep venous thrombosis (DVT) or pulmonary emboli (PE).
   - First episode may occur at age 20 to 30.

4. **Diagnostic Studies**
   - Decreased levels of antithrombin III. **NOTE:** Functional antithrombin III assay should be done to allow evaluation of type I versus type II antithrombin III deficiency.
   - Acute thrombosis may cause decreased levels of antithrombin III, protein C, and protein S; therapy with heparin may reduce antithrombin III levels; therapy with warfarin may decrease levels of protein C and protein S; testing at time of acute thrombosis may affect interpretation of results.
   - Resistance to anticoagulant effects of heparin may be a clinical clue to presence of antithrombin III deficiency.

5. **Management**
   - Asymptomatic patients may require anticoagulation only before surgical procedures.
   - Patients who experience a thrombotic event generally receive IV heparin or low-molecular-weight heparin (LMWH), then oral anticoagulation indefinitely.

B. **Protein C Deficiency**

1. **Etiology**
   - Autosomal dominant disorder.

2. **Pathology**
   - Protein C: vitamin K–dependent liver protein that stimulates fibrinolysis, clot lysis.
   - Deficiency of protein C causes recurrent DVT, PE.

3. **Clinical Features**
   - Patients may have a family history of thromboembolism, DVT.
   - Venous thrombosis may occur in unusual sites; arterial thrombosis is less common.

4. **Diagnostic Studies**
   - Decreased levels of protein C. **NOTE:** Functional protein C assay should be done for the diagnosis of protein C deficiency.
   - Acute thrombosis may cause decreased levels of antithrombin III, protein C, and protein S; therapy with heparin may reduce antithrombin III levels; therapy with warfarin may decrease levels of protein C and protein S; testing at time of acute thrombosis may affect interpretation of results.
   - Normal PT, PTT, bleeding time.
   - **Complications**
     - Warfarin-induced skin necrosis is a medical emergency and may occur in setting of protein C deficiency.

- Newborns may have purpura fulminans or fulminant intravascular coagulation.
- May result in cerebrovascular accident.

5. **Management**
   - Patients who experience a thrombotic event generally receive IV heparin or LMWH, then oral anticoagulation indefinitely.

C. **Protein S Deficiency**

1. **Etiology**
   - Autosomal dominant disorder.

2. **Pathology**
   - Protein S: vitamin K–dependent liver protein that stimulates fibrinolysis, clot lysis.
   - Deficiency of protein S causes recurrent DVT, PE.

3. **Clinical Features**
   - Patients may have a family history of thromboembolism, DVT.
   - Venous thrombosis may occur in unusual sites; arterial thrombosis is less common.

4. **Diagnostic Studies**
   - Decreased levels of protein S. **NOTE:** Total and free protein S levels and protein S activity level should be determined to differentiate among type I, type II, and type III protein S deficiency.
   - Acute thrombosis may cause decreased levels of antithrombin III, protein C, and protein S; therapy with heparin may reduce antithrombin III levels; therapy with warfarin may decrease levels of protein C and protein S; testing at time of acute thrombosis may affect interpretation of results.
   - Normal PT, PTT, bleeding time.
   - **Complications**
     - Warfarin-induced skin necrosis is a medical emergency and may occur in setting of protein S deficiency.
     - May result in cerebrovascular accident.

5. **Management**
   - Patients who experience a thrombotic event generally receive IV heparin or LMWH, then oral anticoagulation indefinitely.

D. **Acquired Hypercoagulability**

1. **Etiology**
   - Four major causes of acquired hypercoagulability need to be recognized and assessed if DVT or PE is suspected or diagnosed.
   - **Pregnancy:** results in increased venous stasis, hyperviscosity, decreased protein S and antithrombin III, decreased fibrinolysis.
   - **Malignancy:** in neoplastic diseases, tumor cells activate platelets. Approximately 15% of patients with DVTs or PEs have cancer. In addition, 5% of patients without cancer who have had DVT or PE will have diagnosis of cancer within 1 year.
   - **Oral contraceptive pills:** increased risk of stroke, DVTs, PEs especially in women older than 40 years and tobacco users.

- **Lupus anticoagulant:** immunoglobulin seen in patients with and without systemic lupus erythematosus, which causes increased risk of thrombosis and spontaneous abortions. Laboratory evaluation: PTT is often elevated; mixing study (50:50 mix of normal plasma and patient plasma) does not completely correct prolonged PTT.

2. **Management**
   - Thorough history, physical examination important.
   - Doppler U/S, impedance plethysmography study, CXR, ventilation/perfusion scans should be ordered, if indicated.
   - Thromboembolism can be treated with heparin, then coumadin.
   - Greenfield filter may have to be placed to prevent recurrent PEs.
   - Women diagnosed with lupus anticoagulant (also known as *antiphospholipid antibody syndrome*) and who have experienced multiple miscarriages previously are generally treated with low-dose aspirin, heparin, or a combination of both during pregnancy, and must be followed up closely for the duration of the pregnancy.

VI. Other Disorders
A. Polycythemia Vera (Primary Erythrocytosis)
1. **Etiology/Pathology**
   - Acquired myeloproliferative disease resulting in overproduction of RBCs.
   - **Epidemiology**
     - Sixty percent of patients are men.
     - Rarely occurs before age 40; peaks at 50 to 60.
2. **Clinical Features**
   - Patients complain of headache, dizziness, blurred vision, pruritus (especially after a hot bath), fatigue, nosebleeds, tinnitus, LUQ pain, GI discomfort, chest pain, claudication. *Erythromelalgia* (burning/throbbing sensation in digits of the hands, feet) may be a prominent symptom.
   - Patients with PV have an increased bleeding tendency, and hemorrhage due to GI bleeding, epistaxis, or gingival bleeding may occur.
   - Patients with PV have increased tendency of thrombosis, and may experience arterial and venous thrombotic events.
   - On physical examination, splenomegaly, plethora, and engorged retinal vessels may be noted.
3. **Diagnostic Studies**
   - Elevated RBC mass (nuclear medicine study using radiolabeled RBCs to determine RBC mass).
   - EPO level is low.
   - Elevated HCT.
   - Elevated WBCs (10,000–20,000 per mm^3); neutrophilia and basophilia may be present.
   - Elevated platelets; the platelet count may exceed 1,000,000 per mm^3 in some patients.

- Elevated serum B_{12} level, elevated LAP, and elevated serum uric acid level may be present.
- Normal arterial O_2 saturation.
- Pseudohyperkalemia may occur because of elevated platelet count.
- Artificial prolongation of PT/PTT may occur in the presence of significantly elevated HCT.
- Genetic testing for Janus kinase 2 (*JAK2*) mutation: (+) in approximately 95% of patients.
- Bone marrow: hypercellular with increased megakaryocytes, absent iron stores.
- **Complications**
  - Thrombosis, bleeding, splenic infarction, peptic ulcer disease, gout.
  - Patients with PV are at increased risk for thrombotic and bleeding complications with surgery.
  - Approximately 15% of all patients with PV enter a "spent phase" characterized by hepatosplenomegaly, anemia, circulating immature WBCs in peripheral blood, and leukocytosis. The bone marrow shows myelofibrosis. Treatment of this phase is supportive, and median survival is approximately 2 years.
  - May progress to secondary AML.
4. **Management**
   - The goals of treatment are to reduce blood volume to normal and to prevent complications such as thrombosis and hemorrhage.
   - Therapeutic phlebotomy is typically continued until HCT <45%. Repeated phlebotomy induces iron deficiency, gradually decreasing the frequency of phlebotomy necessary to maintain target HCT. Administration of iron supplementation, therefore, is not appropriate in these patients and may result in rapid recurrence of the elevated HCT.
   - Myelosuppressive therapy may be indicated instead of, or in addition to, therapeutic phlebotomy, depending on the clinical presentation of the patient. Hydroxyurea is a commonly used myelosuppressive agent and does not appear to be associated with the increased leukemogenic potential associated with alkylating agents (e.g., chlorambucil).
   - IFN-α is also used to treat PV; ruxolitinib (JAK2 inhibitor) is approved as a second-line agent in patients with PV who are intolerant or resistant to hydroxyurea.
   - For patients who require an additional agent for control of thrombocytosis, anagrelide may be a useful option. It inhibits megakaryocyte maturation, thereby decreasing the platelet count. This agent does not appear to be associated with increased leukemogenic potential.
   - Treat gout with allopurinol.
   - Acetylsalicylic acid to reduce the risk of thrombosis; current studies evaluating the efficacy of low-dose

aspirin in reducing thrombotic risk without increasing the risk of bleeding complications suggest that low-dose aspirin may be well tolerated in PV patients.
- Antihistamines are used for the treatment of pruritus.

B. Secondary Erythrocytosis

1. Etiology/Pathology
- **Three major causes:**
  - Reactive (physiologic) as response to hypoxia: high altitude, pulmonary disease, tobacco smokers, high-affinity Hgb, cyanotic heart disease.
  - Pathologic (underlying tissue hypoxia is absent): renal cell carcinoma, renal disease, uterine fibroids, hepatomas, cerebellar hemangiomas, elevated androgen levels.
  - Relative polycythemia characterized by normal RBC mass and decreased plasma volume. Patients are typically overweight, hypertensive men on diuretic therapy, with a history of cigarette smoking.
- **Epidemiology:** major cause of increased red cell mass.

2. Clinical Features
- Patients may have a history of chronic obstructive pulmonary disease, smoking more than two packs of cigarettes a day, congenital heart disease, renal disease.
- On examination, heart murmur, cyanosis, HTN, clubbing (pulmonary osteoarthropathy), ecchymoses, hepatosplenomegaly may be found.

3. Diagnostic Studies
- Elevated RBCs, HCT with normal WBCs, platelets.
- EPO may be normal or high.
- CT scan of abdomen, renal U/S, or IV pyelogram may be indicated in patients with possible renal tumor or other renal cause of secondary polycythemia.
- RBC mass is normal in relative polycythemia and elevated in secondary polycythemia caused by pathologic or reactive condtions (see Etiology/Pathology in section VI. B. 1).
- Hgb electrophoresis.
- Oxygen saturation level.

4. Management
- Treat underlying disorder.
- Smoking cessation.

C. Hereditary Hemochromatosis

1. Etiology/Pathology
- Intestinal iron absorption inappropriately large, leading to increase in plasma iron and increased transferrin saturation.
- Excess iron then deposits in parenchymal cells of the heart, liver, pancreas, and endocrine organs.
- **Epidemiology**
  - Familial genetic iron storage disorder; autosomal recessive inheritance.

- Clinical phenotype of skin pigmentation and organ damage occurs only in homozygotes.
- Among Caucasian population, 1/200 with homozygous C282Y *HFE* genotype.
- Five to 10 times more common in men than in women.

2. Clinical Features
- May be asymptomatic in early stages.
- Patients may then complain of fatigue, weakness, loss of libido, impotence, abdominal pain, and arthritis.
- Diabetes may occur.
- On examination, one may find hepatomegaly in >95% of cases, splenomegaly in >50%.
- Skin may appear metallic or bronze.
- Cardiomyopathy with arrhythmias, congestive heart failure, and heart block can occur.
- Testicular atrophy, synovitis, and polyarthritis may be present.

3. Diagnostic Studies
- Increased plasma iron (>200 μg per dL).
- Increased transferrin saturation (>70% up to 100%).
- Increased SF, normal or low TIBC, increased liver iron, and increased urinary iron after deferoxamine.
- Increased LFTs may be present.
- Increased hepatic iron content demonstrated on CT, MRI; not indicated for routine screening.
- Genetic testing for *HFE* gene mutations consistent with diagnosis.
- Gold standard: liver biopsy with parenchymal hemosiderin.
- **Complications**
  - Cirrhosis of liver can lead to hepatocellular carcinoma.
  - Insulin-dependent diabetes.
  - Peripheral neuropathy, nephropathy, retinopathy.
  - Most important prognostic factor is presence or absence of cirrhosis at time of diagnosis; full life expectancy if treated before clinical symptoms occur; adequate phlebotomy treatment improves prognosis.

4. Management
- Routine phlebotomy to decrease body iron stores and maintain normal iron stores.
- Phlebotomy is typically performed on a weekly basis initially, until depletion of iron is confirmed by laboratory studies (e.g., mild anemia, decreased ferritin, and transferrin saturation <30%). Maintenance phlebotomy regimen is then performed approximately three to four times per year, for the remainder of the patient's life.
- Chelating agents may be indicated if anemia occurs, thus restricting the use of therapeutic phlebotomy (IM injection of deferoxamine).

- Test blood relatives; genetic counseling should be made available.
- Treat complications.
- Dietary restrictions, no iron pills, no alcohol or vitamin C.
- Avoid other potential hepatotoxins.

REVIEW QUESTIONS

1. You are asked to evaluate a 58-year-old male patient who presents for evaluation of recent onset fatigue, early satiety, and LUQ fullness and discomfort. On physical examination, the patient is noted to have splenomegaly with the spleen palpable 6 cm below the left costal margin at the mid-clavicular line. Laboratory findings reveal: WBC 114,000, Hgb 12.0, and Plt 420,000. The differential results include segmented neutrophils: 60%; bands: 4%; metamyelocytes: 10%; myelocytes: 6%; promyelocytes: 4%; blasts: 2%; basophils: 4%; lymphocytes: 6%; monocytes: 1%; eosinophils: 3%. Which of the following test results would support your diagnostic suspicion?

   a) Decreased vitamin B_{12} level
   b) JAK2 mutation: (+)
   c) Presence of Auer rods on peripheral blood smear
   d) Bone marrow aspirate for cytogenetic analysis: (+) Philadelphia chromosome (9;22) translocation

2. You are asked to evaluate a 62-year-old male patient who presents for a yearly physical and is without new complaints. Past medical history (PMH) is significant only for mild HTN, controlled with a diuretic. On examination, you note palpable lymphadenopathy in the cervical and axillary regions bilaterally; there is no splenomegaly noted. The patient denies recent acute illness, fever, night sweats, weight loss, fatigue, or other associated symptoms. Initial CBC results for this patient are as follows:

   WBC: 60,000, Hgb: 14.0, HCT 42%, Plt 168,000
   Differential: 15% segs, 2% bands, 80% lymphs, 1% monos, 1% eos, 1% basos
   Peripheral blood smear: increased number of small, mature-appearing lymphocytes; smudge cells noted; RBCs and Plts appear unremarkable.

   On the basis of this information, which of the following conditions is the most likely diagnosis for this patient?

   a) Chronic myelogenous leukemia (CML)
   b) Acute myelogenous leukemia (AML)
   c) Chronic lymphocytic lymphoma (CLL)
   d) Acute lymphocytic leukemia (ALL)

3. A 48-year-old female patient presents to the Family Medicine clinic for evaluation of recent onset fatigue over past several months. The patient also reports that she has been "having trouble feeling where the floor is" when she gets up at night in the dark to use the bathroom and has to turn on a light "to see where my feet are on the floor" (impaired position sense). The patient has a PMH significant for Hashimoto thyroiditis. She denies other chronic medical conditions and denies use of alcohol, tobacco, or recreational drugs. The patient reports that she follows a healthy, well-balanced diet. Physical examination reveals diminished position and vibration sense, evidence of pallor and glossitis. Examination findings are otherwise unremarkable. Initial CBC results include:

WBC	3,800
Hgb	10.6
HCT	32%
MCV	124
Plt	120,000

   Peripheral blood smear: (+) macroovalocytes and hypersegmented neutrophils ($\geq$5-lobes) are present. When reviewing the patient's chart, you verify that her CBC was normal during her most recent prior physical 1 year ago. On the basis of this information, which of the following conditions is the most likely diagnosis for this patient?

   a) Pernicious anemia
   b) Folate deficiency
   c) Lead poisoning
   d) Iron deficiency anemia

4. A 46-year-old male presented to the Internal Medicine clinic for initial evaluation 1 week ago, complaining of mild shortness of breath on exertion and increasing fatigue. Examination at that time was notable for the presence of conjunctival pallor, koilonychia (*spoon nails*), and angular cheilosis. Rectal examination revealed hemoccult (+) stool. CBC results at the time of most recent annual physical 2 years ago were normal. Initial laboratory testing was ordered, with results as noted (abnormal results are in **bold** type):

   WBC: 7,500 (normal range: 4,500–10,000)
   RBC: **3.4 × 10^6 per μL ($\downarrow$)** (normal range: 4.7–6.1 × 10^6 per μL)
   Hgb: **9.8 g per dL ($\downarrow$)** (normal range: 13.6–17.2 g per dL)
   HCT: **30% ($\downarrow$)** (normal range: 41%–50%)
   MCV: **64 ($\downarrow$)** (normal range: 80–100)
   Plt: **480,000 ($\uparrow$)** (normal range: 150,000–400,000)
   Stool: **Hemoccult (+)**
   SF level: **4 ng per mL ($\downarrow$)** (normal range: 20–270 ng per mL)
   Serum iron level: **15 g per dL ($\downarrow$)** (normal range: 50–175 g per dL)
   TIBC: **520 g per dL ($\uparrow$)** (normal range: 250–460 g per dL)

   On the basis of these results, which of the following interventions is appropriate in the management of this patient?

   a) Begin the patient on oral iron supplementation with ferrous sulfate 325 mg PO TID between meals.

b) Schedule follow-up blood work to include a CBC and reticulocyte count within 7 to 10 days.

c) Refer the patient for urgent GI consultation for further evaluation of hemoccult (+) stool.

d) Each of these interventions is appropriate for this patient.

5. You are asked to evaluate an 8-year-old female patient who presents for evaluation of recent increased bruising and epistaxis during the past several days. PMH is significant for a recent viral infection, from which she is now completely recovered. On examination, she is noted to have multiple bruises and petechiae scattered over her trunk and extremities. Otherwise, she feels entirely well, and, except for several episodes of spontaneous epistaxis and gum bleeding when brushing teeth, she reports no other recent symptoms. Initial laboratory testing was ordered, with results as noted (abnormal results are in **bold** type):

WBC	6,000 (4,000–11,000)
Hgb	13 g per dL (11.5–15.5)
HCT	39% (36–48)
MCV	86 (80–100)
Plt	**24,000 ($\downarrow$)** (150,000–400,000)

On the basis of this information, which of the following additional clinical findings would *support* your diagnostic suspicion for this patient?

a) Normal PT and PTT

b) Presence of splenomegaly on examination

c) Red blood cell fragments on peripheral blood smear

d) Platelet clumping on peripheral blood smear

6. You are evaluating a 24-year-old male patient who was recently diagnosed with Stage II HL following excisional LN biopsy. His initial diagnostic evaluation reveals that there are three areas of LN involvement above the diaphragm. There is no bulky disease, LN involvement below the diaphragm, or evidence of extranodal involvement. He denies recent fever >38° C, weight loss, or night sweats. His ESR is **62 ($\uparrow$)**. On the basis of this information, which of the following statements correctly classifies this patient's disease?

a) The patient has Stage II_A early-stage favorable HL.

b) The patient has Stage II_B early-stage favorable HL.

c) The patient has Stage II_A early-stage unfavorable HL.

d) The patient has Stage II_B early-stage unfavorable HL.

ANSWERS TO REVIEW QUESTIONS

1. **Answer: D**. CML is a myeloproliferative disorder caused by proliferation of myeloid cells, which retain their ability to differentiate. Hematopoietic cells contain reciprocal translocation of the *ABL-1* gene on chromosome 9 to the breakpoint cluster region (*BCR*) gene on chromosome 22, resulting in a *BCR–ABL*1 fusion gene on chromosome 22. The altered chromosome with the presence of the (9;22) translocation is known as the Philadelphia chromosome.

The Philadelphia chromosome is present in approximately 90% of cases of CML on cytogenetic analysis.

WBC differential in CML reveals granulocytes at all stages of maturation, and this helps differentiate it from acute leukemia, which is characterized by WBC differential with maturation arrest and predominance of blast cells in the peripheral blood. Auer rods are eosinophilic needle-like inclusions that may be present in the cytoplasm of leukemic myeloblasts in the peripheral blood and bone marrow of patients with AML. The *JAK2* mutation is an acquired somatic point mutation in the JAK2 protein that is present in the blood and bone marrow of patients with BRC-ABL1–negative myeloproliferative disorders. Nearly all patients with PV and approximately 50% of patients with essential thrombocythemia and idiopathic myelofibrosis are JAK2 (+). Patients with CML do not have the *JAK2* mutation, because CML is a BCR-ABL1–positive myeloproliferative disorder.

Neutrophils contain vitamin B_{12}–binding proteins, and patients with myeloproliferative disorders have an increase in the serum level of vitamin B_{12}–binding capacity, and the source of the protein is primarily in mature neutrophilic granules. Patients with CML have considerably elevated levels of vitamin B_{12}–binding protein, with serum vitamin B_{12} level in patients with CML typically increased to more than 10 times normal. (From Besa EC. Chronic myelogenous leukemia. September 24, 2018. https://emedicine.medscape.com/article/199425; Kaushansky K, Lichtman MA, Prchal JT, et al, eds. *Williams Hematology.* 9th ed. New York, NY: McGraw-Hill Education; 2016; Cashen AF, Wildes TM, eds. *The Washington Manual Subspecialty Consult Series: Hematology and Oncology Subspecialty Consult.* 4th ed. Philadelphia, PA: Lippincott Williams & Wilkins; 2016.) (Using laboratory and diagnostic studies; formulating most likely diagnosis)

2. **Answer: C**. CLL is one of the most common leukemias in the Western hemisphere and is a malignant lymphoid neoplasm characterized by accumulation of small mature B cells. Closely related to SLL, the malignant B cells have similar immunophenotypic features but without the malignant monoclonal B-cell lymphocytosis on assessment of blood or bone marrow. Diagnostic criteria include: absolute lymphocytosis >5,000 per μL with typical morphology of small mature lymphocytes, and characteristic *smudge cells* may be present; flow cytometry of peripheral blood reveals immunophenotype consistent with CLL. Bone marrow biopsy is typically not indicated at time of diagnosis, given that flow cytometry results from peripheral blood or results of excisional LN may confirm diagnosis. Absolute lymphocyte count = Total WBC × (% lymphocytes/100). For this patient, the absolute lymphocyte count = 60,000 × 80/100 = 48,000.

CML is a myeloproliferative disorder and WBC differential in CML reveals granulocytes at all stages of maturation. WBC differential in acute leukemia is characterized by maturation arrest and predominance of blast cells in the peripheral blood. (From Kaushansky K, Lichtman MA, Prchal JT, et al, eds. *Williams Hematology*. 9th ed. New York, NY: McGraw-Hill Education; 2016; Cashen AF, Wildes TM, eds. *The Washington Manual Subspecialty Consult Series: Hematology and Oncology Subspecialty Consult*. 4th ed. Philadelphia, PA: Lippincott Williams & Wilkins; 2016.) (Formulating most likely diagnosis)

3. **Answer: A.** Macrocytic anemia is defined by MCV > 100 fL. Megaloblastic anemia is a subcategory of macrocytic anemia caused by vitamin B_{12} or folate deficiency, and characteristic peripheral blood smear findings include hypersegmented neutrophils and macroovalocytes. Hypersegmented neutrophils is typically defined as >5% of neutrophils with five-lobe or any six-lobe neutrophils. Vitamin B_{12} (cobalamin) deficiency causes a neurologic syndrome, which may present with peripheral neuropathy affecting fingers and toes, and disturbances in position and vibration sense. The most common cause of vitamin B_{12} deficiency is pernicious anemia, which is an autoimmune condition in which the gastric mucosa containing the parietal cells is destroyed. The parietal cells produce IF, and the resultant deficiency of IF caused by pernicious anemia results in impaired absorption of vitamin B_{12}. The coexistence of other autoimmune diseases (e.g., type I DM, Hashimoto thyroiditis, hypoparathyroidism, vitiligo) with pernicious anemia is further evidence of the autoimmune basis of this condition.

   Folate deficiency may also cause megaloblastic anemia with similar peripheral blood smear findings, whereas the neurologic syndrome is limited to vitamin B_{12} deficiency. (From Schick P. Pernicious anemia. 2017. Retrieved from https://emedicine.medscape.com/article/204930; Kaushansky K, Lichtman MA, Prchal JT, et al, eds. *Williams Hematology*. 9th ed. New York, NY: McGraw-Hill Education; 2016; Cashen AF, Wildes TM, eds. *The Washington Manual Subspecialty Consult Series: Hematology and Oncology Subspecialty Consult*. 4th ed. Philadelphia, PA: Lippincott Williams & Wilkins; 2016.) (Formulating Most Likely Diagnosis)

4. **Answer: D.** The patient presents for evaluation and reports increasing fatigue and exertional dyspnea. Physical findings include conjunctival pallor, koilonychia, and angular cheilosis (also known as *cheilosis* or *angular cheilitis*), which are associated with iron deficiency anemia. Laboratory findings consistent with diagnosis of iron deficiency include: low-serum iron, low MCV, anemia, elevated platelet count, elevated TIBC, decreased SF. The presence of hemoccult (+) stool suggests that chronic GI blood loss may be causing the anemia, consistent with a diagnosis of iron deficiency anemia. Chronic blood loss is the most common cause of iron deficiency in adults, and diagnosis of iron deficiency in adults requires evaluation for GI malignancy. Treatment of iron deficiency anemia is 325 mg ferrous sulfate PO TID between meals, with an expected increase in reticulocyte count within 7 to 10 days and correction of the anemia within 6 to 8 weeks.

Treatment with iron supplement should continue for approximately 6 months to ensure adequate repletion of iron stores. (From Schrier SL. Causes and diagnosis of iron deficiency and iron deficiency anemia in adults. 2017. https://www-uptodate-com.dyc.idm.oclc.org/contents/causes-and-diagnosis-of-iron-deficiency-and-iron-deficiency-anemia-in-adults; Kaushansky K, Lichtman MA, Prchal JT, et al, eds. *Williams Hematology*. 9th ed. New York, NY: McGraw-Hill Education; 2016; Cashen AF, Wildes TM, eds. *The Washington Manual Subspecialty Consult Series: Hematology and Oncology Subspecialty Consult*. 4th ed. Philadelphia, PA: Lippincott Williams & Wilkins; 2016.) (Clinical Intervention)

5. **Answer: A.** The clinical presentation is suggestive of immune thrombocytopenia. The process of hemostasis includes *primary hemostasis* and *secondary hemostasis*. Primary hemostasis involves formation of the primary platelet plug, and secondary hemostasis involves activation of the coagulation cascade resulting in formation of cross-linked fibrin and stabilization of the primary platelet plug. Platelet disorders result in defects of primary hemostasis, and characteristic examination findings include petechiae, purpura, and mucosal bleeding (e.g., epistaxis, gingival bleeding). Since immune thrombocytopenia does not involve the process of secondary hemostasis, the PT and PTT would be expected to be normal. The presence of splenomegaly would not be expected in primary immune thrombocytopenia and suggests a secondary cause of thrombocytopenia.

   The presence of platelet clumping on peripheral blood smear may result in *pseudothrombocytopenia*, in which platelet clumping mimics a low platelet count when analyzed. The anticoagulant EDTA is often implicated in cases of pseudothrombocytopenia, and repeating the CBC using a sodium citrate tube may reduce the occurrence of platelet clumping. This condition is not associated with any abnormal clinical findings. RBC fragmentation occurs in conditions that cause microangiopathic hemolysis, such as DIC or TTP, both of which are associated with decreased platelets. This patient's clinical presentation is not consistent with DIC or TTP, and the peripheral blood smear in immune thrombocytopenia typically reveals decreased platelets and otherwise normal RBC and WBC morphology. (From Kaushansky K, Lichtman MA, Prchal JT, et al, eds. *Williams Hematology*. 9th ed. New York, NY: McGraw-Hill Education; 2016; Cashen AF, Wildes TM, eds. *The Washington Manual Subspecialty Consult Series: Hematology and Oncology Subspecialty Consult*. 4th ed. Philadelphia, PA: Lippincott Williams & Wilkins; 2016.) (Formulating most likely diagnosis)

6. **Answer: C.** Staging of HL is based on the Ann Arbor classification to designate Stage I, II, III, and IV; stages may be further classified as "A" (absence of "B" symptoms) and "B" (presence of any of the "B" symptoms). "B" symptoms are defined as (a) unintended weight loss of >10% of body weight in previous 6 months, (b)

drenching night sweats, and (c) recurrent unexplained fever >38° C. The presence of one or more adverse prognostic factors for early-stage (Stages I and II) HL is defined as early-stage unfavorable HL. Adverse prognostic factors for early-stage HL include (a) bulky mediastinal mass exceeding 33% of thoracic width on CXR or >10 cm on CT scan, (b) ESR > 50 mm per hour for "A" stage and >30 mm per hour for "B" stage, (c) extranodal involvement, (d) presence of "B" symptoms, and (e) >3 LN areas of involvement. This patient has Stage II$_A$ early-stage unfavorable HL, due to the elevated ESR > 50 mm per hour and >3 areas of LN involvement. (From National Cancer Institute. Adult Hodgkin lymphoma treatment (PDR⁻): Health professional version. 2018. https://www.cancer.gov/types/lymphoma/hp/adult-hodgkin-treatment-pdq.) (Formulating most likely diagnosis)

SELECTED REFERENCES

Ahya SN, Flood K, Paranjothi S, eds. *Washington Manual of Medical Therapeutics*. 30th ed. New York, NY: Lippincott Williams & Wilkins; 2001.

Barker LR, Burton JR, Zieve PD, et al, eds. *Principles of Ambulatory Medicine*. 3rd ed. Baltimore, MD: Lippincott Williams & Wilkins; 1991.

Berkow R, Fletcher AJ, eds. *The Merck Manual of Diagnosis and Therapy*. 15th ed. Rahway, NJ: Merck, Sharp & Dohme; 1987.

Braunwald E, Fauci AS, Kasper DL, et al, eds. *Harrison's Principles of Internal Medicine*. 17th ed. New York, NY: McGraw-Hill; 2008.

Braunwald E, Fauci AS, Kasper DL, et al, eds. *Harrison's Manual of Medicine*. 17th ed. New York, NY: McGraw-Hill; 2009.

Casciato DA. *Manual of Clinical Oncology*. 6th ed. Philadelphia, PA: Lippincott Williams & Wilkins; 2009.

Casciato DA, Lowitz BB, eds. *Manual of Clinical Oncology*. 4th ed. New York, NY: Lippincott Williams & Wilkins; 2000.

Cashen AF, Wildes TM, eds. *The Washington Manual Subspecialty Consult Series: Hematology and Oncology Subspecialty Consult*. 2nd ed. Philadelphia, PA: Lippincott Williams & Wilkins; 2008.

Dale DC, Federman DD, eds. *Web MD Scientific American Medicine*. New York, NY: WebMD; 2002.

Fauci AS, Braunwald E, Iselbacher KJ, et al, eds. *Harrison's Principles of Internal Medicine*. 14th ed. New York, NY: McGraw-Hill; 1998.

Ferri FF, ed. *Practical Guide to the Care of the Medical Patient*. 4th ed. St Louis, MO: CV Mosby; 1998.

Ferri FF, ed. *Practical Guide to the Care of the Medical Patient*. 5th ed. St Louis, MO: CV Mosby; 2001.

Fischbach F, Dunning MB, eds. *Manual of Laboratory and Diagnostic Tests*. 7th ed. New York, NY: Lippincott Williams & Wilkins; 2004.

Goroll AH, May LA, Mulley AG, eds. *Primary Care Medicine*. 3rd ed. Philadelphia, PA: JB Lippincott; 1995.

Govindan R, Arquette MA, eds. *The Washington Manual of Oncology*. New York, NY: Lippincott Williams & Wilkins; 2002.

Iselbacher KJ, Braunwald E, Wilson JD, et al, eds. *Harrison's Principles of Internal Medicine*. 13th ed. New York, NY: McGraw-Hill; 1994.

Kutty K, Schapira RM, Van Ruiswyk J, et al, eds. *Kochar's Concise Textbook of Medicine*. 4th ed. Philadelphia, PA: Lippincott Williams & Wilkins; 2003.

Lichtman MA, Beutler E, Kipps TJ, et al, eds. *Williams Manual of Hematology*. 6th ed. New York, NY: McGraw-Hill; 2003.

Lichtman MA, Kaushansky K, Kipps TJ, et al. *Williams Manual of Hematology*. 8th ed. New York, NY: McGraw Hill; 2011.

Mazza JJ, ed. *Manual of Clinical Hematology*. 3rd ed. New York, NY: Lippincott Williams & Wilkins; 2002.

McKenzie SB, ed. *Textbook of Hematology*. 2nd ed. Baltimore, MD: Lippincott Williams & Wilkins; 1996.

Pillot G, Chantler M, Magiera H, et al, eds. *The Washington Manual Subspecialty Consult Series: Hematology and Oncology Subspecialty Consult*. New York, NY: Lippincott Williams & Wilkins; 2004.

Tierney LM Jr, McPhee SJ, Papadakis MA, eds. *Current Medical Diagnosis and Treatment (Ambulatory and Inpatient Management)*. Stamford, CT: Appleton & Lange; 1998.

Tierney LM Jr, McPhee SJ, Papadakis MA, eds. *Current Medical Diagnosis and Treatment*. 42nd ed. New York, NY: Lange Medical Books/McGraw-Hill; 2003.

Wagner ND, Bartlett NL. Lymphoma. In: Govindan R, Arquette MA, eds. *The Washington Manual of Oncology*. New York, NY: Lippincott Williams & Wilkins; 2002:278–296:chap 14.

World Health Organization. Classification of neoplastic diseases of the hematopoietic and lymphoid tissues. In: Casciato DA, Lowitz BB, eds. *Manual of Clinical Oncology*. 4th ed. Philadelphia, PA: Lippincott Williams & Wilkins; 2000.

www.cancer.gov.

www.medscape.com.

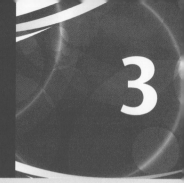

Pulmonary Disorders

3

Robin Risling

I. Pulmonary Thromboembolism

A. Etiology

- Pulmonary thromboembolism (PTE) is considered a major complication of thrombi originating in the venous circulation or the right side of the heart.
- Most commonly affecting but not limited to the femoral and popliteal vessels of the lower extremities.
- Estimated US incidence of venous thromboembolism is 1,000,000 cases annually with 10% (400,000–650,000) developing PTE and 10% (50,000) of those succumbing.
- Mortality is much greater when diagnosis is not established.

B. Pathophysiology

- Nearly all pulmonary emboli originate in the peripheral venous circulation, particularly the pelvis and lower extremities.
- Emboli transported to the pulmonary circulation lodge in vessels relative to their size.
- Emboli predominantly consist of intravascular thrombotic material. Less common embolic sources include fat, foreign bodies, tumor, air, amniotic fluid, and bone marrow.
- "Massive pulmonary emboli" refer to those large enough to lodge near the central pulmonary arterial circulation.
- Pulmonary infarction more typically results from multiple smaller emboli, but is common because of the collateral flow maintained by pulmonary circulation redundancy.
- Hemodynamically, PTE may result in increased pulmonary vascular resistance, pulmonary hypertension, and right ventricular (RV) failure. Local bronchoconstriction and physiologic dead space may also occur.

C. Clinical Features

- Peripheral venous thrombus findings are notoriously nonspecific. Patients with pulmonary embolism (PE) commonly have a history of deep vein thrombosis (DVT). PTE is a consequence of DVT.
- PTE typically presents abruptly with tachypnea, pleuritic chest pain, apprehension, and dyspnea. Other symptoms may include fever, hemoptysis, diaphoresis, cough, and syncope.
- Massive PTE may present as RV failure and systemic hypotension. However, the presentation can be subtle complicating the diagnostic picture.

- The classic triad (Virchow's) of venous stasis, hypercoagulable state, and venous endothelial injury (inflammation) predisposes to venous thrombus development and PTE (Table 3–1).
- History is of critical importance. Physical examination may be normal or reveal a variety of findings or exhibit signs of pulmonary hypertension like RV heaves or increased pulmonary component of S2.
- Clinical risk factors include cancer, oral contraceptives, smoking, prolonged immobility, pregnancy, postpartum state, inflammatory diseases, surgery (specifically, the postoperative state), myocardial infarction, congestive heart failure (CHF), obesity, and orthopedic injury of pelvis, hips, or lower extremities (see Table 3–1).
- Genetic predisposition to hypercoagulability is now recognized in the form of antithrombotic protein deficiencies (rare) including antithrombin III, protein C, and protein S, or abnormal variants of clotting factors. Also consider prothrombin G20210A mutation, antiphospholipid antibody syndrome (Lupus anticoagulant), and dysfibrinogenemia.
- Individuals heterozygous for factor V Leiden have at least three to five times increased risk of developing

TABLE 3–1.	Risk Factors for Thromboembolism

Immobilization
Lower extremity/pelvic trauma or surgery
Malignancy
Pregnancy and postpartum state
Oral contraceptives and estrogens
Obesity
Congestive heart failure
Nephrotic syndrome
Hematologic disorders (polycythemia vera, paroxysmal nocturnal hemoglobinuria, Waldenstrom macroglobulinemia)
Coagulation abnormalities (lupus anticoagulant, anticardiolipin antibodies, protein C or S deficiency, antithrombin III deficiency, factor V Leiden)

Data from Hume HD, ed. *Kelley's Essentials of Internal Medicine*. 2nd ed. Philadelphia, PA: Lippincott Williams & Wilkins; 2001:718.

venous thrombosis, and homozygous patients have even higher risk.

- Because factor V Leiden is so common among known thrombophilic factors, it accounts for 20% of patients with new venous thrombosis incident.
- Patients with elevated levels of plasma homocysteine are also at increased risk. However, in as many as half of the cases, no predominant risk factor is identified.
- The American Heart Association classifies PE into three categories: massive PE, submassive PE, and low-risk PE.
- Failure to diagnose is the most important factor in PTE mortality.

D. Diagnostic Studies

- Ninety percent of patients with proven PTE have a partial pressure of oxygen in arterial blood (PaO_2) <80 mm Hg. However, normal oxygen saturation does not rule out PTE.
- Respiratory alkalosis with hypocapnia is common. In severe cases, profound acidemia, hypercapnia, and hypoxemia may be present.
- Electrocardiographic (ECG) findings include tachycardia, atrial arrhythmias, and nonspecific ST-T wave changes, but are transient and nonspecific.
- Chest X-ray (CXR) abnormalities are frequently nonspecific because of underlying disease state with no pathognomonic findings related to PTE.
- Up to 30% of patients with PTE may have small effusion, which is typically exudative and often hemorrhagic.
- Ventilation/perfusion (V/Q) scan may be useful in low-probability cases and for sparing patients from radiation and contrast exposure.
- The D-dimer test is useful if negative, but nonspecific if positive. It is not recommended for high-probability cases.
- Use of contrast computed tomography (CT) angiography is considered a method of choice for detecting PE.
- Venous thrombosis studies of the lower extremities, including both noninvasive (Doppler, plethysmography, duplex scan, etc.) and invasive (^{125}I fibrinogen scan, venography).
- Pulmonary angiography remains the gold standard but is rarely used because of the less invasive and similar diagnostic accuracy of CT angiography.

E. Management

- Acute-phase management of RV failure and low systemic output requires hemodynamic and respiratory support.
- Measures are aimed at minimizing the risk of early death or the propagation of existing thrombus.
- Anticoagulation is preventative rather than definitive.
- Standard therapy consists of at least 3 months of novel oral anticoagulant therapy (in noncancer patients) or parenteral anticoagulation followed by 3 or more months of oral vitamin K antagonist anticoagulation therapy.
- Low-molecular-weight heparin may be used in place of standard heparin therapy and may also be used prophylactically.
- Thrombolysis is still controversial in clinical practice.
- Surgical or percutaneous (filter) interruption of the inferior vena cava when anticoagulation is contraindicated or for repeated events despite anticoagulation.
- Surgical embolectomy is rarely employed.
- Catheter-based thrombus removal is rarely employed.
- Key feature of management is stabilization and prophylaxis.

II. Bronchogenic Carcinoma (Lung Cancer)

A. Etiology

- Rare in nonsmokers. Other implicated factors include air pollution, ionizing radiation, asbestosis, exposure to secondhand smoke, exposure to heavy metals, and industrial carcinogens.
- Cigarette smoking is the most important etiologic factor in the United States (85% of all cases—87% of male cases and 85% of female cases).
- Lung cancer is the leading cause of cancer death in the United States.
- Risk is proportional to pack-year history with ex-smokers maintaining increased risk throughout life.
- Study of genetic predisposition is ongoing, focusing on smokers who do not develop lung cancer.
- Genetic mutations affecting proteins like k-ras, c-erb, and p53 that function as proto-oncogenes are also being investigated.

B. Pathophysiology

- More than 20 benign or malignant primary lung neoplasms have been identified. Major cell types are small-cell lung cancer (SCLC), representing <20% of reported cases, and non–small-cell lung cancers (NSCLCs) including squamous cell carcinoma (30%–35%), adenocarcinoma (30%–35%), large-cell carcinoma (10%–15%), and bronchioloalveolar cell carcinoma (2%) or BAC, which has been reclassified under adenocarcinoma.
- Squamous cell carcinoma is amenable to early detection (in sputum) because of its tendency to originate in central bronchi. Owing to a slow growth rate, it has lower risk of metastasis, though it is still possible to metastasize to adjacent structures and regional lymph nodes in the hilum or mediastinum.
- Small-cell carcinoma also occurs centrally with widespread metastasis, usually before initial diagnosis.
- Adenocarcinoma has recently equaled or surpassed squamous cell as the most frequent cell type and usually presents in the periphery.

- Adenocarcinoma tends to be glandular and mucus producing and is frequently associated with pleural effusions.
- Large-cell carcinoma tends to originate peripherally and is not amenable to early sputum detection.

C. Clinical Features

- History of cigarette smoking.
- Nonspecific symptoms such as cough, weight loss, dyspnea, chest pain, increased sputum production, and hemoptysis, frequently related to other comorbidities.
- A change in the above symptoms may suggest bronchogenic carcinoma.
- Specific symptoms usually occur late.
- Asymptomatic presentation may be in the form of a solitary pulmonary nodule found incidentally on chest radiograph.
- Physical findings absent or nonspecific.
- Local metastasis may result in symptoms associated with mediastinal structures, such as phrenic nerve, superior vena cava, and recurrent laryngeal nerve.
- Common distant metastatic sites include the bone, brain, adrenal glands, kidney, and liver.
- Cervical and supraclavicular lymphadenopathy occur frequently.
- Presence of paraneoplastic syndromes grouped as endocrine, systemic, neurologic, cutaneous, hematologic, and renal.
- Clubbing is commonly associated with bronchogenic carcinoma.

D. Diagnostic Studies

- CXR, CT, complete blood count (CBC), liver function, electrolytes, calcium, and creatinine.
- CT scan findings suggestive of malignancy include solitary nodule >15 mm, irregular borders, upper lobe location, and thick-walled cavitation.
- Cytology of sputum.
- Analysis of pleural fluid.
- Necessary histologic examination of tissue retrieved by bronchoscopy, lymph node biopsy, metastatic tumor biopsy, open biopsy, needle aspirates, and so on.
- Positron emission tomography (PET) scanning is becoming more commonplace in the evaluation process. It offers good negative predictive value but is less sensitive for small lesions and has high false-positive rate in certain benign lesions that metabolize ^{18}F-fluorodeoxyglucose.
- Screening recommendations: low-dose CT if 55 to 80 years with a 30 or more pack per year smoking history and/or smoking cessation of less than 15 years (USPSTF, Grade B).

E. Management

- Staging by tissue-type diagnosis. NSCLC staged through tumor, node, metastasis classification. SCLC staged through limited (one hemithorax) or extensive disease.

- NSCLC treatment options primarily include surgical resection with considerations for neoadjuvant and adjuvant chemotherapy.
- Five-year survival for SCLC is about 7% with limited-stage disease and 1% for extensive-stage disease. Surgery for bronchogenic carcinoma of all types is most successful in very localized tumors—5-year survival of such patients approaches 50%. The cornerstone of long-term treatment is to prevent smoking.
- Prognosis overall is based on stage of disease, response to therapy, and the overall health status of the patient.

III. Mediastinal Diseases

A. Etiology

- Mediastinal masses are commonly of metastatic origin. Of those originating in the mediastinum, about 75% are benign.
- The most common tumor originating in the mediastinum is thymoma, although lymphatic tumors, teratomatous tumors, and intrathoracic goiters may also appear in the mediastinum. Vascular tumors may also originate in the mediastinum.
- Hernias through the diaphragm may also present as mediastinal masses (Table 3–2).

B. Pathophysiology

- Mediastinum is divided into three compartments—anterior, middle, and posterior.
- Differential of anterior tumors includes thymoma, teratoma, thyroid lesions, parathyroid lesions, lymphoma, germ cell tumor including teratoma, and other miscellaneous mesenchymal tumors.
- Middle mediastinal masses include lymphadenopathy (benign or malignant), pulmonary artery enlargement, great vessel aneurysm, developmental cysts, dilated azygos/hemiazygos vein, some diaphragmatic hernias, and foramen of Morgagni hernias.
- Posterior compartment tumors are primarily neurogenic or diaphragmatic hernias. Most mediastinal masses occupy the anterior or middle compartments. Pheochromocytoma mass can also occupy this compartment.

C. Clinical Features

- Most patients are asymptomatic with incidental findings on CXR.
- Symptoms may be related to the site of original involvement rather than mediastinal condition.
- About 50% of patients with thymoma present initially with myasthenia gravis.
- Physical findings are usually nonspecific.
- There may be a mass effect causing superior vena cava compression with resultant facial and upper extremity edema and prominent venous pattern.

D. Diagnostic Studies

- CXR.
- CT scan helpful in delineating anatomy.

TABLE 3–2.	Clinical Features of Mediastinal Masses			
	Incidence	Peak Age (y)	Common Clinical Findings	Diagnostic Studies
Anterior				
Thymoma	Most common anterior mediastinal mass	40–60	Myasthenia gravis in 35%	CT, needle aspiration, surgical biopsy
Lymphoma	Common	20–30	Cough, pain, fever, and weight loss	CT, needle aspiration, surgical biopsy
Thyroid	Uncommon	Any age	Asymptomatic, airway obstruction, hyperthyroidism, and hypothyroidism	Physical examination: enlarged thyroid, deviated trachea, ^{131}I scan
Teratoma	Uncommon	<35	Asymptomatic	CT, surgical biopsy
Middle				
Hiatal hernia	Very common	>40	Asymptomatic	Esophagram
Metastatic cancer	Very common	>35	Asymptomatic or symptoms of primary tumor	Needle aspiration, surgical biopsy
Sarcoidosis	Common	<35	Asymptomatic or systemic symptoms	Tissue biopsy: skin, lung (transbronchial)
Aortic aneurysm	Common	>50	Asymptomatic or chest pain with dissection	CT or angiogram
Pericardial cyst	Most common mediastinal cyst	Any age	Asymptomatic	CT, surgical resection
Bronchogenic cyst	Rare	<35	Asymptomatic, rare compression, or infection	CT, surgical resection
Posterior				
Neurogenic tumors	20% of all primary mediastinal tumors	Any age	Asymptomatic or rare neurologic symptoms	CT, myelogram, surgical resection

Data from Hume HD, ed. *Kelley's Essentials of Internal Medicine*. 2nd ed. Philadelphia, PA: Lippincott Williams & Wilkins; 2001:713.
CT, computed tomography.

- Angiography and/or venography in suspected vascular conditions.
- Barium swallow if esophageal involvement.
- Magnetic resonance imaging to visualize planes other than axial and to better delineate hilar structures and masses extending into the spinal canal.
- PET/CT can be useful in suspected lymphomas to identify the ideal biopsy site and to monitor treatment.
- Meta-iodobenzylguanidine scans are useful to detect mediastinal pheochromocytoma.
- Anti-acetylcholine receptor antibodies may be produced by the thymus in myasthenia gravis.
- α-Fetoprotein or β-human gonadotropin is associated with germ cell tumors.
- Lactase dehydrogenase (LDH) elevation is associated with lymphomas and seminomas.
- Tissue diagnosis necessary in neoplastic conditions.

E. Management
- Varied depending on underlying cause of mass.

IV. Pleural Effusion
A. Etiology
- Transudative (low-protein) effusions predominantly result from CHF—also cirrhosis and nephrotic syndrome—conditions that do not directly affect the pleural tissue.
- Exudative (high-protein) effusions arise as a result of changes in vascular permeability that results in fluid accumulation, typically result from inflammatory or malignant processes such as tuberculosis, pneumonia, carcinoma, infarction, trauma with possible hemothorax, and the interruption of lymphatic channels and/or the thoracic duct resulting in direct accumulation of lymph (chylothorax) in pleural space and rheumatic disorders.
- Less common etiologies include asbestosis, Meigs syndrome, and uremia. Empyema is a special case in which frank pus is located within the pleural space (Table 3–3).

TABLE 3–3.	Differential Diagnoses of Pleural Effusions

Transudative pleural effusions
Congestive heart failure
Cirrhosis
Nephrotic syndrome
Myxedema
Pulmonary emboli
Urinothorax
Atelectasis
Constrictive pericarditis
Exudative pleural effusions
Neoplastic diseases
Infectious diseases
Bacterial infections
Tuberculosis
Fungal infections
Viral infections
Parasitic infections
Pulmonary emboli
Gastrointestinal disease
Esophageal perforation
Pancreatic disease
Intra-abdominal abscesses
Diaphragmatic hernia
Collagen-vascular disease
Rheumatoid pleuritis
Systemic lupus erythematosus
Drug-induced lupus
Wegener granulomatosis
Churg–Strauss syndrome
Postcardiac injury (Dressler) syndrome
Asbestos exposure
Meigs syndrome
Drug-induced pleural disease
Nitrofurantoin
Dantrolene
Methysergide
Bromocriptine
Procarbazine
Amiodarone
Radiation therapy
Hemothorax
Chylothorax
Uremic pleuritis
Lymphangiomyomatosis

Data from Light RW. *Pleural Diseases*. Philadelphia, PA: Lea & Febiger; 1990.

B. Pathophysiology

- Collection of fluid within the virtual space created by visceral and parietal pleura.
- Pleura consists of two components: visceral (covering the lungs) and parietal (covering the inner surface of the chest wall, diaphragm, and mediastinum).
- Pulmonary circulation supplies blood to the visceral pleura, which has no sensory nerves.
- Systemic circulation supplies parietal pleura, which also contains sensory nerves.
- The two layers create a virtual space, which is normally lubricated by 5 to 10 mL of pleural fluid.
- Pleural fluid is produced in the parietal pleura and resorbed through the lymphatic drainage of the visceral pleura at a rate of 15 to 20 mL per day.
- Pleural fluid is normally drained through the lymphatic channels of the parietal pleura.
- Noninflammatory effusions can occur in any condition that causes ascites, obstruction to venous or lymphatic drainage, or CHF.
- Inflammatory effusions typically result from conditions that cause inflammation of the pleura or adjacent structures.
- Worsened by obstruction of lymphatic drainage.
- Unless iatrogenically introduced, air in the pleural space indicates bronchopleural fistula.
- Empyema is an occasional complication of bacterial pneumonia or lung abscess.

C. Clinical Features

- Depending on the amount of fluid, underlying cause, and ability to compensate, symptoms and physical findings may be absent. Symptoms, when present, may include dyspnea, cough, and pleuritic pain (pleurisy). Dyspnea is related to volume of fluid accumulation.
- Physical examination may reveal decreased breath sounds, decreased diaphragmatic excursion on the affected side(s), decreased tactile fremitus, dullness to percussion, and "E to A" change (egophony).
- Empyema should be suspected in the presence of persistent or recurrent fever after treatment of bacterial pneumonia.

D. Diagnostic Studies

- Light's Criteria Rule for differentiating transudate from exudate.
- CXR with blunting of costophrenic angle (gutter). Up to 300 mL of fluid may be undetectable in posterior/anterior CXR. Lateral decubitus radiograph is more sensitive to smaller fluid amounts. Thoracentesis is both diagnostic and potentially therapeutic in terms of volume reduction.
- Fluid should be evaluated for total protein, LDH, white blood cell with differential, glucose, and/or pH.
- Also include acid-fast, Gram's stain, aerobic and anaerobic cultures, and cytology.

- Other diagnostic studies include pleural biopsy for undiagnosed exudative effusions.
- Larger specimens may be obtained through thoracoscopy or open pleural biopsy.
- Chest CT better at defining pleural space than plain CXR and beneficial in determining anatomical extent of pleural and lung lesions.

E. Management
- Establish cause of effusion and treat appropriately. Thoracentesis for therapeutic reasons should be considered when large effusions result in pulmonary dysfunction. Limit fluid removal to 1,000 to 1,500 mL at a time because of the possibility of pulmonary edema in re-expanded lung.
- Empyema or persistent effusion of other origin may require chest tube to water seal drainage.

V. Pneumothorax
A. Etiology
- Air is not normally present in the pleural space, but can be introduced by a break in either pleural membrane, resulting in a pneumothorax.
- Entry through parietal pleura caused by trauma or iatrogenic means.
- Entry through visceral pleura caused by rupture of bleb, cyst, bulla, and so on, or by necrosis of adjacent lung tissue. Termed *primary spontaneous pneumothorax* when etiology not readily apparent—more common in tall, thin, young adult male smokers.

B. Pathophysiology
- Regardless of etiology, result is positive pleural pressure that compresses the lung tissue reducing lung volume.

C. Clinical Features
- Acute onset of dyspnea and chest pain, although may be asymptomatic, especially if small pneumothorax.
- If large enough, diminished breath sounds, diminished tactile fremitus, and increased resonance on percussion tachycardia, pleural friction rub, and tracheal shift to contralateral side.
- Patient with tension pneumothorax presents in acute distress. Tension pneumothorax is considered a medical emergency.

D. Diagnostic Studies
- CXR confirms the presence of pneumothorax.

E. Management
- Small pneumothorax (<2 cm and no distress in breathing) may resolve spontaneously. Larger pneumothorax may require evacuation of air by catheter or large-bore drainage tube to water seal drainage. Hemodynamic compromise in a tension pneumothorax can be relieved with immediate decompression by placing a needle or catheter in the pleural space.

VI. Chronic Obstructive Pulmonary Disease
- Chronic disorders that disturb airflow either within the airways or within the lung parenchyma.
- Obstruction is generally progressive, may coincide with airway hyperreactivity, and may be partially reversible.
- Generally refers to chronic bronchitis or emphysema; however, patients often exhibit features of both.
- Does not commonly include bronchial asthma.
- Estimated that at least 16 million persons in the United States suffer from chronic obstructive pulmonary disease (COPD), with another 16 million Americans undiagnosed.
- Third leading cause of death and second leading cause of disability in the United States.
- Elderly men are at greatest risk for mortality from the disease.
- Fifteen percent of patients with COPD exhibit progressively disabling symptoms as early as their fifth and sixth decades.
- Up to 15% of patients with established COPD have not been direct consumers of tobacco.
- Owing to the presence of cigarette smoking, the World Health Organization (WHO) predicts that COPD will be the third most common cause of death by the year 2030.

A. Etiology and Pathogenesis
- Risk factors for the development of COPD:
  - Cigarette smoking (80% risk): most important risk factor.
  - The number of cigarettes smoked and the number of smoking years are the main contributors to disease severity.
  - The remaining 20% of patients with COPD frequently are exposed to a combination of environmental tobacco smoke (exposure of nonsmokers to cigarette smoke), occupational dusts and chemicals, indoor air pollution from biomass fuel used for cooking, and heating in poorly ventilated buildings.
  - Genetics (<1% risk); deficiency of the protein α_1-antitrypsin (AAT) may lead to premature emphysema, chronic bronchitis, and, occasionally, bronchiectasis; severity of lung disease varies.
  - Air or environmental pollution: role unclear, low significance, primarily important because of its potential for causing exacerbations of preexisting COPD, pollutants secondary to occupational exposure (i.e., miners).
  - Infection (i.e., viral upper respiratory infection) does not initiate disease, but may lead to a transient worsening of symptoms and pulmonary

functioning in those with preexisting COPD. In those patients with acute viral infection, bacterial infections may lead to superinfection.

- Hyperresponsive airways, Dutch hypothesis (1960): asthma, atopy, nonspecific airway hyperresponsiveness, and serum deficiency of protein AAT may underlie the development of chronic airflow obstruction.
- Presentation types:
  - Type A: emphysema predominates with arterial PO_2 preserved; thus, patient is pink, thin, cachectic appearing. Usually not cyanotic and typically works hard to get air (puffing). Major complaint is often severe shortness of breath. Presentation typically after age 50. Cough is rare, with scant clear, mucoid sputum. No peripheral edema, no adventitious lung sounds.
  - Type B: bronchitis predominates with significant hypoxemia resulting in cyanosis, obesity, and peripheral edema secondary to RV failure. Major complaint is chronic, productive cough with mucopurulent sputum, and frequent exacerbations of disease due to chronic chest infections. Often presents by 30s and 40s. Chest noisy with wheezing and rhonchi common.
  - Most patients do not fall into one category, but rather exhibit symptoms of both.

B. Clinical Features

1. Chronic Bronchitis

- Enlargement of mucus-secreting glands and increased number of goblet cells; quantity of airway mucus is increased.
- Cough and sputum production for 3 months of the year for two consecutive years.
- Rhonchi.
- Wheezing.
- Dyspnea.
- Prolonged expiration.
- Cyanosis and cor pulmonale, consisting of leg edema, elevated jugular venous pressure, RV heave, and tricuspid insufficiency.

2. Emphysema

- Dyspnea on exertion.
- Minimally productive cough.
- Pursed-lip breathing.
- Depressed diaphragm.
- Hyperresonant to percussion.
- Prolonged expiration.
- Diminished breath sounds.
- Wheezing.
- Cor pulmonale.

C. Diagnostic Studies and Approach

1. Chronic Bronchitis

- CXR in chronic bronchitis may reveal increased anteroposterior diameter, thickened bronchial markings, and enlarged right side of heart.

- PFT expected findings are reduced FEV_1 and/or FVC; maybe some reversibility after bronchodilator therapy, normal to elevated TLC/RV; normal diffusing capacity.
- Arterial blood gases (ABGs): hypoxemia and hypercapnia. However, chronic bronchitis diagnosis relies heavily on the clinical picture/history.

2. Emphysema

- CXR in emphysema may reveal low, flat diaphragm; increased retrosternal airspace; "pruning" of vascular markings; long, narrow heart shadow; and bullae (radiolucent, >1 cm, arcuate hairline shadows).
- PFT: fixed reduction in FEV_1 and/or FVC, increased TLC and/or RV, and reduced diffusing capacity.
- ABGs: normocapnia, mild-to-moderate hypoxemia. AAT serum level may be low. Although high-resolution CT is more sensitive as an imaging method for detecting emphysema, it is not routinely performed in the diagnostic evaluation.
- Lung biopsy is not performed to make the diagnosis. True pathologic confirmation is typically obtained through postmortem examination.
- PFT and ABG analyses remain the most useful physiologic adjuncts in evaluating patients with COPD.
- Consider AAT testing in patients who develop emphysema at a young age.

D. Management

- To date, the only treatment strategy shown to reduce mortality is smoking cessation.
- GOLD 2017 advises against supplemental oxygen prescribed to stable COPD patients who are not severely hypoxic.
- Pharmacologic therapy is generally a stepwise approach.
- Assess severity based on symptoms, spirometric abnormality, and complications such as respiratory failure and right-sided heart failure.
- Focus on symptoms and exacerbations.
- Goal: reduce symptoms and reduce frequency and severity of exacerbations; improve quality of life.
- Numerous modalities of treatment available.
- Treatment is individualized and varies from patient to patient.
- Consider referring the patient to a pulmonologist if the COPD onset occurs before the age of 40, there are frequent exacerbations (two or more a year) despite optimal treatment, there is severe or rapidly progressive COPD, symptoms are disproportionate to the severity of airflow obstruction, or there is a need for long-term oxygen therapy.

1. Chronic Bronchitis

- Smoking cessation, exercise (20 minutes, three times weekly), healthy lifestyle, and immunization (pneumococcal and influenza vaccines).

- Pharmacologic intervention:
  - May include β_2-agonist (short-acting β-agonists [SABA] and/or long-acting β-agonists [LABA]).
  - Antimuscarinic drugs (short-acting muscarinic antagonists [SAMAs] and long-acting muscarinic antagonists [LAMAs]).
  - Combination drug use (e.g., LAMA + LABA) is more effective than either medication alone.
  - Short-course corticosteroids (inhaled, oral, or parenteral), although use is controversial and most useful in bronchitis with some reversibility.
  - Antibiotics for acute exacerbations or to treat acute bronchitis and/or prevent acute exacerbations of chronic bronchitis. However, there are little data to support use of prophylactic antibiotics.
  - Supplemental oxygen if $PO_2 > 55$ mm Hg at rest, exercise, nocturnally, or if cor pulmonale is present.
  - Diuretics if cor pulmonale present.
  - Pulmonary rehabilitation focusing on patient education and exercise training.
  - Chest physiotherapy, postural drainage in those patients with excessive amounts of retained secretions who cannot clear by coughing or other methods. To date, outcome data have not supported the use of expectorant and mucolytic therapies.

2. **Emphysema**
  - As mentioned earlier, AAT replacement if deficient.
  - Corticosteroids minimally effective.
  - Lung volume reduction surgery (severe disease only).
  - Lung transplantation (end-stage COPD).
  - Mechanical ventilation to support gas exchange and maintain acceptable ABG values.
  - Bullectomy, an older pulmonary procedure, may prove useful in those patients with severe bullous emphysema.

VII. Asthma

- According to the National Asthma Education and Prevention Program (NAEPP) guidelines, asthma is a chronic inflammatory disease characterized by airway narrowing and obstruction, hyperresponsiveness of airways, and airway inflammation. Airflow obstruction is reversible spontaneously or with pharmacotherapy.
- Can occur at any age. It is one of the most common chronic diseases in children. Fifty to 80% of children with asthma develop symptoms prior to age 5.
- According to the Centers for Disease Control and Prevention, in 2015, 8.4% of children and 7.6% of adults in the United States had asthma.

- Results in over 470,000 hospitalizations per year, with an estimated 3,000 plus deaths in the United States.
  - Hospitalization rates have been highest among blacks and children, and death rates for asthma are consistently highest among blacks aged 15 to 24.
- Health disparities when compared with the general population are experienced by blacks in adulthood and childhood asthma.

A. Etiology
- The strongest identifiable predisposing factor for the development of asthma is atopy; however, obesity is increasingly recognized as a risk factor.
- Potential risk factors for the development of asthma may be classified as inherited or acquired.
- Inherited or allergic asthma is characterized by symptoms that occur with exposure to an allergen to which patients have been previously sensitized.
- Patients exhibit markers for allergic disease (positive skin testing, elevated serum immunoglobulin, IgE, levels), a strong positive family history of allergic conditions (e.g., allergic rhinitis and eczema), and exacerbations based on allergen exposure.
- Acquired or environmental asthma is generally seen in patients who have no history of allergies. There may be no family history of asthma.
- Acquired asthma may be precipitated by exposure to a variety of environmental stimuli such as house dust mites, domestic animals, and cockroaches. These irritants are commonly found indoors, centralized in bedding and carpets, and present throughout the year.
- Maternal cigarette smoking has been implicated as a predisposing factor for the development of childhood asthma.
- Sinusitis, upper respiratory tract infections, influenza, or psychological stress are known to precipitate airway inflammation.
- Exercise-induced bronchoconstriction and inhalation of cold air during winter months may result in asthma exacerbations and/or worsening of symptoms in some patients, as well as aspiration and gastroesophageal reflux.
- Some patients may experience asthma symptoms after ingestion of certain medications such as aspirin, nonselective β-blockers, nonsteroidal anti-inflammatory drugs, or tartrazine dyes.
- There are also reports of women experiencing catamenial asthma at predictable times during menses.
- Occupational asthma is triggered by various agents in the workplace; may occur weeks to years after initial exposure and sensitization.

B. Pathophysiology

- Asthma results from a combination of processes that results in airway obstruction, hyperinflation, and airway limitation.
- Chronic airway obstruction is characterized by infiltration of the airway wall, mucosa, and lumen by activated eosinophils, mast cells, macrophages, and T lymphocytes.
- Bronchial smooth muscle contraction results from mediators released by inflammatory, local neural, and epithelial cells.
- Epithelial damage manifested by denudation and desquamation of the epithelium, leading to mucous plug.
- Airway inflammation underlies disease chronicity and contributes to airway hyperresponsiveness and airflow limitation.
- Airway remolding is characterized by:
  - Subepithelial fibrosis.
  - Smooth muscle hypertrophy and hyperplasia.
  - Goblet cell and submucosal gland hypertrophy and hyperplasia resulting in mucus hypersection.
  - Possible airway wall thickening due to acute edema and cellular infiltration during asthma exacerbations.

C. Clinical Features

- Classified according to frequency of symptoms, FEV_1/FVC, nighttime awakenings, and interference with normal activity.
- Key symptoms include wheezing, cough, dyspnea, and chest tightness. However, these symptoms are highly variable. Symptoms are typically worse at night, may occur spontaneously, or may be precipitated or exacerbated by many different triggers.
- Patients experiencing an asthmatic attack may exhibit tachypnea, prolonged expiratory and/or inspiratory phases of respiration or silent chest, and use of accessory muscles of respiration.
- Symptoms may occur singularly or in combination, and patients may not exhibit a classic presentation with several or all of these complaints.
- Chest may be hyperresonant on percussion.
- Fatigue and pulsus paradoxus (inspiratory decline in systolic blood pressure of at least 10 mm Hg) are late signs and may signal the need for critical types of intervention, including intubation and ventilatory support.
- Wheezing is more pronounced during expiration rather than inspiration. Status asthmaticus (tachycardia, tachypnea, accessory muscle use, pulsus paradoxus, wheezing or silent chest, altered mental status, paradoxic abdominal, and diaphragmatic movement on inspiration) may result from a severe acute asthmatic attack refractory to treatment with bronchodilators.

- Cardiac asthma is defined as wheezing triggered by decompensated CHF.
- Classification of asthma severity for patients ≥12 years of age and recommended treatment:
  - Mild intermittent asthma:
    - Characterized by mild asthma symptoms two or fewer times a week; nocturnal awakening fewer than two times a month; ≤2 days per week use of SABA for symptom control (not prevention of exercise-induced bronchospasm [EIB]); no interference with normal activity; initial peak expiratory flow (PEF) ≥70%, normal or personal best; normal FEV_1 between exacerbations; FEV_1 of >80% predicted and FEV_1/FVC normal.
    - Recommend treatment: Step 1: usually cared for at home; Step 2: prompt relief with an inhaled SABA on an as-needed basis.
  - Mild persistent asthma:
    - This is characterized by asthma symptoms more than 2 days per week, but not daily; three to four times per month of nighttime awakening; PEF 40% to 60% predicted or personal best; FEV_1 > 80% of personal best; >2 days per week use of SABA for symptom control (not for EIB), but not daily and not more than one time on any day; minor interference with normal activity; FEV_1/FVC normal.
    - Recommended treatment: in addition to the SABA, a long-term controller medication is required. A low dose of inhaled corticosteroids (ICSs) is the recommended long-term controller medication for this degree of severity. Alternative treatment (listed alphabetically): cromolyn, leukotriene modifier, nedocromil, or sustained-release theophylline to serum concentration of 5 to 15 g per mL.
  - Moderate persistent asthma:
    - This is characterized by daily asthma symptoms; nighttime awakenings >1 time per week, but not nightly; >1 day per week use of SABA for symptom control (not for EIB daily, but not nightly); impairment; some limited interference with normal activity; FEV_1 >60%, but <80% predicted; FEV_1/FVC reduced 5%; PEF of <60% to <80% of personal best. Recommended treatment: the use of a low to a medium dose of ICS together with a long-acting bronchodilator is the preferred therapy. Alternative treatments include increasing to a medium dose of ICS or adding a leukotriene antagonist such as zafirlukast (Accolate) and montelukast (Singulair) or theophylline to low to medium dose of ICS. ICSs include Fluticasone (Flovent HFA) and Budesonide (Pulmicort Flexhaler). Correct dosing for low and medium therapy depends on age and medication used.

- Severe persistent asthma:
  - This is characterized by asthma symptoms throughout the day; nighttime awakenings often seven times per week; several times per day use of SABA for symptom control (not for EIB) daily; extremely limited interference with normal daily activity; FEV_1 <60%; FEV_1/FVC reduced >5%; PEF of <60 of personal best.
  - Recommended treatment: a high dose of ICS and a long-acting bronchodilator are the preferred therapies. These patients may require long-term oral corticosteroids, although repeated attempts should be made to reduce the dose while they are receiving high-dose ICSs.

D. Diagnostic Studies
- Laboratory studies in asthma may provide both diagnostic and prognostic data. Spirometry (FEV_1, FVC, and FEV_1/FVC) is recommended at initial assessment, when symptoms and peak flow measurements have stabilized, both before and after bronchodilator challenge.

1. **Pulmonary Function Testing**
   - The evaluation of asthma should include spirometry (FEV_1, FVC, and FEV_1/FVC) before and after administration of short-acting bronchodilator.
   - Airflow obstruction is indicated by reduced FEV_1/FVC.
   - Significant reversibility of airflow obstruction is defined by an increase in ≥12% and 200 mL in FEV_1 or ≥15% and 200 mL in FVC after inhaling a short-acting bronchodilator.
   - A positive bronchodilator response strongly confirms the diagnosis. Bronchial provocation testing with inhaled histamine or methacholine is useful when asthma is suspected but spirometry is nondiagnostic.
     - Bronchial provocation test is not recommended if the FEV_1 is <65% of predicted.
     - A positive methacholine test is defined as a ≥20% fall in the FEV_1 at an exposure to a concentration of 8 mg per mL or less.
     - Exercise challenged testing may be useful in patients with symptoms of EIBs.

2. **Peak Expiratory Flow**
   - A 20% change in the PEF values from morning to afternoon or from day to day suggests inadequately controlled asthma.
   - PEF values <200 L per minute indicate severe airflow obstruction.
   - IgE determination: may indicate allergic/inherited asthma, CBC, and sputum cytology showing eosinophilia.
   - Considerations for children with refractory or severe symptoms of asthma: sweat test for cystic fibrosis, immunoglobulins to assess for immunodeficiency, IgE (allergic aspergillosis), evaluate for paranasal or gastroesophageal reflux.

- Skin testing to assess sensitivity to environmental allergens.
- The following may be helpful in acute situations:
  - ABG analysis looking for hypoxemia, normal or increased $PaCO_2$, and acidosis.
  - Chest imaging is indicated when pneumonia or complication of asthma is suspected.
  - Pulse oximetry to monitor oxygen saturation.

E. Management
- The 2007 NAEPP guidelines classify the treatment of asthma into broad categories based on age. The goals of the asthma therapy are as follows: to minimize chronic symptoms that interfere with normal activity (including exercise) guidelines to prevent exacerbations; no missed days at work/school for both the parent and the child; minimal or no chronic symptoms day or night; peak flow measurements >80% of patients personal best; minimal or no adverse effects from medications; and minimal use of short-acting inhaled β_2-agonist (<1 time per day, <1 canister per month) to reduce or prevent underlying airway inflammation and the series of chemical mediators that contribute to bronchospasm. Thus, treatment is geared toward the level of control based on the most severe impairment or risk category. A stepwise approach to diagnose and manage asthma was developed in an effort to assist with clinical decision making to meet individual patient needs and improve patient perceived control of asthma, to reduce or eliminate emergency department visits and hospitalizations.
- The trend has been to use glucocorticoid preparations sooner and more frequently. Inhaled preparations are considered first line and preferred in all patients identified with persistent disease.
- The small risk of delayed growth in children with chronic ICS use is well balanced by the effectiveness of these medications.

1. **Long-Term Control Medications**
   - Anti-inflammatory agents: ICSs are preferred first-line agents for all patients with persistent asthma; systemic corticosteroids (oral or parenteral) most effective in achieving prompt control of asthma during exacerbations or when initiating long-term asthma therapy in patients with severe symptoms.
   - Long-acting bronchodilators: mediator inhibitors, such as cromolyn sodium and nedocromil, are long-term medications that prevent asthma symptoms and improve airway function in patients with mild persistent asthma or exercise-induced symptoms; β-adrenergic agonists, such as salmeterol and formoterol, provide bronchodilation for up to 12 hours after a single dose; phosphodiesterase inhibitors, such as theophylline, provide mild bronchodilation in asthmatic patients.
   - Leukotriene modifiers: zileuton is a 5-lipoxygenase inhibitor that decreases leukotriene production,

and zafirlukast and montelukast are cysteinyl leukotriene receptor antagonists.

- Desensitization immunotherapy for specific allergens can be considered in asthma patients who have exacerbations of asthma symptoms when exposed to allergens to which they are sensitive.
- Vaccination, specifically Pneumovax, annual influenza vaccinations, including seasonal and epidemic influenza A (H1N1). Immunotherapy for specific allergens should be considered in selected asthma patients.

   2. **Quick-Relief Medications**
   - β-Adrenergic agonists: short-acting inhaled β_2-agonists, including albuterol, levalbuterol, bitolterol, pirbuterol, and terbutaline, are effective bronchodilators during exacerbations.
   - Anticholinergic agents (e.g., ipratropium bromide) reverse vagally mediated bronchospasm, but not allergen-induced bronchospasm or EIB, and decrease mucus gland hypersection seen in asthma.
   - Phosphodiesterase inhibitors (e.g., methylxanthines) are not recommended for therapy of asthma exacerbations. Theophylline provides mild bronchodilation in asthmatics. Sustained-release theophylline may be useful in adjunct therapy. It is essential that serum concentrations of theophylline be monitored.
   - Corticosteroids (e.g., methylprednisolone, prednisolone, and prednisone) effective for primary treatment for patients with moderate-to-severe asthma exacerbations and for patients with exacerbations who do not respond promptly and completely to inhaled β_2-agonist therapy.
   - Diet for patients with food allergies, maintain normal exercise and activity except for those patients with exercise-induced asthma, patient education and use of a written action plan regarding the nature of asthma, goals of therapy, warning signs of impending attack, correct use of medication, and peak flow meters are highly recommended, especially for those patients exhibiting moderate or severe persistent asthma, as well as patients with a history of severe exacerbations.
   - Communication with family, school, and work where appropriate.
   - Antibiotics are not recommended for the treatment of acute asthma exacerbations except in cases where the patient has comorbid conditions (i.e., pneumonia and bacterial sinusitis).

VIII. Pulmonary Arterial Hypertension

- Refers to elevation of intravascular pressure within the pulmonary circulation.
- May be acute or chronic.

- Prevalence is estimated at 15 cases per 1 million adults. The development of this disorder is based on right heart catheterization measurements. Defined as mean pulmonary artery pressure >25 mm Hg at rest (normal 8–20 mm Hg) or >30 mm Hg with exercise.
- Classification change: the WHO Functional class (2008 Dana Point classification) is one way of describing the severity of pulmonary arterial hypertension (PAH) and reflects the impact the condition has on a patient's life in terms of physical activity and symptoms.
- There are five classes of PAH based on the underlying pathophysiology associated with the disease: PAH, pulmonary hypertension with left heart disease that is more common than PAH, pulmonary hypertension associated with lung disease and/or hypoxemia, pulmonary hypertension from chronic thrombotic and/or embolic disease, and pulmonary hypertension whose origin is either multifactorial or unclear.
- The WHO also describes four classes of PAH based on patient's ability to function. Class I is the least severe, classified as diseases that localize to small pulmonary muscular arterioles. Class IV is the most complicated. Typically occurs in patients with hematologic disorders, sarcoidosis, glycogen storage disorders, and other miscellaneous causes. Patients with class I PAH are not limited in terms of physical activity. Patients with class IV PAH are unable to perform any physical activity without symptoms and may experience symptoms during rest.
- Central physiologic abnormality of pulmonary hypertension is increased RV afterload caused by elevated pulmonary vascular resistance. The development of RV hypertrophy and intimal proliferation is the consequence of pulmonary hypertension because the pulmonary pressure rises to a level inappropriate for a given cardiac output, despite the etiology. As a consequence, patients may develop atheromatous changes and in situ thrombosis, leading to further narrowing of the arterial bed. Thus, left untreated, pulmonary hypertension has a poor prognosis (15% annual mortality rate) and is considered a life-threatening condition.
- Idiopathic (formerly primary) pulmonary hypertension, or plexogenic pulmonary arteriography, is a rare disorder, occurring mainly in young and middle-aged women. Characterized by histopathologic plexiform lesion found in muscular pulmonary arteries. There may be some genetic history. Typically, no identifiable cardiopulmonary or connective tissue disorder. Risk factors include hepatic cirrhosis, portal hypertension, HIV infection, and use of anorectic drugs. Clinical presentation

consists of progressive shortness of breath with lethal outcome.

- Secondary pulmonary hypertension is caused by varied mechanisms such as emphysema and pulmonary fibrosis and obstruction of the pulmonary vascular bed as seen with chronic pulmonary thromboembolic disease.
- Pulmonary veno-occlusive disease (fibrotic occlusion of pulmonary veins and venules, secondary hypertensive changes in pulmonary arterioles and muscular pulmonary arteries) is a rare cause of postcapillary pulmonary hypertension also seen in children and young adults.
- The etiology is unknown but is associated with conditions such as viral infection, bone marrow transplantation, chemotherapy, and malignancy (Table 3–4).
- Patients exhibit progressive fibrotic occlusion of pulmonary veins and venules coupled with secondary hypertensive changes in the pulmonary arterioles and muscular pulmonary arteries.

A. Etiology

- Causes of PAH can be placed into five broad categories: (1) reduction in cross-sectional area of the pulmonary arterial bed, for example, emphysema, interstitial lung disease (ILD), sickle cell disease, collagen-vascular disease, acidosis, and lung resection hypoxemia from any cause; (2) increased pulmonary venous pressure, for example, constrictive pericarditis, LVF or reduced compliance, mitral stenosis, pulmonary veno-occlusive disease, and mediastinal diseases compressing pulmonary veins; (3) increased pulmonary blood flow, for example, congenital L-R intracardiac shunts; (4) increased blood viscosity, for example, polycythemia; and (5) miscellaneous, for

TABLE 3–4. Classification of Pulmonary Hypertension

Postcapillary
Left-sided heart failure
Aortic or mitral valve disease
Pulmonary venous disease
Left atrial myxoma
Precapillary
Chronic respiratory disease
Congenital heart disease
Pulmonary vasculitis
Primary pulmonary hypertension
Occlusive pulmonary vascular disease

Data from Hume HD, ed. *Kelley's Essentials of Internal Medicine*. 2nd ed. Philadelphia, PA: Lippincott Williams & Wilkins; 2001:136.

example, HIV, PAH in conjunction with hepatic cirrhosis, and portal hypertension.

B. Pathophysiology

- Abnormalities most frequently observed in the small muscular arteries and arterioles include intimal hyperplasia and medial hypertrophy, ensuing destruction of the lumen leading to pulmonary vascular resistance, and a decrease in the number of small vessels (arteries and arterioles).
- Severe pulmonary hypertension leads to further changes in the larger (elastic) pulmonary arteries: thickening of the artery wall, notably the media layer; in situ thrombosis in the pulmonary vasculature; and hypertrophy of RV wall, with or without dilation.

C. Clinical Features

- Symptoms: dyspnea, dull, retrosternal chest pain usually triggered by exertion, exertional fatigue, syncope, or orthopnea. Symptoms of right-sided heart failure (e.g., lower extremity swelling, ascites, and hoarseness caused by impingement of recurrent laryngeal nerve by enlarged pulmonary artery).
- Physical examination findings: narrowing and splitting of S_2, accentuation of the pulmonary component of S_2, cardiac lift/heave in left lower sternal border, right-sided presystolic gallop (S_4), mid-diastolic gallop (S_3), systolic ejection click, jugular venous distension, peripheral edema, occasional pulmonic, or tricuspid insufficiency murmurs.

D. Diagnostic Studies

- CXR and high-resolution CT scans: increased pulmonary artery vasculature, enlarged cardiac silhouette with bulging of the anterior cardiac border, redistribution of blood flow from lower to upper lung zones, interstitial or alveolar edema, and dilation of the right and left main and lobar pulmonary arteries.
- Perfusion lung scan: reveals focal perfusion defects (e.g., recurrent pulmonary emboli).
- PFT: to detect underlying airflow obstruction or restricted lung volumes, and a decreased diffusing capacity.
- ABG analysis: to determine hypoxemia or acidosis.
- Echocardiography and electrocardiography: demonstration of RV hypertrophy and estimation of pulmonary arterial pressure.
- Doppler ultrasonography: a reliable noninvasive means of estimating pulmonary artery systolic pressure.
- Transthoracic echocardiography: to definitively determine the degree of pulmonary hypertension.
- Laboratory analysis should be conducted to assess for secondary pulmonary hypertension—for example, LFTs, HIV, and collagen-vascular serology.
- ECG (EKG) can show right arterial enlargement, right axis deviation, right bundle branch block, and QTc prolongation.

E. Management

- Management of pulmonary hypertension is dependent on the associated specific disorder leading to symptomatology and the severity of disease.
- Focus is placed on correction of cardiac disease and/or decreasing pulmonary venous and capillary pressures.
- **Treatment modalities**
  - For idiopathic PAH without underlying cause, pharmacotherapy is used. The goal is dilation of pulmonary arteries, thereby reducing pulmonary arterial pressures, as well as reducing PAH. Three main categories of drugs are used: (1) prostaglandins, for example, epoprostenol (Flolan), treprostinil (Remodulin), and iloprost (Ventavis); short-acting, intravenous (IV) or inhalation, must be given frequently or on continuous basis; long-term effect suggests a reversal of vascular remodeling and proliferative changes in the pulmonary arterial system in addition to its vasodilator effect; (2) Phosphodiesterase type 5 inhibitor, for example, sildenafil (Revatio, Viagra). Less effective than prostaglandins but have a more favorable dosing regimen of one to three times daily, orally (PO); and (3) endothelium antagonist, for example, bosentan (Tracleer) and Ambrisentan (Letairis). Given PO, one to two times daily. In rare cases, calcium-channel blockers may be of benefit.
  - For PAH with underlying etiology, the goal is treatment of the primary problem, for example, treatment of left-sided heart failure, causes of hypoxia-like COPD, chronic lung disease, and treatment of scleroderma by rheumatologist. Long-term anticoagulation therapy is warranted if patient has some type of clotting disorder such as chronic thromboembolic pulmonary hypertension. Surgical removal of blood clots may be warranted.
  - Continuous IV infusion of prostacyclin (PGI_2) or epoprostenol. There has been therapeutic success with prostacyclin; treatment of polycythemia via repeated phlebotomy, diuretics, salt restriction, and supplemental oxygen for cor pulmonale. For end-stage disease, combined heart–lung transplantation or lung transplantation alone (considered unrealistic for most patients), thromboendarterectomy, and supplemental O_2 for correction of alveolar hypoxia and hypoxemia.
  - Patients are also generally placed on long-term anticoagulation therapy with warfarin.

IX. Sleep Apnea Syndrome

- Repetitive episodes of airflow cessation (apnea) during sleep.
- The syndrome includes three types of sleep apnea: primary central sleep apnea (lack of respiratory drive), obstructive sleep apnea (transient obstruction), and mixed (a combination of both).
- Obstruction occurs at the level of the pharynx.
- Apnea often terminates with short gasps or snorting.
- Typically, a chronic condition that results in excessive daytime sleepiness.

A. Etiology and Epidemiology

- Primary central sleep apnea characterized by the absence of respiratory effort is rare and not well understood.
  - Obstructive sleep apnea caused by narrowing or obstruction of the upper airway may be the result of:
  - Obesity or excessive soft tissue in the soft palate.
  - Alcohol or sedative ingestion prior to sleep.
  - Neuromuscular disorders that cause a loss of normal pharyngeal muscle tone, resulting in the passive collapse of the pharynx.
  - Craniofacial abnormalities such as micrognathia.
  - Macroglossia, adenotonsillar hypertrophy, or enlarged uvula.
  - Nasal obstruction, upper respiratory infections, smoking, or hypothyroidism may precipitate or worsen obstructive sleep apnea.
- Prevalence of primary central sleep apnea is < 1%.
- Prevalence of obstructive sleep apnea is 4% in men and 2% in women.
- Prevalence of obstructive sleep apnea is higher in obese and hypertensive patients.

B. Pathophysiology

- Obstruction of the pharyngeal airway recurring during sleep.
- Sleep induced collapsible airway due to loss of compensatory tonic input to dilatory muscle of the upper airway.

C. Clinical Features

- Disturbed sleep pattern.
- Loud snoring.
- Snorting.
- Agitation during sleep.
- Violent movements during sleep with the sleep partner complaining of being hit or injured because of these random, violent movements.
- Severe headache upon awakening.
- Excessive daytime sleepiness (may fall asleep during daily activities).
- Sore or dry throat.
- Cognitive impairment.
- Personality disorder.
- Morning headaches.
- Decreased libido.
- Depression.

D. Associated Conditions

- Cardiac arrhythmias.
- Conduction disturbances.
- Pulmonary hypertension.

- Unexplained cor pulmonale.
- Systemic hypertension.
- Obesity.
- Type 2 diabetes mellitus.

E. Diagnostic Studies

- Polysomnography, a nighttime sleep study, is the diagnostic test of choice.
- Apneic episodes must last a minimum of 10 seconds and occur 10 to 15 times an hour to be considered clinically significant.
- The apnea/hypopnea index (AHI), total number of apneas and hypopneas divided by the total sleep time, is used to categorize sleep apnea into mild: AHI = 5 to 15; moderate: AHI = 15 to 30; severe: AHI >30.
- Multiple sleep latency test is a diagnostic tool to measure daytime somnolence.
- ABG analysis may reveal daytime hypercapnia.
- CXR and electrocardiography may reveal signs of pulmonary hypertension or cor pulmonale. Serum thyroid-stimulating hormone to detect unsuspected hypothyroidism.
- Erythrocytosis is common; thus, a hemoglobin level should be obtained.
- Other diagnostic studies performed in selected patients include fiber-optic examination of upper airway to rule out obstructing tumors and cephalometric radiography to define the anatomy of the upper airway if surgical treatment is considered.

F. Management

- Treatment is aimed at treating the underlying condition and may include weight loss and avoidance of alcohol, sedatives, and smoking.
  - The most effective treatment for obstructive sleep apnea is nasal continuous positive airway pressure (nasal CPAP).
  - Bilevel positive airway pressure is effective for treating central sleep apnea.
  - Oral and dental appliances such as Snore Guard have been used for obstructive sleep apnea when patients are unable to tolerate CPAP.
  - Various surgical procedures: uvulopalatopharyngoplasty, tracheostomy, and craniofacial surgery may be recommended to patients with obstructive sleep apnea who fail CPAP.
  - Pharmacologic therapy has not proven beneficial for sleep apnea.

X. Pneumonia and Infections of the Lung

A. Etiology

- Pneumonia is an inflammation of the lung parenchyma characterized by consolidation of the affected area and filling of the alveolar air spaces with exudate, inflammatory cells, and fibrin.
- Pneumonias are grouped into two categories: community-acquired pneumonias and health care–related pneumonias (hospital-acquired and ventilator-associated).
- Age, environmental exposure(s), underlying disease processes, and seasonal factors may affect etiology and pathology of pneumonia.
- Infection by bacteria or viruses is the most common cause; however, trauma to the chest wall, inhalation of chemicals, or infection by other infectious agents such as rickettsia, fungi, parasites, and yeasts can occur (Table 3–5).
- In addition to the above causes, events surrounding September 11, 2001, have brought to light organisms uncommonly seen in clinical practice.

B. Pathophysiology

- Factors that may affect the lung's defenses include age; chronic lung diseases such as cystic fibrosis,

TABLE 3–5.	Organisms That Cause Pneumonia
Common	**Uncommon**
Outpatient pneumonia	
Streptococcus pneumoniae	*Legionella* species
Mycoplasma pneumoniae	*Staphylococcus aureus*
Respiratory viruses	*Mycobacterium tuberculosis*
Chlamydia pneumoniae	Fungi
Haemophilus influenzae	*Klebsiella pneumoniae*
Community-acquired pneumonia requiring hospitalization	
S. pneumoniae	*M. pneumoniae*
H. influenzae	*Moraxella catarrhalis*
Polymicrobial	*M. tuberculosis*
Anaerobic bacteria	Fungi
Aerobic Gram-negative bacilli	
Legionella species	
S. aureus	
C. pneumoniae	
Respiratory viruses	
Severe community-acquired pneumonia requiring hospitalization	
S. pneumoniae	*H. influenzae*
Legionella species	*M. tuberculosis*
Aerobic Gram-negative bacilli	Fungi
M. pneumoniae	
Respiratory viruses	

Data from Fauci AS, Harrison TR, eds. *Harrison's Principles of Internal Medicine*. 17th ed. New York, NY: McGraw-Hill; 2008.

asthma, and COPD; immunocompromised states such as chemotherapeutic medications and HIV/AIDS; cigarette smoking; allergens; anesthesia; and alcohol abuse.

- Two main routes of infection of the lungs are aspiration of oropharyngeal flora and inhalation of airborne pathogens.
- Two other less common routes of infection include systemic bacteremia (bloodborne) and direct extension from a focus of infection adjacent to the lung.
- Previously, pneumonias were classified by the anatomic structure invaded, but the current classification system categorizes them by etiologic agent: bacterial, mycoplasma, pneumocystic, viral, and so on.
- Necrotizing pneumonia or lung abscesses or both occur when necrotic lung tissue is released into small, adjacent airways, creating multiple abscesses (<2 cm in diameter), or into larger airways or bronchopulmonary segments, creating larger abscesses (>2 cm in diameter).

C. Clinical Features

- Depending on the pathogen, route of exposure, age of the patient, and environment, presentation of a patient with pneumonia may be classified as typical or atypical.

- A typical (obvious or classical) presentation might include sudden onset of fever, single shaking chill, productive cough (usually with purulent sputum), and pleuritic chest pain.
- Signs of consolidation may include egophony, dullness to palpation, and increased fremitus.
- Auscultatory findings may include bronchial breath sounds and crackles over the affected areas.
- An atypical (obscure or unusual) presentation may be characterized by a gradual onset of nonspecific symptoms (headache, myalgia, fatigue, nausea, vomiting, diarrhea, loss of appetite), and a dry cough.
- Physical findings tend to be minimal (crackles or scattered rhonchi) without overt signs of consolidation.

1. **Signs and Symptoms of Pulmonary Disease Caused by Bioterrorism (Table 3–6)**
   - Pulmonary anthrax (etiologic agent, *Bacillus anthracis*): patients are first seen with flu-like illness. Symptoms can include malaise, low-grade fever, myalgia, nonproductive cough, and chest discomfort. Several days after the initial presentation, patients become acutely ill and can have high fever, severe respiratory distress, shock, and coma.
   - Pneumonic plague (etiologic agent, *Yersinia pestis*): patients become acutely ill after a 2- to 3-day incubation period. High fever, rigors, tachycardia,

TABLE 3–6.	Historic Clues to Unusual Pneumonias	
Type of Pneumonia	**Exposure History**	**Occupational or Risk Population**
Anthrax	Cattle, horses, swine, wools, hides	Butchers, tanners, wool carders, agricultural workers
Brucellosis	Cattle, swine, goats, raw milk products	Abattoir workers, recent Mexican immigrants, veterinarians, agricultural workers
Coccidioidomycosis	Travel to San Joaquin Valley, southern California, southwest Texas, New Mexico, Arizona	Agricultural workers, construction workers
Cryptococcosis	Pigeon droppings, HIV	AIDS
Histoplasmosis	Chicken or bat droppings, travel to Ohio or Mississippi River valley	Agricultural workers, construction workers
Legionnaires disease	Contaminated air coolers or hospital water supply	Office workers, maintenance workers, hospitalized patients
Melioidosis	Travel to southeast Asia, Australia, South and Central America, Guam	Military personnel
Plague	Ground squirrels, prairie dogs, rabbits, rats in endemic areas (western United States)	Hunters, campers, agricultural workers
Psittacosis	Budgerigars, cockatoos, parrots, parakeets, pigeons, turkeys	Bird fanciers, agricultural workers
Q fever	Cattle, sheep, or goat milk, placentas, or feces	Agricultural workers
Sporotrichosis	Rose thorns	Gardeners, florists
Tularemia	Tissue of rabbits or squirrels, bite of infected ticks or flies	Hunters, campers

Data from Fauci AS, Harrison TR, eds. *Harrison's Principles of Internal Medicine.* 17th ed. New York, NY: McGraw-Hill; 2008.

headache, myalgias, dyspnea, cough, malaise, and/ or cyanosis are common features.

- Pulmonary tularemia (etiologic agent, *Francisella tularensis*): patients clinically complain of fever, chills, drenching sweats, severe weakness, cough, and/or headache.
- Bioterrorism has become a reality after spores of *B. anthracis* sent through the mail caused skin lesions or lung infections or both in some citizens of the United States.
- Other organisms the Pentagon recognizes as agents of bioterrorism that can infect the skin or lung or both include *Y. pestis* (etiologic agent of the plague) and *F. tularensis* (etiologic agent of tularemia).
- Pneumonias are classified by infecting or causative agents, each of which will have differing etiology, clinical manifestation, clinical course, and treatment regimen.

2. **Pathophysiology**
- Pneumonia typically occurs when host defense mechanisms are incapable of contending with a pathogenic challenge by bacteria, fungus, rickettsia, etc.
- Defense mechanisms include the mucociliary lining of lung, phagocytic cells (alveolar macrophages, neutrophils), lung surfactant, specific antibodies (IgG), and chemoattractive/tactic agents (C5a, interleukin-8).

3. **Complications of Pneumonia**
- The inflammatory process of pneumonia can have the potential to extend from the parenchyma to the pleural surface. If this occurs, an empyema, or collection of pus in the pleural space, develops.
- CXR shows a pleural effusion, and empyema is diagnosed when a thoracentesis demonstrates pleural fluid containing significant amounts of leukocytes or bacterial organisms or both.
- Staphylococci also have been implicated along with other aerobic organisms in cases of empyema.
- Treatment includes antibiotics and placement of a chest tube into the pleural space for drainage.
- Another complication of pneumonia is the formation of a lung abscess, or a localized collection of pus, which typically causes tissue destruction and complicates pneumonia.
- CXR will generally reveal the lung abscess.
- Treatment consists of prolonged antibiotic treatment. Surgical intervention is rarely needed because the abscess usually drains through the tracheobronchial tree.

D. Diagnostic Studies
- CXRs are used most often to confirm the presence and extent of involvement of the inflammatory process. Findings may include infiltrates, consolidation, and cavitation.

- CXRs may not be diagnostic if patients are unable to mount an inflammatory response (e.g., patients with HIV/AIDS, agranulocytosis) or if CXR is taken at an early phase of an infiltrative process (pneumocystis pneumonia in a patient with HIV/AIDS).
- The American Thoracic Society consensus panel recommends sputum gram stain and culture for suspected resistant organisms.
- Techniques (such as transtracheal aspiration, transthoracic lung puncture, and bronchoscopically obtained specimens) through use of protected brush or bronchoalveolar lavage can yield noncontaminated results for viral, aerobic, anaerobic, and mycobacterium cultures, as well as Gram, acid-fast, Gomori, and fluorescent antibody staining.
- Open-lung biopsy is reserved for suspicious (cancerous) focal lesions that cannot be reached through bronchoscopy, or when a definitive diagnosis is not forthcoming after other techniques have been used, or both.
- Two blood cultures from different venipuncture sites should be obtained when evaluating patients with pneumonia.
- Culture of pleural fluid should be obtained if empyema is suspected.
- Antibody titer (IgG, IgM, *Legionella*) can be helpful for diagnosing *Mycoplasma pneumoniae*, *Chlamydia pneumoniae*, and *Legionella pneumophila*.
- A urine antigen test highly specific and sensitive for *L. pneumophila* can also be obtained, as appropriate.
- Viral studies are available to detect influenza A and B as well as severe acute respiratory syndrome coronavirus (SARS-COV).

E. Management
- In general, pharmacologic treatment of patients with pneumonia begins empirically.
- The following microbes are important to detect because they require different treatment: *Legionella* species, Middle Eastern respiratory syndrome coronavirus, SARS-COV, community-associated methicillin-resistant *Staphylococcus aureus*, influenza A and B, and agents of bioterrorism.
- Patient history, medication allergies, mechanism, as well as environmental site of exposure, age, and underlying disease states guide the clinical decision-making process.
- Common empiric oral antibiotics used to treat community-acquired pneumonia can include macrolide antibiotics such as azithromycin or clarithromycin, amoxicillin + clavulanate, second- or third-generation cephalosporins, fluoroquinolones, cotrimoxazole, and erythromycin in combination with either a cephalosporin or an amoxicillin + clavulanate.
- Antibiotics used to empirically treat hospital-acquired pneumonia are usually given IV and can include choices from the following classes: penicillins, cephalosporins, and aminoglycosides.

- Other drugs used for this type of pneumonia are metronidazole, chloramphenicol, fluoroquinolones, clotrimazole, clindamycin, and vancomycin.
- Rickettsial infections are commonly treated with doxycycline, and fungal infections are treated with either fluconazole or amphotericin B.
- Influenza A or B can be treated with oseltamivir or zanamivir within the first 48 hours, but these drugs are only effective in reducing symptoms and duration of illness. No treatment has proven efficacious for respiratory syncytial virus in adults, parainfluenza virus, adenovirus, metapneumovirus, SARS-COV, or hantavirus. Treatment is supportive care (oxygen and ventilator support).
- Current treatment recommendations for pathogens used in bioterrorism
  - *B. anthracis*: ciprofloxacin or doxycycline.
  - *Y. pestis*: streptomycin or doxycycline.
  - *F. tularensis*: streptomycin.

XI. Diffuse Parenchymal Lung Disease (Also Called ILD)

A. Etiology
- Diffuse parenchymal lung disease, also known as ILD, is a clinical term for a heterogeneous group of lower respiratory tract disorders that affect the alveolar interstitium: capillaries, alveolar spaces, connective tissue, larger blood vessels, lymphatics, and airways.
- Incidence has been estimated as high as 80.9 per 100,000 men and 67.2 per 100,000 women in the United States.
- Causes of ILD are diverse and range from idiopathic to genetic. Drugs, environmental factors, alveolar-filling disorders, rheumatologic disorders, and vasculitides are included as possible causes.
- Classifying the diseases into clinical categories can aid in the clinical decision-making process and narrow of the differential diagnosis (Table 3–7).

B. Pathophysiology
- Although causes of ILD are numerous (~150 separate diseases are characterized by some interstitial diffuse parenchymal lung tissue damage), the reason so many diseases are couched under that title is the common pathophysiologic, radiographic, and clinical features of the affected patients.
- The basis for these common findings is extensive disruption of alveolar tissue, loss of functional alveoli, and replacement of functional tissue by scar tissue (fibrosis).
- Immunopathologic response of lung tissue to irritants causes an initial inflammation that heals by scar tissue formation. If the irritant/disease is persistent, a chronic phase of the disorder causes disruption of pulmonary function and gas exchange.

- Larger airways, such as the bronchioles, can be involved in the inflammatory process, leading to bronchiolitis obliterans and an organizing pneumonia. This occurrence also is thought to be a part of interstitial diffuse parenchymal lung disease.

C. Clinical Features
1. **Assessment**
   - The most common presenting complaint is development of progressive dyspnea. Initially, the shortness of breath is felt only with exertion and worsens as the inflammatory process progresses.
   - Nonproductive (dry) cough and fatigue are common complaints of patients with ILD.

TABLE 3–7.	Etiologic Classification of Interstitial Lung Disease
Idiopathic interstitial pneumonias	**Associated with collagen-vascular disease**
Idiopathic pulmonary fibrosis	Progressive systemic sclerosis
Desquamative interstitial pneumonia	Ankylosing spondylitis
Acute interstitial pneumonia (Hamman–Rich syndrome)	Rheumatologic and autoimmune diseases
Respiratory bronchiolitis–associated ILD	Systemic lupus erythematosus
Cryptogenic organizing pneumonia (idiopathic bronchiolitis obliterans with organizing pneumonia)	Rheumatoid arthritis
	Progressive systemic sclerosis
	Sjögren syndrome
	Polymyositis and dermatomyositis
Occupational and environmental exposures	Mixed connective tissue disease
Alveolar-filling disorders	**Associated with pulmonary vasculitis**
Goodpasture syndrome	Wegener granulomatosis
Pulmonary alveolar proteinosis	Churg–Strauss syndrome
Pulmonary hemosiderosis	
Pulmonary hemorrhage	
Chronic eosinophilic pneumonia	
Inherited forms	**Hypersensitivity pneumonitis**
Familial idiopathic pulmonary fibrosis	Occupational and environment ILD
Tuberous sclerosis	Drug-induced/iatrogenic ILD
Neurofibromatosis	
Gaucher disease	**Other forms**
Niemann–Pick disease	Sarcoidosis
Hermansky–Pudlak syndrome	Langerhans cell histiocytosis

ILD, interstitial lung disease.
Data from Goldman L, Ausiello D, eds. *Cecil Medicine.* 23rd ed. Philadelphia, PA: Saunders Elsevier; 2008:641.

- If pneumonia is present (as with bronchiolitis obliterans), cough will be a major complaint.
- In patients with ILD diffuse parenchymal lung disease from a rheumatic source, a common complaint may be pleuritic chest pain.
- Any symptom that worsens or is out of the ordinary must be taken seriously.
- If pleuritic chest pain and sudden worsening of shortness of breath should occur, spontaneous pneumothorax in association with lymphangioleiomyomatosis, neurofibromatosis, tuberous sclerosis, or Langerhans cell histiocytosis could be suspected.
- Hemoptysis should alert the clinician to malignancy, diffuse alveolar hemorrhage syndromes, pulmonary embolus, and superimposed infection.

2. **History**
- Obtaining a thorough history with specific attention to duration and progression of illness is of utmost importance in discovering the cause.
- Obtaining and reviewing prior patient records will help toward this end. Evaluation should include a detailed, lifelong occupational and environmental history; known exposures to inhaled agents (including hobbies); specific questions related to medications that induce ILD; smoking history; and family history.

3. **Physical Findings**
- Physical examination can disclose findings ranging from a normal pulmonary examination to bilateral crackles, wheezing, rhonchi, or coarse rales. Clubbing (pulmonary osteoarthropathy) of the nails (both fingers and toes) may be present, but physical examination findings rarely aid in establishing the diagnosis.

D. Diagnostic Studies
1. **CXR**
- Usually has an important role in establishing the diagnosis of interstitial diffuse parenchymal lung disease.
- As with patient history, evaluation of previous CXRs to ascertain disease progression in a given patient is most important.
- Infiltrates in lower lung zones provide a clue to the presence of an ILD process; they will have a "ground-glass" appearance in the early stage of the disease, and a nodular, linear, and/or honeycombed appearance in the later stages.

2. **High-Resolution CT**
- High-resolution CT scan can distinguish reversible lung disease from irreversibly damaged areas and thus establish a diagnosis and provide staging of the disease.

3. **More Invasive Procedures**
- Fiber-optic bronchoscopy and open-lung biopsy are reserved for disease processes that remain undiagnosed (malignancy, sarcoidosis, infection, etc.), despite other less invasive procedures.

4. **Laboratory and Other Studies**
- Laboratory studies rarely point to a specific diagnosis and more often suggest a diagnosis.
- Erythrocyte sedimentation rate is usually elevated in ILD diffuse parenchymal lung disease.
- Tests for cryo-Igs and serologic tests for collagen-vascular disease, rheumatoid factor, antinuclear antibodies, and complement levels offer clues to the presence of underlying disease processes.
- ECG may show RV and atrial strain.
- ABG measurements can show mild hypoxemia, although arterial blood pH is usually normal unless the patient is exercising, in which case it will fall.
- In most cases, PFT can provide useful information when trying to document physiologic changes associated with ILD diffuse parenchymal lung disease and responses (or lack thereof) to treatment.
- PFT should be used with caution, especially in current or former smokers who might have ILD and emphysema.

E. Management
Goals of Treatment
- Remove/discontinue exposure of pulmonary irritants such as smoke, dust, and medication.
- Prevent destruction of lung tissue by inhibiting the inflammatory reaction within the lung.
- Relieve symptoms of these disease processes.
- Every effort should be made to ascertain the underlying disease process and treat accordingly; otherwise, corticosteroids are the mainstay of treatment for ILD diffuse parenchymal lung disease.
- In patients who cannot tolerate corticosteroids, or whose symptoms progress despite steroid treatment, cyclophosphamide or azathioprine can be tried.
- Supplemental oxygen can be administered in patients whose oxygen tension is < 55 mm Hg at rest or with exercise.
- Pneumococcal and influenza vaccines should be administered prophylactically.
- When therapeutic measures fail, lung transplantation has been authorized as a treatment in patients with end-stage ILD diffuse parenchymal lung disease.
- Selection guidelines and relative contraindications for transplantation are fairly stringent.
- Two-year survival rates are currently between 60% and 80%, with failures usually occurring from infections that complicate immunosuppressive therapy or from tissue rejection.

XII. Respiratory Failure
A. Etiology
- Respiratory failure can be divided into acute or chronic stages, depending on evolution of the process; each stage has specific physiologic, pathogenic, and therapeutic characteristics.

- Respiratory failure can be further categorized into (a) type I—hypoxemic respiratory failure (a failure of gas exchange) and (b) type II—hypercapnic with or without hypoxemic respiratory failure (a failure of ventilation).
- It is important to note that respiratory failure can be the result of extrapulmonary processes, such as sepsis, shock, or trauma.
- Increased dead space: refers to conditions that cause areas of the lung to be ventilated but not perfused, or when the decrease in perfusion exceeds decreases in ventilation, as in COPD, asthma, cystic fibrosis, or interstitial lung fibrosis.
- Decreased minute ventilation: refers to processes or diseases that affect the patient's normal ventilation/metabolism of gases, specifically CO_2, and may be the result of chest wall abnormalities, neurologic abnormalities, metabolic abnormalities, drug overdose, or airway obstruction.
- Patients usually have more than one disease or process that precipitates respiratory failure.
- Age at onset and overall patient health are two important prognostic factors for recovery from respiratory failure.
- The most common cause of death in patients with respiratory failure is multisystem organ failure.

B. Pathophysiology

1. Hypoxic Respiratory Failure

- Any acute or chronic condition that produces PaO_2 <60 mm Hg or arterial oxygen saturation (SaO_2) <90% is considered hypoxic respiratory failure.
- Acute lung injury and acute respiratory distress syndrome (ARDS) both fall into this category. The most common risk factor for developing ARDS is sepsis. Other risk factors for developing ARDS include systemic inflammatory response syndrome, shock, trauma, aspiration, near-drowning, pancreatitis, disseminated intravascular coagulation, and burns.
- Can occur as a result of:
  - Shunting: refers to anatomic- or physiologic-acquired defect that causes venous blood to mix with arterial blood after bypassing functional pulmonary architecture such as can be seen with vascular lung tumors, congenital heart disease, and pulmonary arteriovenous fistulas.
  - Ventilation/perfusion mismatch: refers to diseases that decrease or inhibit normal ventilation-to-perfusion ratios such as COPD, interstitial inflammation, and vascular inflammation.
  - Low inspired oxygen tension: refers to a *combination* of conditions that can lead to hypoxia (e.g., low oxygen levels such as those seen at high altitudes or inhalation of toxic gases in combination with cardiopulmonary disease processes).

- Hypoventilation: refers to processes that might elevate the $PaCO_2$, thus displacing the alveolar oxygen.
- Diffusion impairment: refers primarily to patients who have ILD that decreases the diffusion of gases in the alveoli.
- Low mixed venous oxygenation: refers to factors that cause a decrease in mixed venous oxygen tension, which, in turn, affects the PaO_2, especially in the presence of intrapulmonary shunting or ventilation/perfusion mismatch.

2. Hypercapnic-(Hypoxic) Respiratory Failure

- Any disease or process (e.g., COPD, sedatives) that causes acute CO_2 retention in which the $PaCO_2$ tension is 45 mm Hg or higher and respiratory acidosis (pH < 7.35) is present is considered hypercapnic (hypoxic) respiratory failure.
- Increased $PaCO_2$ is the result of increased CO_2 production, decreased tidal ventilation, or increased dead space ventilation. Hypermetabolic states such as exercise, fever, sepsis, trauma, burns, excessive carbohydrate intake, and hyperthyroidism can increase CO_2 production.

C. Clinical Features

- Depending on the pathogenesis of respiratory failure (hypoxia vs. hypercapnia), patients can have specific symptomatology. The severity of symptoms (a patient's ventilatory response) depends on the degree of the patient's physiologic ability to sense and respond to hypoxia or hypercapnia (Table 3–8).
- Typical initial presentations of both types can include complaints of sudden breathlessness, palpitations, dizziness, anxiety, hypersomnolence, headaches, delirium and confusion.
- Physical examination may disclose diffuse crackles, signs of consolidation, decreased breath sounds, weakness, hypotension, tachycardia, wheezing, altered mental status, and lower extremity edema.

D. Diagnostic Studies

1. Hypoxia

- Pulse oximetry.
- Arterial blood gas (ABG).
- CXR may show small "white" lungs, patchy, diffuse infiltrates, signs of consolidation, and/or lobar atelectasis.

2. Hypercapnia

- CXR may show hyperinflation, large "black" lungs, bullae, and increased vascular markings (COPD); in addition, hypoinflation and small "black" lungs with neuromuscular disease or drug toxicity may be present.

3. ECG findings can range from sinus tachycardia, acute myocardial infarction, and left ventricular hypertrophy to normal ECG, RV hypertrophy, and low voltage.

TABLE 3–8.	Pulmonary and Extrapulmonary Causes of Acute Lung Injury and Acute Respiratory Distress Syndrome

Direct or primary pulmonary causes

Aspiration of gastric contents

Diffuse pneumonia

Pulmonary contusion

Inhalation injury

Chest trauma

Near-drowning

Extrapulmonary causes

Sepsis

Bacteremia without sepsis

Severe sepsis/systemic inflammatory response syndrome

Major trauma

Hypertransfusion

Postcardiopulmonary bypass

Shock and hypotension

Drug overdose

Severe burns

Pancreatitis

Data from Goldman L, Ausiello D, eds. *Cecil Medicine*. 23rd ed. Philadelphia, PA: Saunders Elsevier; 2008:778.

4. Blood studies are also cause-dependent and range from nonspecific findings to elevated hemoglobin, respiratory acidosis, mixed metabolic and respiratory acidosis, and hypokalemia.

E. Management

- Treatment is etiology dependent. A thorough patient history is essential and should include events leading up to and after the onset of respiratory problems, and past and present pulmonary diseases/conditions. The physical examination and laboratory/radiographic findings are necessary to pinpoint a diagnosis.
- Treatment is then based on the condition identified and type of failure (hypoxia vs. hypercapnia).
- Hypoxic respiratory failure treatment includes treating the predisposing condition and administering supportive therapy, including maintaining an open airway (possible intubation), administering O_2, and ventilator support (placing patients on a mechanical ventilator).
- No increase in survival rates have been demonstrated in randomized controlled clinical trials with the use of early administration of high-dose corticosteroids, prostaglandin E_1, nonsteroidal anti-inflammatory drugs, antiendotoxin and anticytokine therapy, inhaled nitric oxide, surfactant therapy, antioxidant therapy, positional changes, or partial liquid ventilation.

- The main goal of therapy is to maintain adequate PaO_2 levels while remaining aware of therapeutic complications such as O_2 toxicity, volume overload, gastrointestinal (GI) bleeding, malnutrition, sepsis, thromboembolism, and mechanical ventilator-associated problems.
- Weaning patients from mechanically assisted ventilation devices should be accomplished as soon as possible after they are stabilized.
- Treatment of hypercapnic respiratory failure is similar to hypoxic respiratory failure with some slight variation in ventilatory support. The main goal continues to be maintenance of adequate PaO_2 and decreasing the elevated levels of $PaCO_2$.
- In patients who have high baseline $PaCO_2$ (such as patients with COPD), normalization of $PaCO_2$ should not be the primary goal; rather, adequate PaO_2 levels should be maintained. Patients with COPD can be difficult to wean from ventilatory devices.
- Complications such as infection, thromboembolism, GI bleeding, agitation, and volume overload become accentuated because of the prolonged time on mechanical ventilatory support.
- Antibiotics, heparin, H_2-blockers, antianxiolytics, and maintenance of electrolyte balance are strategies to use as the situation warrants.

XIII. Pulmonary Function and Diagnosis (Figure 3–1)

A. Pulmonary Function Testing

1. **Pathology**
   - A group of tests designed to measure the lungs capacity to take in and release air, as well as the volume and rate of air on inspiration and expiration.
   - Objective method to evaluate functional change in a patient with known or suspected lung disease.
   - In addition, pulmonary function testing (PFT) allows for the determination of whether the patient has lung disease significant enough to result in respiratory impairment and dysfunction.
   - PFT provides three main categories of information:
     - Lung volumes.
     - Measurement of the size of the assorted compartments within the lung.
     - Flow rates, measurement of maximal flow within the airways and diffusing capacity, measurement of gas transfer between alveoli and pulmonary capillary blood.
   - PFT varies based on a patient's age, gender, height, weight, and ethnicity.
   - During the testing, maximal respiratory effort is required because suboptimal respiratory effort may result in difficulty with test interpretation.

2. **Indications**
   - Although indications for PFT are varied, it is indicated in the basic evaluation of lung function pattern.

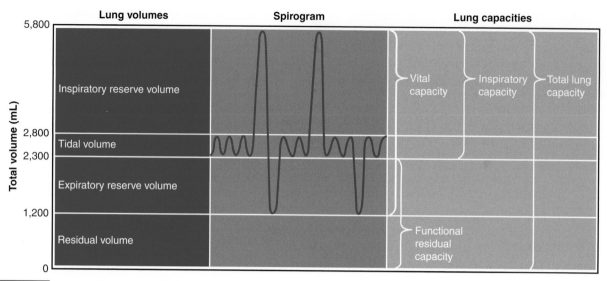

FIGURE 3–1. **Lung volumes and capacities.** (Adapted from Cohen BJ, Taylor JJ. *Memmler's the Human Body in Health and Disease.* 10th ed. Baltimore, MD: Lippincott Williams & Wilkins; 2005.)

- Serial PFT allows for quantification of improvement/deterioration in functional lung status, evaluation for initiation and response to therapeutic interventions, disability evaluations, longitudinal surveillance in the occupational setting, and determination of possible significant pre- and postoperative respiratory problems.

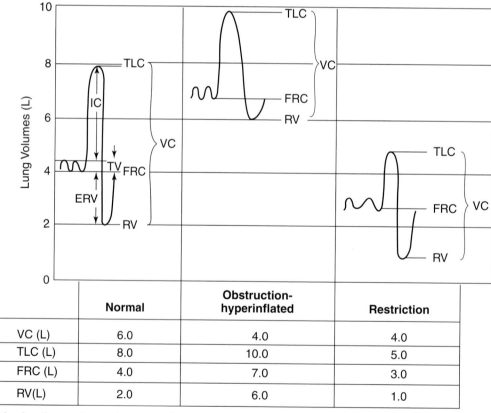

	Normal	Obstruction-hyperinflated	Restriction
VC (L)	6.0	4.0	4.0
TLC (L)	8.0	10.0	5.0
FRC (L)	4.0	7.0	3.0
RV(L)	2.0	6.0	1.0

FIGURE 3–2. **Absolute lung volumes in a normal person, a patient with hyperinflation secondary to obstructive airway disease, and a patient with restrictive lung disease.** VC, vital capacity, the volume expired from a maximal inspiration (TLC, total lung capacity) to full expiration (RV, residual volume); FRC, functional residual capacity, volume at the end of a normal tidal breath; IC, inspiratory capacity; TV, tidal volume; ERV, expiratory reserve volume. In obstruction, FRC and RV are both increased at the expense of the VC; thus, TLC is only minimally increased. In restriction, FRC, RV, and VC are all decreased proportionally, resulting in a decrease in the TLC, which defines restriction. (From Hume ED, ed. *Kelley's Essentials of Internal Medicine.* 2nd ed. Philadelphia, PA: Lippincott Williams & Wilkins; 2001:632.)

3. Contraindications

- There are certain medical conditions where PFT may be contraindicated: acute severe—asthma, respiratory distress, angina aggravated by testing, pneumothorax, ongoing hemoptysis, and active pulmonary tuberculosis.

B. Patterns of Impairment

- Spirometry: documentation of exhaled volume versus time during a forced exhalation (with or without response to an inhaled bronchodilator for possible reversible airflow), allows for the basic assessment of obstructive and restrictive pulmonary dysfunction.
- In a restrictive pattern (i.e., neuromuscular and chest wall diseases), there is a reduction in lung volumes—total lung capacity (TLC), residual volume (RV), vital capacity (VC), and functional residual capacity (FRC)—and normal expiratory airflow—maximum midexpiratory flow rate (MMFR) and forced expiratory volume in 1 second (FEV_1) to forced vital capacity (FVC) ratio. With severe disease, MMFR is decreased.
- An obstructive pattern (i.e., asthma, chronic bronchitis, and emphysema) results in a decrease in rates of expiratory airflow (decrease FEV_1/FVC and MMFR) with high RV and increased RV/TLC ratio depicting air trapping (Figure 3–2).
- A mixed obstructive/restrictive pattern results in difficulty in test interpretation and would show decreased FEV_1 and FVC, decreased FEV_1/FVC ratio, and decreased TLC.
- Interpretation:
  - Normal standards (predicted value) have been established.
  - As aforementioned, normality is based on patient demographic variables and may vary between laboratories.
  - Normal values are defined between 95% and 80% of predicted value.
  - FEV_1/FVC, however, confers a normal test if value is >80% of predicted value.

REVIEW QUESTIONS

1. A 58-year-old man with a 35-pack-per-year smoking history comes to the clinic asking for antibiotics. He states that he has a chronic cough, which makes him susceptible to recurrent pneumonia with the last infection being about 2 months ago. He complains of being short of breath more than usual and is having some back pain. He says that he notices a little blood in the sputum when he coughs as well. You obtain a chest radiograph and note a solitary pulmonary nodule. You suspect that the patient has a bronchogenic carcinoma. Of the following, what would be the most likely histology?
   a) Large cell
   b) Small cell
   c) Oat cell
   d) Carcinoid
   e) Adenocarcinoma

2. Which of the following symptoms would strongly indicate the diagnosis of PE in a patient with a known deep venous thrombosis?
   a) Chest pain and tachypnea
   b) Cough and fever
   c) Facial and truncal edema
   d) Loss of leg hair and claudication
   e) Pitting edema and cough

3. Which of the following pneumonias can be prevented by administration of a vaccine?
   a) *Pseudomonas*
   b) *Legionella*
   c) *Mycobacteria*
   d) Pneumococcal
   e) Staphylococcal

4. A 55-year-old man comes to the clinic with a 6-month history of persistent cough, hemoptysis, night sweats, and weight loss. He has smoked two packs per day for 30 years and also complains of bilateral shoulder and chest pain. On examination, he is pale, febrile, and dyspneic upon minimal exertion. The CXR shows perihilar adenopathy. What is the most likely diagnosis?
   a) Asthma
   b) Sarcoidosis
   c) COPD
   d) Pulmonary tuberculosis
   e) Bronchogenic carcinoma

5. A patient is determined to have normal airflow when the FEV_1/FVC ratio is above which threshold level of predicted value?
   a) 50%
   b) 60%
   c) 70%
   d) 80%
   e) 90%

6. Which of the following tests will be most diagnostic in determining the etiology of ILD?
   a) Pulmonary arteriogram
   b) C-reactive protein (CRP)
   c) PFT
   d) Lung biopsy
   e) Spiral CT scan of the chest

7. The etiology for PE is best described by which of the following?

    a) Lack of ventilatory effort, hypercoagulability, decreased platelet count
    b) Smoking history, birth control therapy, sedentary lifestyle
    c) Venostasis, hypercoagulability, vessel wall inflammation
    d) Cardiac arrhythmia, low-dose aspirin therapy, venostasis

8. The primary pathogenesis of asthma is which of the following?

    a) Allergy-mediated bronchospasm
    b) Chronic inflammation
    c) Excess secretion of viscid mucus
    d) Irritant-mediated bronchospasm
    e) Bronchodilation

9. Patients with COPD characteristically present with clinical symptoms of which of the following?

    a) Cough, sputum production, and shortness of breath
    b) Fever, night sweats, and unintentional weight loss
    c) Nonproductive cough, myalgias, and fatigue
    d) Hemoptysis, chest discomfort, and fever
    e) Productive cough, chest tightness, and fatigue

10. The drug of choice in the treatment of an acute asthma exacerbation is which of the following?

    a) ICS
    b) Anticholinergic (ipratropium)
    c) Mast cell stabilizer (cromolyn)
    d) Short-acting β_2-agonist (albuterol)
    e) Leukotriene inhibitor (montelukast)

11. The most effective way to slow the progression of COPD in a patient who is stable and adequately managed is to do which of the following?

    a) Prescribe daily use of ICSs
    b) Administer the influenza vaccination
    c) Noninvasive positive pressure ventilation
    d) Lung volume reduction surgery
    e) Stop smoking

12. A 28-year-old woman complains of fever, chills, productive cough, and malaise for the past 48 hours. Physical examination shows crackles in the left lung base on auscultation and dullness to percussion over the same area. Which of the following will be most helpful in making an initial diagnosis?

    a) CBC with differential
    b) CXR
    c) Sputum culture
    d) PFT
    e) Ventilation/perfusion lung scan

13. A 65-year-old woman presents complaining of a chronic cough that started 6 months ago getting worse. The cough was a dry cough at the beginning but is now a productive cough and sometimes there is blood in the sputum. She reports 10 lb unintentional weight loss and fatigue. Which of the following may also be true?

    a) She also complains of an itchy rash.
    b) She also complains of sneezing.
    c) She also complains of itchy watery eyes.
    d) The CXR will probably show hyperinflation of lungs.
    e) She also complains of night sweats and low-grade fever.

14. What would be the best test to order to rule out PE in patients with low renal function?

    a) CT pulmonary angiography (CTPA)
    b) CXR
    c) D-Dimer
    d) A V/Q scan
    e) Thoracic ultrasound

ANSWERS TO REVIEW QUESTIONS

1. **Answer: E.** About 85% of lung cancers are classified as NSCLCs. Of the NSCLC forms of cancers, there are three main types: adenocarcinoma, squamous cell, and large cell. In both male and females, adenocarcinoma is the most common of these forms of lung cancer in the United States. The least common of these three types of NSCLC is large cell. SCLC accounts for about 15% of lung cancers and usually has a more rapid onset. Oat cell is a type of small-cell carcinoma. Lung carcinoid tumors are even rarer in occurrence than either NSCLC or SCLC.

2. **Answer: A.** PE can be difficult to diagnose because its symptoms can be nonspecific. However, the most common presenting symptoms in PE are tachypnea and chest pain, which makes the suspicion of PE highly likely in individuals with a known history of DVT. Cough and fever are nonspecific symptoms of PE that can have other causes such as underlying infection. Facial and truncal edema can be a cause of endocrine and lymph disorders not associated with PE. Loss of leg hair and claudication are typical findings associated with peripheral artery disease. Pitting edema and cough are common findings of CHF.

3. **Answer: D.** Pneumonias are caused by fungi, bacteria, and viruses. The influenza vaccine can help prevent pneumonia caused by a virus. For bacterial causes of pneumonia such as *Pseudomonas*, *Legionella*, *Mycobacteria*, staphylococcal, and pneumococcal, the only vaccine currently available is the pneumococcal vaccination.

4. **Answer: E.** Individuals who smoke have the greatest risk for developing lung cancer. Smoking is also the main cause of COPD, which affects smokers and carries a high risk of developing lung cancer. While lung cancer and COPD can have similar symptoms, cancer should be suspected in those with weight loss, fever, night sweats, and hemoptysis. Lymph node metastases to the hilar regions are common findings of lung cancer. Asthma is a chronic

disease characterized by inflammation and narrowing of the bronchial tubes manifesting in shortness of breath and wheezing. Sarcoidosis is an autoimmune disorder causing inflammation in the lungs and other organ systems. Tuberculosis is an infection of the lung tissue causing coughing, fever, and hemoptysis. Chest radiograph shows lobar consolidation and/or cavitation.

5. **Answer: D**. Spirometry is a standard test used to assess and measure lung function. Normal results of a spirometry test vary from person to person depending on age, sex, gender, and height. In general, a normal score is considered to be 80% or more of the predicted value.

6. **Answer: D**. Although CRP, PFT, and CT of the chest are all measures for diagnosing ILD, they are not as specific in identifying etiology of disease as is an actual biopsy of lung tissue. The decision to obtain a lung biopsy, however, should be made on a case-by-case basis with careful consideration of risk versus benefit and patient preferences.

7. **Answer: C**. Thrombus formation and proliferation fall under three broad categories: circulatory stasis, vessel wall injury, and a hypercoagulable state.

8. **Answer: B**. Asthma is a chronic inflammatory condition of the airways. Inflammation of the airways causes hyperresponsiveness and limitation of airflow. Atopy is a predisposing factor for developing asthma. Excess secretion of viscid mucous is a consequence of inflammation, and bronchoconstriction occurs as a result of the inflammatory process. Bronchodilation is involved in the treatment of asthma.

9. **Answer: A**. COPD is a chronic inflammation process of the lungs causing airway obstruction, usually as a result of tobacco smoking. The primary symptoms are chronic cough, sputum, and shortness of breath. Fever, night sweats, and unintentional weight loss are signs of malignancy. Nonproductive cough, myalgia, and fatigue are nonspecific symptoms that can be associated with other disease states. Hemoptysis, chest discomfort, and fever should raise suspicion for an infectious process such as tuberculosis. Productive cough, chest tightness, and fatigue can be associated with other disorders such as asthma and CHF.

10. **Answer: D**. The first-line treatment for an acute asthma exacerbation is the administration of a short-acting β_2-agonist (albuterol). Depending on the severity, systemic corticosteroids may also be administered. ICSs, ipratropium, cromolyn, and leukotriene inhibitors are not indicated for first-line treatment of an asthma flair but can be used as adjunct therapies.

11. **Answer: E**. COPD is a progressive condition without a cure. Early diagnosis and intervention, primarily by smoking cessation, is critical to halt disease progress. The use of daily ICSs can improve quality of life by helping to abate symptoms leading to further lung deterioration; however, without smoking cessation deterioration continues. Administering the influenza vaccination can help prevent complications of COPD caused by the flu. Noninvasive positive pressure and lung volume reduction surgery improve symptomology but do not slow progression of disease.

12. **Answer: B**. The clinical presentation points to pneumonia as the most likely cause of the patient's symptoms. The gold standard for diagnosing pneumonia is the presence of lung infiltrates on a chest radiograph. A CBC and PFT are not specific for pneumonia. A ventilation/perfusion scan measures air and blood flow in the lung used primarily to help detect PE. A sputum culture is not always routinely ordered, but can be helpful once the diagnosis of pneumonia has been made to determine the causative pathogen.

13. **Answer: E**. A chronic cough that has worsened in an older patient and produces blood should raise suspicion of a malignant respiratory system lesion. An itchy rash, sneezing, and itchy watery eyes suggest allergies, which are not typically associated with the presentation. Hyperinflation of the lungs suggests air trapping associated with emphysema.

14. **Answer: D**. Both CTPA and V/Q scans are used to diagnose PE. However, the contrast dye that is used in CT scan can cause kidney problems in susceptible patients. V/Q scanning is generally preferred over CT scan in patients with kidney disease. D-Dimer has low specificity for PE and when positive is followed by CT or V/Q scanning. A CXR can be useful to rule out differential diagnoses for PE symptoms but is not diagnostic for PE. A thoracic ultrasound can be helpful in diagnosing a PE but is not considered first-line imaging.

SELECTED REFERENCES

American Thoracic Society. Interstitial lung disease. https://www.thoracic.org/patients/patient-resources/breathing-in-america/resources/chapter-10-interstitial-lung-disease.pdf

American Thoracic Society. Statements, guidelines, and reports. http://www.thoracic.org/statements/resources/copd/179full.pdf. Accessed June 2, 2017.

American Thoracic Society: Medical Section of the American Lung Association. Standards for the diagnosis and care of patients with chronic obstructive pulmonary disease. *Am J Respir Crit Care Med.* 1995;152:S77–S120.

Ball WC Jr. Pleural effusions. In: Stobo JD, Hellmann DB, Ladenson PW, Petty BG, Traill TA, eds. *The Principles and Practice of Medicine.* 23rd ed. Stamford, CT: Appleton & Lange; 1996:184–188.

Beers MH, ed. *Merck Manual.* 18th ed. Whitehouse Station, NJ: Merck Research Laboratories; 2006.

Bell WR. Venous thrombosis and pulmonary embolism. In: Stobo JD, Hellmann DB, Ladenson PW, Petty BG, Traill TA, eds. *The Principles and Practice of Medicine.* 23rd ed. Stamford, CT: Appleton & Lange; 1996:171–176.

Benjamin IJ, Griggs RC, Wing EJ, eds. *Cecil Essentials of Medicine.* 8th ed. Philadelphia, PA: Saunders Elsevier; 2010:241–243.

Berry MF. Approach to the adult patient with a mediastinal mass. In: Mulle RNL, Friedberg JS, Midthun DE, eds. *UpToDate.* https://goldcopd.org/wp-content/uploads/2018/11/

GOLD-2019-v1.7-FINAL-14Nov2018-WMS.pdf. Accessed June 2017.

Celli BR. Diseases of the diaphragm, chest wall, pleura, and mediastinum. In: Bennett JC, Plum F, eds. *Cecil Textbook of Medicine*. 20th ed. Philadelphia, PA: WB Saunders; 1996:442–448.

Centers for Disease Control and Prevention. Chronic obstructive pulmonary disease. https://www.cdc.gov/copd/index.html. September 16, 2016. Accessed June 2, 2017.

Centers for Disease Control. Data, statistics, and surveillance. https://www.cdc.gov/asthma/asthmadata.htm. September 8, 2016. Accessed March 9, 2018.

Dempsey JA, Veasey SC, Morgan BJ, O'Donnell CP. Pathophysiology of sleep apnea. Physiol Rev. 2010;90(1):47–112. https://www.ncbi.nlm.nih.gov/pmc/articles/PMC3970937/. Accessed December 10, 2018.

Domino FJ, ed. *The 5-Minute Clinical Consult*. 19th ed. Philadelphia, PA: Lippincott Williams & Wilkins; 2011.

Drazen JM, Weinberger SE, McFadden ER. Disorders of the respiratory system. In: Fauci AS, Braunwald E, Isselbacher KJ, et al, eds. *Harrison's Principles of Internal Medicine*. 14th ed. New York, NY: McGraw-Hill; 1998:1407–1491.

Expert Panel Report 2. Clinical practice guidelines. Guidelines for the diagnosis and management of asthma. National Institutes of Health. National Heart, Lung and Blood Institute; 1997 October. Report No.: NIH 97-4051.

Fauci AS, Harrison TR, eds. *Harrison's Principles of Internal Medicine*. 17th ed. New York, NY: McGraw-Hill; 2008.

Feller-Kopman DJ, Schwartzstein RM. The evaluation, diagnosis, and treatment of the adult patient with acute hypercapnic respiratory failure. In: Stoller JK, ed. *UpToDate*. Waltham, MA: UpToDate. Accessed June 2017.

Global Initiative for Chronic Obstructive Lung Disease (GOLD). Global strategy for the diagnosis, management and prevention of COPD, 2017. http://goldcopd.org. Accessed June 5, 2017.

Goldman L, Ausiello D, eds. *Cecil Medicine*. 23rd ed. Philadelphia, PA: Saunders Elsevier; 2008:641.

Heffner JE. Diagnostic evaluation of a pleural effusion in adults: initial testing. In: Broaddus FC, ed. *UpToDate*. Waltham, MA: UpToDate. Accessed June 2017.

Isada CM, Kasten BL Jr, Goldman MP, Gray LD, Aberg JA, eds. Disease syndromes. In: *Infectious Disease Handbook*. 2nd ed. Ohio, OH: Lexi-Comp; 1996:42–44.

Jankowich MA, Aliotta JM. Neoplastic disorders of the lung. In: Andreoli TE, Benjamin IJ, Griggs RC, Wing EJ, eds. *Cecil Essentials of Medicine*. 8th ed. Philadelphia, PA: Saunders Elsevier; 2010:266–270.

Johanson WG Jr. Overview of pneumonia. In: Bennett JC, Plum F, eds. *Cecil Textbook of Medicine*. 20th ed. Philadelphia, PA: WB Saunders; 1996:411–413.

Kim V, Criner GJ. Chronic bronchitis and chronic obstructive pulmonary disease. *Am J Respir Crit Care Med*. 2013;187:228–237.

Kollef MH. Critical care. In: Carey CF, Lee HH, Woeltje KF, eds. *The Washington Manual of Medical Therapeutics*. 29th ed. Philadelphia, PA: Lippincott-Raven; 1998:170–188.

Marrie TJ. Epidemiology, pathogenesis, and microbiology of community-acquired pneumonia in adults. In: Bartlett JG, ed. *UpToDate*. Waltham, MA: UpToDate. Accessed June 2017.

McCool FD. Disorders of the pleura, mediastinum, and chest wall. In: Andreoli TE, Benjamin IJ, Griggs RC, Wing EJ, eds. *Cecil Essentials of Medicine*. 8th ed. Philadelphia, PA: Saunders Elsevier; 2010:266–270.

Midthun DE. Overview of the risk factors, pathology and clinical manifestations of lung cancer. In: Lilenbaum RC, ed. *UpToDate*. Waltham, MA: UpToDate. Accessed June 2017.

Miller YE. Pulmonary neoplasms. In: Bennett JC, Plum F, eds. *Cecil Textbook of Medicine*. 20th ed. Philadelphia, PA: WB Saunders; 1996:436–441.

Qaseem A, Wilt TJ, Weinberger SE, et al. Diagnosis and management of stable chronic obstructive pulmonary disease: A clinical practice guideline update from the American College of Physicians, American College of Chest Physicians, American Thoracic Society, and European Respiratory Society. *Ann Intern Med*. 2011;155:179–191. doi:10.7326/0003-4819-155-3-201108020-00008.

Rounds S, Jankowich MD. Chapter 13: Lung in health and disease. In: Benjamin IB, Fitz GJ, Wing EJ, Griggs RC, eds. *Andreoli and Carpenter's Cecil Essentials of Medicine*. 9th ed. Philadelphia, PA: WB Saunders; 2016:182–184.

Runge MS, Greganti MA, eds. *Netter's Internal Medicine*. 2nd ed. Philadelphia, PA: Saunders Elsevier; 2009.

Schapira RM, Varkey B, Kutty K. Bronchogenic carcinoma. In: Kutty K, Schapira RM, Ruiswyk JV, eds. *Kochar's Concise Textbook of Medicine*. 4th ed. Philadelphia, PA: Lippincott Williams & Wilkins; 2003:953–955.

Schuller D. Pulmonary disease. In: Carey CF, Lee HH, Woeltje KF, eds. *The Washington Manual of Medical Therapeutics*. 29th ed. Philadelphia, PA: Lippincott-Raven; 1998:190–211.

Selvakumar S, Casserly B, Rounds S. Chapter 21: Infectious diseases of the lung. In: Benjamin IB, Fitz GJ, Wing EJ, Griggs RC, eds. *Andreoli and Carpenter's Cecil Essentials of Medicine*. 9th ed. Philadelphia, PA: WB Saunders; 2016:254–258.

Senior RM. Pulmonary embolism. In: Bennett JC, Plum F, eds. *Cecil Textbook of Medicine*. 20th ed. Philadelphia, PA: WB Saunders; 1996:422–429.

Stauffer JL. Lung. In: Tierney LM Jr, Mcphee SJ, Papadakis MA, eds. *Current Medical Diagnosis and Treatment*. 36th ed. Stamford, CT: Appleton & Lange; 1997:236–319.

Summer WR. Respiratory failure. In: Bennett JC, Plum F, eds. *Cecil Textbook of Medicine*. 20th ed. Philadelphia, PA: WB Saunders; 1996:452–459.

Tautz TJ, Urwyler A, Antogninni JF. Case scenario: increased end-tidal carbon dioxide: a diagnostic dilemma. *Anesthesiology*. 2010;112(2):440–446. doi:10.1097/ALN.0b013e3181ca7c38.

Terry PB. Nodules and masses in the lung and mediastinum. In: Stobo JD, Hellmann DB, Ladenson PW, Petty BG, Traill TA, eds. *The Principles and Practice of Medicine*. 23rd ed. Stamford, CT: Appleton& Lange; 1996:177–183.

Toews GB. Interstitial lung disease. In: Bennett JC, Plum F, eds. *Cecil Textbook of Medicine*. 20th ed. Philadelphia, PA: WB Saunders; 1996.

U.S. Preventative Services Task Force. Final update summary: lung cancer: screening. https://www.uspreventiveservicestaskforce.org/. July 2015. Accessed June 5, 2017

Wender R, Fontham ETH, Barrera E, et al. American Cancer Society lung cancer screening guidelines. *CA Cancer J Clin*. 2013;63(2):107–117. doi:10.3322/caac.21172.

World Health Organization. Chronic respiratory diseases. http://www.who.int/respiratory/en/. 2017. Accessed May 30, 2017.

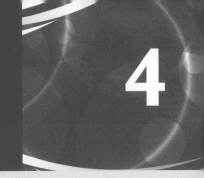

Gastrointestinal Disorders

Julie J. Kinzel • Rosalie G. Coppola

I. Disorders of the Esophagus
A. Gastroesophageal Reflux Disease
1. **Etiology**
   - Etiology multifactorial.
   - Multiple defects contribute to the development of gastroesophageal reflux disease (GERD).
2. **Pathology**
   - Major pathogenesis appears to be transient or sustained inappropriate relaxation of the lower esophageal sphincter (LES), not associated with swallowing.
   - Results in retrograde flow of gastric contents with or without esophageal tissue damage.
   - Contributing factors: abnormal esophageal epithelial resistance, abnormal gastric emptying, and characteristics of gastric reflux.
   - Other factors influencing LES tone include foods, increased intra-abdominal pressure, and medications.
   - Foods decreasing LES tone include fatty foods, chocolate, alcohol, peppermint, tomato sauces, coffee, tea, and onions.
   - Factors increasing intra-abdominal pressure include pregnancy, obesity, truncal obesity, bending, lifting, straining, coughing, vomiting, and tight-fitting clothes.
   - Common drugs or medications known to decrease LES tone include caffeine, nicotine, calcium channel blockers, nitrates, theophylline, and some sedatives.
   - When associated with a hiatal hernia, delayed esophageal clearance can lead to significant esophageal tissue damage and Barrett esophagus.
3. **Clinical Features**
   - Heartburn and/or regurgitation: hallmark symptom.
   - Pain: often described as burning, substernal, radiating upward, usually worse 30 to 60 minutes after meals, and when lying supine, and typically relieved with sitting up and antacids.
   - Ten percent of patients present with atypical "anginal"-type chest pain or extraesophageal manifestations.
   - Sour taste in mouth, sore throat, laryngitis, hoarseness, cough, and wheezing may be presenting symptoms.
   - Dysphagia, odynophagia, weight loss, iron deficiency anemia, advanced age, and family history of gastrointestinal (GI) cancers are alarm signs and necessitate further diagnostic evaluation of GERD. Esophagitis may result in peptic stricture, esophageal obstruction, esophageal perforation, or Barrett metaplasia.
   - Severity of symptoms does not correlate well with the degree of esophageal mucosal damage.
   - Physical examination findings are nonspecific in uncomplicated cases.
4. **Diagnostic Studies**
   - Indicated in patients with atypical symptoms such as dysphagia, regurgitation, or vomiting, or in those unresponsive to empiric therapy.
   - Upper endoscopy with biopsy documents type and extent of esophageal tissue damage.
   - Barium esophagography is of limited value and may fail to identify reflux disease or esophageal mucosal damage. May be useful in patients with severe dysphagia to evaluate for peptic stricture before endoscopy.
   - Esophageal pH or combined esophageal pH–impedance testing can be used to document pathologic reflux and is indicated in patients with normal endoscopy results and symptoms nonresponsive to proton pump inhibitors (PPIs), when considering antireflux surgery in patients with normal endoscopy results, and with atypical symptoms such as noncardiac chest pain and cough nonresponsive to antireflux therapy.
   - Esophageal manometry is useful in documenting evidence of motility disorders and LES pressures, and recommended when surgical intervention is planned.
5. **Management**
   - Mild, intermittent symptoms (symptoms less than once weekly) may be treated with trial of antacids and histamine-2 receptor antagonists (H$_2$RAs) along with lifestyle modifications.
   - Lifestyle modifications should include weight loss, low-fat diet, and smaller serving portions.
   - Avoidance of foods (citrus fruits, tomatoes, and soft drinks) or medications known to decrease LES tone or cause direct mucosal irritation.
   - Avoidance of cigarette smoking and limited alcohol intake.

- Elevation of head of bed, refraining from lying down after meals, not eating at least 3 hours before bedtime, and avoiding tight-fitting clothes.
- Pharmacologic therapy indicated in moderate-to-severe disease and when attempts at lifestyle modification fail.
- H_2RAs decrease gastric acid secretion; in higher doses, they facilitate esophagitis healing.
- Promotility agents enhance esophageal clearance, increase LES pressure, and are more effective in patients with nocturnal symptoms and predominantly dyspeptic symptoms (e.g., abdominal bloating, nausea, early satiety).
- PPIs are the drugs of choice in moderate-to-severe cases, documented esophagitis, or failure with H_2RAs, and are frequently used as a first-line choice because of ease of dosing, availability, and efficacy.
- Once symptomatic relief ensues, daily PPI use can be discontinued after 8 to 12 weeks. PPI side effects, although uncommon, include headache, diarrhea, and abdominal pain.
- Long-term use of PPI has been associated with potential risk of community-acquired pneumonia, *Clostridium difficile*, hip fractures, iron and vitamin B_{12} deficiency anemias, hypomagnesemia, and fundic gland polyps.
- Surgical fundoplication indicated when medical therapy fails.

B. Barrett Esophagus

1. Etiology/Epidemiology

- Prolonged exposure to gastric acid in the refluxate from GERD results in metaplastic changes to esophageal mucosa in the distal esophagus.
- Presence of bile salts in the refluctate, obesity, and genetic and environmental factors may also play a contributing role.
- Prevalence in U.S. adults with severe GERD is approximately 5% to 10% and reaches almost 30% in patients with peptic strictures.
- Disease typically affects middle-aged Caucasian males more than females at a ratio of 3:1.
- Uncommon in Asians and blacks.

2. Pathogenesis

- Injury sustained from acid reflux results in changes from normal squamous epithelium to metaplastic columnar epithelium (specialized intestinal metaplasia) in the distal esophagus.
- Over time, dysplastic changes can lead to the major complication of esophageal adenocarcinoma.

3. Clinical Presentation

- Disease is typically asymptomatic. Symptoms arise from the severity of GERD symptoms and the degree of esophageal tissue inflammation.

4. Diagnostic Studies

- Esophagogastroduodenoscopy (EGD) with endoscopic biopsies at the squamocolumnar junction (SCJ) at the top of the gastric folds is the diagnostic gold standard.
- Recommendations for screening remain controversial. Currently, only patients with multiple risk factors for adenocarcinoma (chronic GERD, hiatal hernia, obesity, white race, male gender, and age 50 or older) should be screened.
- It is recommended that patients diagnosed with Barrett esophagus undergo surveillance endoscopy every 3 to 5 years.

5. Management

- All patients with Barrett esophagus should be placed on PPI therapy indefinitely.
- Ablative therapies should be reserved for patients with high-grade dysplasia or intramucosal adenocarcinoma.

C. Functional or Nonulcer Dyspepsia

1. Etiology

- Prevalence ranges from 25% to 40%.
- Estimated to be 27% in children.

2. Risk Factors

- Smoking.
- Use of aspirin or high-dose acetaminophen.
- History often includes:
  - Postprandial fullness.
  - Early satiety.
  - Epigastric pain or burning.
  - No documented structural disease or damage.

3. Management

- Evaluate for predominant symptom.
- Trial of PPI or H_2 blocker.
- Avoid exacerbating foods such as caffeine and alcohol.
- Counseling, psychological interventions.

D. Infectious Esophagitis

1. Etiology

- Common in immunosuppressed patients (e.g., in patients with AIDS, solid organ transplants, leukemia, and lymphoma).
- Candidal infections often associated with uncontrolled diabetes and systemic antibiotic, corticosteroid, and radiation therapies.
- Eosinophilic esophagitis is a rare idiopathic disorder seen in children and adults. Results in esophageal infiltrates of eosinophils associated with food allergies, asthma, and other atopic diseases.

2. Pathology

- Common opportunistic pathogens include *Candida albicans*, herpes simplex, and cytomegalovirus (CMV).
- Herpes simplex may be seen in immune-competent patients.

3. Clinical Features
- Odynophagia, dysphagia, and retrosternal chest pain.
- Oral thrush may be seen in 75% of patients with candidal esophagitis and in 25% to 50% of patients with viral esophagitis.
- Physical examination may disclose signs of underlying immune deficiency (e.g., fever, generalized lymphadenopathy, skin lesion, or rashes).

4. Diagnostic Studies
- Endoscopy with biopsy yields high diagnostic accuracy.
- Endoscopic findings suggestive of candidal esophagitis include linear or diffuse yellow–white plaques.
- Endoscopic findings suggestive of CMV include single and multiple large superficial ulcers.
- Endoscopic findings consistent with herpes simplex include multiple small deep ulcers.

5. Management
- Dependent on the pathogen isolated, severity of illness, and immune status of the patient.
- Candidal esophagitis in immune-competent patients may be treated with topical antifungal agents; in immunosuppressed patients, oral or intravenous (IV) antifungal agents are required.
- Initial treatment of choice for CMV esophagitis is IV ganciclovir; when side effects are intolerable or response is poor, IV foscarnet is indicated.
- Eosinophil esophagitis treatment: topical steroids swallowed ± esophageal dilatation.

E. Pill-Induced Esophagitis

1. Etiology
- Commonly implicated drugs include nonsteroidal anti-inflammatory drugs (NSAIDs), iron, antibiotics, vitamin C, potassium chloride, quinidine, zalcitabine, zidovudine, and alendronate.

2. Pathology
- Inflammation of esophageal mucosa presumed secondary to direct prolonged contact with various medications.
- Risk factors include swallowing pills without water or while lying supine, hospitalized or bedridden patients, and concurrent intestinal motility disorders.

3. Clinical Features
- Sudden retrosternal chest pain, odynophagia, and dysphagia typically occurring several hours after taking a pill.
- Elderly more often present with dysphagia and minimal pain.
- Complications include esophagitis with stricture, hemorrhage, and perforation.
- Physical examination findings are nonspecific in uncomplicated cases.

4. Diagnostic Studies
- Endoscopy typically discloses one or more discrete ulcers.

5. Management
- Remove offending agent.
- Drink at least 4 oz of water with medications.
- Remain upright at least 30 minutes after ingestion of medication.

F. Esophageal Achalasia

1. Etiology
- Progressive motor disorder of unknown etiology.

2. Pathology
- Thought to result from degeneration of the myenteric plexus and enteric nervous system, along with defective LES innervation.
- LES remains tonically contracted, failing to relax during swallowing.
- Often associated with loss of normal peristalsis in distal two-thirds of esophageal smooth muscle.

3. Clinical Features
- Symptoms typically seen between the ages of 25 and 60.
- Gradual progressive dysphagia for solids and liquids.
- Regurgitation of undigested food.
- Nocturnal regurgitation results in cough and possible aspiration pneumonia.
- Substernal discomfort and fullness after eating.
- Anorexia and weight loss.
- Complications include esophageal dilation, ulceration, infection, and rupture.
- Physical examination findings are typically nonspecific in uncomplicated cases.

4. Diagnostic Studies
- Esophageal manometry confirmatory. Findings on manometry include absence of peristalsis, low-amplitude waves associated with swallowing, and incomplete relaxation of the LES on swallowing.
- Barium esophagography may disclose esophageal dilation "sigmoid esophagus," absent peristalsis, and classic "bird's beak" narrowing of distal esophagus.
- Endoscopy should be performed to evaluate the presence of esophageal inflammation, carcinoma, or other possible causes of obstruction.
- Chest X-ray may disclose enlarged dilated esophagus.

5. Management
- Endoscopic-guided injections of botulinum toxin into the LES result in relaxation of LES and symptomatic relief in two-thirds of patients for 6 to 12 months.
- Fluoroscopic-guided pneumatic dilation of gastroesophageal junction results in symptomatic relief in over two-thirds of patients.
- Surgical myotomy is indicated when conservative methods have failed.

G. Diffuse Esophageal Spasm

1. Etiology
- Uncommon motility disorder seen equally in all ages and sexes.

2. Pathology
- Motor disorder of the esophageal smooth muscle characterized by high-amplitude nonperistaltic spontaneous esophageal contractions.

3. Clinical Features
- Nonprogressive, mild intermittent dysphagia to solids and liquids.
- Dysphagia may be provoked by stress, extremes in temperature of liquids, or large food boluses.
- Intermittent chest pain described as dull, stabbing, or crushing that may radiate to neck, back, or arms and may be provoked by certain foods and hot or cold beverages, often unrelated to meals.
- Chest pain may last minutes to hours and may awaken patient from sleep.
- Pain may be confused with angina, although typically not exertional.

4. Diagnostic Studies
- Barium esophagography discloses uncoordinated simultaneous contractions below the aortic arch, taking on characteristic "corkscrew" or "rosary bead" appearance.
- Esophageal manometry may show characteristic prolonged large-amplitude intermittent simultaneous esophageal contractions.

5. Management
- Goal of therapy: reassurance and reduction of symptoms.
- Sublingual nitroglycerin, longer-acting nitrates, and calcium channel blockers are effective in eliminating symptoms in some patients.
- Dilation with Maloney bougies reported to relieve symptoms, and a long surgical myotomy may be required in debilitated patients with intractable symptoms.

H. Scleroderma Esophagitis

1. Etiology
- Commonly associated with progressive systemic sclerosis or calcinosis, Raynaud phenomenon, esophageal dysmotility, sclerodactyly, and telangiectasia (CREST) syndrome.
- May be the presenting patient complaint, leading to diagnosis of scleroderma.

2. Pathology
- Atrophy and fibrosis of the esophageal smooth muscle lead to low-amplitude peristaltic waves and eventual aperistalsis.
- Marked decrease in LES pressures results in free gastroesophageal reflux and severe esophagitis.
- Some studies suggest neural defect rather than primary myogenic disorder.

3. Clinical Features
- Major symptoms include heartburn and dysphagia.
- Complications include severe erosive esophagitis, peptic stricture, and Barrett metaplasia.

4. Diagnostic Studies
- Barium esophagography discloses loss of peristalsis in distal esophagus and patulous LES.
- Esophageal manometry discloses low LES pressures and decreased or absent peristalsis in distal two-thirds of the esophagus.
- Upper endoscopy with biopsy confirms degree of esophagitis, presence of Barrett metaplasia, or peptic stricture.

5. Management
- Antireflux therapy including H_2RAs, PPIs, and promotility agents to prevent reflux complications.
- Dilation may be required in the presence of peptic stricture.

I. Esophageal Webs and Rings

1. Etiology
- Webs are thin, web-like constrictions typically located in the proximal esophagus.
- Webs associated with iron deficiency common in middle-aged women constitute Plummer–Vinson syndrome.
- Schatzki ring: lower web-like constriction located at the SCJ.

2. Pathology
- Exact pathogenesis is unclear; lesions are typically congenital or inflammatory in nature.
- Some evidence suggests GERD may be a predisposing factor for the development of Schatzki ring.

3. Clinical Features
- Usually asymptomatic, unless marked esophageal narrowing occurs.
- Intermittent dysphagia to solid foods may occur as large boluses of food lodge.
- Obstructing food may spontaneously clear with ingestion of liquids or regurgitation.
- Occasionally, impacted food may require endoscopic extraction.

4. Diagnostic Studies
- Barium esophagography may disclose esophageal stricture.
- Upper endoscopy may differentiate other causes of obstruction.

5. Management
- Reassurance.
- Instruct patients to chew food well.
- Webs associated with iron deficiency anemia resolve well with treatment of anemia.
- Mechanical disruption of the web or ring with bougienage dilation.

J. Zenker Diverticulum

1. Etiology
- Esophageal diverticula.

2. Pathology
- Weakness in posterior pharyngeal wall at pharyngoesophageal junction, possibly due to loss of elasticity of the upper esophageal sphincter.

3. Clinical Features
- Symptoms result when undigested food particles lodge in the diverticula.
- Gradual onset dysphagia.
- Spontaneous regurgitation of undigested food particles.
- Halitosis.
- Nocturnal choking.
- Neck mass on physical examination may be noted.
- Complications include obstruction, aspiration pneumonia, bronchiectasis, and lung abscess.

4. Diagnostic Studies
- Video esophagography: diagnostic procedure of choice to visualize diverticula.
- Upper endoscopy: should be used cautiously due to risk of perforation.

5. Management
- Cricopharyngeal myotomy with or without diverticulectomy or surgical excision may be required.

K. Esophageal Varices

1. Etiology
- Dilated submucosal veins.

2. Pathology
- Venous collateral circulation secondary to portal hypertension seen in approximately 50% of patients with cirrhosis.
- One-third of patients with varices develop upper GI bleeding.
- Bleeding commonly occurs in varices located in gastroesophageal junction.
- Factors believed to be related to bleeding include size of the varix, presence of red weal markings on endoscopy, current alcohol abuse, and severity of liver disease.

3. Clinical Features
- Typically present with painless, massive upper GI bleeding.
- Bright red or "coffee ground" hematemesis.
- Melena: massive bleeds may present with hematochezia.
- Postural hypotension, tachycardia, and shock.

4. Diagnostic Studies
- Upper endoscopy localizes bleeding.
- Complete blood cell (CBC) count, platelet count, prothrombin time (PT), partial thromboplastin time (PTT), electrolytes, liver function tests (LFTs), and albumin.
- Evaluate for coagulopathies, liver function, and hemodynamic state.

5. Management
- Emergency stabilization of patients.
- Treat underlying coagulopathy, if present.
- Endoscopic evaluation with therapeutic banding or sclerotherapy of varix.
- When hemorrhage is too vigorous or endoscopy is unavailable, balloon tube tamponade may be used.
- Pharmacologic management includes use of vasoconstrictive drugs (e.g., somatostatin, octreotide infusion).
- Antibiotic prophylaxis (oral or IV fluoroquinolones or third-generation cephalosporins).
- When endoscopic or pharmacologic therapy fails, portal decompressive procedures or transvenous intrahepatic portosystemic shunts (TIPSs) may be necessary.

L. Mallory–Weiss Syndrome

1. Etiology
- Superficial mucosal tear at the gastroesophageal junction.

2. Pathology
- Presumed to occur secondary to sudden elevation of intra-abdominal pressure, as seen in vomiting or retching.

3. Clinical Features
- Acute upper GI bleeding with hematemesis and occasionally melena.
- Accounts for 5% to 10% of acute upper GI bleeding.
- History of preceding vomiting, retching, or alcohol abuse may be obtained.

4. Diagnostic Studies
- Upper endoscopy confirms the tear.

5. Management
- Emergency stabilization, if necessary.
- Bleeding typically resolves spontaneously.

II. Disorders of the Stomach and Intestines

A. Peptic Ulcer Disease

1. Etiology
- Common disorders include gastric and duodenal ulcers.
- Approximately 10% of adults develop peptic ulcer disease (PUD) in their lifetime.
- Ulcers are slightly more common in men than in women, in the ratio of 1.3:1.
- Duodenal ulcers are five times more common than gastric ulcers and typically seen in younger patients.
- Gastric ulcers are more common in the elderly and have a high association with gastric cancer.
- PUD is the most common cause of acute upper GI bleeding.

2. Pathology
- Ulcers are typically 5 mm in diameter and extend through the muscularis mucosae.
- Peptic ulcers result from disruption of gastric or duodenal mucosa secondary to an overproduction of acid or defects in the protective mucous barrier of the stomach.
- Three major causes have been implicated in the development of PUD: *Helicobacter pylori*, NSAIDs, and hypersecretory peptic states.
  - *H. pylori*: noninvasive spiral gram-negative bacillus, residing in the mucous gel coating the epithelial cells of the stomach, seen in approximately one in six patients with PUD. Exact pathogenesis of ulcer formation remains unclear, but may reflect disruption of the protective mucous barrier.
  - NSAIDs inhibit prostaglandin synthesis. Prostaglandins are known to increase mucosal blood flow, increase bicarbonate and mucus secretion, and stimulate mucosal repair. Aspirin is the most ulcerogenic NSAID.
  - Zollinger–Ellison (ZE) syndrome: benign gastrin-secreting tumor usually located in the pancreas that results in uninhibited secretion of gastrin and constant acid production.

3. Clinical Features
- Hallmark symptom: epigastric pain (dyspepsia).
- Dyspepsia: often characterized as gnawing, dull, "hunger-like" discomfort localized to the epigastrium.
- Pain typically fluctuates in intensity throughout the day and night (rhythmicity) and may last for weeks with long intervals of pain-free periods (periodicity).
- Pain relieved with food or antacids, recurring 2 to 4 hours after meals, with strong nocturnal component, suggestive of duodenal ulcers.
- Pain aggravated by food and associated with weight loss, suggestive of gastric ulcers.
- Many patients deny provocative or palliative relationship with food or antacids.
- Associated symptoms include nausea, anorexia, and abdominal bloating.
- Vomiting, weight loss, early satiety, hematemesis, melena, hematochezia; change in intensity, quality, radiation, rhythmicity, or periodicity; may indicate complicated PUD.
- Complications include bleeding, perforation, penetration, and obstruction.
- Physical examination findings may disclose epigastric tenderness.
- Rigid, board-like abdomen and rebound tenderness—suggestive of perforation; pallor, weakness, dyspnea, orthostatic changes—suggestive of bleeding; abdominal distension with positive "succussion" splash—suggestive of gastric outlet obstruction; change in quality and radiation of pain to the back may indicate penetration.

4. Diagnostic Studies
- Upper endoscopy provides optimal visualization and opportunity for biopsy and is a procedure of choice.
- Barium esophagography limited because of poor visualization of ulcers hidden in duodenal folds and inability to differentiate between benign and malignant ulcers. When used to screen uncomplicated dyspepsia, follow-up endoscopy should be performed.
- Computed tomography (CT) imaging is reserved for patients with suspected perforation, penetration, or obstruction.
- Tests to diagnose *H. pylori* include endoscopic gastric mucosal biopsy for rapid urease testing and histology, noninvasive urease breath test, and serology.
- Laboratory studies: usually normal in uncomplicated PUD.

5. Management
- Pharmacotherapy directed at reduction of acid secretion, preserving mucosa defenses, and eradication of *H. pylori* infection.
- PPIs inactivate acid-secreting enzymes.
- PPIs are currently the treatment of choice for PUD, given their high safety and efficacy profile.
- H_2RAs bind to H_2 receptors on gastric parietal cells and inhibit cyclic adenosine monophosphate and acid secretion.
- Sucralfate, bismuth, antacids, and prostaglandin analogs enhance mucosal barrier defenses and promote ulcer healing.
- Combination antibiotic regimes with bismuth or PPIs are most effective in eradication of *H. pylori* and decrease the incidence of antibiotic resistance associated with monotherapy.
- Regular, well-balanced diets.
- Discontinuation of smoking increases the rate of healing.

B. Erosive and Hemorrhagic Gastritis
1. Etiology
- Commonly associated with stress seen in critically ill, hospitalized patients; patients taking medications such as aspirin and NSAIDs; and heavy alcohol consumption.
- Also associated with portal hypertension and, less commonly, radiation, ingestion of caustic agents, drugs such as potassium chloride, iron supplements.

2. Pathology
- Characterized by superficial inflammation and erosions of gastric mucosa without penetration into the submucosa and muscularis.

- Multiple factors implicated in the development of gastritis include hypersecretion of acid, diminished mucus secretion, epithelial growth, tissue mediators, decreased intramucosal pH, and intramucosal energy deficits.

3. Clinical Features

- Usually asymptomatic.
- When symptomatic, hematemesis and melena are often the presenting symptoms, indicating upper GI bleeding.
- Bleeding: usually minimal and results in <5% of upper GI bleeding.
- Associated symptoms may include anorexia, nausea, vomiting, and dyspepsia.

4. Diagnostic Studies

- Upper endoscopy discloses classic mucosal erythema, subepithelial hemorrhages, and erosions.

5. Management

- Pharmacologic prophylaxis for patients at high risk for stress-related gastritis, including trauma, burns, sepsis, coagulopathy, respiratory failure, central nervous system injury, and liver and renal failure.
- Prophylactic agents such as IV PPIs, sucralfate, or H_2RAs given routinely to high-risk patients have been shown to reduce incidence of significant bleeding by 50%.
- Discontinuation of NSAIDs, aspirin, and alcohol.
- Reduction of portal hypertension.

C. Malabsorption

1. Etiology

- Comprises multiple disease entities.
- May result from pancreatic enzyme deficiency, pancreatic enzyme inactivation, primary mucosal disease, celiac disease, extensive intestinal resections, defective bile formation, disruptive enterohepatic circulation, ingestion of nutrient-binding agents, bacterial overgrowth, and lymphatic obstruction.

2. Pathogenesis

- Impaired intraluminal digestion prevents adequate digestion of dietary fats, proteins, and carbohydrates as seen in pancreatic insufficiency and liver and biliary tract disorders.
- Disruption of the intestinal mucosal function due to inadequate absorptive surface area as seen in short-bowel syndrome; primary mucosal absorptive defects as in Crohn disease, tropical sprue, and celiac disease; isolated brush border enzyme deficiency as seen in lactase deficiency, prevents fats, proteins, amino acids, and specific nutrients from being absorbed.

3. Clinical Features

- Symptoms vary depending on etiology, pathogenesis, severity, location, and length of intestines involved. Celiac disease is thought to be widely undiagnosed in the adult population.
- Diarrhea may reflect increased secretion and decreased absorption of water and electrolytes; malabsorption of fatty acids and bile salts.
- Steatorrhea reflects malabsorption of fats.
- Weight loss, malnutrition, and weakness reflect malabsorption of fats, proteins, and carbohydrates.
- Anemia may reflect defects in absorption of iron, vitamin B_{12}, or folic acid.
- Paresthesia, tetany, and bone pain may denote malabsorption of calcium, vitamin D, and magnesium.
- Muscle cramps and weakness may reflect excess potassium loss.
- Bleeding tendency may reflect malabsorption of vitamin K–dependent coagulation factors.
- Edema and muscle wasting reflect hypoalbuminemia secondary to malabsorption of protein.
- Classical presentation of celiac disease is malabsorption and failure of infants to thrive after cereal is added to their diet. In adults, more nonspecific symptoms such as fatigue, iron deficiency anemia, change in bowel habits, infertility, and bone weakness may be presenting signs or symptoms.

4. Diagnostic Studies

- Routine studies for suspected malabsorption: CBC, serum iron studies, vitamin B_{12} and folate levels, serum calcium, alkaline phosphatase (ALK-P), albumin, β-carotene (a precursor to vitamin A; deficiencies may lead to malabsorption of vitamin A), and PT (may be prolonged due to vitamin K malabsorption). Initial serologic tests for celiac disease should be performed in all patients with malabsorptive-type symptoms. The recommended test is tissue transglutaminase immunoglobulin A (IgA), which has a 95% specificity and sensitivity for celiac disease (Papadakis 2017, p. 634) with distal duodenal mucosal biopsy for confirmation.
- Specific studies: excretion of >7 g per day of fat by way of quantitative 72-hour stool collection is a more sensitive means of detecting fat malabsorption than qualitative studies. If the 72-hour fecal fat collection is positive, a D-xylose test is used to determine the integrity of the intestinal mucosa. Urinary excretion would be lower than normal due to intestinal mucosal damage or changes (http://emedicine.medscape.com/article/180785-workup#c5). Schilling test may determine malabsorption of vitamin B_{12} due to a deficiency of intrinsic factor (e.g., pernicious anemia, gastric resection), pancreatic insufficiency, bacterial overgrowth, ileal resection, or disease.
- Hydrogen breath test: readily available for the diagnosis of lactase deficiency.
- Elevated serum amylase and lipase may indicate pancreatic insufficiency. Further specialized direct

testing can be performed at specialized centers using stimulation with secretin or cholecystokinin to determine exocrine pancreatic insufficiency.
- Plain films or CT scan of abdomen may disclose calcification of the pancreas.
- Endoscopic retrograde cholangiopancreatography shows visualization of the ductal system and can evaluate the pancreas for dilated ducts, intraductal stones, strictures, or pseudocyst.

5. Management
- Treatment: dependent on etiology of the malabsorption.
- Dietary restriction of gluten: essential in the treatment of celiac disease.
- Avoidance of lactose-containing products or the use of lactase enzyme supplements dramatically decreases symptoms associated with lactase deficiency.
- Malabsorption secondary to short-bowel syndrome may require supplementation with total parenteral nutrition (TPN), teduglutide (a glucagon-like peptide-2 analog), antidiarrheal agents, parenteral vitamins, and lactose restriction.
- Malabsorption secondary to chronic pancreatic disease requires supplementation with pancreatic enzymes and concurrent bicarbonate administration; H_2RAs or PPIs reduce steatorrhea by decreasing acid and uninhibiting the activity of lipase.

D. Irritable Bowel Syndrome

1. Etiology
- Chronic functional intestinal disorder characterized by abdominal pain, altered bowel habits not related to a detectable organic pathology.
- Symptoms typically begin in late teens or early 20s.
- More common in women than in men.

2. Pathology
- Multiple pathophysiologic mechanisms have been identified: dysmotility in both the small bowel and the colon, heightened visceral nociception, alterations in intestinal microbiome, noncardiac chest pain, and psychosocial disorders such as anxiety or depression. About 10% of patients will report an episode of bacterial gastroenteritis within the year preceding the symptoms.

3. Clinical Features
- Symptoms should be present 3 to 6 months before diagnosis is considered.
- Abdominal pain may be characterized as intermittent, crampy, sharp, burning, often aggravated by stress and worse 1 to 2 hours after meals, not interfering with sleep, and often relieved by defecation. Usually associated with a change in stool frequency.
- Constipation, diarrhea, or alternating constipation and diarrhea.

- Characteristic stool patterns: first morning stool is usually normal followed by frequent episodes of increasingly loose stool; formed pencil-sized, hard pellet stools reflect rectosigmoid spasms.
- Explosive defecation is seen in 20% of patients with irritable bowel syndrome (IBS).
- Mucus may cover stools or pass separately.
- Abdominal bloating and flatulence are common.
- Physical examination may disclose mild lower abdominal tenderness.
- Presence of "alarm symptoms" including hematochezia, weight loss, fever, and nocturnal diarrhea—inconsistent with IBS—warranting further investigation.

4. Diagnostic Studies
- In patients whose symptoms fulfill the diagnostic criteria, no further diagnostic testing needs to be performed.
- CBC, serologic test, serum albumin, erythrocyte sedimentation rate (ESR), and stool for occult blood are normal in patients with IBS.
- When diarrhea predominates thyroid functions, stool for ova and parasites, and possibly a 24-hour stool collection is warranted.
- Hydrogen breath test or a lactose-free diet trial for patients with symptoms of excess bloating or gas.
- Endoscopic evaluations are often performed in patients who have not shown clinical improvement with initial management.

5. Management
- Patient reassurance and education on the functional and chronic nature of the disease process is essential.
- Daily record of specific food intake, concurrent psychosocial stressors, along with symptoms, may be helpful for some patients.
- Dietary therapy: foods found to provoke symptoms should be avoided. Common flatulogenic foods: apples, pears, brown beans, cabbage, Brussels sprouts, raisins, coffee, red wine, and beer.
- Trial of high-fiber diet.
- Pharmacotherapy targeted at specific symptoms reserved for refractory cases.
- Antispasmodic agents: dicyclomine given 30 to 60 minutes before meals may relieve postprandial bloating. Alosetron, loperamide for diarrhea, specifically symptom-targeted pharmacologic agents such as linaclotide, lubiprostone, or polyethylene glycol 3350 may benefit constipation refractory to fiber supplementation. Probiotics may reduce IBS symptoms.
- Psychotropic agents: amitriptyline may be helpful in patients with intractable pain.
- Behavioral modification, biofeedback, and hypnotherapy benefit some patients.

E. Antibiotic-Associated Colitis

1. Etiology
- Diarrhea related to antibiotic use. Common culprits: ampicillin, clindamycin, tetracycline, and cephalosporins.

2. Pathogenesis
- Diarrhea is often mild, dose related, and rarely occurring up to 3 weeks after discontinuation of antibiotic and is more often resolving after discontinuation of antibiotic.
- Significant diarrhea most often caused by intestinal proliferation of *C. difficile* and elaboration of its toxin.

3. Clinical Features
- Mild-to-moderate foul-smelling watery diarrhea. Nocturnal symptoms possible.
- Crampy, lower abdominal pain.
- Profuse, watery, bloody diarrhea and fever may be seen in more severe cases.
- Complications: dehydration, electrolyte imbalance, toxic megacolon, perforation, and death.

4. Diagnostic Studies
- Demonstration of cytotoxin B in stool: definitive but takes 24 hours.
- Rapid enzyme-linked immunosorbent assays for both enterotoxin A and cytotoxin B are faster, but less sensitive.
- Cultures are expensive and timely and do not differentiate from toxigenic strains.
- Fecal leukocytes may be seen in 50% of patients.
- Flexible sigmoidoscopy may disclose nonspecific inflammation; yellow adherent colonic plaques (pseudomembranes) may be noted in severe disease. Pseudomembranes localized in the proximal colon may be missed by sigmoidoscopy.

5. Management
- Discontinue antibiotics, if possible.
- Drug of choice for severe cases: metronidazole.
- Vancomycin is equally effective, more expensive, and associated with the development of antibiotic-resistant organisms.
- In case of multiple relapses, consider tapering and pulsed antibiotic therapy.
- Twenty percent of patients may relapse within 1 to 2 weeks of discontinuation of therapy. Relapses respond well to second course of metronidazole or vancomycin. Newer fecal transplants are also effective for failed courses of antibiotics.

F. Crohn Disease

1. Etiology
- Idiopathic chronic inflammatory bowel disease (IBD) of unknown etiology.
- More common in Caucasians than African Americans and Asians.
- Men and women are affected equally.
- Peak incidence between the ages of 15 and 35.
- Evidence suggests some familial basis along with environmental component.

2. Pathogenesis
- Transmural inflammatory process involving any area of the GI tract from the mouth to the anus. One-third of the cases involve only the small bowel and about half involve the proximal colon, also known as ileocolitis.
- Characterized by exacerbations and periods of remission.
- Chronic inflammation results in ulceration, stricture, fistula, and abscess formation.

3. Clinical Features
- Symptoms and signs are dependent on the site and severity of inflammation.
- Low-grade fever, malaise, weight loss, and generalized fatigability.
- Abdominal pain may be steady, localized to the right lower quadrant.
- Usually nonbloody diarrhea.
- Associated perianal fissures, fistulas, and abscesses.
- Extraintestinal infestations: oral aphthous ulcers, erythema nodosum, pyoderma gangrenosum, episcleritis, iritis, uveitis, nondeforming arthritis, pericholangitis, and sclerosing cholangitis.
- Extensive ileal disease results in malabsorption of bile salts, increasing incidence of gallstones, steatorrhea, deficiency in fat-soluble vitamins, and increased colonic oxalate absorption increasing the incidence of nephrolithiasis.
- Anemia of chronic disease, iron deficiency, and vitamin B_{12} or, rarely, folate deficiency.
- Increase in colon cancer has been noted in the presence of colonic disease.
- Physical findings may show right lower quadrant tenderness with palpable mass. Other findings vary depending on severity of involvement and degree of inflammation.

4. Diagnostic Studies
- Laboratory findings correlate poorly with patient's clinical status.
- CBC may disclose anemia, leukocytosis; serum albumin may show hypoalbuminemia secondary to intestinal protein loss or malabsorption; ESR or C-reactive protein (CRP) may be elevated during active inflammation.
- Stool for occult blood, white blood cells (WBCs), culture, ova and parasites, and *C. difficile* toxin.
- Upper GI series with small bowel follow through may show ulcerations, strictures, or fistulas.
- Colonoscopy to evaluate colonic disease. Colonoscopy allows for mucosal biopsies and may disclose ulcers, alternating with area of normal mucosa, giving the mucosa a cobblestone appearance and rectal sparing.

- CT scanning may distinguish thickened, matted bowel loops, intra-abdominal abscess.
- Presence of granulomas on biopsy: highly suggestive of Crohn disease.

5. Management

- Well-balanced diet; high-fiber supplementation is helpful in patients with mainly colonic involvement; patients with obstructive symptoms do best with low-roughage diet; and a trial lactose-free diet is helpful because lactose deficiency is common.
- Four-week course of enteral therapy may induce remissions; TPN may be required in the presence of severe malnutrition or preoperatively to improve nutritional status.
- Pharmacotherapy includes antispasmodics and antidiarrheals for symptomatic relief. Patients with ileal resection may require medications such as cholestyramine to bind bile salts. Once used as initial therapy, 5-aminosalicylic acid (5-ASA) agents such as mesalamine are no longer recommended in Crohn disease. Corticosteroids such as prednisone 40 to 60 mg daily are effective in suppressing both small- and large-bowel inflammation in more severe cases. Entocort 9 mg daily for up to 4 months will often lead to remission. Immunomodulating drugs such as azathioprine or mercaptopurine (6-MP) indicated in patients for maintenance. Patients on 6-MP require frequent CBCs to evaluate for neutropenia. Tumor necrosis factor (TNF) inhibitors (anti-TNF therapy) adalimumab, certolizumab, and infliximab IV infusion promote rapid symptom improvement and are more often preferred as first-line agents to induce remission in patients with moderate-to-severe disease and those with fistula disease.
- Indications for surgery: intractability, abscess, stricture, and severe bleeding.

G. Ulcerative Colitis

1. Etiology

- Idiopathic chronic IBD of unknown etiology.
- Occurs in all age groups with peaks in both the third and the seventh decades.
- More common and may be more severe in non-smokers and former smokers.

2. Pathogenesis

- Inflammation of mucosal surface of the colon and rectum resulting in erosions, friability, and bleeding.
- Lesions typically involve the rectum and extend proximally in a continuous process.
- Characterized by exacerbations and periods of remission.
- Approximately 50% of patients have disease localized to the rectosigmoid colon; approximately 10% to 15% of patients have extensive pancolitis.

3. Clinical Features

- Although the clinical picture is highly variable, certain clinical features appear to correlate with the extent of disease.
- Disease may be classified as mild, moderate, and severe (Table 4–1).
- Bloody diarrhea is hallmark of severe disease. Patients with mild-to-moderate disease may have a gradual onset of diarrhea with intermittent rectal bleeding.
- Mucus and pus in stools.
- Crampy abdominal pain.
- Fecal urgency, constipation, and tenesmus with predominately rectal involvement.
- Fever, weight loss, anemia, hypovolemia, and hypoalbuminemia in severe disease.
- Extracolonic manifestations: erythema nodosum, pyoderma gangrenosum, episcleritis, thromboembolism, and oligoarticular nondeforming arthritis.
- Complications: fulminant colitis, toxic megacolon; risk of colon cancer after 10 years increases from 0.5% to 1% per year.

4. Diagnostic Studies

- Test of choice in evaluation of acute disease is sigmoidoscopy. Endoscopic findings: mucosal edema, friability, mucopus, and erosions.
- Colonoscopy should not be performed during acute severe illness because of the risk of bowel perforation. When symptoms improve, colonoscopy is useful to evaluate disease extent and cancer surveillance.
- Plain film radiographs identify colonic dilation in acute severe disease.
- Barium enemas are contraindicated in evaluation of acute disease and may precipitate toxic megacolon.
- Low hemoglobin and hematocrit reflect anemia; elevated ESRs indicate inflammation; decreased albumin in the presence of protein loss indicates enteropathy.

5. Management

- Regular diet, avoidance of caffeine and flatulogenic foods. Fiber supplementation decreases diarrhea and rectal symptoms. Antidiarrheals contraindicated during acute disease, but may be helpful in patients with mild chronic symptoms.
- Goals of pharmacotherapy: symptomatic relief, suppression of inflammation, termination of acute exacerbation, and prevention of relapse.
- Acute disease: topical mesalamine rectal suppositories or enemas are the recommended treatment of choice for distal colitis. Topical corticosteroids are less effective. Systemic corticosteroids or immunosuppressive agents are recommended when topical therapy fails.

TABLE 4–1. Spectrum of Clinical Severity of Ulcerative Colitis

Feature	Mild	Moderate	Severe or Fulminant
Bowel movements per day	≤5	>5	Hourly
Rectal bleeding	Intermittent	Usual	Continuous and severe
Weight loss	Minimal	<10 lb	10–20 lb
"Toxic" appearance	No	No	Yes
Fever	No	Perhaps	Yes
Tachycardia	No	Frequently	Yes
Abdominal tenderness	No	Frequently	Yes
Bowel sounds	Normal	Normal or increased	Reduced or silent
Anemia	No	Hematocrit > 30	Hematocrit < 25–30
Leukocytosis	No	Yes	Yes
Left shift	No	Yes	Yes
Albumin	Normal	Normal	Reduced
Bacteremia	No	Seldom	Frequently

Data from Yamada T, Hasler W. Inflammatory bowel disease. In: Kelly WN, ed. *Inflammatory Bowel Disease*. Philadelphia, PA: JB Lippincott Company; 1994:128.

- Acute disease extending above the sigmoid colon: oral sulfasalazine and oral mesalamine are recommended.
- Failure to respond after a 2- to 3-week course of oral agent: consider an adjunctive 2-week trial of topical corticosteroid foam or enemas. Continued failure requires systemic corticosteroids such as prednisone. Budesonide 9 mg orally daily may provide some relief. Patients who do not respond to corticosteroids may show some improvement with mercaptopurine or azathioprine. A better option for remission is the initiation of anti-TNF agents such as infliximab, adalimumab, and golimumab. Used as an outpatient when unresponsive to oral prednisone, oral 5-ASA and rectal medications should be considered before colectomy.
- Anti-integrin therapy: vedolizumab, a monoclonal antibody directed against the $\alpha_4\beta_7$ heterodimer, is U.S. Food and Drug Administration (FDA) approved for treatment in moderate-to-severe ulcerative colitis (UC) in patients who have not responded to other therapies.
- Surgical therapy recommended in severe disease unresponsive to systemic corticosteroids.

H. Microscopic Colitis
- Typically more common in women in the fifth or sixth decade.
- Unknown etiology.
- Patients present with symptoms of persistent watery diarrhea.
- On endoscopic evaluation, the colonic mucosa appears normal.
- Histologic mucosal biopsies reveal either lymphocytic or collagenous colitis.
- Antidiarrheal treatment with loperamide is first line. Budesonide 9 mg daily for 6 to 8 weeks has also shown high rates of remission.

I. Diverticular Disease
1. Etiology
- Herniations of colonic mucosa through the muscularis, typically at a site of least resistance, usually where the nutrient artery penetrates the muscularis. Diverticula vary in sizes and numbers and are most often located in sigmoid colon with approximately one-third present in proximal colon.
- Incidence increases with age. More than one-third of patients older than 60 years have diverticular disease.

2. Pathogenesis
- High prevalence in Western countries and low incidence in underdeveloped countries, and vegetarians suggest a strong dietary influence in the pathogenic development. However, the etiology of diverticulosis is uncertain.
- It is believed that decreased fecal bulk, a narrowed and contracted bowel, and high intraluminal pressures to move along smaller hard fecal mass over time result in thickening, hypertrophy, and fibrosis of the colonic musculature and herniation of the colonic mucosa.

- Inherited weakness in colonic wall; intestinal dysmotility and patients with abnormal connective tissue diseases such as Marfan syndrome, scleroderma, and Ehlers–Danlos syndrome may also have a role in the development of diverticulosis.
- Hardened fecaliths within the diverticula may erode through the nutrient vessel, resulting in hemorrhage.
- Fecaliths, invasion of colonic bacteria, may result in inflammation of the diverticular sac with subsequent microperforation, pericolic abscess, or generalized peritonitis.

3. Clinical Features

- Uncomplicated diverticulosis is most often asymptomatic. Complaints of nonspecific chronic constipation, alterations in bowel habits, and abdominal pain may be noted.
- Bleeding diverticulosis typically presents with an acute onset of painless, large-volume hematochezia.
- Bleeding complicates diverticulosis in 3% to 5% of the cases and is the most common cause of acute lower GI bleeding.
- Diverticulitis, a macroscopic inflammation of a diverticulum, presents as aching left lower quadrant abdominal pain, tenderness, and palpable mass; fever, nausea, vomiting, constipation, or loose stools. Hematochezia—rare; occult blood loss—common.

4. Diagnostic Studies

- Plain films may be used for evaluation of free abdominal air.
- CT scan of the abdomen and pelvis can be diagnostic as well as document the presence of an abscess and inflammation.
- Colonoscopy and sigmoidoscopy (although contraindicated during acute diverticulitis) may be helpful in confirming presumptive diagnosis and excluding others.
- Diverticular hemorrhage may be evaluated by colonoscopy after bleeding subsides. Continued active bleeding may be evaluated with ^{99m}Tc-labeled red blood scan, mesenteric angiography, and scintigraphy.

5. Management

- Uncomplicated diverticulosis should be treated with high-fiber diet or fiber supplements.
- Patients with mild diverticulitis may be treated as outpatients with low-residue diet, metronidazole, in addition to ciprofloxacin or trimethoprim/sulfamethoxazole DS.
- Patients unresponsive to outpatient therapy require hospitalization, nothing by mouth, IV antibiotics.
- Severe disease or failure to respond within 72 hours necessitates surgical consultation.

- Massive diverticular bleeding with hypovolemia requires emergent hospitalization, evaluation, and resuscitation.
- Bleeding ceases spontaneously in 90% of patients.
- Therapeutic options for unresponsive bleeding: surgery or intra-arterial vasopressin.

J. Vascular Ectasis (Angiodysplasia and Arteriovenous Malformations)

1. Etiology

- Etiology unknown.
- Associated with congenital disorders.
- Hereditary hemorrhagic telangiectasias and scleroderma.
- May result in acute or chronic upper or lower GI bleeding.
- Located throughout the GI tract, most commonly in the cecum and ascending colon.
- One-fourth of patients older than 60 years have lower GI bleeding secondary to angiodysplasia.
- Responsible for 5% to 10% cases of lower GI bleeding.

2. Pathology

- Degenerative lesion consisting of distorted, dilated vessels lined with vascular endothelium.

3. Clinical Features

- Hematochezia, typically massive, resolving spontaneously, often recurring.
- Occult blood in chronic bleeds.
- Iron deficiency anemia.
- Hematemesis and melena may be seen with upper GI tract involvement.

4. Diagnostic Studies

- Panendoscopy and small bowel capsule endoscopy are the diagnostic studies to identify lesions in the colon, stomach, and duodenum.
- Occasionally, laparotomy and intraoperative endoscopy of the small bowel are required to control bleeding.

5. Management

- Chronic bleed: iron supplements, intermittent transfusions; hormonal therapy with estrogen and progesterone is currently under investigation.
- Minor active bleeding lesions may be treated by way of endoscopic cauterization or laser therapy.
- Severe active bleeding may require angiography with vasopressin to control bleeding.
- Uncontrolled or recurrent bleeding may require right hemicolectomy.

III. Anorectal Disorders
A. Hemorrhoids
1. Etiology

- Hemorrhoids are seen in 50% of persons older than 50 years and are uncommon in persons younger than 25 to 30 years.

- Five percent of persons above age 50 have symptoms.
- Hemorrhoids may become symptomatic secondary to increased systemic venous pressures as seen with pregnancy, prolonged sitting, straining, constipation, obesity, and increased portal pressure associated with congestive heart failure and cirrhosis.

2. Pathology
- Hemorrhoidal venous plexuses, along with arterial plexuses, smooth muscle, and connective tissue, comprise anal cushions that allow variable stool sizes to pass without damaging the rectal mucosa. Hemorrhoidal disease is believed to arise when the internal or external hemorrhoidal plexus enlarges, resulting in venous swelling and displacement of vascular anal cushions.
- Enlargement and redundancy of anal cushions over time may result in protrusion or bleeding.

3. Clinical Features
- Internal hemorrhoids: most often present with intermittent rectal bleeding described as painless bright red, seen on toilet paper, coating stool, or dispersed in toilet water following defecation.
  - If occult bleeding occurs, massive bleeding is rare.
  - Vague anal discomfort may be associated.
  - Discomfort increases with progressive enlargement or prolapse through the anus.
  - Prolapse can become chronic, leading to soiling, mucoid anal discharge, pruritus ani, infection, thrombosis, and strangulation.
  - Presence of rectal pain associated with internal hemorrhoids suggests complication and requires surgical consult.
- External hemorrhoids: covered by pain-sensitive skin most commonly manifest as perianal pain aggravated by defecation.
  - A tender anal mass may be palpated.
  - Thrombosis may be precipitated by coughing and heavy lifting and result in a perianal hematoma or thrombosis of an external hemorrhoid.

4. Diagnostic Studies
- Typically made on perianal inspection, digital examination, and direct visualization by way of anoscope or proctoscope.
- Proctosigmoidoscopy or colonoscopy should be performed in all patients with hematochezia, especially in the presence of anemia, to rule out disease proximal to the sigmoid colon.
- Colonoscopy is preferred in patients older than 40 years with anemia.
- External hemorrhoids appear as soft, painless mass outside the anal verge; when thrombosed, they appear as firm, tender, bluish mass.

- Internal hemorrhoids are typically not visible, but may protrude through the anus with straining.
- Prolapsed hemorrhoids appear as purple nodules covered by mucosa.
- Uncomplicated internal hemorrhoids on digital rectal examination are neither palpable nor tender.

5. Management
- Often, hemorrhoidal symptoms, even associated with thrombosis, abate spontaneously within days to weeks.
- Symptoms often recur.
- Conservative therapy: high-fiber diet, increased fluid intake, warm sitz baths, and topical rectal hydrocortisone preparations for relief of pruritus and discomfort.
- Analgesic rectal preparation or systemic analgesics are useful when pain is problematic.
- Injection sclerotherapy and rubber-band ligation are the options for treatment.
- Surgical referral: failure to respond to conservative treatment, chronic severe bleeding, debilitating pain, evidence of infection, strangulation, or ulceration.

B. Perianal Abscess and Fistulas

1. Etiology
- Anorectal abscesses are more common in men.
- Often result from a bacterial infection of anal glands and ducts.
- Typical organisms isolated: *Staphylococcus aureus*, *Escherichia coli*, Bacteroides, Proteus, and *Streptococcus* species.
- Most abscesses are located in the posterior rectal wall.
- Most anorectal fistulas result from abscesses of the anal glands.
- Some are not pyogenic in nature and are due to IBD, tuberculosis, diverticular or neoplastic disease, and trauma.

2. Pathology
- Abscesses result when discharge from anal glands is inhibited because of anal muscle tone causing stasis, dilation, and eventual infection.

3. Clinical Features
- Anorectal abscess: sudden onset of throbbing perianal pain aggravated by sitting, coughing, defecating, and walking.
- Draining abscess produces mucopurulent discharge and scant blood.
- Fever, malaise, and chills may be present.
- Complication: systemic and necrotizing infection.
- Uncomplicated fistulas most commonly present with intermittent painful perianal swelling, followed by relief with onset of purulent discharge.
- Tenesmus and painful defecation may occur with high intramuscular fistulas.

4. Diagnostic Studies
- Diagnosis is frequently made by inspection and digital rectal examination.
- Anoscopy also allows for better visualization.

5. Management
- Surgical referral for incision and drainage.

IV. Disorders of the Liver and Pancreas

A. Viral Hepatitis

1. Etiology
- Hepatitis A virus (HAV), an RNA virus primarily transmitted by way of the oral-fecal route, typically by contamination of food or water.
  - Risk factors include poor sanitation; closed communities sharing toilet and eating facilities—schools, daycare facilities, or military bases; ingestion of raw, contaminated shellfish.
  - Children younger than 6 years in a household have been reported to be the most common source of infection in adults without other identifiable risk factors. Most likely because 70% of children with hepatitis A are asymptomatic.
  - Incubation period is 2 to 6 weeks—average 30 days.
  - Mortality rate is 0.1%, fulminant course uncommon, and carrier state and chronic disease absent.
- Hepatitis B virus (HBV) is a double-stranded DNA virus with eight different genotypes.
  - Transmitted by way of inoculation of infected blood or body fluids: transfusions; unprotected sexual intercourse; needle sharing; and, in children, close personal contact in endemic areas through open cuts or sores.
  - High-risk populations include health care workers, men who have sex with men, and IV drug abusers.
  - Incubation period: 6 weeks to 6 months; average 12 to 14 weeks.
  - Mortality rate: up to 60%; fulminant disease: less than 1%; chronic disease and cirrhosis occur in 3% to 5% of patients with hepatitis B.
  - Acute illness usually subsides in a few weeks, with complete clinical recovery by 16 weeks.
  - Chronic hepatitis B has become more prevalent in the United States because of immigration from more endemic countries. Chronic HBV is defined as persons with a positive hepatitis B surface antigen (HBsAg) for >6 months. They are at increased risk for developing cirrhosis and hepatocellular cancer.
- Hepatitis C virus (HCV) is a single-stranded RNA virus, transmitted by infected blood and body fluids with six major genotypes identified.
  - Approximately 50% of cases are related to IV drug use, 4% attributed to blood transfusions, 6% by sexual or household exposure, and 4% by way of occupational exposure to contaminated blood; in the remaining cases, the source is unclear.
  - Additional risk factors identified include intranasal cocaine use, hemodialysis, and body piercing. Maternal–perinatal transmission is low.
  - Incubation period: 6 to 7 weeks.
  - Mortality rate: 1%, with chronic disease seen in approximately 50% of patients.
- Hepatitis D (δ agent) is defective RNA virus requiring association with hepatitis B, specifically the presence of HBsAg, to illicit infection.
- Hepatitis E virus is an RNA virus typically transmitted by the fecal-oral route, responsible for epidemic outbreaks in developing countries.
- It may be spread by swine or consuming undercooked organ meats.
- No carrier state exists.

2. Pathogenesis
- The exact pathogenesis remains unclear and may be more a result of immunologic host response than direct cytopathic effect of the virus.
- Histologic findings include focal liver necrosis, mononuclear infiltration, hyperplasia of Kupffer cells, and cholestasis.

3. Clinical Features of Viral Hepatitis
- Variable ranging from asymptomatic disease, chronic progressive symptoms, fulminant disease, to death.
- Prodromal phase (2–14 days) characterized by malaise, fatigue, migratory arthralgias, anorexia, coryza, low-grade fever, skin rash, right upper quadrant (RUQ) pain, pruritus, nausea, and abdominal fullness; amber-colored urine; acholic stools appear 1 to 4 days before the onset of jaundice. Hepatitis A is the only viral hepatitis causing spiking fevers.
- Icteric stage often absent; peaks approximately during the second week, but may persist 6 to 8 weeks. Onset of jaundice typically signals clinical improvement.
- Convalescent stage with improvement of appetite, resolution of jaundice, and abdominal pain.
- Physical findings include hepatomegaly seen in 50% of patients; splenomegaly in 15%; posterior cervical and epitrochlear lymphadenopathy.
- Sequelae: acute fulminant disease characterized by encephalopathy, coagulopathy, jaundice, edema, ascites, electrolyte abnormalities, asterixis, spasticity, hyperreflexia, fetor hepaticus. Chronic hepatitis characterized by a prolonged course (>3-6 months) of persistent elevated serum

aminotransferase levels, with hepatic inflammation, necrosis, fibrosis, and eventual cirrhosis.
- Hepatitis B and C viruses carry a high risk of hepatocellular cancer.

4. Diagnostic Studies
- WBC count usually low or normal, with occasional predominance of large atypical lymphocytes.
- Mild proteinuria and bilirubinuria.
- Elevated aspartate aminotransferase (AST) and alanine aminotransferase (ALT).
- Elevated bilirubin (Bil) and ALK-P.
- Prolonged PT, hypoalbuminemia, and elevated blood ammonia levels in severe or end-stage disease.
- Serologic markers for hepatitis A–fecal HAV rarely present beyond the first week of illness. Immunoglobulin M (IgM) antibodies to HAV (anti-HAV) indicate acute hepatitis; immunoglobulin G (IgG) antibodies peak after 1 month and may persist for years; presence of IgG anti-HAV alone indicates previous exposure, noninfectivity, and future immunity.
- Several serologic markers are associated with hepatitis B.
- HBsAg indicates infection with HBV and denotes infectivity.
- Antibody to HBsAg (anti-HBs) appears after the antigen is cleared and with successful immunization, signaling recovery from acute disease.
- Serologic gap between the time HBsAg clears and antibody to the surface antigen (anti-HBs)

becomes detectable is referred to as the window period.
- IgM antibody to the HBV core (anti-HBc) may be the only marker detectable during the window period, indicating acute infection or relapse in chronic disease.
- IgG antibody to the HBV core also appears during acute infection, but persists indefinitely. IgG antibody in the presence of HBsAg indicates chronic infection, and in the absence of HBsAg indicates recovery.
- Hepatitis B envelop antigen (HBeAg) appears shortly after HBsAg is detected, indicating viral replication and infectivity.
  - Persistence beyond 3 months suggests chronic disease.
  - Clearance of HBeAg followed by antibody to the HBV envelop (anti-HBe) denotes decreased replication and decreased infectivity.
- HBV DNA closely corresponds with the presence of HBeAg in serum, but is a more precise marker of infectivity and viral replication.
- Common serologic patterns and interpretation are listed in Table 4–2.
- Hepatitis D virus (HDV) may be diagnosed by detection of hepatitis D antigen, HDV antibody (anti-HDV), or HDV RNA in serum.
- HCV may be diagnosed by enzyme immunoassay detecting antibodies to HCV. Supplemental recombinant immunoblot assay is more sensitive and specific to confirm the diagnosis, or polymerase chain reaction to detect HCV RNA.

TABLE 4–2. Serologic Screening Tests for the Diagnosis of Acute Viral Hepatitis

Anti-HAV IgM	HBsAg	Anti-HBc IgM	Anti-HCV	Interpretation
Positive	Negative	Negative	Negative	Acute hepatitis A
Positive	Positive	Negative	Negative	Acute hepatitis A in a chronic HBsAg carrier
Negative	Positive	Positive	Negative	Acute hepatitis B
Negative	Negative	Positive	Negative	Recent hepatitis B; "serologic window" between disappearance of HBsAg and appearance of anti-HBs
Negative	Negative	Negative	Positive or negative	Acute hepatitis C[a]
Negative	Positive	Negative	Negative or positive	Chronic HBsAg carrier[b] with a superimposed hepatitis (hepatitis C, delta[c], alcohol, or drug related); possible reactivation of HBV infection

[a]Positive test may be delayed for 2 to 4 weeks; current assays may not detect all cases.

[b]Minority of HBsAg carriers with active disease exhibit low-titer IgM anti-HBc.

[c]Reflex testing with antibody to delta virus is appropriate.

HAV, hepatitis A virus; HBsAg, hepatitis B surface antigen; HBV, hepatitis B virus; HCV, hepatitis C virus; Ig, immunoglobulin.

Data from Perillo RP, Regenstein FG. Viral and immune hepatitis. In: Kelly WN, ed. *Essentials of Internal Medicine*. Philadelphia, PA: JB Lippincott Company; 1994:822–833.

- Liver biopsy in patients with chronic disease evaluates the extent of hepatocellular damage. HCV FibroSURE test is a six biochemical marker blood test that correlates well with liver biopsy Metavir fibrosis scoring and necroinflammation and could be substituted for liver biopsy to minimize risks associated with biopsy.

5. Management
- Treatment during the acute phase is primarily supportive: hydration, rest, restricted physical activity, high-calorie diet, avoidance of hepatotoxic drugs, and evaluation for complications.
- Follow-up LFTs and seromarkers until return to normal.
- Treatment of fulminant hepatitis requires intensive care with maintenance of fluid balance, support of circulation and respiration, correct control bleeding and hypoglycemia, restriction of protein intake, and liver transplantation.
- Chronic hepatitis B: standard therapy is treatment with a nucleoside or nucleotide analog or with pegylated interferon. The available nucleoside and nucleotide analogs are entecavir and tenofovir preferred as first-line drugs and lamivudine and telbivudine when short courses of treatment may be required because of their higher rate of resistance with long-term use.
- General preventative guidelines: universal precaution when handling all blood and body fluids; strict attention to hand washing when in contact with contaminated linens, clothing, and eating utensils; careful screening of all donated blood; routine hepatitis screening for all pregnant women; careful disposal of all contaminated needles; immunization against hepatitis A and B; and safe sexual practices.
- Immune globulin should be administered to all household personnel and close contacts of patients with hepatitis A. Vaccines are recommended for all patients living or traveling to endemic areas.
- Hepatitis B immunoglobulin (HBIG) may provide protection if given within 7 days of exposure.
  - Newborns of HBV-infected mothers should receive HBIG and HBV vaccine at delivery.
  - Subsequent HBV vaccine should be started.
  - Currently, universal vaccinations of all infants and children are recommended.

B. Nonalcoholic Fatty Liver Disease
1. Etiology
- Affects up to 45% of the U.S. population mainly due to obesity, diabetes mellitus (DM), and hypertriglyceridemia.
- Other causes of fatty liver disease include certain medication such as corticosteroids, amiodarone, diltiazem, certain occupational toxins, and endocrinopathies.

- Pathogenesis: macrovesicular steatosis, focal infiltration by polymorphonuclear neutrophils and Mallory hyalin.
- Physical activity helps prevent against nonalcoholic fatty liver disease (NAFLD).
- Most patients are asymptomatic, and initial findings are a result of routine labs showing mild elevations in aminotransferase and ALK-P levels.

2. Diagnostic Studies
- Ultrasound (U/S) or abdominal CT may reveal hepatomegaly or macrovesicular steatosis.
- Liver biopsy is diagnostic and can differentiate the degree of inflammation and fibrosis and progression to nonalcoholic steatohepatitis (NASH), a worsening progression of NAFLD.
- Treatment consists of lifestyle modification including the initiation of regular exercise, weight loss, and dietary fat restriction. Vitamin E 800 IU daily appears to be beneficial in patients with NASH without DM.

C. Cirrhosis
1. Etiology
- In the United States, causes of cirrhosis include chronic viral hepatitis, alcohol, drug toxicity, and autoimmune and metabolic liver diseases.

2. Pathogenesis
- Irreversible liver destruction characterized by hepatocellular injury, fibrosis, and nodular regeneration.

3. Clinical Features
- Onset of symptoms is typically gradual, rarely abrupt.
- Weight loss, weakness, disturbed sleep, muscle cramps, and fatigue are common.
- Abdominal discomfort.
- Anorexia, nausea, and vomiting are noted in advanced disease.
- Menstrual disorders, impotence, testicular atrophy, gynecomastia, loss of pubic and axillary hair, spider telangiectasias, and palmar erythema.
- Hepatomegaly, splenomegaly, jaundice, and bleeding esophageal varices result from portal hypertension.
- Late manifestations: coagulopathy, ascites, dilated superficial abdominal veins, peripheral edema, and pleural effusions.
- Hepatic encephalopathy characterized by alterations in consciousness, disruption in the sleep–awake cycle, asterixis, tremor, hyperreflexia, eventual coma, and death.

4. Diagnostic Studies
- WBC count may be low, normal, or elevated. Anemia, typically megaloblastic reflecting folate deficiency. Thrombocytopenia secondary from alcoholic bone marrow suppression, splenic sequestration, or sepsis. Prolonged PT and PTT reflect

inability of liver to produce clotting factors. Elevated bilirubin, AST, ALT, and ALK-P. Decreased serum albumin and increased γ-globulin.
- U/S discloses hepatomegaly, splenomegaly, liver nodularity, or atrophy.
- Upper endoscopy or barium swallow identifies esophageal varices.
- CT scan may delineate nodules consistent with hepatocellular carcinoma.
- Paracentesis in the presence of ascites.
- Liver biopsy identifies characteristic histologic features.

5. Management
- Vaccinate against hepatitis A.
- Screen for esophageal varices.
- Abstinence from alcohol is the most important aspect of therapy.
- Low protein diet: 1 to 1.5 g per kg.
- Sodium restriction, fluid restriction, and diuretics for ascites and edema.
- Avoidance of drugs metabolized in the liver.
- Multivitamins, folic acid, and iron supplements for anemia.
- Evaluate and treat complications such as spontaneous bacterial peritonitis, hepatorenal syndrome, variceal bleeding, and hepatic encephalopathy.
- Evaluation for liver transplantation.

D. Acute and Chronic Pancreatitis
1. Etiology
- Causes of acute pancreatitis include alcohol ingestion, gallstones, trauma, metabolic diseases such as renal failure, infectious agents, cystic fibrosis, certain drugs, vasculitis, penetrating peptic ulcer, congenital anomaly, and conditions that result in obstruction of the ampulla of Vater such as Crohn disease.
- Heavy alcohol intake or biliary tract (gallstones) disease are main causes. Other causes include cystic fibrosis, severe malnutrition, pancreatic and duodenal cancer, hyperparathyroidism, ZE syndrome, trauma, hematochromatosis, postsurgery, enzyme deficiencies; frequently idiopathic.

2. Pathology
- Exact pathogenesis of acute pancreatitis is unclear.
- Thought to result from direct injury to the pancreatic acinar cells, possibly from reflux of bile into the pancreas.
- Activated pancreatic enzymes from damaged acinar cells leak into surrounding tissue, resulting in inflammation.
- Exact pathogenesis of chronic pancreatitis is unclear.
- Chronic inflammation results in progressive fibrosis and destruction of the pancreas.

3. Clinical Features
- Acute pancreatitis: sudden onset of epigastric pain, radiating to the back or sides; described as

severe, constant, boring, aggravated by walking and lying supine, and relieved by leaning forward.
- Associated symptoms include nausea and vomiting.
- Physical examination shows epigastric tenderness, abdominal distension, low-grade fever, decreased or absent bowel sounds with associated paralytic ileus, ascites, and mild jaundice.
- Inflamed pancreas is occasionally palpable.
- Tachycardia, pallor, hypotension, and shock may be noted.
- In severe necrotizing pancreatitis with hemoperitoneum, a bluish discoloration of the skin around the umbilicus (Cullen sign) and an ecchymotic discoloration of the flanks (Turner sign) from tissue catabolism of hemoglobin may be noted.
- Ten to 20% of patients have pulmonary findings including basilar rales and pleural effusion.
- Complications: acute renal failure, pancreatic infection or abscess, acute respiratory distress syndrome, pseudocysts, chronic pancreatitis (10% of patients), and DM rarely after single acute attack.
- Chronic pancreatitis: may present similar to acute pancreatitis.
  - Typically, with persistent epigastric pain referred to the upper left lumbar region associated with anorexia, nausea, vomiting, bowel changes, and weight loss; lasting hours to weeks.
  - Malabsorption symptoms or signs such as weight loss and steatorrhea are also common.
  - Physical findings are minimal, including low-grade fever and abdominal tenderness.
  - Complications: DM, pancreatic abscess, pseudocyst, common bile duct stricture, steatorrhea, malnutrition, PUD, and narcotic addiction.

4. Diagnostic Studies

ACUTE PANCREATITIS
- Elevated serum amylase and lipase greater than three times the upper limit of normal. Lipase is the most accurate enzyme for acute pancreatitis.
- Leukocytosis (10,000–30,000 per μL) in acute pancreatitis.
- Hyperglycemia, hypocalcemia, hyperbilirubinemia, hypertriglyceridemia, proteinuria, glycosuria, abnormal coagulation studies, elevated blood urea nitrogen (BUN), and serum ALK-P.
- Pancreatic insufficiency suggested by excess fecal fat in stool and confirmed by response to pancreatic enzyme supplements or direct or indirect stimulation of pancreatic enzymes in chronic pancreatitis.
- Plain films of the abdomen may show nonspecific findings including gallstones, "sentinel loop," a segment of gas-filled small bowel in the left upper

quadrant or a "colon cutoff sign" where the gas-filled transverse colon ends abruptly because of pancreatic inflammation, although normal in >50% of patients with pancreatitis.

- Upper GI series may identify thickened duodenal folds, displaced stomach suggestive of pancreatic mass.
- CT scan is excellent for detailed visualization of the pancreas and surrounding tissue. Dynamic bolus CT scan can identify areas of pancreatic necrosis. CT-guided biopsy of necrotic area may disclose infection or malignancy.

5. Management

ACUTE PANCREATITIS

- Often responds well to bed rest, restricted solid or liquid oral feeding, nasogastric suctioning for patients with ileus or severe pain, and narcotics such as meperidine for pain control.
- Diet may be advanced to clear liquids when pain or ileus resolves.
- Surgical consult for all patients.
- Severe acute disease may require large amounts of IV fluids, infusions of serum albumin, or fresh frozen plasma.
- Monitor and treat complications.
- Antibiotics for documented infection.

CHRONIC PANCREATITIS

- Management is directed at controlling pain and malabsorption.
- Nonnarcotic drugs for pain relief, avoidance of alcohol and meals rich in fat, and pancreatic enzyme replacement.
- Endoscopic U/S is the most sensitive study to detect structural changes in chronic pancreatitis.
- Treat associated diabetes.
- Surgery consult for possible surgical or endoscopic treatment of persistent draining.

REVIEW QUESTIONS

1. A 35-year-old woman presents to the office with a 2-month history of recurrent postprandial substernal burning discomfort and sour regurgitation, usually in the morning. It is aggravated by bending forward and lying supine after eating. Her body mass index (BMI) is 31% and the rest of her physical examination is normal. What is the likely pathogenesis of her symptoms?

a) Gastric acid hypersecretion
b) New onset of a hiatal hernia
c) Decreased acid clearance; impaired peristalsis
d) LES relaxation
e) *H. pylori* infection

2. A 24-year-old overweight man presents with symptoms of heartburn over the past 2 weeks. Initial attempts to relieve the symptoms with Tums have not been successful. His history is negative for change in bowel habits, rectal bleeding, hematemesis, nausea, vomiting, and weight loss. On physical examination, there are no significant findings. Which of the following would include the next step in managing his symptoms?

a) EGD to exclude Barrett esophagus
b) Lifestyle modification
c) Initiation of a PPI medication
d) A, B, and C are correct
e) B and C are correct

3. A 75-year-old woman presents with substernal chest pain and odynophagia occurring over the past 2 days. She denies exertional dyspnea, nausea, vomiting, fever, chills, regurgitation, and change in bowel habits. Her medications include alendronate for osteoporosis and levothyroxine for hypothyroidism. Her physical examination is unremarkable. What is the likely cause of her symptoms?

a) Reflux esophagitis
b) Medication-induced esophagitis
c) Eosinophilic esophagitis
d) Esophageal spasm
e) Perforated esophagus

4. A 35-year-old patient presents to her primary care provider with gnawing epigastric pain and nausea occurring intermittently over the past 2 weeks. She reports taking ibuprofen daily for back pain. She notes that she feels better after eating. She denies melena, hematochezia, vomiting, and weight loss. Which of the following would be the next best step in the management of this patient?

a) Admit to hospital for monitoring
b) Start sucralfate and PPI medication
c) Urgent referral to GI for endoscopic evaluation
d) Change ibuprofen to Tylenol
e) Test for *H. pylori* infection

5. A 34-year-old woman presents with dysphagia occurring intermittently over several years. She feels the symptoms are progressively worsening occurring at times when swallowing liquids. Palliative factors include sitting up straighter while eating and moving her head back when swallowing. She admits to 10-lb weight loss over the last year, but denies hematochezia and melena. On physical examination, her vital signs are normal and there are no other significant findings. Which of the following would be the initial diagnostic test to further evaluate her symptoms?

a) EGD with esophageal brushings
b) Esophageal manometry
c) Upper GI barium swallow X-ray
d) A 24-hour esophageal pH monitor
e) Gastric emptying scan

6. An 18-year-old male college student presents with symptoms of bloody stools occurring intermittently over the past several weeks. He admits to loose stools, mucus, and crampy abdominal pain typically after eating. He denies fever, chills, nausea, vomiting, and significant weight loss. Laboratory studies reveal mild elevations in CRP and ESR, and a slight decrease in hemoglobin. Stool studies are negative for culture, *C. difficile*, ova, and parasites. Sigmoidoscopy reveals proctosigmoid bleeding, erythema, and friability. What is the most likely diagnosis?

   a) Infectious diarrhea
   b) Crohn disease
   c) IBS
   d) Internal hemorrhoidal flare
   e) UC

7. An elderly patient presents with a new onset of dysphagia with solids over the past month. He reports occasionally having to wait several minutes or drink water for food to move down into his stomach and describes food feeling stuck in his mid-sternum. He denies regurgitation, nausea, vomiting, abdominal pain, chest pain, and weight loss. Which of the following is the best initial test to evaluate his symptoms?

   a) EGD
   b) Barium esophagram
   c) Chest X-ray
   d) Videofluoroscopy

8. Which statement is true about *H. pylori* infection?

   a) It is a spiral gram-positive bacteria
   b) It is more common in industrialized societies
   c) It is a major cause of duodenal ulcers
   d) It is not associated with gastric cancer
   e) It causes increased acidity of the stomach

9. An 18-year-old woman presents with crampy abdominal discomfort and loose stools occurring intermittently for as long as she can remember. She was diagnosed with anxiety-related functional GI symptoms in the past. Family history includes a cousin with Crohn disease and her mother has IBS. Her thyroid workup was normal. Which is the definitive test to evaluate for celiac disease?

   a) Tissue transglutaminase IgA blood test
   b) Anti-gliadin antibody blood test
   c) Barium study with small bowel follow through
   d) A 72-hour stool test for fecal fat
   e) EGD with duodenal biopsy

10. A 52-year-old patient presents with left lower abdominal pain over the past 24 hours. She admits to feeling feverish and having chills. She has modified her diet and is eating more bland foods. She reports a slight alteration in bowel habits and mild dysuria but denies rectal bleeding. On physical examination, her vitals are as follows: temperature 101, pulse 90, respiratory rate (RR) 16, and blood pressure (BP) 146/85. She appears in mild distress. Abdominal examination reveals hypoactive bowel sounds and exquisite tenderness over the left lower abdomen with guarding. CBC reveals leukocytosis. Upper abdomen is clear with mildly increased WBCs, negative proteinuria, no hematuria. Which is the most likely diagnosis?

    a) IBS
    b) Crohn disease
    c) Ischemic bowel
    d) Urinary tract infection
    e) Diverticulitis

11. A patient is hospitalized with acute pancreatitis. Which of the following factors contribute to a more severe course and poorer patient outcomes?

    a) Elevated blood pressure
    b) Serum amylase levels higher than lipase
    c) Elevated BUN
    d) Age younger than 40
    e) Perceived intensity of abdominal pain

12. A 35-year-old woman presents with acute RUQ abdominal pain, nausea, and vomiting. On physical examination, her weight is 175 lb, height 64 in, temperature 99, heart rate 102, and BP 162/90, RR 18. She appears in distress. Her abdominal examination reveals normal bowel sounds in four quadrants and, tenderness in RUQ with a positive Murphy sign. Which of the following is the best test to confirm the diagnosis of acute cholecystitis?

    a) Abdominal U/S
    b) CT scan of abdomen and pelvis
    c) Kidney, ureter, and bladder (KUB) X-ray
    d) Abdominal flat plate
    e) Endoscopic retrograde cholangiopancreatography

ANSWERS TO REVIEW QUESTIONS

1. **Answer: D.** Three dominant mechanisms of esophagogastric junction incompetence are recognized: (1) transient LES relaxations (a vagovagal reflex in which LES relaxation is elicited by gastric distension), (2) LES hypotension, and (3) anatomic distortion of the esophagogastric junction inclusive of hiatus hernia. Factors tending to exacerbate reflux regardless of mechanism are abdominal obesity, pregnancy, gastric hypersecretory states, delayed gastric emptying, disruption of esophageal peristalsis, and gluttony. This patient has a high BMI adding to her risk factors for GERD. (From Kahrilas PJ, Hirano I. Diseases of the esophagus. In: Jameson J, Fauci AS, Kasper DL, Hauser SL, Longo DL, Loscalzo J, eds. *Harrison's Principles of Internal Medicine*. 19th ed. New York, NY: McGraw-Hill; 2014.) (Applying basic science concepts)

2. **Answer: E.** Aimed at eliminating the conditions noted in the differential diagnosis and documenting the type and extent of tissue damage. Generally, when symptoms

of GERD are typical and the patient responds to therapy, there is no need for further diagnostic tests to verify the diagnosis. (From Ferri FF. Gastroesophageal reflux disease. In: *Ferri's Clinical Advisor*. Edinburgh, Scotland: Elsevier; 2018:511–512, Figure E2.) (Clinical intervention)

3. **Answer: B**. Medication-induced esophagitis. Symptoms are usually acute and can occur immediately after ingestion of medication to as long as several hours later. Most patients present with retrosternal chest pain, odynophagia, and dysphagia, although hematemesis and melena have been reported from drug-induced esophageal damage. The sudden onset of severe retrosternal pain clearly exacerbated by swallowing should raise the possibility of pill esophagitis, even if medication has been taken correctly. When potentially caustic medications fail to rapidly transit into the stomach and remain in the esophagus, dissolving and releasing their noxious contents and damaging the esophageal wall, the resulting injury is called medication-induced esophagitis. To date, close to 100 different medications have been reported to induce esophageal disorders. Antibacterials such as doxycycline, tetracycline, and clindamycin are the offending agents in more than 50% of cases. Other commonly prescribed drugs that cause esophageal injury include naproxen, aspirin (acetylsalicylic acid), potassium chloride, ferrous sulfate, quinidine, alprenolol, alendronate, and various steroidal and nonsteroidal anti-inflammatory agents. (From Ferri FF. Gastroesophageal reflux disease. In: *Ferri's Clinical Advisor*. Edinburgh, Scotland: Elsevier; 2018:511. e3–512.e3.) (Formulating most likely diagnosis)

4. **Answer: B**. Disease: Peptic ulcer disease (PUD). Sucralfate is a complex aluminum salt of sulfated sucrose. When exposed to gastric acid, the sulfate anions can bind electrostatically to positively charged proteins in damaged tissue. Sucralfate (1 g four times daily) is equally effective for H_2RAs in healing duodenal ulcers (DUs) and is approved by the FDA in the United States for this indication. Very little (<5%) of sucralfate is absorbed owing to its poor solubility, and the drug is excreted in the feces. Because of its lack of systemic absorption, sucralfate appears to have no systemic toxicity. Current evidence indicates that PPIs are superior to standard-dose H_2RAs in healing NSAID-induced peptic ulcers. EGD is the procedure of choice for diagnosis of uncomplicated PUD. EGD is more sensitive and specific than radiologic studies, such as upper GI series with barium. In addition, it is necessary to stop the NSAID use. (From Chan FKL, Lau JYW. Peptic ulcer disease. In: Feldman M, Friedmand LS, Brandt LJ, eds. *Sleisenger and Fordtran's Gastrointestinal and Liver Disease*. Philadelphia, PA: Elsevier; 2016:884.e5–900.e5.) (Clinical intervention)

5. **Answer: C**. Achalasia is diagnosed by barium swallow X-ray and/or esophageal manometry; endoscopy has a relatively minor role other than to exclude pseudoachalasia. The barium swallow X-ray appearance is of a dilated esophagus with poor emptying, an air-fluid level, and tapering at the LES giving it a beak-like appearance.

Achalasia is a rare disease caused by loss of ganglion cells within the esophageal myenteric plexus with a population incidence of about 1:100,000 and usually presenting between ages 25 and 60. Long-standing achalasia is characterized by progressive dilatation and sigmoid deformity of the esophagus with hypertrophy of the LES. Clinical manifestations may include dysphagia, regurgitation, chest pain, and weight loss. Most patients report solid and liquid food dysphagia. (From Friedman S, Blumberg RS. Inflammatory Bowel Disease. In: Kasper D, Fauci A, Hauser S, Longo D, Jameson J, Loscalzo J, eds. *Harrison's Principles of Internal Medicine*. 19th ed. New York, NY: McGraw-Hill; 2014.) (Using laboratory and diagnostic studies)

6. **Answer: E**. UC. The major symptoms of UC are diarrhea, rectal bleeding, tenesmus, passage of mucus, and crampy abdominal pain. The severity of symptoms correlates with the extent of disease. Although UC can present acutely, symptoms usually have been present for weeks to months. Occasionally, diarrhea and bleeding are so intermittent and mild that the patient does not seek medical attention. Active disease can be associated with a rise in acute-phase reactants (CRP), platelet count, and ESR, and a decrease in hemoglobin. Fecal lactoferrin is a highly sensitive and specific marker for detecting intestinal inflammation. Sigmoidoscopy is used to assess disease activity and is usually performed before treatment. (From Friedman S, Blumberg RS. Inflammatory bowel disease. In: Kasper D, Fauci A, Hauser S, Longo D, Jameson J, Loscalzo J, eds. *Harrison's Principles of Internal Medicine*. 19th ed. New York, NY: McGraw-Hill; 2014.) (Formulating most likely diagnosis)

7. **Answer: B**. This patient is suffering from esophageal dysphagia. Since he is elderly, and this is the first experience with dysphagia, the initial test of choice would be the barium esophagram to exclude any obstructing lesions causing these symptoms. If there is only dysphagia to solids, this is more likely a result of a mechanical obstruction. With dysphagia to both solids and liquids, this suggests a motility disorder such as achalasia or diffuse esophageal spasm. If there is first dysphagia to solids and then to liquids, this can be caused by an obstruction such as a peptic stricture or a growing esophageal tumor. If there is intermittent dysphagia, particularly with certain foods, this is suggestive of a peptic stricture or a Schatzki ring. (From Sands BE. *Gastroenterology*. Chichester, England: John Wiley & Sons, Incorporated; 2014. ProQuest Ebook Central. https://ebookcentral-proquest-com.ezproxy2.library.drexel.edu.) (Using laboratory & diagnostic studies)

8. **Answer: C**. *H. pylori* is a spiral gram-negative urease-producing bacterium that can be found in the mucus coating the gastric mucosa or between the mucus layer and gastric epithelium. Multiple factors enable the bacterium to live in the hostile stomach acid environment, including its ability to produce urease, which helps alkalinize the surrounding pH. Infection with *H. pylori*

increases the risk of peptic ulcers and GI bleeding from 3- to 7-fold. *H. pylori* has been associated with the development of gastric adenocarcinoma and gastric mucosa–associated lymphoid tissue lymphoma. In 1994, the International Agency for Research on Cancer classified *H. pylori* as a group 1 carcinogen and a definite cause of gastric cancer in humans. (From Lew E. Peptic ulcer disease. In: Greenberger NJ, Blumberg RS, Burakoff R, eds. *Current Diagnosis & Treatment: Gastroenterology, Hepatology, & Endoscopy*. 3rd ed. New York, NY: McGraw-Hill; 2015.) (Applying basic science concepts)

9. **Answer: E**. Celiac disease is an immune-mediated gluten intolerance in genetically predisposed individuals in whom exposure to wheat, barley, rye, or triticale induces a characteristic, although not specific mucosal lesion that responds to dietary gluten withdrawal. Serologic tests are useful screening tests for celiac disease. Both the enzyme-linked immunosorbent assay–based IgA anti-tTGA and the immunofluorescent IgA anti-EMA tests are useful and have reported sensitivities of 90% to 98% and specificities of 90% to 98%. Mucosal intestinal biopsy of the bulb, the distal duodenum, or proximal jejunum, coupled with a clinical response to the dietary withdrawal of gluten, remains the gold standard for the diagnosis of celiac disease. (From Trier JS. Intestinal malabsorption. In: Greenberger NJ, Blumberg RS, Burakoff R, eds. *Current Diagnosis & Treatment: Gastroenterology, Hepatology, & Endoscopy*. 3rd ed. New York, NY: McGraw-Hill; 2015.) (Using laboratory & diagnostic studies)

10. **Answer: E**. Diverticulitis. Diverticula are acquired herniations of the colonic mucosa and submucosa through the muscularis propria. They occur most commonly in the sigmoid colon. Diverticular disease is the most common structural abnormality of the colon. Acute diverticulitis can be either complicated or uncomplicated. Diverticulitis should be suspected in a patient presenting with lower abdominal pain, fever, and leukocytosis and sometimes with urinary complaints if abscess is near the bladder. In the West, left lower quadrant pain is the most common complaint (70%). The onset is usually gradual, and the pain may be present for several days before the patient seeks medical attention. (From Travis AC. Diverticular disease of the colon. In: Greenberger NJ, Blumberg RS, Burakoff R, eds. *Current Diagnosis & Treatment: Gastroenterology, Hepatology, & Endoscopy*. 3rd ed. New York, NY: McGraw-Hill; 2015.) (Formulating most likely diagnosis)

11. **Answer: C**. Elevated BUN. Traditional severity indices such as acute physiologic assessment and chronic health evaluation (APACHE II) and Ranson criteria have not been as useful clinically because they are cumbersome, require collection of a large number of clinical and laboratory variables over 48 hours, and do not have acceptable positive and negative predictive value for severe acute pancreatitis. A more recently developed and widely validated clinical scoring system for use during the initial 24 hours of hospitalization for acute pancreatitis is the bedside index of severity in acute pancreatitis (BISAP). This five-factor scoring system assigns one point for the presence of each of the following, either at admission or during the initial 24 hours of hospitalization: **B**UN > 25 mg per dL, **I**mpaired mental status, **S**IRS, **A**ge > 60, and a **P**leural effusion. A score of ≥3 points has been associated with increased risk of mortality and complications such as necrosis as well as organ dysfunction. Patient-related risk factors for severe acute pancreatitis include older age (>60), obesity (basal metabolic index ≥ 30), and comorbid disease. In terms of prognostic indices, the persistence of systemic inflammatory response syndrome for >48 hours or any rise in BUN during the initial period of resuscitation indicate a poor prognosis marked by increased risk of in-hospital mortality. (From Conwell DL, Banks PA. Acute pancreatitis. In: Greenberger NJ, Blumberg RS, Burakoff R, eds. *Current Diagnosis & Treatment: Gastroenterology, Hepatology, & Endoscopy*. 3rd ed. New York, NY: McGraw-Hill; 2015.) (Health maintenance)

12. **Answer: A**. Ultrasonography of the RUQ is the method of choice for the diagnosis of gallbladder stones. Its sensitivity is greater than 95% for the detection of gallstones 1.5 mm or more in diameter. Complete imaging of the gallbladder in various planes or in at least two positions of the patient is mandatory. The characteristic finding is a mobile echogenic focus with an acoustic shadow within the gallbladder lumen that moves in a gravity-dependent manner with the patient's position. The gravity-dependent mobility of the echogenic foci allows differentiation from gallbladder polyps or carcinoma. Ultrasonography also offers information about the size of the gallbladder, the presence of a thickened gallbladder wall, and pericholecystic fluid (signs of acute cholecystitis). Ultrasonography has high sensitivity (94%) and specificity (78%) for the diagnosis of acute cholecystitis. (From Paumgartner G, Greenberger NJ. Gallstone disease. In: Greenberger NJ, Blumberg RS, Burakoff R, eds. *Current Diagnosis & Treatment: Gastroenterology, Hepatology, & Endoscopy*. 3rd ed. New York, NY: McGraw-Hill; 2016; 2015.) (Using laboratory and diagnostic studies)

SELECTED REFERENCES

Cheskin LJ. Constipation and diarrhea. In: Barker LR, Burton JR, Zieve PD, eds. *Principles of Ambulatory Medicine*. 4th ed. Baltimore, MD: Lippincott Williams & Wilkins; 1995:476–491.

Cheskin LJ. Diverticular disease of the colon. In: Barker LR, Burton JR, Zieve PD, eds. *Principles of Ambulatory Medicine*. 4th ed. Baltimore, MD: Lippincott Williams & Wilkins; 1995:499–502.

Cheskin LJ. Gastrointestinal bleeding. In: Barker LR, Burton JR, Zieve PD, eds. *Principles of Ambulatory Medicine*. 4th ed. Baltimore, MD: Lippincott Williams & Wilkins; 1995:469–476.

Dienstag JL, Isselbacher KJ. Acute hepatitis. In: Isselbacher KJ, Braunwald E, Wilson JD, et al, eds. *Harrison's Principles of Internal Medicine*. 13th ed. New York, NY: McGraw-Hill Inc; 1994:1458–1477.

Dienstag JL, Isselbacher KJ. Chronic hepatitis. In: Isselbacher KJ, Braunwald E, Wilson JD, et al, eds. *Harrison's Principles of Internal Medicine*. 13th ed. New York, NY: McGraw-Hill Inc; 1994:1478–1483. http://dynaweb.ebscohost.com/.

Friedman LS. Liver, biliary, and pancreas. In: Tierney LM, McPhee SJ, Papadakis MA, eds. *Current Medical Diagnosis and Treatment*. 46th ed. New York, NY: Lange Medical Books, McGraw-Hill; 2007.

Glickman RM. Inflammatory bowel disease. In: Isselbacher KJ, Braunwald E, Wilson JD, et al, eds. *Harrison's Principles of Internal Medicine*. 13th ed. New York, NY: McGraw-Hill Inc; 1994:1403–1416.

Goyal RK. Diseases of the esophagus. In: Isselbacher KJ, Braunwald E, Wilson JD, et al, eds. *Harrison's Principles of Internal Medicine*. 13th ed. New York, NY: McGraw-Hill Inc; 1994:1355–1363.

Greenberger NJ, Isselbacher KJ. Disorders of absorption. In: Isselbacher KJ, Braunwald E, Wilson JD, et al, eds. *Harrison's Principles of Internal Medicine*. 13th ed. New York, NY: McGraw-Hill Inc; 1994:1386–1403.

Greenberger NJ, Toskes PP, Isselbacher KJ. Acute and chronic pancreatitis. In: Isselbacher KJ, Braunwald E, Wilson JD, et al, eds. *Harrison's Principles of Internal Medicine*. 13th ed. New York, NY: McGraw-Hill Inc; 1994:1520–1532.

Huether SE. Structure and function of the digestive tract. In: McCance KL, Huether SE, Brashers VL, et al, eds. *Pathophysiology: The Biologic Basis for Disease in Adults and Children*. 6th ed. Maryland Heights, MO: Mosby Inc; 2010.

Katz PO. Disorders of the esophagus. In: Barker LR, Burton JR, Zieve PD, eds. *Principles of Ambulatory Medicine*. 4th ed. Baltimore, MD: Lippincott Williams & Wilkins; 1995:435–446.

Katz PO. Peptic ulcer disease. In: Barker LR, Burton JR, Zieve PD, eds. *Principles of Ambulatory Medicine*. 4th ed. Baltimore, MD: Lippincott Williams & Wilkins; 1995:456–468.

Kimmey MB, Silverstein FE. Gastrointestinal endoscopy. In: Isselbacher KJ, Braunwald E, Wilson JD, et al, eds. *Harrison's Principles of Internal Medicine*. 13th ed. New York, NY: McGraw-Hill Inc; 1994:1350–1355.

LaMont JT, Isselbacher KJ. Diseases of the small and large intestine. In: Isselbacher KJ, Braunwald E, Wilson JD, et al, eds. *Harrison's Principles of Internal Medicine*. 13th ed. New York, NY: McGraw-Hill Inc; 1994:1417–1424.

Lingappa VR. Gastrointestinal disease. In: McPhee SJ, Lingappa VR, Ganong WF, et al, eds. *Pathophysiology of Disease: An Introduction to Clinical Medicine*. 1st ed. Stamford, CT: Appleton & Lange; 1995:215–244.

Lingappa VR. Liver disease. In: McPhee SJ, Lingappa VR, Ganong WF, et al, eds. *Pathophysiology of Disease: An Introduction to Clinical Medicine*. 1st ed. Stamford, CT: Appleton & Lange; 1995:245–277.

Lok ASF, McMahon BJ. AASLD practice guidelines chronic hepatitis B: update 2009. *Hepatology*. 2009;50:661–662, 1–38.

Loyd RA, McClellan DA. Update on the evaluation and management of functional dyspepsia. *Am Fam Physician*. 2011;83(5):547–552.

McGuigan JE. Peptic ulcer and gastritis. In: Isselbacher KJ, Braunwald E, Wilson JD, et al, eds. *Harrison's Principles of Internal Medicine*. 13th ed. New York, NY: McGraw-Hill Inc; 1994:1363–1382.

McQuaid KR. Alimentary tract. In: Tierney LM, McPhee SJ, Papadakis MA, eds. *Current Medical Diagnosis and Treatment*. 46th ed. New York, NY: Lange Medical Books, McGraw-Hill; 2007.

McQuaid KR. Gastrointestinal disorders. In: Tierney LM, McPhee SJ, Papadakis MA, eds. *Current Medical Diagnosis and Treatment*. 50th ed. New York, NY: Lange Medical Books, McGraw-Hill; 2011.

Mezey E. Diseases of the liver. In: Barker LR, Burton JR, Zieve PD, eds. *Principles of Ambulatory Medicine*. 4th ed. Baltimore, MD: Lippincott Williams & Wilkins; 1995:507–517.

Papadakis MA, McPhee SJ, Rabow MW. eds. *Current Medical Diagnosis & Treatment*. New York, NY: McGraw-Hill; 2017:634.

Wong, RJ, Ayoub, WS. *Current Treatment Strategies for the Management of Chronic Hepatitis B Hospital Physician Gastroenterology*. 14th ed. Part 2. Wayne, Pennsylvania: Turner-White Communications Inc. http://www.hospitalphysician.com/pdf/brm_Gast_V14P2.pdf

Environmental Emergencies

5

Colleen M. Kennedy • Charles Stream

I. Venomous Bites and Stings
A. Reptile Bites
- An estimated 3 million bites and 150,000 deaths occur worldwide each year from venomous snakes.
- Approximately 6,000 bites each year, with approximately 2,000 of them from venomous snakes.
- The major venomous snakes of the world can be divided into three groups: Viperidae (vipers), Elapidae, and Hydrophiinae (sea snakes).
- Approximately 20 of the 120 snake species indigenous to North America are venomous and include pit vipers (Crotalinae subfamily of Viperidae) and coral snakes (Elapidae family). The crotaline snakes are represented by the rattlesnakes (*Crotalus* species), pygmy rattlesnakes, massauah (*Sistrurus* species), and the copperheads and water moccasins (*Agkistrodon* species).

1. Crotaline (Pit Viper) Bites
- The crotaline snakes are called pit vipers because of depressions or pits located midway between and below the level of the eye and nostril; the pits function as heat receptors that guide strikes at warm-blooded prey or predators.

a. Pathophysiology
- Crotaline venom is a complex enzyme mixture that causes local tissue injury, systemic vascular damage, hemolysis, fibrinolysis, and neuromuscular dysfunction.
- Hypovolemia, coagulopathy, cranial nerve weakness, respiratory failure, and altered mental status.

b. Clinical Features
- Fang marks; localized pain; and progressive edema, nausea, and vomiting; weakness; oral numbness or tingling of tongue and mouth; tachycardia; dizziness; and muscle fasciculation.
- Systemic effects with tachypnea, tachycardia, hypotension, and altered level of consciousness. In general, local swelling at the bite site becomes apparent within 15 to 30 minutes; but in some cases, it may not start for several hours.
- Edema may progress to involve an entire limb within an hour. Edema near an airway or in a muscle compartment may threaten life or limb without the presence of systemic effects.

c. Diagnosis
- Presence of fang marks and a history consistent with exposure to a snake plus evidence of tissue injury.
- Clinically, the injury may be manifested in three ways: local injury, coagulopathy, or systemically.
- The absence of any of these manifestations for a period of 8 to 12 hours after the bite indicates a dry bite.

d. Treatment
- Immediate transport to the emergency department.
- Tourniquets are contraindicated.
- Constriction bands may be of some use: an elastic bandage or a Penrose drain, rope, or a piece of clothing wrapped circumferentially above the bite, applied with enough tension to restrict superficial venous and lymphatic flow while maintaining distal pulses.
- Advanced life support as indicated.
- Rapid intravenous (IV) isotonic fluid infusion for hypotension.
- Supplemental oxygen.
- Limb immobilization continued during transport to reduce further venom absorption.
- Cleanse the wound area.
- Tetanus prophylaxis.
- Antivenom is the mainstay of therapy.

2. Coral Snake (Elapid) Bite
- North American coral snakes include the eastern coral snake (*Micrurus fulvius fulvius*), the Texas coral snake (*Micrurus fulvius tener*), and the Arizona (Sonoran) coral snake (*Micruroides euryoxanthus*).
- The eastern coral snake is found primarily in the southeast United States.
- The Texas and Arizona coral snakes are found primarily in the states that bear their names.
- Venom is primarily composed of neurotoxic components.

a. **Clinical Features**
  - Primary neurologic effects: salivation, dysarthria, diplopia, bulbar paralysis with ptosis, fixed and contracted pupils, dysphagia, dyspnea, and tremors and seizures.
  - Cause of death is paralysis of respiratory muscles. Signs and symptoms may be delayed up to 12 hours.

b. **Diagnosis**
  - Presence of fang marks and a history consistent with exposure to a snake.

c. **Treatment**
  - Hospital admission for observation.
  - Antivenin (*Micrurus fulvius*), administered to patients who have definitely been bitten because it may not be possible to prevent further effects or reverse effects that have already developed.
  - Respiratory monitoring.
  - Bites by the Sonoran coral snake are mild, and antivenom is not usually needed.

B. **Spider Bites**
 1. **Brown Recluse Spider Bites**
  a. **Etiology**
    - The brown recluse spider (*Loxosceles reclusa*) is one of the most common species found in the United States, with an endemic range in the south-central United States, from Texas to Georgia and Iowa to Louisiana.
    - Approximately 1-cm body, a tan to brown coloration, and a violin-shaped mark on its dorsal cephalothorax.
    - Prefers warm, dry areas such as abandoned buildings, woodpiles, and cellars.
  b. **Pathophysiology**
    - The venom of the brown recluse has multiple enzymes (hyaluronidase, alkaline phosphate, 5′-ribonucleotide phosphohydrolase, and sphingomyelinase D).
    - Sphingomyelinase D is the major enzyme responsible for necrosis.
    - Necrotic wounds are possible through neutrophil activation, platelet aggregation, and intravascular thrombosis.
  c. **Clinical Features**
    - Initial bite is painless, usually prohibiting definitive identification of the spider.
    - Most common manifestation is mild erythematous lesion that will become firm and heal over several days to weeks.
    - Occasionally, a more severe local reaction occurs, starting with mild to severe pain for several hours with discoloration within the first 24 hours.
    - This lesion may become necrotic over the next 3 to 4 days, with eschar formation by the end of the first week.

d. **Management**
  - Tetanus prophylaxis.
  - Analgesics.
  - Antibiotics when appropriate.
  - Surgery consult for lesions >2 cm.
  - Dapsone and hyperbaric treatment controversial.
  - Hospitalization for system reactions.

2. **Black Widow Spider Bites**
  a. **Etiology**
    - The black widow spider (*Latrodectus mactans*) is found in woodpiles, basements, garages, and sheds.
    - Classic orange-red hourglass-shaped marking.
    - Female spiders range in body size up to 1.5 cm in length, with leg spans of 4 to 5 cm.
    - The female spider will aggressively defend her web, particularly when guarding her eggs.
    - Most bites occur between April and October and are usually seen on the hands and forearm.
    - The male spider is approximately one-third the size of the female, lighter in color, and bite cannot penetrate human skin.
  b. **Pathophysiology**
    - Active component of the venom is α-latrotoxin, acting through a calcium-mediated mechanism leading predominately to the release of acetylcholine and norepinephrine from nerve terminals.
  c. **Clinical Features**
    - Initial bite is felt as a pinprick sensation at the bite site, followed by increasing local pain that may spread quickly to include the entire bitten extremity.
    - Erythema appears 20 to 60 minutes after the bite.
    - In two-thirds of bites, a small <5-mm erythematous macule develops.
    - In one-third of bites, initial erythema evolves into a larger "target lesion" with blanched center and surrounding erythema.
    - Patients may complain of cramping of the larger muscle groups (trunk, back, and abdomen), which becomes generalized and may be mistaken for a surgical abdomen.
    - Confirmatory testing is not available; however, the presence of the characteristic lesion in association with severe pain and muscle spasms is pathognomonic.
    - Patients may develop hypertension, and symptoms such as headache, nausea, diarrhea, diaphoresis, photophobia, and dyspnea.
  d. **Management**
    - Supportive care of airway, breathing, and circulation.
    - Cleanse the bite site.

- Pain and muscle spasm can be controlled with opioids and benzodiazepines.
- Severe envenomation admission is required for continued analgesia.
- Administration of *Latrodectus* antivenin often causes rapid resolution of symptoms and can shorten the course of illness.
- *Latrodectus* antivenin is administered by intramuscular (IM) injection. It is derived from horse serum and hypersensitivity reactions are possible.

C. Bee Stings (Hymenoptera)

1. Etiology
- Most allergic reactions occur from wasp, hornet, and yellow jacket stings.

2. Pathophysiology
- Venom composed of many substances.
- Histamine.
- Melittin causes degranulation of basophils and mast cells.

3. Clinical Features
- Local reaction:
  - Urticaria.
  - Pain.
  - Erythema.
  - Edema.
  - Pruritus.
- Systemic/anaphylactic reaction:
  - Urticaria.
  - Itchy eyes.
  - Cough.
  - Bronchospasm.
  - As the reaction progresses, patients may experience respiratory and cardiovascular failure.

4. Management
- Oral antihistamines.
- Analgesics.
- Steroids.
- Bronchospasm responds to inhaled albuterol.
- Hypotension should be treated with crystalloids; may require dopamine and epinephrine.
- Severe reactions require treatment with 1:1,000 epinephrine subcutaneously; 0.3 to 0.5 mL for an adult and 0.01 mL per kg for a child (0.3 mL maximum).
- Patients who experience hymenoptera reactions should be referred to an allergist and prescribed an EpiPen.

D. Marine Fauna Stings, Trauma, and Envenomation

1. Epidemiology
- There is little information on the epidemiology of marine injuries and envenomation.
- The most common envenomation incidents occurred with jellyfish stings.

- In the United States, thousands of cases of minor jelly fish stings occur yearly from *Physalia* (Portuguese man-of-war) and *Chrysaora* species.
- Of the 373 species of shark, 32 have been described in attacks on humans.
- Minor trauma is most frequently caused by coral cuts sustained underwater, usually involving the extremities.

2. Clinical Features
- Abrasions, puncture wounds, lacerations, and crush injuries.
- Shark bites are associated with substantial tissue loss, hemorrhagic shock, hypothermia, and near-drowning fatalities.
- Coral cuts are associated with local stinging, erythema, pruritus, and urticaria, which may progress to cellulitis secondary to potentially pathogenic bacteria.

3. Treatment
- Copious irrigation of the affected area and exploration and debridement of tissue.
- Supportive care for hemorrhagic shock, hypothermia, and anaphylaxis.
- Soft-tissue X-rays should be ordered to identify foreign bodies.
- Tetanus prophylaxis.
- Aerobic and anaerobic cultures should be obtained.
- Patients with grossly contaminated soft-tissue injuries should be started on antibiotic therapy that covers *Staphylococcus* and *Streptococcus* species; *Vibrio* species should be covered with a third-generation cephalosporin.

II. Near-Drowning

1. Definition
- Near-drowning is defined as survival longer than 24 hours after a submersion event.

2. Epidemiology
- In the United States, drowning is the fourth leading cause of accidental death overall and is the second leading cause of death in those younger than 15 years.
- There are an estimated over 500,000 submersion events per year in the United States.
- Near-drowning events also occur in pools, open bodies of water, toilets, buckets, and bathtubs.

3. Pathophysiology
- "Dry-drowning," occurs when there is laryngospasm, followed by hypoxia leading to loss of consciousness.
- "Wet-drowning," occurs more commonly, with aspiration of water into the lungs causing washout of pulmonary surfactant and resulting in diminished gas transfer across the alveoli, atelectasis, and ventilation perfusion mismatch. This leads to hypoxemia and metabolic acidosis.

4. Prehospital Treatment
- Rapid, cautious rescue.
- C-spine immobilization.
- Cardiopulmonary resuscitation.
- Supplemental oxygen.

5. Emergency Department
- Secure the airway, provide oxygen, and assist ventilation as necessary.
- Administer warmed isotonic IV fluids.
- Warming adjuncts (e.g., blankets, overhead warmers, and warming devices) should be used.
- If after 4 to 6 hours the patient still requires oxygen, has an abnormal pulmonary examination (rales, rhonchi, wheeze retractions, etc.), or deteriorates in the emergency department, reassessment and admission or transfer to a monitored bed is needed.
- All near-drowning victims who require emergency department resuscitation should be admitted to an intensive care unit for continuous cardiopulmonary and frequent neurologic monitoring.

III. Lightning Injuries

1. Epidemiology
- Approximately 300 lightning injuries occur each year in the United States, of which there are about 100 deaths; the U.S. locations with the greatest numbers of incidents include Arizona, Arkansas, Florida, Mississippi, New Mexico, and Wyoming.

2. Pathophysiology
- Lightning is a high-voltage direct current (DC) discharge of energy.
- Mechanisms of lightning strikes: direct strike, side flash—when a nearby object is struck and current passes through the air; contact strike—when an object the person is carrying is struck; ground current—when lightning hits the ground and is transferred to a person.
- Cardiac arrest from DC depolarization of the myocardium causing asystole and respiratory arrest secondary to depolarization of the medullary respiratory center.

3. Clinical Features
- Varying level of mental status.
- Dysrhythmias.
- Burns.
- Cataracts, retinal detachment, corneal lesions, macular degeneration.
- Myoglobinuria.
- Fetal death, placental abruption.

4. Treatment
- Advanced cardiac life support (ACLS) resuscitation for cardiac and respiratory arrest and cardiac dysrhythmias.
- C-spine immobilization.
- IV access.

- Tetanus prophylaxis.
- Hospital admission for close cardiac and neurologic monitoring.

IV. Carbon Monoxide Poisoning

1. Epidemiology
- Carbon monoxide (CO) poisoning is responsible for greater morbidity and mortality than any other toxin.
- CO is formed from the incomplete combustion of any fossil fuel.
- Exposure is more common in northern climates during colder months.

2. Pathophysiology
- CO is an odorless, colorless, nonirritating gas.
- Clinical manifestations can develop with levels as low as 200 parts per million.
- CO binds to hemoglobin about 240 times greater than oxygen.
- Poisoning of the myocardial myoglobin causes decrease in contractility, cardiac output, and oxygen delivery.

3. Clinical Features
- Fatigue.
- Malaise.
- Flu-like symptoms; nausea, vomiting.
- Altering variances of level of consciousness.
- Seizures.
- Hypotension.
- Respiratory arrest.
- Myocardial ischemia/arrest.

4. Diagnosis
- Elevated COHb levels.
- Pulse oximetry.
- Chest radiographs.

5. Emergency Department Treatment
- Attention to airway, breathing, and circulation.
- High-flow 100% oxygen with a tight-fitting mask and reservoir.
- Hyperbaric oxygen therapy is indicated for severe poisoning.

V. Burns

A. Thermal Burns

1. Epidemiology
- There are more than 1 million burn injuries each year in the United States.
- Burn injuries account for:
  - 700,000 emergency department visits.
  - 45,000 hospitalizations.
  - 4,500 deaths.

2. Pathophysiology
- Severity of burn injury is related to the rate at which heat is transferred to the skin, resulting in varying degrees of coagulation, stasis, and hyperemia.

3. Clinical Features

- Burn size is calculated as the percentage of body surface area, either with the "rule of nines" or the Lund and Browder burn diagram.
- Burn depth is described in degrees: first, second, third, and fourth.
- Clinically, burns are classified as superficial partial-thickness, deep partial-thickness, and full-thickness burns.
- Superficial partial-thickness burns develop blisters and are painful; capillary refill is intact.
- Deep partial-thickness burns are white to yellow in color; two-point discrimination is diminished; capillary refill and pain sensation are absent.
- Full-thickness burns are charred, pale, and leathery in appearance.
- Smoke inhalation can develop into upper airway edema indicated by singed nasal hair, soot in the nose or mouth, carbonaceous sputum, and wheezing.
- CO poisoning should be suspected in all patients.

4. Diagnosis

- Chest radiograph for smoke inhalation–related injuries; may need to perform flexible fiber-optic bronchoscopy to confirm the diagnosis.
- COHb levels should be obtained.

5. Management

- Secure airway, breathing, and circulation.
- High-flow oxygen should be administered.
- Endotracheal intubation should be performed for patients who present with perioral burns, stridor, circumferential neck burns, altered mental status, or respiratory distress.
- Two large-bore IV lines.
- Fluid resuscitation directed by the Parkland formula.
- Foley catheter.
- Narcotic analgesia.
- Burns should be cooled either with cold water or with application of cool compresses.
- Escharotomy may need to be performed for circumferential burns.
- Hyperbaric oxygen therapy for those patients who have suffered smoke inhalation.
- Tetanus toxoid prophylaxis.

B. Chemical Burns

1. Epidemiology

- It is estimated that 5% to 10% of all U.S. burn center admissions are related to chemical burns.
- Common household offending agents are lye, disinfectants, paint removers, bleach, and sulfuric acid.

2. Pathophysiology

- Acid burns cause a coagulation necrosis with formation of a leathery eschar.
- Alkali burns result in a liquefaction necrosis that creates passage of hydroxyl ions into deep tissues.

3. Clinical Features

- Skin damage is dependent on the type of agent.
- Pain and tissue destruction.
- Acid burns produce dark brown or black skin discoloration.
- Alkali burns produce soft, gelatinous, brownish eschars; may progress to full-thickness burns.
- Chemical burns of the eye cause redness, pain, and tearing and are considered a medical emergency.

4. Diagnosis

- pH paper can help differentiate the difference between acid and alkali exposure to the eye.

5. Management

- Copious irrigation to the involved area.
- Ocular irrigation with 1 to 2 L of normal saline for a minimum of 1 hour, and a return of the pH to neutral (pH 7.4).
- Gluconate gel applied topically to skin.
- IV fluid resuscitation.
- Analgesia.
- Tetanus toxoid prophylaxis.

C. Electrical Burns

1. Epidemiology

- Electrocution is the fifth leading cause of fatal occupation injuries in the United States.
- Responsible for approximately 800 deaths annually.
- Household accidents are most common in children.

2. Pathophysiology

- Electricity causes damage by direct effects of current on cells, and thermal damage from the heat generated by the resistance of tissues.

3. Clinical Features

- Thermal burns.
- Cardiac arrest, ventricular fibrillation, arrhythmias.
- Hemorrhage, arterial and venous thrombosis, ischemia.
- Loss of consciousness, suppression of respiratory center, seizures, paralysis.
- Rhabdomyolysis.
- Myoglobinuria, renal failure.
- Cataracts.

4. Diagnosis

- Diagnosis is based on history of event and exposure.
- Elevated creatine kinase due to myocardial damage.
- Computed tomography (CT) scan of the head for those patients with severe head injury, coma, or varying altered mental status changes.
- Electrocardiogram (ECG) to rule out cardiac abnormalities.

5. Emergency Department Treatment

- Secure airway, breathing, and circulation.

- High-flow oxygen through air mask.
- Continuous cardiac monitoring.
- Blood pressure monitoring.
- Two large-bore IV lines; IV crystalloid fluid.
- ACLS as needed.
- Tetanus prophylaxis.
- Seizures are treated with standard therapy.
- General surgery consult for evidence of deep tissue injury.

VI. Mushroom and Plant Poisoning

1. Epidemiology
- Children account for 80% of all plant-related exposures, and mushroom poisonings are the most common.
- Ninety-five percent of fatalities associated with mushrooms in the United States are due to the *Amanita* species.

2. Pathophysiology
- The toxins in plants and mushrooms produce physiologic symptoms, ranging from gastrointestinal (GI) and neurologic to organ failure and death.
- Toxins
  - Psilocybin and psilocin: neuroactive chemicals producing hallucinogenic effects similar to lysergic acid diethylamide.
  - Ricin: cytotoxin causing multiple organ failure.
  - Gyromitrin: causes hepatic necrosis and inhibits the cytochrome P450 system.
  - Amatoxins: bind to hepatocytes and inhibit messenger RNA.
  - Amygdalin: metabolized to hydrocyanic acid leading to acute cyanide poisoning.

3. Clinical Features
- Toxicity from mushroom poisoning occurring within 1 hour of ingestion usually indicates a benign course.
- Toxicity caused by mushroom poisoning >6 hours following ingestion indicates a more severe prognosis.
- GI: abdominal pain, nausea, vomiting, hematemesis, and chemical burns to the oropharynx.
- Neurologic: seizures, delirium, hallucinations, and death.
- Cardiovascular: dysrhythmias, hypotension, and conduction defects.
- Dermatologic: contact dermatitis.
- Muscarinic and cholinergic effects.
- SLUDGE (*s*alivation, *l*acrimation, *u*rination, *d*efecation, *g*astrointestinal hypermobility, and *e*mesis) syndrome.

4. Diagnosis
- On the basis of history of ingestion and symptom onset.
- Cholinergic, anticholinergic involvement should be assessed on physical examination.

- Laboratory analysis should include electrolytes, creatinine, blood urea nitrogen, liver enzymes, and coagulation studies if poisoning is suspected.

5. Treatment
- Supportive care with attention to airway, breathing, and circulation.
- Activated charcoal to decontaminate the GI tract.
- High-dose penicillin or cimetidine therapy to block amatoxin uptake into the liver.
  - Penicillin G: 0.3 to 1.0 million units/kg/day.
- Cimetidine: 10 g per day.
- Bowel irrigation.
- Liver transplant when aspartate aminotransferase is >2,000 IU, prothrombin time >50 seconds, or grade 2 hepatic encephalopathy.
- High-dose pyridoxine (25 mg per kg) with neurologic symptoms associated with exposure to gyromitrin.
- Atropine for severe muscarinic effects.
- Orellanine toxicity requires fluid and electrolyte replacement and hemodialysis.
- Amatoxin, gyromitrin, or orellanine exposure requires admission for at least 48 hours; otherwise, if asymptomatic after 4 to 6 hours of treatment, can be discharged.

VII. Cold Emergencies

A. Hypothermia

1. Epidemiology
- Defined as a core temperature of <35° C (95° F).
- More than 700 people die each year in the United States as a result of hypothermia.

2. Pathophysiology
- Hypothermia is a result of heat loss by conduction, convection, radiation, or evaporation.
- Exposure to cold environments, slowed metabolic rate, sepsis, depressed central nervous system (CNS), and drug use can predispose hypothermia.

3. Etiology
- Environmental.
- Metabolic.
- Hypothalamic and CNS dysfunction.
- Drug induced.
- Sepsis.

4. Clinical Features
- Abnormally low body temperature.
- Drowsiness that may progress to confusion, lethargy, and coma.
- Bradycardia.
- Bradypnea.
- Shivering.
- Weakness.
- Discolored (purple) fingers and toes.
- ECG changes in hypothermia:
  - T-wave inversions.
  - PR, QRS, QT prolongation.
  - Osborn (J) wave.

- Dysrhythmias: sinus bradycardia, atrial fibrillation or flutter, nodal rhythms, atrioventricular block, premature ventricular contraction (PVCs), ventricular fibrillation, asystole.

5. Treatment
- Gentle rewarming techniques.
- Aggressive handling can precipitate ventricular fibrillation.
- Airway and cardiac support as necessary.
- Warmed IV fluids.
- Thiamine-depleted patients (alcoholics) should be administered IV thiamine 50 mg.
- Respiratory and cardiac monitoring.

B. Frostbite

1. Epidemiology
- Elderly, alcoholic abuse, homeless, and the psychiatric populations are at increased risk.

2. Pathophysiology
- Hypothermia causes increased blood viscosity, extracellular ice formation, intracellular dehydration, and lysis leading to progressive tissue loss.

3. Clinical Features
- Early symptoms: shivering, weakness, fatigue, drowsiness, lethargy, and impaired coordination.
- Later findings: bradycardia, hypotension, and hypoventilation.
- Rhabdomyolysis, acute renal failure.
- ECG may show PR, QRS, and QT interval prolongations and Osborn J waves.
- First-degree frostbite: edema, burning, erythema, stinging, and burning.
- Second-degree frostbite: same as above plus blistering.
- Third-degree frostbite: involves deeper layers of skin; hemorrhagic blisters, necrosis, and blue-gray discoloration.
- Fourth-degree frostbite: involves deep tissue injuries of the subcutaneous tissue, muscle, and bone.

4. Diagnosis
- Hypothermia is diagnosed when the core body temperature is below 35° C or 95° F.

5. Emergency Department Treatment
- Rapid rewarming with water at 107° F.
- Narcotic pain control.
- Penicillin G 500,000 units every 6 hours for 48 to 72 hours.
- Clear blisters can be debrided; hemorrhagic blisters should be left intact.
- Airway, breathing, and circulation.
- ECG.
- Suspected thiamine depletion should receive thiamine 100 mg IV or IM.
- Suspected hypothyroidism should receive IV thyroxine and hydrocortisone 100 mg.
- More aggressive rewarming may need to be performed through gastric, bladder, peritoneal, and pleural lavage.

- Hospital admission for any patient suffering more than superficial frostbite and hypothermia.

VIII. Heat Emergencies

1. Epidemiology
- Four hundred deaths annually in the United States.
- Children and elderly individuals are at an increased risk.

2. Pathophysiology
- Evaporation is the primary mechanism for heat dissipation in a hot environment.
- Exposure to heat stress augments cardiac output, circulation is shifted to the peripheral circulation, vasodilatation occurs, and sweating is enhanced.
- Heat stroke causes endothelial injury, coagulation disorders, circulatory failure, and, ultimately, multiorgan failure.

3. Clinical Features
- Core temperature ranges from 40° to 47° C.
- Neurologic abnormalities: ataxia, confusion, agitation, seizures, coma.
- Anhidrosis may be present.
- Lactic acidosis.

4. Diagnosis
- Diagnosis should be considered in the setting of heat stress, hyperthermia, and altered mental status.

5. Emergency Department Treatment
- Airway, breathing, and circulation.
- High-flow supplemental oxygen.
- Monitor core temperature.
- Rehydrate with normal saline or lactated Ringer.
- Cooling of the patient with fans and spraying the body with tepid water.
- Benzodiazepines for seizures.
- Check electrolytes every few hours.
- Hospital admission.

A. Heat Cramps
- Painful spontaneous contraction of the skeletal muscles.
- Occur during physical activity or after vigorous activity.
- Treatment includes oral or IV fluid and salt replacement in a cool location.

B. Heat Exhaustion
- Can occur by two different means, but is often a combination of water depletion and sodium depletion.
- Water depletion occurs when it is hot and there is insufficient water intake or supply.
- Sodium depletion occurs when fluid losses are replaced with significant amounts of isotonic fluids.

1. Clinical Features
- Core body temperature is normal or below 40° C.

- Nausea, vomiting, lightheadedness, headache, tachycardia, and orthostatic hypotension.
- Neurologically intact.
- Electrolyte and hematologic findings are variable depending on the degree of fluid and electrolyte losses.

2. Emergency Department Treatment

- Fluid and electrolyte replacement either orally or intravenously.
- Admission is recommended when critical electrolyte imbalances exist or in patients with congestive heart failure secondary to the time needed to amend the electrolyte and/or fluid deficiencies.
- May progress to heat stroke; therefore, if symptoms do not improve after 30 minutes of treatment, core temperature should be cooled to 39° C.

C. Heat Stroke

- Mortality rates as high as 80%.
- Fatal if untreated.
- Differentiation between exertional and nonexertional heat stroke is not necessary because treatment is identical and urgent.

1. Clinical Features

- Core body temperature >40° C.
- Include those seen in heat exhaustion along with confusion, inappropriate behaviors, hallucinations, seizures, hemiplegia, decorticate and decerebrate posture, and coma.
- Laboratory studies including complete blood count, comprehensive metabolic panel, creatine phosphokinase, arterial blood gas, coagulation profile, ECG, urinalysis chest radiographs, and head CT can assist in identifying end organ damage and ruling out other causes of the altered mental status.

2. Emergency Department Treatment

- Resuscitation including airway, breathing, and circulation. High-flow oxygen and rehydration with normal saline or lactated Ringer.
- Cooling of the patient with fans and spraying the body with tepid water.
- Hospital admission.

IX. Infectious Diseases

A. American Trypanosomiasis (Chagas Disease)

1. Etiology

- Protozoan *Trypanosoma cruzi*.
- Prevalent in Latin America northward to Texas.
- Vector is the assassin bug that is active in the evening hours.
- Leading cause of congestive heart failure in Latin America.

2. Clinical Features

- Acute illness lasts for 3 weeks to 3 months with fever, unilateral periorbital edema, lymphadenopathy, edema at the site of the bite, and hepatosplenomegaly.
- Latent phase with destruction of nerve cell ganglia causing cardiomyopathy, congestive heart failure, arrhythmias, and decreased GI performance.
- Peripheral blood smear or culture identifies the parasite in acute illness.
- Serology or muscle biopsy in the latent phase.

3. Treatment

- Nifurtimox orally four times daily for 90 to 120 days depending on age.

B. Human African Trypanosomiasis (African Sleeping Sickness)

1. Etiology

- Protozoan *Trypanosoma brucei gambiense* and *T. brucei rhodesiense*.
- Prevalent in South/Central America and sub-Saharan Africa.
- Vector is the tsetse fly.

2. Clinical Features

- Painless chancre 2 to 3 days after bite that increases in size and resolves after 2 to 3 weeks.
- Fever, fatigue, wasting, changes in behavior, encephalitis, anemia, pancarditis, coma, and death.
- Diagnosis is completed with peripheral blood smears, aspiration of lymph nodes, bone marrow and cerebral spinal fluid examination.

3. Treatment

- Infectious disease consult.

C. Leishmaniosis

1. Etiology

- Protozoan.
- Prevalent in Central/South America, Africa, Asia, and the Mediterranean.
- Vector is the sand fly.

2. Clinical Features

- Chronic, systemic disease including fever, wasting, pancytopenia, hepatosplenomegaly, and hypergammaglobulinemia.
- High fatality due to secondary infections including pneumonia, dysentery, and tuberculosis.

3. Treatment

- Infectious disease consult.

REVIEW QUESTIONS

1. Which of the following is contraindicated in the treatment of a pit viper bite?

   a) Tourniquet
   b) Constriction bands
   c) Rapid IV isotonic fluid infusion for hypotension
   d) Cleansing the wound area
   e) Tetanus prophylaxis

2. Which of the following should be completed for the management of marine fauna stings?

 a) Aerobic and anaerobic cultures
 b) Constriction bands
 c) Hyperbaric oxygen therapy
 d) Monitoring of liver enzymes

3. Which of the following accounts for 80% of all plant-related exposures and mushroom poisonings?

 a) Children
 b) Adults
 c) Adolescents
 d) Geriatrics

4. Which of the following is associated with SLUDGE syndrome?

 a) Plant poisonings
 b) Electrical burns
 c) Hypothermia
 d) Black widow bite
 e) Pit viper bite

5. Which of the following presents with latent phase cardiomyopathy, congestive heart failure, arrhythmias, decreased GI performance?

 a) American Trypanosomiasis
 b) Human African Trypanosomiasis
 c) Leishmaniosis
 d) Brown recluse spider bite
 e) Marine fauna sting

ANSWERS TO REVIEW QUESTIONS

1. **Answer: B**. Constriction bands, such as a piece of clothing or thick rope wrapped above the bite, restrict superficial venous and lymphatic flow without sacrificing distal pulses and capillary flow and allow for delay in venom penetration. Tourniquets block arterial flow. (From Dart RC, White J. Reptile bites. In: Tintinalli JE, Stapczynski J, Ma O, Yealy DM, Meckler GD, Cline DM, eds. *Tintinalli's Emergency Medicine: A Comprehensive Study Guide*. 8th ed. New York, NY: McGraw-Hill; 2016. ISBN: 978-0-07-179476-3.)

2. **Answer: A**. Culture results can refine antibiotic treatment. Marine-associated infections are frequently diagnosed late because the history of marine exposure or injury is poorly recalled, and patients are often initially given inappropriate antibiotics, which potentially increase the morbidity of an already virulent infection. Patients with underlying conditions such as liver disease, immunosuppression, and diabetes are more susceptible to halophilic *Vibrio* infections. (From Devlin JJ, Knoop K. Marine trauma and envenomation. In: Tintinalli JE, Stapczynski J, Ma O, Yealy DM, Meckler GD, Cline DM, eds. *Tintinalli's Emergency Medicine: A Comprehensive Study Guide*. 8th ed. New York, NY: McGraw-Hill; 2016. ISBN: 978-0-07-179476-3.)

3. **Answer: A**. Mushrooms are a common toxic exposure, with >6,600 poisonous mushroom exposures and 6 deaths reported to poison control centers in 2012. More than half occur in children younger than 6 years. (From Brayer AF, Froula L. Mushroom poisoning. In: Tintinalli JE, Stapczynski J, Ma O, Yealy DM, Meckler GD, Cline DM, eds. *Tintinalli's Emergency Medicine: A Comprehensive Study Guide*. 8th ed. New York, NY: McGraw-Hill; 2016. ISBN: 978-0-07-179476-3.)

4. **Answer: A**. SLUDGE syndrome is a product of plant/mushroom ingestion. Patients with muscarinic ingestions can develop diaphoresis, muscle fasciculations, miosis, bradycardia, and bronchorrhea. Symptoms typically present within 30 minutes of ingestion and spontaneously resolve in 4 to 12 hours. (From Brayer AF, Froula L. Mushroom poisoning. In: Tintinalli JE, Stapczynski J, Ma O, Yealy DM, Meckler GD, Cline DM, eds. *Tintinalli's Emergency Medicine: A Comprehensive Study Guide*. 8th ed. New York, NY: McGraw-Hill; 2016. ISBN: 978-0-07-179476-3.)

5. **Answer: A**. During a long latent phase, nerve ganglia are destroyed, leading to cardiac complications including myocarditis, dysrhythmias, cardiomyopathy, and sudden death. Chagas-induced heart disease is the leading form of congestive heart failure in much of Latin America. GI complications are megaesophagus or megacolon. (From Venugopal R, D'Andrea S. Global travelers. In: Tintinalli JE, Stapczynski J, Ma O, Yealy DM, Meckler GD, Cline DM, eds. *Tintinalli's Emergency Medicine: A Comprehensive Study Guide*. 8th ed. New York, NY: McGraw-Hill; 2016. ISBN: 978-0-07-179476-3.)

SELECTED REFERENCE

Tintinalli JE, Stapczynski JS, Ma O, et al, eds. *Tintinalli's Emergency Medicine: A Comprehensive Study Guide*. 8th ed. New York: McGraw-Hill; 2016.

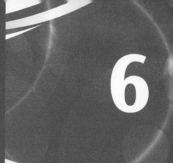

Geriatric Update

6

Matt Dane Baker • Michele Zawora

I. Demography of Aging
- Life expectancy in the United States has increased remarkably in the past century.
- Average life expectancy in 1900 was 47 years; current life expectancy is about 79 years. In 1947, about 4% of the population was ≥65 years; today, it is approximately 13%; and by 2020 it is estimated to be 25%.
- The elderly population is growing rapidly as a proportion of the U.S. population and is becoming more ethnically diverse.
- The fastest growing subgroup of the elderly population is the "oldest old," those older than 85 years.
- Women live approximately 5 years longer than do men.

II. Health Status of Seniors
- The majority of elderly individuals live in the community.
- The proportion of those ≥65 years living in nursing homes is small, around 5%.
- On average, older people visit a physician more often than do the general population.
- Seniors are hospitalized three times as often as the younger population, and their hospital stays are longer.
- Heart disease is the leading cause of death, followed by cancer.
- The rate of injury rises with aging, especially fall-related injury.
- Older people use twice as many prescription medications than do the general population.
- Many seniors have multiple chronic conditions: arthritis, hypertension, heart disease, diabetes, and hearing impairments.
- Most hospital admissions of older adults are for acute episodes of chronic conditions, such as heart failure.

III. Age-Related Changes
- Age changes the human body.
- Medical problems often present differently in seniors.

A. Physiologic Changes of Aging
- The rate of aging varies among individuals.
- Organs in the same person age at different rates.

1. **Homeostasis**
   - Deficits associated with aging are more apparent when an elderly person is challenged.
   - Seniors have limited physiologic reserve and, thus, can rapidly develop complications when they sustain injuries, develop common illnesses such as influenza, and are hospitalized.
2. **Control of Body Temperature**
   - Increased susceptibility to hypothermia and hyperthermia.
3. **Blood Pressure Regulation**
   - Higher risk for orthostatic (postural) hypotension (especially in those being treated for hypertension).
4. **Volume Regulation**
   - Higher risk for both volume depletion and volume overload.
   - Decreased reserves of body water.
   - Decreased thirst drive.
   - Renal impairments associated with aging.
5. **Renal System**
   - The number and size of nephrons and renal mass are decreased by 25% to 30% between ages 30 and 80.
   - Fat and fibrosis partly replace renal parenchyma.
   - Glomerular filtration rate (GFR) and creatinine clearance decrease with age (1 mL/minute/year after 40 years).
   - Serum creatinine does not change with age, but elderly people produce less creatinine because of decreased muscle mass. Therefore, serum creatinine is not a reliable measure of creatinine clearance because it underpredicts renal function.
   - For the purposes of estimating renal function or prescribing drugs, it is best to use the Modification of Diet in Renal Disease (MDRD) method to estimate GFR.
6. **Respiratory System**
   - Partial pressure of oxygen in arterial blood (PaO_2) decreases with age. Estimate of $PaO_2 = (100 - age)/3$.
   - Decreased chest wall compliance.
   - Increased usage of abdominal muscles.
   - Enlarged alveolar ducts due to loss of elastic tissue result in decreased surface area.

- Decreased forced vital capacity and forced expiratory volume.
- Decreased maximum consumption of oxygen (VO_{2max}) with age reflecting cardiac, respiratory, and peripheral muscle changes; and decreased level of fitness.

7. **Cardiovascular System**
   - Increased left ventricular wall mass.
   - Increased ventricular wall and aortic stiffness.
   - Decreased number of pacemaker cells in sinoatrial (SA) node.
   - Decreased ionotropic and chronotropic response adrenergic stimulation and exercise.

8. **Musculoskeletal**
   - Decreasing muscle and bone mass.

9. **Neurologic**
   - Brain atrophy.
   - Slowed reaction, learning, and retrieval time.

B. Host Defenses
1. **Aging Skin**
   - Skin is thinner, and more likely to sustain abrasions or pressure ulcers.
   - Skin changes can lead to infections or bacteremia.

2. **Respiratory**
   - Impairments in swallowing and cough reflex increase risk of aspiration and pneumonia.
   - Ciliary action is less effective. Decreased pulmonary functional reserves.

3. **Genitourinary**
   - Less prostatic fluid is present in urine, and prostatic fluid has fewer antibacterial antibodies.
   - Incomplete bladder emptying: permits bacterial overgrowth.

4. **Immune Responses**
   - Up to 25% of seniors who are clinically septic are afebrile.
   - Decreased response to vaccines.
   - Humoral antibody-mediated response is decreased.
   - Increased autoantibodies, not associated with autoimmune disease, which can cause false-positive tests for syphilis, rheumatoid arthritis, and lupus erythematosus.
   - Erythrocyte sedimentation rate increases with age.

IV. Geriatric Assessment
- Evaluation of biopsychosocial problems and functional disabilities to improve quality of life and functional status.
- **Assessment**
  - Physical assessment
    - Medical history.
    - Vision.
    - Hearing.
    - Continence.
    - Osteoporosis (OP).
    - Medications.
    - Nutritional assessment.
  - Cognitive assessment
    - Dementia.
    - Delirium.
  - Functional assessment
    - Mobility.
    - Fall risk and history.
  - Psychological assessment
    - Depression.
    - Anxiety.
  - Social assessment
    - Social supports/networks.
    - Quality-of-life assessment.
    - Goals of care and advanced care planning.
    - Home safety evaluation.
    - Elder abuse/neglect.
    - Economic factors, insurance coverage/benefits.
- Katz activities of daily living (ADLs): six basic ADLs—bathing, dressing, toileting, transferring, continence, and feeding.
- Instrumental activities of daily living (IADLs): six intermediate activities involving executive function—ability to use telephone, prepare meals, do housework, take medicine, use transportation, and manage own money. These are impaired earlier in the disease process than are ADLs in dementia.

V. Geriatric Syndromes
- Definition and description
  - Syndromes or diseases associated with elderly adults.
  - These conditions may affect quality of life as well as treatment of other morbidities, and lead to loss of independence.
  - Management: geriatric syndromes are often due to several problems and require a multidisciplinary health-team approach to be treated with success.

A. Hearing Loss
1. **Presbycusis: "Elderly Hearing" Loss; Age-Related Hearing Loss**
   - Common health problem in geriatric medicine.
   - Approximately 39% of those aged 65 or older report some hearing loss. Prevalence increases with each decade.
   - Bilateral high-frequency sensorineural hearing loss and decreased ability to understand speech secondary to hair cell degeneration.
   - Hearing loss is associated with social and emotional problems and cognitive impairment.

2. **Hearing Loss Types**
   a. **Sensorineural**
      - Due to damage to cochlea or fibers of eighth cranial nerve.
      - **Causes**
        - Presbycusis: most common in aging (loss begins in the higher frequencies).

- Noise exposure–related loss is also common.
- Less common: viral infection, trauma, vascular event, neoplasm (acoustic neuroma), autoimmune, Ménière syndrome, and certain drugs (aminoglycosides, chemotherapy, nonsteroidal anti-inflammatory drugs [NSAIDs], etc.).

  b. **Conductive**
  - Sound transmission through external or middle ear space damage.
  - Cerumen impaction is most common external ear cause in aging and is often the result of using cotton-tipped swabs to clean ear.
  - Other causes are otosclerosis, otitis media, and otitis externa.

  c. **Central Auditory Dysfunction**
  - Less common (loss of speech understanding in excess of that from hearing loss).
  - Involves the central nervous system (CNS): seen in dementia, Alzheimer, stroke, and neoplasm.

3. **Evaluation**
   - Ask about hearing problems.
   - Examine ear canal and tympanic membrane.
   - Whisper test: stand behind patient, 2 ft from the ear, cover the ear that is not tested, fully exhale, and whisper a question easy to answer or two-syllable words to be repeated.
   - Weber and Rinne tests can help distinguish between conductive and sensorineural hearing loss.
   - Audiometry: helps establish type and degree of loss of hearing.
   - Hearing is evaluated in decibels (dB) across a range of frequencies with tests of air and bone conduction.
   - Normal hearing (-10 to 15 dB), mild hearing loss (26–40 dB), moderate loss (41–55 dB), severe loss (56–90 dB), and profound loss (>90 dB).

4. **Management**
   - Avoid loud noises.
   - Cerumen removal.
   - Refer to ear, nose, and throat (otolaryngology/ENT) department and/or audiology.
   - Hearing aids: amplification improves communication and reduces hearing handicaps.
   - Assistive listening devices: small, portable pocket amplifiers are helpful in medical situations, especially in hospital setting.
   - Telephone devices.

B. Vision and Aging

1. **Definition and Description**
   - Vision impairment: visual acuity of 20/40 or worse.
   - Legal blindness (severe impairment): visual acuity 20/200 or worse.
   - Aging is associated with increased prevalence of visual impairment.

- **Leading causes of visual impairment**
  - Presbyopia: inability to focus on near items. Commonly begins in the mid-40s.
  - Cataract.
  - Age-related macular degeneration (ARMD).
  - Diabetic retinopathy.
  - Glaucoma.
- Vision impairment can cause loss of independence and decrease quality of life.

2. **Cataracts**
   - Definition: clouding and opacification of lens.
   - Seen on ophthalmoscopic examination.
   - Initial symptoms: decreased glare tolerance.
   - Eventual loss of color vision.
   - Risk factors: age, sun exposure, corticosteroids, diabetes mellitus (DM).
   - Management: refer to ophthalmology for surgical evaluation (extraction with intraocular lens implant).

3. **Age-Related Macular Degeneration**
   - Definition: damage and atrophy of cells in central (macular) region of retinal pigmented epithelium.
   - Prevalence: leading cause of blindness in elderly Caucasians.
   - Risk factors: age, sun exposure.
   - Results in loss of central vision.

   a. **Classification**
   - **Dry or atrophic ARMD**
     - Eighty percent of cases.
     - Patients see blurry dark spot in the center of visual field.
     - Degree of loss variable.
     - Only 10% experience severe loss or legal blindness.
     - Dry ARMD may change to wet ARMD.
   - **Wet or exudative ARMD**
     - Associated with more severe vision loss.
     - Due to subretinal neovascularization.
     - May lead to partial retinal detachment.
     - Suspect subretinal hemorrhage if individual with ARMD has sudden loss of vision, blurred vision, or new scotoma.

   b. **Management**
   - Refer to ophthalmologist.
   - Vitamin, zinc, and antioxidant supplements for dry ARMD.
   - Wet type: anti–vascular endothelial growth factor (VEGF) intraocular injections, photocoagulation.

4. **Glaucoma**
   - Definition: increased intraocular pressure (>21 mm Hg), cupping and atrophy of optic nerve head, and peripheral visual field loss.
   - Prevalence: leading cause of blindness in elderly African Americans.
   - Risk factors: age, African American race, and diabetes.

a. **Classification**
  - **Open-angle glaucoma**
    - Chronic low-level impairment to the drainage of aqueous flow from anterior chamber that leads to increased intraocular pressure and optic nerve damage.
    - More than 80% of cases of glaucoma.
    - Insidious disease.
  - **Narrow-angle glaucoma (acute angle-closure)**
    - Aqueous humor outflow is obstructed by narrow anterior chamber angle between the iris and the cornea.
    - Ten percent of cases of glaucoma.
    - Symptoms can include ocular erythema and pain, headache, nausea, visual distortion-halos, and steamy cornea.
    - Ocular pressures can rapidly become very high. This is an emergency situation.

b. **Management**
  - Open angle: medical—β-adrenergic blockers, sympathomimetics, and carbonic anhydrase inhibitors (not recommended in renal failure).
  - Narrow angle: emergency referral to ophthalmology. Surgical—laser trabeculoplasty, peripheral iridotomy, and iridectomy.

5. **Diabetic Retinopathy**
  - Definition: chronic disorder of retinal microvasculature.

  a. **Types**
    - Background retinopathy: microaneurysms, flame, and dot-and-blot hemorrhages.
    - Proliferative retinopathy: ischemia, neovascularization, retinal detachment, and vitreous hemorrhage.

  b. **Management**
    - Maximize long-term glycemic control.
    - Refer to ophthalmologist for annual checkup.
    - Prompt treatment of neovascularization with laser therapy.
    - Photocoagulation to avascular retinal areas to prevent neovascularization.

6. **Keratoconjunctivitis Sicca**
  - Definition: dry eyes.
  - Produces symptoms of burning, discomfort, or foreign-body sensation.

  a. **Etiology**
    - Tear secretion decreases with age.
    - Medications with anticholinergic side effects can cause dry eyes.
    - Connective tissue disorders, Sjögren syndrome, and lupus erythematosus are associated with dry eyes.

  b. **Management**
    - Discontinue unneeded medications with this adverse effect.

  - Adequate lubrication: artificial tears. Cyclosporine ophthalmic (Restasis) can be used.
  - New medication: Xiidra (lifitegrast) ophthalmic solution.

C. **Falls and Gait Disorder**
  1. **Definition and Description**
    - Falls: a person unintentionally descends to the ground or lower level; excludes falls associated with a major event such as a stroke or seizure.
    - Gait disorder: limitation in walking.
    - One in three adults ≥65 years will fall each year.
    - Complications from falls represent the leading cause of death from injury in those >65 years.
    - Falls and gait disorders are commonly caused by multiple factors.
    - Falls can be a nonspecific presentation for an acute illness in an elderly person.
    - Seventy-five percent of falls occur in the home.
    - **Falls can lead to:**
      - Death.
      - Fractures.
      - Immobility.
      - Subdural hematoma.
      - Nursing home admission.
      - Fear of falling and self-imposed functional limitations.
      - Decreased quality of life.
      - Increased social isolation and depression.
      - Increased direct and indirect costs of care.
      - Soft-tissue injury.
      - Accidental hypothermia.
  2. **Risk Factors for Falls**
    - Medications
      - Taking more than four medications.
      - Recent changes in medication.
      - Psychotropics: medication class most associated with falls (benzodiazepines, sedatives, antidepressants, and antipsychotics).
      - Class Ia antiarrhythmic medications.
      - Digoxin.
      - Diuretics.
      - Hypoglycemic.
      - Analgesics (especially narcotics).
    - Risk factors other than medications
      - History of previous falls.
      - Balance and gait abnormalities.
      - Dementia, cognitive impairment, or Parkinson disease.
      - Postural hypotension.
      - Cerebrovascular disease/accidents (CVAs and transient ischemic attacks [TIAs]).
      - Lower-extremity (LE) disabilities/weakness and foot disorders.
      - Proprioceptive deficiency.
      - Medical diseases.
      - Pain.

- Syncope.
- Vestibular dysfunction: vertigo.
- Visual disorders.
- Upper-extremity disabilities or weakness.
- High anxiety or depression.
- Arthritis.
- Vitamin D deficiency.
- B_{12} deficiency.
- Type of task preformed.
- Acute illness (e.g., sepsis).
- Environmental issues.

3. **Evaluation**
   - History: all elderly patients should be screened.
     - Ask about any falls in the past year, consider annual screening.
     - Specific questions:
     - Any history of falls?
     - Mechanism of fall?
     - Prodromal signs/symptoms?
     - Home evaluation: loose rugs, lighting, clutter?
     - Footwear?
   - Medications, particularly new medications or dose adjustments.
   - Vision and hearing.
   - Neurologic, to include strength, tone, sensation, proprioception, coordination, gait station.
   - Cardiovascular.
   - Lower-limb joints.
   - **Gait disorder and functional ability**
     - Observe patient's ability to get up from chair, turn, gait stability, mobility, and speed.
     - Tinetti gait evaluation and the "Get Up and Go Test" can be used: directly observe and time patient's ability to stand up from chair without using arms, walk 10 ft, turn, and then return to chair. Strong association between performing this task and person's ability to retain functional independence. Most adults can perform in 10 seconds or less. Consider referral for physical therapy (PT) evaluation if >14 seconds.
   - Functional Reach test: patient instructed to stand next to wall, with arm at 90° of flexion at shoulder with closed fist. Patient then reaches as far forward as possible without taking a step. Measure distance between end position and starting position. Most adults should score >10 in; 6 to 7 in represent limited functional balance.
4. **Management**
   - Decrease risk factors.
   - Review medications; if possible, decrease number and dosages.
   - Treat underlying diseases.
   - Address vision and hearing impairment.
   - Proper footwear.
   - Initiate physical therapy: balance and gait training, proper usage of assistive devices, request home physical therapy if needed by patient.

- Exercise program: Tai chi or a balance and gait training exercise.
- Treat OP: strengthen bone, but only for patients with Vitamin D Deficiency. USPSTF now does not recommend routine use of Vitamin D for this purpose.
- Vitamin D supplementation has been shown to decrease subsequent falls in those with a history of falls in patients in nursing homes.
- Hip protectors no longer recommended.
- Reduce environmental risks: consider home safety evaluation by home care nursing or occupational therapy.
  - Assess and make appropriate changes, such as removing electrical cords from walking areas, adding grab bars, raising toilet seats, improving lighting, reducing use of restraints.
  - **NOTE:** Restraints *do not* prevent serious injuries from falls.
- The American Geriatrics Association has produced updated guidelines (http://www.americangeriatrics. org/health_care_professionals/clinical_practice/ clinical_guidelines_recommendations/prevention_ of_falls_summary_of_recommendations).

D. Osteoporosis
1. **Definition and Description**
   - Loss of bone mass and deterioration of microarchitecture of bone tissue, which lead to increased fragility and increased risk of fractures.
   - Definition based on bone mineral density (BMD) measurements via dual energy X-ray absorptiometry (DEXA) scan.
     - T score > -1 reflects normal bone density.
     - T score between -1 and -2.5 is termed osteopenia
     - T score < -2.5 is termed osteoporosis.
   - Most common systemic skeletal disease. Up to two-thirds of patients may go undiagnosed.
   - Huge public health problem, associated with approximately 2 million fractures annually, loss of independence, psychological distress, and increased morbidity and mortality, decreased quality of life, increased rates of falls.
   - Bone is live tissue: we are always making bone (osteoblasts) and destroying bone (osteoclasts).
   - Bone is strongest and least likely to fracture at age 30 (peak bone density).
   - Rate of bone formation changes with age, with balance favoring increased resorption and decreased formation.
   - **Two types of bone—trabecular and cortical**
     - Spine: mostly trabecular bone.
     - Wrist (distal radius): mostly trabecular bone.
     - Hip (femur): trabecular and cortical bone.
     - **NOTE:** *Trabecular bone is very sensitive to estrogen loss.*

2. **Two Types of Primary Osteoporosis (Clinically Overlap)**
   - Type I: postmenopausal (~age 50) rapid loss of trabecular bone 3% to 5% per year during first 10 to 15 years following menopause. First site of bone loss is spine and wrist—distal radius.
   - Type II: aging-associated OP (less rapid bone loss)—0.5% to 3% per year in women and men approximately 65 years and older.
   - Associated with fractures of the hip (trabecular and cortical bone).
   - Mixed types I and II is common.

3. **Clinical Presentation**
   - OP is asymptomatic and does not cause pain until fractures occur.
   a. **Spinal Fractures**
      - Microfractures of spine: common, cause no pain or minimal pain.
      - Larger fractures can lead to collapse of vertebral bodies (compression fractures) and more pain.
      - Patients are rarely hospitalized for vertebral fractures.
      - Lead to loss of height of 2 or more inches.
      - Fractures heal irregularly: lead to dorsal kyphosis and scoliosis, and can cause discomfort or pain.
      - Cause gait abnormality, exhaustion, increased risk of falls; can decrease forced expiratory volume in 1 second (FEV_1) and increase risk of lung disease.
   b. **Wrist Fractures**
      - Fracture after a fall.
      - Wrist usually has a deformity confirmed by X-ray.
      - Orthopedic referral.
   c. **Hip Fractures**
      - Usually associated with a fall, but some fractures occur with weight bearing only.
      - Associated with pain, usually in groin with radiation to buttock.
      - External rotation and shortening of involved LE are common.
      - If clinically suspicious and negative X-ray, then magnetic resonance imaging (MRI) or computed tomography (CT) is indicated.
      - There is a 14% to 36% mortality rate 1 year after hip fracture.

4. **Risk Factors**
   - Intrinsic factors: increasing age, postmenopausal state in females, age >70 for males, decrease of 10% of weight, physical inactivity, previous fragility fracture Caucasian/Asian, thin (low body mass index [BMI]), family history, and early menopause (before age 45).
   - Behavioral/environmental: heavy alcohol consumption, smoking, excessive caffeine, excessive carbonated drinks (sodas), low calcium and vitamin D intake, malnutrition including anorexia, immobilization, and exercise-induced amenorrhea.
   - Medications: anticonvulsants (phenytoin, phenobarbital), corticosteroids, thyroid hormone, isoniazid (INH), aluminum containing antacids, loop diuretics, vitamin A and D excess, and methotrexate, heparin, calcineurin inhibitors, PPIs, selective serotonin-reuptake inhibitors (SSRIs).
   - Medical conditions (secondary OP): diabetes, renal disease, hyperthyroidism, primary hyperparathyroidism, Cushing disease, liver failure, gastrointestinal (GI) malabsorption, multiple myeloma, male hypogonadism, vitamin D insufficiency, idiopathic hypercalciuria, solid organ transplantation.

5. **Screening**
   - National Osteoporosis Foundation recommendations: assess risk factors for all postmenopausal females and all men ≥50 years.
   - USPSTF recommendations: BMD testing in all females ≥65 years with risk factors, "I" recommendation for men—insufficient evidence.

6. **Diagnosis**
   - Early recognition and prevention are important.
   - Consider diagnosis in any older adult with a fracture.
   - Conventional X-rays are insensitive: do not detect OP until 30% to 50% bone mass has been lost.
   - BMD is the best predictor of future fracture risk.
   - BMD can diagnose asymptomatic OP in women with risk factors.
   - **DEXA absorptiometry**
      - Diagnostic measure of choice.
      - Very low dose of radiation is used to measure spine, hip, and forearm.
      - DEXA results are reported in T- and Z-score.
      - Usually, lumbar spine and total hip are measured.
      - T score defines OP and its severity.
      - Density is compared with peak bone density (young healthy adult, 30 years old), same gender, and race.
   - **For each standard deviation below the peak mean, there is an approximate 2-fold increase in fracture risk:**
      - Normal bone density: T score—1 or more is better.
      - Mild osteopenia: T score—1 to 2.5 is below normal.
      - OP: T score—2.5 or more is below normal (2.5 standard deviations below peak).
   - Z-score: comparison of any given patient's bone density with mean age-matched bone density (comparison with same-age peers).

- Z-score does not define OP, but if patient deviates from his or her same-age peers, may need further evaluation for secondary OP.
- Quantitative CT scan can also be used.
- **Bone turnover markers (optional)**
  - Examples: urine *N*-telopeptide, pyridinium cross-links, and serum osteocalcin.
  - Used to monitor response to therapy; should decrease at least 35% within 3 months.
- Tests to exclude secondary cause of OP: electrolytes, blood urea nitrogen (BUN), creatinine, calcium, thyroid-stimulating hormone (TSH), liver function tests (LFTs), complete blood count (CBC), calcium, vitamin D 25-OH level, and alkaline phosphatase (ALP), serum phosphorus. If appropriate, serum and urine protein electrophoresis, parathyroid hormone (PTH), serum testosterone.
- Physical examination: height, weight, BMI, posture, mobility, functional status, nutritional status, signs of fracture, signs of secondary causes of OP.
- The Fracture Risk Assessment Tool (FRAX): free online tool to assess the 10-year fracture risk. There are some limitations on age, race, and ethnicity.

7. **Management**
   - When possible, decrease risk factors (alcohol, tobacco).
   - Exercise: weight-bearing and resistance exercises such as walking, dancing, running, jumping, and tennis. Goal = improve muscle mass, balance, and strength.
   - Sunlight 15 minutes, two times per week.
   - Nutritional: diet with 1,500 mg of elemental calcium for women after menopause and men aged 65 and older (includes food sources and calcium supplements if needed).
   - Calcium food sources: milk (1 cup = 300 mg calcium), yogurt, cheese, canned fish, broccoli, soy, kale, tofu, turnip, greens, some beans, orange juice with calcium supplementation.
   - **Calcium supplements**
     - Dosage depends on dietary intake.
     - Recommended: 1,000 mg daily premenopausal and 1,200 to 1,500 mg daily postmenopausal of elemental calcium in divided doses of 500 to 600 mg per dose.
     - Do not give to patients with hypercalcemia or hyperparathyroidism.
   - Vitamin D: most multivitamins contain 400 IU of vitamin D.
     - Men and women 51 to 70 years = goal is 600 IU daily.
     - Men and women > 70 years = goal is 800 IU daily.

8. **Therapies**
   a. **Bisphosphonates**
      - Examples: alendronate, risedronate, etidronate, ibandronate, pamidronate, and zoledronic acid.
      - Approved for prevention in postmenopausal women and treatment in both men and women.
      - Alendronate decreases fracture risk by 50% in women with preexisting fractures. Relatively contraindicated in gastroesophageal reflux disease (GERD). Adverse effects: nausea, heartburn, esophagitis, dysphagia, ulcers, constipation/diarrhea, atypical femur fractures, musculoskeletal pain, bisphosphonate-related osteonecrosis of the jaw (BRONJ), and question of increased risk of esophageal cancer. Many of the serious adverse effects are seen with the IV preparations (BRONJ) and with long-term use of 3 to 5 years or greater (BRONJ, atypical femur fractures, cancer of the esophagus).
   b. **Selective Estrogen Receptor Modulators**
      - Example: raloxifene.
      - Approved for OP prevention and treatment in postmenopausal women.
      - Estrogen agonist in bone and heart; estrogen antagonist in breast and uterine tissue.
      - Does not stop hot flashes. Does not increase risk of breast cancer. Increases risk of deep venous thrombosis (DVT).
      - Effect on mortality or other risks is not yet known.
   c. **Salmon Calcitonin**
      - Hormonal inhibitor of bone resorption.
      - Available intranasally, intravenously, or subcutaneously. May have analgesic effect in OP, particularly in compression fractures. Intranasal—alternate nostrils daily. Adverse effects: rhinitis and epistaxis. Injectable—adverse effects: allergic reactions—skin test.
      - U.S. Food and Drug Administration (FDA) recommends **against** use in postmenopausal women for treatment of OP due to increased breast cancer risk.
   d. **Hormone Replacement Therapy**
      - Estrogen replacement decreases fracture risk: associated with adverse effects such as increased risk of DVT, stroke, endometrial cancer, breast cancer, and so on.
      - Postmenopausal women taking estrogen and progesterone for 5 years have increased risk of DVT, stroke, invasive breast cancer, myocardial infarction, and pulmonary emboli (WHI—Women's Health Initiative).
      - Because of these risks, hormone replacement therapy (HRT) is not generally recommended for this indication.
      - USPSTF advises against use for prevention and treatment of OP.

e. **Teriparatide (Forteo)**
   - Recombinant human PTH. Indicated for moderate-to-severe disease (second-line agent).
   - Increases both bone formation and resorption.
   - Adverse reactions: nausea, HA, dizziness, leg cramps, hypercalcemia, and hypotension (seated first doses).
   - Risk osteosarcoma: rats. Black box warning. Avoid in Paget, with increased ALP, children and prior X-radiation therapy (XRT).

f. **Denosumab (Prolia)**
   - Monoclonal antibody, inhibition of RANKL.
   - Second-line agent; decreases bone turnover and increases BMD.
   - Adverse reactions: back/musculoskeletal pain, urinary tract infection (UTI), and increased cholesterol.

E. **Urinary Incontinence**
1. **Definition and Description**
   - Involuntary loss of urine.
   - Prevalence increases from age 65 and above: over 43% on noninstitutionalized adults >65 reporting some urinary leakage.
   - Can cause morbidity: cellulitis, sleep deprivation, falls, UTI, and increased long-term care (LTC) placement.
   - Associated with psychological distress and embarrassment, which can lead to social isolation.
   - Symptoms can range from occasional dribbling to continuous loss of urine.
   - Aging predisposes to incontinence, but does not cause incontinence.
   - **Age-related changes (present in both continent and incontinent elderly)**
     - Bladder capacity decreases.
     - Bladder (detrusor) smooth muscle replaced by fibrous connective tissues.
     - Bladder residual volume increases from impaired emptying.
     - Prostate size increases.
     - Estrogen decreases.
     - Urine output at night increases.
     - Involuntary contractions (detrusor overactivity) are common.
     - Urethral length in women decreases.
   - **Risks**
     - Female gender.
     - Aging.
     - Hospitalization.
     - Nursing home.
     - Other diseases (e.g., DM, CVA).
     - Impaired cognition, trouble with ADLs.
     - Chronic constipation.
     - Impaired mobility.
     - Cigarette smoking.

- **Acute incontinence etiologies (mnemonic DI-APPERS, usually reversible and multifactorial)**
  - **D**elirium and dementia.
  - **I**nfection (UTI).
  - **A**trophic vaginitis (urethritis).
  - **P**sychiatric.
  - **P**harmacologic. Examples: diuretics and narcotics.
  - **E**xcess output or endocrine: DM, diabetes insipidus, congestive heart failure (HF), LE edema, and hypercalcemia.
  - **R**estricted mobility.
  - **S**tool impaction.

2. **Types of Incontinence (Alone or in Combination) and Symptoms**
   a. **Stress Incontinence (Outlet Incontinence, Sphincter Incompetence)**
      - Female gender, small amount of urine loss with sneeze, laugh, and cough; sphincter/pelvic relaxation (estrogen loss, parity).
   b. **Urge or Urgency Incontinence (Detrusor Instability, "Overactive Bladder," Reflex or Spastic Incontinence)**
      - Urgency, frequency, moderate amount of urine loss, and abnormal stimulation.
      - Caused by inflammation, brain inhibitory dysfunction, and diuresis.
      - Most common type of incontinence.
   c. **Overflow Incontinence**
      - Decreased detrusor contractility (atonic or hypotonic bladder) or bladder outlet/urethral obstruction.
      - Reduced stream, difficult void: benign prostatic hyperplasia (BPH), neuropathy, fecal impaction, neoplasm, and anesthesia.
      - A postvoid residual volume of more than 400 mL indicates overflow incontinence is likely.
   d. **Functional Incontinence (Inability or Unwillingness)**
      - "Normal" genitourinary.
      - Mobility problems.
      - Delirium and dementia.
      - Medications or environmental factors.
   e. **Nocturnal Enuresis: Not Common in Elderly**
   f. **Mixed**
3. **Evaluation**
   - History: medical history (LUTS—lower urinary tract symptoms), voiding record.
   - Medications, including over the counter and alcohol.
   - Environmental evaluation.
   - **Physical**
     - Mental status/mobility: ADLs.
     - Neurologic.
     - Abdominal/gynecologic/genitourinary/rectal.

- Stress testing (standing with full bladder, single strain)—ask patient to cough.
- Postvoid residual: bedside. Can be done by straight catheter or ultrasound methods.
- Laboratory: urinalysis (UA), BUN, creatinine, electrolytes, glucose, calcium, vitamin B_{12}, consider prostate-specific antigen (PSA).

4. **Management**
  a. **General Management**
    - Treat transient causes first.
    - Avoid coffee, alcohol, and cigarettes.
    - Correct constipation.
    - **Kegel exercises: pelvic muscle exercises**
      - Pelvic floor muscles are squeezed for 10 seconds, squeeze is released, and exercise is repeated 10 to 20 times.
      - Exercise is performed three times a day.
      - Effective treatment if done consistently.
      - Good for all menopausal and postmenopausal women.
      - Also may help men with urinary leakage after prostate surgery.
      - Decrease evening intake of fluids.
  b. **Management by Type of Incontinence**
    - **Stress incontinence**
      - Kegel exercises: pelvic muscle exercises.
      - Drugs (be aware of side effects): adrenergics (pseudoephedrine) and estrogen.
      - Duloxetine (Cymbalta).
      - Imipramine (be aware of side effects—use low dose).
      - Pessaries: women with vaginal or uterine prolapse.
      - Surgery to reestablish angle.
    - **Urge incontinence**
      - Behavioral: bladder training and scheduled toileting.
      - Biofeedback.
      - Treat UTI.
      - Drugs (anticholinergics): be aware of side effects (e.g., confusion, constipation, and dry mouth).
      - Oxybutynin (Ditropan, Oxytrol Patch).
      - Tolterodine (Detrol).
      - Solifenacin succinate (Vesicare).
      - Darifenacin (Enablex).
      - Trospium (Sanctura).
      - Fesoterodine fumarate (Toviaz).
      - Mirabegron (Myrbetriq)
      - Tricyclic antidepressants: imipramine (low dose).
    - **Overflow/atonic obstruction incontinence**
      - Discontinue offending agent.
      - Drugs for atonic bladder (be aware of side effects): α-antagonists and cholinergics—bethanechol (Urecholine).
      - Drugs for BPH: α-blockers and 5α-reductase inhibitors.

- Catheter: as briefly as possible—can cause significant morbidity.
  - **Functional incontinence**
    - Treat psychological/alcohol/medical/mobility problems.
    - Pain relief if needed.
    - Physical/occupational therapy: assistive device, commode, and lighting.
    - Refer to urology or uro-gynecology as needed.

F. Dementia and Memory Loss
1. **Definition and Description**
  - Significant decline in two or more areas of cognitive functioning.
  a. **Alzheimer Dementia (AD) the Most Common Dementia**
    - Constitutes 60% to 70% of dementias (including mixed).
    - Affects possibly 5.3 million U.S. residents. By year 2040, number may rise as high as 14 million.
    - Disease prevalence increases after age 60.
    - Prevalence of 5% to 10% in people 65 years and older and nearly 50% in those 85 years and older.
    - Has a gradual onset and is slowly progressive.
    - Causes deterioration of memory, speech, judgment, and executive function. Motor function rarely affected.
    - Patient usually dies within 5 to 10 years: recent studies indicate survival of some up to 20 years.
    - Pathogenesis: amyloid plaques, tau neurofibrillary tangles.
  b. **Dementia with Lewy Bodies**
    - Second most common dementia.
    - Brain histology: Lewy bodies as seen in Parkinson disease.
    - Typically gradual onset and progression.
    - Pathogenesis: α-synuclein inclusion bodies.
    - Rigidity simultaneous with dementia.
    - Visual hallucinations and paranoid delusions are key features.
    - Affects memory and visuospatial function.
    - Changes in alertness and cognition.
    - Wandering.
    - Treatment: avoid neuroleptics/antipsychotics.
  c. **Vascular Dementia**
    - Fifteen to 20% of dementia cases often coexist with AD.
    - Due to multiple occlusions of small cerebral arteries causing small lacunar infractions.
    - May have sudden onset and progresses in stepwise increments.
    - Often causes abnormal gait and other focal neurologic abnormalities.

d. **Frontotemporal Dementia**
  - Gradual onset, earlier presentation in <60-year-olds.
  - Executive disinhibition, apathy, language deficits.
  - Memory is less of a concern in this type of dementia.
  - Pathogenesis: tau or ubiquitin plaques.

e. **Other Less Common Causes of Irreversible Dementia**
  - Parkinson disease, Pick disease, Huntington chorea, and Creutzfeldt–Jakob disease.

f. **Mild Cognitive Impairment, Mild Neurocognitive Disorder**
  - Memory impairment that is mild, and patient is able to function well.
  - Most will develop full dementia. Some believe that this as an early stage of dementia.
  - Recognize and monitor for cognitive decline.

2. **Risk Factors for Dementia**
  - Absolute risk factors: increasing age, family history, APOE4 allele and several other recognized genetic mutations, and Down syndrome.
  - Possible risk factors: past head trauma, fewer years of formal education, depression, cardiovascular risk factors (HTN, HL, DM, obesity).
  - APOE4 is associated with increased risk of late-onset AD, but also is present in many people without the disease.
  - Early-onset dementia: amyloid precursor proteins and presenilin proteins.

3. **Evaluation of Dementia**
  - History: from patient and informant.
    - Include: onset, comorbidities, medications, substance use/abuse, psychological history, living arrangements.
  - Physical and neurologic examination.
  - Assessment of functional status.
  - Assessment of mental status and cognition.
    - **Montreal cognitive assessment (MoCA) test**
      - Twelve items: orientation, recall, attention, naming, repetition, verbal fluency, abstraction, executive function, and visuospatial.
      - Assesses the following domains: orientation, recall, attention, naming, repetition, verbal fluency, abstraction, executive function, and visuospatial.
      - Available as a free download, in several different languages.
      - Normalizes for educational levels.
    - **Saint Louis University mental status (SLUMS) test**
      - Eleven items: orientation, recall, calculation, naming, attention, and executive function.

  - Assesses the following domains: orientation, recall, calculation, naming, attention, and executive function.
  - Available for free download.
- **Mini-cog test**
  - Quick, validated screening test for use in office.
  - Combines three-item delayed recall with a clock drawing test.
  - Evaluates visuospatial and executive function, along with recall.
  - Abnormal screen may be assessed with additional tests.
- **Mini-mental status examination (MMSE)**
  - Nineteen items: assess orientation, registration, attention, calculation, recall, three-step command, repetition, visuospatial, and language.
  - Assesses the following domains: orientation, registration, attention, calculation, recall, three-step command, repetition, visuospatial, and language.
  - Proprietary tool, cost for use.
  - Scores <24 of a possible 30 are highly correlated with cognitive loss.
  - MMSE results are influenced by prior educational level. If highly educated, patient will score higher than if lower level of education.
- **Animal naming test**
  - Name as many animals as you can in 1 minute.
  - Scoring equals number named in 1 minute.
  - Average performance is 18 in 1 minute.
  - Less than 12 is abnormal.
- **Clock drawing test**
  - Draw a 3-in circle and put numbers on clock.
  - Score by quadrants.
  - Ability to complete fourth quadrant is most sensitive for predicting dementia.
- **Seven-minute neurocognitive screen for AD**
  - Identifies patients with AD with MMSE of 24 or more as early AD.
  - Age and education are not significant factors. Screen for depression—common treatable morbidity in patients with dementia.
  - Laboratory testing to rule out reversible causes of dementia: CBC, vitamin B_{12}, TSH, serum calcium, ESR, RPR, electrolytes, and liver function and renal function tests.
  - Neuroimaging: noncontrast CT or MRI scan, when indicated (see below).
  - Neuropsychological testing: referral can be helpful if diagnosis is not clear; for example, early dementia or to distinguish from depression.
  - Newer biomarkers for β-amyloid accumulation and neuronal degeneration involving PET

scanning and lumber puncture, and genetic testing are available and used for investigation and predictive purposes, but are not yet widely recommended.

- **Signs and symptoms of AD:** Cognitive dysfunction (memory impairment, apraxia, and agnosia), aphasia, functional impairment (incontinence and inability to perform ADLs), behavioral manifestations (hallucinations, delusions, and agitation).
- **Imaging (noncontrast CT or MRI)**
  - Majority of patients do not require neuroimaging.
  - Consider in the following:
    - Onset of dementia < 65 years.
    - Sudden onset or rapidly progressive.
    - Focal/asymmetric findings on neurologic examination.
    - Findings consistent with normal pressure hydrocephalus.
    - Fall or head trauma.
    - Concern for tumor or CVA.

4. Management
- Goal: improve functional level, behavior, and mood.
- Treat medical conditions to maximize functioning. Example: control hypertension and hypercholesterolemia.
  a. **Cholinesterase Inhibitors for Mild-to-Moderate AD—Small Average Degree of Benefit**
    - Donepezil, galantamine, and rivastigmine.
    - May delay or slow progression.
    - No indication for widespread use in vascular dementia.
    - Rivastigmine may be beneficial with attention and behavioral symptoms in dementia with Lewy bodies.
    - Side effects increase with higher dosing.
    - Possible adverse effects: nausea/vomiting, diarrhea, dyspepsia, and anorexia.
  b. **Memantine—for Moderate to Advanced AD**
    - *N*-methyl-D-aspartate (NMDA) receptor antagonist.
    - Monotherapy or in combination with donepezil.
    - Modest benefit in agitation, ADLs, and behaviors in patients with AD.
    - Possible adverse effects: dizziness, confusion, headache, and constipation.
    - Not recommended in patients with severe renal impairment.
    - Follow patients' cognitive and functional status by caregiver reports and by test scores—MoCA, SLUMS, and MMSE.

  c. **Nonpharmacologic Management**
    - Moderate stimulation (overstimulation may cause confusion and agitation; understimulation may cause withdrawal).
    - Familiar surroundings: avoid changing residences.
    - Daily routines.
    - Cognitive rehabilitation/therapy.
    - Increase physical therapy.
    - Scheduled toileting and prompted voiding to reduce urinary incontinence.
    - Soothing music.
    - Family members providing reassurance to patients.
    - Regular health maintenance visits.
    - Family and caregiver support and education.
    - Environmental and home safety evaluation.
    - Discussion about driving and limitation.
    - Advanced care planning, living wills, durable power of attorney.

5. **Behavior Problems**
- Agitation: aggressive behavior, combativeness, and hyperactivity.
- Almost half of patients will experience periods of agitation.
- Less common is psychosis: paranoia, delusions, and hallucinations.
- First try nonpharmacologic management: environmental manipulation, focus on orientation.
- Always rule out delirium.
- Antipsychotic and antiseizure medications have been used. Need to use in very small doses, titrate up slowly, and watch for adverse reactions (extrapyramidal side effects, sedation, and CVA). Atypical antipsychotic agents (olanzapine and risperidone) may be better tolerated, but now carry an FDA black box warning that they are not approved for use in dementias and are to be used with caution because of possible increase in mortality from cardiovascular events and infection. Avoid benzodiazepines if possible.
- Antidepressants are used to treat patients with AD who have depressive symptoms.

6. **Caregiver Issues**
- Work closely, communicate, and educate family caregivers.
- Improve patient support services to avoid caregiver burnout. Refer to social worker if available.
- Recognize caregiver stress: 30% to 50% of caregivers for patients with dementia meet criteria for major depression as defined in *Diagnostic and Statistical Manual of Mental Disorders*, 5th edition (*DSM-5*). (Most are daughters and spouses.)
- Refer to AD support group.

G. Delirium

1. **Definition and Description**
   - Acute change in mental status characterized by inattention, fluctuating course in the day, altered level of consciousness, and disorganized thinking, confusion.
   - In 70-year-old hospitalized patients, delirium is experienced by:
     - One-third of those on general medical floor.
     - Three-fourth of those in intensive care unit (ICU) settings.
     - Almost 85% of those at end of life, termed "terminal delirium."
   - Fifteen to 41% of hospitalized elderly individuals have delirium.
   - Hospitalized patients with delirium have higher mortality rates than those without delirium.
   - Delirium is often not recognized in elderly patients. Less than 50% are properly identified, documented, and managed.
   - Postoperative delirium is common among elderly patients (up to 50%).
   - Intraoperative meperidine increases risk of delirium compared with other opioids.
   - Delirium in an elderly person can be a nonspecific presentation of an acute problem or illness (e.g., UTI and acute myocardial infarction).
   - Increases hospital length of stay by 60%.
   - Two-fold increase in mortality risk.
   - A 2.4-fold increased LTC placement.
   - A 12.5-fold increase in future dementia.

2. **Reversible Causes of Delirium**
   - Fever/infections.
   - Fluids/electrolyte imbalance.
   - Neurologic events: subdural hematoma and CVA.
   - Endocrine: diabetic ketoacidosis (DKA), hyperthyroidism, hypothyroidism, and Cushing disease.
   - Drugs: especially drugs with anticholinergic effects.
   - Organ dysfunction, for example, myocardial infarction, liver failure with hepatic encephalopathy, and uremia.
   - Nutrition: vitamin B_{12} and folate deficiency.
   - Trauma: fractures.
   - Sleep deprivation and environmental change.
   - Fecal impaction.
   - Urinary retention.
   - Hypoxia.
   - Perioperative hypotension.
   - Sensory deprivation and environmental change.
   - Alcohol: acute toxicity and withdrawal.
   - Medications.
   - Restraints.
   - Sensory impairment.

3. **Irreversible Risk Factors for Developing Delirium**
   - Dementia.
   - Advanced age.
   - Brain disease. Examples: stroke and Parkinson disease.
   - Functional impairments.
   - Comorbidities.

4. **Evaluation**
   - Recognition of syndrome is important.
   - **Obtain history**
     - Ask family members or caregivers if there is an acute change in patient's mental status and behavior.
     - Obtain baseline cognitive and functional levels.
     - Establish time course of symptoms, along with fluctuations.
     - Perform complete medication and substance review, check specifically for alcohol and benzodiazepine use.
     - Ask family members to bring all pill bottles patient uses.
     - Assess whether pain management is sufficient, especially in postoperative elderly patient with dementia.
   - Physical examination: include pulse oximetry, vital signs, neurologic evaluation, mental status examination, and rectal examination (rule out fecal impaction).
   - Routine laboratory studies (CBC, chemistry panel), electrocardiogram, pulse oximetry, chest X-ray, and, if indicated, vitamin B_{12}/folate, TSH, LFTs, CT (if suspect trauma or focal neurologic deficits), electroencephalogram, drug levels, and blood cultures.

5. **Management**
   - Treat underlying medical problem(s).
   - Keep patient in quiet, well-lit room.
   - Family members at bedside to provide reassurance and orientation.
   - Orientation: clock and calendar.
   - Use of personal eyeglasses and hearing aids.
   - Increase socialization and physical activity, as tolerated.
   - Ensure proper hydration and nutrition.
   - Identify and correct underlying causes: pain, infection, cardiac and pulmonary conditions.
   - **Pharmacologic**
     - For agitation and psychosis, low-dose Haldol PO or IM.
     - Start with 0.5 mg PO for most elderly patients.
     - Sedation is rapid, but full antipsychotic effect takes longer.
     - May cause hypotension and extrapyramidal effects.
     - If delirium because of alcohol or benzodiazepine withdrawal, use of benzodiazepines, such as lorazepam, may be indicated (in addition to thiamine and folic acid if alcohol problem).
     - Benzodiazepines may themselves cause delirium, and therefore it is desirable to taper them off slowly.

H. Depression

1. **Definition and Description**
   - Major depressive disorder: *DSM-5* criteria—five or more associated symptoms which are:
     - Depressed mood or irritable
     - Weight loss or gain (appetite).
     - Fatigue.
     - Guilt.
     - Psychomotor agitation or retardation.
     - Insomnia or hypersomnia.
     - Suicidal ideation.
     - Impaired ability to think or make decisions.
     - Mnemonic SIGECAPS: **S**leep disturbance; **I**nterest—decreased (anhedonia); **G**uilt; **E**nergy—fatigue; **C**oncentration—reduced; **Ap**petite—anorexia; **P**sychomotor—retardation or agitation; **S**uicide.
   - Minor depressive disorder: provisional category of *DSM-IV-TR* ("subsyndromal depression"—depressive symptoms, but not sufficient criteria for "major depressive disorder").
   - Particularly common in persons older than >75 years.
   - Clinical presentation may include medical complaints, preoccupation with poor health or functional disabilities, fatigue, poor concentration, and loss of interest or pleasure.
   - Older people are less likely to report disability.
   - Dysthymic disorder: chronic mild depressive disorder—present on more days than not for 2 years.
     - Less depressed mood and two associated symptoms: impaired ability to think or make decisions, fatigue, low self-esteem, appetite disturbance, insomnia or hypersomnia, or hopelessness.
   - Lifetime risk for major depressive disorder is 10% to 25% for women and 5% to 12% for men.
   - **Community-living older adults—15% have depressive symptoms:**
     - Major depressive disorder: 2% to 4%.
     - Minor depressive disorder: 10%.
     - Dysthymic disorder: remainder.
   - Minor depressive disorder accounts for greatest percentage of depression in older persons.
   - **Elderly depressed adults compared with younger depressed adults are more likely to:**
     - Not report depressed mood.
     - Not report feelings of guilt.
     - Express somatic complaints.
     - Suffer from comorbid conditions or cognitive disorder, which can interfere with the diagnosis and recognition of depression by health care providers.
   - Caucasian males 60 years and older are the group with highest rate of successful suicide in the United States.
   - One-third of older persons report loneliness as the main reason for considering suicide.
   - **Medical conditions associated with increased incidence of depression:**
     - Cerebrovascular disease: left frontal lobe is the location of strokes most often associated with depression.
     - AD.
     - Parkinson disease.
     - Endocrine.
     - Vitamin B_{12}/folate deficiency.
     - Autoimmune disorders.
     - Viral: HIV and hepatitis.
     - Chronic pain.
   - **Drugs associated with increased incidence of depression:**
     - β-Blockers, CNS drugs, benzodiazepines, major tranquilizers, steroids, NSAIDs, cimetidine, and centrally acting α_2-agonists (clonidine, methyldopa).
     - Alcohol.
   - Some elderly patients develop depression that mimics dementia ("pseudodementia") and improves completely or partially when depression is treated.
   - In 3 years, 43% of patients with pseudodementia are truly demented.

2. **Diagnosis**
   - History: include reports from family or caregivers.
   - Ask patient if he or she often feels sad or depressed.
   - Check if considered harming himself or herself.
   - Assess support systems available to patient.
   - **Physical**
     - Include evaluation of cognition: MMSE.
       - Neuropsychological testing can help distinguish depression from dementia, especially early AD.
       - Patients can have both depression and dementia at the same time.
     - Functional assessment: ADL and IADL.
     - Depression: Geriatric Depression Scale (GDS)—15 questions, a score of 5 or more suggests depression.
   - Review medications, including over-the-counter medication, medication borrowed from friends, and alcohol.
   - Laboratory studies.

3. **Management**
   - Treat comorbid conditions.
   - Review and adjust drugs as necessary.
   - If appropriate, bright light treatment.
   - Exercise: example, aerobic exercise.
   - Request physical therapy if appropriate.

- Social worker support services, evaluate need for home assistance, community centers.
- Psychotherapy.
- Pharmacotherapy (see Table 8–1).
- SSRIs, mixed serotonin/norepinephrine inhibitors, and tricyclic antidepressants are equally effective for treating major depression, although SSRIs may have fewer side effects, may be safer in overdose, and may be easier to titrate. These are generally recommended as first-line therapy.
- Saint John's wort is more efficacious than placebo.
  - Efficiency compared with tricyclic antidepressants needs to be established.
  - This treatment is not approved by the FDA. Dosages may vary.
  - Saint John's wort affects plasma concentration of drugs metabolized by cytochrome P450 system.
- Selection of antidepressant is based on side effects and tolerance.
- Adequate trial of an antidepressant in geriatric patient is 12 weeks of treatment.
- Titrate dose every 2 to 3 weeks.
- Tricyclic antidepressant therapy must be titrated more than SSRIs.
- If, however, patient shows no response or poor response at 6 weeks, antidepressant should be changed.
- Tricyclic antidepressant side effects (anticholinergic): dry mouth, constipation, blurred vision, dizziness, tremors, urinary retention.
  - Rarer adverse effects: orthostatic hypotension, cardiac arrhythmias, neuroleptic syndrome, decreased seizure threshold.
- SSRI side effects: GI upset, nausea, vomiting, diarrhea, headache insomnia.
- Approximately 35% of patients who discontinue antidepressant therapy will relapse within 6 months.
- Antidepressant therapy should be continued at same dose for at least 4 months after patient improves to avoid relapse.
- Electroconvulsive therapy (ECT) indications: severe depression requiring rapid improvement, severe depression that does not respond to antidepressants, inability to tolerate antidepressants, previous positive response to ECT, psychotic depression, depression in patients with Parkinson disease.
- Possible adverse effects: memory loss and confusion, arrhythmias, falls, aspiration, bronchospasm.
- Contraindications: increased intracranial pressure or tumor, recent myocardial infarction or CVA.

I. Pressure Ulcers

1. **Definition**
   - Lesions caused by pressure over bony prominences.
   - Also called decubitus ulcers or bed sores (old terms).
   - Sites will vary depending on the position of patient (e.g., sitting in wheelchair vs. supine).
   - Decreased local blood flow to area of contact causing ischemia and eventual necrosis.
   - Occurs in areas of bony prominences.

2. **Etiology**
   - **Factors that impair normal tissue perfusion, repair, and regeneration:**
     - Pressure.
     - Friction.
     - Shear.
     - Moisture.
     - Time in same position.
     - Anaerobic waste products.

3. **Epidemiology**
   - Affects 1 to 3 million adults annually.
   - Hospitalized patients: 8% to 25% over 3 weeks in bed- or chair-bound patients. Up to 50% in hip fracture and ICU.
   - Nursing facility residents: 1 year incidence of 13.2%, 2 year incidence of 21.6%. Mortality rate is two to six times greater than for a nursing home resident without a pressure ulcer.
   - Seventy percent of lesions develop in patients >70 years.

4. **Costs/Outcomes**
   - Decreased quality of life.
   - Increased hospital length of stay.
   - Increased risk of readmission.
   - Increased LTC use.
   - Increased mortality.

5. **Risk Factors**
   - Age.
   - Immobility.
   - Paralysis.
   - CVA.
   - Orthopedic problems.
   - Malnutrition: protein and calorie.
   - Dehydration.
   - Iron and vitamin deficiency.
   - Moisture: urinary incontinence, fecal incontinence, and perspiration.
   - Sensory impairment: neuropathy and dementia.
   - Depression.
   - Thin body habitus.
   - Dermatitis.
   - Edema.
   - Hypoperfusion (peripheral vascular disease).
   - Long-term corticosteroid use.
   - Friction/shear forces.
   - Use of medical devices.

6. **Risk Assessment**
   - Braden Scale Tool.
   - Validated tool to identify risk factors.
   - Includes: sensory perception, moisture, activity, mobility, friction, shear.

7. **Complications**
   - Cellulitis: *Pseudomonas aeruginosa, Providencia, Staphylococcus aureus, Bacteroides.*
   - Osteomyelitis.
   - Septicemia.
   - Abscess.
   - Sinus tracts and fistulas.
   - Tetanus.
   - Infestations.
   - Necrotizing fasciitis.
   - Fevers.
   - Pain.
   - Non-healing wounds.
8. **Evaluation**
   - History and physical examination.
   - Dietary history.
   - **Ulcer**
     - Location.
     - Size, length, width, depth, undermining, tunneling, odor, discharge.
     - Exudate: serous, sanguineous, and purulent.
     - Tissue/wound bed assessment: epithelial, granulation, necrotic, and eschar.
9. **Staging**
   - Stage I: nonblanchable erythema of intact skin.
   - Stage II: partial-thickness skin loss involving epidermis and/or dermis. Superficial. Vesicle, bulla, shallow open ulcer, intact or open blister, or abrasion.
   - Stage III: full thickness. Damage or necrosis of subcutaneous tissue may extend down to, but not through, fascia. Subcutaneous fat often visible. Deep crater. Eschar, exudate.
   - Stage IV: full-thickness skin loss with extensive necrosis or damage to muscle, tendon, or bone. Eschar. Exudate.
   - Unstageable: full-thickness loss with base of ulcer covered by eschar.
   - Suspected deep tissue injury: intact skin with ecchymosis or blood-filled vesicle.
10. **Prevention**
    - Reduce tissue pressure.
    - Use lifting devices.
    - Patient positioning: change frequently, at least Q15 minutes sitting and Q2 hours supine.
    - Avoid direct trochanteric and heel pressure.
    - Do not drag, raise head of bed, massage, or use donut cushions.
    - Skin care: keep clean and dry, barrier creams and continence care important.
    - Pressure-reducing devices: pillows—heel, sheepskin, wheelchair cushions, static flotation mattress—static, low air loss mattress—dynamic/alternating excellent, air fluidized mattress—dynamic excellent.
11. **Management**
    - Assess overall health and nutrition status of patient.
    - Assess and address psychosocial needs.
    - Treat underlying chronic diseases.
    - Address pain.
    - Reduce pressure and shear forces.
    - Control infection.
    - Control moisture: prevent maceration of surrounding tissue.
    - Dressings: many different types. Should be selected depending on the presence/absence of exudate/necrotic tissue and underlying wound bed assessment.
      - Types include: wet-to-dry gauze, hydrocolloid, semipermeable films, hydrogels, foams, alginates, collagen, silver dressings, enzymatic debridements, honey, and antiseptics.
    - Debridement: all necrotic tissue and eschar should be debrided.
      - One exclusion: eschar over heel wounds should be left in place.
    - Avoid cytotoxic agents (Betadine, hydrogen peroxide).
    - Keep wound moist, but surrounding skin dry.
    - Protect skin, prevent infection, and promote granulation.
    - Dry gauze: protection and absorbs exudate.
    - Nutritional support: albumen >3.5 g per dL, 30 to 35 kcal/kg/day with 1 to 2 g protein. Vitamins: zinc and vitamin C. Tube feedings, TPN.
    - Antibiotics: only in infection. No routine culture.
    - Agency for Healthcare Research and Quality guidelines.
    - Electrical stimulation therapy.
    - Negative pressure wound care.
    - Hyperbaric oxygen therapy.
12. **Prognosis**
    - Stages I and II: good.
    - Stages III and IV: poor.
13. **Referral**
    - Ostomy or wound care registered nurse (RN).
    - Occupational therapy for preventative devices.
    - General surgeon for debridement. Plastic surgeon for grafting.
    - Wound care center.

REVIEW QUESTIONS

1. Which of the following statements is true about the geriatric population?
   a) Average life expectancy is over 80 years old.
   b) Women and men are now living to about the same age.
   c) The majority of elderly people live in retirement communities.

d) Many elderly have multiple chronic conditions.

e) Most hospital admissions for older adults are due to falls.

2. Over the past several months, Mrs. Jones, an 85-year-old woman, has shown signs of missing meals, forgetting about pots on the stove, and difficulty managing her daily schedule. Her family members have reported these things to you as her health care provider. Your next step in her evaluation would be which of the following?

a) Refer her to neurology for follow up.

b) Order a CT of the brain to evaluate for space-occupying lesions.

c) Perform a cognitive assessment without the family present.

d) Evaluate her diet to ensure she is getting proper nutrition.

e) Arrange for in-home assistance with ADLs.

3. Mr. Frank is a 68-year-old Caucasian man who presents with symptoms of blurred vision over the past 3 weeks. He states that this is fairly constant and is worse when reading the newspaper to the point that he has not been reading the paper lately. He also notes that faces seems more blurry to him. His past medical history includes hypertension, COPD, GERD, and basal cell carcinoma on the nose. He takes lisinopril 20 mg, albuterol inhaler prn and pantoprazole daily. What is the most likely cause of his vision changes?

a) Presbyopia.

b) ARMD.

c) Medication causes.

d) Hypertensive retinopathy.

e) Glaucoma.

4. Mr. Melendez, a 72-year-old Hispanic man, presents to your office accompanied by his wife who complains that her husband is not participating in conversations with friends and has trouble hearing the television at a "normal" volume. He is a retired large equipment operator and has a past medical history of hypertension, type 2 diabetes, and obesity. His symptoms are most consistent with which of the following?

a) Sensorineural hearing loss.

b) Central hearing loss.

c) Conductive hearing loss.

d) Presbycusis.

e) Long-term use of Q-tips.

5. Mrs. Jackson, a 78-year-old African American woman, presents to the emergency department with right hip pain following a fall in her home. She reports a fairly active lifestyle, walking 2 to 3 miles daily and using the weight machines at her gym 2 to 3 days a week. She has a past medical history of asthma, hypertension, hypothyroidism, hyperlipidemia, and major depressive disorder. Her medications include albuterol inhaler prn, lisinopril 40 mg, amlodipine 10 mg, levothyroxine 75 μg, aspirin 81 mg, and sertraline 50 mg. She denies tobacco and

alcohol use. What is the most likely risk factor contributing to her fall?

a) Age.

b) More than four medications.

c) Living alone.

d) Thyroid condition.

e) Hypotension.

6. Mrs. Jones, a 76-year-old woman, returns to discuss the results of her recent test. Her DEXA T score was −3.0. What is the next step in management of this patient?

a) Ensure that she is following a regular exercise routine.

b) Encourage her to have adequate sun exposure for vitamin D.

c) Begin HRT.

d) Prescribe 1,500 mg of daily calcium supplement.

e) Begin bisphosphonate medication.

7. Mrs. Murphy, a 73-year-old woman, is brought to the primary care office by her daughter for evaluation of an acute change in mental status. She states she is confused and did not know who her daughter was or the time of day. Her daughter said she had an "accident" and soiled her clothing before coming to the office, which is new for her. She notes that her mother has also been having more problems with constipation lately. She denies substance use, new medications, fever, chills, nausea, and pain. On examination, she is a pleasant but disoriented elderly woman who appears her stated age. UA dipstick reveals cloudy urine with increased white cells, likely a UTI. What type of urinary incontinence would this causing her symptoms?

a) Stress.

b) Transient.

c) Urge.

d) Mixed.

e) Overflow.

8. Which of the following is an abnormal physiologic change associated with aging?

a) Development of actinic keratosis.

b) Reduced cognitive ability to perform two tasks at once.

c) Decline in maximal oxygen consumption or VO_{2max}.

d) Increased gastric-emptying time.

e) Less ability to tolerate extremes in temperature.

ANSWERS TO REVIEW QUESTIONS

1. **Answer: D**. Many seniors have multiple chronic conditions: arthritis (49%), hypertension (40%), heart disease (31%), diabetes, and hearing impairment.

2. **Answer: C**. "The use of cognitive screening instrument allows the clinician to demonstrate the presence and with longitudinal administrations, the course of deficits, objectively. Cognitive assessment should be conduction without the family present to avoid distractions and any potential embarrassment over failed items." (From

Soriano RP. *Fundamentals of Geriatric Medicine: A Case-Based Approach*. New York, NY: Springer Science and Business Media, LLC; 2007:217.) (Dementia; diagnostic evaluation)

3. **Answer: B**. There are two types of ARMD: the dry or atrophic type accounts for 90% of the new cases diagnosed, whereas the wet type accounts for the remaining 10%. Risk factors include smoking, light-colored irises, women over 60, family history, individuals taking antihypertensive drugs, and hyperlipidemia. Typical symptoms include blurred vision and dark spots in the center of the visual field. (From Soriano RP. *Fundamentals of Geriatric Medicine: A Case-Based Approach*. New York, NY: Springer Science and Business Media, LLC; 2007:149.) (ARMD; diagnosis)

4. **Answer: D**. Age-related hearing loss is manifested by deterioration in each of the two critical dimensions of hearing: reduction in threshold sensitivity and reduction in the ability to understand speech. The most common complaint with presbycusis is "I can't understand." The high-frequency hearing impairment causes certain consonants to be unintelligible. (From Soriano RP. *Fundamentals of Geriatric Medicine: A Case-Based Approach*. New York, NY: Springer Science and Business Media, LLC; 2007:153.) (Geriatric hearing loss; diagnosis)

5. **Answer: B**. Risk factors for falls include older age (>75), white race, housebound status, living alone, use of cane or walker, previous falls, acute illness, chronic conditions (especially neuromuscular disorders), medications (especially the use of four or more prescription drugs), cognitive impairment, reduced vision, difficulty rising from a chair, foot problems, neurologic changes, environmental hazards, decreased hearing, and risky behaviors. (From Fuller GF. Falls in the elderly. *Am Fam Physician*. 2000;61(7):2159–2168. https://www.aafp.org/afp/2000/0401/p2159.html.) (Falls in geriatric population; risk factors/etiology of falls)

6. **Answer: E**. "Alendronate, risedronate, zoledronic acid, and denosumab, which have been shown to reduce vertebral, nonvertebral, and hip fractures, should be offered to women with OP to help decrease their risk of experiencing a hip or vertebral fracture. This recommendation is supported by high-quality evidence of effectiveness in postmenopausal women. Calcium and vitamin D can be added as dietary supplements, but their effectiveness for preventing fractures is not known." (From Hauk L. Treatment of low BMD and OP to prevent fractures: updated guideline from the ACP. *Am Fam Physician*. 2018;97(5):352–353. https://www.aafp.org/afp/2018/0301/p352.html.) (Osteoporosis; diagnosis and treatment)

7. **Answer: B**. The first step in the evaluation is to identify transient or reversible causes of urinary incontinence. Reversible incontinence usually has a sudden onset and has been present for <6 weeks at the time of evaluation. The mnemonic DIAPPERS is useful for recalling the common reversible causes of urinary incontinence.

DIAPPERS stands for delirium, infection, atrophic vaginitis, pharmaceuticals, psychological disorder, excessive urine output (hyperglycemia), reduced mobility, stool impaction. (From Khandelwal C, Kistler C. Diagnosis of urinary incontinence. *Am Fam Physician*. 2013;87(8):543–550. https://www.aafp.org/afp/2013/0415/p543.html.) (Urinary incontinence; diagnosis)

8. **Answer: A**. Actinic keratoses are scaly lesions that develop mostly in sun-exposed areas of the skin. They are thought to be carcinoma in situ and can progress to squamous cell carcinoma. (From Mcintyre WJ, Downs MR, Bedwell SA. Treatment options for actinic keratoses. *Am Fam Physician*. 2007;76(5):667–671. https://www.aafp.org/afp/2007/0901/p667.html.) (Physiologic changes with aging; scientific concepts)

SELECTED REFERENCES

Agency for Healthcare Research and Quality. *Osteoporosis Guidelines*. Rockville, MD: National Guideline Clearinghouse. http://www.guideline.gov.

Alexopoulous GS, Meyers BS, Young RC, et al. The course of geriatric depression with "reversible dementia": a controlled study. *Am J Psychiatry*. 1993;150:1693–1699.

American Geriatrics Society; British Geriatrics Society; American Academy of Orthopedic Surgeons Panel on Falls Prevention. Guidelines for prevention of falls in older persons. *J Am Geriatr Soc*. 2001;49(5):666.

Beckman AT, Copeland JR, Prince MJ. Review of community prevalence of depression in later life. *Br J Psychiatry*. 1999;174:307–311.

Capezuti E, Stumpf NE, Evans LK, et al. The relationship between physical restraint removal and falls and injuries among nursing home residents. *J Gerontol A Biol Sci Med Sci*. 1998;53(1):M47–M52.

Cassel CK, Leipzig RM, Carson EB, et al, eds. *Geriatric Medicine: An Evidence-Based Approach*. 4th ed. New York, NY: Springer-Verlag; 2003.

CDC Steadi guidelines: Older Adult Fall Prevention. https://www.cdc.gov/steadi/index.html

Doody RS, Stevens, JC, Beck C, et al. Practice parameter: management of dementia (an evidence-based review). Report on the quality standards subcommittee of the American Academy of Neurology. *Neurology*. 2001;56:1154–1166.

Fantl J, Fanti JA, Kaschaknenman D, et al, eds. *Urinary Incontinence in Adults: Acute and Chronic Management*. Clinical Practical Guideline No. 2. AHCPR Publication No 96-0682. Rockville, MD: U.S. Department of Health and Human Services, Public Health Service, Agency for Healthcare Policy and Research; 1996.

Fillit HM, Kenneth K, Young J, eds. *Brocklehurst's Textbook of Geriatric Medicine and Gerontology*. 8th ed. Philadelphia, PA: Elsevier; 2017.

Folstein MF, Folstein SE, McHugh PR. Mini-mental state: a practical method for grading the cognitive state of patients for the clinician. *J Psychiatr Res*. 1975;12(3):189–198.

Glass RM. Treating depression as a recurrent or chronic disease [Editorial]. *JAMA*. 1999;281:83–84.

Hay-Smith EJC, Bø K, Berghmans LCM, et al. Pelvic floor muscle training for urinary incontinence in women (Cochrane Review). In: *The Cochrane Library*. Issue 3. Oxford, UK: Update Software; 2003.

Knopman DS, DeKosky ST, Cummings JL, et al. Practice parameter: diagnosis of dementia (an evidence-based review). Report on the Quality Standards Subcommittee of the American Academy of Neurology. *Neurology*. 2001;56:1143–1153.

Koenig HG, Meador KG. Dosing recommendations and prescribing patterns for depressed, medically ill, hospitalized older patients. *J Am Geriatr Soc.* 1997;45:1409.

Laveretsky H, Kumar A. Clinically significant non-major depression. *Am J Geriatr Psychiatry.* 2002;10(3):239–255.

Leipzig RM, Cumming RG, Tinetti MEI. Drugs and falls in older people: a systematic review and meta-analysis: I. Psychotropic drugs. *J Am Geriatr Soc.* 1999;47:30–39.

Lonergan E, Luxenberg J, Colford J. Haloperidol for agitation in dementia (Cochrane Review). In: *The Cochrane Library.* Issue 3. Oxford, UK: Update Software; 2003.

Mathias S, Nayak USL, Isaacs B. Balance in elderly patients: the "get-up and go" test. *Arch Phys Med Rehab.* 1986;67:387–389.

Mulrow CD, Williams JW Jr, Trivedi M, et al. Treatment of depression: newer pharmacotherapies. Evidence Report/Technology Assessment No. 7. AHCPR Publication No. 99-E014. Rockville, MD: Agency for Health Care Policy and Research; 1999. http://www.ahcpr.gov/clinic/depresumm.htm.

Nevitt MC. Falls in the elderly: risk factors and prevention. In: Masdeu JC, Sudarsky L, Wolfson L, eds. *Gait Disorders of Aging: Falls and Therapeutic Strategies.* Philadelphia, PA: Lippincott-Raven; 1997:13–36.

Petersen RC, Stevens JC, Ganguli M, et al. Practice parameter: early detection of dementia: mild cognitive impairment (an evidence-based review). Report on the Quality Standards Subcommittee of the American Academy of Neurology. *Neurology.* 2001;56:1133–1142.

Pfeffer RI, Kuroski TT, Harrah H Jr, et al. Measurement of functional activities in older adults in the community. *J Gerontrol.* 1982;37:323–329.

Podiallo D, Richardson S. The timed "up & go": a test of basic functional mobility for frail elderly persons. *J Am Geriatr Soc.* 1991;39:142–148.

Reisberg B, Doody R, Stoffler A, et al. Memantine in moderate-to-severe Alzheimer's disease. *N Engl J Med.* 2003;348(14):1331–1341.

Reuben DB. *Geriatrics at Your Fingertips.* Belle Mead, NJ: Excerpta Medica, for the American Geriatrics Society; 2001.

Reynolds CF III, Frank E, Perel JM, et al. Nortriptyline and interpersonal psychotherapy as maintenance therapies for recurrent major depression: a randomized controlled trial in patients older than 59 years. *JAMA.* 1999;281:39–45.

Snow V, Lascher S, Mottur-Pilson C. Pharmacological treatment of acute major depression and dysthymia. ACP-ASIM Clinical Practice Guidelines. *Ann Intern Med.* 2000;132(9):738–742.

Solomon PR, Hirschoff A, Felly B, et al. A seven minute neurocognitive screening battery highly sensitive to Alzheimer's disease. *Arch Neurol.* 1998;55:349–355.

Steffens DC, Skoog I, Norton MC, et al. Prevalence of depression and its treatment in an elderly population: the Cache County study. *Arch Gen Psychiatry.* 2000;57:601–607.

Tennstedt S, Cafferata GL, Sullivan L. Depression among caregivers of impaired elders. *J Aging Health.* 1992;4:58–76.

U.S. Census Bureau. *Population Projections for the United States by Age, Race, and Hispanic Origin: 1993–2050.* Washington, DC: U.S. Census Bureau; 1993.

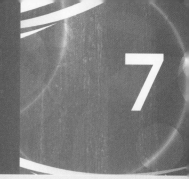

Heart and Blood Vessel Disorders

Matt Dane Baker • Jesse Coale

I. Heart Failure (HF)

A. Etiology

1. **High-Output HF (Less Common than Low-Output HF)**
   - Anemia.
   - Hyperthyroidism.
   - Arteriovenous (A-V) fistula with shunting.
   - Beriberi (thiamine deficiency).
   - Paget disease.

2. **Low-Output HF**
   - Chronic hypertension: common etiology.
   - Ischemic heart disease: common etiology.
   - Cardiomyopathies.
   - Valvular heart disease (VHD).
   - Dysrhythmias.

3. **Right-Sided HF**
   - Pulmonary disease (chronic obstructive pulmonary disease with cor pulmonale).
   - Pulmonary hypertension.
   - Right ventricular infarction.
   - Mitral stenosis (MS).
   - Simultaneous with left-sided HF: common etiology.

4. **Left-Sided HF**
   - Myocardial infarction (MI) with left ventricular (LV) infarction: common etiology.
   - Systemic hypertension: common etiology.
   - Cardiomyopathy.
   - Endocarditis.
   - Aortic valve disease and mitral regurgitation (MR).

5. **HF with Reduced Ejection Fraction, Systolic**
   - Dilated cardiomyopathies.
   - MI: common etiology.
   - Chronic hypertension: common etiology.

6. **HF with Normal or Preserved Ejection Fraction, Diastolic**
   - Restrictive, infiltrative cardiomyopathies (amyloidosis, sarcoidosis).
   - Pericardial effusion.
   - Hypertrophic cardiomyopathy.
   - Myocardial ischemia and infarction: common etiology.
   - Hypertension: common etiology.

B. Pathology

- HF refers to an abnormal state characterized by failure of the heart to pump enough blood to meet the metabolic demands of the body tissues. It is described by the American Heart Association (AHA) and American College of Cardiology (ACC) as "a complex clinical syndrome that results from any structural or functional impairment of ventricular filling or ejection of blood."
- Congestive heart failure (CHF) is the state of circulatory congestion secondary to HF, which can be divided into high- or low-output failure, left- or right-sided failure, and systolic or diastolic failure. Often, substantial crossover exists between these pathophysiologic categories because left- and right-sided failure, and systolic and diastolic dysfunction, often occurs simultaneously.
- High-output failure results from excessive demand for cardiac output (CO) or abnormally high tissue demands. Myocardial function itself may be normal but inadequate to meet increased demands. This is uncommon.
- Low-output failure occurs secondary to disorders of the heart that result in diminished cardiac output.
- Right-sided failure involves impairment of the right side of the heart and, thus, leads to systemic venous congestion seen in the liver and periphery.
- Left-sided failure results from insults to the left atrium and ventricle and, consequently, results in pulmonary congestion.
- Simultaneous left- and right-sided failure is often referred to as biventricular failure.
- Systolic failure or heart failure with reduced ejection fraction involves a decrease in cardiac contractility and ejection fraction (EF), whereas diastolic dysfunction or heart failure with normal or preserved ejection fraction results from poor ventricular compliance and relaxation, and impaired ventricular filling. Diastolic failure is now referred to as HF with normal or preserved EF.
- Diminished cardiac output can be caused by conditions that alter preload, afterload, and contractility; most therapies are designed to correct these physiologic derangements or address the compensation mechanisms.

128

- Compensation mechanisms in HF include adrenergic autonomic stimulation; activation of the rennin–angiotensin–aldosterone system; ventricular hypertrophy, then remodeling; secretion of antidiuretic hormone; and secretion of atrial or brain natriuretic peptides (BNPs) and cytokines.
- Obesity is now known to be an independent risk factor for HF, as is obstructive sleep apnea.

C. Precipitating Factors
- Myocardial ischemia or infarction.
- Dysrhythmia, especially atrial fibrillation due to loss of atrial kick (contraction).
- Infection.
- Shock/trauma.
- Thyroid disease (hyper or hypo).
- Pulmonary embolism.
- Dietary indiscretion (excess salt intake).
- Medication nonadherence.
- Drugs: β-blockers, nonsteroidal anti-inflammatory drugs (NSAIDs), calcium channel blockers (CCBs), and thiazolidinediones.

D. Epidemiology and Demographics
- Over 5 million (5.1) persons have HF in the United States, with 650,000 new cases being diagnosed each year.
- Most common admitting diagnoses in hospitalized elderly individuals; and second largest expense for Medicare.

E. Clinical Features
1. **History**
   - Fatigue.
   - Anorexia.
   - Dyspnea, initially dyspnea on exertion.
   - Orthopnea.
   - Paroxysmal nocturnal dyspnea (PND).
   - Coughing (pink, frothy sputum), wheezing.
   - Minimal right upper quadrant abdomen discomfort.
   - Ankle edema.
   - Nocturia.
   - **Symptoms classified using New York Heart Association (NYHA) scale:**
     - Class I: cardiac disease but no limitations. Asymptomatic on ordinary activities.
     - Class II: slight limitation. Comfortable at rest but experience symptoms with ordinary activities.
     - Class III: marked limitation. Comfortable at rest, but symptomatic with less than ordinary activities.
     - Class IV: inability to perform any physical activity without symptoms. Symptoms at rest.
   - HF is also classified using the AHA/ACC staging system. This system acknowledges HF as a progressive disorder that should be addressed from a preventative perspective with intervention before structural damage or symptoms appear.
     - Stage A: at high risk of HF but without structural heart disease or symptoms of HF.
     - Stage B: structural heart disease but without signs or symptoms of HF.
     - Stage C: structural disease with prior or current symptoms of HF.
     - Stage D: refractory HF requiring specialized interventions.

2. **Physical Findings**
   - Early or mild HF may have no signs.
   - Tachypnea.
   - Jugular venous distention (JVD).
   - Hepatojugular reflux.
   - Pulmonary rales or crackles (bibasilar).
   - Wheezing ("cardiac asthma").
   - Pleural effusion with diminished breath sounds and dullness to percussion (bilateral or right).
   - Lateral displacement of apical impulse.
   - Third heart sound (S_3 gallop).
   - Cardiac murmurs as etiology or MR murmur from dilated ventricle.
   - Paradoxical splitting of second heart sound (S_2).
   - Hepatomegaly.
   - Ascites.
   - Cyanosis.
   - Peripheral edema (ankle, pedal, pretibial, sacral if bedfast patient, anasarca).
   - Hypotension, cool extremities, and mental status changes (in severe CHF).
   - Cheyne–stokes respiration (in severe failure).

F. Diagnostic Studies
- Chest X-ray (CXR): cardiomegaly, pleural effusions (right or bilateral), Kerley B lines, increased pulmonary vascular markings and cephalization of pulmonary vascular markings (increase in upper lobes), interstitial edema, and butterfly or batwing pattern of pulmonary edema (Figure 7–1).
- Echocardiography (two-dimensional [2-D] and cardiac Doppler): this is the most useful test in diagnosis. Can see wall/chamber hypertrophy or dilatation, ventricular wall akinetic or dyskinetic areas, and reduced estimated LVEF (<50%) in systolic failure, valvular lesions.
- BNP or N-terminal pro-BNP: elevated. Used in emergency department and inpatient settings.
- Multigated acquisition (MUGA) scan (nuclear ventriculography): reduced LVEF. Used if echocardiogram (echo) results are not optimal.
- Cardiac catheterization with ventriculography: reduced LVEF. Used if concurrent coronary artery disease (CAD) is suspected.
- Electrocardiogram (ECG): sinus tachycardia, LV hypertrophy (LVH), and evidence of MI (not specific for HF).

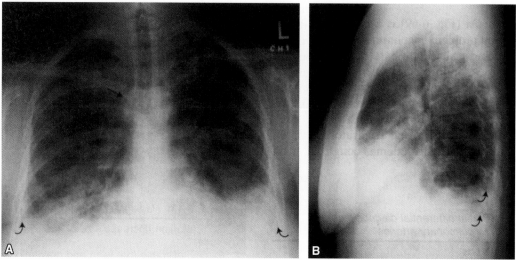

FIGURE 7–1. **Chest PA (A) and lateral (B) radiographs.** Congestive heart failure with pulmonary edema. (From Erkonen WE. Diagnostic radiology chest. In: Erkonen WE, ed. *Radiology 101: The Basics and Fundamentals for Imaging.* Philadelphia, PA: Lippincott-Raven; 1998:122, with permission.)

- Arterial blood gas studies: respiratory alkalosis. Used in emergency department and inpatient settings.
- Cardiac computed tomography (CT) or magnetic resonance imaging (MRI) sometimes used.
- Blood urea nitrogen (BUN): mild azotemia.
- Creatinine: mildly increased.
- Electrolyte: dilutional hyponatremia.
- Complete blood cell (CBC): anemia.
- Aspartase aminotransferases (ASTs; alanine aminotransferase): sometimes increased.
- Urine analysis (UA): proteinuria.
- Albumin and thyroid-stimulating hormone (TSH): to look for underlying etiology.

G. Management (Based on AHA/ACC System)

1. **Stage A: Prevention in High-Risk Patients**
   - Treat hypertension: thiazide diuretics, angiotensin-converting enzyme (ACE) inhibitors, or angiotensin receptor blockers (ARBs) are good choices: lipid disorders, diabetes, obstructive sleep apnea, and metabolic disorder.
   - Treat diabetes, metabolic syndrome, obstructive sleep apnea, dyslipidemia, and dysrhythmia.
   - Fish oil may provide some benefit.
   - **Lifestyle changes**
     - Salt (sodium) restriction.
     - Smoking cessation.
     - Exercise: avoid deconditioning or overexercise.
     - Weight reduction, if appropriate.
     - Alcohol avoidance.
     - Tobacco cessation.

2. **Stage B: Prevention of Progression in Patients with Structural Damage but No Symptoms**
   - **All measures in Stage A plus:**
     - ACE inhibitor or ARB.

- Consider β-blocker in CAD patients with angina or past MI.
- Revascularization and valve repair when indicated.

3. **Stage C: Symptomatic HF**
   - Lifestyle changes (e.g., sodium reduction; see earlier).
   - Daily weight monitoring.
   - Assessment for precipitating, treatable causes.
   - Antiembolism stockings.
   - ACE inhibitors (ACE-I): the mainstay of therapy because these have been proved to reduce mortality *or*
   - Angiotensin II (AII) receptor antagonists (e.g., valsartan, candesartan); consider if patient develops cough on ACE inhibitors. Have been shown to decrease mortality *or*
   - Sacubitril and valsartan (Entresto is now considered by many to be first line therapy replacing ACE.): neprilysin inhibitor and ARB.
   - Diuretics, especially loop diuretics (furosemide) initially; can add metolazone. These are for symptomatic control.
   - β-Blockers: carvedilol, extended release metoprolol succinate, bisoprolol (use when stable, start with low dose, and increase slowly). Have been shown to decrease mortality.
   - All Stage C patients should be on an ACE-I or ARB, and a β-blocker if tolerated.
   - **Can then add:**
     - Combination of hydralazine and isosorbide dinitrate. Shown to be effective in African American patients.
     - Spironolactone–aldosterone antagonist or eplerenone (Inspra; G.D. Searle, Peapack, NJ), a

selective aldosterone receptor antagonist. Has been shown to decrease mortality.
- Digoxin: in systolic failure, especially in patients with atrial fibrillation. Keep digoxin level between 0.5 and 0.8 ng per mL.
- Implantable cardioverter defibrillators (ICDs) in patients with NYHA Class II or III and LVEF < 35%.
- Biventricular pacemaker in patients with cardiac dyssynchrony and QRS duration > 0.12 ms; LVEF ≤ 35%; and NYHA Class III or IV.
- Nitroglycerin (NTG) intravenously (IV). Used only in inpatient or emergency department setting.
  - Anticoagulants: useful in atrial fibrillation.
- In severe HF hospitalized patients: nitroprusside, IV morphine, amrinone, milrinone, dopamine, dobutamine, and LV assist devices (LVADs).
- **NOTE:** CCB may be helpful in HF with normal EF.
  4. **Stage D: Refractory HF**
- Younger patients and patients of all ages with few comorbidities should be referred for LVADs and transplant.
- Older patients with significant comorbidities and poor prognosis should be considered for hospice care and ICD deactivation.

H. Monitoring
- Weights.
- Electrolytes (especially potassium because of diuretic-induced hypokalemia).
- BUN, creatinine.
- CXR.

II. Hypertension
A. Etiology
1. **Primary Essential Hypertension**
- Idiopathic: has genetic component and environmental precipitating factors such as salt intake, obesity, stress, sedentary lifestyle, and alcohol intake. This is by far the most common etiology for hypertension. Sympathetic hyperactivity, the renin–angiotensin–aldosterone system, and defects in natriuresis play a role.
2. **Secondary Hypertension**
- Glomerulonephritis.
- Pyelonephritis.
- Polycystic kidney disease.
- Renal artery stenosis or renovascular hypertension.
- Coarctation of the aorta.
- Hyperaldosteronism.
- Cushing disease.
- Hyperthyroidism.
- Pheochromocytoma.
- Acromegaly.
- Hyperparathyroidism.
- Preeclampsia.
- Obstructive sleep apnea.
- Drugs: cocaine, oral contraceptives, NSAIDs, decongestants, corticosteroids, and sympathomimetics.

B. Pathology
- Hypertension: defined as a state of sustained elevated systemic arterial blood pressure (BP).
- Primary essential hypertension: idiopathic disorder without established etiology.
- Secondary hypertension: less common and caused by disorders in other organ systems (see Section II.A).
- Hypertensive emergency: presents with severe elevation of BP (diastolic > 130 mm Hg); can have funduscopic changes (hemorrhages, exudates, papilledema), often with manifestations of hypertensive encephalopathy such as confusion and stupor.
- Systolic hypertension is a greater risk of cardiovascular disease (CVD) than diastolic in those over the age of 50.

C. Complications and End-Organ Damage from Hypertension
- Retinopathy.
- CAD.
- HF.
- Peripheral vascular disease (peripheral arterial disease [PAD]).
- Nephropathy, chronic renal disease, and end-stage renal disease (ESRD).
- Cerebrovascular disease: transient ischemic attack (TIA), cerebrovascular accident (CVA), and vascular dementia.
- Aortic dissection.

D. Demographics and Epidemiology
- About one-third of U.S. population; 50% of those not controlled.
- Increased frequency with aging.

E. Clinical Features
- Silent or mostly asymptomatic disease. History, physical examination, and laboratory evaluation designed to establish diagnosis, rule out secondary etiologies, identify end-organ damage, and uncover concurrent atherosclerosis risk factors.
1. **History**
- Occipital headache with high BP.
2. **Physical Findings**
- BP: two or more readings on two or more office visits (2017 ACC/AHA Guidelines: Systolic ≥ 130 mm Hg and diastolic ≥ 80 mm Hg.).
- Staging:
  - Stage 1: Systolic 130–139; diastolic 80–89 mm Hg
  - Stage 2: Systolic 140 or >; diastolic 90 or > mm Hg
- Hypertensive Crisis: Systolic >180 mm Hg; diastolic >120 mm Hg

- Eye: funduscopic-narrowed arteries, A-V nicking, copper or silver wiring of arterioles, hemorrhages, exudates, and papilledema.
- Heart: increased S_2.
- Also should do neck, lung, heart, abdomen, peripheral pulses, extremity, and neurologic examinations to identify end-organ damage.

F. Diagnostic Studies
- None needed for diagnosis: ambulatory BP monitoring may be useful.
- CBC count or hemoglobin/hematocrit.
- UA (assess for proteinuria).
- Electrolytes (sodium, potassium).
- Creatinine.
- Lipids: cholesterol—total, high-density lipoprotein (HDL-C), low-density lipoprotein (LDL-C), triglycerides.
- Twelve-lead ECG (assess for LVH).
- BUN.
- Fasting blood glucose.
- Calcium.
- CXR and echo looking for cardiomegaly and ventricular hypertrophy may be helpful.
- Can order renal ultrasound (U/S) if renovascular hypertension or polycystic kidney disease suspected.

G. Management
- Salt restriction: 2.4 g sodium (Na) or 6 g sodium chloride per day. Dietary Approaches to Stop Hypertension (DASH) diet with increased fruits and vegetables and decreased salt.
- Weight reduction.
- Decreased alcohol (<1 oz per day).
- Tobacco cessation.
- Adequate potassium, magnesium, and calcium intake.
- Aerobic exercise program.
- Stress reduction: biofeedback, relaxation exercises.
- **Pharmacologic management**
  - Goal: <140/90 (or <150/90 in those >60 years old per the Eighth Joint National Committee [JNC-8]).
  - Most will need at least two agents for optimal control.
  - Diuretics: thiazides such as hydrochlorothiazide (HCTZ), potassium sparing, and loop. Low-dose thiazides (e.g., HCTZ 12.5–25 mg) are excellent starting agents.
  - ACE inhibitors (e.g., captopril, enalapril, lisinopril). Useful in patients with concurrent diabetes mellitus (DM), HF, or old MI.
  - Angiotensin (AII) receptor antagonists (e.g., losartan, valsartan, candesartan).
  - β-Blockers (e.g., metoprolol, propranolol). Useful in patients with old MI or with concurrent tachycardia.
  - α-Blockers (e.g., prazosin, terazosin, doxazosin). Useful in male patients with concurrent benign prostatic hyperplasia (BPH).
  - Mixed α- and β-blockers (e.g., labetalol).
  - CCBs (e.g., amlodipine). Verapamil and diltiazem useful in patients with concurrent supraventricular tachycardia (SVT).
  - Vasodilators (e.g., hydralazine, minoxidil).
  - Centrally and peripheral-acting adrenergic inhibitors (e.g., clonidine, methyldopa, reserpine).
  - Selective aldosterone receptor antagonists (e.g., eplerenone).
  - Renin inhibitors (e.g., aliskiren).
  - Diuretics, ACE-I, ARBs, and CCBs are good first-line therapy, with diuretics; CCBs preferred first-line therapy for African American patients.

H. Monitoring
- BP: home, office, and ambulatory monitors.
- Potassium level if on diuretics.
- Periodic UA, creatinine.

III. Coronary Heart Disease (CHD) or CAD with Angina Pectoris

A. Etiology
- Atherosclerotic stenosis of coronary arteries: most common.
- Coronary artery spasm.
- Congenital coronary artery anomalies.
- Aortic stenosis (AS), regurgitation.
- Hypertrophic cardiomyopathy.
- Myocardial muscle bridge.
- Pulmonary hypertension.
- Severe systemic hypertension.
- Collagen vascular disease.
- Syndrome X (possible microvascular disease).

B. Pathology
- Symptom complex of chest discomfort or equivalent secondary to myocardial ischemia because of mismatch of supply and demand.
- Classic stable angina: substernal pressure or heaviness sensation precipitated by exertion or anxiety; relieved in a predictable pattern by rest.
- Unstable angina: chest discomfort at rest, or new and severe (within 2 months and brought on by minimal exertion), or has changed in pattern with increased frequency, duration, and intensity.
- Crescendo angina: angina occurring with increasing frequency.
- Variant angina (Prinzmetal): rest or nocturnal chest pain with ST segment elevation on ECG; thought to be caused by coronary artery spasm.
- Postprandial angina: angina occurring after meals.

- Anginal equivalent: dyspnea on exertion caused by myocardial ischemia.
- Syndrome X: typical exertional or stress-induced angina in the absence of coronary artery stenosis on angiography.
- Silent ischemia: evidence of myocardial ischemia on stress ECG, thallium, or echocardiography without chest discomfort; thought to be more common in patients with diabetes.

C. Risk Factors for Atherosclerosis
- Advancing age.
- Male gender (female begins to equal male after menopause).
- Smoking tobacco.
- Hypertension.
- Genetic (family history: CHD in male first-degree relative <55 years; CHD in female first-degree relative <65 years).
- Increased total cholesterol and LDL-C, decreased HDL-C, increased apolipoprotein (a) (Lp[a]), increased small, dense LDL particles, and increased triglycerides.
- DM.
- Obesity.
- Metabolic syndrome.
- Sedentary lifestyle.
- Increased homocysteine.
- Increase C-reactive protein (inflammation).
- Low-glutathione peroxidase (antioxidant enzyme).
- Proteinuria.

D. Clinical Features
1. History
- Precordial pressure or heaviness radiating to back, neck, shoulders, arms, lower jaw, or teeth brought on by exertion, eating large meal, cold air exposure, or emotional stress and relieved by rest or NTG; usually lasts minutes.
- May present as dyspnea on exertion.
- Levine sign: patient describes pain using clenched fist over his or her anterior chest (sternum).
- May be accompanied by dyspnea, dizziness, palpitations, and infrequently syncope.

2. Physical Findings
- May be normal.
- Fourth heart sound (S_4) and sometimes S_3.
- Paradoxical splitting of S_2 during angina episode.
- May have signs of atherosclerosis (e.g., xanthelasma, decreased peripheral pulses).
- May have signs of hypertension as risk factor (e.g., increased BP, retinopathy).
- Murmur of AS or aortic regurgitation (AR) as etiology, or MR from papillary muscle dysfunction.
- Signs of HF as complication.

E. Diagnostic Studies
- ECG: can frequently be normal or may show ST segment depression or T-wave inversion during attack; Q waves seen in patients with previous MI.
- Cholesterol may be elevated with elevated LDL-C, increased Lp(a), decreased HDL-C, and increased triglycerides.
- C-reactive protein: increased.
- Homocysteine: increased.
- Ambulatory ECG may show transient ST segment depression with exertion.
- Stress testing is usually done as the second step after the resting ECG and can include the following:
  - Stress or exercise ECG: may disclose temporary ST segment depression.
  - Myocardial perfusion scintigraphy after exercise (or pharmacologic stress testing with IV dipyridamole or adenosine) with thallium-201, technetium-99m, tetrofosmin, or sestamibi using planar or single-photon emission CT imaging: may show reversible perfusion defects.
  - Stress echocardiography using exercise or pharmacologic agents (dipyridamole, dobutamine, adenosine): may show stress-induced global or regional wall motion abnormalities.
  - Stress gated blood-pool scintigraphy (technetium-99m) using exercise or pharmacologic agents: may show stress-induced global or regional wall motion abnormalities.
- Positron emission tomography.
- Cardiac MRI.
- Cardiac CT.
- Ultrafast electron-beam CT scan for coronary artery calcification (high sensitivity but low specificity).
- Cardiac arteriography: cardiac catheterization with angiography is a definitive study to diagnose, quantify, and anatomically define CAD ("gold standard").

F. Management
- Smoking cessation.
- Weight reduction, low-fat/low-cholesterol diet.
- Cardiac rehabilitation or supervised exercise program to improve exercise capacity.
- Treat hypertension and diabetes.
- Aggressive hypercholesterolemia treatment (goal—LDL <100 mg per dL, ideal would be <70 mg per dL); hydroxymethylglutaryl coenzyme A (HMG-CoA) reductase inhibitors (statins) preferred.

1. Pharmacologic Management
- Aspirin: 81 to 325 mg per day, or clopidogrel.
- Sublingual (SL) NTG spray or tablets: as needed or before exertion.
- Long-acting oral nitrates (e.g., isosorbide dinitrate and isosorbide 5-mononitrate) with 8- to 12-hour nitrate-free period to avoid tolerance.

- Long-acting transdermal nitrates by way of paste or patches with 8- to 12-hour nitrate-free period to avoid tolerance.
- IV NTG in unstable angina.
- IV heparin in unstable angina.
- β-Adrenergic blockers.
- CCBs (i.e., diltiazem or verapamil): not first line. Avoid short-acting nifedipine because this may increase the risk of cardiac event.
- Ranolazine (Ranexa): can cause QT prolongation.
- Folic acid to decrease homocysteine. This has not been proved to yield absolute benefit.
- Statin to decrease LDL and C-reactive protein.

2. **Invasive Revascularization Procedures (Percutaneous Coronary Interventions)**
   - Percutaneous transluminal coronary angioplasty (PTCA).
   - Directional coronary atherectomy.
   - Coronary laser angioplasty.
   - Coronary stenting, including drug-eluting stents (used with PTCA).

3. **Surgical Procedures**
   - Coronary artery bypass grafting surgery.

4. **Others**
   - Mechanical extracorporeal counterpulsation: limited data.

IV. Acute Myocardial Infarction

A. Etiology/Pathology
- Most acute myocardial infarction (AMI) events occur in patients with preexisting atherosclerotic coronary artery stenosis when endothelial plaque becomes unstable by rupturing or fissuring, which stimulates adhesion of platelets and deposition of fibrin. Platelets release vasoconstrictors such as thromboxane A2. These factors lead to occlusion of coronary vessels and subsequent myocardial ischemia and necrosis. A small percentage (2% or less) of AMIs are secondary to pure vasospasm, congenital anomalies, vasculitis, or embolism.

B. Demographics
- Age: usually over age 40.
- Gender: age 40 to 70: men > women; age > 70: men = women.

C. Complications
- HF.
- Cardiogenic shock.
- Papillary muscle dysfunction or rupture with MR.
- Ventricular aneurysm.
- Ventricular rupture, ventricular septal defect (VSD).
- Dysrhythmias, heart blocks.
- Pericarditis.
- Dressler syndrome: post-MI pericarditis, fever, pulmonary infiltrates.
- Mural thrombus.

D. Clinical Features
1. **History**
   - Severe squeezing retrosternal pain or tightness lasting >30 minutes. Radiation of pain to neck, jaw, and left arm is common. Radiation to right arm or back occurs less frequently. Unrelieved by NTG or rest.
   - Dyspnea.
   - Anxiety.
   - Generalized weakness.
   - Lightheadedness.
   - Nausea, vomiting.
   - Diaphoresis.
   - Syncope: occasional.
   - Silent AMIs are rare but do occur; elderly patients and patients with diabetes can have atypical presentations.

2. **Physical Findings**
   - May be normal.
   - Clammy skin.
   - Increased or decreased BP.
   - JVD with HF.
   - S_4.
   - S_3 with CHF.
   - Apical systolic murmur of MR with papillary muscle dysfunction.
   - Dysrhythmias.
   - Wheezing or rales.

E. Diagnostic Studies
- ST segment elevation MI (STEMI): inverted T waves, elevated ST segments (concave downward), Q waves usually within 12 to 36 hours, dysrhythmias common (Q wave MI). ECG in non-STEMI: ST segment depression. All MIs can have dysrhythmias, atrioventricular (AV) blocks, and bundle branch blocks.
- Elevated cardiac enzymes: creatine kinase-MB (CK-MB) isoenzymes rise within 4 to 8 hours, peak at 12 to 20 hours, and return to normal in 2 to 3 days. Lactase dehydrogenase isoenzymes rise within 14 to 24 hours, total lactate dehydrogenase (LDH) peak at 2 to 3 days, and return to normal in 8 to 14 days. AST rises within 12 hours, peaks at 36 hours, and returns to normal in 3 to 4 days.
- Troponin T and I rise within 4 hours, and return to normal in 7 days for I, and 10 to 14 days for T; can also be elevated in unstable angina.
- Most MIs are diagnosed with ECG, CK-MB, and troponin.
- Leukocytosis: nonspecific.
- Plasma myeloperoxidase (inflammation marker): can detect early AMI before necrosis, but not widely.
- Elevated erythrocyte sedimentation rate (ESR): nonspecific.

- Elevated myoglobin: nonspecific.
- Technetium-99m infarct imaging and thallium perfusion imaging.
- Echo to evaluate valve and LV function.
- MRI with gadolinium.

F. Management

- Oxygen.
- Nitrates: SL and IV.
- Morphine sulfate.
- Aspirin: 162 to 325 mg.
- Clopidogrel (Plavix) or Prasugrel (Effient).
- β-Adrenergic blocking agents (metoprolol or carvedilol) PO if no HF.
- ACE inhibitors (captopril, enalapril, and lisinopril).
- Emergency or primary percutaneous transluminal intervention (percutaneous coronary interventions; PTCA with drug-eluting stent) if center equipped properly (preferred treatment).
- Thrombolytic therapy: if patient has pain ≤12 hours (some studies have shown benefit up to 24 hours), ST segment elevation, and no contraindications (e.g., recent bleed). *Drugs*: Tissue plasminogen activator, streptokinase, reteplase, tenecteplase, anistreplase, or anisoylated plasminogen-streptokinase activator complex with heparin.
- Glycoprotein IIb/IIIa antagonists or inhibitors: abciximab (ReoPro; Eli Lilly, Indianapolis, IN), tirofiban (Aggrastat; Merck, West Point, PA), eptifibatide (Integrilin; Millennium, San Francisco, CA, and Schering, Kenilworth, NJ): used for unstable angina, and AMI sometimes with thrombolytics or PTCA.
- Heparin: unfractionated or low-molecular-weight heparin (LMWH): enoxaparin and others or fondaparinux or direct thrombin inhibitor bivalirudin. Usually used in conjunction with thrombolytics or PTCA.
- Cardiac monitoring.
- **Post-AMI care**
  - Submaximal stress test within 1 to 3 weeks.
  - Holter monitoring.
  - Echocardiography and MUGA to determine LVEF.
  - Cardiac rehabilitation.
  - Address high lipids with statin (LDL < 100 mg per dL, ideal < 70), glucose, or BP.
  - Stop smoking.
  - Continue aspirin, clopidogrel, or both, and β-blocker or ACE inhibitor as prophylaxis against recurrent AMI.
  - Folic acid if homocysteine level is high. Benefit not fully established.

V. Pericarditis

A. Etiology

- Idiopathic.
- Viral: coxsackie virus, echovirus, HIV, adenovirus, Epstein-Barr virus, mumps virus.
- Bacterial: *Staphylococcus*, *Pneumococcus*, *Mycoplasma*, tuberculosis.
- Fungal.
- Lyme disease.
- Parasites.
- Collagen vascular diseases: rheumatoid arthritis (RA), systemic lupus erythematosus (SLE), scleroderma.
- AMI.
- Postcardiac surgery.
- Post-MI; Dressler syndrome.
- Uremia.
- Neoplasm (lung, lymphoma, mesothelioma).
- Trauma.
- Radiation.
- Myxedema.
- Sarcoidosis.
- Pancreatitis.
- Inflammatory bowel disease.
- Aortic dissection.
- Drugs: procainamide, hydralazine, minoxidil, bleomycin, phenytoin, and mesalamine.

B. Pathology

- Inflammation of pericardial sac. Can cause effusion. When effusion is large enough to decrease cardiac output, it is called cardiac tamponade and is a medical emergency. Constrictive pericarditis: caused by chronic pericardial inflammation leading to fibrosis, scarring, and calcification.

C. Demographics

- Men > women.

D. Clinical Features

1. **History**
   - Sharp retrosternal chest pain with radiation to back and shoulder, intensifies with inspiration and lying supine, relieved by sitting up and leaning forward.
   - Odynophagia.
   - Anorexia.
   - Anxiety.
   - Myalgia.
2. **Physical Findings**
   - Fever.
   - Splinted breathing.
   - Pericardial friction rub (three components—systolic, early diastolic, and late diastolic).
   - Dysrhythmias: SVT.
   - Tachypnea.
3. **Pericardial Tamponade**
   - Dyspnea.
   - Tachycardia.

- Cyanosis.
- JVD.
- Hypotension.
- Pulsus paradoxus.
- Muffled heart tones.
4. **Constrictive Pericarditis**
   - Can be asymptomatic early in course.
   - Dyspnea.
   - Fatigue.
   - JVD.
   - Peripheral edema.
   - Hepatomegaly, ascites.

E. Diagnostic Studies
- ECG: acute phase with concave-up ST elevation in precordial leads, especially with absence of reciprocal ST depression seen in AMI. Intermediate phase ST segment returns to baseline and T waves invert. In late phase, ECG can return to normal. In constrictive pericarditis and cardiac tamponade, ECG may disclose low QRS voltage. In cardiac tamponade, electrical alternans may be seen.
- Echo to detect pericardial effusion.
- Leukocytosis.
- Elevated ESR or CRP.
- BUN and creatinine to rule out uremia.
- CXR may show large effusion, but not nearly as sensitive or specific as echo.
- May see mildly elevated cardiac enzymes, especially CK-MB.
- Viral titers, antinuclear antibody, rheumatoid factor, purified protein derivative, antistreptolysin O (ASO) titers, BUN, creatinine, and blood cultures may be helpful in elucidating the cause.
- Some use CT or MRI.
- Cardiac catheterization should be considered in constrictive pericarditis.

F. Management
1. **Uncomplicated Acute Pericarditis**
   - Acetylsalicylic acid (ASA), NSAIDs (if no AMI), or prednisone.
   - Colchicine; need to use for 6 months.
   - Analgesia (e.g., codeine).
   - Rest.
   - Observation for signs/symptoms of evolving tamponade.
   - Treat underlying etiology (e.g., infection, ESRD).
2. **Chronic Constrictive Pericarditis**
   - Cardiothoracic surgery referral for possible stripping.
3. **Cardiac Tamponade**
   - Immediate pericardiocentesis.
   - Cardiothoracic surgery referral for pericardial window drainage, if recurrent.

VI. Valvular Heart Disease
A. Pathology
- Cardiac valves maintain unidirectional forward flow of blood through the heart. VHD presents with cardiac and pulmonary symptoms or with heart murmur. It causes cardiac murmurs, although all murmurs do not reflect VHD. All VHDs cause derangement of blood flow in the heart. This derangement causes turbulent flow across valves, which often leads to fibrosis and calcifications of valves that can eventually cause hemodynamic compromise. When confronted with the possibility of VHD, five questions must be asked.
  - *What valve is affected?* Disorders of aortic and mitral valve are more common, although pulmonic and tricuspid lesions do occur.
  - *What is the hemodynamic derangement?* VHD usually presents as either stenosis or regurgitation. In stenosis, the valve fails to open completely, and subsequent outflow obstruction can occur, often causing backflow circulatory congestion. In regurgitation or insufficiency, the valve fails to remain completely closed when it should, thus allowing for backward reflux of blood.
  - *How severe is the hemodynamic compromise?* Lesions in VHD can vary from minimal to severely life threatening.
  - *What is the etiology of the lesion?*
  - *How has the VHD lesion affected the patient's circulation, especially in regard to ventricular function and pulmonary circulation?*

B. Aortic Stenosis
- Valvular narrowing with resistance to LV outflow.
1. **Etiology**
   - Congenital unicuspid, bicuspid, or tricuspid valve with commissural fusion.
   - Rheumatic fever: was the most common cause 50 years ago; now congenital and degenerative are more common. Usually involves both aortic and mitral valves, but AS can occur alone.
   - Degenerative calcific disease in elderly patients, which may be an autoimmune reaction.
2. **Clinical Features**
   a. **History**
      - Angina pectoris (occurs in 50%–70% of patients with severe AS).
      - Syncope and presyncope (with severe AS).
      - Dyspnea on exertion.
      - PND.
      - Orthopnea.
      - Fatigue.
      - Palpitations.
      - Sudden death.
   b. **Physical Findings**
      - Narrowed pulse pressure.
      - Hypertension in elderly patients with AS.
      - Delayed and diminished carotid upstroke (pulsus parvus et tardus).

- Systolic thrill felt over base or carotids.
- LV heave or lift.
- Crescendo-decrescendo systolic murmur best heard at right second intercostal space (ICS), right sternal border with radiation into carotids, down left parasternal border to the apex.
- Early systolic ejection click.
- Paradoxical splitting of S_2 may occur (suggests severe disease).
- Delayed, decreased intensity or absent aortic second sound (A_2).
- S_4 gallop.
- Early diastolic murmur of AR.
- Can have irregular–irregular cardiac rhythm if atrial fibrillation is present.

3. **Diagnostic Studies**
   - Echo/Doppler: decreased valve excursion or aortic valve area, ARA (<1.0 cm^2 severe stenosis, <0.8 cm^2 indicates severe AS compromising cardiac output), calcification of valve, LVH, decreased LVEF ($<50\%$), increased valve gradient (>40 mm Hg mean valve gradient high, >55 mm Hg severe).
   - ECG: LVH, dysrhythmias, conduction defects.
   - CXR: normal or cardiomegaly.
   - Elevated BNP reflects LV failure and increased severity.
   - Cardiac catheterization.

4. **Management**
   - Cardiothoracic surgery referral for valve replacement in patients with symptomatic disease.
   - Transcatheter aortic valve replacement is an option for some patients.
   - Balloon valvuloplasty may be considered for pediatric congenital disease and for elderly patients who may not tolerate valve replacement surgery.

C. Aortic Regurgitation
- Incompetent valve causing retrograde flow from aorta into left ventricle that may lead to HF. There are both acute and chronic forms of AR.

1. **Etiology**
   - Congenital bicuspid valve.
   - Bacterial endocarditis (acute AR).
   - Rheumatic fever.
   - Valve injury from pacemaker lead placement.
   - Syphilis.
   - Dissecting aortic aneurysm.
   - Marfan syndrome.
   - Ankylosing spondylitis.
   - Giant cell arteritis.
   - Osteogenesis imperfecta.
   - SLE.
   - RA.
   - Reiter syndrome.
   - Aneurysm of sinus of Valsalva.
   - Severe systemic hypertension.

2. **Clinical Features**
   a. **History**
      - May be asymptomatic in mild and moderate disease.
      - Dyspnea on exertion.
      - Orthopnea.
      - PND.
      - Palpitations.
      - Fatigue.
   b. **Physical Findings**
      - Widened pulse pressure with increased systolic BP and reduced diastolic BP.
      - Korotkoff sounds persisting until zero.
      - Abrupt rise of upstroke, quick collapse of peripheral pulses (water hammer or Corrigan pulse).
      - Bisferious pulse with double pulsation.
      - Pistol shot sounds over femoral artery (Traube sign).
      - Thrill felt at carotids, base of heart.
      - Single S_2 (A_2 absent).
      - S_3 may be heard.
      - Early decrescendo high-frequency blowing diastolic murmur best heard at left sternal border/third and fourth ICS; accentuated by having patient sit up, lean forward, and hold breath after deep expiration, or by squatting, or isometric exercise such as handgrip. Some can be heard at right parasternal border. In severe disease, murmur may be holodiastolic or an Austin Flint murmur (rumbling mid- and late-diastolic heard at apex) may be identified.
      - Midsystolic murmur may be heard at base due to augmented stroke volume and rates of ejection.

3. **Diagnostic Studies**
   - Echo/2-D and Doppler: regurgitation, aortic leaflet thickening, calcification of valve, and decreased LVEF.
   - ECG: left axis deviation (LAD) and/or LVH.
   - CXR: normal or cardiomegaly.
   - Elevated BNP in LV dysfunction.
   - MRI or CT may be helpful.
   - Cardiac catheterization.

4. **Management**
   - Endocarditis treatment if required in acute AR.
   - Cardiothoracic surgery referral for annuloplasty valve repair valve replacement in patients with symptomatic disease.

D. Mitral Stenosis
- Valvular narrowing with resistance to LV filling causing left atrial enlargement, dysthymias (atrial fibrillation), HF with pulmonary edema, and eventually right-sided symptoms.

1. **Etiology**
   - Rheumatic fever most common; most commonly develops in third or fourth decades.

2. **Clinical Features**
   a. **History**
      - Fatigue.
      - Dyspnea on exertion.
      - Orthopnea.
      - PND.
      - Palpitations.
      - Cough.
      - Hoarseness due to compression on left recurrent laryngeal nerve by dilated left atrium.
      - Hemoptysis due to rupture of bronchial vein.
      - Chest pain.
      - Edema.
   b. **Physical Findings**
      - Early- to mid-diastolic low-pitch rumble murmur best heard at apex in left lateral decubitus position; presystolic murmurs also may be present.
      - Apical diastolic thrill can sometimes be felt in patients with loud murmurs in left lateral decubitus position.
      - Right ventricular lift in pulmonary hypertension.
      - Accentuated S_1 early in disease.
      - Single or closely split and accentuated S_2 can occur later in disease.
      - Opening snap after S_2.
      - Malar flush over cheeks.
      - Clubbing.
      - Rales.
      - Peripheral edema.
      - JVD.
      - Irregular–irregular rhythm of atrial fibrillation.
      - Graham Steell murmur (high-pitched decrescendo diastolic murmur at left sternal border) of pulmonic regurgitation (PR) can be heard in patients with severe pulmonary hypertension.
3. **Diagnostic Studies**
   - Echo/2-D and Doppler: thickening and calcification of valve, reduced leaflet excursion and doming, decreased mitral orifice (severe if valve area is <1.5 cm^2), enlarged left atrium, increased valve gradient.
   - ECG: left atrial enlargement, atrial fibrillation, right axis deviation (RAD) may be seen.
   - CXR: left atrial enlargement, cephalization of pulmonary markings, Kerley B lines, pulmonary edema with CHF.
   - Cardiac catheterization.
4. **Management**
   - Patient should avoid unnecessary stress or exertion.
   - Treat atrial fibrillation, usually with digoxin.
   - Treat HF as needed.
   - Balloon valvuloplasty and commissurotomy (percutaneous balloon mitral commissurotomy) may be considered in younger symptomatic patients.

   - Cardiothoracic surgery referral for valve replacement in patients with severe disease.

E. **Mitral Regurgitation**
   - Disorders of leaflets, chordae tendineae, papillary muscles, annulus, and LV myocardium can cause failure of complete valve closure with reflux into left atrium during systole. Acute pulmonary edema occurs less frequently with MR than with MS.
   1. **Etiology**
      - Mitral valve prolapse (MVP).
      - Rheumatic fever.
      - Ruptured chordae tendineae from endocarditis, MVP, rheumatic disease, and trauma.
      - Infective endocarditis (IE).
      - Papillary muscle dysfunction or rupture from ischemic heart disease and AMI.
      - Calcified mitral annulus.
      - Congenital heart disease.
      - Marfan syndrome.
      - Dilated cardiomyopathy.
   2. **Clinical Features**
      a. **History**
         - May be asymptomatic in mild and sometimes moderate disease.
         - Fatigue.
         - Dyspnea on exertion.
         - Orthopnea.
         - PND.
         - Palpitations.
         - Symptoms of MVP (see Section VI.F.2).
      b. **Physical Findings**
         - High-frequency blowing holosystolic murmur best identified at apex with radiation to axilla in chronic MR; can be accentuated by squatting; can be decrescendo in acute MR; and can have late-systolic murmur with click in MVP.
         - Soft S_1.
         - S_3.
         - Irregular–irregular rhythm of atrial fibrillation.
         - JVD in long-standing disease.
         - Pulmonary rales can occur.
         - Peripheral edema in severe disease.
   3. **Diagnostic Studies**
      - Echo/2-D and Doppler: MR, decreased LVEF.
      - ECG: left atrial enlargement, atrial fibrillation.
      - CXR: left atrial and ventricular enlargement and increased pulmonary markings can be seen.
      - Cardiac catheterization.
   4. **Management**
      - Treat atrial fibrillation usually with digoxin.
      - Functional MR can sometimes be treated with biventricular pacing.
      - Cardiothoracic surgery referral for valve repair or replacement in patients with progressive disease.

F. MVP Syndrome

- Bulging or billowing of mitral valve leaflets into left atrium during systole with or without MR. Many patients have benign course but some have significant MR, dysrhythmias, and rare cases of sudden death have been reported. Women > men under age 20, and women = men over age 20.

1. Etiology
- Primary: genetic, autosomal dominant with variable expression.
- Primary: Marfan syndrome and other connective tissue diseases.
- Secondary to CAD, rheumatic heart disease, or cardiomyopathies.

2. Clinical Features

a. History
- May be totally asymptomatic.
- Can have left precordial atypical chest pain.
- Palpitations.
- Dyspnea.
- Panic attacks/anxiety.
- Fatigue.
- Dizziness, presyncope, rarely syncope.
- Rare transient cerebral ischemic episodes

b. Physical Findings
- Low BP and orthostasis.
- Midsystolic click.
- Late-systolic murmur best heard at apex, increases in intensity with standing and handgrip.
- Thoracic skeletal abnormalities such as scoliosis, pectus excavatum, and straight thoracic spine.
- Dysrhythmias such as SVT sometimes noted.

3. Diagnostic Studies
- Echo/2-D and Doppler: MVP and determine whether MR is present.
- ECG: usually normal; can show ST segment depression or T-wave inversion in inferior leads III and aVF.
- Cardiac catheterization may be needed in patients with significant MR.

4. Management
- Most patients require only education.
- β-Blockers are helpful if palpitations are problematic.
- Cardiothoracic surgery referral for valve replacement in patients with severe MR.

G. Pulmonic Stenosis

- Narrowing of pulmonic valve leading to right ventricular outflow obstruction and right-sided HF.

1. Etiology
- Almost always congenital and disease of the young.
- Severe disease may present as HF in neonatal period. Disease may also progress with time and become symptomatic in late childhood and adolescence.
- Rubella embryopathy.

2. Clinical Features

a. History
- Fatigue.
- Dyspnea on exertion.
- Dizziness.
- Occasional syncope.
- Chest pain.
- Edema.

b. Physical Findings
- Harsh midsystolic crescendo-decrescendo murmur loudest at left upper sternal border with radiation to neck, increased with inspiration. The longer the murmur, the more severe the stenosis.
- Right ventricular heave felt at epigastrium.
- Thrill with louder murmurs (IV/VI or greater).
- Pulmonic ejection sound.
- Wide split S_2 with soft delayed pulmonic second sound (P_2).
- S_4 can be heard.
- JVD may be present.
- Hepatomegaly and ascites with right-sided HF.
- Peripheral edema later in course.

3. Diagnostic Studies
- Echo/2-D and Doppler: pulmonic stenosis (PS), thickened valve.
- ECG: RAD and right ventricular hypertrophy (RVH) may be seen.
- CXR: right ventricular enlargement can be seen.
- Cardiac catheterization.

4. Management
- Balloon valvuloplasty is the preferred treatment.
- Cardiothoracic surgery referral for valve replacement in patients with progressive disease.

H. Pulmonic Regurgitation

- Incomplete valve closure with retrograde flow into right ventricle during systole.

1. Etiology
- Pulmonary hypertension from left VHD.
- Pulmonary hypertension from pulmonary disease.
- Congenital.
- Idiopathic pulmonary artery dilatation.
- Complication of corrective surgery for tetralogy of Fallot.
- Infectious endocarditis.

2. Clinical Features
- Most cases well tolerated with few, if any, symptoms. Can see decreased exercise tolerance in patients with severe disease.
- Graham Steell murmur (high-pitched decrescendo early diastolic murmur at second left ICS and mid-left sternal border) in patients with PR secondary to severe pulmonary hypertension.

- PR secondary to congenital etiology may be lower-pitched, late-diastolic best heard at third and fourth left ICS.
- Loud P_2 with pulmonary hypertension.
- Right ventricular heave.
  3. **Diagnostic Studies**
  - Echo/2-D and Doppler: PR, look for RV enlargement.
  - Cardiac catheterization.
  4. **Management**
  - Many patients do not require specific treatment for PR, but pulmonary hypertension should be treated.
  - Cardiothoracic surgery referral in patients with severe progressive disease.

I. Tricuspid Stenosis
- Narrowing of valvular orifice obstructing flow from right atrium to right ventricle.
  1. **Etiology**
  - Rheumatic fever most common; mostly seen in conjunction with mitral and aortic lesions.
  - Congenital.
  - Right atrial myxoma.
  - Carcinoid syndrome.
  - Endomyocardial fibroelastosis.
  - Bacterial endocarditis.
  2. **Clinical Features**
    a. **History**
    - Fatigue.
    - Pulsation or fluttering sensation in neck.
    b. **Physical Findings**
    - Low-pitched mid-diastolic or presystolic rumbling murmur best heard at fourth and fifth ICS left sternal border or below xiphoid process. Intensified by inspiration (Carvallo sign). Also can be higher pitched and can be identified at apex.
    - Sometimes opening snap can be heard.
    - Diastolic thrill can sometimes be palpated.
    - Split S_1 with loud tricuspid first sound (T_1).
    - Single S_2.
    - S_3 can be heard over the jugular veins.
    - Prominent presystolic venous wave and JVD.
    - Hepatomegaly and hepatic pulsations.
    - Peripheral edema.
  3. **Diagnostic Studies**
  - Echo/2-D and Doppler: tricuspid stenosis.
  - ECG: right atrial hypertrophy.
  - CXR: right atrial enlargement.
  - Cardiac catheterization.
  4. **Management**
  - Sodium restriction.
  - Diuretics.
  - Valvotomy.
  - Cardiothoracic surgery referral in patients with severe progressive disease.

J. Tricuspid Regurgitation
- Inadequate closure of valve with retrograde flow from right ventricle into right atrium.
  1. **Etiology**
  - Dilatation of annulus secondary to right ventricular dilation (functional).
  - Rheumatic fever.
  - Congenital.
  - Myxoma.
  - Carcinoid syndrome.
  - Bacterial endocarditis especially in IV drug abuse.
  - Tricuspid valve prolapse.
  2. **Clinical Features**
    a. **History**
    - Dyspnea.
    - Pulsation sensation in neck.
    - Abdominal pain and bloating.
    - Peripheral edema.
    b. **Physical Findings**
    - Parasternal lift.
    - High-pitched blowing holosystolic or pansystolic murmur best heard at left sternal border fourth ICS. Intensified by inspiration and squatting. Decreases with standing and Valsalva.
    - Right ventricular S_3.
    - Irregular–irregular rhythm of atrial fibrillation.
    - JVD and pulsatile neck veins.
    - Palpable liver pulsations.
    - Ascites.
    - Peripheral edema.
  3. **Diagnostic Studies**
  - Echo/2-D and Doppler: tricuspid regurgitation, right atrial enlargement.
  - ECG: right atrial hypertrophy.
  - CXR: right atrial and ventricular enlargement.
  - Cardiac catheterization.
  4. **Management**
  - Treat underlying condition.
  - Annuloplasty.
  - Cardiothoracic surgery referral for valve replacement in patients with severe disease.

VII. Aortic Aneurysm
A. Etiology
- Atherosclerosis: most common etiology.
- Marfan syndrome, especially with thoracic aneurysms.
- Aortitis: mycotic, salmonella, and other infections.

B. Pathology
- Aneurysm: localized area of dilatation or increased diameter of vessel. Most aortic aneurysms are located in abdominal aorta just below the level of renal arteries. Aneurysms can also be located in ascending aorta, aortic arch, and descending aorta. Complications of aortic aneurysms include rupture (chance higher if >5.5 cm), thromboembolism, and distal ischemia.

C. Clinical Features

1. History

- Most cases are asymptomatic until large or rupturing.
- Abdominal fullness or pulsation sensation.
- Back pain.

2. Physical Findings

- Pulsatile mass in epigastric area if abdominal with aortic width >3 cm; 80% can be detected by palpation if 5 cm or more.

D. Diagnostic Studies

- U/S.
- CT scan with contrast.
- Aortography used before surgical intervention.
- CXR may disclose calcifications.

E. Management

- If abdominal aortic aneurysm is <4 cm and asymptomatic, can watch and follow with serial U/Ss.
- If >4 cm, surgical referral warranted; consider elective surgery if >5.5 cm; open or endovascular.

VIII. Aortic Dissection

A. Etiology

- Hypertension.
- Marfan syndrome.
- Cystic medial necrosis.
- Iatrogenic complication of catheterization.
- Coarctation of the aorta and bicuspid AV risk factors.

B. Pathology

- Aortic dissection: caused by tear in intima with formation of false channel in media by hematoma. Mostly occur in ascending aorta several centimeters from aortic valve or descending aorta just distal to origin of left subclavian. Ascending aortic dissections have high mortality rate without treatment as opposed to dissections of descending aorta that have a much better prognosis.
- Classification
  - Type A: involves the aortic arch proximal to the left subclavian artery.
  - Type B: involves the proximal descending thoracic aorta just beyond the left subclavian artery.

C. Demographics

- Most common between the sixth and eighth decade; men > women.

D. Clinical Features

1. History

- Sudden onset of tearing, severe anterior chest pain with radiation to interscapular region.
- Back pain.
- CHF symptoms: dyspnea.
- Syncope.

- Abdominal pain.
- CVA symptoms.

2. Physical Findings

- Increased BP or hypotension.
- Wide pulse pressure.
- Aortic insufficiency murmur in dissections of ascending aorta.
- Diminished or asymmetric peripheral pulses.
- Left pleural effusion sometimes seen with decreased breath sounds and dullness at left base.
- Focal neurologic deficits may be seen.

E. Diagnostic Studies

- CXR: widening of superior mediastinum, displacement of trachea, left pleural effusion, enlargement of aortic knob.
- Transesophageal echocardiography (TEE).
- CT scan with contrast.
- Aortic angiogram ("gold standard").
- MRI.

F. Management

- Immediate BP lowering with IV β-blocker labetalol
- or esmolol; can use nitroprusside if further lowering is required.
- Immediate surgical referral for all type A or type B dissections with aortic branch compromise.

IX. Rheumatic Fever and Heart Disease

A. Etiology

- Group A: β-hemolytic streptococcal pharyngitis.

B. Pathology

- An inflammatory immunologic response to streptococcal infection affecting the heart (endocardium and valves, myocardium, pericardium), skin, joints, and central nervous system (CNS); recurrences are common.

C. Demographics

- Children of ages 5 to 15.
- Incidence in United States dropping.

D. Clinical Features

- Symptoms of rheumatic fever commonly occur 1 to 3 weeks after pharyngitis episode.
- Symptoms of VHD from childhood infection can be delayed until third or fourth decade.

1. Revised Jones Criteria for Diagnosis of Initial Attack (2015)

- With documented preceding group A streptococcal infection (throat culture, throat rapid antigen detection test, elevated or rising strep antibody titers), two major manifestations or one major and two minor manifestations.

2. Major Manifestations
- Carditis (pericarditis, myocarditis, VHD that can affect any valve, but mitral and aortic lesions are most common).
- Polyarthritis (medium-to-large joints; knees, ankles, wrists). Migratory and disappear within 3 to 4 weeks.
- Chorea; Sydenham (late finding).
- Erythema marginatum.
- Subcutaneous nodules (painless over bony prominences).

3. Minor Manifestations
- Polyarthralgia (this cannot be used as minor criterion a part of the modified Jones criteria, if polyarthritis is used as a major criterion).
- Fever (101°–104° F).
- Prolonged PR interval.
- Elevated acute phase reactants; ESR > 60 mm per hour or CRP ≥3.0 mg per dL.

4. Other Manifestations Outside of Jones Criteria
- Abdominal pain.
- Facial tics or grimace.
- Epistaxis.

E. Diagnostic Studies
- Acute phase reactants (e.g., ESR, C-reactive protein) elevated.
- ASO, antideoxyribonuclease-B, rapid strep antigen test, or throat culture bacteriologic or serologic evidence group A strep infection.
- ECG: prolonged PR interval.
- Echo: pericardial effusion or valvular lesions (cannot use as a sole diagnostic method).
- CBC: anemia.

F. Management
- Penicillin IM to treat streptococcal infection.
- Prednisone.
- Aspirin if no cardiomegaly.
- Haloperidol to treat chorea.

X. Infective Endocarditis
A. Etiology
1. Acute Bacterial Endocarditis
- *Staphylococcus aureus*: most common.
- Group A, B, C, and G streptococci.
- *Haemophilus influenzae*.
- *Streptococcus pneumoniae*.
- *Neisseria gonorrhea*.
- *Enterococcus*.

2. Subacute Bacterial Endocarditis
- *Streptococcus viridans* and *Streptococcus bovis*: most common.
- *Streptococcus fecalis* and *Streptococcus faecium* (i.e., enterococci).

- *S. aureus*.
- *Haemophilus, Actinobacillus, Cardiobacterium, Eikenella, Kingella* organisms.

3. Endocarditis with IV Drug Abuse
- *S. aureus*: frequently methicillin-resistant *S. aureus*.
- *Pseudomonas aeruginosa* and *Pseudomonas cepacia*.
- *Enterococcus*.
- *Candida* fungal species.

4. Prosthetic Valve Endocarditis
- *S. aureus* (within first 2 months).
- *Staphylococcus epidermidis* (within first 2 months).
- *Candida* and *Aspergillus* fungal species.
- *S. viridans*.
- *Enterococcus*.

B. Pathology
- Infection with inflammation affecting valvular endocardium and occasionally mural endocardium. May lead to vegetations, valve destruction, and systemic embolization.
- Can be classified into acute bacterial endocarditis (ABE), subacute bacterial endocarditis (SBE), endocarditis with IV drug abuse, and early (within 60 days of implantation) or late (60 days or longer after implantation) prosthetic valve endocarditis. ABE is caused by virulent organisms and has an aggressive course. SBE usually occurs in patients with preexisting VHD and has a slower, more indolent course. Endocarditis in IV drug abusers has predilection for tricuspid valve.

C. Risk Factors
- Prosthetic cardiac valves.
- Congenital cardiac anomalies.
- Previous IE.
- Rheumatic heart disease.
- Any VHD, including MVP when with MR.
- Hypertrophic cardiomyopathy.
- Indwelling intravascular devices.
- Dental or surgical procedures that cause transient bacteremia.
- IV drug abuse.

D. Clinical Features
- Classic triad: fever, heart murmur, and positive blood culture; however, all of these do not have to be present.

1. History
- Fever.
- Anorexia and weight loss.
- Night sweats.
- Fatigue.
- Arthralgias, myalgias.
- Cephalgia.
- Delirium.
- Muscle weakness, paralysis.
- Cold painful extremity with embolism.

- Gross hematuria.
2. **Physical Findings**
   - Murmurs: mostly mitral and aortic involvement, but tricuspid lesions seen in IV drug abuse.
   - Fever (ABE: 102°–105° F; SBE: 99°–100° F).
   - Conjunctival hemorrhage.
   - Petechiae (particularly oropharynx, lower extremity).
   - Splinter hemorrhages (on nail beds).
   - Osler nodes (subcutaneous nodules of fingers).
   - Janeway lesions (small nonpainful hemorrhagic patches on palms, soles of feet).
   - Roth spots (oval white areas surrounded by hemorrhage) on funduscopy.
   - Pericardial friction rub.
   - JVD, rales, and gallops with HF.
   - Cold, pale extremity with absent pulse in septic emboli.
   - Focal neurologic signs in septic emboli with CVA.

E. Diagnostic Studies
- Positive blood cultures (multiple 2–3; 2 by modified Duke criteria) for typical organisms.
- Echo disclosing vegetations; TEE may be especially sensitive.
- Leukocytosis.
- Elevated ESR or C-reactive protein.
- Microscopic hematuria and/or proteinuria on UA.
- Anemia (normocytic) in SBE on CBC.
- Positive rheumatoid factor in SBE.
- Circulating immune complexes, decreased C3 and C4.
- CXR: infiltrates, pleural effusion.
- ECG: conduction abnormalities.

F. Management
- Empiric awaiting culture and sensitivity results: vancomycin and ceftriaxone.
- IV antibiotics for 4 to 6 weeks; penicillin G for penicillin-susceptible *S. viridans*, and others as indicated by culture and sensitivity results.
- Surgical consultation for valve replacement should be considered in complicated cases (e.g., with HF, emboli, dehiscence of prosthetic valve, or resistance to antibiotics).
- Prophylaxis: in 2007, the AHA, in conjunction with the professional organizations representing dentistry (ADA), infectious disease (IDSA), and pediatrics (AAP), published updated recommendations for the prevention of IE. The new guidelines recommend that antibiotic prophylaxis be administered only to patients undergoing dental procedures who are at the highest risk of adverse outcomes from IE (see Section X.G). They no longer recommend prophylaxis for lower-risk patients (such as those with most types

of VHD including MVP) or for patients undergoing genitourinary or gastrointestinal (GI) procedures. Patients at highest risk should receive antibiotic prophylaxis—amoxicillin 2 g PO 60 minutes prior to the procedure (cephalexin, clindamycin, azithromycin, or clarithromycin may be used for penicillin-allergic patients.)

G. Cardiac Conditions Requiring IE Prophylaxis
- Adapted from Wilson W, Taubert KA, Gewitz M, et al. Prevention of infective endocarditis. *Circulation*. 2007;116:1736–1754.
- Prosthetic cardiac valves.
- Previous IE.
- Cardiac transplantation recipients who develop VHD.
- **Congenital Heart Disease**
  - Unrepaired cyanotic congenital heart disease, including palliative shunts and conduits.
  - Completely repaired congenital heart disease defects with prosthetic material or device during the first 6 months after the procedure.
  - Repaired congenital heart disease with residual defects at the site or adjacent to the site of the patch or device.

XI. Chronic Occlusive Arterial Disease/PAD
A. Etiology
- Atherosclerosis (arteriosclerosis obliterans): most common etiology.
- Thromboangiitis obliterans (Buerger disease): occurs in young (<50 years) male smokers.
- Trauma.
- Arteritis.
- Extrinsic compression.

B. Pathology
- Obstruction or narrowing of lumen of peripheral arteries, most commonly in lower extremity, causing interruption of blood flow. These patients are at high risk of CAD.

C. Risk Factors
- Advancing age.
- Smoking tobacco.
- DM.
- Hypertension.
- Hyperlipidemia.
- Obesity.

D. Demographics
- Increases with age.
- Men > women.

E. Clinical Features

1. **History**
   - Intermittent claudication: reproducible exercise-induced pain, commonly in calf with femoral obstruction, relieved with rest.
   - Foot ulcers.
   - Rest pain in severe disease.
   - Erectile dysfunction.

2. **Physical Findings**
   - Diminished or absent peripheral pulses.
   - Absent hair on toes, feet.
   - Atrophic skin changes.
   - Lower-extremity rubor on dependency, pallor on elevation.
   - Decreased temperature of affected limb.
   - Ischemic ulcers on toes, heels, or foot.
   - Gangrene in severe disease.

F. Diagnostic Studies

- Doppler U/S.
- Arteriography.
- Magnetic resonance angiography.

G. Management

- Control of diabetes, hypertension, and dyslipidemia.
- Smoking cessation.
- Low-fat/low-cholesterol/low-calorie diet.
- Optimal diabetes, hypertension control.
- Foot care.
- Graduated exercise program.
- Aspirin: 162 to 325 mg per day.
- Cilostazol (Pletal; Otsuka America, Rockville, MD). Now the mainstay of drug therapy.
- Pentoxifylline (Trental; Aventis, Bridgewater, NJ). Not widely used but may help.
- Clopidogrel (Plavix; Sanofi-Synthelabo, New York, NY, and Bristol-Myers Squibb, New York, NY).
- Propionyl-L-carnitine may be helpful.
- Surgical and invasive measures (e.g., angioplasty, bypass grafting, arthrectomy, stents) for rest pain, intolerable or disabling claudication, or changes that may lead to gangrene (e.g., nonhealing ulcers) especially in patients with diabetes.

XII. Acute Arterial Occlusion

A. Etiology

- **Embolism**
  - VHD.
  - Atrial fibrillation.
  - IE.
  - AMI.
  - Cardiomyopathy.
  - Myxoma.
  - Myocardial aneurysm.
  - Proximal atherosclerotic plaques.
  - Proximal arterial aneurysms.
  - Thrombosis.

B. Pathology

- Acute arterial occlusions may be caused by all the same etiologies as chronic disease (see Section XI) but may also be caused by embolic events from thrombi in heart disease or aneurysms, arterial spasm, myeloproliferative disorders (polycythemia vera), or hypercoagulability states (neoplastic disease).

C. Clinical Features

1. **Five Ps**
   - Pain.
   - Pallor.
   - Paresthesia.
   - Pulselessness.
   - Paralysis.

2. **Other Manifestations**
   - Livedo reticularis (with arteriolar occlusions).
   - Cyanosis.

D. Diagnostic Studies

- Arteriography.

E. Management

- Embolism: heparin.
- Thrombosis: thrombocytosis (e.g., alteplase).
- Surgical referral: embolectomy.
- Treat underlying cause.

XIII. Varicose Veins

A. Etiology

- Hereditary faulty or incompetent venous valves and weak vein walls. Incompetence at saphenofemoral junction common.
- Congenitally absent venous valves.
- Deep vein thrombophlebitis (DVT).
- Increased with dependency, obesity, right-sided HF, pregnancy.

B. Pathology

- Dilated, torturous superficial veins mostly in lower extremities; medial fibrosis and valve atrophy in veins are noted.

C. Clinical Features

1. **History**
   - Often asymptomatic other than cosmetic concerns.
   - Lower-extremity muscle cramps, aching.

2. **Physical Findings**
   - Dilated, torturous superficial veins in lower extremities.
   - Edema of affected limb.
   - Varicose, stasis ulcers.
   - Trendelenburg test.

D. Diagnostic Studies

- None helpful.

E. Management

- Elevate legs.
- Elastic compression stockings.
- Avoid girdles.

- Surgical treatment with ligation, stripping, stab evulsion phlebectomy, or sclerotherapy.
- Encourage ambulation.

XIV. Chronic Venous Insufficiency
A. Etiology
- Hereditary faulty or incompetent venous valves, weak vein walls.
- DVT.
B. Pathology
- Dysfunction or incompetence of venous valves in both superficial and deep venous systems.
C. Clinical Features
1. **History**
   - Lower-extremity aching.
2. **Physical Findings**
   - Edema of lower extremities.
   - Stasis skin changes including hyperpigmentation (often brownish), dermatitis, and ulceration.
   - Stasis ulcers.
   - Trendelenburg test.
D. Diagnostic Studies
- Venous Doppler studies of lower extremities.
E. Management
- Elevate legs.
- Elastic compression stockings.
- Avoid girdles.
- Treat ulcers with dressings, skin grafting, or hyperbaric oxygen when large and nonhealing.
- Encourage ambulation.

XV. Superficial Thrombophlebitis
A. Etiology
- Septic: *S. aureus*, *Klebsiella*, *Candida*, cytomegalovirus in HIV.
- Malignancy.
- Oral contraceptives.
- Pregnancy.
- Hypercoagulability states.
- Behçet disease.
- Buerger disease.
B. Pathology
- Inflammation of superficial veins with thrombosis.
C. Risk Factors
- Immobilization.
- Obesity.
- Advanced age.
- IV catheter in place for >2 days.
- Burns.
- Steroids.
- AIDS.
- Varicose veins.

- Postoperative.
- Pregnancy.
D. Clinical Features
- Fever.
- Local pain.
- Edema, erythema, warmth, tenderness along course of vein.
- Tender palpable cord.
E. Diagnostic Studies
- In septic etiology: leukocytosis, culture blood, and IV site.
- Duplex Doppler U/S.
F. Management
- Extremity elevation.
- Apply heat.
- In aseptic: NSAIDs also consider heparin, warfarin.
- In septic: IV synthetic penicillin, aminoglycoside; consider excision of vein.

XVI. DVT and Thrombophlebitis/ Venous Thromboembolic Disease
A. Etiology
- Venous stasis.
- Coagulopathies.
- Genetic.
B. Pathology
- Thrombosis in deep veins of lower extremities or pelvis causing inflammation. Major complication: pulmonary embolism.
C. Risk Factors
- Virchow triad (stasis, vascular injury, hypercoagulable state).
- Immobility, prolonged bed rest.
- Pregnancy.
- Oral contraceptives.
- Surgery, especially hip surgery.
- Long bone fractures of legs.
- Increased age.
- Varicose veins.
- Cancer.
- Central venous pressure lines.
- Antiphospholipid antibodies.
- Protein C deficiency.
- Protein S deficiency.
- Factor V Leiden mutation and activated protein C resistance.
- Antithrombin III deficiency.
- Connective tissue disorders.
- Polycythemia vera.
- Family history of VTE or IBD.
- Obesity.
- Previous person history of VTE.
- Stroke with hemiplegia or immobility.

D. Clinical Features
- Lower-extremity pain.
- Lower-extremity edema.
- Calf tenderness.
- Erythema, warmth in some cases.
- Positive Homans sign (pain on dorsiflexion of foot).

E. Diagnostic Studies
- Venogram ("gold standard").
- Noninvasive venous studies: duplex Doppler U/S and B-mode U/S or impedance plethysmography.

F. Management
- Heparin (unfractionated or LMWH: e.g., enoxaparin) followed by outpatient warfarin for 3 to 6 months. Consider lifetime warfarin if protein C or S or anti-thrombin III deficient or for factor V Leiden mutation.
- New oral anticoagulants: rivaroxaban and apixaban can be used as initial therapy. Dabigatran can be used after initial therapy with heparin (unfractionated or LMWH).
- Monitor for pulmonary embolus.

XVII. Hyperlipidemia and Dyslipoproteinemia

A. Etiology
1. **Primary**
   - Dietary.
   - Genetic.
   - Obesity.
   - Sporadic.
2. **Secondary**
   - DM.
   - Uremia.
   - Metabolic syndrome.
   - Nephrotic syndrome.
   - Hypothyroidism.
   - Pregnancy.
   - Acromegaly.
   - Cushing disease.
   - Drugs: β-blockers (nonintrinsic sympathomimetic activity, ISA), diuretics, corticosteroids, oral contraceptives, progestins, alcohol for triglyceride.

B. Pathology
- Plasma lipids (triglyceride, cholesterol ester): transported in blood by lipoproteins, classified by their density; chylomicrons are largest and least dense and carry mostly triglycerides, very low-density lipoprotein (VLDL) carry mostly triglycerides, LDL transports cholesterol as its major function, and HDL transports cholesterol from peripheral tissues to the liver.
- Lipoproteins: composed of lipids and protein (called apoproteins). Lp(a) is an LDL-like particle. Increased total cholesterol, LDL, Lp(a), small dense LDL particles, and decreased levels of HDL have been associated with atherosclerosis and CAD.

- High triglyceride levels have been associated with increased risk of CAD in women and patients with DM. High triglyceride levels (>1,000) can cause pancreatitis.

C. Types
- The six types of dyslipoproteinemia are shown in Table 7–1.

D. Clinical Features
- Usually asymptomatic until atherosclerosis develops (CAD, TIA/CVA, PAD).
- Xanthelasma, xanthomas.
- Corneal arcus before age 50.

E. Diagnostic Studies
- Fasting lipid studies. Some also now test for Lp(a) and LDL particle size.
- Triglycerides.
- TSH if hypothyroidism suspected.
- Fasting glucose if DM suspected.
- BUN, creatinine, UA if nephrotic syndrome suspected.

F. Management
- Weight-loss diet.
- Low-fat/low-cholesterol diet: AHA or National Cholesterol Education Program (NCEP) Step I diet <30% total calories from fat with 8% to 10% saturated fat. Cholesterol intake should be ≤300 mg per day. Dietary changes should be initiated in all patients with elevated lipid levels.
- Aerobic exercise program.
- 2018 ACC/AHA Guidelines:
  - Stress primary prevention & treatment of Metabolic Syndrome.
  - Patients with past ASCVD aim to lower LDL-C by 50% or >
  - Goal for patients at very high ASCVD risk or diabetes is 70 mg/dL or lower.
  - Moderate- or high-intensity statin for patients 40 to 75 years old with ≥7.5% 10-year CVD risk.

TABLE 7–1.   Types of Hyperlipidemia

Type	Lipid Elevation	Coronary Artery Disease Risk
I	Triglyceride (chylomicrons)	Normal
IIA	Cholesterol (LDL)	Very high
IIB	Cholesterol and triglyceride (LDL and VLDL)	Very high
III	Cholesterol and triglyceride (β-VLDL and LDL)	Very high
IV	Triglycerides (VLDL)	Varied
V	Triglycerides (VLDL and chylomicrons)	Moderate

β-VLDL, β-very low-density lipoproteins; LDL, low-density lipoproteins.

- HMG-CoA reductase inhibitors or statin drugs are excellent for reduction of LDL-C. They can also cause modest reduction in triglycerides and small increase in HDL-C. Hepatic toxicity and myositis are major side effects, and liver enzymes should be monitored.
- Fibric acid derivatives (e.g., gemfibrozil) are used primarily to lower triglycerides and increase HDL-C and are effective in this regard. They only show small reductions in LDL-C and should not be used primarily to treat elevated LDL-C. Major side effects of these agents are GI. Liver function abnormalities may occasionally be noted.
- Nicotinic acid (niacin) is effective at lowering triglycerides and elevating HDL-C. It can also lower LDL-C moderately. This medication is inexpensive but use is limited due to side effects such as severe flushing. Flushing can be limited if started at low doses (50 mg TID), increasing slowly and gradually, and by giving aspirin simultaneously. GI side effects and hyperuricemia are also reported with this agent.
- Bile acid sequestrants or resins (e.g., cholestyramine, colestipol) can lower LDL-C effectively. These agents are not widely used since the introduction of statin drugs because this class is unpalatable and causes significant annoying GI side effects (e.g., bloating, constipation).
- Probucol: related to antioxidants; can lower LDL-C modestly but may also lower HDL-C; not widely used currently.
- If target cannot be reached on statin alone, add ezetimibe. If target not reached consider a PCSK9 inhibitor.
- Ezetimibe (Zetia; Merck, Schering-Plough, North Wales, PA): inhibits intestinal cholesterol absorption.

XVIII. Cardiomyopathy
A. Pathology
- Primary cardiomyopathies: disorders of myocardium that negatively affect its pumping capability and can lead to HF.
- They can be classified into three types: dilated cardiomyopathy, hypertrophic cardiomyopathy, and restrictive cardiomyopathy.
- Myocardial dysfunction caused by ischemic heart disease (CAD), hypertensive disease, or VHD is classified as secondary cardiomyopathies.

B. Dilated Cardiomyopathy
- Damage to myocardium causing dilated left ventricle, decreased EF, systolic HF. HF, emboli, dysrhythmia, and sudden death are major complications.
1. Etiology
- Idiopathic (to 50% of cases).
- Infective myocarditis: commonly caused by enterovirus, specifically coxsackie virus group B; can also be caused by Lyme disease and HIV.
- Drugs: cocaine, Adriamycin.
- Alcohol.
- Autoimmune: SLE, scleroderma.
- Peripartum.
- Hemochromatosis.
- Thyroid dysfunction (hypo or hyper).
2. Clinical Features
a. History
- Flulike symptoms a few weeks before cardiac failure symptoms in viral myocarditis.
- Dyspnea on exertion and rest in severe disease.
- Orthopnea.
- PND.
- Fatigue.
- Syncope.
- Palpitations.
b. Physical Findings
- Tachycardia.
- Tachypnea.
- Pulsus alternans.
- Cyanosis.
- Cool extremities.
- JVD, hepatojugular reflux.
- Bibasilar rales.
- S_3 gallop.
- S_4 gallop.
- Hepatomegaly.
- Ascites.
- Peripheral edema.
- Systolic murmur of functional MR.
3. Diagnostic Studies
- Echo, cardiac Doppler: chamber size dilation, reduced LVEF.
- ECG: nonspecific ST-T wave abnormalities, LVH, left bundle branch block (LBBB).
- CXR: cardiomegaly, pulmonary congestion, and pleural effusions.
- Nuclear ventriculography (MUGA scan): reduced LVEF.
- Catheterization.
- Myocardial biopsy.
4. Management
- Rest.
- Sodium restriction.
- Diuretics.
- ACE inhibitors or ARBs.
- Nitrates.
- Hydralazine.
- Digoxin.
- Consider warfarin.
- Dopamine in hospital.
- Treat arrhythmias carefully.
- Surgery referral: transplant.

C. Hypertrophic Cardiomyopathy
- Massive hypertrophy of left ventricle, often more pronounced at septum, leads to delayed cardiac relaxation, impaired ventricular filling, diastolic

dysfunction, small LV cavity, and often LV outflow obstruction. Hypertrophy may be asymmetric or concentric. Usually presents in young adulthood.

1. **Etiology**
   a. **Primary**
      - Genetic (autosomal dominant) familial hypertrophic cardiomyopathy (previously called idiopathic hypertrophic subaortic stenosis).
   b. **Secondary**
      - Hypertension.
      - AS.
2. **Clinical Features**
   a. **History**
      - Dyspnea on exertion.
      - Angina pectoris.
      - Presyncope and syncope on exertion.
      - Fatigue.
      - Palpitations.
      - PND.
      - Sudden death.
   b. **Physical Findings**
      - Bisferious carotid pulsation.
      - Prominent A wave of jugular vein.
      - S_4 gallop.
      - Harsh crescendo-decrescendo systolic murmur best heard at left sternal border, apex; increases with Valsalva and standing; decreases with squatting.
      - May have concurrent MR.
3. **Diagnostic Studies**
   - Echo: often diagnostic.
   - ECG: LVH, nonspecific ST-T abnormalities, deep septal Q waves in inferior leads, or tall narrow R waves in V1 and V2.
   - Twenty-four-hour Holter monitor to assess for ventricular tachycardia (VT) if syncope or palpitations present.
   - Cardiac catheterization.
4. **Management**
   - Avoid overly vigorous exercise.
   - β-Blockers.
   - Verapamil, a CCB.
   - Surgical referral for myectomy in refractory cases.
   - Digoxin: contraindicated except for atrial fibrillation with uncontrolled rate.
   - Nitrates and diuretics should usually be avoided.

D. Restrictive Cardiomyopathy
- Decreased elasticity and compliance of ventricles usually from infiltrative process, causing high filling pressures and diastolic dysfunction, and failure.
- Less common than hypertrophic or dilated type.
1. **Etiology**
   - Amyloidosis.
   - Sarcoidosis.
   - Hemochromatosis.
   - Scleroderma.
   - Friedreich ataxia.
2. **Clinical Features**
   a. **History**
      - Dyspnea on exertion.
      - Fatigue.
      - PND.
      - Orthopnea.
      - Edema.
   b. **Physical Findings**
      - JVD.
      - S_3 gallop.
      - S_4 gallop: occasional.
      - Pulmonary rales.
      - Pedal, ankle edema.
3. **Diagnostic Studies**
   - Echo: often diagnostic.
   - Cardiac biopsy: occasionally necessary.
4. **Management**
   - Diuretics (loop).
   - Vasodilators (ACE inhibitors, nitrates).
   - Digoxin may be of benefit.
   - Referral or transplant if refractory.

XIX. Congenital Heart Disease
- There are a variety of congenital structural abnormalities of the heart. Many are diagnosed in infancy, but some do not become symptomatic until adulthood. Etiology of most is unknown. Some are caused by known genetic factors, intrauterine rubella syndrome, and medications (e.g., lithium with Ebstein anomaly).

A. Atrial Septal Defect
1. **Pathology**
   - Except for MVP and bicuspid aortic valve, atrial septal defect (ASD) is the most common type of congenital heart disease.
   - Defect in atrial septum causing opening between left and right atria.
   - Shunting: typically left to right.
   - Symptoms may not appear until adulthood.
   - Ostium secundum: most common type of ASD.
2. **Clinical Features**
   - Usually minimal in childhood, but can exhibit failure to thrive.
   - Adults may have dyspnea on exertion and fatigue.
   - Right ventricular lift.
   - Fixed widely split S_2.
   - Early systolic flow murmur can be heard at left second to third ICS. Later, a low-pitched diastolic murmur at upper left sternal border can sometimes be identified.
   - Clubbing.
   - Cyanosis.
3. **Diagnostic Studies**
   - Echocardiography.

- ECG: RAD, RVH, and RSR′ pattern.
- Cardiac catheterization.
  4. **Management**
- Surgical repair.

B. Ventricular Septal Defect
1. **Pathology**
- Defect in ventricular septum causing opening between left and right ventricles.
- Mostly congenital in origin, but may be acquired as a complication of AMI.
- Shunting: typically left to right.
- Can lead to pulmonary hypertension.
- Symptoms may not appear until adulthood.
2. **Clinical Features**
- Failure to thrive in infancy.
- Dyspnea.
- JVD.
- Left lower sternal thrill.
- S_3.
- High-pitched holosystolic murmur at left sternal border.
- Diastolic murmur of PR.
- Clubbing.
- Cyanosis.
3. **Diagnostic Studies**
- Echocardiography.
- ECG: LVH, RVH, and atrial enlargement.
- CXR: may have enlarged heart.
- Cardiac catheterization.
4. **Management**
- Endocarditis prophylaxis.
- Surgical repair in significant impairments.

C. Coarctation of the Aorta
1. **Pathology**
- An area of narrowing of aorta usually located distal to left subclavian artery.
2. **Clinical Features**
- Failure to thrive in infancy.
- Bilateral claudication.
- Headache.
- Hypertension.
- Delayed femoral pulse compared with brachial pulse.
- Decreased leg BP.
- Murmurs (AS, AR).
- S_4.
3. **Diagnostic Studies**
- Echocardiography (transthoracic, TEE).
- ECG: LVH.
- CXR: rib notching.
- Cardiac catheterization, angiogram.
4. **Management**
- Balloon angioplasty.

- Surgical correction.

D. Patent Ductus Arteriosus
1. **Pathology**
- Failure of ductus arteriosus (shunt from pulmonary artery to aorta) to close as it usually does in the first or second day of life.
- Common in infants and children, but relatively rare in adults.
- Can occur as a result of maternal rubella.
2. **Clinical Features**
- Failure to thrive in infancy.
- Recurrent respiratory infections.
- Fatigue.
- Dyspnea on exertion.
- Angina and syncope can occur in adults.
- With left-to-right shunt: continuous machine murmur or systolic murmur, thrill can occur.
- With right-to-left shunt: cyanosis, clubbing, diastolic Graham Steell murmur.
3. **Diagnostic Studies**
- Echocardiography/cardiac Doppler.
- ECG: LVH, left atrial hypertrophy.
- Cardiac catheterization, angiogram.
4. **Management**
- Catheter plug procedure.
- Surgical correction.

E. Tetralogy of Fallot
1. **Pathology**
- Most common cyanotic congenital heart disease in older children and adults.
- Can have five characteristics including large VSD, right ventricular infundibular stenosis and obstruction, PS, RVH, overriding aorta.
- Right-to-left shunting typical.
2. **Clinical Features**
- Cyanosis, retarded growth in childhood.
- **Adults without correction**
  - Clubbing.
  - Fatigue.
  - Dyspnea on exertion.
  - Edema and syncope can be late findings.
  - Thrill at left sternal border.
  - Single S_2.
  - Systolic ejection murmur.
3. **Diagnostic Studies**
- CBC: polycythemia.
- Echocardiography/cardiac Doppler.
- ECG: RVH, RAD.
- CXR: in children, a small boot-shaped heart may be seen.
- Cardiac catheterization, angiogram.
4. **Management**
- Good dental hygiene.
- Endocarditis prophylaxis.
- Surgical repair.

XX. Giant Cell Arteritis (Also Called Cranial Arteritis and Temporal Arteritis)

A. Etiology
- Idiopathic may be autoimmune.

B. Pathology
- Systemic granulomatous inflammation of medium and large arteries, mostly affecting cranial arteries.
- Blindness: significant complication if untreated.
- Usually occurs in people older than 60 years and associated with polymyalgia rheumatica.

C. Clinical Features
1. **History**
   - Headache: usually unilateral temporal.
   - Jaw claudication with mastication.
   - Visual disturbances (scotoma, diplopia, amaurosis fugax, blindness).
   - Sore throat.
   - Fever.
   - Arthralgias, myalgias.
   - TIA/CVA symptoms.
2. **Physical Findings**
   - Swollen, tender temporal artery.
   - Scalp tenderness.
   - Focal neurologic signs with TIA/CVA.

D. Diagnostic Studies
- Elevated ESR: sometimes >100.
- Temporal artery biopsy: diagnostic.
- May have to biopsy contralateral side if initially negative.

E. Management
- Prednisone: high dose (60 mg) for approximately 6 weeks, then taper over months to years, guided by symptoms and ESR.

XXI. Conduction Disorders
A. Etiology
- Drugs (digoxin, β-blockers, and some CCBs such as diltiazem and verapamil).
- Ischemia, AMI.
- Congenital heart disease.
- Thyroid disorders.

B. Pathology
- Interruptions in cardiac conduction pathways that can occur between atria and ventricles (AV blocks) or at ventricular bundle branches (bundle branch blocks [BBB]).
- These conditions are often related to fibrosis of conduction tissue.

C. Clinical Features
- Many, such as first-degree AV block, second-degree AV block (type I), right bundle branch block (RBBB), and LBBB, may be asymptomatic.
- Some second-degree type II AV blocks and third-degree AV blocks with significant bradycardia can cause lightheadedness, angina, and syncope.

D. Diagnostic Studies
- Most diagnosed on 12-lead ECG.

E. Management
- First-degree AV blocks frequently require no treatment.
- Underlying causes should be determined and treated.
- Offending drugs should be discontinued, when possible.
- Second-degree type II AV block and third-degree AV block require temporary pacemaker; if persistent, require permanent pacemaker.

F. Types
1. **AV Blocks**
   - First-degree AV block: impulse from SA node delayed conducting to ventricles at AV node. PR interval on ECG >0.20 seconds. Every P wave followed by normal ventricular impulse (QRS) complex (Figure 7–2).
   - Second-degree AV block type I (Mobitz type I or Wenckebach): characterized by progressively lengthening PR intervals until complete block occurs and QRS complex dropped, and cycle repeats itself. QRS complexes are normal (Figure 7–3).

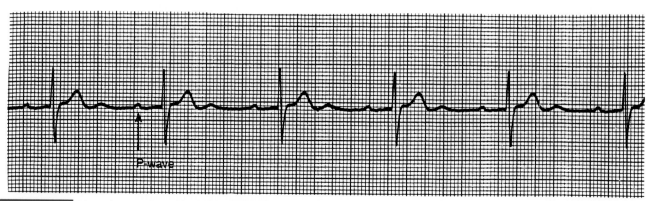

FIGURE 7–2. **First-degree atrioventricular block electrocardiogram.** (From Huff J. AV junctional arrhythmias and AV blocks. In: Huff J, ed. *ECG Workout: Exercises in Arrhythmia Interpretation.* 3rd ed. Philadelphia, PA: Lippincott-Raven; 1997:58, with permission.)

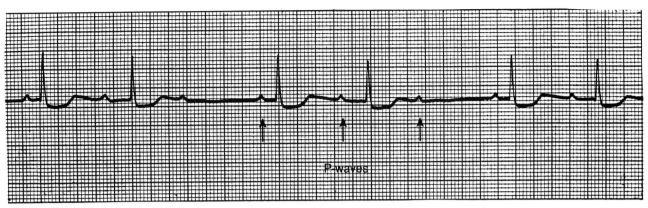

FIGURE 7–3. **Second-degree atrioventricular block, type I or Wenckebach.** (From Huff J. AV junctional arrhythmias and AV blocks. In: Huff J, ed. *ECG Workout: Exercises in Arrhythmia Interpretation.* 3rd ed. Philadelphia, PA: Lippincott-Raven; 1997:59, with permission.)

- Second-degree AV block type II (Mobitz type II): this rhythm involves intermittent complete block with dropped QRS complex without lengthening PR interval. PR intervals are uniform, but atrial rate faster than ventricular rate. This often has a regular pattern with one QRS for every two or three atrial impulses (P wave), as in a 2:1 or 3:1 block. This type of AV block can progress to complete or third-degree AV block (Figure 7–4).
- Third-degree AV block: complete AV block or complete disassociation between atria and ventricles with no atrial impulses reaching ventricles. Independent atrial and ventricular rates are present. Ventricle must pace itself independently through an ectopic pacemaker in nodal areas or ventricles. If ectopic pacemaker is ventricular, QRS complexes are wide (Figure 7–5).

2. **BBBs and Pre-excitation**
   - RBBB: interruption of cardiac impulse at right bundle branch causing left ventricle to be depolarized slightly before right ventricle, which causes widened QRS (>0.12 seconds) with the RSR′ configuration seen in right precordial leads (V_1 and V_2) on ECG (Figure 7–6). Biphasic QRS with broad S wave is also seen in lead I.

- LBBB: interruption of cardiac impulse at left bundle branch causing right ventricle to be depolarized slightly before left ventricle, which causes widened QRS (>0.12 seconds) with RSR′ configuration seen in left precordial leads (V_5 and V_6) on ECG. BBB almost always related to pathologic condition. LBBB may interfere with interpretation of ischemia and AMI on ECG.
- Left anterior hemiblock or left anterior fascicular block: interruption of conduction at anterior division or fascicle of left bundle branch, which has the following characteristics on ECG:
  - **Left anterior hemiblock**
    - LAD (lead I positive, lead aVF negative).
    - Normal or slightly widened QRS (0.08–0.11).
    - Small Q waves can be seen in leads I and aVL.
    - Small R waves and deep S waves seen in leads II, III, and aVF.
  - **Left posterior hemiblock**
    - RAD (lead I negative, lead aVF positive).
    - Small R waves with deep S waves in leads I and aVL.
    - Small Q waves with tall R waves in leads II, III, and aVF.
    - Normal or slightly widened QRS (0.08–0.11).

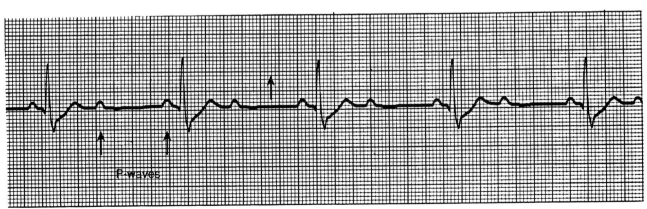

FIGURE 7–4. **Second-degree atrioventricular block type II electrocardiogram.** (From Huff J. AV junctional arrhythmias and AV blocks. In: Huff J, ed. *ECG Workout: Exercises in Arrhythmia Interpretation.* 3rd ed. Philadelphia, PA: Lippincott-Raven; 1997:59, with permission.)

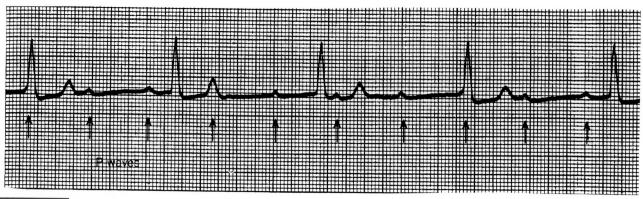

FIGURE 7–5. **Third-degree atrioventricular block electrocardiogram.** (From Huff J. AV junctional arrhythmias and AV blocks. In: Huff J, ed. *ECG Workout: Exercises in Arrhythmia Interpretation.* 3rd ed. Philadelphia, PA: Lippincott-Raven; 1997:59, with permission.)

- Wolff–Parkinson–White (WPW): condition characterized by accessory conduction pathway or bypass tract that may bypass normal conduction delay to ventricles occurring at AV node, which can lead to pre-excitation and paroxysmal tachycardias. ECG features of WPW are as follows:
  - δ Wave, slurred upstroke of QRS (Figure 7–7).
  - Widened QRS of >0.10 seconds (Figure 7–7).
  - Shortened PR interval of <0.12 seconds.
  - Symptomatic WPW with tachycardia can be treated with catheter ablation of accessory pathways.

XXII. Cardiac Dysrhythmias

A. Etiology

- Ischemia and AMI.
- Drugs.
- Electrolyte imbalances (especially potassium).
- Thyroid disease.
- Congenital heart diseases.
- Inflammatory conditions (myocarditis, endocarditis).
- Cardiomyopathies.
- VHD.

B. Pathology

- Cardiac dysrhythmias: abnormalities of cardiac rhythm and can include ectopic beats, slow heart rates (bradycardias), rapid heart rates (tachycardias), and disorganized or erratic rhythms (fibrillation).
- These disturbances can arise from abnormalities of impulse formation, abnormalities of impulse conduction, triggered activity, or reentry phenomenon.

C. Clinical Features

- Many dysrhythmias (e.g., sinus arrhythmia, sinus bradycardia, mild sinus tachycardia) can be asymptomatic.
- Many dysrhythmias (e.g., tachycardias, atrial fibrillation, ectopic beats) present with palpitations.
- Severe bradycardias (with rate <40 per minute) and tachycardias may cause decreased cerebral perfusion with mental status changes, dizziness, and syncope.
- Severe bradycardias and tachycardias may lead to decreased cardiac output and CHF symptoms and signs; atrial fibrillation may also cause CHF due to loss of atrial contraction or "kick."
- Severe bradycardias and tachycardias can cause diminished coronary perfusion in patients with CAD and may precipitate angina pectoris.

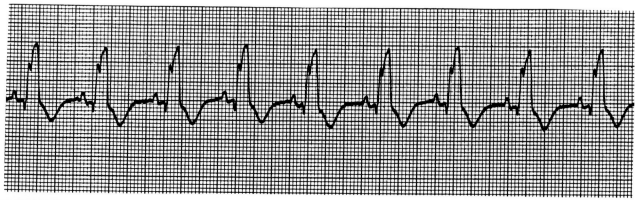

FIGURE 7–6. **Bundle branch block electrocardiogram.** (From Huff J. AV junctional arrhythmias and AV blocks. In: Huff J, ed. *ECG Workout: Exercises in Arrhythmia Interpretation.* 3rd ed. Philadelphia, PA: Lippincott-Raven; 1997:60, with permission.)

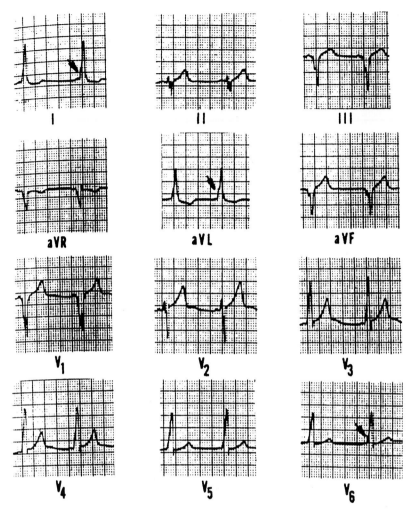

FIGURE 7–7. **Wolff–Parkinson–White electrocardiogram.** (From Zipes DP. Cardiac arrhythmias. In: Kelley WN, ed. *Textbook of Internal Medicine.* 3rd ed. Philadelphia, PA: Lippincott-Raven; 1997:60, with permission.)

- Lethal dysrhythmias (e.g., ventricular fibrillation) cause sudden death.
- Cardiac auscultation is the major step in diagnosing.

D. Diagnostic Studies
- ECG: 12-lead ECG and rhythm strips are the main studies used to diagnose dysrhythmias.
- Twenty-four-hour ambulatory Holter monitoring; event recorders may be needed to disclose intermittent dysrhythmias.
- Signal-averaged ECGs are used to uncover late potentials seen in patients susceptible to VT.
- Autonomic tilt-table testing can be performed for syncope of unknown etiology.
- Electrophysiologic studies (EPS) use electrode catheters in the heart to stimulate and map dysrhythmias; these can also be used to test the effectiveness of certain medications and ablate accessory pathways.
- Other studies (e.g., serum electrolytes, thyroid function tests [TFTs], echocardiography, stress testing, cardiac catheterization) may be needed to delineate the etiology of dysrhythmia.

E. Types
1. **Sinus Tachycardia**
   - Sinus rhythm originating from SA node with resting heart rate of >100 per minute but almost always <160 per minute (can rarely go as high as 200 per minute).
   - Normal for infants and young children, and often caused by noncardiac conditions in adults such as drugs (cocaine, sympathomimetics, decongestants, bronchodilators, nicotine, caffeine), anxiety, anemia, fever, hypovolemia, hypoxemia, exercise, and thyrotoxicosis.
   - Management: usually aimed at delineating and treating cause.
2. **Sinus Bradycardia**
   - Sinus rhythm originating from SA node with a rate of <60 per minute, which can be caused by vagal stimulation, hypothyroidism, medications (β-blockers), high levels of aerobic fitness, and inferior AMI.
   - Management: usually no treatment required unless CNS symptoms develop secondary to cerebral

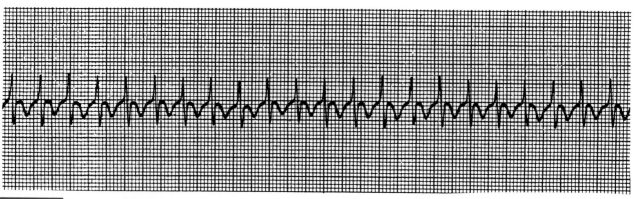

FIGURE 7–8. **Paroxysmal supraventricular tachycardia electrocardiogram.** (From Huff J. Post-test. In: Huff J, ed. *ECG Workout: Exercises in Arrhythmia Interpretation*. 3rd ed. Philadelphia, PA: Lippincott-Raven; 1997:62, with permission.)

hypoperfusion; in those cases, IV atropine and pacing can be used.

3. Paroxysmal Supraventricular Tachycardia

- Characterized by abrupt onset of increased heart rate of 200 to 250 per minute from atrial or junctional foci; common presentation of WPW and reentry phenomenon (Figure 7–8).
- **Management**
  - Carotid sinus massage.
  - Vagal stimulation.
  - Synchronized direct current (DC) electrical cardioversion for hemodynamically unstable patients.
  - Adenosine IV.
  - Calcium channel blockers (i.e., verapamil or diltiazem).
  - β-Blockers (e.g., propranolol, metoprolol, esmolol).
  - Amiodarone.
  - Digoxin IV (unless caused by digoxin toxicity).
  - Overdrive pacing.
  - Radiofrequency ablation can be used in pre-excitation syndromes with an accessory pathway such as WPW.

4. Atrial Flutter

- Tachycardia with atrial rate of 250 to 350 per minute and some AV block causing ventricular rate usually half or one-third of atrial rate (2:1, 3:1 AV block). P waves occur in rapid succession and form characteristic "sawtooth" pattern or "flutter waves." These flutter waves may not be apparent until rate is slowed by carotid sinus massage. Atrial flutter can be caused by HF and pulmonary disease and sometimes seen alternating with atrial fibrillation ("fib-flutter"; Figure 7–9).
- **Management**
  - Rate control: β-blockers, CCBs, or digoxin.
  - Cardioversion: use with anticoagulation if >48 hours. Synchronized DC cardioversion. Can use with ibutilide.
  - Chronic: amiodarone, dofetilide, or EPS with ablation.

5. Atrial Fibrillation

- Dysrhythmia caused by rapid erratic atrial impulse firing from multiple foci. Ventricular response irregular–irregular and may have slow, normal, or fast rate. Distinct P waves usually not discernible; can be caused by chronic hypertension, HF, WPW,

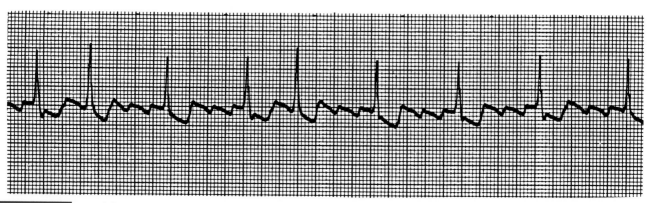

FIGURE 7–9. **Atrial flutter electrocardiogram.** (From Huff J. Post-test. In: Huff J, ed. *ECG Workout: Exercises in Arrhythmia Interpretation*. 3rd ed. Philadelphia, PA: Lippincott-Raven; 1997:62, with permission.)

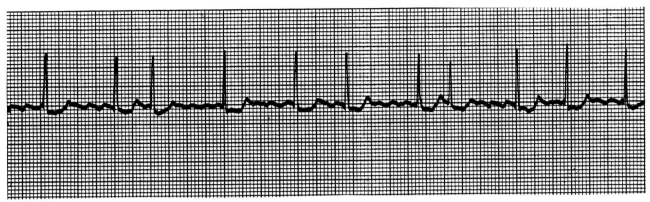

FIGURE 7–10. **Atrial fibrillation electrocardiogram.** (From Huff J. Post-test. In: Huff J, ed. *ECG Workout: Exercises in Arrhythmia Interpretation*. 3rd ed. Philadelphia, PA: Lippincott-Raven; 1997:63, with permission.)

pericarditis, S/P cardiac surgery, heavy alcohol use, sick sinus syndrome, rheumatic heart disease, pulmonary disease, thyrotoxicosis, VHD/mitral valve disease, hypokalemia, CAD/AMI, or pulmonary embolus (Figure 7–10). Can also be seen in normal heart (lone atrial fibrillation).

- **Management**
  - Search for cause TFTs, echo, cardiac enzymes, and electrolytes.
  - Control rate: digoxin, β-blockers, verapamil, or diltiazem can be given to control ventricular response rate.
  - Cardioversion can be attempted using drugs such as amiodarone. If unstable, synchronized electrical cardioversion should be done with or without ibutilide, followed by anticoagulation. If stable and in atrial fibrillation >48 hours, a TEE should be performed prior to cardioversion to look for an atrial thrombus. If present, the patient should be treated with anticoagulant for 4 weeks prior to cardioversion followed by 4 weeks after.
  - Anticoagulation with warfarin to the international normalized ratio of 2:3 will reduce the risk of embolic stroke. Dabigatran (Pradaxa), Rivaroxaban (Xarelto), and Apixaban (Eliquis) can also be used in nonvalvular atrial fibrillation and

may have lower risk of bleeding. For lone atrial fibrillation in young (<65 years old) patients with no history of heart disease, hypertension, or diabetes ASA can be used.
  - Dronedarone (Multaq), amiodarone, propafenone, flecainide, and dofetilide have been used to maintain patients in normal sinus rhythm (NSR).
    - Recent studies show rate control with anticoagulation may be as efficacious as cardioversion.
    - Radiofrequency ablation also has been successful in refractory cases.

6. **Ventricular Tachycardia**
  - Characterized by a rapid rate (150–250 per minute) originating from ectopic ventricular focus. Can be caused by CAD, AMI, or antiarrhythmic drugs. Antiarrhythmic drugs (e.g., quinidine, procainamide, disopyramide, flecainide, encainide, amiodarone, Stadol) can cause polymorphic form of VT (called torsades de pointes) usually by prolonging the QT interval. VT can cause hemodynamic instability and even pulseless state. Even when the patient appears hemodynamically stable, VT is an emergent condition because it can progress to ventricular fibrillation and death. Important to differentiate VT from SVT with aberrancy, although sometimes difficult without slowing the rate (Figures 7–11 and 7–12).

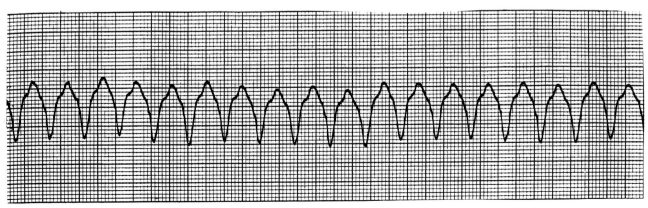

FIGURE 7–11. **Ventricular tachycardia electrocardiogram.** (From Huff J. Ventricular arrhythmias and bundle branch blocks. In: Huff J, ed. *ECG Workout: Exercises in Arrhythmia Interpretation*. 3rd ed. Philadelphia, PA: Lippincott-Raven; 1997:63, with permission.)

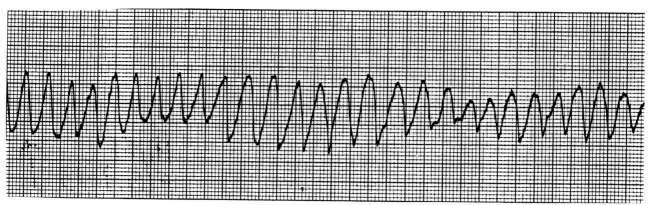

FIGURE 7–12. **Torsades de pointes electrocardiogram.** (From Huff J. Ventricular arrhythmias and bundle branch blocks. In: Huff J, ed. *ECG Workout: Exercises in Arrhythmia Interpretation.* 3rd ed. Philadelphia, PA: Lippincott-Raven; 1997:63, with permission.)

- **Management**
  - Unstable and pulseless VT should be defibrillated.
  - Synchronized DC cardioversion for stable VT.
  - Lidocaine IV can also be used in stable VT.
  - Magnesium can be given to treat torsades de pointes.
  - Overdrive pacing also can be used in VT.
7. **Ventricular Fibrillation**
  - Totally, disorganized rapid ventricular firing from multiple ectopic foci causing no effective cardiac output, pulseless state, and death (Figure 7–13).
  - **Management**
    - Immediate cardiopulmonary resuscitation.
    - Defibrillation.
    - Automatic ICDs can be surgically installed in patients at high risk of ventricular fibrillation.
8. **Premature Atrial Contractions (PAC, APC, APB)**
  - Caused by impulse originating in ectopic focus in atrium outside of SA node that occurs earlier than expected in cardiac cycle. P wave has different morphology than normal sinus beats, but QRS usually appears normal. These can be idiopathic or related to caffeine, tobacco, or myocardial ischemia (Figure 7–14).

- **Management**
  - PACs usually require no treatment other than correcting potential underlying etiologies.
  - Persons with no underlying heart disease can have PACs.
  - Patients should be instructed to avoid tobacco, alcohol, and caffeine products.
9. **Premature Ventricular Contractions (PVC, VPC, VPB)**
  - Caused by ectopic focus in ventricle with impulse that occurs earlier than expected in cardiac cycle. QRS complex appears wide; they can occur in pairs (couplets), can occur after every other normal beat (bigeminy), can originate from one ectopic focus with a similar morphology (unifocal), or can originate from multiple foci with different morphology (multifocal). They can be idiopathic and occur in people without disease, or can be caused by myocardial ischemia, cardiomyopathy, or structural abnormalities (Figure 7–15).
  - **Management**
    - In patients with no underlying heart disease, PVCs are usually not treated. The Cardiac Arrhythmia Suppression Trial study disclosed higher mortality in patients with ventricular ectopy treated with class IC antiarrhythmic drugs in comparison with placebo groups.

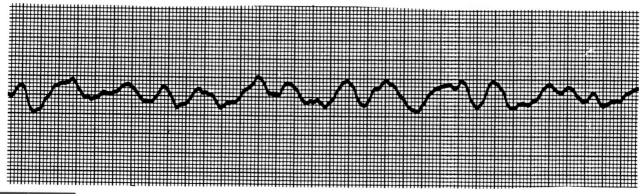

FIGURE 7–13. **Ventricular fibrillation electrocardiogram.** (From Huff J. Ventricular arrhythmias and bundle branch blocks. In: Huff J, ed. *ECG Workout: Exercises in Arrhythmia Interpretation.* 3rd ed. Philadelphia, PA: Lippincott-Raven; 1997:64, with permission.)

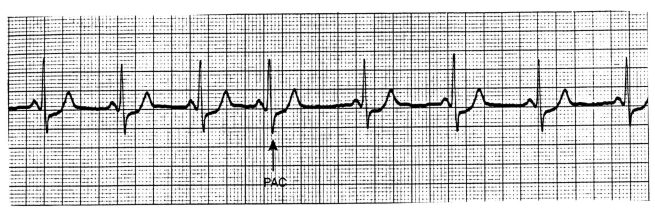

FIGURE 7–14. **Premature atrial contraction electrocardiogram.** (From Huff J. Atrial arrhythmias. In: Huff J, ed. *ECG Workout: Exercises in Arrhythmia Interpretation*. 3rd ed. Philadelphia, PA: Lippincott-Raven; 1997:64, with permission.)

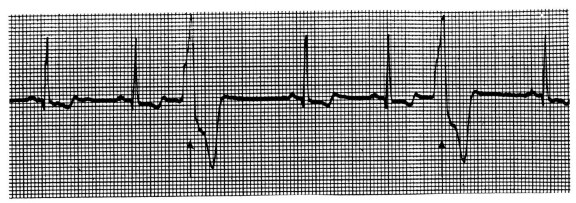

FIGURE 7–15. **Premature ventricular contraction electrocardiogram.** (From Huff J. Ventricular arrhythmias and bundle branch blocks. In: Huff J, ed. *ECG Workout: Exercises in Arrhythmia Interpretation*. 3rd ed. Philadelphia, PA: Lippincott-Raven; 1997:65, with permission.)

- Patients with ventricular ectopy and LV dysfunction with an EF < 30% may also benefit from antiarrhythmic medication.
- Patients should be instructed to avoid caffeine, tobacco, and alcohol.
- β-Blockers can be used in low-risk patients with symptoms.

10. **Premature Junctional Contractions**
- Ectopic premature beats originating from AV node or AV junction; characterized by retrograde conducted P waves that may be inverted, buried in the QRS, or appear after the QRS and narrow QRS complex.

11. **Escape Beats and Rhythms**
- At times when SA node fails to function properly or AV conduction is interrupted, as seen with pauses, severe bradycardia, and higher level AV blocks (second-degree type II or third degree), an ectopic pacemaker takes over. If pacemaker is at the AV junction, the patient exhibits premature junctional contractions or develops junctional escape or idiojunctional rhythm with rate usually about 60 per minute, retrograde P wave, and

narrow QRS. They also have accelerated junctional rhythm with a rate of 70 to 130 per minute that can occur after cardiothoracic surgery, with digoxin toxicity, or with myocarditis. If pacemaker is in the ventricles, PVCs, ventricular escape rhythm, or idioventricular rhythm is seen with wide QRS complex and at a rate of about 30 to 40 per minute. Accelerated ventricular rhythms can also occur.
- **Management**
  - Treat underlying cause.
  - Symptomatic bradycardias can be treated temporarily with IV atropine.
  - Second-degree type II or third-degree AV blocks require pacemaker insertion.

12. **Sick Sinus Syndrome**
- Includes various disorders affecting SA node and conduction system. Occurs commonly in elderly persons and can cause sinus arrest or intermittent episodes of bradycardia alternating with tachycardia ("brady–tachy syndrome"). Pacemaker insertion is sometimes required.

REVIEW QUESTIONS

1. Which of the following studies can be used to determine ventricular wall motion, wall size/dimensions, and approximate LVEF?

   a) Thallium stress testing
   b) N-terminal pro-BNP
   c) Echo/cardiac Doppler
   d) Cardiac CT

2. What is the mechanism of action for sacubitril and valsartan (Entresto) in HF?

   a) Neprilysin inhibitor and AII receptor antagonist
   b) Diuretic and angiotensin-converting enzyme inhibitor
   c) Positive inotropic agent
   d) Aldosterone antagonist and diuretic

3. Which of the following drugs would be the best first-line agent to treat hypertension in a patient with a history of HF?

   a) Terazosin
   b) Propranolol
   c) Verapamil
   d) Enalapril

4. A decreased level of which of the following blood tests is a risk factor for coronary artery/heart disease?

   a) C-reactive protein
   b) HDL
   c) Homocysteine
   d) VLDL

5. What is the ideal level for LDL in a patient with a previous MI?

   a) Below 70 mg per dL
   b) Below 100 mg per dL
   c) Below 130 mg per dL
   d) Below 160 mg per dL

6. A 38-year-old man comes to the emergency department with complaint of 6 hours of sharp retrosternal chest pain with radiation to back and shoulder that increases with inspiration and lying supine. There is no complaint of dyspnea. Physical exam reveals a fever and friction rub. What is the most appropriate treatment for this patient?

   a) SL NTG
   b) Immediate cardiac catheterization and angioplasty
   c) NSAIDs
   d) IV Furosemide

7. A 78-year-old woman comes to the office complaining of chest pain with exertion and dizziness. Her cardiac exam reveals a grade IV/VI crescendo-decrescendo systolic murmur best heard at right second ICS, right sternal border with radiation into carotids, and down left parasternal border to the apex. What is the most likely diagnosis?

   a) AS
   b) AR
   c) MS
   d) MR

8. A 28-year-old man presents to the office for evaluation after a syncopal episode after his usual exercise routine at the gym. He denies chest pain, SOB, dizziness, palpitations, headache, or other neurologic symptoms. Family history is significant for sudden cardiac death of an uncle at age 36, and his brother has had syncopal spells. He is on no meds, and his physical exam is unremarkable. The ECG revealed an NSR with no sinus pauses or ectopy, normal axis, no LVH, and a QTc of 0.470 second. In formulating a treatment plan, what medicines should this patient be counseled to avoid?

   a) Erythromycin
   b) Amoxicillin
   c) Doxycycline
   d) Macrodantin

9. A 22-year-old patient presents to the office complaining of progressive dyspnea over the past 2 years to the point that he cannot complete his exercise routine, and palpitations and orthopnea over the last 2 months. On two occasions, the patient has experienced near syncope related to exercise and dizziness upon standing from a seated position. On examination, the patient is found to have a systolic ejection crescendo-decrescendo murmur heard best along the apex and left sternal boarder and radiates to the suprasternal notch, but not to the neck, a prominent jugular venous pulse a wave, and a laterally displaced, double apical impulse. A cardiac echo revealed a septal wall thickness, and asymmetrical septal hypertrophy with diastolic dysfunction with reduced LV compliance, LVH, and color Doppler reveal an MR. What is a common dysrhythmia associated with this condition?

   a) Sinus dysrhythmia
   b) Multifocal atrial tachycardia
   c) Wandering atrial pacemaker
   d) Atrial fibrillation

10. A 46-year-old patient with no significant PMH presented to the emergency room after suddenly developing pleuritic chest pain, dyspnea, orthopnea, and ankle swelling. Review of systems was unremarkable except for some recent nasal congestion and scratchy throat, which the patient attributed to allergies, and some arthralgias in the hips and knees that are worse with prolonged sitting and associated with stiffness. What laboratory studies would be included in the workup of this patient?

   a) Complete metabolic panel
   b) Hepatitis screening
   c) Rheumatologic screening
   d) Thyroid screening

ANSWERS TO REVIEW QUESTIONS

1. **Answer: C**. Echo/cardiac Doppler is an excellent test in HF diagnosis in that it is used to determine ventricular wall motion, wall size/dimensions, and approximate left ventricular ejection fraction. Thallium stress testing is an effective diagnostic perfusion study used to test for coronary artery/heart disease. N-terminal pro-BNP (B-type natriuretic peptide) is a blood test that is sensitive for ventricular stretch and fluid overload. Cardiac CT can be used to visualize wall dimensions but is mostly now used to obtain coronary calcium scoring.

2. **Answer: A**. Entresto (sacubitril and valsartan) is a highly effective drug with a unique mechanism of action. It is the first neprilysin inhibitor (sacubitril) combined with an existing AII receptor antagonist (valsartan). Sacubitril degrades vasoactive and natriuretic peptides. The PARADIGM-HF study revealed that Entresto was superior to an ACE-I in HF.

3. **Answer: D**. An angiotensin-converting enzyme inhibitor such as enalapril would be an excellent choice to treat both hypertension and HF and indicated in both disease states. Terazosin is an α-blocker that can be used in hypertension or BPH. Propranolol is a β-blocker not used in HF because of its negative inotropic effects. Carvedilol and metoprolol are β-blockers also indicated for HF. Verapamil is a CCB with negative inotropic effects. Diuretics and AII receptor antagonists can also be useful in both disorders.

4. **Answer: B**. Low HDL is a risk factor for CAD/CHD. Elevated C-reactive protein, LDL, homocysteine, triglycerides, Lp(a), and VLDL are CAD/CHD risk factors.

5. **Answer: A**. Recent data reveal that <70 mg per dL is the ideal level for LDL in a patient with a previous MI.

6. **Answer: C**. This patient is showing the signs and symptoms of pericarditis. After the appropriate diagnostic studies, these cases are often treated with NSAIDs, analgesics, and rest.

7. **Answer: A**. This patient is showing the typical symptoms and murmur of AS.

8. **Answer: A**. Long QT syndrome most often is a congenital disorder that can cause ventricular tachyarrhythmias that lead to cardiac manifestations—syncope and cardiac arrest often times after a precipitating event like exercise and emotional stress. It is characterized by a long QTc on ECG (QTc varies with age and sex but generally >0.46 seconds indicates prolongation). Patients with long QTc syndrome need to avoid medications that can further prolong the QT interval which include diphenhydramine, erythromycin, trimethoprim and sulfamethoxazole, pentamidine, quinidine, procainamide, disopyramide, sotalol, probucol, bepridil, dofetilide, ibutilide, cisapride, ketoconazole, fluconazole, itraconazole, tricyclic antidepressants, phenothiazines, butyrophenones, and benzisoxazole.

9. **Answer: D**. Hypertrophic cardiomyopathy (HCM) is associated with a variety of cardiac dysrhythmias including atrial fibrillation, atrial flutter, PVCs, ventricular tachycardia, and ventricular fibrillation. Patients with HCM are at an extremely high risk of developing ventricular fibrillation.

10. **Answer: C**. Myocarditis has several different etiologies including infection, infiltrative processes, autoimmune processes, acute rheumatic fever, hypersensitive/eosinophilic, giant cell and peripartum among others. Viral causes are the most common. The laboratory workup should include a CBC, ESR, C-reactive protein, rheumatologic screening, cardiac enzymes, and possibly serum viral antibody titers to rule out other causes. Viral titers are rarely indicated.

SELECTED REFERENCES

Abbott JA, Cheitlin MD. Cardiac arrhythmias. In: Saunders CE, Ho MT, eds. *Current Emergency Diagnosis and Treatment*. 6th ed. Stamford, CT: Appleton & Lange; 2008:578–607.

American Heart Association. *ACLS Provider Manual*. Dallas, TX: American Heart Association; 2001:123–144.

Armstrong C; Joint National Committee. JNC 8 guidelines for the management of hypertension in adults. *Am Fam Physician*. 2014;90(7):503–504.

Bashore TM, Granger CB, Hranitzky P, Patel MR. Heart disease. In: McPhee S, Papadakis M, Rabow MW, eds. *2011 Current Medical Diagnosis and Treatment*. New York, NY: McGraw-Hill; 2017:322–498.

Bates B. The cardiovascular system. In: Bates B, ed. *A Guide to Physical Examination and History Taking*. 6th ed. Philadelphia, PA: Lippincott-Raven; 1995:259–312.

Blankenberg A, Rupprecht HJ, Bickel C, et al. Glutathione peroxidase 1 activity and cardiovascular events in patients with coronary artery disease. *N Engl J Med*. 2003;349:1605–1613.

Branch WT, Alexander RW, Schlant RC, et al. *Cardiology in Primary Care*. New York NY: McGraw-Hill; 2000.

Braunwald E, Goldman L. *Primary Cardiology*. 2nd ed. Philadelphia, PA: WB Saunders; 2003.

Brennan ML, Penn MS, Van Lente F, et al. Prognostic value of myeloperoxidase in patients with chest pain. *N Engl J Med*. 2003;349:1595–1604.

Caruso AC. Arrhythmias. In: Noble J, Greene HL, Levinson W, Modest GA, Young MJ, eds. *Textbook of Primary Care Medicine*. 2nd ed. St. Louis, MO: Mosby; 1996:199–210.

Chobanian AV, Bakris GL, Black HR, et al; National Institutes of Health, National Heart, Lung, and Blood Institutes. Seventh report of the Joint National Committee on prevention, detection, evaluation, and treatment of high blood pressure: the JNC 7 report. *JAMA*. 2003;289:2560–2572.

Dambro MR. Aortic dissection. In: Dambro MR, ed. *Griffith's 5 Minute Clinical Consult*. Baltimore, MD: Lippincott Williams & Wilkins; 1998:66–67.

Dambro MR. Aortic valvular stenosis. In: Dambro MR, ed. *Griffith's 5 Minute Clinical Consult*. Baltimore, MD: Lippincott Williams & Wilkins; 1998:68–69.

DeGowin EL, DeGowin RL. The thorax and cardiovascular system. In: DeGowin EL, DeGowin RL, eds. *Bedside Examination*. 4th ed. New York, NY: Macmillan; 1981:229–471.

Dipiro JT, Talbert RL, Yee GC, et al. *Pharmacotherapy: A Pathophysiologic Approach*. 5th ed. New York, NY: McGraw-Hill; 2002:chaps 15 and 17.

Dubin D. Infarction. In: Dubin D, ed. *Rapid Interpretation of EKG'S*. 3rd ed. Tampa, FL: Cover Publishing; 1981:204–245.

Geraets DR. The heart and myocardial infarction. In: Traub SL, ed. *Basic Skills in Interpreting Laboratory Data*. 2nd ed. Bethesda, MD: American Society of Health-System Pharmacists; 1996:187–212.

Gotto AM. Hyperlipidemia. In: Rakel RE, ed. *Conn's Current Therapy*. Philadelphia, PA: WB Saunders; 1998:567–574.

Huff J. Atrial arrhythmias. In: Huff J, ed. *ECG Workout, Exercises in Arrhythmia Interpretation*. 3rd ed. Philadelphia, PA: Lippincott-Raven; 1997:89–132.

Huff J. AV junctional arrhythmias and AV blocks. In: Huff J, ed. *ECG Workout, Exercises in Arrhythmia Interpretation*. 3rd ed. Philadelphia, PA: Lippincott-Raven; 1997:133–180.

Huff J. Post-test. In: Huff J, ed. *ECG Workout, Exercises in Arrhythmia Interpretation*. 3rd ed. Philadelphia, PA: Lippincott-Raven; 1997:247–284.

Huff J. Ventricular arrhythmias and bundle branch blocks. In: Huff J, ed. *ECG Workout, Exercises in Arrhythmia Interpretation*. 3rd ed. Philadelphia, PA: Lippincott-Raven; 1997:181–226.

Johnson JA, Lalonde RL. Congestive heart failure. In: Dipiro JT, Talbert RL, Yee GC, Matzke GR, Wells BG, Posey LM, eds. *Pharmacotherapy: A Pathophysiologic Approach*. 3rd ed. Stamford, CT: Appleton & Lange; 1997:219–256.

Lowering plasma homocysteine. *Med Lett Drugs Ther*. 2003;45(1168):85–86.

Margolis S. Disorders of plasma lipids and lipoproteins. In: Stobo JD, Traill TA, Hellman DB, Ladenson PW, Petty BG, eds. *The Principles and Practice of Medicine*. 23rd ed. Stamford, CT: Appleton & Lange; 1996:338–347.

Michael TAD. Systolic and diastolic murmurs. In: Tap M, ed. *Auscultation of the Heart: A Cardiophonetic Approach*. New York, NY: McGraw-Hill; 1998:161–218.

Miles NM, Williams ES, Zipes DP. Acquired valvular heart disease. In: Andreoli TE, Bennett JC, Carpenter CCJ, Plum F, eds. *Cecil Essentials of Medicine*. 4th ed. Philadelphia, PA: WB Saunders; 1997:45–52.

Miles NM, Williams ES, Zipes DP. Congestive heart failure. In: Andreoli TE, Bennett JC, Carpenter CCJ, Plum F, eds. *Cecil Essentials of Medicine*. 4th ed. Philadelphia, PA: WB Saunders; 1997:40–44.

Pagana KD, Pagana TJ. *Manual of Diagnostic and Laboratory Tests*. 2nd ed. St. Louis, MO: Mosby; 2002:123.

Pederson D. Infectious endocarditis. In: Labus JB, ed. *The Physician Assistant Medical Handbook*. Philadelphia, PA: WB Saunders; 1995:378–388.

Rahimtoola SH. Valvular heart disease. In: Stein JH, ed. *Internal Medicine*. 5th ed. St. Louis, MO: Mosby; 1998:239–262.

Schwartz B, O'Brien KL. Streptococcal infections. In: Kelly WN, ed. *Textbook of Internal Medicine*. 3rd ed. Philadelphia, PA: Lippincott-Raven; 1997:1614–1622.

Segal BL. Clinical recognition of rheumatic heart disease. In: Chizner MA, ed. *Classic Teachings in Clinical Cardiology: A Tribute to W. Proctor Harvey*. Cedar Grove, NJ: Laennec Publishing; 1996:991–1016.

Spittell PC, Spittell JA. Diseases of the peripheral arteries and veins. In: Stein JH, ed. *Internal Medicine*. 5th ed. St. Louis, MO: Mosby; 1998:305–312.

Stanley VR. Fascicular blocks. In: Stanley VR, ed. *12-Lead ECG Interpretation for Emergency Personal: A Systematic Analytical Approach*. Fayetteville, WV: Independently Published; 1995:71–75.

Stone NJ, Robinson JG, Lichtenstein AH, et al. 2013 ACC/AHA Guideline on the treatment of blood cholesterol to reduce atherosclerotic cardiovascular risk in adults. *Circulation*. 2014;129:S1–S45. doi:10.1161/01.cir.0000437738.63853.7a.

Thompson T, Hallan SD. Behavioral and cognitive-behavioral interventions. In Tierney LM, McPhee SJ, Papadakis MA, eds. *Lange Current Medical Diagnosis and Treatment*. New York, NY: McGraw-Hill; 2004:chap 10.

Yancy CW, Jessup M, Bozkurt B, et al. 2017 ACC/AHA/HFSA focused update of the 2013 ACCF/AHA guideline for the management of heart failure: a report of the American College of Cardiology/American Heart Association Task Force on Clinical Practice Guidelines and the Heart Failure Society of America. *Circulation*. 2017;136:e137–e161. doi:10.1161/CIR.0000000000000509.

Zipes DP. Cardiac arrhythmias. In: Kelly WN, ed. *Textbook of Internal Medicine*. 3rd ed. Philadelphia, PA: Lippincott-Raven; 1997:410–435.

Zipes DP. Management of cardiac arrhythmias: pharmacological, electrical, and surgical technique. In: Braunwald E, ed. *Heart Disease: A Textbook of Cardiovascular Medicine*. Philadelphia, PA: WB Saunders; 1992:628–666.

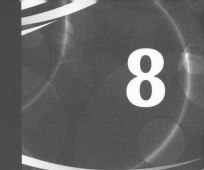

Behavioral Disorders

Ann McDonough Madden • Ryan J. Clancy

This chapter is not an exhaustive review of the extensive array of behavioral and mental health disorders that may present across all populations and various demographics of individuals. Rather, the selection of clinical disorders is based on those that the physician assistant may most likely encounter during the course of his or her practice. The summaries of the disorders are meant as quick synopses of the disorder in question, differential diagnoses, common symptomatology, and potential treatment considerations. As with all areas of medical and psychiatric practice, providers are advised to consult with their colleagues and specialty-specific professionals for additional guidance when the possibility of several different diagnostic and subsequent treatment pathways exists.

Be advised that the most recent data and available information have been gleaned from the clinical literature on these disorders. However, changes and updates in prevalence rates and other statistical considerations are continuous and ongoing. As a result, recent changes may not be reflected in this chapter at this time.

I. Childhood Disorders

A. Autism Spectrum Disorder

1. Definition

- Autism spectrum disorder (ASD) is characterized by persistent deficits in social communication and interaction and repetitive, restricted patterns of behavior or areas of interest. The symptoms of ASD are often recognized in the second year of life (12–24 months). The prevalence in the United States is estimated to be 1%, with boys diagnosed four times more often than girls.

2. Etiology

- Although not completely certain, a combination of biologic factors including prenatal viral exposure, immune system abnormality, and/or genetic factors are involved.
- Studies demonstrate a concordance rate of 36% in monozygotic twins compared to 0% in dizygotic twins.
- Biomarkers in ASD include elevated serotonin in the blood (particularly in the platelets).

3. Clinical Features

- Clinical features of the disorder are typically evidenced between the ages of 12 and 24 months, generally with onset observed before 36 months.

a. Primary Signs

- Social interactions: infant or toddler exhibits physical signs of significant emotional discomfort, if not detachment (i.e., may not cuddle or respond to affection and touching; may not make eye contact).
- Communication difficulties: typically demonstrates language difficulties (i.e., appears to be unable to communicate or has ability to communicate, but fails to communicate with others across a variety of settings, such as home, school, and social environments).
- Repetitive behaviors: may engage in repetitive, self-stimulating behavior (i.e., repetitive face scratching, head rubbing, and other behavioral tics/movements).
- May exhibit impulsivity.

b. Other Signs and Symptoms

- *Persistent failure* to develop sufficient and appropriate mutual social relationships in many, if not most, interactions and social situations.
- Failure to show preference for parents over other adults.
- Failure to develop friendships with other children.
- May display severe anxiety when the usual routine is disrupted.
- May exhibit an exquisite, if not unusual, sensitivity (even possibly extreme responses) to various visual, auditory, and olfactory stimuli, and either an avoidance or a preoccupation with such (e.g., child overreacts when fire alarm or school bell rings).
- May also express exquisite tactile sensitivity to certain food.
- May form unusual attachments to ordinary objects (e.g., paper or rubber bands).
- Possible spinning and repetitive body movements (e.g., arm flapping).
- Extreme cases may include evidence of potential self-injurious or even self-destructive behavior.
- May experience gastrointestinal (GI) symptoms and higher than usual number of upper respiratory infection.
- Insomnia is common.

4. Diagnostic Studies

- Multidisciplinary team evaluation as possible (psychiatrist, psychologist, neurologist, speech

pathologist, pediatrician, etc.). Evaluations to include structured psychiatric interview, and, as possible, psychological/neuropsychological testing, and neurologic and speech evaluations. Using a standardized assessment tool such as *Autism Diagnostic Observation Schedule-Generic* (ADOS-G) is beneficial.
- Extensive family and social history.
- Physical examination.

5. Management/Treatments
- Referral to child psychiatrist, psychologist, or neuropsychologist to establish accurate autism diagnosis and degree of severity, and to determine appropriate interventions, including intensive multidisciplinary learning support (LS) services. Behavior therapy and school-based interventions/options.
- Pharmacotherapy: plays a minor role at this stage, and is used only for specific symptoms (e.g., atypical antipsychotics for aggression and stimulants for comorbid attention-deficit/hyperactivity disorder [ADHD]).
- Resources and supports for family.

B. Conduct Disorder
1. Definition
- Conduct disorders include a group of behavioral and emotional problems in children and adolescents characterized by repetitive, disruptive, and persistent age-inappropriate patterns of behavior that violate the rights of others and/or grossly violate societal rules and boundaries.
- Children and adolescents with these disorders exhibit great difficulty perceiving, acknowledging, and abiding by socially acceptable rules of behavior and interaction.
- Children with conduct disorder exhibit behaviors in the following four categories: physical aggression toward people and/or animals; destruction of property/violation of property rights of their own or others; theft or acts of deceit; chronic and consistent violation of age-appropriate rules (imposed by adults such as parents or other formal agents).
- Such patterns of behavior cause significant impairment in social, academic, and occupational arenas of functioning and development.
- A minority of patients with this disorder may eventually develop an antisocial personality (ASP) disorder or develop substance abuse and/or other addictive disorders in adulthood, if left untreated.

2. Etiology and Epidemiology
- A number of causal factors implicated, including parental, genetic, sociocultural, psychological, and neurobiologic, along with a history of child abuse/maltreatment, but there is no known single cause.
- Potential causal interactive factors:
  - Temperament.
  - Parenting style focused on problem behavior, ignoring good behavior, and indirectly reinforcing problem behavior.

- Parental modeling of impulsivity and rule-breaking behavior.
- Parental/marital conflict may exist in the home.
- Placement in institutional settings as infant or toddler (e.g., nonparental and nonfamilial custodial care) may coincide with such diagnoses.
- Lower socioeconomic status.
- Prevalence rates in the United States are 6% to 16% for males and 2% to 9% for females. Conduct problems are usually referred to child and adolescent mental health professionals.

3. Clinical Features
- Persistent repetitive pattern of inappropriate behaviors that have the violation of the basic rights of others and/or age-appropriate rules of society as an essential feature.
- **Demonstrates at least three of the following:**
  - Stealing.
  - Persistent lying.
  - Property destruction of varying degrees (including vandalism).
  - Running away from home.
  - Violating curfew set by parents and caregivers.
  - Deliberate fire setting.
  - Repeated truancy (beginning before age 13).
  - Cruelty to animals.
  - "Bullying" behaviors (i.e., physical and verbal aggressive behavior with other children or adults).
  - Initiating physical fights.
  - Weapon use (e.g., bat, brick, knife, gun).
  - Forced someone into sexual activity.

4. Diagnostic Determinations and Differentiation
- Reports from parent, child, and/or other social/community agents (e.g., teachers and coaches).
- **Rule out of common concurrent diagnosis, especially:**
  - ADHD.
  - Anxiety and mood disorders (depression, mania, and psychosis).
  - Substance abuse.
  - Developmental disorders (especially developmental reading and expressive language disorder).
  - Intellectual disability (ID).
  - Complex partial seizures (especially children with violent conduct disorders).

5. Management/Treatment
- Multimodal treatment approach that uses all available family and community resources provides best results.
- Individual psychotherapy.
- Behavior modification.
- Parental counseling.
- Environmental intervention, including special education programs and hospitalization, for severely aggressive presentations.
- Residential treatment as indicated.

- Legal assistance/intervention as necessary to enforce cooperation with treatment.
- **Psychopharmacologic intervention for aggressive behavior as follows:**
  - Antidepressants (selective serotonin-reuptake inhibitors [SSRIs] for irritability, impulsivity, and mood).
  - Atypical antipsychotics (Table 8–1).

TABLE 8–1. Pharmacotherapeutics

Generic (Brand Name)	Maximum Daily Dose (mg)
Typical antipsychotic agents	
Chlorpromazine (Thorazine)	1,000
Thioridazine (Mellaril)	800[a]
Perphenazine (Trilafon)	64
Fluphenazine (Prolixin)	40 (10 mg/d IM)
Trifluoperazine (Stelazine)	40
Thiothixene (Navane)	60
Haloperidol (Haldol)	100
Molindone (Moban)	225
Atypical antipsychotic agents	
Clozapine (Clozaril)	900[a]
Olanzapine (Zyprexa)	20[a]
Quetiapine (IR, XR)	800[a]
Risperidone (Risperdal)	16[a]
Ziprasidone (Geodon)	80 mg BID[a]
Aripiprazole (Ability)	30[a]
Paliperidone (Invega)	12[a]
Mood stabilizers	
Lithium	1,800[a]
Valproic acid (Depakote, Depakene)	60 mg/kg/d[a]
Carbamazepine (Tegretol)	1,600[a]
Lamotrigine (Lamictal)	200[a]
Sedatives and hypnotics	
Chloral hydrate (Noctec)	200 (rarely used)
Flurazepam (Dalmane)	30 (rarely used)
Zolpidem (Ambien)	10
Temazepam (Restoril)	30
Estazolam (Prosom)	2
Eszopiclone (Lunesta)	2
Ramelteon (Rozerem)	8
Antianxiety agents and benzodiazepines	
Alprazolam (Xanax)	4
Chlordiazepoxide (Librium)	100–300 for alcohol withdrawal
Clonazepam (Klonopin)	20
Clorazepate (Tranxene)	90
Diazepam (Valium)	40
Lorazepam (Ativan)	10
Oxazepam (Serax)	120
Hydroxyzine HCI (Atarax/Vistaril)	600
Buspirone (BuSpar)	60
Diphenhydramine (Benadryl)	400

Generic (Brand Name)	Maximum Daily Dose (mg)
Tricyclic antidepressants/other	
Amitriptyline (Elavil)	300[a]
Clomipramine (Anafranil)	250[a]
Doxepin (Sinequan)	300[a]
Imipramine (Tofranil)	300[a]
Amoxapine (Asendin)	400[a]
Desipramine (Norpramin)	300[a]
Nortriptyline (Pamelor)	150[a]
Maprotiline (Ludiomil)	225[a]
Trazodone (Desyrel)	600[a]
Mirtazapine (Remeron)	45[a]
Selective serotonin-reuptake inhibitors	
Fluoxetine (Prozac)	80[a]
Sertraline (Zoloft)	200[a]
Paroxetine (Paxil)	40[a]
Citalopram (Celexa)	60[a]
Escitalopram (Lexapro)	20[a]
Selective norepinephrine reuptake inhibitors	
Bupropion (Wellbutrin, SR and XL, Zyban)	450
Venlafaxine (Effexor, XR)	225
Duloxetine (Cymbalta)	120
Desvenlafaxine (Pristiq)	50
Antiparkinsonian drugs	
Trihexyphenidyl (Artane)	15
Diphenhydramine (Benadryl)	400 (also used in adjunct with neuroleptics for EPSs)
Benztropine (Cogentin)	6 (also used in adjunct with neuroleptics for EPSs)
Carbidopa/levodopa (Sinemet)	200/2,000
Amantadine (Symmetrel)	400
Alzheimer drugs	
Memantine (Namenda)	20
Donepezil (Aricept)	10
Stimulants and nonstimulants	
Methylphenidate HCI (Ritalin)	60[a]
Methylphenidate transdermal (Daytrana)	30[a]
Methylphenidate (Concerta)	72[a]
Lisdexamfetamine (Vyvanse)	70[a]
Dextroamphetamine sulfate (Dexedrine)	60[a]
Amphetamine (Adderall)	60[a]
Atomoxetine (Strattera)	100[a]
Drugs used in chemical dependency	
Acamprosate (Campral)	1,998
Naltrexone (ReVia)	50

Note: This list is not meant to be inclusive of all psychiatric medications. Doses will need to be adjusted for elderly persons, children (where indicated), and for hepatic and renal function.

[a]Black Box warnings.

C. Oppositional Defiant Disorder

1. Definition

- Milder form of chronic behavior problems than seen in conduct disorder.
- Frequent and persistent pattern of angry mood, argumentative behavior, and vindictiveness.
- Behavior problems are usually worse at home, but may extend to school and peers.

2. Etiology and Epidemiology

- Although unknown with certainty, hypothesized factors may include inherited predisposition, modeling of parental oppositional and defiant behavior, and parental inability to reward good behavior or set firm, fair, and consistent limits.
- Prevalence rates range from 2% to 16%.
- Before puberty, the condition is more common in boys. Post puberty, rates have an equal sex ratio.
- May begin as early as age 3, but usually manifests by age 8 and no later than early adolescence.

3. Clinical Features

- Chronic pattern of stubborn, negativistic, provocative, hostile, and defiant behavior. No typical violation of others' rights.
- Often irritable, resentful, and quick to take offense.
- Loss of temper.
- Frequent arguments with adults.
- Difficulty and outright refusal to follow directives.
- Tendency to *blame others* for his or her own inappropriate actions.
- Exhibiting a tendency toward vindictiveness when he or she perceives "injury" to sense of self.
- Symptoms tend to be more prominent as familiarity of the patient with others increases.

4. Diagnostic Studies

- Structured psychiatric interview.
- Critical parent and teacher reports. (**NOTE:** Behavior may not seem abnormal or evidence itself during a diagnostic interview.)
- Psychological testing to rule out low intelligence quotient (IQ) or learning disabilities.

5. Management

- Psychotherapy: behavioral therapy, individual therapy, family counseling, and behavior modification.

D. Attention-Deficit/Hyperactivity Disorder

1. Definition

- A persistent pattern of inattention and/or hyperactivity-impulsivity.
- Symptoms typically are evidenced before age 12 and present for at least 6 months.
- To meet criteria for ADHD, these symptoms must occur *in more than one setting* (e.g., school and home for children, and work and home for adults).
- Symptoms cause impairment in social, academic, or occupational setting.

2. Etiology and Epidemiology

- No clear etiology; but evidence from twin and adoptive family studies suggests a strong genetic component. Other factors include neurochemical, neurophysiologic, neuroanatomic, psychosocial, and developmental factors.
- ADHD occurs in 5% of children and is more prevalent in boys than in girls. Male-to-female ratio ranges from 2:1 to 9:1.

3. Clinical Features

- Must have *six or more* symptoms of *hyperactivity* or *inattention* for at least 6 months. Symptoms were seen before age 12.

a. Inattention

- Difficulty following instructions.
- Short attention span at work and play.
- Does not appear to be listening.
- May appear to be "daydreaming."
- Loses things.
- Makes careless mistakes.
- Difficulty organizing.
- Forgetful.
- Avoids engaging in "effortful" mental activities, particularly when "not interested" (again, this may suggest an avoidance tactic when called on to demonstrate something that he or she does not know what to do, given a lack of attention to instructions and directions initially).
- Attention to an agent or an item is easily distracted by an extraneous stimuli.

b. Hyperactivity and Impulsivity

- Fidgety or restless.
- Difficulty staying seated.
- Difficulty waiting in lines or awaiting his or her turn.
- Impulsive or intrusive speech.
- Difficulty playing quietly.
- Running about or climbing excessively in situations in which these activities are inappropriate.
- Talks incessantly.
- Interrupts or intrudes on others.
- Often blurts out an answer before a question has been completed.

4. Diagnostic Studies

- Structured psychiatric interview. Consider neuropsychological assessment.
- Comprehensive medical history with attention to prenatal, perinatal, and toddler information.

- Diagnosis based on specific criteria and ruling out of other causes of behavior.
- Cognitive testing is very useful in confirming inattention and impulsivity.

5. Management
- Pharmacologic treatment, specifically central nervous system (CNS) stimulants, is the first line of treatment. Stimulants are contraindicated in patients with cardiac risks and abnormalities.
- Methylphenidate, short acting and/or long acting (Ritalin, Concerta).
- Dextroamphetamine sulfate (Vyvanse).
- Nonstimulant medication such as atomoxetine (Strattera).
- Behavioral interventions at home and school.
- School programs and LS systems designed to address this disorder.
- Cognitive behavioral therapy.

E. Intellectual Disability
1. Definition
- Significant limitations in intellectual functioning and adaptive behavior and associated difficulties in a variety of skill domains, most typically involving communication, self-care, social/interpersonal skills, self-direction, academic skill acquisition, and occupational, leisure, and safety concerns.
- Qualified as mild, moderate, severe, or profound.
- Accompanied by significant limitations in adaptive functioning.
- Must manifest itself before age 18.

2. Etiology and Epidemiology
- Etiology derives from genetic chromosomal and inherited conditions.
- Prenatal exposure to infections and toxins may be implicated in fetal alcohol syndrome (FAS)/fetal alcohol effect (FAE), as would be perinatal trauma (i.e., prematurity).
- Genetic, environmental, biologic, and psychosocial factors appear to work additively in ID.
- Prevalence is 1% in the United States.
- Males are more likely than females to be diagnosed with ID.

3. Clinical Features
- *Concurrent deficits in age-appropriate adaptive functioning expected for his or her age and cultural group in at least two of the following areas:*
  - Communication.
  - Self-care.
  - Home living.
  - Social/interpersonal skills.

- Use of community resources.
- Self-direction.
- Functional academic skills.
- Work.
- Leisure.
- Health.
- Safety.
- Varied physical examination presentations depending on underlying cause.
- Craniofacial, skeletal, cardiovascular (CV), neurologic, and stature abnormalities may also present as markers in this disorder.
- Associated psychiatric disorders may be three to four times as common in patients with an ID as in the general population.

a. Down Syndrome
- General hypotonia.
- Oblique palpebral fissures.
- Abundant neck skin.
- Small, flattened skull.
- Slanted eyes and flat nose.
- High cheekbones.
- Protruding tongue.
- Broad, thick hands with short, inward-curving fingers.
- Single palmar transversal crease.
- Moro reflex: weak or absent.
- Language function: weak.
- Muted affect.

b. Fragile X Syndrome
- Large, long head and ears.
- Short stature.
- Hyperextensible joints.
- Postpubertal macroorchidism.
- Intellectual function declines in the pubertal period.
- High rates of comorbid ADHD.

c. Prader–Willi Syndrome
- Compulsive eating behavior.
- Hyperphagia.
- Obesity.
- Hypogonadism.
- Small stature.
- Hypotonia.
- Small hands and feet.

d. Phenylketonuria
- Hyperactive.
- Erratic, unpredictable behavior: difficult to manage.
- Eczema.
- Vomiting.
- Convulsions.
- Temper tantrums.
- Bizarre movements of bodies and upper extremities.

- Twisting hand movements.
- Verbal and nonverbal communication is usually severely impaired or nonexistent.
- Poor coordination.
- Perceptual difficulties.

4. Diagnostic Studies
- Structured psychiatric interview.
- Intelligence testing and psychological evaluation.
- Hearing and speech evaluation.
- History and physical examination.
- Clinical observation.
- Assessment of adaptive functioning (i.e., Vineland Adaptive Behavior Scales).
- Urine and blood tests to rule out metabolic disorders.
- Chromosome analysis.
- Amniocentesis (during pregnancy).
- Chorionic villi sampling (CVS).
- Electroencephalography (EEG).

5. Management
  a. Primary, Secondary, and Tertiary Actions
    - May assist in the prevention, if not alter the course of the disorder, as well as its eventual management.
    - **Primary: actions to eliminate or reduce the conditions that lead to the development of the disorders associated with ID may include the following:**
      - Genetic counseling.
      - Family counseling.
      - Proper prenatal and postnatal medical care.
      - Immunization.
    - **Secondary: treatment to diminish the course of the complications of ID**
      - Early screening for and treatment of metabolic and endocrine disorders (e.g., phenylketonuria [PKU] and hypothyroidism).
    - **Tertiary:** treatment to minimize the sequelae or consequent disabilities.
  b. Psychotherapy
    - Modified psychiatric treatment for specific disorders depending on the child's level of intelligence.
    - Individual psychotherapy or parental counseling to deal with developmental or situational crises, or in the treatment of coexisting psychiatric disorders.
    - Parents may need assistance in dealing with their grief over having a "defective" child.
    - Specific behavioral programs to teach adaptive behaviors and reduce stereotypic behaviors, aggression, and self-injury.
  c. Pharmacotherapy
    - Same medications are used for treating psychiatric disorders in children and adolescents with normal IQs (i.e., stimulants for ADHD symptoms) (see Table 8–1).
  d. Environmental Interventions
    - Special education programs.
    - Specialized infant stimulation and preschool programs.

II. Eating Disorders
A. Anorexia Nervosa
  1. Definition
    - The three essential criteria for anorexia nervosa are self-induced starvation, relentless drive for thinness accompanied by a morbid fear of fatness, and the presence of medical signs and symptoms resulting from starvation.
  2. Etiology, Epidemiology, and Comorbidity
    - Biologic, social, and psychological factors.
    - Midteens (age 14–18) is the most common age at onset.
    - Prevalence is 0.5% to 1% of adolescent girls.
    - Female-to-male ratio of 10:1.
    - Frequently seen in athletes and in professions requiring thinness.
    - Depression is seen in 65% of cases, and social phobia and obsessive–compulsive disorder (OCD) in 35% and 24%, respectively.
  3. Clinical Features
    - Refusal to maintain body weight at or above a minimally normal weight for height, body mass index (BMI) <17.
    - Intense fear of gaining weight even though underweight.
    - Disturbance in perception of one's weight and shape and/or denial of the seriousness of current low weight.
    - If postmenarchal, the absence of at least three consecutive menstrual cycles.
    - May be restricting intake or binge eating/purging, or both. Behaviors include misuse of laxatives, enemas, diuretics, or other medications; excessive exercise; self-induced vomiting; and drinking excessive amounts of water.
    - Physical signs may include bradycardia, hypothermia, hypotension, dependent edema, and lanugo.
  4. Diagnostic Studies
    - Full psychiatric and physical examination; vital signs (VS) may reveal hypotension and bradycardia, significant skin and hair changes.
    - Complete blood count (CBC): may show leukocytosis, leukopenia, or anemia.
    - Electrolytes: hypokalemia.
    - Thyroid-stimulating hormone (TSH): hypothyroidism.
    - Electrocardiogram (ECG): ST segment and T-wave changes.
    - Hypercholesterolemia.

5. Treatment

- Hospitalization, depending on patient's medical condition. Generally, inpatient hospitalization is required for <75% below expected body weight. Goal is to stabilize medically.
- Psychotherapy: cognitive behavioral therapy (CBT) and family therapy.
- Pharmacotherapy: if there is underlying depression, treat with SSRIs. Cyproheptadine (Periactin) may increase appetite.

B. Bulimia Nervosa

1. Definition

- Episodic binge eating with inappropriate ways of preventing weight gain.

2. Etiology and Epidemiology

- Bulimia is more prevalent than anorexia nervosa. One to 4% of young women are diagnosed with bulimia nervosa. It is more common in females than in males.
- May occur in later adolescence and in early adulthood.
- Etiologic factors vary and include biological, social, and psychological factors.

3. Clinical Features

- Recurrent episodes of binge eating characterized by eating within a 2-hour period, or eating more than most people would in a similar period, a sense of lack of control over eating during the episode.
- Behaviors include misuse of laxatives, enemas, diuretics, or other medications; excessive exercise; self-induced vomiting; drinking excessive amounts of water; and fasting. Patients may present with GI complaints of abdominal pain, constipation, or bloating.
- Behaviors occur at least once a week for 3 months.
- Most patients are within their normal weight range.
- Comorbid psychiatric conditions include depression, anxiety, and personality disorders.

4. Diagnostic Studies

- Full psychiatric and physical examination; VS may reveal hypotension and bradycardia; examination of teeth may reveal pitting or erosion of tooth enamel; calluses may be present on finger used to induce vomiting.
- Electrolytes: hypokalemia and hypomagnesemia.
- Serum amylase: hyperamylasemia.
- Dexamethasone suppression test: nonsuppression.

5. Treatment

- Psychotherapy: CBT and family therapy.
- Pharmacotherapy: as with anorexia nervosa, treat underlying mood disorders if present. Fluoxetine (Prozac) has been shown to be effective in doses ranging from 60 to 80 mg daily. Tricyclic antidepressants (TCAs) have also been effective in

reducing the binge–purge cycle. These are to be used with caution in view of the increased risk of CV side effects, especially if electrolyte abnormalities are present.

III. Personality Disorders

OVERVIEW

A. Definition

- Personality disorders are patterns of affect and behavior characterized not only by their deviations from what are considered typical ranges seen within the general population but especially by their pervasiveness, their enduring features, and their inflexibility toward change. Over time, these disorders result in significant distress and psychosocial impairments for the individuals challenged by them, as well as major disruptions in their social, occupational, and other interpersonal relationships. Individuals with these disorders present as major challenges for caregivers and treating providers.

B. Etiology and Epidemiology

- Genetic factors may play a role in the etiology and development of such disorders, as well as other psychogenic and environmental factors.
- Ten to 20% of the U.S. population meets the *Diagnostic and Statistical Manual of Mental Disorders*, 5th edition (*DSM-5*) criteria for a personality disorder.

C. Clinical Features

- Inflexible, maladaptive behavior patterns/traits and characteristic responses to life events, which exceed the range of variation, present in most people.
- Results in significant impairments in social, interpersonal, and occupational functioning.
- Manifests fully by late adolescence or early adulthood.
- Influences all aspects of personality including cognition, mood, behavior, and interpersonal style of relating to others.
- Disordered thoughts/behavior must be stable and of long duration; chronic, not just in response to a limited event/stressor.
- Cannot be explained as a result of another adult mental disorder.
- Brain disease, injury, or dysfunction must be excluded as the cause of the disorder.
- Grouped into three major subtypes/clusters (Cluster A, Cluster B, and Cluster C) based on predominant symptoms. See below for more detail.

D. Diagnostic Studies

- Unless otherwise noted, no specific laboratory test or radiologic examinations are used to make the diagnosis of a personality disorder.

- **Assessment and diagnosis of a personality disorder are made through the use of the following:**
  - Clinical interviews.
  - Self-report inventories (e.g., the Minnesota Multiphasic Personality Inventory [MMPI-2], Personality Diagnostic Questionnaire).
  - Semistructured interviews (e.g., Structured Interview for Diagnosis of Personality Disorders, Personality Disorder Examination, Structured Clinical Interview).
  - Routine history and physical and laboratory tests to rule out any other underlying physiologic disorders (e.g., hyperthyroidism).
  - Various diagnostic studies (e.g., sleep studies, EEG, dexamethasone suppression) have been used to study different disorders, but their clinical use continues to be evaluated.

E. Management
- Psychotherapy with/without pharmacotherapy is the cornerstone of treatment.
- Type of psychotherapy (i.e., psychodynamic, supportive, interpersonal, behavioral, cognitive, dialectical behavior therapy [DBT]) varies according to the disorder and other conditions affecting the patient.
- Pharmacotherapy often focuses on symptom management/relief to allow for better psychotherapeutic/behavioral response.
- **NOTE:** In each subtype of the personality disorder that follows, at least three to four of the specific subtype criteria and the general personality disorder clinical features listed previously must be met to make the diagnosis.

CLUSTER A DISORDERS (INCLUDE THOSE WHO APPEAR ODD OR ECCENTRIC)

A. Schizoid Personality Disorder
1. Definition
- The essential characteristic of this disorder is a lifelong pattern of withdrawal, inhibition, if not absence of emotional expression, and shyness.
- Apparent bland and constricted affect.

2. Etiology and Epidemiology
- Onset: usually early childhood.
- Prevalence: may affect 5% of the general population.
- Sex ratio: unknown, but some studies report a 2:1 male-to-female ratio.

3. Clinical Features
- Central characteristic: inability to form relationships or respond to others in a meaningful way, typically resulting in a lifelong pattern of social withdrawal.
- Appears indifferent to others; lack of response to praise, criticism, or any feelings expressed by others.

- Often seen by others as eccentric, isolated, or lonely.
- People with the disorder tend to gravitate toward solitary jobs/activities involving little or no contact with others; many prefer night work to day for this reason.
- Neither desires nor enjoys close relationships, including being part of a family.
- Takes pleasure in few, if any, activities.
- May appear to be cold and aloof.
- The absence of a clearly diagnosed thought disorder or delusional thinking and a normal capacity to recognize reality and respond appropriately, and an absence of relatives with schizophrenia differentiate it from schizophrenia.
- May have successful, if isolated, work histories, differentiating it from schizotypal personality disorder and schizophrenia.

4. Diagnostic Studies
- Generally diagnosed through a solid structured psychiatric interview, and possibly additional psychosocial assessment.

5. Management
- Psychotherapy.
- Pharmacotherapy: small doses of antipsychotics, antidepressants, and psychostimulants are effective in some patients (see Table 8–1).
- It remains unclear what proportion of individuals with this diagnosis will eventually manifest and develop symptoms of schizophrenia.

B. Schizotypal Personality Disorder
1. Definition
- A disorder characterized by patterns of thought and behaviors suggestive of schizophrenia without classic symptoms suggestive of psychosis (e.g., delusions).
- An acute discomfort with and reduced capacity for close relationships.

2. Etiology and Epidemiology
- Three percent of the general population is believed to suffer from this disorder, with a greater association evidenced among biologic relatives of patients with schizophrenia.
- Sex ratio: unknown.

3. Clinical Features
- Strikingly odd, "obtuse," and/or peculiar behaviors or appearance, even discernible by laypersons.
- Constricted or inappropriate affect (e.g., laughs inappropriately during conversations).
- Peculiar notions, ideations, ideas of reference, and illusions.
- Episodes of derealization.
- May evidence suspiciousness and/or paranoid ideation.

- Lack of close friends or confidants other than first-degree relatives.
- Speech may be distinctive or peculiar; may have meaning only to the person and may need interpretation.
- Exquisitely sensitive to and aware of the feelings of others, especially negative feelings such as anger.
- Excessive social anxiety.
- Some involvement in cults, engagement in strange religious practices, or even in the occult.
- Under stress may decompensate and have psychotic symptoms of brief duration.
- Oddities in behavior, thinking, perception, and communication, as well as a clear family history of schizophrenia may differentiate this disorder from schizoid personality disorder.
- Absence of psychosis, except rare "fragmented" episodes of psychosis while under stress, differentiates this disorder from schizophrenia, although chronicity of such patterns may suggest that this disorder may be a "precursor personality" of schizophrenia.

4. Diagnostic Studies
- Structured psychiatric interview.
- Psychological testing may provide additional diagnostic indications as well as assist in differential diagnosis.

5. Management
- Psychotherapy.
- Pharmacotherapy: antipsychotics may be useful in dealing with ideas of reference, illusions, and other symptoms of the disorder (see Table 8–1).
- Antidepressants are helpful with a comorbid diagnosis of depression.

C. Paranoid Personality Disorder
1. Definition
- A disorder characterized by suspiciousness, systemized delusions of persecution, or grandeur without hallucinations.
- A tendency toward global, excessive, or irrational suspiciousness.

2. Etiology and Epidemiology
- Two to 4% of the population, with men exhibiting the disorder more frequently than women.
- No familial pattern, although a higher incidence appears in those patients with family members having schizophrenia.

3. Clinical Features
- Long-standing patterns of suspiciousness and mistrust of people in general.
- Begins by early adulthood and appears in a variety of contexts.
- Interprets other people's actions as deliberately demeaning or threatening.
- Refuses responsibility for own feelings and assigns them to others.

- Expects to be exploited or harmed by others in some way.
- Can be affectively restricted, appearing unemotional or, conversely, may exhibit intense and situation-inappropriate affect given an exquisite sensitivity to nuances of potential threat.
- Ideas of reference and logically defended illusions are common.
- Rarely seeks treatment voluntarily; if treatment is requested by family or employer, can "pull themselves together" sufficiently to appear "intact" and not under any apparent distress.
- "Reads" hidden, demeaning, or threatening meanings into benign remarks or events.
- Persistently bears grudges (i.e., is unforgiving of insults, injuries, or slights).
- Perceives attacks on his or her character or reputation not apparent to others, and is quick to react angrily or counterattack.
- May have recurrent suspicions, without justification, regarding fidelity of spouse or sexual partner.
- Differentiated from paranoid schizophrenia by absence of hallucinations or formal thought disorders.
- Differentiated from schizoid personality disorder by absence of interactivity with other people and presence of paranoid ideation.

4. Diagnostic Studies
- Structured psychiatric interview.
- Psychological testing.

5. Management
- **Psychotherapy:** treatment of choice (1:1); avoid "interpersonal closeness/contact"; remain professional.
- **Pharmacotherapy**
  - Benzodiazepines may be useful in dealing with agitation and anxiety (for very brief periods). Consider addictive potential.
  - Severe agitation/quasi-delusional thinking may be addressed through the use of antipsychotics, such as thioridazine or haloperidol, in small doses/brief periods.

CLUSTER B DISORDERS (INCLUDE THOSE WHO APPEAR ERRATIC, DRAMATIC, OR OVERIRRATIONAL)
A. Antisocial Personality Disorder
1. Definition
- A disorder characterized by behaviors deviating sharply from norms, rules, and laws of society. Such behaviors can be hostile or harmful to society.

2. Etiology and Epidemiology
- Prevalence rate of 0.2% to 3%; more common in males than in females.
- Most common in poor urban areas and among transient residents within these areas and other geographic areas.

- Evidence of conduct disorder with onset is present before 15 years of age.
- Familial pattern: disorder is five times more common in first-degree relatives of men with the disorder than in controls.

3. Clinical Features
- Inability to conform to the social norms that govern accepted behavior; repeated infractions of the law and actions leading to arrest may be common (e.g., lying to police if questioned, use of aliases, truancy, running away from home as a child/adolescent, frequent thefts, frequent fights, and substance abuse, drug trafficking).
- A significant feature is a lack of remorse for their inappropriate actions and violation of rules, norms, the rights of others, etc., typically being indifferent or rationalizing their actions. Appear to lack what most consider a "conscience."
- As the disorder progresses, it may be increasingly characterized by the commission of serious antisocial, if not criminal acts.
- Such patients can often seem normal, even charming or ingratiating; but underneath, tension, hostility, irritability, and rage are present.
- May appear seductive with opposite sex clinicians and manipulative with same-sex clinicians.
- Impulsivity; failure to plan ahead.
- Irritability and aggressiveness.
- Reckless disregard for safety of self or others.
- Consistent irresponsibility: repeated failure to honor work demands, rules, and financial obligations.
- Exhibit no anxiety or depression: incongruous with their behavior.
- Promiscuity, spouse abuse, child abuse, and drunk driving common in their history—"con men."
- Patient must be at least 18 years old to receive a diagnosis of ASP disorder.

4. Diagnostic Studies
- Structured psychiatric interview.
- Thorough neurologic examination: often shows abnormal electroencephalogram results, soft neurologic signs.
- History of brain damage in childhood.

5. Management
- Psychotherapy: limits must be established.
- Pharmacotherapy: used for incapacitating symptoms only.

B. Borderline Personality Disorder
1. Definition
- A disorder characterized by a pervasive pattern of excessive, impulsive behaviors, extreme attitudes, chaotic relationships, chronic anger, suicidal threats, depression, and impaired social and vocational functioning.

2. Etiology
- One to 2% of population, with a preponderance of women exhibiting the disorder (2:1) over men.
- Diagnosis is usually made before age 40.
- Prevalence of major depressive disorder, alcohol and other substance abuse disorders, and substance abuse in first-degree relatives of people with borderline personality disorder (BPD).

3. Clinical Features
- The essential feature of this disorder is a pervasive pattern of instability in relationships, affect, and self-image, accompanied by chronic impulsivity in response to such. As a result, individuals with this disorder frequently present as being in a "state of crisis."
- Mood swings are common. Short-lived psychotic episodes may be possible, although the symptoms are typically circumscribed, fleeting, or doubtful.
- Transient, stress-related paranoid ideation or severe dissociative symptoms.
- May evidence highly unpredictable behavior.
- Achievements are rarely at the level of their abilities or self-expectations.
- Recurrent suicidal behavior, gestures, or threats, especially at times of perceived or actual stress.
- Repetitive self-destructive acts (e.g., wrist slashing, self-mutilation) to elicit help from others, express anger, or numb themselves to overwhelming effect. Such self-injury gestures are typically nonsuicidal self-injury (NSSI).
- Tumultuous interpersonal relationships are common markers of this disorder.
- "Cannot tolerate being alone": may accept strangers as "friends" rather impulsively, with poor judgment, or act promiscuously, placing themselves in precarious, if not episodic, dangerous situations.
- Frantic efforts to avoid real or imagined abandonment. A sense of abandonment is a persistent feature and complaint associated with this disorder (i.e., "no one understands or cares about me," despite evidence to the contrary from caregivers, family, and friends).
- See people as either "good or bad," nurturant, or hateful. Such "splitting" results in idealized versions of what is perceived as "good" and devalued versions of what is "bad."
- Inappropriate, intense anger, and/or difficulty controlling anger.
- Often complains of chronic feelings of emptiness, depression, and boredom.
- Lack of consistent sense of identity.
- Markedly and persistently unstable self-image or sense of self.
- Impulsivity in potentially self-damaging areas: spending, sex, substance abuse, reckless driving, and binge eating.

4. Diagnostic Studies and Differentiation
- Psychiatric interview.
- Psychological testing.
- Diagnosis is typically made by early adulthood.
- Biologic studies may aid in diagnosis, but are rarely used clinically.
- Some sleep studies have shown shortened rapid eye movement (REM) latency and sleep continuity disturbances in individuals with this disorder.
- Dexamethasone suppression: abnormal test results.
- Thyrotropin-releasing hormone: abnormal.

5. Management
- **Psychotherapy:** treatment of choice. Structured and directive treatment is shown to have better results, with firm limit setting of dramatic and intense behaviors. Dialectical behavior therapy should be considered as a first-line choice among therapy options.
- **Pharmacotherapy: to deal with specific personality features that interfere with overall functioning**
  - Antipsychotics for control of anger, hostility, and brief psychotic episodes.
  - Antidepressants to improve depressed moods.
  - Mood stabilizers may improve global functioning.
  - Benzodiazepines for short periods. (Consider addictive potential in use of these medications with this particular personality disorder.)

C. Histrionic Personality Disorder
1. Definition
- A pervasive pattern of excessive emotionality, self-absorption, and attention-seeking behavior. May be characterized by frequent quasi or actual "temper tantrums," efforts to draw attention to oneself (such as by being flirtatious and vain, and overly dramatic).
- May also be characterized by endless verbalizations of their fantasies and experiences.

2. Etiology
- Unknown. Limited data suggest 1% to 3% of population; more frequently diagnosed in women than in men.

3. Clinical Features
- Excitable, emotional, and behave in a colorful, dramatic, extroverted manner.
- Inability to maintain deep, long-lasting attachments, and develop truly intimate relationships (despite the fact that they may consider relationships to be more intimate than they actually are).
- High degree of attention-seeking behavior: tend to exaggerate their thoughts and feelings and make everything sound more important than it actually is.
- Display temper tantrums, tears, and accusations when not the center of attention or receiving praise or approval.

- Seductive behavior is common, but may have psychosexual dysfunction elements.
- Displays rapidly shifting and shallow expressions of emotions.
- May utilize physical appearance as a way to draw attention to self.
- Style of speech is excessively impressionistic and lacking in detail.
- Can be very suggestible and easily influenced by others or circumstances.
- Typically unaware of, if not confused about, their true feelings and unable to explain their motivations.
- Reality testing becomes impaired under stress.
- Gestures and dramatic punctuation are common in conversations—colorful language, may make frequent slips of the tongue.
- Individuals with this disorder may develop a sensation-seeking pattern, resulting in possible legal difficulties, substance abuse, and promiscuity.
- Is uncomfortable in situations where he/she is not the center of attention.

4. Diagnostic Studies
- Structured psychiatric interview. (In interviews, generally cooperative and eager to provide a detailed history.)
- Psychological testing.
- Rule out alcohol or drug use.

5. Management
- Psychotherapy: psychoanalytically oriented psychotherapy (group or person) is the treatment of choice.
- Pharmacotherapy: adjunctive when symptoms are targeted (antianxiety medicines for anxiety, antidepressants for depression, etc.).

D. Narcissistic Personality Disorder
1. Definition
- A disorder that can be characterized as excessive sense of self-importance, lack of empathy, and grandiose sense of self.

2. Etiology
- One to 6% of general population, with a higher risk than normal among children of parents with the same disorder.

3. Clinical Features
- Grandiose sense of self-importance: consider themselves special and expect special treatment.
- Striking sense of entitlement.
- Preoccupied with fantasies of unlimited success, power, brilliance, beauty, or ideal love.
- Believes he or she is "special" and unique and can only be understood by, or should associate with, other special or high-status people (or institutions).
- Seeks and expects excessive admiration.
- May be interpersonally exploitative, taking advantage of others to achieve own ends.

- Typically lacks or is unable to express empathy, being unwilling (or unable) to recognize or identify with the feelings of others.
- Often envious of others or believes others are envious of him or her.
- Demonstrates arrogant behaviors or attitudes.
- Does not tolerate or manage perceived or actual rejection well and is prone to depression.

4. Diagnostic Studies
- Structured psychiatric interview.

5. Management
- **Psychotherapy**
  - Patients must modify or alleviate their narcissism to make progress—difficult.
  - Chronic and difficult to treat.
  - Aging handled poorly: may be more vulnerable to midlife crises.
- **Pharmacotherapy**
  - Lithium used in patients who have mood swings.
  - Antidepressants, especially serotonergic drugs, may be useful.

CLUSTER C DISORDERS (INCLUDE THOSE WHO APPEAR ANXIOUS OR FEARFUL)

A. Avoidant Personality Disorder

1. Definition
- A disorder characterized by a pervasive pattern of inhibited social behaviors, exquisite sensitivities to perceived or actual negative evaluations, feelings of inadequacy and insufficiency, and attendant nervousness regarding personal status and how others perceive the individuals.
- Highlighted by a turning away or withdrawing from relationships because of a fear of humiliation and failure.

2. Etiology
- Prevalence is 2% to 35% of the general population.
- Information is not available regarding sex ratio or familial patterns.

3. Clinical Features
- Hypersensitivity to rejection.
- Reluctance to get involved with people unless certain of being liked.
- Timidity and shyness.
- Although may have a great desire for companionship, tend to have difficulty with acquiring and maintaining social relationships, given their expressed need for unusually strong guarantees of uncritical and unconditional acceptance.
- Sometimes referred to as having an "inferiority complex."
- When talking with someone, the person expresses uncertainty, shows a lack of self-confidence, and may speak in a self-deprecating manner.
- Avoids occupational activities that involve significant interpersonal contact because of fear of criticism, disapproval, or rejection.

- Preoccupied with being criticized or rejected in social situations.
- Shows restraint within intimate relationships because of fear of being abandoned or ridiculed.
- Inhibited in new interpersonal situations because of feelings of inadequacy.
- Views self as socially inept, personally unappealing, or inferior to others.
- Is unusually reluctant to take personal risks or engage in new activities because they fear that they may prove embarrassing.
- Rarely attains much personal advancement or exercises much authority, although eager to please and will take directions from others in authority.
- Typically, the person has no close friends or confidants; over time, phobic patterns (such as social phobia) and other avoidance patterns may develop and broaden.

4. Diagnostic Studies
- Structured psychiatric interview.

5. Management
- **Psychotherapy**
  - Individual and group psychotherapy works well in alleviating some of the distress of individuals with this diagnosis.
  - CBT may include social skills training, assertiveness training, and cognitive restructuring to help individuals improve their assessment and appraisal of social events, particularly as they pertain to self-appraisals.
- **Pharmacotherapy**
  - Treat anxiety and depression if associated.
  - β-Blockers (e.g., atenolol) to manage autonomic nervous system.
  - Serotonergic agents to help rejection sensitivity.

B. Dependent Personality Disorder

1. Definition
- A disorder characterized by a pervasive pattern of dependent/submissive behavior.
- Usually have a long-standing pathologic relationship with one person on whom they are dependent, rather than on a series of people.

2. Etiology
- Estimated prevalence is 0.6%. Occurs more in women than in men.
- More common in younger than in older children.
- People with chronic physical illness in childhood may be most prone to this disorder.
- Little is known about the etiology of dependent personality disorder.

3. Clinical Features
- Pervasive and excessive expressed need to be cared for, nurtured, and emotionally protected.
- Subordinates own needs to those of others.

- Allows others to assume responsibility for major areas of their lives.
- Lacks self-confidence.
- May experience intense discomfort when alone for more than a brief period.
- Difficulty making everyday decisions without an excessive amount of advice and reassurance from others.
- Has difficulty expressing disagreement with others, unrealistically fearing a loss of support or approval.
- Difficulty initiating projects or doing things on their own (because of lack of self-confidence in judgment or abilities rather than a lack of motivation or energy).
- Goes to excessive lengths to obtain nurturance and support from others, to the point of volunteering to do unpleasant things.
- Urgently seeks another relationship as a source of care and support when a close relationship ends (fear of emotional abandonment).
- Unrealistically preoccupied with fears of being left to take care of himself or herself.
- Avoids positions of responsibility and becomes anxious if asked to assume a leadership role.
- Experiences difficulty in task completion on own accord, but may find it easier to perform these tasks for someone else when directed to do so.
- Relationships are distorted and undermined by their expressed intense attachment needs.
- Pessimism, self-doubt, passivity, and fears of expressing sexual and aggressive feelings typify the behavior of people with dependent personality disorder.
- Tends to have impaired occupational functioning and limited social relationships.
- Many suffer physical or mental abuse because they cannot assert themselves.

4. Diagnostic Studies
- Structured psychiatric interview.
- Although dependent personality disorder may occur in patients with agoraphobia, it is differentiated from agoraphobia by the high level of overt anxiety or even panic displayed in the latter.

5. Management
- **Psychotherapy**
  - Insight-oriented therapies.
  - Behavioral therapy, assertiveness training, family therapy, and group therapy have all been used successfully.
- **Pharmacotherapy**
  - Used to deal with specific symptoms such as anxiety and depression (common associated features of dependent personality disorder).
  - Imipramine is helpful in patients who experience panic attacks or have high levels of separation anxiety.
  - Benzodiazepines and serotonergic agents also have been useful.

- Psychostimulants have successfully been used in some cases to treat a patient's depression or withdrawal symptoms.

C. Obsessive–Compulsive Personality Disorder
1. Definition
- The defining characteristic of this disorder is an intense preoccupation with effecting orderliness in their lives, expressed perfectionism, and control over both mental thoughts (internal stimuli) and interpersonal (external) events and environments. The disorder itself creates inefficiency and disruption in the lives of individuals by reducing flexibility and undermining true control over events and task conditions.
- Can be characterized as constriction of the entire personality and affect.

2. Etiology an Epidemiology
- Prevalence is 2% to 8%. It is more common in males than in females, with a ratio of 2:1.
- Diagnosed most often in oldest children.
- Occurs more frequently in first-degree biologic relatives of people with the disorder than in the general population.
- Patients often have backgrounds characterized by harsh discipline.

3. Clinical Features
- Characterized by emotional constriction, orderliness, perseverance, stubbornness, and rigidity.
- Pervasive pattern of perfectionism and inflexibility.
- Preoccupation with orderliness, perfectionism, and mental and interpersonal control at the expense of flexibility, openness, and efficiency.
- Preoccupation with details, rules, lists, orderliness, neatness, organization, or schedules to the extent that the major point of the activity is lost.
- Perfectionism that interferes with task completion demonstrated (e.g., inability to complete a project because own overly strict standards are not met).
- Excessively devoted to work and productivity to the exclusion of leisure activities and friendships.
- Overly conscientious, scrupulous, and inflexible about matters of morality, ethics, or values (not accounted for by culture or religious identification).
- Unable to discard worn-out or worthless objects even when they have no sentimental value.
- Reluctant to delegate tasks or work with others unless others submit to exactly their way of doing things.
- Adopt a miserly spending style toward both self and others; money is viewed as something to be hoarded for future catastrophes.
- Shows rigidity, stubbornness, and intolerance.
- Limited interpersonal skills.
- Formal and serious, and often lacks a sense of humor.
- May alienate others, given their inflexibility and difficulty with compromise.

- Eager to please those whom they see as more powerful than themselves, and they carry out these people's wishes in an authoritarian manner.
- Indecisive and ruminates about making decisions.
- Lacks spontaneity.
- Diagnosis of personality disorder when significant impairment occurs in their occupational or social effectiveness.
- May be anxious about not being in control of the patient interview; their answers to questions are unusually detailed.

4. Diagnostic Studies
- Structured psychiatric interview.
- Rule out delusional disorders that may co-occur.

5. Management
- **Psychotherapy**
  - Unlike those with other personality disorders, those with obsessive–compulsive personality disorder (OCPD) tend to be aware of the disorder and its negative impact on their lives, and may often seek treatment on their own.
  - Group therapy can be helpful in facilitating shared experiences and shared skill enhancement.
  - Behavioral therapy can be helpful for symptom management and situational control.
- **Pharmacotherapy**
  - Benzodiazepines can reduce symptoms in patients with severe OCD (short term); unknown whether useful in treating the personality disorder.
  - Clomipramine and serotonergic agents may be useful if obsessive–compulsive signs and symptoms break through or persist.

IV. Mood Disorders
A. Adjustment Disorder
1. Definition
- An emotional reaction to an identifiable stressor (e.g., job loss, physical illness) or event that represents a disproportionate response to what would be expected normally in the general population, resulting in markedly impaired social and occupational functioning.
- Symptoms occur within 3 months of onset of stressor.
- Remission of symptoms occurs within 6 months of termination of the stressor, or of its consequences (i.e., stress reaction diminishes when individuals find another job after losing the one that resulted in the reaction).
- Reaction is not an exacerbation of some other mental disorder.

2. Etiology and Epidemiology
- Prevalence is 2% to 8%; higher in females than in males at a ratio of 2:1.

- Acute medical condition is a risk factor in developing adjustment disorder.
- Can occur in adults and in children.
- Adolescent population has the most frequent rate of diagnosis.
- Persons with poor coping skills and inadequate social supports are more prone to develop the disorder.
- Etiologic factors include psychodynamic, family, and genetic factors.

3. Clinical Features
- External stressful event is linked to the development of symptoms.
- Symptoms can vary widely—severity does not parallel the intensity of precipitating event.
- May present primarily as anxiety, depression, or mixed features.
- Sadness may be evident.
- Social isolation.
- Difficulty concentrating.
- Preoccupation with the stressful event.
- Sleep disturbance.
- Appetite disturbance.
- Symptoms expected to resolve over time (6 months), but can be associated with severe dysphoria, despondency, and suicidal ideations and attempts.
- Usually do not have same major cognitive deficits as in major depressions (i.e., patients feel bad about their situation, but not about themselves).
- Symptoms do not represent normal bereavement.

4. Diagnostic Studies
- Structured psychiatric interview.

5. Management
- Supportive psychotherapy.
- Crisis-oriented psychosocial intervention.
- Short-term, symptom-focused pharmacotherapy (e.g., for insomnia or anxiety) (see Table 8–1).

B. Major Depressive Disorder
1. Definition
- Depressed mood and anhedonia with five or more associated symptoms (see section IV.B.3).
- Symptoms occur almost every day, for most of the day, for 2 weeks.
- Symptoms represent a change from previous level of functioning.
- Symptoms cause clinically significant distress or impairment in social, occupational, or other important areas of functioning.
- Symptoms are not due to a general medical condition, drug or alcohol abuse, or side effects of prescribed medication.
- Symptoms are not accounted for by bereavement.
- Absence of symptoms of mania or hypomania.
- Qualified as "single episode" or "recurrent."

2. Etiology

- Lifetime prevalence is 5% to 17%.
- More prevalent in females than in males at a ratio of 2:1.
- Fifty percent onset between ages 20 and 50, although onset can also be observed in childhood and later in life. Mean age is 40.
- Although exact etiology remains unknown, numerous theories may account for its development and course, including:

  a. **Biologic Factors**
    - **Alterations in neurotransmitters**
      - Serotonin.
      - Epinephrine: norepinephrine.
      - Dopamine.
      - Acetylcholine.
      - Histamine.
    - **Alterations of hormonal regulation**
      - Adrenal axis.
      - Thyroid axis.
      - Growth hormone axis.
      - Genetic factors: family history of clinical depression.

  b. **Psychosocial Factors**
    - Life events or environmental stressors preceding first episode.
    - History of family dysfunctional patterns and/or psychopathology.
    - Learned helplessness (i.e., sense of powerlessness over conditions and life).
    - Limited coping mechanisms.

3. Clinical Features

- Depressed mood.
- Anhedonia.
- **At least five of the following for the same 2-week period:**
  - Sleep (insomnia or hypersomnia).
  - Decreased interest.
  - Guilt and decreased self-esteem, worthless feelings.
  - Energy and vegetative symptoms (fatigue and constipation).
  - Concentration (impaired and indecisiveness).
  - Appetite (decreased or increased with weight loss or gain).
  - Psychomotor (retardation or agitation).
  - Suicide (frequent thoughts of death with or without a plan).
  - Somatic complaints (headache, backache, GI complaints, dizziness, numbness, lethargy).
- Often undiagnosed or misdiagnosed in elderly individuals.

4. Diagnostic Studies and Differential Diagnosis

- Structured psychiatric interview. (Key to diagnosis: careful depression history and mental status examination.)
- Psychological evaluation and assessment.
- Complete history and physical examination.
- Medication review, appropriate laboratory screening tests, or both, to rule out underlying medical conditions (Table 8–2).
- **Some "bedside measures" used for evaluating depression are as follows:**
  - Beck Depression Inventory.
  - General Health Questionnaire.
- Need to rule out other causes of major depression.

5. Management

- Treat any underlying medical conditions.
- Psychotherapy and pharmacotherapy for persistent depressive symptoms.

TABLE 8–2.	Nonpsychiatric Causes of Depression		
Neurologic Disorders	**Endocrine/Metabolic**	**Pharmacologic**	**Other**
All dementias	Cushing syndrome	Benzodiazepines	Acquired immune deficiency syndrome
Huntington disease	Addison disease	Barbiturates	Malignancies
Parkinson disease	Thyroid disease	Chloral hydrate	Vitamin deficiencies
Narcolepsy	Parathyroid disorders	Amantadine	Systemic lupus erythematosus
CNS tumors—infections	Diabetes mellitus	Antipsychotics	
Cerebral vascular accident, especially left frontal	Renal disease	Bromocriptine	
Neurosyphilis		Levodopa	
Multiple sclerosis		Carbamazepine	
Traumatic brain injury		Diltiazem	
		Ethanol	
		Cocaine or other stimulants	
		Steroids	

- **Pharmacotherapeutic agents**
  - SSRIs.
    - Add selective norepinephrine reuptake inhibitors (SNRIs).
  - TCAs (contraindicated in patients with active suicidal ideation).
  - Monoamine oxidase inhibitors (MAOIs).
  - Benzodiazepines, carbamazepine, valproic acid, and lithium may all be used for the treatment of major depressive disorder if clinically indicated on the basis of patient's presentation; however, they are not first-line medications.
- Electroconvulsive therapy (ECT) or combination of ECT, psychotherapy, and pharmacotherapy if other measures have been unsuccessful.
- Medications need to be maintained a minimum of 6 to 12 months or longer after clinical improvement.
- Current theory recommends lifelong, daily pharmacologic maintenance for those with recurrent depressive episodes.
- Cessation of psychopharmacologic interventions before 6 months may result in relapse.
- Patient must be continually assessed for symptoms of mania and hypomania that would change the diagnosis and suicidality.

6. Suicide and Other Information
- Fifteen percent of depressed patients commit suicide.
- Depressive disorders are associated with 80% of suicidal events.
- Fifty percent of those with a first major depressive episode have a recurrence.
- **Risk factors for recurrence**
  - Incomplete recovery.
  - Previous recurrences.
  - Strong family history of recurrent affective disorders.
  - History of major depression superimposed on dysthymia.
  - Substance dependence.
- **Patients with a depressive disorder should be referred to a psychiatrist in the following situations:**
  - Increased suicidal risk whether verbal or actual gestures, intimations, or patient's lack of response to interventions.
  - Need for hospitalization for worsening of symptoms or evidence of emergent comorbid conditions.
  - Failure of an adequate antidepressant trial.
  - Complicated medical or psychiatric comorbidity.
  - Evaluation for pharmacotherapy.
  - Provision of psychotherapy and pharmacotherapy.

C. Persistent Depressive Disorder (Dysthymia)
1. Definition
- Chronically depressed mood (or possibly irritable mood in children or in adolescents) for a period of 2 years (1 year in children and adolescents), with an observed presence of depressed mood for most days.
- Severity of mood disturbance does not meet criteria for major depression.
- Periods without depressed mood may have occurred during the 2 years, but failed to last more than 2 months.

2. Etiology
- Biological and psychosocial factors are involved.
- Five to 6% of the general population is affected. Males and females are equally affected.
- Often coexists with other psychiatric illnesses.

3. Clinical Features
- Poor appetite.
- Insomnia.
- Low self-esteem.
- Feelings of hopelessness.
- Pessimism.
- Guilt feelings or brooding over the past.
- Social withdrawal.
- Decreased productivity or activity.
- Low energy.
- Difficulty with concentration and memory.
- Irritability or excessive anger.
- Difficulty making decisions.
- Generalized loss of interest or pleasure.
- Greater risk for substance abuse and suicide.

4. Diagnostic Studies
- Structured psychiatric interview.
- Psychological evaluation and assessment.

5. Management
- **Psychotherapy**
  - Cognitive therapy.
  - Behavioral therapy.
  - Family and group therapy.
- **Pharmacotherapy**
  - Antidepressants (SSRIs, SNRIs).

D. Bipolar Disorder: Type I
1. Definition
- One or more manic episodes, and sometimes, major depressive episodes. Mania is defined by an abnormally and persistently elevated, expansive, or irritable mood lasting at least 1 week (or less if hospitalization is required).
- History of depression or hypomania also may be present, but is not essential for the diagnosis—only documentation of manic episode is needed.
- Symptoms are not due to another mental disorder, substance abuse, medication, or general medical condition (e.g., hyperthyroidism).

- Mood disturbance is sufficiently severe to cause marked impairment in occupational functioning, social activities, and relationships with others.
- May necessitate hospitalization to prevent harm to self or others.
- Psychotic features can be present.

2. Etiology and Epidemiology
- May be linked to biologic, genetic, and/or psychosocial factors.
- Prevalence of 0% to 2.4%.

3. Clinical Features for Mania
- **Abnormally and persistently elevated, expansive, or irritable mood plus three (or more) of the following:**
  - Grandiosity/inflated self-esteem.
  - Decreased need for sleep.
  - More talkative than usual, or pressured speech.
  - Flight of ideas or racing thoughts.
  - Distractibility.
  - Increase in goal-directed activity (social behaviors, sexual behaviors, work, or school) or psychomotor agitation.
  - Excessive involvement in pleasurable activities that have a high potential for painful outcome (e.g., unrestrained buying sprees and gambling).
- Symptoms have been present for at least 1 week or any duration if hospitalization is necessary.
- Symptoms range from mild to psychotic.
- Mood: can be euphoric, irritable, labile, or dysphoric.
- Thinking: includes racing, disorganized, expansive, or grandiose thoughts.
- Behavior: can include physical hyperactivity, pressured speech, decreased need for sleep, hypersexuality, increased impulsivity, and risk taking.

4. Diagnostic Studies
- Structured psychiatric interview.
- Diagnosis is based on history and physical findings. Must rule out other causes of mania or bipolar presentation (Table 8–3).
- **Laboratory tests**
  - CBC.
  - Thyroid function tests (TFTs).
  - Urine toxicology screen.
  - Chemistry profile.
  - Hepatic and renal function: blood urea nitrogen (BUN) and creatinine.
  - ECG.

5. Management
  a. **Acute**
  - Maintain a secure environment that prevents flight or self-harm.
  - Evaluate patient for signs of medical disorders, drug intoxication, or side effects of prescribed medication.
  - **Hospitalization and pharmacologic treatment (see Table 8–1):**
    - Lithium.
    - Antipsychotics if psychotic symptoms are present or to treat symptoms of mania.
    - Benzodiazepines (e.g., clonazepam, lorazepam): short term for hyperactivity, controlling agitation, decreasing anxiety, and improving sleep.
    - In patients with intolerance or unresponsiveness to lithium—valproate or carbamazepine alone or in conjunction with neuroleptic.
  - **NOTE:** Neuroleptics generally result in rapid improvement, but patients with bipolar disorder are at increased risk for neuroleptic malignant syndrome and tardive dyskinesia.

TABLE 8–3.   Nonpsychiatric Causes of Secondary Mania

Metabolic	Neurologic	Pharmacologic	Other
Electrolyte abnormalities	Traumatic brain injury	Amphetamines	Herpes simplex
Thyroid disorders	Central nervous system tumors—infection	Cocaine	Acquired immune deficiency syndrome
Adrenal disorders	Seizure disorders	Monoamine oxidase inhibitors	Menses related
Vitamin B_{12} deficiency	Huntington disease	Sedatives	Postpartum
	Neurosyphilis	Hypnotics	
	Multiple sclerosis	Antipsychotics	
	Migraines	Steroids	
	Cerebral vascular accident	Excessive thyroxine	
		Isoniazid	
		Disulfiram	
		Cimetidine	

b. **Chronic**
- Preventive treatment with antimanic agents (lithium, valproic acid, and carbamazepine).
- Serum level monitoring to avoid toxicity. More frequently at the beginning of treatment.
- Therapeutic lithium level range is between 0.5 and 1.5. (Laboratory ranges may differ.)
- Lithium blood levels are increased by thiazide diuretics, nonsteroidal anti-inflammatory drugs (NSAIDs), neuroleptic agents, and dehydration.
- Assessment of thyrotropin (TSH), BUN, and creatinine every 6 months.
- Addition of or replacement with valproic acid or carbamazepine when lithium alone is ineffective.
- Use of benzodiazepines during periods of sleep deprivation (i.e., times of increased stress) to decrease the risk of manic episodes.
- Antidepressants may precipitate a manic episode.

c. **Signs and Symptoms of Lithium Toxicity**
- Lethargy and fatigue.
- Ataxia and clumsiness.
- Weakness.
- Nausea.
- Vomiting.
- Marked tremor.
- Blurred vision.
- Confusion.
- Nystagmus.
- Increased deep tendon reflexes (DTRs).
- Mental status change.
- Seizures.
- Coma.
- Cardiac arrhythmias.
- **NOTE:** Lithium toxicity is a medical emergency—needs to be managed in intensive care setting. Treatment includes discontinuing the lithium and treating the dehydration.

E. **Bipolar Disorder: Type II**
1. **Definition**
- One or more episodes of a major depressive episode and a hypomanic episode.
- Presence (or history) of one or more major depressive episodes.
- Presence (or history) of at least one hypomanic episode, but never a manic episode.
- Symptoms cause clinically significant distress or impairment in social, occupational, or other important areas of functioning.

2. **Etiology**
- May be linked to biologic, genetic, or psychosocial factors.
- Prevalence is 0.8%.

3. **Clinical Features**
- Symptoms of a major depressive disorder together with the clinical features of a hypomanic episode.
- Hypomania symptoms: distinct period of persistently elevated, expansive, or irritable mood, clearly different from the usual nondepressed mood. **Plus three to four of the following:**
  - Inflated self-esteem or grandiosity.
  - Decreased need for sleep (i.e., feels rested after only 3 hours of sleep).
  - More talkative than usual, or pressured speech.
  - Flight of ideas/racing thoughts.
  - Distractibility.
  - Increase in goal-directed activity, socially, at work, or in school; or sexual or psychomotor agitation.
  - Excessive involvement in pleasurable activities that have a high potential for painful consequences (e.g., unrestrained buying sprees, sexual indiscretions, and foolish business investments).
- Hypomanic symptoms last throughout 4 consecutive days.
- Symptoms are present to a significant degree.
- Symptoms are associated with an unequivocal change in functioning, uncharacteristic of the person when not symptomatic.
- Disturbance in mood and change in functioning are observable by others.
- Symptoms of hypomania are not severe enough to cause marked impairment in social or occupational functioning, or require hospitalization. Key in differentiating hypomania from mania.
- No psychotic features.
- Symptoms are not due to another mental illness, substance abuse, medication, treatment, or general medical condition (e.g., hyperthyroidism).

4. **Diagnostic Studies**
- Diagnosis is based on structured psychiatric interview, history, physical examination, and ruling out other conditions that can cause similar symptoms.

5. **Management**
- Similar to bipolar I pharmacologically (lithium). There is a role for anticonvulsant mood stabilizers such as lamotrigine (Lamictal), Tegretol, and Depakote.
- Antidepressants may precipitate a manic episode.
- Medication compliance is a major concern with bipolar disorder. A collaborative relationship between provider and patient is crucial.
- Suicide is common if untreated.

F. **Cyclothymic Disorder**
1. **Definition**
- Symptomatically, a mild form of bipolar II disorder.
- Characterized by episodes of hypomania and mild depression.

- Numerous periods of hypomanic symptoms and depressive symptoms exist for at least 2 years (1 year in children and adolescents) and no absence of symptoms for more than 2 months.

2. Etiology

- May be linked to biologic and/or psychosocial factors.
- Biologic factors: 30% have positive family histories of bipolar disorder type I.
- Psychosocial factors: trauma/interpersonal loss triggers symptoms.
- Onset of symptoms: insidious; teens or early 20s.
- Prevalence of 1% in the United States.

3. Clinical Features

- Symptoms are identical to those of bipolar II, except they are less severe in intensity, duration, or both.
- Changes in mood are irregular and abrupt, and sometimes occur within hours.
- Episodes of mixed (hypomania and depressive) symptoms with marked irritability are common.
- Alcohol and substance abuse are common—patients use substances to self-medicate or achieve further stimulation.
- Often have a history of multiple geographic moves and involvement in religious cults and other subcultures.
- Often not successful in professional and social lives because of this disorder.

4. Diagnostic Studies

- Structured psychiatric interview.
- Psychological evaluation and assessment.

5. Management

- **Psychotherapy:** CBT assists the patient with regaining control over cognitions and behavioral patterns associated with the disorder.
- **Pharmacotherapy**
  - Mood stabilizers.
  - Antidepressants should be used with caution; they pose the same danger of inducing hypomania or manic episodes as in patients with bipolar I and II.
  - One-third of patients subsequently develop major mood disorders—most often bipolar disorder type II.

V. Anxiety Disorders

A. Generalized Anxiety Disorder

1. Definition

- Excessive anxiety and worry about several events for most days for at least a 6-month period.
- Anxiety is difficult to control and is often associated with somatic symptoms—fatigue, muscle tension, irritability, difficulty sleeping, and restlessness. These symptoms frequently lead them to

multiple other specialists, seeking treatment for their somatic complaints.

- Symptoms cause clinically significant distress in social, occupational, or other areas of functioning.

2. Etiology and Epidemiology

- May have biologic or psychosocial links.
- Likely familial pattern.
- Prevalence rate of 3% to 8%.
- In the general population, women may present over men with this disorder in the ratio of 2:1, which rises to approximately 60% of more women than men with this disorder over a lifetime (National Institute of Mental Health).
- Fifty to 90% of patients often have another coexisting mental disorder.

3. Clinical Features

- **Anxiety and worry are associated with three or more of the following symptoms:**
  - Restlessness or feeling keyed up/on edge.
  - Easily fatigued.
  - Difficulty concentrating or mind going blank.
  - Irritability.
  - Muscle tension.
  - Sleep disturbance.
- **Other symptoms**
  - Headaches, dizziness, and tinnitus.
  - Autonomic hyperactivity: shortness of breath, excessive sweating, palpitations, and GI symptoms—nausea, vomiting, dysphagia, diarrhea.

4. Diagnostic Studies

- Psychological evaluation and assessment.
- Structured psychiatric interview.

5. Management

- **Psychotherapy**
  - CBT.
  - Supportive therapy.
  - Insight-oriented therapy.
- **Pharmacotherapy (see Table 8–1)**
  - Antidepressants, primarily SSRIs.
  - Benzodiazepines, used temporarily for <4 weeks while waiting for SSRIs to achieve efficacy. They should be slowly tapered and eventually discontinued altogether.
  - Buspirone.
- Supportive measures.

B. Panic Attack (Specifier Only and Not a Codable Disorder)

1. Definition

- A discrete period of intense fear or discomfort, accompanied by at least four (or more) somatic or cognitive symptoms, that develops abruptly and reaches a peak within 10 minutes.
- Can occur in mental disorders other than panic disorder.
- May or may not be associated with any identifiable situational stimulus.

2. Etiology and Epidemiology
- May be linked to biologic, genetic, and/or psychosocial factors.
- Prevalence of 11.2%.

3. Clinical Features
- Presentation: patients often present at an emergency department (ED) with somatic symptoms and fears that are suggestive of a heart attack.
- **Intense fear or discomfort plus four or more of the following:**
  - Palpitations, pounding heart, or increased heart rate.
  - Sweating.
  - Trembling or shaking.
  - Sensation of shortness of breath or smothering.
  - Choking feeling.
  - Chest pain or discomfort.
  - Nausea or abdominal distress.
  - Feeling dizzy, unsteady, lightheaded, or faint.
  - Derealization (feelings of unreality) or depersonalization (being detached from oneself).
  - Fear of losing control or going crazy.
  - Fear of dying (e.g., a heart attack).
  - Paresthesias (numbness or tingling).
  - Chills or hot flashes.

4. Diagnostic Studies
- Structured psychiatric interview.
- Detailed history is a critical factor in the evaluation of panic attacks.
- Focused physical assessment.
- Disease-specific set of laboratory tests (i.e., TSH, cardiac monitoring).
- **Common medical disorders that can look like panic attacks:**
  - Hyperthyroidism.
  - Hyperparathyroidism.
  - Pheochromocytoma.
  - Vestibular dysfunctions.
  - Cardiac arrhythmias.
  - Seizure disorders.
  - Medication toxicity (i.e., CNS stimulants, bronchodilators, caffeine).
  - Mitral valve prolapse.
  - Pulmonary embolus.
  - Asthma.
  - Chronic obstructive pulmonary disorder.
  - Hypoglycemia.
  - Stimulant use (amphetamines, cocaine, caffeine).
  - Medication withdrawal.

5. Management/Treatment
- **Psychotherapy:** CBT is generally viewed as the most effective form of treatment for panic attacks, panic disorder, and agoraphobia. CBT focuses on the thinking patterns and behaviors that are sustaining or triggering the panic attacks and helps individuals review their fears in a more realistic light.

- **Pharmacotherapy (see Table 8–1)**
  - Benzodiazepines are effective in managing panic attacks.
  - Start with low dose and increase dosage until clearly effective treatment is noted.
  - Refer to psychiatrist for long-term follow-up and care.

C. Panic Disorder

1. Definition
- Spontaneous, unexpected occurrence of a number of panic attacks. The *DSM 5* does not specify a minimum number of attacks or a time frame.
- Occurrence can vary from several attacks in 1 day to a few attacks during a year.
- **Intense fear or discomfort plus four or more of the following that reach peak intensity in minutes:**
  - Palpitations, pounding heart, or increased heart rate.
  - Sweating.
  - Trembling or shaking.
  - Sensation of shortness of breath or smothering.
  - Choking feeling.
  - Chest pain or discomfort.
  - Nausea or abdominal distress.
  - Feeling dizzy, unsteady, lightheaded, or faint.
  - Derealization (feelings of unreality) or depersonalization (being detached from oneself).
  - Fear of losing control or going crazy.
  - Fear of dying (e.g., a heart attack).
  - Paresthesias (numbness or tingling).
  - Chills or hot flashes.
- **At least one of the attacks has been followed by 1 month or more of the following:**
  - Persistent concern about having additional attacks.
  - Worry about the implications of the attack or its consequences (e.g., losing control, having a heart attack, or "going crazy").
  - A significant change in behavior related to the attacks.
- Initial attacks must be "uncued" (unexpected) to meet diagnostic criteria.

2. Etiology
- May be linked to biologic (drugs, mitral valve prolapse, etc.), genetic, or psychosocial factors.

3. Epidemiology
- Twelve-month prevalence is 2.0% to 3.0%.
- Twice as prevalent in women than in men.
- Most commonly develops in young adulthood (mean age: 25), but can occur at any time.

4. Clinical Features
- Symptoms of panic attack.
- Associated frequently with major depression, other anxiety disorders, and alcohol and substance dependence.

- Normal desire to engage in activities, but avoids because of phobias/triggers of panic symptoms; may have personality changes.
- Frequent use of alcohol or sedative to get rid of anxiety/panic symptoms or prevent occurrence, resulting in substance-abuse problems.
- Agoraphobia, if present, is given its own separate diagnosis—anxiety about being in places or situations from which escape may be difficult or in which help may be unavailable, leading to avoidance or marked distress.

5. Diagnostic Studies
- Structured psychiatric interview.
- Rule out possible medical causes for panic symptoms.
- Include detailed physical examination, ECG, chemistry profile, including electrolytes, calcium, magnesium, TFTs, urine toxicology screen, CBC, and liver and renal function tests.
- Other tests as indicated.
- Detailed symptom history, medication history, and social history; especially, use of caffeine, alcohol, drugs, sedative–hypnotics, nicotine, bronchodilators, CNS stimulants, or withdrawal from CNS depressants.
- Full psychological evaluation.

6. Management (See Table 8–1)
- Benzodiazepines briefly, to stop panic attacks.
- Start with low dose and increase dosage as needed until clearly effective.
- Dosage needed may be higher than the range needed for other conditions.
- Reassurance.
- Referral to psychiatrist for further evaluation/treatment.
- SSRIs are first-line treatment. SNRIs and TCAs can be considered second-line treatments. MAOIs have a limited role because of their side effects.

D. Specific Phobia
1. Definition
- Irrational and persistent fear or anxiety of a specific situation (e.g., elevators, heights), certain activities, or clearly identifiable objects (e.g., spiders, needles).
- Fear out of proportion to the inherent danger.
- Fear cannot be reasoned or explained away.
- People feel no voluntary control over their fears and avoid the situation or object to control the fear.
- Typically, the fear has lasted at least 6 months.
- Causes marked distress in all levels of functioning, whether in social or occupational setting.
- Anxiety experienced when in contact or imagined contact with object of fear.
- Patients realize fear is unrealistic.
- Children do not realize their fear is unrealistic.

2. Types of Phobias
- **Specific phobia**
  - Animal: dogs, snakes, spiders.
  - Natural environment: water, heights, storms.
  - Blood–injection–injury: seeing blood, venipuncture, medical procedures.
  - Situational: closed spaces, flying, bridges, tunnels.
- **Social anxiety disorder**
  - Social interactions: speaking in public, using public restrooms, speaking to a date, or any activity drawing attention to themselves.
  - Alcohol dependence is common in patients with phobia—may medicate their anxiety with alcohol.
  - Alcohol withdrawal may worsen their anxiety.

3. Etiology
- Prevalence is 7% to 9% in the United States.
- Prevalence is 16% in 13- to 17-year-olds.
- A 2:1 ratio of females > males.
- Unknown: probable biologic, genetic, environmental interactions.
- Genetics: first-degree relatives of people with social phobia are three times more likely to be affected.

4. Clinical Features
- Severe anxiety.
- **Physiologic symptoms secondary to anxiety**
  - Restlessness.
  - Diarrhea.
  - Dizziness.
  - Palpitations.
  - Excessive sweating.
  - Tremor.
  - Syncope.
  - Tachycardia.
  - Urinary frequency.
- Some patients may engage in risky behaviors in an attempt to overcome the fear (e.g., hang gliding by a person afraid of heights).
- Children may express their fear by clinging, freezing, crying, or tantrums.
- A 60% greater risk of suicide attempt.

5. Diagnostic Studies
- Structured psychiatric interview.

6. Management/Treatment
- Specific phobia: consider exposure therapy, cognitive therapy.
- Social anxiety disorder: consider behavioral and cognitive therapy.
- Hypnosis: supportive and family therapy.
- **Pharmacotherapy**
  - β-Adrenergic receptor antagonists shortly before exposure to stimulus (atenolol 25–50 mg or propranolol 20–40 mg).
  - SSRIs.
  - Benzodiazepines.
  - Buspirone: may be used as an additive agent with SSRIs.

E. Obsessive–Compulsive Disorder

1. Definition

- An anxiety disorder manifested by obsessions, compulsions, or both, severe enough to be time consuming (>1 hour per day) or cause marked distress or significant impairment in daily functioning.
- Obsession: recurrent and intrusive thought, feeling, idea, or sensation/urge.
- Compulsion: a conscious, standardized recurring pattern of behavior or thought (e.g., counting, checking, or avoiding).
- Obsessions increase anxiety; carrying out compulsion reduces anxiety.
- Failure to carry out a compulsion increases anxiety.
- Responsive to treatment.
- Symptoms have usually existed for many years before person comes in for treatment.
- Symptom onset is generally gradual, but can be abrupt.
- Often have other coexisting disorders: major depressive disorder, social phobia, alcohol use disorders, specific phobia, panic disorder, and eating disorders.

2. Etiology and Epidemiology

- Dysregulation of serotonin has been involved in the symptom formation.
- Significant genetic component, with a 10-fold increase if a first-degree relative also has the disorder.
- Biologic, behavioral, psychosocial component.
- Affects 2% to 3% of the population. Fourth most common psychiatric diagnosis.
- Onset at any age: most commonly evident in early adulthood (average 19.5 years) with one-fourth of cases by 14 years of age.
- Childhood: more common in males than in females.
- Adulthood: slightly higher rate in females than in males.
- Up to 25% will attempt suicide at some point.

3. Clinical Features

- Anxiety: central feature.
- Repetitive mental acts or behaviors/rituals to reduce anxiety.
- Depressive symptoms.
- Specify if insight classified as:
  - Good or fair.
  - Poor.
  - Absent with delusional beliefs.
- **Major symptom patterns listed in order of commonality:**
  - Contamination.
  - Pathologic doubt.
  - Symmetry (precision).

- Other obsessive-compulsive and related disorders:
  - Religious obsessions.
  - Compulsive hoarding.
  - Trichotillomania (compulsive hairpulling).
  - Excoriation disorder: compulsive skin picking.
- Onset of symptoms for 50% to 70% of patients occurs after a stressful event (e.g., pregnancy, sexual problem, death of a relative).

4. Diagnostic Studies

- Structured psychiatric interview with extensive history (e.g., Yale–Brown Obsessive Compulsive Scale [Y-BOCS]) and physical examination to rule out similar conditions: major neurologic disorders—tic disorders, temporal lobe epilepsy, trauma, and postencephalitic complications.
- **Clinical considerations**
  - Tourette syndrome: two-thirds of people with Tourette syndrome meet the diagnostic criteria for OCD.
  - Common in certain other disorders such as schizophrenia and schizoaffective disorder, with a 12% occurrence rate.
  - OCPD does not have the same degree of functional impairment as does OCD.
  - OCPD is more pervasive and lacks the obsessions, compulsions, rituals, and severe anxiety of OCD.
  - OCD personality traits tend not to disturb the patient, whereas OCD compulsions and obsessions are disturbing and time consuming.

5. Management/Treatment

- Behavior therapy.
- Family therapy.
- Group therapy.
- **Pharmacotherapy (see Table 8–1)**
  - SSRI, first line. TCAs (clomipramine), mood stabilizers, atypical antipsychotics, buspirone, and SNRIs are among the other drugs used if SSRIs are ineffective.
  - Higher doses are often necessary for a beneficial effect.
  - SSRI dosing must be titrated upward over 2 to 3 weeks to avoid GI adverse effects and orthostatic hypotension.
  - Initial therapeutic effects are usually seen after 4 to 6 weeks of treatment; 8 to 16 weeks are needed for maximum therapeutic benefit.
- Significant proportion of patients seems to relapse if drug therapy is discontinued.
- **Other clinical considerations**
  - ECT is used in cases of severely treatment-resistant patients.
  - Treatment efficacy for patients with OCD varies greatly from minimal improvement to significant improvement in symptoms.

- One-third of patients with OCD have major depressive disorder.
- Suicide is a risk factor for all patients with OCD.
  - **Poor prognostic predictors**
    - Yielding to compulsions.
    - Childhood onset.
    - Bizarre compulsions.
    - Need for hospitalization.
    - Coexisting major depressive disorder.
    - Delusional beliefs.
    - Presence of a personality disorder.
  - **Good prognostic predictors**
    - Positive social and occupational adjustment.
    - Presence of a precipitating event.
    - Episodic nature of symptoms.

F. Posttraumatic Stress Disorder (PTSD)
1. Definition
- Group of symptoms that develop after the person experiences or witnesses a traumatic event that involves a response of intense fear, helplessness, or horror.
- Exposure happens in one of four ways:
  - Direct trauma to individual.
  - Direct witness as events unfold to others.
  - Direct trauma to close member of family or close friend.
  - Repeated exposure to adverse event and details.
- Symptoms persist for >1 month.
- May not manifest until months or years after the traumatic event.
- **Common situations precipitating PTSD response are as follows:**
  - Experiences in war, particularly combat but also as a civilian.
  - Torture, terrorist attack, prisoner of war.
  - Natural catastrophes: hurricanes, flooding, earthquakes.
  - Physical or sexual assault (e.g., single or multiple occurrences of trauma).
  - Serious accidents.
2. Etiology and Epidemiology
- By definition, the stressor is the prime causative factor; not everyone experiences the disorder after a traumatic event.
- Other contributing factors may be individual preexisting biologic and psychosocial factors and events occurring immediately after the trauma.
- Lifetime prevalence is 8.7%.
- Prevalence in females > males.
- Eighty percent more likely to have a comorbid disorder such as depression, anxiety, bipolar, or a substance-use disorder.
- **Predisposing vulnerability factors:**
  - Presence of childhood trauma by age 6.

- Borderline, paranoid, dependent, or ASP disorder traits.
- Inadequate support system.
- Genetic: constitutional vulnerability to psychiatric illness.
- Recent stressful life changes.
- Perception of an external loss of control rather than an internal one.
- Recent excessive alcohol intake.
3. Clinical Features
- Intrusion symptoms:
  - Recurrent, intrusive, distressing recollections of the event, including images, thoughts, and perceptions.
  - Recurrent, distressing dreams of event—nightmares.
  - Acting or feeling as if the trauma/event were recurring (i.e., hallucination), flashbacks.
  - Intense psychological distress at exposure to internal or external cues that resemble or symbolize an aspect of the traumatic event.
  - Physiologic reactivity distress at exposure to internal or external cues that resemble or symbolize an aspect of the traumatic event.
- Avoidance: persistent avoidance of stimuli is associated with the trauma.
  - Efforts to avoid activities, places, or people that arouse recollections of the trauma.
  - Efforts to avoid thoughts, feelings, or conversations associated with the trauma.
- Negative mood and cognition: Numbing of general responsiveness is not present before the trauma.
  - Inability to recall an important aspect of the trauma.
  - Markedly diminished interest or participation in significant activities.
  - Feelings of detachment or estrangement from others.
  - Restricted range of affect.
  - Sense of a foreshortened future (does not expect to have a career, marriage, children, or normal life span).
- **Arousal change: persistent symptoms of increased arousal are not present before the trauma (two or more of the following)**
  - Difficulty falling or staying asleep.
  - Irritability or outbursts of anger.
  - Difficulty concentrating.
  - Hypervigilance.
  - Exaggerated startle response.
- **Common feelings are expressed:**
  - Fear of a repetition of the trauma.
  - Fear of sharing the fate of others who died or were injured.
  - Rage at those responsible.

- Resentment toward those who were not harmed.
- Remorse over what the person thought or did during the event.
- Guilt because person survived and others did not.
- Acute: symptoms lasting < 3 months.
- Chronic: symptoms lasting 3 months or more.
- Delayed expression: symptoms frequently present right away, but there is delay for at least 6 months after a trauma in meeting full diagnostic criteria.

4. Diagnostic Studies
- Structured psychiatric interview.
- **Rule out**
  - Acute stress disorder.
  - Major depressive disorder.
  - Psychotic disorders.
  - Adjustment disorder.
  - Head injury secondary to trauma.
  - Epilepsy.
  - Alcohol use disorders.
  - Other substance-abuse disorders.

5. Management
- May require different types of help at different stages.
- **Acute**
  - Support.
  - Protection/reassurance of safety.
  - Help with decisions and plans.
  - Encouragement to discuss the event.
  - Education about a variety of coping mechanisms (i.e., relaxation, deep-breathing techniques).
  - Education of family members/support persons regarding disorder and how to support patient.
  - Benzodiazepines prn (1–7 days) until normal sleep patterns return.
  - Referral to a psychiatrist for additional pharmacotherapy and psychotherapy.
- **Chronic/delayed**
  - Support.
  - Education about the disorder and its treatment (pharmacologic and psychotherapeutic).
- **Pharmacologic treatment (see Table 8–1)**
  - SSRIs are first-line treatment.
  - Eight-week trial: good response, continue for at least 1 year.
  - Other drugs (alternates): SNRIs, TCAs, trazodone, anticonvulsants (carbamazepine, valproate), clonidine, and propranolol.
- **Psychotherapeutic interventions**
  - Must be individualized: some patients overwhelmed by reexperiencing traumas.
  - Exposure therapy: eye movement desensitization and reprocessing (EMDR), systematic desensitization. Evidence-based procedures, such as prolonged exposure (PE) therapy and cognitive processing therapy (CPT).

- Some forms of behavior therapy.
- Cognitive therapy.
- Hypnosis.
- Group therapy and family therapy are also helpful.
- Hospitalization: when symptoms are particularly severe or when the risk of suicide or other violence is significantly elevated.

G. Acute Stress Disorder

1. Definition
- Acute anxiety symptomatology accompanied by dissociative symptoms brought on by exposure to a traumatic event.
- **Symptoms**
  - Occur within 1 month of exposure to an extremely traumatic stressor.
  - Last at least 3 days.
  - Resolve within 4 weeks. (Key in differentiating between this disorder and PTSD.)
  - Disturbance causes significant distress and impairment in social, occupational, or other areas of functioning *or* prevents person from performing some necessary task such as obtaining medicine or legal assistance or mobilizing personal resources by telling family members about the traumatic experience.
  - Must have nine symptoms from the following categories:
    - Negative mood.
    - Dissociative symptoms.
    - Avoidance symptoms.
    - Arousal symptoms.

2. Etiology
- **Exposure to a traumatic event.**
- **The person experienced, witnessed, or was confronted with an event or events involving:**
  - Actual or threatened death.
  - Serious injury.
  - A threat to the physical integrity of the person or of others (i.e., sexual violation).
  - In which the person's response involved intense fear, helplessness, or horror.

3. Epidemiology
- Less than 20% prevalence in cases not including interpersonal assault.
- Twenty to 50% in severe interpersonal cases such as rapes or mass shooting.

4. Clinical Features
- **Either during or immediately after the distressing event, the patient develops at least nine symptoms from the below five categories:**
  - Subjective sense of numbing, detachment, or absence of emotional responsiveness.
  - Decreased awareness of surroundings (being in a daze).
  - Derealization (environment seems unreal or dreamlike).

- Depersonalization (feeling detached—an outside observer of one's own mental processes or body, or like an automatic machine).
  - Dissociative amnesia (inability to recall an important aspect of the trauma).
- **Persistent reexperiencing of the traumatic event in one of the following ways:**
  - Recurrent images, thoughts, dreams, illusions, flashbacks, or a sense of realizing the experience.
  - Distress when exposed to reminders of the traumatic event.
  - Marked avoidance of thoughts, feelings, conversations, activity, places, or people that arouse recollections of the trauma.
- **Marked symptoms of anxiety or increased arousal:**
  - Difficulty sleeping.
  - Irritability.
  - Poor concentration.
  - Hypervigilance.
  - Exaggerated startle response.
  - Motor restlessness.
  - Hard to enjoy activities previously thought pleasurable.
  - Feelings of guilt resuming their usual routine.
  - Hopelessness and despair.

5. **Diagnostic Studies**
   - Structured psychiatric interview.
6. **Management**
   - **Crisis intervention**
     - Protection.
     - Consolation.
     - Assurance of safety.
   - **Assistance with decisions and plans** (i.e., Greatest help may be the support of those closest as soon as possible; preferably before going to sleep the night after the trauma, talking about what happened with an empathic person or someone who has shared the same or similar experience).
   - **Therapy**
     - Supportive psychotherapy: focused on working through emotional responses to trauma or stress.
     - Relaxation techniques: for example, progressive muscle relaxation and biofeedback.
     - Group therapy.
     - Benzodiazepines (short term, 1–7 days) to assist with sleep until normal sleep patterns return.
     - Persons with acute stress disorder are at increased risk for developing PTSD when not treated.

H. **Somatic Symptom and Related Disorders**
   - Characterized by somatic complaints causing significant impairment without objective physical findings or presence of a significant medical condition to adequately explain the symptoms.

1. **Somatic Symptom Disorder (No Longer Called Somatization Disorder)**
   - A fixed false belief of having factitious medical disorder.
   - Interferes markedly with activities of daily living.
   - Anxiety and persistent thoughts regarding health and is preoccupied with the health problem and symptoms.
   - Time frame of main symptom is usually > 6 months.
   - Epidemiology:
     - Equally effects both genders.
     - Most common in second and third decades but can happen at any age.
     - Prevalence 4% to 7% of general population.

2. **Conversion Disorder**
   - One or more unintentional symptoms affecting motor or sensory function.
   - Specified by symptom type such as weakness or paralysis, tremors, slurred speech or difficulty swallowing, seizures, sensory loss, vision, smell or hearing loss.
   - Associated with psychological factors preceded by a conflict or other stressor.
   - May account for up to 5% of neurology referrals.

3. **Illness Anxiety Disorder (No Longer Called Hypochondriasis)**
   - Preoccupation and fear of having a severe medical illness based on misinterpretation of symptoms in spite of appropriate medical care and reassurance, lasting >6 months.
   - May be classified as care-seeker type or care-avoidant type
   - Epidemiology: 1.3% to 10% of the population and similar male:female ratio.

4. **Factitious Disorders**
   - Intentional physical or psychological symptoms produced by patients to assume the sick role. No objective physical finding explanation for the symptoms.
   - Can be imposed on self or another person.
   - No external motivation.
   - Treatment is focused on good communication among the health care team to avoid unnecessary diagnostic procedures. The patient will rarely agree to psychotherapy.

5. **Malingering (Removed As a Diagnosis from the *DSM 5*)**
   - Intentional production of false or exaggerated physical or psychological symptoms.
   - Patient has a motive of secondary gain (avoid responsibilities or punishment; to receive free housing, drugs, or monetary compensation; retaliation for perceived loss or injustice).
   - Treatment is essentially to do a thorough evaluation and treat the patient based on objective data without negative emotions. This will preserve the patient–provider relationship.

VI. Psychotic Disorders

A. Psychosis

1. Definition

- A major mental disorder characterized by gross impairment in perception of reality and ability to communicate/interact with others.

2. Etiology

- Multiple causes; can be biologic or emotional in origin (Table 8-4).

3. Clinical Features

- **Common symptoms of psychosis**
  - Delusions.
  - Hallucinations.
  - Bizarre behavior.
  - Ideas of reference.
  - Paranoia.
  - Disorganized speech.
  - Illogical thinking.
- Psychotic symptoms can occur as part of a primary psychiatric diagnosis (e.g., schizophrenia) or be secondary to multiple medical, neurologic, or substance-abuse disorders.

4. Diagnostic Studies

- Structured psychiatric interview.
- Psychological evaluation and assessment.
- **Laboratory studies**
  - CBC with differential.
  - Serum electrolytes.
  - Fasting blood glucose, lipid profile. (Important to have a baseline due to the role of atypical antipsychotics in treatment.)
- Renal function (BUN/creatinine).
- Calcium.
- Phosphate.
- Liver function tests (LFTs).
- TFTs.
- Rapid plasma reagin (RPR).
- HIV antibody test in high-risk patients.
- Urinalysis.
- Urine toxicology screen: may need to specify specific drugs; routine urine toxicology screens usually monitor for only a limited number of substances.
- ECG.
- Chest X-ray (CXR).
- Head computed tomography (CT) scan or magnetic resonance imaging (MRI).
- Sleep-deprived EEG.
- Blood levels of therapeutic medications—when appropriate.
- Lumbar puncture.

5. Management

- **Pharmacotherapy** (see Table 8-1): antipsychotics; typical (haloperidol), atypical (clozapine, olanzapine, risperidone, etc.).

TABLE 8-4.	Medical and Neurologic Conditions That Include Psychosis	
Neurologic	**Pharmacologic**	**Others**
Delirium	Amphetamines	Acquired immune deficiency syndrome
Dementia	Hallucinogens	Acute intermittent porphyria
Central nervous system tumor—infections	Belladonna	Carbon monoxide poisoning
Huntington disease	Alkaloids	Heavy metal poisoning
Parkinson disease	Cocaine	Systemic levels
Temporal arteritis	Alcohol	Vitamin deficiency (i.e., vitamin B_{12})
Migraine	Barbiturates	Thyroid disorders
Wernicke–Korsakoff syndrome	Benzodiazepines	Adrenal disorders
Neurosyphilis	Steroids	Wilson disease
Herpes encephalitis	Designer drugs (i.e., Ecstasy)	
Sensory deprivation	Ephedrine	
	Antihistamine	
	Cimetidine	
	Digoxin	
	β-Blockers	
	L-Dopamine	
	Metronidazole	
	Anticholinergics	
	Thyroid hormone	

- Hospitalization (if required).
- **Therapy**
  - Supportive therapy.
  - Group therapy.
  - Individual therapy.
  - Behavioral therapy.

B. Schizophrenia

1. Definition

- **A fundamental disturbance of personality characterized by distorted thinking:**
  - Delusions.
  - Altered perceptions.
  - Inappropriate emotional responses.
- Onset, time course, and nature of disturbances in emotion, personality, cognition, and motor activity vary widely in patients with schizophrenia.
- Person's sense of external and internal reality is profoundly distorted.
- Chronic, relapsing, remitting, debilitating psychotic disorder.
- Affects every aspect of psychological functioning, including all the ways people think, feel, perceive, decide, view themselves, and relate to others.
- Diagnostic requisites: symptoms that last a minimum of at least 6 months; 1 month with a minimum of two positive or negative symptoms; deterioration noted in functioning at work, school, and home, or in relationships. The symptoms must not be from any drug or substance use.

2. Etiology

- Schizophrenia is a clinical syndrome that probably comprises several disease processes.
- Exact cause is unknown.
- Considerable evidence exists that it is a brain disease and is neurobiologic in origin.
- **Leading theories**
  - Chemical imbalance: level of dopamine.
  - Genetics: biologic relatives of patients with schizophrenia are at greater risk for the disorder.
  - Gestational and birth complications: increased prevalence of winter births; 5% to 15% excess of winter births among people who develop schizophrenia.
  - Statistical association only: not predictive for any person.

3. Epidemiology

- Most develop symptoms between 17 and 24 years of age, but can develop up to age 45.
- Affects both men and women equally.
- Men tend to develop symptoms earlier (17–30 years) and suffer more chronic and severe symptoms.
- A 0.03% to 0.07% lifetime prevalence.

4. Clinical Features

- Idiopathic: some patients develop only minimal symptoms; others have extreme impairment.
- Symptoms often vary: patient may appear calm and rational at times, then agitated and incoherent a few hours later.
- Typically consists of several stages.

  a. **Prodromal Phase**
  - Usually precedes onset of illness by 1 year.
  - Behavior changes gradually.
  - Begins to withdraw from social interaction.
  - Less attention to personal hygiene/dressing appropriately.
  - Acts peculiarly.
  - Length of phase is extremely variable.

  b. **Acute/"Active" Phase**
  - Development of "positive symptoms" (i.e., abnormal mental activity causing grossly abnormal behavior).
  - Delusions.
  - Hallucinations (auditory most common).
  - Thought-process disorders.
  - Disorganized speaking.
  - Disorganized behavior requiring medical intervention, including hospitalization, typically necessary.

  c. **Residual Phase**
  - Positive symptoms subside and negative "deficit" symptoms develop (i.e., signs of a deficiency in certain mental functions and absence of normal behaviors).
  - Less dramatic than positive symptoms, but can be disabling.

  d. **Negative Symptoms**
  - Affective flattening.
  - Inappropriate affect.
  - Apathy.
  - Alogia (lack of logic).
  - Anhedonia (inability to experience pleasure).
  - Impaired attention and concentration signs.
  - Impaired capacity in relating to others; may lead to complete withdrawal and avoidance.
  - Clinical subtypes of schizophrenia were removed from *DSM 5* because of the lack of ability to improve clinical outcomes using these subtypes.

5. Diagnostic Studies

- Structured psychiatric interview.
- Psychological evaluation and assessment.
- Diagnosis by exclusion (does not easily meet criteria for other types).

6. Management

- No known cure.
- Psychopharmacology: antipsychotics—typical or atypical (see Table 8-1).

- **Current therapy goals**
  - Eliminate or reduce symptoms.
  - Minimize the often severe side effects of antipsychotic drugs—extrapyramidal symptoms (EPSs), tardive dyskinesia, neuroleptic malignant syndrome, agranulocytosis. Monitor for metabolic syndrome with routine blood work, fasting blood sugar, and lipid profile.
  - Prevent relapse.
  - Socially and occupationally rehabilitate the patient.
- During acute phase, medical intervention and hospitalization are often needed.
- People with schizophrenia, especially >55 years, have mortality rates eight times greater than those who do not.
- **Persons with schizophrenia are at an increased risk for suicide:**
  - Twenty-five to 50% of persons with schizophrenia attempt suicide, and 1 in 10 succeeds.
  - Persons often do not express their suicidal intent and act impulsively, making prevention difficult.
- Aggressive behavior or violence at home is a common problem for parents and other family members of patients with schizophrenia. However, rather than being perpetrators, schizophrenic patients are more commonly victims of violence.
- Substance abuse, especially alcohol abuse, is common and can exacerbate symptoms.
- Schizophrenic persons, especially young men, may use drugs or alcohol to relieve anxiety or depression.
- Sleep disturbances are common.

C. Schizophreniform Disorder

1. Definition
- Identical to schizophrenia, but duration of symptoms is shorter.
- Relationship between two conditions is unclear.

2. Etiology and Epidemiology
- All symptoms of schizophreniform disorder last 6 months (these include those of the prodromal, active, and residual phases).
- Persons have a better prognosis than do those with schizophrenia.
- Greater percentage of patients recover completely.
- Similar incidence as schizophrenia, but lower in developed countries.
- Higher risk of blood relations to develop schizophrenia.
- **Characteristics of those most likely to recover quickly:**
  - Developed psychotic symptoms quickly (change in behavior within 4 weeks).
  - Confused or disoriented during the psychotic episode.

- Functioned well before the onset of symptoms.
- Maintained a normal range and display of emotions rather than blunted feelings.

3. Clinical Features
- Schizophrenia.

4. Diagnostic Studies
- Structured psychiatric interview.
- **Rule out**
  - Temporal lobe epilepsy.
  - CNS tumors.
  - Cerebrovascular disease.
  - Human immunodeficiency virus (HIV).

5. Management
- Treatment: same as for schizophrenia including pharmacotherapy (see Table 8–1).
- Psychosocial care.

D. Schizoaffective Disorder

1. Definition
- Disorder characterized by a combination of symptoms of both schizophrenia and a mood or "affective" disorder (either major depression or bipolar illness).

2. Etiology
- Less common than schizophrenia.
- Onset in late adolescence or in early adulthood.
- The combination of a depressive disorder and psychosis greatly increases the risk of suicide with a 5% lifetime risk.

3. Clinical Features
- Clinical signs and symptoms of schizophrenia, mania, and depressive disorders.
- Must have two of the following symptoms for at least 1 month:
  - Delusions, hallucinations, disorganized speech, disorganized behavior, and negative symptoms.
- The major depressive episode must include depressed mood.
- Schizophrenia and mood disorders may be present together or in an alternating sequence.
- Course may vary from acute exacerbations with remissions or present with a long-term deteriorating course.
- Timing of symptoms of delusions or hallucinations must last for 2 weeks or more in the absence of any severe mood disorder.

4. Diagnostic Studies
- Structured psychiatric interview.
- Completed medical examination.
- Meets criteria for major depression or mania concurrently with the diagnostic criteria seen in schizophrenia.

5. Management
- Treatment should be individualized.
- Pharmacotherapy is the cornerstone of treatment (see Table 8–1).
- Occasionally, dysphoric symptoms subside with antidepressant medication alone—if not, add

antipsychotic agent to antidepressant. Caution in mania or hypomania.
- If mania—mood-stabilizing agent (i.e., lithium plus antipsychotic).
- ECT in some treatment-resistant patients.
- Psychotherapy may be beneficial for some patients.
- Long-term outlook is better than for those with schizophrenia.
- Some improve significantly between episodes of depression or mania.
- Others suffer chronic residual symptoms and never recover completely or function normally.

E. Brief Psychotic Disorder

1. Definition
- **Sudden onset of at least one (active) positive symptom of psychosis:**
  - Delusions.
  - Hallucinations.
  - Disorganized speech.
  - Grossly disorganized or catatonic behavior.
- Can specify whether it occurs with or without a major stressor, whether it occurs during pregnancy, or whether the episode involves catatonia.

2. Etiology and Epidemiology
- Symptoms last hours to 1 day, but no more than 30 days.
- Symptoms may appear after an event or series of events that would be extremely stressful to almost anyone in similar circumstances (e.g., combat, a violent attack, or a loved one's death).
- Two times greater risk in females than in males.
- Greater prevalence in developing countries.
- Up to 9% of all patients present with initial psychosis episode.

3. Clinical Features
- Onset: late adolescence, early adulthood (late 20s to early 30s).
- Increased risk in persons with personality disorders.
- Anyone in a situation with overwhelming stress can develop psychotic symptoms.
- Can be extremely frightening for affected persons and those around them.
- May behave bizarrely, screaming and refusing to speak; may repeat nonsense phrases or speak gibberish.
- Often disoriented and unable to remember recent events.
- Some become aggressive and suicidal.

4. Diagnostic Studies
- Structured psychiatric interview.
- Toxicology screens.
- Rule out CNS pathology.
- Rule out cerebrovascular disease.

5. Management
- Initially, close observation in a safe setting to rule out general medical condition or substance abuse.
- Symptoms may resolve on their own, and person recovers quickly.
- **If symptoms persist:**
  - Sedatives or antipsychotics are prescribed (see Table 8–1).
  - Antipsychotics are tapered as soon as symptoms subside.
- Patients then recover fully from psychosis, but some may be troubled by secondary effects (e.g., diminished self-esteem and mild depression) for some time.
- In some patients, symptoms persist, requiring continuing treatment with antipsychotics.
- If symptoms persist for more than 30 days or have increasing severity, diagnosis is changed to schizophreniform or schizophrenia.
- Brief hospitalization may be required—suicide is a concern.

F. Delusional Disorder

1. Definition
- A psychotic disorder whose chief feature is a nonbizarre delusion presents for at least 1 month.
- Several types of delusions: predominant type identified used to specify and to make the diagnosis.
- Patient has minimal deterioration in personality or function and no other psychopathologic symptoms, and this helps distinguish it from schizophrenia and other psychotic conditions.
- Subtypes are specified as erotomanic, grandiose, jealous, persecutory, or somatic types.
- These subtypes are usually nonbizarre delusions involve situations that occur in real life (e.g., being followed, poisoned, or deceived by a lover or spouse, having a disease), but could be specified as having bizarre content that is entirely unbelievable or farfetched.
- Often do not come to psychiatrist's attention—more often underdiagnosed/misdiagnosed—seen by internists, dermatologists, police, and lawyers.

2. Etiology and Epidemiology
- Paranoid, schizoid, or avoidant personality disorders may increase likelihood.
- Relatively uncommon with 0.2% lifetime prevalence.
- Persecutory subtype most commonly diagnosed.
- One to 2% of all annual admissions to psychiatric hospitals.
- Prevalence same in both genders.

3. Clinical Features
- **Main types of delusional disorders:**
  - Grandiose: belief in inflated worth, power, knowledge, identity, or special relationship to a duty or an important famous person.

- Jealous: belief that one's sexual partner is unfaithful.
- Persecutory: belief that someone to whom one is close is being treated poorly and unjustly in some way.
- Somatic: belief that person has some physical defect, disorder, or disease.
- Erotomanic: belief that person, usually of a higher status, is in love with them (obsession-stalker situation).
- Mixed: more than one of the above types is present, but no theme is predominant.
- Unspecified: delusions do not fit into any of the categories.
- May appear normal with no overt symptoms unless talking about or acting on their delusions.
- Many are angry, hostile, and suspicious.
- Some become reclusive and socially isolated or behave in eccentric ways.
- Most have little or no insight into their problems and refuse to admit anything is wrong with them.
- Sexual problems and depressive symptoms are common complications of delusional disorder.
- Violence is rare; but it can occur, especially in erotomania.
- Stalker's significant others are more likely to be targets of violence than the fantasy love object.

4. Diagnostic Studies
- Structured psychiatric interview.
- Toxicology screens.
- Rule out CNS pathology.
- Rule out cerebrovascular disease.

5. Management
- Usually do not admit that they have a problem or seek therapy unless forced to by family members or legal action.
- **Pharmacotherapy (see Table 8–1)**
  - Antipsychotic medications (typical or atypical) may decrease delusions and anxiety.
  - Symptoms may not dissipate completely.
  - May relieve somatic delusions.
- **Psychotherapy:** Individual.
  - Brief hospitalization may be required because of risk and safety issues.

VII. Delirium and Major Neurocognitive Disorder (Dementia)

A. Delirium
1. Definition
- A syndrome characterized by the impairment of consciousness and the global impairment of cognitive function that develops over a short period of time (i.e., hours to days). Evidence suggests that this condition can develop in response to a general medical condition, substance intoxication withdrawal, toxicity, or a combination of such factors.

2. Etiology and Epidemiology
- **Multiple etiologies may exist, with major causes possibly including:**
  - CNS disease (e.g., epilepsy).
  - Systemic disease, congestive heart failure (CHF), fever, or HIV.
  - Endocrine dysfunction (hypo or hyper).
  - Intoxication or withdrawal from pharmacologic or toxic agents, alcohol, or street drugs.
- **Postoperative causes**
  - Stress of surgery.
  - Postoperative pain.
  - Use of pain medication.
  - Insomnia.
  - Electrolyte imbalance.
  - Infections.
  - Fever.
  - Blood loss.
- **Trauma**
  - Previous brain injury.
  - Burns.
- Can occur at any age.
- Low prevalence of 1% to 2% in general population.
- Advanced age is a major risk factor because of metabolic changes in elderly individuals; 40% of hospitalized patients older than 65 years have an episode of delirium.
- Patients with a history of prior episodes of delirium are at an increased risk for recurrence under similar conditions.
- Delirium tends to be an underrecognized and underdiagnosed disorder in elderly individuals.
- Prevalence of around 80% of people who are nearing the end of their lives.

3. Clinical Features
- Sudden onset of symptoms. (**NOTE:** In the absence of any history or psychological dysfunction or other comorbid disorders, the rapid onset of symptomatology should be a major clue in evaluating medical condition and other possible precipitants of this presentation.)
- Reduced clarity or awareness of the environment.
- Decreased ability to focus, sustain, or shift attention.
- Inability to concentrate.
- Disorganized thinking (not due to other factors or syndromes).
- May not be able to follow a normal conversation or respond to questions.
- Lucid periods alternate with symptomatic periods. (**NOTE:** This is another feature that aids in differential diagnosis with dementia or other cognitive disorder.)
- Abnormal arousal.
- Disorientation.
- Rambling, irrelevant, or incoherent speech.

- Impaired comprehension.
- Memory impairment (recent memory most affected).
- Impaired perception: delusions and hallucinations (auditory and visual most common).
- Most lucid in the morning with symptoms worsening as day progresses.
- Affective (mood) changes not accounted for by premorbid or comorbid conditions—fear, anger, rage, apathy, dysphoria, euphoria, and combativeness.
- Sleep disturbances: reversal of sleep–wake cycles. Sleep patterns are almost always short and fragmented.
- Exacerbation of symptoms at bedtime (sundowning).
- Associated neurologic symptoms: dysphasia, tremor, asterixis, incoordination, and urinary incontinence. Focal neurologic signs may also be evident.
- **May have a prodromal phase of symptoms:**
  - Anxiety.
  - Drowsiness.
  - Insomnia.
  - Restlessness.
  - Nightmares.
  - Transient hallucinations.

4. Diagnostic Studies
  - Structured psychiatric interview.
  - Cognitive evaluation.
  - Face-hand test: used to document cognitive impairment.
  - Physical examination.
  - Neurologic evaluation.
  - Laboratory studies (standard tests).
  - Thyroid profile.
  - Additional or specific studies based on clinical indicators:
    - EEG.
    - CT scan or MRI of brain.
    - Blood, urine, and cerebrospinal fluid (CSF) cultures.
    - Vitamin B_{12} and folic acid levels.
    - Lumbar puncture and CSF analysis.
    - Blood and urine toxicology.

5. Management
  - Treat the underlying medical cause(s). Resolution of concurrent medical conditions may result in a more rapid resolution of the symptoms associated with delirium.
  - Provide physical, sensory, and environmental support.
  - **Pharmacotherapy**
    - Transient symptoms of psychosis, if evident, may be treated with antipsychotics, but should be carefully monitored, evaluated for efficacy,

and modulated. Evaluation of psychotic symptoms should continue throughout to determine their association with the medical condition instigating the symptomatology.
    - Insomnia: benzodiazepines with short half-lives or hydroxyzine.
  - Symptoms usually recede over a 3- to 7-day period following the identification and removal of causative agent or condition.
  - Some symptoms can take up to 3 weeks to resolve completely.
  - The older the patient and the longer the patient has been delirious, the longer delirium takes to resolve.
  - Delirium has a poor prognosis because of the potentially serious underlying medical conditions.

B. Major and Minor Neurocognitive Disorders
  1. Definition
  - A syndrome characterized by increasingly and multiple cognitive impairments affecting memory, language, thinking, emotion, and personality without impairment in consciousness, typically due to multiple etiologies, such as progressive medical conditions, persistent and pervasive effects of long-term substance abuse, and other medical condition/events—for example, multiple cerebrovascular accidents, cerebrovascular disease, and Alzheimer disease.
  - Alzheimer dementia: now more commonly recognized as occurring across a continuum of stages: (a) Alzheimer itself with clear symptoms, (b) mild cognitive impairment (MCI) with mild symptoms, and (c) a "preclinical" stage, when there are no dramatic symptoms, but when recognizable brain changes may already be observed.
  - New guidelines suggest and incorporate the use of so-called biomarkers (e.g., such as protein levels in blood or spinal fluid) to diagnose the disease and assess its progress, although the latter is used mostly for research purposes at this stage. The new guidelines also make a clearer distinction between Alzheimer dementia and vascular dementia (such as that caused by stroke). Another stage, MCI, can represent an earlier phase of dementia and consists of modest impairments, primarily in memory, which can be a precursor of a more complete Alzheimer presentation later in a person's life.
  - The syndrome can represent a meaningful decline in social, environmental, and occupational activities.
  - Cognitive changes are not an aspect of normal aging or the result of congenital brain deficits and represent a significant decline from a previous level of functioning.
  - Disorder may be progressive or static, permanent or reversible, depending on underlying cause.

2. Etiology
- Multiple causes: more than 50 disorders may result in dementia.
- Thirteen percent of individuals >65 years and 50% of individuals >85 years will be observed with dementia of the Alzheimer type (most common), with women demonstrating symptomatology more frequently than men.
- Fifteen to 30% of all patients have vascular dementia, with a preponderance of men over women in this form of dementia.
- **Other causes**
  - Hypertension: predisposes to dementia.
  - Parkinson disease.
  - Pick disease.
  - HIV.
  - Drugs, toxins, and alcohol abuse.
  - Intracranial masses.
  - Head injury.
  - Huntington disease.
  - Nutritional disorders.
  - Metabolic disorders.
  - Endocrinopathies.
- Generally considered an illness of elderly people, given their general decline and sometimes dramatic changes in physical status and overall state, as well as other accumulated causes, such as long-term effects of other conditions noted above.
  - Five percent of persons >65 years have severe dementia (Alzheimer type).
  - Fifteen percent of persons >65 years have mild dementia.
  - Twenty percent of persons >80 years have severe dementia.
  - Ten to 15% of patients with dementia are treatable because dysfunctional brain tissue may retain capacity for recovery if treatment is timely.

3. Clinical Features
- Usually begins with subtle signs of cognitive dysfunction.
- Gradual onset of symptoms is commonly associated with dementia of the Alzheimer type, vascular dementia, endocrinopathies, brain tumors, and metabolic disorders.
- Signs and symptoms vary greatly depending on the cause, course, and severity; the part of the brain most affected; and on the person's personality before the dementia.
- Memory impairment is an early feature and most prominent characteristic.
- **Early stages of dementia**
  - Recent memory impairment.
  - Confabulation: language problems.
  - Difficulty in sustaining mental performance.
  - Fatigue.
  - Tendency to fail when a task is different and complex, or requires a shift in problem-solving strategy.

- Disturbance in orientation.
- Compromised abstract reasoning.
- Impaired insight and judgment.
- Personality changes: apathy, disinterest, labile affect, impaired social skills, exaggerated premorbid personality.
- Attempts to hide performance and cognitive deficit.
- Depression, anxiety, excessive orderliness, social withdrawal, and tendency to relate events in minute detail can be characteristic.
- Sudden outbursts of anger or sarcasm.
- Paranoia/delusions.
- **Middle–late stages of dementia**
  - Remote memory loss: confabulation.
  - Mood changes: depression, anxiety, and apathy.
  - Personality changes.
  - Emotional lability with no apparent provocation.
  - Loss of orientation.
  - Advanced intellectual impairment.
  - Grossly impaired insight judgment.
  - Perceptual distortion: hallucinations and delusions.
  - Aphasia.
  - Apraxia.
  - Agnosia.
  - Urinary then fecal incontinence.
  - Primitive reflexes may be present on neurologic examination.

4. Diagnostic Studies
- Structured psychiatric interview.
- Complete medical history from patient and family.
- Physical examination.
- Neurologic examination.
- Neuropsychological testing.
- Rule out pseudodementia.
- Detect reversible causes of dementia.
- EEG, MRI, or CT scan of brain.
- Laboratory studies (standard tests).
- Blood and urine toxicology.
- Thyroid profile.
- Vitamin B_{12} and folic acid levels.
- Additional laboratory testing as clinically indicated.
- HIV testing.
- Lumbar puncture.
- ECG.
- Liver profile.

5. Management
- Treat any underlying causes.
- **Use all available resources to provide appropriate intervention/care:**
  - Medical.
  - Supportive and educational psychotherapy.
  - Family counseling.

- Community resources (local support groups for both patient and family/caregivers specific to the type of dementia and stage, such as support groups for caregivers of patients with Alzheimer disease).
- **Pharmacotherapy (see Table 8–1): treat specific symptom complex including:**
  - Depression.
  - Anxiety.
  - Agitation.
  - Combativeness.
  - Aggression.
  - Insomnia.
  - Perceptual distortion.
- Therapeutics: antipsychotics in low doses (i.e., haloperidol); antidepressants (SSRIs); benzodiazepines, short acting in small doses.
- **Symptomatic treatment**
  - Provide a supportive environment.
  - Nutritional.
  - Proper exercise.
  - Recreational and activity therapies.
  - Attention to visual and auditory problems.
  - Treatment of associated medical problems.

VIII. Substance-Related Disorders

A. Disorders Arise from 10 Different Drug Classes
- Alcohol.
- Caffeine.
- Cannabis.
- Hallucinogens.
- Inhalants.
- Opioids.
- Sedatives/hypnotics/anxiolytics.
- Stimulants.
- Tobacco.
- Other.

B. Two Classifications of Substance-Related Disorders
- Substance-use disorders.
- Substance-induced disorders
  - Intoxication.
  - Withdrawal.
  - Substance/medication-induced mental disorders.

C. Definition
1. Substance-Use Disorder
- Characterized by the presence of at least two or more specific symptoms, indicating the use of a substance has interfered with a person's life and may lead to impairment or distress manifested by one or more symptoms occurring within a 12-month period:
  - Continued use of a substance despite significant cognitive and behavioral problems.

- Loss of control: the person uses more of the substance or for a longer period of time.
- Craving.
- Persistent desire or unsuccessful efforts to cut down or control use.
- Spends a majority of time obtaining, using, and recovering from substance abuse.
- Substance is used to change a mood or feeling.
- Tolerance.
- Withdrawal.
- Giving up or reducing involvement in important social, occupational, or recreational activities because of substance use.
- Substance use is continued despite knowledge of having a persistent or recurrent physical, psychological, or social problem caused by or worsened by the substance.

2. Severity Classification
- Mild: two to three symptoms.
- Moderate: four to five symptoms.
- Severe: >six symptoms.

3. Remission Classification
- Early: 3 months but <1 year without meeting criteria except for having cravings.
- Sustained: >12 months with above.

D. Etiology
- No definitive etiology is known.
- Genetic, psychodynamic, and neurochemical.
- **Numerous risk factors**
  - Genetics: children of alcoholics are more likely to develop alcoholism.
  - More men tend to develop this disorder than do women, although this trend has been changing in recent years.
  - Family dynamics includes a pattern of regular and intense family stress, parenting problems, history of physical or sexual abuse, and permissive attitude toward substance use can be a contributing factor.
- **Environmental dynamics**
  - Peer group drug use.
  - Poverty.
  - Social isolation.
  - Drug trafficking.
  - Drug accessibility (e.g., physician, physician assistant, pharmacist, nurse).
- **Other psychodynamics/pathology**
  - Low self-esteem.
  - Poor self-image.
  - Mood disorders.
  - Schizophrenia.
  - Self-medication.
  - Alcohol and nicotine are the most commonly abused substances.
  - Increased prevalence of substance abuse 18 to 22 years of age.

- Greater risk of substance abuse when onset is before 15 years of age.
- Recent evidence indicates the use of "gateway drugs" (i.e., alcohol, nicotine, marijuana, inhalants) has increased among children and adolescents.
- Predictive factors for the progression to substance dependence remain unclear.

E. Epidemiology
- Increased prevalence of substance abuse 18 to 22 years of age.
- Greater risk of substance abuse when onset is before 15 years of age.
- Recent evidence indicates increased use of "gateway drugs" (i.e., alcohol, nicotine, marijuana, and inhalants) among children and adolescents.
- Genetics/psychosocial: children of alcoholics are more likely to develop alcoholism.
- Prevalence in Men > Women.

F. Clinical Features
- These features are outlined under the description of the specific substance (see section IX).

G. Diagnostic Studies
- Structured psychiatric interview.
- Detailed substance-use history.
- Detailed family history.
- Medical history.
- Social history.
- Complete physical examination.
- **Standard laboratory tests**
  - Blood and urine toxicology screens.
  - HIV testing (intravenous [IV] drug use).
  - Liver profile: hepatitis screening.
- Other diagnostic studies based on pertinent physical and historic findings.

H. Management
- **Treatment of substance abuse involves two major goals:**
  - Abstinence.
  - Physical, psychiatric, and psychosocial well-being of the patient.

IX. Specific Substance-Use and Substance-Induced Disorders

A. Specific Substance-Use Disorder
- Screening tools: CAGE (Cut down, Annoyed, Guilty, and Eye-opener) and AUDIT (Alcohol Use Disorders Identification Test).
- Intoxication or impairment from specific substance: recent ingestion accompanied by detoxification.
  - Withdrawal from the specific substance and the management of associated withdrawal symptoms.
  - Primary use of symptom-specific pharmacotherapy.
  - Support and reassurance.
  - Assessment and treatment of medical complications.

- Rehabilitation/treatment:
  - Inpatient treatment programs.
  - Outpatient treatment programs.
  - Relapse prevention.
- **Self-help groups**
  - Alcoholics Anonymous (AA).
  - Narcotics Anonymous (NA).
- **Family therapy**
  - Alcoholics Anonymous (ALANON).
  - Is a recovery group for adolescents ages 9–19 (ALATEEN).
  - Adult Children of Alcoholics (ACOA).
- Individual psychotherapy/group therapy.
- Support and reassurance.
- Assessment and treatment of medical complications.
- Pharmacotherapy
  - Primary use of symptom-specific pharmacotherapy.
    - Disulfiram: provokes severe reaction with ingestion of alcohol.
    - Naltrexone: an opioid antagonist; blocks pleasurable effects of opioids and alcohol.
    - Acamprosate (Campral): seems to reduce craving of alcohol.
    - Buprenorphine/naloxone (Suboxone): opioid antagonist/agonist.
    - Methadone: an opioid agonist; is given to replace heroin and suppress withdrawal symptoms.

B. Specific Substance-Induced Disorders
1. Alcohol Intoxication
a. **Recent Alcohol Ingestion Accompanied by:**
- Maladaptive behaviors.
- Aggression.
- Sexual activity.
- Psychological changes.
- Impaired judgment.
- Mood changes.
- Impaired occupational and social functioning.
- **One or more of the following symptoms:**
  - Slurred speech.
  - Incoordination.
  - Unsteady gait.
  - Nystagmus.
  - Memory impairment.
  - Stupor of coma.
  - Duration is variable.
  - Blood alcohol level usually >0.10%.

b. Epidemiology
- Prevalence greatest during college years with average age of first episode in mid to late teens.

c. Management
- Secure, safe, structured environment.
- Reassurance.
- Intramuscular (IM) haloperidol may be useful for controlling assaultiveness.
- Condition should be differentiated from other causes of abrupt behavioral change.

- If severe, can lead to respiratory depression, coma, or death.
- May receive mechanical ventilatory support and monitoring.
- Attention to patient's acid–base, electrolytes, and temperature.

2. **Alcohol Withdrawal**
   a. **Cessation or Reduction of Alcohol Use That Was Heavy or Prolonged, As Well As the Presence of the Following Specific Physical and/or Psychiatric Symptoms:**
      - Autonomic hyperactivity.
      - Tremor.
      - Insomnia.
      - Nausea or vomiting.
      - Transient visual, tactile, or auditory hallucinations.
      - Psychomotor agitation.
      - Anxiety.
      - Seizures.
      - Delirium.
      - Symptoms may last from several hours to several days.
      - These symptoms can lead to delirium tremens (DTs), a medical emergency.
      - If delirium is present, it may indicate the presence of other general medical conditions.
      - Can occur with or without perceptual disturbances.
   b. **Diagnostic Studies**
      - Structured psychiatric interview.
      - Substance-use history.
      - Physical examination.
      - **Rule out**
        - Lateralizing seizures.
        - Head trauma.
        - CNS pathology.
        - Hepatic failure.
        - Hypoglycemia.
        - Hyponatremia.
        - Hypomagnesemia.
        - Thiamine deficiency and anemias.
        - Blood and urine toxicology screens.
        - Routine laboratory evaluation.
        - LFTs, electrolytes, serum ammonia (if indicated), lipid profile, and CBC.
   c. **Management**
      - Cessation of alcohol use.
      - Provide a calming psychotherapeutic environment with safety precautions, nutritional support, and hydration.
      - Benzodiazepines in titrating doses. Phenobarbital can also be used as second line.
      - Diazepam and chlordiazepoxide have a poor IM absorption ratio.
      - Carbamazepine.

- Clonidine.
- β-Adrenergic receptor antagonists.
- Symptomatic treatment of nausea, vomiting, diarrhea, and insomnia.
- Thiamine, folate, magnesium, and other vitamin supplements as indicated.
- Anticonvulsants if indicated.

3. **Alcohol Intoxication Delirium (Also Known As Delirium Tremens)**
   - Delirium tremens (DTs) is one of the most serious alcohol withdrawal symptoms and should always be considered a medical emergency.
   - About 5% of individuals with severe alcohol intoxication will experience DTs. Left untreated, it is estimated that up to 35% of individuals experiencing DTs will die.
   - Withdrawal seizures commonly precede development of alcohol withdrawal delirium, but can occur throughout.
   - Delirium can also appear unheralded.
   - The *essential feature* of the syndrome is delirium that occurs *within 1 week* after cessation or reduction of alcohol intake.
   - **Accompanied by:**
     - Autonomic hyperactivity.
     - Tachycardia.
     - Fever.
     - Diaphoresis.
     - Hypertension.
     - Anxiety and insomnia.
     - Perceptual distortion (visual/tactile hallucinations are common).
     - Fluctuating levels of psychomotor activity.
   - Usually begins in a patient's 30s or 40s after 5 to 15 years of heavy drinking.
   - Can result in significant morbidity and mortality if untreated.
   - **Management**
     - Cessation of alcohol use.
     - Provide a calming psychotherapeutic environment.
     - Benzodiazepines in titrating doses.
     - May use lorazepam IV if oral route is not available.
     - Antipsychotics may reduce seizure threshold, but may be necessary to treat a superimposed psychosis.
     - Fluids to control dehydration.
     - Skillful verbal support is imperative.
     - Anticonvulsants until seizure etiology is determined.
     - Seclusion is an alternative for combative and uncontrollable patients.
     - High-caloric, high-carbohydrate diet.
     - Thiamine, folate, magnesium, and other vitamin supplements as indicated.

4. **Alcohol-Induced Persisting Amnestic Disorder**
   a. **Wernicke Encephalopathy**
      - Definition: an acute neurologic disorder characterized by ataxia, vestibular dysfunction, ocular abnormalities, and confusion.
      - Etiology: caused by thiamine deficiency.
      - **Management**
         - Reversible with treatment.
         - May clear spontaneously in a few days or weeks or progress into Korsakoff syndrome.
         - Thiamine 100 mg PO two to three times daily for 1 to 2 weeks. May initially use IM.
   b. **Korsakoff Syndrome**
      - Definition: a chronic amnestic syndrome characterized by impaired mental functioning, including recent memory, anterograde amnesia in an alert and responsive patient. The hallmark is confabulation.
      - Etiology: caused by thiamine deficiency.
      - **Management**
         - Thiamine 100 mg PO two to three times daily for 3 to 12 months.
         - Twenty percent recovery rate with some improvement in cognitive abilities.

5. **Blackouts**
   a. **Definition**
      - Experience of specific short-term memory impairment with an inability to recall recent events.
      - Similar to episodes of transient global amnesia in that discrete episodes of anterograde amnesia are present.
   b. **Etiology**
      - Blackouts occur in association with alcohol intoxication or severe alcohol abuse.
   c. **Clinical Features**
      - Remote memory is relatively intact.
      - Intellectual functioning is preserved, allowing performance of complicated tasks.
      - The person may appear normal to the casual observer.
   d. **Management**
      - Cessation of alcohol use. Management of withdrawal if indicated. Rehabilitation.

6. **Stimulant Intoxication (Amphetamine Type Substance, Cocaine or Other Unspecified Simulant)**
   a. **Symptoms**
      - Euphoria.
      - Affective instability.
      - Aggression.
      - Hypervigilance.
      - Impulsive sexual behavior.
      - Impaired judgment.
      - Anxiety.
      - Tension.
      - Anger.
      - Impaired social, occupational, and interpersonal functioning.
      - **With at least two or more of the following physical symptoms:**
         - Tachycardia or bradycardia.
         - Pupillary dilatation.
         - Elevated or lower blood pressure.
         - Perspiration or chills.
         - Nausea or vomiting.
         - Weight loss.
         - Psychomotor agitation.
         - Muscular weakness.
         - Respiratory depression.
         - Chest pain.
         - Cardiac arrhythmias.
         - Confusion.
         - Seizures.
         - Dyskinesias.
         - Dystonias.
         - Coma.
   b. **Clinical Features**
      - Cocaine use has numerous adverse effects outside of the diagnostic criteria:
         - Nasal congestion.
         - Inflammation, swelling, bleeding, and ulceration of the nasal mucosa.
         - Perforation of nasal septum.
      - IV use of cocaine is associated with local and systemic infections, embolism, and transmission of HIV and hepatitis B and C. Can also be transmitted intranasally if mucosa is compromised.
      - Effects are almost immediate.
      - Duration is relatively brief.
      - Metabolites of cocaine may be present in blood for up to 10 days and in urine for up to 4 days.
   c. **Major Complications of Cocaine Use:**
      - Cerebral vascular accidents.
      - Nonhemorrhagic cerebral infarction.
      - Hemorrhagic cerebral infarction including subarachnoid, intraparenchymal, and intraventricular.
      - Seizures.
      - Myocardial infarction.
      - Cardiac arrhythmia.
      - Cardiomyopathies can develop with long-term use.
   d. **Diagnostic Studies**
      - Structured psychiatric interview.
      - Substance-use history.
      - Extensive physical examination.
      - Blood and urine toxicology screens.
      - Appropriate laboratory studies.
      - ECG.

e. Management
- Cessation of cocaine use.
- Hospitalization if required.
- Structured, safe, secure environment. Sleep is primary supportive treatment.
- Treat withdrawal symptoms.
- Screen and manage any cardiac or CNS complications.
- Broad treatment approach including social, biologic, and psychological strategies.
- Involvement in support groups, 12-step programs.
- Inpatient or outpatient rehabilitation.
- Individual and family counseling.
- After cessation of cocaine use or acute intoxication, postintoxication depression may occur and may last up to 1 week.
- Pharmacotherapy to reduce craving.
- **Dopaminergic agonists**
  - Bromocriptine.
  - Amantadine.
- Tricyclics.
- Carbamazepine.
- Off-label use of bupropion, modafinil, and topiramate. Studies are ongoing.

7. **Opiate Withdrawal**
- Heroin.
- Prescription drugs: morphine, OxyContin, Dilaudid, fentanyl, Percocet, etc.
  a. **Clinical Features**
  - Symptoms develop after discontinuation of drug following a period of heavy use or administration of opioid antagonist.
  - Three or more of the following symptoms: dysphoric mood, nausea/vomiting/diarrhea, muscle aches, lacrimation and/or rhinorrhea, pupillary dilation, piloerection, sweating, yawning, fever, and insomnia.
  - Symptoms cause clinically significant distress in social, occupational, or other important area of functioning.
  b. **Treatment**
  - Treat any medical condition: cellulitis, sepsis, subacute bacterial endocarditis, HIV, hepatitis.
  - Psychotherapy/group therapy: treat mood disorders.
  - **Pharmacotherapy**
    - Symptomatic relief; Phenergan, NSAIDs, clonidine, trazodone, fluids. nutritional support.
    - Suboxone.
    - Methadone.
    - Naltrexone as prophylaxis. Slight chance of overdosing on heroin if relapse occurs.

8. **Tobacco Use Disorder**
  a. **Diagnosis**
  - Increasing need and marked tolerance of increased amounts of tobacco products containing nicotine.
  - Marked diminished satisfaction with continued use of the same volume of nicotine products, requiring increased and continued use of greater amounts of the product.
  - The product is taken over larger amounts over time and beyond what was intended ("I'll only smoke one pack, or I'll quit before I become pregnant...").
  - Persistent desire and unsuccessful efforts to decrease or control the amount used.
  - Incorporation of tobacco use into many domains of personal and social functioning.
  - Continuation of usage despite knowledge or awareness of harmful effects and/or negative impacts on physiologic, psychological, social, and possibly occupational domains of personal functioning.
  b. **Epidemiology**
  - Thirteen percent of adults in the United States.
  - Greatest use in Native Americans on those native to Alaska.
  c. **Risk Factors**
  - **Comorbid conditions**
    - Genetics.
    - Mental illness.
    - Substance abuse.
  d. **Possible Physiological Complications**
  - Lung cancer and other lung diseases.
  - Heart and circulatory system problems.
  - Additional cancers (e.g., esophageal, laryngeal, throat [pharynx] and mouth, bladder, pancreas, kidney and cervix, and some leukemias).
  - Physical appearance (e.g., changes in structure of skin causing premature aging and wrinkles. Yellowing of teeth, fingers, and fingernails).
  - Possible changes in fertility. Chance of impotence in men.
  - Pregnancy and newborn complications.
  - Cold, flu, and other illnesses. (Smokers are more prone to respiratory infections, such as colds, flu, and bronchitis.)
  - Diabetes (i.e., increase in insulin resistance, possible development of type II diabetes; possible acceleration and progression of extant diabetes process, including progression of complications, such as kidney disease and eye problems).
  - Weakened senses (e.g., alterations in senses of taste and smell, so food is not as appetizing).
  - Family risks (i.e., family members of smokers are at a higher risk for lung cancer and heart disease, compared with people who do not live with a smoker).

e. Tobacco Withdrawal
  - **Symptoms (four or more in a 24-hour period)**
    - Dysphoric or depressed mood.
    - Irritability and anxiety.
    - Difficulty concentrating.
    - Restlessness.
    - Problems falling asleep or frequent waking.
    - Craving for tobacco.
    - Tingling sensations and dizziness.
    - Coughing.
    - Appetite changes.
  - **Management/treatment**
    - Nicotine replacement therapy (patches, gum, lozenges, nasal spray, and inhaler).
    - Non-nicotine medications (combinations of medications shown as more effective).
    - Combine a longer-acting medication (e.g., nicotine patch or bupropion [Zyban, Wellbutrin] or varenicline [Chantix]) with a short-acting nicotine replacement product, such as nicotine gum, lozenge, nasal spray, or inhaler.

REVIEW QUESTIONS

1. Which of the following personality disorders is characterized by a pervasive pattern of excessive, impulsive behaviors, suicidal threats, avoidance of abandonment, unstable relationships, and impaired social and vocational functioning?
   a) OCPD
   b) Paranoid personality disorder
   c) BPD
   d) Avoidant personality disorder

2. Which of the following is a nonstimulant option for the treatment of ADHD?
   a) Dextroamphetamine (Dexedrine)
   b) Methylphenidate (Ritalin)
   c) Atomoxetine (Strattera)
   d) Amphetamine salts (Adderall)

3. Which of the following medications is most likely to cause depression in an elderly adult?
   a) Levodopa
   b) Metformin
   c) Colchicine
   d) Amlodipine

4. Which of the following include clinical features of schizophrenia?
   a) Elevated heart rate
   b) Flat affect
   c) Fruity breath
   d) Organized speech patterns

5. Predisposing vulnerability factors for a diagnosis of post-traumatic stress disorder include:
   a) Absence of childhood trauma
   b) Family history of schizophrenia
   c) Inadequate support system
   d) Internal locus of control

ANSWERS TO REVIEW QUESTIONS

1. **Answer: C.** These symptoms are some of the diagnostic criteria for borderline personality disorder. OCPD is characterized by rigid perfectionism and a preoccupation with order, details, and organization. Avoidant personality disorder is characterized by feelings of inferiority, diminished social interactions, low self-esteem, and decreased intimacy.

2. **Answer: C.** There are a variety of pharmacologic options for the treatment and management of ADHD. Strattera is the nonstimulant option choice listed.

3. **Answer: A.** Dopamine, along with serotonin and norepinephrine, is a neurotransmitter associated with mood. Levodopa affects the amount of dopamine in the brain and may cause depression in a patient. The risks and benefits of levodopa (and all drugs) should be carefully weighed on a case-by-case basis.

4. **Answer: B.** Symptoms of schizophrenia include disorganized thoughts and behavior, delusions, and hallucinations. Physical examination findings include flat or blunted affect, lack of attention to grooming and hygiene, odd or rigid postures, and disorganized speech.

5. **Answer: C.** A small percentage of people who experience trauma will be diagnosed with PTSD. Risk factors for PTSD include presence of childhood trauma, abuse in childhood, family instability, and lower levels of income and education.

SELECTED REFERENCES

American Psychiatric Association. *Diagnostic and Statistical Manual of Mental Disorders.* 4th ed. Text rev. Washington, DC: American Psychiatric Association; 2000.

Ebert M, Loosen P, Nurcombe B, eds. *Current Diagnosis & Treatment in Psychiatry.* New York, NY: McGraw-Hill/Appleton & Lange; 2000.

Epocrates Essentials. www.epocrates.com.

Kaplan HI, Sadock BJ, eds. *Synopsis of Psychiatry, Behavioral Sciences, Clinical Psychiatry.* 10th ed. Baltimore, MD: Lippincott Williams & Wilkins; 2007.

Lewis M, ed. *Child and Adolescent Psychiatry: A Comprehensive Textbook.* 3rd ed. Philadelphia, PA: Lippincott Williams & Wilkins; 2002.

National Institute on Child Health and Human Development. http://NICHD.NIH.GOV. Accessed May 15, 2011.

National Institute of Mental Health. http://NIMH.NIH.GOV. Accessed May 20, 2011.

National Institute of Aging. http://NIA.NIH.GOV. Accessed May 2011.

Tierney LM, McPhee SJ, Papadakis MA, eds. *Current Medical Diagnosis & Treatment.* Stamford, CT: Appleton & Lange, 2003.

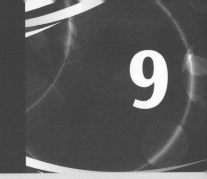

Endocrine Disorders

Ellen D. Feld • Daniela Cheles-Livingston

I. Pituitary Disorders
A. Anterior Pituitary
1. **Pituitary Tumors**
   a. **Etiology**
      - Several cell types comprise the pituitary gland; each cell type may give rise to pituitary adenomas.
      - Clinical consequences are associated commonly with hypersecretion of one of the pituitary gland's products or by compression of nearby anatomic structures (mass effect). The latter may manifest with headaches, optic nerve damage (bitemporal hemianopia to complete blindness), and seizures.
      - Pituitary tumors also can be "nonfunctioning," secreting biologically inactive hormones.
   b. **Pathology**
      - Formerly classified as chromophobic, eosinophilic, and basophilic; usually benign neoplasms.
      - **Six types have been defined, according to secretory characteristics:**
        - Prolactin secreting (prolactinomas are the most common secretory pituitary tumors). Other than prolactinomas, there are other causes for hyperprolactinemia: physiologic (pregnancy, lactation), medication (metoclopramide, anti-psychotic agents, opiates, verapamil), and chronic disorders (cirrhosis, kidney disease, hypothyroidism).
        - Growth hormone (GH) secreting.
        - Adrenocorticotropic hormone (ACTH) secreting.
        - Melanocyte-stimulating hormone (MSH) secreting.
        - Thyroid-stimulating hormone (TSH) secreting; follicle-stimulating hormone (FSH)/luteinizing hormone (LH) secreting—all rare.
      - Anterior pituitary anatomic features with clinical consequences: relationship with the hypothalamus, which secretes the releasing factors, location in the sella turcica, below the optic chiasm.
      - Mass effects of pituitary tumors cause disruption in the optic chiasm with typical visual field defect—bitemporal hemianopsia.
   c. **Clinical Features**
      - Manifestations: headache, visual field defect, and cranial nerve III palsy.
      - **Hormonal abnormalities are characterized by specific effects:**
        - Excess prolactin: symptoms of hypogonadism and infertility.
        - Oligomenorrhea, amenorrhea, or galactorrhea is more common in women; decreased libido and impotence in men.
        - Excess GH results in acromegaly in adults and gigantism in children and also produces clinical findings of diabetes mellitus (DM) or glucose intolerance.
        - Excess ACTH: Cushing disease and pigmentation caused by association of increased MSH.
        - Excess TSH: rare tumors.
        - Excess gonadotropins: rare tumors.
   d. **Diagnostic Studies**
      - Endocrinologic studies: to determine the type(s) of pituitary hormone(s) hypersecreted.
      - Hypersecretion of prolactin: increased serum prolactin level.
      - ACTH hypersecretion (see Chapter 16, Section II.B.1.).
      - Excess GH: diagnosed by association with increased insulin-like growth factor I levels and glucose suppression test.
      - Primary hypersecretion of TSH is rare, accompanied by increased T_3 and T_4; secondary hypersecretion of TSH, due to hypothyroidism, is common.
      - LH and FSH hypersecretion (secondary) occurs in the primary gonadal failure accompanied by low gonadal hormone concentrations; primary hypersecretion of LH and FSH is rare.
      - Visual field testing and neurologic testing if mass effect is considered.
      - Magnetic resonance imaging (MRI) has become the study of choice in the evaluation of sellar lesions.
   e. **Management**
      - For prolactinomas, dopamine agonist (bromocriptine) as pharmacologic therapy has partially replaced the need for surgery.

- Surgery is a preferred treatment for all pituitary tumors, except prolactinoma.
- Surgery is a primary treatment for micro- or macroadenomas secreting excess GH; radiation therapy, somatostatin analogs may be used as an adjuvant therapy. Patients with acromegaly have to be monitored for lipid abnormalities, DM type 2, cardiac dysfunction, sleep apnea, arthropathy, and colon polyps.
- Cushing disease is treated by transsphenoidal tumor resection (may be curative or pituitary tumor can recur). After surgery, glucocorticoid replacement therapy is necessary while the hypothalamic–pituitary–adrenal axis is recovering the endogenous function. Radiation or medical therapy (ketoconazole) is beneficial in surgically untreatable cases of Cushing disease.

2. **Hypopituitarism**
   a. **Etiology**
   - Hypopituitarism results from either anterior pituitary destruction or deficient hypothalamic regulatory function.
   - Can be caused by pituitary tumors, postsurgery and radiation therapy for pituitary tumors, infiltrative disorders, trauma, and vascular lesions (Sheehan syndrome caused by postpartum pituitary infarction).
   b. **Pathology**
   - Hypopituitarism is often slow appearing and may result in single or multiple hormone deficiencies.
   - GH deficiency has the strongest impact when it appears in childhood.
   c. **Clinical Features**
   - GH deficiency: during infancy and childhood manifests as growth retardation, short stature (dwarfism with normal mental development), and fasting hypoglycemia. Adults with GH deficiency have mild-to-moderate central obesity, increased systolic blood pressure, increased low-density lipoprotein (LDL) cholesterol, and reduced cardiac output as well as reduced muscle and bone mass, reduced physical and mental energy, impaired concentration and memory, and depression.
   - TSH deficiency: results in secondary thyroid gland hypofunction. Symptoms include fatigue, weakness, weight change, and hyperlipidemia. In infants, dwarfism with delayed mental development—cretinism (see Section II.A.3.).
   - Gonadotropin deficiency: during childhood manifests as delayed puberty and causes failure of epiphyseal closure; the resulting clinical picture is that of tall adolescents with eunuchoid features. Adult features are amenorrhea, loss of secondary sexual characters, infertility, decreased libido, and impotence.

- ACTH deficiency (see Section V.A.4.).
- Prolactin deficiency: failure of lactation.
   d. **Diagnostic Studies**
   - Imaging: MRI studies.
   - GH deficiency: no established "gold standard" test. Evaluation—levodopa test should be performed for patients with known hypothalamopituitary disease, cranial irradiation, or childhood onset of GH deficiency.
   - TSH deficiency: low TSH with low T_4 and T_3.
   - ACTH deficiency (see Section V.A.4.).
   - Gonadotropin deficiency can be evaluated by concurrent measurement of serum gonadotropins and gonadal hormone production.
   e. **Management**
   - TSH and ACTH deficiencies require thyroid hormone and corticosteroid replacement, respectively.
   - In GH deficiency: hormone replacement, important in children and adults who are symptomatic or have severe deficiency.
   - For FSH and LH deficiencies: replacement with end-organ hormones—estrogen, progesterone, and testosterone.

B. **Posterior Pituitary**
   1. **Diabetes Insipidus**
      a. **Etiology**
      - Diabetes insipidus (DI) is caused by the deficiency of the peptide arginine vasopressin (AVP), also called antidiuretic hormone (ADH).
      - **Causes of DI can be categorized as:**
        - Central/neurogenic deficiency of AVP owing to autoimmune destruction of AVP-secreting cells, pituitary neoplasms, trauma, surgery, infections, and infiltrative sarcoid granuloma.
        - Nephrogenic: less common, caused by intrinsic renal disease, abnormal receptors sensitivity.
        - Other causes: sickle cell anemia and long-term lithium therapy.
      b. **Pathology**
      - Cause of central DI is AVP absence.
      - Nephrogenic DI is caused by the loss of renal sensitivity to AVP.
      c. **Clinical Features**
      - Polyuria (excretion of >3 L per day of dilute urine; up to 20 L per day), polydipsia, nocturia, intense thirst, with craving for ice water.
      - Children may have enuresis.
      - If water intake is limited, hypovolemia and dehydration with hypotension and vascular collapse develop rapidly.
      - Associated manifestations of anterior pituitary or hypothalamic defects may be present.
      - Signs and symptoms are aggravated by administration of high-dose glucocorticoids (increased renal clearance of free water).

d. **Diagnostic Studies**
  - **No single diagnostic lab test:**
    - Twenty-four-hour urine collection for volume (<2 L per day rules out DI) and creatinine (to ensure accurate collection).
    - Serum for osmolality, glucose, potassium (hypokalemia causes polyuria), sodium, and uric acid.
    - Urinalysis: low specific gravity, but is otherwise normal, no glucosuria.
    - Serum osmolality is greater than urine osmolality (evidence of inability to concentrate urine).
    - Hypernatremia if access to water is restricted or if hypothalamic thirst center is damaged.
    - In nephrogenic DI, serum vasopressin is high during modest fluid restriction.
    - Hyperuricemia implicates central DI.
    - Dehydration test followed by "vasopressin challenge test" to differentiate between neurogenic and nephrogenic causes; in central DI, urine osmolality increases above plasma osmolality, whereas in nephrogenic DI, urine osmolality barely shows an increase.
  - MRI of brain to evaluate hypophysis/hypothalamus.
e. **Management**
  - Neurogenic DI can be treated with vasopressin analog desmopressin acetate, aqueous vasopressin subcutaneously and intranasally.
  - Treatment of nephrogenic DI is difficult; mainly, salt restriction and thiazide diuretics.

2. **Syndrome of Inappropriate ADH Secretion**
  a. **Etiology**
    - Excess ADH produces hypotonic, euvolemic hyponatremia.
    - The most common causes of syndrome of inappropriate antidiuretic hormone (SIADH): stroke, meningitis, central nervous system (CNS) tumors.
    - Other causes: ectopic ADH—small cell lung cancer, drugs, HIV.
  b. **Pathology**
    - ADH is inappropriately high for plasma osmolality. Consequence: water retention leading to hyponatremia and decreased plasma osmolality.
    - Important to distinguish SIADH from adrenocortical insufficiency and hypervolemic hyponatremia syndromes: congestive heart failure (CHF), nephrotic syndrome, and renal insufficiency.
  c. **Clinical Features**
    - Symptoms are usually seen with serum sodium levels <120 mEq per L.
    - Patients with mild or slowly developing hyponatremia may have no symptoms.
    - Weakness, anorexia, nausea with or without vomiting, headaches, irritability, muscle cramps, lethargy, confusion, seizures, coma, and eventually death.
    - Despite water retention, patients with SIADH have *no* edema.
    - In the brain, if extracellular fluid is low in sodium, osmosis occurs, leading to fluid shift into intracellular spaces and cellular edema; mentation changes may be difficult to distinguish from the brain metastasis.
  d. **Diagnostic Studies**
    - Diagnosis *cannot* be made in the presence of renal, adrenal, pituitary, and thyroid disorders and diuretic treatment because all of them can alter free-water clearance.
    - Serum Na^+ concentration <130 mEq per L (<130 mmol per L).
    - Decreased serum osmolality (<280 mOsm per kg) with inappropriately increased urine osmolality (>150 mOsm per kg).
    - Low blood urea nitrogen (<10 mg per dL) and hypouricemia (<4 mg per dL) are not only dilutional but result from increased urea and uric acid clearances in response to the volume-expanded state.
  e. **Management**
    - Mainstay of therapy, water restriction (500–1,000 mL per day), and adequate sodium in the diet.
    - If sodium is between 125 and 134, fluid restriction allows homeostasis to occur.
    - If due to chronic disease or age, or if patient is unable to restrict fluids, treat with demeclocycline, a tetracycline derivative, which inhibits ADH at renal tubular level.
    - Furosemide, combined with saline, for symptomatic hyponatremia can lead to balance through increased excretion of free water.
    - Only in life-threatening circumstances, hypertonic (3% saline) infusion may be necessary. Infuse along with diuretics, to avoid pulmonary edema secondary to fluid overload. Do not correct hyponatremia too rapidly because of the risk of contraction of the brain cells resulting in demyelination.

II. Thyroid Disorders
A. Hypothyroidism
1. Etiology
  - Primary: in the United States—Hashimoto (autoimmune) thyroiditis, idiopathic atrophy, antithyroid medications, lithium, excessive iodine in susceptible people, and iatrogenic (postthyroidectomy/postradioiodine ablation/posthead and neck irradiation). Worldwide—iodine deficiency.

- Secondary/tertiary: owing to pituitary/hypothalamic disorders.

2. **Pathology**
   - Primary hypothyroidism results in TSH elevation (lack of negative feedback); serum-free thyroxine levels are usually reduced.
   - Less commonly, secondary hypothyroidism is characterized by decreased serum TSH and free thyroxine.

3. **Clinical Features**
   - **Symptoms**
     - Lethargy and fatigue.
     - Intolerance to cold.
     - Impaired memory and decreased cognitive function.
     - Constipation.
     - Weight gain.
     - Decreased libido and fertility, irregular anovulatory cycles, and menorrhagia.
     - Depression.
   - **Physical examination**
     - Coarse, dry skin; atrophy of dermis; brittleness of nails; thinning of hair and lateral eyebrows; nonpitting peripheral edema; and facial puffiness.
     - Thyroid gland may be enlarged, decreased in size, or absent (e.g., postthyroidectomy).
     - Muscle strength is decreased; deep tendon reflexes are delayed.
     - Slow, hoarse speech.
     - Hypothermia (in severe forms).
     - Bradycardia, cardiomegaly, and diastolic hypertension.
     - Myxedema: most severe presentation.
     - Subclinical hypothyroidism: subtle and difficult to recognize without high level of clinical suspicion.
     - Congenital hypothyroidism: associated with severe intellectual disability and dwarfism ("cretinism").

4. **Diagnostic Studies**
   - Elevated TSH by radioimmunoassay (except in the secondary hypothyroidism).
   - Decreased total T_4 and, especially, decreased free T_4 (except in subclinical hypothyroidism).
   - Subclinical hypothyroidism: increased TSH and normal T_3 and T_4.
   - Hashimoto thyroiditis: high titers of antibodies against thyroperoxidase and thyroglobulin.
   - Other tests: increased cholesterol, creatinine phosphokinase (CPK), and hepatic enzymes.

5. **Management**
   - Thyroid hormone replacement (synthetic levothyroxine): mainstay of management. Monitor TSH levels at 6-week intervals after starting/changing doses. Slow, small, increasing dosages for patients with cardiovascular risks.

- Occasional patients may respond better to a combination of levothyroxine and L-triiodothyronine.
- Elderly patients and those with angina, myocardial infarction, or CHF must be monitored carefully for adverse reactions as metabolism increases, or not treated at all until cardiovascular status is stabilized.
- Anticoagulants, insulin, and oral hypoglycemics may need to be decreased. Carbamazepine, phenytoin, and tyrosine kinase inhibitors (and others) may increase T_4 requirements.

B. **Thyroiditis**
   - Group of disorders associated with inflammation of the thyroid gland; most of them associated with hypothyroidism.

1. **Hashimoto Thyroiditis (Chronic Lymphocytic Thyroiditis)**
   a. **Etiology**
      - Most common form of thyroiditis and hypothyroidism.
      - Autoimmune etiology.
      - Occurs six times more commonly in women than in men.
   b. **Pathology**
      - Immune-mediated destruction of thyroid parenchyma.
      - Hashimoto thyroiditis can be associated with other autoimmune diseases (adrenal insufficiency, vitiligo).
   c. **Clinical Features**
      - Patients may be euthyroid or hypothyroid.
      - Thyroid gland may be symmetrically, diffusely enlarged, firm, or rubbery, and is usually nontender; surface is irregular or nodular.
      - Complication: slow progression to hypothyroidism.
   d. **Diagnostic Studies**
      - Thyroid function tests (TFTs) disclose hypothyroidism.
      - Antithyroid antibodies are present.
   e. **Management**
      - Thyroid hormone replacement (shrinks gland even in euthyroid patients).

2. **Painful Subacute Thyroiditis (de Quervain Thyroiditis)**
   a. **Etiology**
      - Probably, viral may be preceded by upper respiratory infection.
   b. **Pathology**
      - Thyroid enlargement and inflammation.
      - Self-limited disease presents with thyrotoxicosis in early stage, followed by several months of hypothyroidism.
      - Young and middle-aged women are most commonly affected.

c. **Clinical Features**
- Gland is moderately enlarged, exquisitely tender, and firm; one or both lobes may be affected.
- Pain in the thyroid region radiating to the jaw or the ear.
- Fever, sweating, heat intolerance, malaise, and myalgias.
- No ophthalmopathy.
- Thyrotoxicosis develops in 50% of patients and lasts several weeks.
- Subsequent hypothyroidism lasts 4 to 6 months; 10% remain hypothyroid after 1 year.

d. **Diagnostic Studies**
- Lymphocytosis and elevated erythrocyte sedimentation rate (ESR).
- T_3 or T_4 levels are elevated initially and may fall later.
- Low thyroid radioiodine uptake (RAIU).

e. **Management**
- Acute illness subsides in 3 to 8 weeks.
- Aspirin or other nonsteroidal anti-inflammatory drugs (NSAIDs).
- Initial stage: β-blockers; antithyroid medication is not effective.
- Longer, hypofunctional stage: hormone replacement.

3. **Painless Thyroiditis (Silent, Postpartum)**
a. **Etiology**
- Characterized by thyrotoxic phase, then hypothyroid phase; occurs more frequently in women. About 50% of the patients eventually develop permanent hypothyroidism.
- Postpartum thyroiditis is Hashimoto disease occurring within 12 months after delivery.

b. **Pathology**
- Enlargement, followed by atrophy.

c. **Clinical Features**
- Thyrotoxic phase typically lasts 2 to 6 weeks, followed by hypothyroid phase.
- Malaise, fatigue, and weight loss.
- Nontender thyroid enlargement.

d. **Diagnostic Studies**
- TFTs can be normal; or mild hyperfunction initially, followed by hypofunction.
- ESR is normal or slightly elevated.

e. **Management**
- Most patients need no initial treatment because of short duration and mild manifestations of the initial phase. Antithyroid medication is not effective.
- For the second (hypofunctional) stage, thyroid replacement therapy.

C. **Hyperthyroidism (Thyrotoxicosis)**
1. **Etiology**
- Graves disease: the most common cause of hyperthyroidism in the United States.

- Autoimmune: hyperthyroidism is caused by TSH receptor-stimulating antibodies.
- Female:male ratio, 8:1.
- Additional causes of hyperthyroidism:
  - Toxic multinodular goiter (Plummer disease).
  - Solitary hyperfunctioning nodule.
  - Early stage of subacute (de Quervain) thyroiditis or of postpartum thyroiditis.
  - Exogenous thyroid hormone.
  - Rarely, secondary hyperthyroidism due to pituitary tumor-secreting TSH.

2. **Pathology**
- Normally, the thyroid gland secretes thyroxine (T_4) and triiodothyronine (T_3) under pituitary TSH stimulation, which in turn is stimulated by thyrotropin-releasing hormone (TRH) from the hypothalamus. The secretion of TRH and TSH is controlled by negative feedback from free thyroid T_4 and T_3.
- In hyperthyroidism, the production of thyroid hormones is unregulated or autonomous.
- Graves disease is caused by a thyroid-stimulating immunoglobulin.
- Another way to classify and understand hyperthyroidism is to evaluate the gland's activity, directly, by radioimmunoassay. When the thyroid's production and secretion activities are high (Graves disease, toxic goiter, solitary "hot" nodule), the RAIU is elevated. In subacute thyroiditis, RAIU is low; the gland is not actively producing hormone, and the excess T_4 is due to the leakage of hormone caused by the inflammatory process. With exogenous thyroid hormone, RAIU also is low.

3. **Clinical Features**
- **Symptoms**
  - Anxiety, irritability, restlessness, difficulty concentrating, insomnia, emotional lability, and tremor.
  - Weight loss despite increase in appetite; loose stools.
  - Dyspnea and palpitations.
  - Patients with underlying cardiovascular disease may develop angina and heart failure.
  - Increased sweating and heat intolerance.
  - Fatigue and weakness.
  - Excessive lacrimation and diplopia.
  - In elderly individuals, thyrotoxicosis can be asymptomatic; also, it may present only with atrial fibrillation or as apathetic hyperthyroidism.
- **Physical examination**
  - Hyperactivity, rapid speech, and anxious appearance.
  - Skin moist, warm, smooth; hair often fine in texture, alopecia may occur; pretibial myxedema.
  - Eye findings: retraction of upper lid (lid lag), exophthalmos (in Graves only), and eye irritation; all may be asymmetric.

- Fine tremor.
- Hyperactive deep tendon reflexes proximal muscle weakness.
- Thyroid gland is usually enlarged (goiter); however, goiter may not be apparent in elderly patients or if thyroid gland is substernal. Absence of goiter does not rule out hyperthyroidism.
  - **Characteristics of goiter vary with etiology**
    - Graves disease: symmetrically enlarged, soft or firm, with smooth surface, possibly slight tenderness, venous hum, arterial bruit, or palpable thrill.
    - Toxic multinodular goiter: the gland may be larger than in Graves, asymmetric, firm, and irregular, with two or more discrete nodules.
    - Subacute thyroiditis: gland is moderately enlarged, tender, and asymmetric.
    - Absence of goiter suggests possibility of exogenous thyroid hormone.
4. **Diagnostic Studies**
   - TSH is suppressed.
   - Increased serum thyroid hormones (T_3, T_4, or both), increased free T_4 and T_3 (free T_3 is a better indicator of hyperthyroidism than free T_4).
   - In conditions with increased serum estrogen (pregnancy, estrogen therapy, acute hepatic process), thyroid-binding globulin is increased, possibly resulting in high serum T_4 or T_3; however, free thyroid hormone levels will be normal.
   - RAIU is elevated or low (see Section II.C.2.).
   - In Graves disease, TSH receptor antibodies and antimicrosomal antibodies are usually elevated.
5. **Management**
   - **Medical treatment**
     - Good response in patients with increased RAIU.
     - For symptom relief: β-adrenergic blockers (to decrease catecholamine effect).
     - Radioactive iodine therapy (ablative): the treatment of choice in nonpregnant adults. Also safe in adolescents.
     - Propylthiouracil (PTU) and methimazole. Methimazole is generally preferred (less likely to cause hepatic necrosis). However, PTU is preferred in the first trimester of pregnancy because of methimazole's association with fetal anomalies.
   - **Surgical treatment**
     - Indicated for patients not responding to medical therapy, having contraindication to radioactive iodine (pregnancy), or not willing to take medication; also for patients with large goiters and local symptoms (compression).

D. Thyroid Storm
1. **Etiology**
   - Uncommon form of thyrotoxicosis, life-threatening emergency.

- Generally, precipitating factor is a major stress or illness (e.g., surgery, infection, delivery, or trauma), or RAI therapy.
- Mortality rate is high.
2. **Pathology**
   - Graves disease, multinodular goiter, or solitary hyperfunctioning nodule.
3. **Clinical Features**
   - Exaggerated signs and symptoms of thyrotoxicosis, including high fever, delirium, nausea, vomiting, dehydration, tremulousness, and anxiety.
   - Cardiovascular manifestations include atrial fibrillation with rapid ventricular response, hypotension, and death.
4. **Diagnostic Studies**
   - Highly elevated serum T_3 and T_4.
   - Electrocardiogram (ECG) may show sinus tachycardia, atrial fibrillation, or flutter.
5. **Management**
   - Aggressive approach using antithyroid medical therapy (methimazole or PTU).
   - Oral or intravenous (IV) sodium iodide to decrease thyroid hormone release.
   - Propranolol to block the peripheral cardiovascular effects of excess thyroid hormone.
   - Glucocorticoids to inhibit peripheral conversion of T_4 to T_3.
   - Supportive therapy and treatment of underlying illness.

E. Thyroid Nodules
1. **Etiology**
   - Common, increasing prevalence with increasing age.
   - Nodularity may be caused by any number of thyroid disorders as well as some nonthyroid conditions.
   - Must consider cancer in 10% to 20% of cases.
2. **Pathology**
   - Adenomas, cysts, colloid nodules (the most common nodules), localized thyroiditis, and cancer (mostly papillary and follicular carcinoma).
3. **Clinical Features**
   - Most nodules, regardless of pathology, are asymptomatic; symptoms may arise from the compression of surrounding structures and may range from sensation of pressure to dysphagia.
   - Signs and symptoms of hyperthyroidism or hypothyroidism may occur.
   - Characteristics vary: smooth, firm, irregular, sharply outlined, discrete, multinodular, and usually painless.
   - Suspect cancer if rapid growth, fixed in place, with no movement on swallowing; other risk factors: prior head and neck irradiation, male gender, and extremes of age.

4. **Diagnostic Studies**
   - TSH, free T_4, to assess thyroid function.
   - Fine-needle aspiration cytology: the best method to assess for malignancy.
   - Ultrasound: baseline and follow-up.
   - Consider MRI or CT scanning for larger nodules/multinodular goiters to assess for tracheal compression, local extension, and/or pathologic lymph nodes.
   - Consider RAIU of low TSH, or if ectopic thyroid tissue or retrosternal goiter is suspected.
5. **Management**
   - Most important: exclude malignancy.
   - Treatment according to specific diagnosis, patient's age, presence or absence of symptoms, and suspicion of cancer.
   - For malignancy, surgery followed by thyroid radio-iodine ablation.

III. Parathyroid Disorders
A. Primary Hyperparathyroidism
1. **Etiology**
   - Mostly adenoma of parathyroid glands, less frequently diffuse hyperplasia.
   - Occurs in some patients as part of multiple endocrine neoplasia (MEN) and in 20% of patients taking lithium.
2. **Pathology**
   - Parathyroid hormone (PTH) is oversecreted because of diminished inhibitory feedback from a reduced number of calcium-sensing receptors.
   - Excess PTH results in hypercalcemia directly (bone and renal action) and indirectly, by stimulating the synthesis of 1,25-dihydroxy-vitamin D.
   - By contrast, secondary hyperparathyroidism is caused by calcium and vitamin D deficiency (for renal causes see Section IV.C) or by skeletal resistance to PTH action.
3. **Clinical Features**
   - Hypercalcemia (see Chapter 10, Section XX.C.3).
4. **Diagnostic Studies**
   - Serum calcium (total and/or ionized) elevated and also increased urinary calcium.
   - Serum phosphorus decreased.
   - PTH (radioimmunoassay) elevated.
   - 1,25-Dihydroxy-vitamin D elevated.
   - Renal imaging may show renal stones.
   - Bone radiography: osteopenia.
5. **Management**
   - Treatment of hypercalcemia (see Chapter 10, Section XXI.C.5).
   - Criteria for surgical removal of the parathyroid gland or glands: symptomatic hypercalcemia, younger age, high level of hypercalcemia, osteoporosis, and kidney stones; parathyroidectomy is curative in 90% of patients.

- Recent guidelines support a closer monitoring of asymptomatic patients with hyperparathyroidism using extensive evaluation of the skeletal and renal systems.

B. Hypoparathyroidism
1. **Etiology**
   - Follows parathyroid or thyroid surgery.
   - Can be autoimmune, caused by damage from radiation to the neck or induced by hypomagnesemia.
2. **Pathology**
   - Reduced PTH secretion results in hypocalcemia (decreased mobilization from bone, reduced renal reabsorption, and diminished 1,25-dihydroxy-vitamin D activation).
   - Pseudohypoparathyroidism: PTH level elevated, but tissues are resistant to its effect.
3. **Clinical Features**
   - Hypocalcemia (see Chapter 1, Section XXI.B.3).
4. **Diagnostic Studies**
   - Hypocalcemia (corrected for albumin), hyperphosphatemia, and low PTH level: diagnostic triad.
   - If magnesium is low, it indicates a reversible hypoparathyroidism.
5. **Management**
   - Treatment of hypocalcemia (see Chapter 1, Section XXI.B.5).

IV. Metabolic Bone Disorders
A. Osteoporosis
1. **Etiology**
   - Osteoporosis may be primary (postmenopausal and senile) or secondary, following a chronic disease.
   - Causes of secondary osteoporosis: hypogonadism in both genders, Cushing syndrome, thyrotoxicosis, hyperparathyroidism, immobilization, malignancy, multiple myeloma, DM, liver disease, celiac disease, heparin therapy, and anticonvulsant treatment.
   - Risk factors for postmenopausal osteoporosis: thin body habitus, Caucasian or Asian race, smoking, heavy alcohol use, low calcium and vitamin D diets, and physical inactivity.
2. **Pathology**
   - Osteoporosis is characterized by bone mass reduction in both mineral component and protein matrix.
   - Primary postmenopausal osteoporosis: mostly trabecular bone loss; results in vertebral compression fractures and fractures of the distal wrist.
   - Primary senile osteoporosis: age related, affecting both men and women—characterized by trabecular and cortical bone loss; increased risk of hip fractures.
3. **Clinical Features**
   - Usually asymptomatic; first symptom can be a fracture, back pain, or deformity.

- Vertebral, hip, and distal radius (Colles) fractures (may occur with no trauma).
- When spine compression occurs (mostly upper lumbar and middle thoracic), it results in shortening of stature, bowing of back (kyphosis), and forward thrust of head.
- Chronic pain from vertebral body collapse is common and disabling.

4. **Diagnostic Studies**
- Fracture risk assessment with the Fracture Risk Assessment Tool (available as an app) should be included in the initial history and physical.
- Vitamin D deficiency is very common.
- Serum calcium, phosphate, and PTH: normal.
- Alkaline phosphatase: usually normal, but may be slightly elevated, especially following fracture.
- Testing for thyrotoxicosis and hypogonadism may be required.
- Screen for celiac disease with serum IgA, anti-tissue transglutaminase IgA and anti-endomysial IgA antibodies.
- X-ray of spine may show demineralization or compression of vertebrae.
- X-ray of pelvis may show demineralization.
- Dual-energy X-ray absorptiometry (DEXA) is quite accurate and delivers negligible radiation.
- Osteoporosis: bone densitometry T score ≤ -2.5; osteopenia: T score ≤ -1.0 to -2.5.
- Quantitative CT delivers more radiation but is highly accurate.

5. **Management**
- True prophylaxis begins in adolescents, at the time of bone-density formation, with adequate calcium intake, vitamin D, and exercise.
- Maintain adequate dietary intake of calcium, to a total intake (including diet plus supplement, if needed) of 1,200 mg per day for women ≥ 50 years.
- Maintain serum vitamin D at ≥ 30 ng per mL in pts with osteoporosis.
- Supplement with vitamin D_3 if needed; 1,000 to 2,000 IU daily PO.
- Bisphosphonates: mainstay of treatment.
- Estrogen or raloxifene for women with hypogonadism.
- Teriparatide; subQ bone forming agent.
- Adequate diet/smoking cessation/avoid alcohol/increase exercise.
- Discontinue or reduce corticosteroids.
- Fall avoidance education.
- Periodic measurements of patient's height and bone mass to assess disease progression.

B. **Osteomalacia and Rickets**
1. **Etiology**
- Most frequently caused by inadequate levels of calcium and inorganic phosphorus because of vitamin D deficiency.

- **Vitamin D deficiency**
  - Lack of vitamin D (poor diet, malabsorption, pollution).
  - Defective activation of vitamin D (liver and renal disease, hypoparathyroidism).
  - Tissue resistance to 1,25-dihydroxy-vitamin D (phenytoin).
- Other causes include calcium malabsorption, chronic hypophosphatemia, and systemic acidosis.
- Homebound elderly patients, who are unlikely to eat dairy products (inadequate dietary vitamin D) or go out in the sun, are at increased risk for osteomalacia.

2. **Pathology**
- In contrast to osteoporosis in which the decrease in bone mineral and matrix is proportional, osteomalacia is characterized by only decreased mineralization.
- Decreased deposition of calcium and phosphorus in the bone matrix leads to changes in the epiphyses (increased width) and the bone (cortical thinning).
- When defective mineralization occurs in childhood, before the closing of epiphyseal growth plates, the disease is called rickets. Osteomalacia develops in adults.

3. **Clinical Features**
- Manifestations depend on age of onset and severity.
- **Infants and young children**
  - Features include irritability, delayed closure of fontanelles, growth retardation, and delayed dentition.
  - Enlargement of costal cartilages (rachitic rosary), bowing of long bones.
- **Adults**
  - Osteomalacia is typically asymptomatic at first.
  - Symptoms include diffuse skeletal pain and proximal muscular weakness; pain may be localized to hip and result in antalgic gait.
  - Hypocalcemia leads to tetany, muscle wasting, and hypotonia.
  - Fractures occur with little or no trauma.

4. **Diagnostic Studies**
- Studies aimed at possible etiologies (i.e., renal function and serum PTH).
- Serum calcium and phosphate are low; alkaline phosphatase is high.
- 1,25-Dihydroxy-vitamin D may be low.
- In adult patients, radiographic images show osteopenia, transverse radiolucent markings (pseudofractures).

5. **Management**
- Treat underlying cause.
- Vitamin D (50,000–100,000 U per week) and calcium; monitor urinary calcium for adjustment of doses.

- Oral calcium supplements with meals.
- Calcitriol for cases of inactive vitamin D (patients with renal failure).
- Vitamin D resistance requires treatment with large doses of calcium and phosphorus.
- A 25-hydroxyvitamin D level than 30 ng per dL is appropriate for good bone health. In the United States, in adults between 19 and 70 years of age, vitamin D deficiency is 30% to 60%; experts suggest nonserial screening.

C. Renal Osteodystrophy

1. Etiology
- Group of bone disorders (osteitis fibrosa and osteomalacia) present in patients with chronic renal failure.
- Bone disorders are caused by secondary hyperparathyroidism.

2. Pathology
- Failing kidneys do not eliminate phosphate properly and, at the same time, poorly synthesize 1,25-dihydroxy-vitamin D; these trigger a compensatory increase in PTH.
- Mineralization disorders such as subperiosteal erosions and osteoid production are features of pathologic PTH action on bone.

3. Clinical Features
- Bone and proximal muscle pain in a uremic context.
- Pathologic fractures especially of vertebrae, ribs, and long bones.

4. Diagnostic Studies
- Increased serum phosphate and decreased serum calcium; serum vitamin D level depends on the degree of renal failure.
- Bone turnover markers are not reliable because of altered renal clearance.
- Radiographic: subperiosteal erosion, cystic (brown tumor), and fibrous anomalies of long bones.

5. Management
- Goal is to normalize serum phosphate and calcium levels and indirectly PTH.
- Phosphate binders are used to decrease phosphate level.
- When phosphate level is controlled, calcium supplements can also include vitamin D.
- Correction of acidosis is also important.

D. Paget Disease

1. Etiology
- Possible consequence of a slow viral infection; genetic analyses support autosomal dominant inheritance.
- Mainly affects persons of western European descent.
- Clinical presentation before age 40 is unusual.

2. Pathology
- Characterized by increased formation and resorption of bone (rapid turnover).

- The lysed bone is replaced by the formation of dense trabecular bone with abnormal architecture. This process can remain localized or extend to an entire bone or multiple bones.
- The remodeled bone has areas of weakening producing fractures and, due to its enlargement, compresses neural structures (i.e., cranial nerve VIII).

3. Clinical Features
- Asymptomatic patients are usually discovered as a result of an elevated alkaline phosphatase on screening or during routine radiographic procedures.
- Symptomatic patients experience pain (predominant complaint) in the back or lower extremities, gait disturbances, increasing head size, and hearing loss.
- Common bones involved are pelvis, femur, skull, tibia, and lumbosacral spine.
- Complications: hypercalcemia, hypercalciuria, nephrolithiasis, high-output cardiac failure secondary to the increased skeletal vascularity, and osteosarcoma.

4. Diagnostic Studies
- Marked elevated serum alkaline phosphatase due to increased osteoblastic activity. Serum calcium and phosphorous typically normal.
- Increased urinary excretion of hydroxyproline due to increased bone resorption; this test has been replaced with the detection of urinary pyridinolines or N-telopeptide.
- Increased uptake on technetium bone scan, even before diagnostic changes are visible on X-ray.
- Radiographic changes: initially—lytic lesions; later—coarser, chaotic, and denser cortical bone with deformity and possible fractures.
- X-ray abnormalities are most often seen in the pelvis, femur, and skull.

5. Management
- Main therapy for Paget disease of bone: bisphosphonates. Asymptomatic patients do not seem to benefit from the use of antiresorptive medication.
- Indications for treatment include pain, neurologic complications, fractures, hypercalcemia, and high cardiac output.
- Aspirin and NSAIDs are used for mild-to-moderate bone pain and joint discomfort.
- Bone resorption can be decreased with bisphosphonates and calcitonin, ensuring longer remissions.
- Orthotic and orthopedic measures.

V. Adrenal Cortex Disorders

A. Adrenocortical Insufficiency (Addison Disease)

1. Etiology
- Primary disease (Addison disease): insufficiency of the adrenal cortex.
- Secondary adrenal insufficiency is due to deficient ACTH; tertiary form of disease is produced by low levels of corticotropin-releasing factor.

2. **Pathology**
   - Progressive destruction of the adrenal gland.
   - Primary adrenocortical insufficiency is usually autoimmune process, involving all zones of the cortex, and can be associated with other autoimmune diseases. Secondary adrenocortical insufficiency appears commonly when glucocorticoid therapy is interrupted abruptly.
   - Deficiency of all adrenocortical hormones: glucocorticoids, mineralocorticoids, androgens in primary adrenocortical insufficiency, and only glucocorticoids in secondary insufficiency.
   - Main glucocorticoid hormone: cortisol; its deficiency affects intermediary metabolism, vascular tone, water balance, and inflammation.
   - Most important mineralocorticoid: aldosterone (part of renin–angiotensin–aldosterone system); its decrease leads to changes in sodium and potassium balance. In secondary adrenocortical insufficiency, aldosterone is relatively normal.

3. **Clinical Features**
   - Weakness, fatigue, anorexia, nausea and vomiting, abdominal pain, and weight loss.
   - Hypotension with postural drop and hypoglycemia may occur.
   - Cortisol insufficiency may cause inability to withstand surgical stress, trauma, and infection, and result in vascular collapse.
   - Aldosterone deficiency manifests by increased renal sodium loss, failure to adequately excrete potassium (neuromuscular and cardiac dysfunction), and associated volume depletion (dehydration) with salt craving.
   - Adrenal androgen deficiency may cause decreased libido.
   - Hyperpigmentation is an important characteristic, typical to primary adrenocortical insufficiency, and present on extensor surfaces of extremities, buccal mucosa, genitalia, nipples, palmar creases, and knuckles.

4. **Diagnostic Studies**
   - Cosyntropin stimulation is the major test for diagnosis.
   - Low morning plasma cortisol, low aldosterone levels, and elevated plasma ACTH levels in Addison disease.
   - Also in primary adrenal insufficiency—hyponatremia, hyperkalemia, and metabolic acidosis.
   - Eosinophilia, normochromic normocytic anemia.
   - Secondary adrenocortical insufficiency: low level of ACTH and cortisol.

5. **Management**
   - Adrenal crisis: acute, emergent phase with cardiovascular collapse: high-dose glucocorticoid therapy (hydrocortisone, 100–300 mg IV along with saline solution), followed with IV hydrocortisone 50 to 100 mg per 6 hours; because bacterial infection frequently precipitates an adrenal crisis, broad-spectrum empirically administered antibiotics are required; manage also hypoglycemia, electrolyte abnormalities, and dehydration
   - Addison disease requires long-term management: glucocorticoid replacement therapy (prednisone and hydrocortisone), mineralocorticoid replacement (fludrocortisone), and adrenal androgens supplied in DHEA.

B. **Hypercortisolism (Cushing Syndrome)**
   1. **Etiology**
      - Results from excessive levels of glucocorticoids.
      - Endogenous causes include ACTH-secreting pituitary tumor (Cushing disease), autonomous adrenal adenoma or hyperplasia, adrenal carcinoma, ectopic production of ACTH, and ectopic production of corticotropin-releasing hormone.
      - Exogenous cause: the most common—is the result of chronic glucocorticoid treatment. Exogenous glucocorticoids with longer half-lives are more apt to produce suppression of hypothalamo-pituitary–adrenal axis; commonly used prednisone, in doses of 10 to 20 mg per day, after 3 weeks of therapy may have similar effect.

   2. **Pathology**
      - Usually, the endogenous cause is bilateral adrenal hyperplasia secondary to an ACTH pituitary–secreting tumor.
      - Sustained increase in cortisol with loss of diurnal rhythm.
      - Hypercortisolism results in decreased protein synthesis, increased protein catabolism, nitrogen wasting, glucose intolerance, and changes in mineral metabolism.

   3. **Clinical Features**
      - Hypertension.
      - Weight gain with central obesity, but slender extremities, "moon" facies, "buffalo hump," and fat pads in supraclavicular and dorsocervical areas.
      - Easy fatigue, muscle weakness, and wasting.
      - Easy bruising, poor wound healing, and purple abdominal striae.
      - Thinning of scalp hair, temporal balding, acne, and hirsutism.
      - Diminished libido, menstrual irregularities, and infertility in men.
      - Associated conditions: emotional disturbances (e.g., depression, psychosis, mania), osteoporosis, DM, hypokalemia, nephrolithiasis, and venous thromboembolism.

   4. **Diagnostic Studies**
      - Baseline 24-hour urinary-free cortisol elevation.
      - ACTH level, overnight low-dose dexamethasone suppression test (LDST), and late-night (LN) salivary cortisol level (loss of physiologic dip) are additional screening tools.

- Diagnostic: high-dose overnight dexamethasone suppression test.
- After Cushing syndrome is confirmed biochemically, it is necessary to establish if the syndrome is ACTH-dependent or ACTH-independent.
- Radiologic studies (MRI) for pituitary gland and ectopic site; chest X-ray (CXR) for ectopic site, and DEXA scan for the evaluation of bone involvement. Imaging of the adrenal gland may use thin section CT or MRI—both with equal sensitivity.
- Also impaired glucose tolerance testing, glycosuria.
- Often leukocytosis with relative granulocytosis and lymphopenia.

5. Management
- If exogenous: removal of agent or use of lowest dose possible.
- If endogenous: surgical intervention on source, medication if inoperable (metyrapone, ketoconazole), or both.

C. Hyperaldosteronism
1. Etiology
- Aldosterone-producing adrenal adenomas (40%) and bilateral adrenal hyperplasia (60%) cause primary hyperaldosteronism (Conn syndrome).
- Secondary hyperaldosteronism is caused by increased renin.

2. Pathology
- Primary hypersecretion of aldosterone causes hypertension and hypokalemia.
- Elevated aldosterone increases sodium reabsorption by the kidneys, resulting in the expansion of plasma volume.
- Sodium reabsorption in exchange for potassium and hydrogen ions results in hypokalemia and metabolic alkalosis, respectively.
- Secondary hyperaldosteronism appears in the context of high renin secretion due to renal artery stenosis and any clinical situation with decreased renal perfusion (CHF, hypovolemia), although in the latter, there is no hypertension.

3. Clinical Features
- Usually, no specific symptoms.
- Hypokalemia and hypertension.
- Patients with primary hyperaldosteronism, despite vascular expansion, have no edema.
- Paresthesias, proximal muscle weakness, fatigue, and decreased or absent deep tendon reflexes due to hypokalemia.

4. Diagnostic Studies
- Hypokalemia with metabolic alkalosis; ECG changes consistent with hypokalemia (e.g., prominent U waves).
- Midmorning plasma aldosterone concentration (PAC) and plasma renin activity (PRA); PAC/PRA >20 typical for primary hyperaldosteronism.

- Hypomagnesemia.
- CT scan and MRI to assess adrenal or extra-adrenal mass.
- Adrenal vein sampling is a sensitive localization technique for the measurement of aldosterone.
- Testing for primary hyperaldosteronism should be considered in all patients with difficult to control hypertension.

5. Management
- Surgical intervention: treatment of choice for aldosterone-producing adenomas; angioplasty in renal artery stenosis.
- Antihypertensive medication: spironolactone, angiotensin-converting enzyme (ACE) inhibitors, and calcium channel blockers.
- Correct electrolyte abnormalities.

VI. Disorders of Adrenal Medulla
A. Pheochromocytoma
1. Etiology
- Benign: 90%; malignant: 10%.
- 0.1% to 0.5% of hypertensive patients.
- Can be part of MEN syndromes.

2. Pathology
- Tumor of chromaffin tissue from adrenal medulla that secretes catecholamines.
- Synthesizes norepinephrine and epinephrine autonomously.
- Paroxysmal catecholamine release may be triggered by surgery, exercise, pregnancy, and medication (tricyclic antidepressants [TCAs], opiates, and metoclopramide).

3. Clinical Features
- Hypertension: most consistent finding—may be sustained or acutely elevated. Hypertension due to pheochromocytoma is classically associated with paroxysmal headaches, profuse sweating, and palpitations.
- Other symptoms: chest and abdominal pain, nausea, weakness, fatigue, weight loss (despite increased appetite).

4. Diagnostic Studies
- Screening: measuring of increased 24-hour urinary excretion of catecholamines or their metabolites—metanephrines and vanillylmandelic acid.
- Plasma catecholamines are particularly increased during a hypertensive episode.
- MRI to visualize the tumor.

5. Management
- Surgical excision, unless widespread metastases or patients with unacceptable surgical risk.
- Before surgery, α-adrenergic blockade (phenoxybenzamine and phentolamine), *followed* by β-adrenergic blocking agents; calcium channel blockers (nifedipine) may be used to control hypertension.

VII. DM and Hypoglycemia
A. Diabetes Mellitus
1. **Etiology**
   a. **Type 1 Diabetes**
      - Pancreatic islet β-cell destruction by an auto-immune process, resulting in complete lack of insulin.
      - Type 1 diabetes is part of human leukocyte antigen–associated immune-mediated diseases; not genetically predetermined but increased susceptibility may be inherited.
      - Disease of juveniles, usual onset before age 30.
      - Environmental factors: viruses, chemicals, toxins—may act as triggers in genetically predisposed persons.
   b. **Type 2 Diabetes**
      - About 95% of patients with diabetes in the United States have type 2 DM.
      - Epidemiologic data suggest a strong genetic influence and a familial character.
2. **Pathology**
   a. **Type 1 Diabetes**
      - Autoimmune process destroys pancreatic islet β-cells' secretion; absolute deficiency of insulin results in the accumulation of circulating glucose and fatty acids, associated with hyperosmolality and hyperketonemia.
      - Hyperglycemia induces osmotic diuresis; also, without insulin, accelerated breakdown of muscle mass and fat.
      - Dehydration and metabolic acidosis (ketoacidosis).
   b. **Type 2 Diabetes**
      - Tissue insensitivity to insulin; other contributing mechanisms: β-cell dysfunction, abnormality in postprandial glucose metabolism (impaired glucose tolerance), and excessive hepatic glucose production.
      - Obesity appears to be a cofactor in 60% to 70% of patients.
      - Maturity-onset diabetes of the young is a rare disorder, characterized by onset before age 25 years, in nonobese patients of non–insulin-dependent DM secondary to impaired glucose-induced secretion of insulin.
      - Insulin resistance = syndrome X = metabolic syndrome: chronic hypertension, atherosclerosis, abdominal obesity—is seen in patients with glucose intolerance, hyperinsulinemia, and dyslipidemia. This syndrome is a precursor of diabetes; it carries a greatly increased cardiovascular risk.
3. **Clinical Features**
   a. **Type 1 Diabetes**
      - Manifestations may have acute or subacute presentation.
      - During exacerbations: anorexia, nausea and vomiting, alteration of consciousness, diaphoresis.
   b. **Type 2 Diabetes**
      - Often asymptomatic.
      - Occasionally, with prolonged "occult" DM (blood sugars not high enough to cause symptoms), patients may already have vascular or neuropathic complications at the time of diagnosis.
      - Obesity with increased waist-to-hip ratio.
   c. **Common Features**
      - Polyuria, polydipsia, and polyphagia (3 Ps).
      - Weakness.
      - Peripheral neuropathy: paresthesia and neuropathic ulcers.
      - Autonomic neuropathy: nausea, vomiting, diarrhea, constipation, and impotence.
      - Eruptive xanthomas (when triglycerides reach high levels) on flexor surfaces of limbs and buttocks; chronic skin infections.
      - Loss of subcutaneous fat and muscle wasting, especially in poorly controlled type 1 DM.
      - Blurred vision.
      - Recurrent candidiasis (vulvovaginitis, cheilitis).
4. **Diagnostic Studies**
   a. **Diagnostic Criteria**
      - Fasting plasma glucose (FPG) <100 mg per dL (5.6 mmol per L) is normal; FPG 100 to 125 mg per dL indicates prediabetes; FPG ≥126 mg per dL (7.0 mmol per dL) shows the presence of diabetes.
      - Random plasma glucose ≥200 mg per dL and the presence of symptoms indicate DM.
      - Glycosylated hemoglobin (HbA1c) measurements reflect the state of glycemia over the preceding 8 to 12 weeks. HbA1c <5.7 is normal. HbA1c 5.7 to 6.4 indicates impaired glucose tolerance ("prediabetes"). HbA1c ≥6.5% indicates DM.
      - Urinalysis may show ketonuria or glucosuria.
   b. **Criteria for Screening for Type 2 Diabetes in High-Risk Populations**
      - Screen overweight/obese adults; those ≥45 years; and those with cardiovascular disease, hypertension, dyslipidemia, or other risk factors for cardiovascular disease.
      - Screen patients who, on previous tests, had impaired glucose tolerance or impaired fasting glucose (prediabetes).
      - Screen adults with risk factors for type 2 DM (family history of DM, obesity, gestational DM, polycystic ovarian syndrome, or membership in high-risk ethnic groups—African Americans, Hispanic Americans, American Indians, and Asian and Pacific Islanders).

c. **Other Studies**
- Urine albumin excretion; albumin/creatinine ratio for glomerular evaluation. Assess electrolytes.
- Lipid profile, in insulin-resistance syndrome, shows elevated triglycerides, decreased high-density lipoprotein (HDL), and elevated LDL levels.
- Evaluate cardiac function and peripheral vessels.
- TSH (type 1 DM only): higher incidence of autoimmune thyroid disease in these patients.
- Eye examinations: annual from the time of diagnosis for type 2 DM, and beginning 5 years after the diagnosis of type 1 DM.
- Refer to podiatrist for the treatment of calluses and deformities and for advice on footwear.

5. **Management**
   a. **Goals of Therapy**
   - Relieve symptoms due to hyperglycemia (3 Ps), and prevent/delay progression of complications; importance of early therapeutic intervention and aggressive follow-ups.
   - To prevent morbidity and mortality, management in diabetes involves teamwork: primary provider, nutritionist, podiatrist, ophthalmologist, social worker, and psychologist.

   b. **Diet**
   - Major part of the treatment.
   - Personalized according to the type of diabetes (type 2, due to obesity, usually needs low-calorie diet), age of the patient (adolescents need increased protein intake), and cultural background.
   - Carbohydrates should provide about 45% of total calories, proteins—10% to 35%, and the remainder should be from fat.
   - A Mediterranean-style diet is recommended.

   c. **Insulin Therapy**
   - Absolute requirement in type 1 and sometimes used in type 2 diabetes.
   - Insulin replacement using the regimen most appropriate to the patient.
   - Insulin preparations include: rapid-acting (lispro, aspart, glulisine), short-acting (regular), intermediate-acting Neutral Protamine Hagedorn, or Isophane Insulin (NPH), long acting (detemir, glargine), and mixed, short/intermediate acting (70/30, 75/25, 50/50).
   - Insulin is delivered subcutaneously, by injection or by infusion pumps.
   - Self-monitoring of blood glucose is recommended for all patients with type 1 diabetes and should be strongly considered for patients with type 2 diabetes on insulin.
   - Patient education about insulin-induced hypoglycemia.

- Other insulin therapy complications include:
  - Somogyi phenomenon: rebound hyperglycemia following hypoglycemia; due to activation of counterregulatory systems for hypoglycemia.
  - Dawn phenomenon: early morning rise in glycemia not preceded by hypoglycemia; mediated by nocturnal secretion of GH; correct with later evening administration of slow-acting insulin.

   d. **Oral Antihyperglycemic Agents**
   - Insulin secretagogues: sulfonylureas (glyburide and others), meglitinides (repaglinide), and amino acid derivatives (nateglinide).
   - Insulin sensitizer: thiazolidinediones (pioglitazone and rosiglitazone).
   - Decreased hepatic glucose output: biguanides. (Metformin is usually considered the first-line drug for most patients.)
   - Decreased glucose absorption: α-glucosidase inhibitors (acarbose, miglitol).

   e. **Incretins**
   - GLP-1 receptor agonists: these drugs amplify glucose-induced insulin release—exenatide and liraglutide (and others) are given by subcutaneous injection.
   - DPP-4 inhibitors (incretins): these drugs prolong the action of endogenous GLP-1—sitagliptin and saxagliptin (and others) are given PO.

   f. **Others**
   - A synthetic analog of the human β-cell hormone, amylin—pramlintide is given subcutaneously and may be used by patients with type 1 or type 2 DM.
   - Sodium-glucose cotransporter-2 inhibitors (canagliflozin and others) lower plasma glucose by increasing glucosuria.

   g. **Additional Therapy**
   - As important as treating hyperglycemia is the treatment of dyslipidemia (statins) and hypertension (especially with ACE inhibitors, which are also beneficial for patients with microalbuminuria).

   h. **Patient Education**
   - How to administer insulin and how to do home glucose monitoring (patient should maintain a log and bring it to each appointment).
   - Signs or symptoms of hyperglycemia or hypoglycemia.
   - Pathogenesis and progression of the disease and its complications.
   - Lifestyle changes: exercise program, diet, weight loss (especially for patients with type 2 diabetes), and smoking cessation.

6. **Chronic Complications**
   a. **Macrovascular Complications**
      - Cardiovascular: hypertension, myocardial ischemia, and infarction.
      - Cerebrovascular: stroke and transient ischemic attacks.
      - Peripheral vascular disease.
      - In type 2 diabetes, clinical manifestations of macrovascular complications can appear even before three Ps.
      - Risk factors: duration of disease, increased age, hypertension, hyperinsulinemia, obesity, hypertriglyceridemia, proteinuria, increased LDL, and low HDL.
      - Pathologic mechanism: accelerated atherosclerosis and vascular thrombosis.
      - Imperative to treat early and aggressively to decrease the severity of complications.
      - Hypertension: ACE inhibitors or angiotensin receptor blockers (also for kidney protection); all other antihypertensive classes including β-blockers (also secondary prevention of myocardial infarction). Target blood pressure: <130/80.
      - Procoagulation state may benefit from low dose of aspirin.
      - Statins for dyslipidemia. LDL goal <100 (<70 if multiple cardiovascular risk factors).
      - Smoking cessation, treat obesity.
   b. **Microvascular Complications**
      - Diabetic retinopathy affects nearly all patients with type 1 diabetes and 80% with type 2, leading cause of blindness in highly developed countries.
        - Diabetic eye disease can present as nonproliferative/proliferative retinopathy, macular edema, and premature cataracts.
        - Annual ophthalmologist appointments (dilated examination and laser therapy).
      - Diabetic nephropathy is the leading cause of premature death in young patients and the most common cause of end-stage renal disease in developed countries.
        - Pathologic mechanisms: glomerular damage (sclerosis) and ischemic changes in the nephron's vasculature.
        - Earliest sign: microalbuminuria (at this stage, renal function is still normal).
        - The stage of persistent proteinuria can progress to nephrotic syndrome with peripheral edema, hypoalbuminemia, and decline in glomerular filtration rate.
        - Frequently associated with normochromic, normocytic anemia, and hypertension.
        - Importance of regular checkups; ACE inhibitors when microalbuminuria appears.
        - Women with diabetes have an increased risk of developing ascending urinary tract infections (bladder stasis due to autonomic neuropathy).
      - Diabetic neuropathy presents in several varieties: distal symmetric, mainly sensorial polyneuropathy ("stocking-glove"); acute painful neuropathy; mononeuropathy (cranial nerves, isolated peripheral nerve); and autonomic neuropathy.
        - Autonomic neuropathy clinically manifests as postural hypotension, gastroparesis (nausea, vomiting), diarrhea, bladder stasis, and erectile dysfunction.
        - Diabetic foot: peripheral neuropathy, ischemia, and infection combine in producing tissue necrosis. Podiatrist appointments; careful feet examination at home.
   c. **Other Chronic Complications**
      - Diabetic amyotrophy: especially in older men, painful wasting of quadriceps.
      - Skin: necrobiosis diabetica, *Candida* infections; sometimes vitiligo, acanthosis.
      - Chronic infections are a marker of poor glycemic control; can affect skin, gastrointestinal tract, urinary tract, and lungs.
      - Bone and joints: signs of osteopenia; osteoporosis can develop in both genders.
7. **Acute Complications**
   a. **Diabetic Ketoacidosis**
      - **Etiology**
        - Results from uncontrolled diabetes, and presents most commonly in patients with DM type 1; also can be seen in type 2 diabetes, during acute illness.
        - If hyperglycemia is not present, other causes of anion gap metabolic acidosis—uremia, salicylates, poisoning with alcohols (i.e., methanol), and lactic acidosis—must be considered.
      - **Pathology**
        - Hyperglycemia associated with ketosis and high anion gap metabolic acidosis.
      - **Clinical features**
        - Recent onset of polyuria, polydipsia, nocturia, fatigue, weight loss, abdominal pain and tenderness, nausea, and vomiting.
        - Decreased level of consciousness.
        - Kussmaul breathing due to acidosis and acetone breath.
        - Orthostatic hypotension with tachycardia, poor skin turgor, indicating dehydration.
        - Signs and symptoms of precipitating illness.
      - **Diagnostic studies**
        - Elevated serum glucose level (>250 mg per dL).
        - High anion gap metabolic acidosis, elevated serum acetone, elevated serum phosphate, mild-to-moderate hyperkalemia (despite total body potassium depletion), and mild-to-moderate hyponatremia (if thirst is maintained).

- Volume depletion, associated with elevated hematocrit and azotemia.
- Urine, blood, and throat cultures.
- Diagnostic studies are appropriate for the precipitating illness.
- **Management**
  - Fluid replacement: first priority; with monitoring of pH and glucose.
  - Therapy with regular insulin: should be initiated as needed, either by infusion or intramuscular (IM); monitor and replenish potassium level.
  - Treatment of underlying cause (e.g., infection) is essential.

b. **Hyperglycemic Hyperosmolar State**
- **Etiology**
  - Hyperglycemic hyperosmolar state occurs almost exclusively in type 2 DM.
  - Severe hyperglycemia in the absence of ketosis/acidosis.
  - Profound dehydration due to intense osmotic diuresis from high-level hyperglycemia.
  - Often, precipitating factor, such as infection; elderly and physically impaired patients with limited access to free water.
- **Pathology**
  - Main mechanism: severe hyperosmolality and intense dehydration.
  - Minimal levels of insulin prevent appearance of ketosis.
- **Clinical features**
  - Insidious onset (days to weeks).
  - Polyuria, polydipsia, nocturia, weight loss, and malaise.
  - Altered sensorium, progressing to coma.
  - Patients appear severely ill and dehydrated (dry mucous membranes and poor skin turgor).
  - Mortality rate > 50%.
- **Diagnostic studies**
  - Serum glucose levels demonstrate severe hyperglycemia (600–2,000 mg per dL).
  - Significantly elevated serum osmolality (>320 mOsm per L).
  - Absence of ketones (blood pH > 7.3).
  - Low levels of potassium.
  - Lactic acidosis indicates a poor prognosis.
  - Complete blood count, arterial blood gases, blood and urine cultures, CXR, and other studies should be incorporated to find underlying precipitant and guide therapy.
- **Management**
  - Fluid and electrolyte replacement: mainstay of management.
  - Insulin is required.
  - Antibiotics: if underlying infection exists.

B. **Hypoglycemia**
1. **Etiology**
   - Hypoglycemia occurs when insulin is highly relative to the level of endogenous or exogenous supply of glucose.
   - Common cause is iatrogenic: in type 1 DM, excessive administered dose of insulin; in type 2 DM, sulfonylurea side effect.
   - Reactive (postprandial) hypoglycemia develops a few hours after eating is characterized by the presence of adrenergic symptoms, and is a rare condition.
   - Fasting hypoglycemia can be caused by hepatic failure, adrenocortical insufficiency, ethanol, insulinomas, and surreptitious administration of insulin or sulfonylureas.
2. **Pathology**
   - Body tissues require glucose to maintain integrity and function.
   - Without adequate glucose levels, organ dysfunction develops acutely (especially CNS).
3. **Clinical Features**
   - Symptoms begin at plasma levels of 60 mg per dL; brain function is impaired at approximately 50 mg per dL.
   - Coma and death can develop rapidly.
   - Sympathetic response is characterized by:
     - Hunger, diaphoresis, and anxiety.
     - Palpitations and tachycardia.
     - Tremulousness, weakness, and tingling around the mouth/fingers.
   - Neuroglycopenic symptoms
     - Altered mental status and focal neurologic deficits.
     - Blurred vision and headaches.
     - Incoordination and difficulty speaking.
     - Seizure and coma.
4. **Diagnostic Studies**
   - Low plasma glucose levels.
   - Elevated insulin level indicates insulinoma or exogenous insulin source. In endogenous source (insulinoma), C-peptide is elevated.
   - High levels of sulfonylureas may be detected when these drugs are the cause.
5. **Management**
   - Hypoglycemia is life-threatening.
   - Emergency treatment for symptomatic hypoglycemia requires IV infusion of glucose or sublingual glucose (if patient is unable to take oral glucose), or glucagon given subcutaneously or IM.
   - Glucagon stimulates endogenous glucose production.
   - When patient is stable, high carbohydrate meal may be given.
   - Assess for the cause of episode, including medications, diet, physical activity, and alcohol.
   - Small, frequent meals (minimal amount of simple sugars) for reactive hypoglycemic patients.

- Treat underlying disorders (e.g., liver and renal disease), if present.
- Adjust oral hypoglycemic agents/insulin as required.
- Surgery for pancreatic tumor.

VIII. Obesity
A. Etiology
- One of the most common disorders in medical practice.
- Multifaceted disorder in which energy intake exceeds expenditure; lipid storage enhanced, mostly in adipose tissue.
- Obesity has a strong genetic predisposition and is influenced by sedentary lifestyle.

B. Pathology
- Increased total body fat; enlarged fat cells.
- Several mechanisms involved: enzymatic (lipoprotein lipase), hormonal (leptin), neuromediators in hypothalamus.

C. Clinical Features
- The most used indicator of obesity is the body mass index (BMI): weight/(height)^2. Values are measured in kg per m^2.
- BMI 25 to 29.9—overweight; BMI 30 to 34.9—class I obesity; BMI 35 to 39.9—class II obesity; BMI >40—class III (extreme/morbid) obesity.
- Patients may complain of:
  - Fatigue, shortness of breath, large joint pain, and ambulating difficulty.
  - Recurrent fungal infection under the skin folds (e.g., breast and groin).
  - Excessive accumulation of subcutaneous adipose tissue, with occasional "yellow striae."
  - Pattern of obesity may vary from truncal distribution without limb involvement to involvement of every segment of the body.
  - Fat deposition pattern affects health risks (e.g., increased abdominal fat correlates with the risk of heart disease).
  - In severe/morbid obesity, chronic hypoventilation, left ventricular dysfunction, and arrhythmias.
  - Serious psychosocial consequences.

D. Diagnostic Studies
- Laboratory abnormalities may include hyperlipidemia and glucose intolerance.
- Pertinent studies to rule out other causes may be warranted (i.e., glucocorticoid excess, tumors of hypothalamus and pituitary, hypothyroidism).

E. Management
- If assessment reveals excessive intake, nutritional factors and exercise are mainstays of therapy.
- Investigate insulin resistance and treat accordingly.
- Anorectic medications should be used cautiously.
- Underlying causes or complications should be identified and managed.

- Aggressive health care provider monitoring and support.
- For morbid obesity, bariatric surgery may be indicated.

IX. Multiple Endocrine Neoplasia
A. Etiology
- A group of familial disorders that affect multiple endocrine organs.

B. Pathology
- Autosomal dominant chromosomal abnormalities lead to hyperplasia or neoplasms.
- Types of MEN (by organ affected).
  - MEN1: Wermer syndrome: parathyroids (90% of patients with this disorder), pituitary adenoma, and pancreatic tumors—secreting insulin, gastrin, vasoactive intestinal polypeptide, and serotonin.
  - MEN2 (MEN2a): Sipple syndrome: thyroid (medullary carcinoma producing calcitonin), parathyroids, adrenals (pheochromocytoma), and Hirschsprung disease.
  - MEN3 (MEN2b): same tumors as type 2a, but less preponderance of parathyroid hyperplasia; also patients with MEN 2b have a marfanoid habitus and multiple mucosal and GI ganglioneuromas.
  - MEN4 (MENX): pituitary, parathyroid and pancreas, as well as adrenal, renal, testicular, and cervical.

C. Clinical Features
- Clinical manifestations depend on the endocrine dysfunctions.

D. Diagnostic Studies
- Patients who have neoplasms in one of these glands should be evaluated for MEN syndromes (also review family history).
  - Type 1: measure PTH and calcium levels; image pancreas and pituitary.
  - Type 2 (2a): measure PTH, urinary catecholamines, and calcitonin; image adrenals.
  - Type 3 (2b): same as type IIa plus mucosal neuromas and marfanoid features.
  - Type 4: same as type 1 also image adrenals and reproductive organs.

E. Management
- Treat identified neoplasia with surgery if possible—for example, parathyroidectomy.
- Cinacalcet orally is effective for hyperparathyroidism (MEN 1).
- Prevention is aimed toward screening first-degree relatives.

X. Paraneoplastic Endocrine Syndromes
A. Etiology
- Paraneoplastic endocrine syndromes are consequences of remote effects of cancer due to ectopic hormone secretion (approximately 10% of patients with advanced malignancies).

B. Pathology
- Most common ectopic hormones:
  - ACTH produced by small cell lung cancer and other carcinoids.
  - ADH secreted in primary lung cancers (small cell); rarely, prostate and cervical cancers.
  - PTH-related protein from squamous cell lung cancer.

C. Clinical Features
- Cushing syndrome (see Section V.B.3).
- SIADH (see Section I.B.2.c).
- Hypercalcemia of malignant disease; in cases of breast cancer and myeloma, hypercalcemia is produced by local osteolytic factors.

D. Diagnostic Studies
- Diagnosis is suggested by new endocrine symptoms in patients with known cancers.
- The most common cause of hypercalcemia, after primary hyperparathyroidism, is malignancy; therefore, if hypercalcemia is present, but serum PTH is low, malignancy must be sought.

E. Management
- Treatment of underlying cause is the main objective.
- Symptomatic relief with medications specific to each hormonal disorder.

REVIEW QUESTIONS

1. A 32-year-old woman presents to the office with complaints of frequent headaches and now she is noticing visual changes. She notes abnormal menstrual cycle, which she attributes to her difficulty in becoming pregnant. Laboratory studies in this patient would likely reveal which of the following?

   a) Elevated prolactin levels
   b) Decreased thyrotropin hormone
   c) Elevated T_4 and T_3 levels
   d) Decreased GH
   e) Elevated cortisol levels

2. A 24-year-old man presents with symptoms of excessive thirst and urination. He reports having to urinate every hour but he attributes that to drinking so much water lately. He states his urine is light in color. His past medical history is significant for bipolar disorder, asthma, and eczema. His medications include lithium, albuterol inhaler prn, and topical steroid cream prn. Which of the following would be the best diagnostic test to confirm your suspicion of this patient's diagnosis?

   a) Serum electrolytes and glucose
   b) Plasma ADH

   c) Twenty-four-hour urine collection
   d) Insulin-like growth factor
   e) Hemoglobin A1c

3. Which of the following is a typical lab finding in a patient with syndrome of inappropriate ADH secretion?

   a) Decreased urine osmolality
   b) Hyponatremia
   c) Excess cortisol
   d) Elevated blood urea nitrogen (BUN)
   e) Increased serum osmolality

4. A 45-year-old woman presents to the office with complaints of weight gain and fatigue occurring over the past several months. She reports associated symptoms of dry hair and scalp and mild edema of her ankles. Her past medical history is significant for hypertension and inflammatory bowel disease. Her medications include Lisinopril 20 mg and a maintenance dose of mesalamine. On examination, her vital signs are temp 98.5, pulse 62, R 12, BP 120/74, BMI 28. Significant findings on examination include thinning of her lateral eyebrows, +1 ankle edema, hypoactive bowel sounds, and a mass on examination of the thyroid. Which of the following would be a likely finding in her evaluation?

   a) Elevated T_3 and T_4
   b) Thyroperoxidase and thyroglobulin antibodies
   c) Decreased cholesterol
   d) Low TSH
   e) Decreased thyroid-releasing hormone

5. A 14-year-old girl is brought to the PCP office by her mother with complaints of acne. Her mother noticed that her daughter eats a lot but never gains any weight. She also notes more excessive perspiration, being fidgety, and a light menstrual flow. On examination, her vital signs are temp 99, pulse 104, BP 128/88, R 16, BMI 20. Eye examination reveals mild proptosis, skin is warm and moist, slight tachycardia with no murmur, lungs are clear to auscultation, abdomen is flat, nontender, with hyperactive bowel sounds. You suspect hyperthyroidism. Which of the following would confirm your diagnosis of Graves?

   a) Elevated TSH
   b) Decreased T_3 and T_4
   c) Elevated free T_3
   d) TSH receptor and antimicrosomal antibodies
   e) Presence of thyroid nodules

ANSWERS TO REVIEW QUESTIONS

1. **Answer: A.** Prolactinomas can cause symptoms secondary to the hormonal effects of excess PRL and to the space-occupying effects of the tumor itself. Reproductive-aged females can present with menstrual disturbance and/or infertility. The usual menstrual aberration in these women is oligomenorrhea, amenorrhea, or the occurrence of irregular menstrual cycles. Larger tumors are frequently associated with headache secondary to stretching of the pain-sensitive structures around the

pituitary gland. Encroachment of surrounding tissues may result in visual problems in the form of field defects. Visual problems range from bitemporal hemianopsia (from compression of the optic chiasm), which is common, to total vision loss and ophthalmoplegia (from compression of cranial nerves III, IV, or VI). Serum PRL—measure serum PRL levels on one or more occasions, especially if the elevation is modest. Do not measure the PRL level directly after performing a breast examination because the breast examination may cause a physiological PRL elevation. (From Segu VB, Khardori R. Prolactinoma clinical presentation. *Medscape*. Updated March 25, 2018.) (Formulating most likely diagnosis)

2. **Answer: C**. In a patient whose clinical presentation suggests DI, laboratory tests must be performed to confirm the diagnosis. A 24-hour urine collection for determination of urine volume is required. In addition, the clinician should measure the following:

 • Serum electrolytes and glucose
 • Urinary specific gravity
 • Simultaneous plasma and urinary osmolality
 • Plasma ADH level

 (From Khardori R, Griffing GT. Diabetes insipidus workup. *Medscape*. Updated February 21, 2018. https://emedicine.medscape.com/article/117648-workup#cl.) (Using laboratory and diagnostic studies)

3. **Answer: B**. SIADH typically occurs in the presence of stroke, CNS tumors, meningitis, small-cell lung cancer, drugs, or HIV. Clinical features are weakness, anorexia, nausea, muscle cramps, lethargy, confusion, seizures, and coma. Patients have low serum sodium, serum osmolality, and increased urine osmolality. BUN is usually low. Treatment is adequate sodium intake and restriction of water. (Using laboratory and diagnostic studies)

4. **Answer: B**. This woman has Hashimoto thyroiditis, the most common form of thyroiditis and hypothyroidism. It is an autoimmune etiology, occurring more commonly in women and often associated with other autoimmune diseases. The thyroid gland may be diffusely enlarged and is usually nontender. Antithyroid antibodies are present. (Using laboratory and diagnostic studies)

5. **Answer: D**. The patient is experiencing signs and symptoms of hyperthyroidism. Additional exam findings would include hyperreflexia, proximal muscle weakness, fine hair, lid lag, and fine tremor. Graves disease includes exophthalmos. TSH is suppressed; free T_3 is a better indicator of hyperthyroidism; and in Graves disease, TSH receptor antibodies and antimicrosomal antibodies are elevated (using laboratory and diagnostic studies).

SELECTED REFERENCES

American College of Physicians. *MKSAP 17: Medical Knowledge Self-assessment Program*. Philadelphia, PA: American College of Physicians; 2015.

American Diabetes Association. Standards of medical care in diabetes—2010 [position statement]. *Diabetes Care*. 2010;33:S11–S61. doi:10.2337/dc10-S011.

Bahn RS, Burch HB, Cooper DS, et al. Hyperthyroidism and other causes of thyrotoxicosis: management guidelines of the American Thyroid Association and American Association of Clinical Endocrinologists. *Endocr Pract*. 2011;17(3):456–520.

Bushardt RL, Turner JL, Ragucci KR, Askins DG Jr. Non-estrogen treatments for osteoporosis: an evidence-based review. *JAAPA*. 2006;19(12):25–30.

Camacho PM, Petak SM, Binkley N, et al. American Association of Clinical Endocrinologists and American College of Endocrinology clinical practice guidelines for the diagnosis and treatment of postmenopausal osteoporosis—2016 update. *Endocr Pract*. 2016; 22(suppl 4):1111–1118.

Fatourechi V. Subclinical hypothyroidism: an update for primary care physicians. *Mayo Clin Proc*. 2009;84(1):65–71.

Fitzgerald PA. Endocrine disorders. In: Tierney LM Jr, McPhee SJ, Papadakis MA, eds. *Current Medical Diagnosis & Treatment*. 56th ed. Stamford, CT: Lange; 2017:1108–1209.

Gaitonde DY, Rowley KD, Sweeney LB. Hypothyroidism: an update. *J Clin Endocrinol Metab*. 2012;97(12):4287–4292.

Garber JR, Cobin RH, Gharib H, et al. Clinical practice guidelines for hypothyroidism in adults: cosponsored by the American Association of Clinical Endocrinologists and the American Thyroid Association. *Endocr Pract*. 2012;18(6):988–1028.

Gharib H, Papini E, Garber JR, et al. AACE/ACE/AME medical guidelines for clinical practice for the diagnosis and management of thyroid nodules—2016 update. *Endocr Pract*. 2016;22(suppl 1):622–639.

Handelsman Y, Bloomgarden ZT, Grunberger G, et al. American Association of Clinical Endocrinologists and American College of Endocrinology—clinical practice guidelines for developing a diabetes mellitus comprehensive care plan. *Endocr Pract*. 2015;21(suppl 1):1–87.

Jochen AL, O'Shaughnessy IM. Diseases of parathyroid glands, vitamin D metabolism, and calcium homeostasis; metabolic bone disease. In: Kutty K, Shapira RM, Van Ruiswyk J, eds. *Kochar's Concise Textbook of Medicine*. 4th ed. Philadelphia, PA: Lippincott Williams & Wilkins; 2003:380–392.

Jonklaas J. Update on the treatment of hypothyroidism. *Curr Opin Oncol*. 2016;28(1):18–25.

Katznelson L, Atkinson JL, Cook DM, et al. AACE acromegaly guidelines. *Endocr Pract*. 2011;17(suppl 4):1–44.

Masharani U. Diabetes mellitus and hypoglycemia. In: Tierney LM Jr, McPhee SJ, Papadakis MA, eds. *Current Medical Diagnosis & Treatment*. 56th ed. Stamford, CT: Lange; 2017:1210–1258.

McAdams BH, Rizvi AA. An overview of insulin pumps and glucose sensors for the generalist. *J Clin Med*. 2016;5(1). doi:10.3390/jcm5010005.

Neumann HPH. Pheochromocytoma. In: Fauci AS, Braunwald E, Kasper DL, et al, eds. *Harrison's Principles of Internal Medicine*. 17th ed. New York, NY: McGraw Hill; 2008:chap 337:2269–2275.

Peeters RP. Subclinical hypothyroidism. *N Engl J Med*. 2017;376:2556–2565. doi:10.1056/NEJMcp1611144.

Potts JT Jr. Diseases of the parathyroid gland and other hyper- and hypocalcemia disorders. In: Fauci AS, Braunwald E, Kasper DL, et al, eds. *Harrison's Principles of Internal Medicine*. 17th ed. New York, NY: McGraw Hill; 2008:chap 347:2377–2396.

Powers AC. Diabetes mellitus. In: Fauci AS, Braunwald E, Kasper DL, et al, eds. *Harrison's Principles of Internal Medicine*. 17th ed. New York, NY: McGraw Hill; 2008:2275–2304.

Raisz LG. Is steroid osteoporosis preventable? *N Engl J Med*. 1993;328(24):1781–1782.

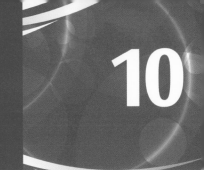

Musculoskeletal Disorders

10

10

Allison S. Rusgo • Patrick C. Auth

I. Infections
A. Acute Osteomyelitis
1. Etiology
- Bone marrow infection caused by blood-borne pathogens.
- Commonly affects children (boys more than girls).
- Be aware with intravenous (IV) drug users.
- High prevalence in patients with diabetes mellitus (DM) because of vascular insufficiency.
- Caution with patients after traumatic injuries and those with orthopedic hardware.

2. Pathology
- May be triggered by trauma or obvious primary focus of infection (e.g., abscess and sore throat); usually seeding is hematogenous, anaerobic, or aerobic.
- *Staphylococcus aureus*: most common offender.
- Group A streptococci: common in children.
- Group B streptococci and *Escherichia coli*: neonates.
- *Haemophilus influenzae* bone infections have almost completely been eliminated with recent immunizations.
- *S. aureus, Pseudomonas aeruginosa, Serratia,* and *Candida albicans* bone infections are common in IV drug users.
- After an open fracture or open reduction with internal fixation (ORIF): *S. aureus, P. aeruginosa,* and coliforms are common pathogens.
- Patients with sickle cell anemia: *Salmonella.*
- *P. aeruginosa* is associated with puncture wounds of the foot.
- *Pasteurella multocida* infection commonly follows cat bites.

3. Clinical Features
- Patient identified by refusal to bear weight or move extremity.
- Acute onset with high fever, chills, malaise, and sometimes soft-tissue abscess.
- Early radiographic changes include soft-tissue swelling, periosteal elevation, and demineralization (10 days to 2-week time frame).
- Late radiographic changes include sequestra (dead bone with surrounding granulation tissue) and eventual new bone growth.
- Bone scan shows focal increased activity.

- Plain film radiography is the initial imaging test of choice, but evidence of osteomyelitis can take up to 10 days to manifest on radiography and thus cannot rely on early radiographic changes to confirm diagnosis.
- Magnetic resonance imaging (MRI) can show changes in bone and bone marrow before plain radiographs.
- Computed tomography (CT) scan shows a radiolucent area in cancellous bone and signs of periosteal elevation—limited role in acute osteomyelitis.
- Elevated white blood cell (WBC) count and erythrocyte sedimentation rate (ESR); blood cultures are usually positive.
- C-reactive protein (CRP) is the most sensitive monitor for the course of infection.

4. Management
- Infectious disease (ID) consultation.
- Identification of the organism(s).
- Aspiration is helpful for antibiotic determination.
- Initial use of IV antibiotics followed by a course of oral antibiotics once patient is afebrile (total 6 weeks or until ESR and CRP return to normal).
- Limb should be immobilized.
- Indications for surgery: drainage of abscess, debridement of tissue, or if refractory to medications.

B. Chronic Osteomyelitis
1. Etiology
- May result from inappropriate treatment of acute osteomyelitis, trauma to bone, hematogenous spread, soft-tissue spread, or complication of surgery.
- Infected host may be immunocompromised (e.g., immunosuppressed, diabetic, and IV drug abuse).

2. Pathology
- *S. aureus* anaerobes are frequent offending organisms.
- In IV drug users: *P. aeruginosa.*
- Skin and soft tissue are often involved.
- Fistulous tracts develop into epidermoid carcinoma.

3. Clinical Features
- Patient presentation is characterized by flares of infection with associated pain, swelling, and

pus formation, which alternates with periods of quiescence.
- Radiographs demonstrate abnormal bone texture with thickening, diffuse cavity formation.
- Sequestrum appears as localized mass of bone, denser than its surroundings.
- Nuclear medicine scans further disclose activity of disease; as increased osteoblast activity results in increased uptake of the radioactive tracer in the surrounding bone.
- CT scan: excellent for detection of sequestra, cortical destruction, soft-tissue abscesses, and sinus tracts.
- Operative sampling of deep specimens from multiple foci is the most accurate means of identifying the pathologic organism.
- WBC may show moderate leukocytosis.
- ESR is usually elevated; positive blood cultures.

4. **Management**
- Combination of IV antibiotics based on deep cultures, surgical debridement, bone grafting, stabilization, soft-tissue coverage (flaps), and amputations.
- Empiric therapy is not indicated in chronic osteomyelitis.
- Refractory patients may require surgical intervention.

II. Inflammatory Disorders
A. Rheumatoid Arthritis (RA)
1. **Etiology**
- The most common form of inflammatory arthritis.
- Affects females more than males.
- Peak age of onset, 25 to 55 years of age.

2. **Pathology**
- Most likely related to cellular-mediated immune response (T cell); incites inflammatory response initially against soft tissues and later against cartilage and bone, and this leads to joint destruction.

3. **Clinical Features**
- Insidious onset of morning stiffness, fatigue, low-grade fever, and polyarthritis.
- Most commonly, hands and feet are affected early.
- Involvement of knees, elbows, shoulders, ankles, and cervical spine (usually C1-C2) is also common.
- Chronic swelling, thickening of metacarpophalangeal (MCP) joint and proximal interphalangeal (PIP) joint, and the pannus ingrowth gradually denude articular cartilage and lead to chondrocyte death.
- Range of motion (ROM) is limited, and ulnar deviation of the MCP joint is present.
- Interosseous atrophy and rheumatoid nodules of the bony prominences.
- Hand deformities: swan-neck deformity and boutonniere deformity.

- There may be systemic involvement of other organ systems: for example, lung, heart, skin, eye, gastrointestinal (GI), and genitourinary system.
- Sjögren syndrome: associated with RA. Symptoms include decreased salivary and lacrimal gland secretion; dryness affects conjunctiva, cornea, and mouth.
- Felty syndrome: RA with splenomegaly and leukopenia.
- Still disease: acute-onset RA with fever, rash, splenomegaly, and lymphadenopathy.

4. **Diagnostic Studies**
- Laboratory studies may show elevated ESR and CRP, positive rheumatoid titer, and the presence of anti-cyclic citrullinated protein antibodies (ACPAs); hypochromic, normocytic anemia is usually present.
- Radiographs include periarticular erosions and osteopenia of the hand (i.e., MCPs, PIPs), joints, wrist (i.e., carpal bones), and cervical spine (C-spine) (Figure 10–1).
- Synovial fluid analysis findings are shown in Table 10–1.

5. **Classification Criteria**
- The American College of Rheumatology and European League against Rheumatism created new classification criteria for RA in 2010.
- Score-based algorithm: adding categories A to D with a score ≥6 of 10 to diagnose RA (Table 10–2).
- Target population: patients who have at least one joint with definite synovitis that is not defined by another disease.

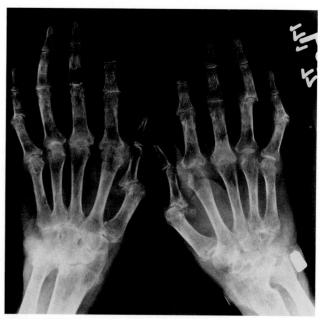

FIGURE 10–1. **Rheumatoid arthritis of the hands and wrists.** Note the involvement of the wrist joints, metacarpophalangeal joints, and interphalangeal joints. (From Daffner RH, ed. *Clinical Radiology: The Essentials.* 2nd ed. Baltimore, MD: Lippincott Williams & Wilkins; 1999:436, with permission.)

TABLE 10–1.   Synovial Fluid Analysis

	Normal	Noninflammatory	Inflammatory	Septic
Clarity	Transparent	Transparent	Transparent	Turbid
Color	Clear	Clear-Slightly Turbid	Turbid	Yellow
WBC/mm³	0–200	50–2,000	2,000–160,000	5,000–250,000
Percent of PMNs	<10%	<30%	~70%	~90%
Diagnosis example		Osteoarthritis	Rheumatoid arthritis	Bacterial infection

PMNs, polymorphonuclear leukocytes; WBC, white blood cell.

6. **Management**
   - Treatment goal: controlling synovitis and pain, maintaining joint function, and preventing deformities.
   - Drug therapy: disease-modifying antirheumatic drugs (DMARDs) started once diagnosis is confirmed and adjusted with the goal of suppressing disease activity. Synthetic DMARDs such as methotrexate, sulfasalazine, leflunomide, antimalarials, and minocycline can be used. Biologic DMARDs including tumor necrosis factor (TNF) inhibitors, abatacept, rituximab, and tocilizumab are additional treatment options. Nonsteroidal anti-inflammatory drugs (NSAIDs) provide symptomatic relief and should be used in conjunction with DMARDs; low-dose corticosteroids produce prompt anti-inflammatory effect, but multiple side effects limit their long-term use.
   - Artificial tears: used to treat dryness of eyes.
   - Physical and occupational therapy may be used to improve patient function.
   - Exercise to preserve joint motion, muscular strength, and endurance. ROM exercises need to be done daily.
   - Weight loss for overweight patients to reduce generalized wear and tear on arthritic joints of the lower extremities.
   - Splints and braces can be used on affected joints to prevent destruction.
   - Synovectomy adjunct to medical therapy.
   - When joint pain and swelling interfere with function and joints do not respond to conservative therapy, total joint replacement may be indicated.

B. **Reactive Arthritis**
   1. **Definition**
      - Common features including oligoarticular arthritis, mouth ulcers, conjunctivitis, urethritis, or cervicitis (can't pee, can't see, and can't climb a tree).
   2. **Etiology**
      - Most patients develop within days or weeks of either dysenteric or sexually transmitted disease (occurs most commonly in young males).
      - *Chlamydia trachomatis*: usual causative organism of postvenereal variety.
      - Need to determine whether *Ureaplasma* is a causative organism.
      - Dysenteric form following enteric bacterial infection (e.g., *Shigella, Salmonella, Yersinia*, and *Campylobacter*).
   3. **Pathology**
      - Epidemiologically similar to other reactive arthritis syndromes, characterized by sterile inflammation of joints from infections originating at nonarticular sites.

TABLE 10–2.   Classification of Rheumatoid Arthritis

A. Joint Involvement	B. Serology	C. Acute-Phase Reactants	D. Duration
1 large joint (0 pt)	Negative RF and negative ACPA (0 pt)	Normal CRP and normal ESR (0 pt)	<6 wk (0 pt)
2–10 large joints (1 pt)	Low positive RF *or* low positive ACPA (2 pts)	Abnormal CRP or normal ESR (1 pt)	>6 wk (1 pt)
1–3 small joints (with or without involvement of large joints) (2 pts)	High positive RF *or* high positive ACPA (3 pts)		
4–10 small joints (with or without involvement of large joints) (3 pts)			
>10 joints (at least one small joint) (4 pts)			

ACPA, anti-citrullinated protein antibody; CRP, C-reactive protein; ESR, erythrocyte sedimentation rate; RF, rheumatoid factor.

4. **Clinical Features**
   - Fever, malaise, anorexia, and weight loss.
   - Buccal ulceration or balanitis (it is possible for only two features to be present).
   - Uveitis.
   - Arthritis: most commonly asymmetric and frequently involves large weight-bearing joints (usually knee, ankle, and foot).
   - Can appear seriously ill (fever, rigors, tachycardia, and exquisitely tender joints).
   - Mucocutaneous symptoms can include balanitis, stomatitis, and keratoderma blennorrhagica (hyperkeratotic skin lesions of palms, soles, and around nails).
   - Most symptoms disappear within days to weeks.

5. **Diagnostic Studies**
   a. **Blood**
      - Human leukocyte antigen B27 (HLA-B27): positive in 60% to 80% of patients in non–human immunodeficiency virus–related reactive arthritis.
      - WBC: 10,000 to 20,000 with neutrophilic leukocytosis.
      - Elevated ESR, moderate normochromic anemia, and hypergammaglobulinemia.
   b. **Synovial Fluid**
      - In reactive arthritis, expect WBC 1,000 to 8,000 cells per mm^3 with negative bacterial cultures.
      - Collaborative tests: culture or serology positive for *C. trachomatis* or stools positive for *Salmonella*, *Shigella*, *Yersinia*, and *Campylobacter* support the diagnosis.
   c. **Imaging: X-Ray**
      - Periosteal proliferation, thickening, spurs, erosions at articular margins, residual joint destruction, syndesmophytes (spine), and sacroiliitis.

6. **Management**
   - Treatment: symptomatic.
   - No treatment is necessary for conjunctivitis or mucocutaneous lesions; iritis will require treatment.
   - NSAIDs: mainstay of therapy.
   - Patients who do not respond to NSAIDs may respond to sulfasalazine or methotrexate.
   - Physical therapy is important during recovery phase.
   - Prompt treatment of precipitating infections reduces the chance of developing reactive arthritis.

C. Septic Arthritis

1. **Etiology**
   - May be hematogenous (e.g., secondary to upper respiratory infection and impetigo), contiguous spread from an adjacent infection, or through direct inoculation (e.g., puncture wound).
   - May also develop as a complication of a diagnostic or therapeutic procedure.
   - Most commonly affects knee, hip, shoulder, and ankle.
   - Most commonly affects hip joints in infants.
   - Predominantly monoarticular (90%).
   - Medical emergency because delay in treatment may lead to joint destruction.

2. **Pathology**
   - *S. aureus* is the most common cause of nongonococcal septic arthritis, accounting for about 50% of all cases.
   - Methicillin-resistant *S. aureus* (MRSA) and group B *Streptococcus* have become increasingly frequent causes of septic arthritis.
   - In newborns and infants up to 3 months of age, the most common causative organisms are *S. aureus* and group B *Streptococcus*.
   - In infants and children (3 months to 14 years), the most common causative organisms are *S. aureus*, *Streptococcus pyogenes*, and *Streptococcus pneumonia*. *H. influenzae* has decreased with vaccination.
   - In sexually active adults aged 15 to 40 years with acute monoarticular septic arthritis, the most common causative organisms are *Neisseria gonorrhoeae*, *S. aureus*, streptococci, and aerobic Gram-negative bacilli.
   - In sexually active adults aged 40 years and older with acute monoarticular septic arthritis, the most common causative organisms are *N. gonorrhoeae* and *S. aureus*.

3. **Clinical Features**
   - Failure to use involved joint, swelling, tenderness, and localized warmth.
   - Sudden onset of monoarticular arthritis should be considered septic until proven otherwise.
   - Fever occurs in 90% of patients.
   - Patient also resists passive movement of joint.
   - Toddler may refuse to walk if lower extremity is involved.
   - Constitutional signs are helpful in suggesting an infection, but not pathognomonic.

4. **Diagnostic Studies**
   - Diagnosis: confirmed by direct arthrocentesis with synovial fluid analysis and culture (aerobic and anaerobic).
   - Definitive diagnosis requires the demonstration of causative bacteria on Gram stain or culture or both.
   - Complete blood counts (CBCs) and ESR should also be checked.
   - Plain radiographs: usually normal early, but provide baseline evaluative tool for subsequent study of joint changes.
   - Later examination shows joint space narrowing and destruction without appropriate treatment.

- Certain gas-producing organisms (e.g., *E. coli* anaerobes) may generate articular gas.
- MRI and CT scans are sensitive in detecting fluid in joints that are not accessible to physical examination (e.g., the hip), and ultrasound (U/S) can also be used; need to image joints, especially the hip, to confirm there is an effusion.
- Radionuclide imaging techniques may aid the diagnosis of septic arthritis in joints difficult to aspirate.

5. **Management**
   - Treatment must be initiated before available culture results.
   - Begin with broad-spectrum antibiotic; may require change based on Gram stain; vancomycin should be used if MRSA is likely.
   - Length of parenteral therapy is usually 10 days to 6 weeks.
   - CBC and blood cultures should be monitored routinely.
   - Consider open drainage if loculation is suspected.
   - Joint rest encouraged until inflammation subsides, then physical therapy may be introduced slowly.

D. Psoriatic Arthritis

1. **Etiology**
   - Male:female ratio, 1:1.
   - Onset: 40 to 50 years of age.
   - Affects approximately 5% to 20% of patients with psoriasis.
   - Psoriasis precedes the onset of arthritis in 80% of patients.
   - More common in patients with severe skin disease than those with mild skin findings.

2. **Pathology**
   - Emerges long after or commensurate with cutaneous psoriasis.

3. **Clinical Features**
   - Forms of psoriatic arthropathy include psoriatic nail disease and distal interphalangeal (DIP) involvement, asymmetric oligoarthropathy, symmetric polyarthropathy, arthritis mutilans, and psoriatic spondylitis.
   - Insidious onset, usually peripheral arthritis asymmetric, with "sausage" appearance of fingers and toes.
   - Joint swelling, tenderness, warmth, and decreased ROM.
   - Nail changes include pitting, traverse ridging, onycholysis, keratosis, yellowing, and destruction of nails.
   - Sacroiliac joint involvement is common.
   - May be associated with ankylosing spondylitis.
   - Dry erythematous papular skin lesions, conjunctivitis.

4. **Diagnostic Studies**
   - Serum rheumatoid factor (RF) negative.

- Elevated ESR.
- Elevated uric acids.
- HLA-B27 present: spondylitis.
- Radiographic findings include osteolysis, DIP pencil-in-cup deformity, lack of osteoporosis, bony ankylosis, asymmetric sacroiliitis, and atypical syndesmophytes, which are pathologically similar to osteophytes and found in the ligaments of the intervertebral joints of the spine.

5. **Management**
   - Treat symptomatically.
   - Encourage exercise to maintain strength and flexibility.
   - Treatment of skin lesions may be accompanied by improvement in peripheral articular symptoms.
   - NSAIDs are usually sufficient for mild cases; methotrexate is the drug of choice for patients who do not respond to NSAIDs; cases that are refractory to methotrexate usually respond to the addition of TNF inhibitors.
   - Other agents that may benefit are cyclosporine, retinoic acid derivatives, and psoralen plus ultraviolet.
   - Corticosteroids are not as effective as in psoriatic arthritis compared with other forms of inflammatory arthritis and may precipitate pustular psoriasis during tapers; antimalarials may exacerbate psoriasis.

E. Systemic Lupus Erythematosus (SLE)

1. **Etiology**
   - Chronic inflammatory autoimmune disease of unknown origin that affects multiple organs.
   - Affects women more than men, mainly young women.
   - Higher prevalence in African Americans, Hispanics, Asians, and Native Americans than Caucasian women.
   - Greatest cluster between ages 20 and 40 years.

2. **Pathology**
   - Clinical manifestations thought to be secondary to trapping of antigen–antibody complexes in the capillaries of visceral structures, leading to inflammation and tissue damage and affecting multiple organs.
   - B-cell hyperactivity with overproduction of autoantibodies is present.

3. **Clinical Features (Table 10–3)**
   - Course and severity of SLE varies widely: fever, anorexia, malaise, weight loss, skin lesions, oral ulcers, eye pain, and arthritic pain.
   - Malar (butterfly) rash, discoid rash, photosensitivity, arthritis, serositis, oral/nasopharyngeal ulcer, pleuritis, pericarditis, nephritis, psychosis, and seizures.
   - Joint involvement: most common feature, affecting 75% of patients with SLE.

TABLE 10–3.	Clinical Features of Systemic Lupus Erythematosus	
Organ System	**ARA Criteria for Classification of SLE**	**Other Features**
Constitutional		Fever, malaise, anorexia, weight loss
Cutaneous	1. Malar rash	Alopecia
	2. Discoid rash	Raynaud phenomenon
	3. Photosensitivity	Other rashes: subacute cutaneous LE, urticaria, bullous lesions
	4. Oral/nasopharyngeal ulcers	Vasculitis
		Panniculitis (lupus profundus)
Musculoskeletal	5. Nonerosive arthritis	Arthralgia/myalgia
		Myositis
		Ligamentous laxity
		AVN of bone
Cardiopulmonary	6. Pleuritis	Pleural effusions
		Pericarditis myocarditis
		Pneumonitis
		Verrucous endocarditis (Libman–Sacks syndrome)
		Interstitial fibrosis
		Pulmonary hypertension
Renal	7. Proteinuria (>500 mg/dL)	Nephrotic syndrome
	Urinary cellular casts	Renal insufficiency
		Renal failure
Neurologic	8. Psychosis	Organic brain syndrome
	Seizure	Cranial neuropathies
		Peripheral neuropathies
		Cerebellar signs
Gastrointestinal		Serositis
		Ascites
		Vasculitis (bleeding/perforation)
		Pancreatitis
		Elevated levels of liver enzymes
Hematologic	9. Hemolytic anemia	Anemia of chronic disease
	Leukopenia (<4,000/mL)	Lupus anticoagulant
	Lymphopenia (<1,500/mL)	Thrombosis
	Thrombocytopenia (<100,000/mL)	Splenomegaly
		Lymphadenopathy
Other systems		Sicca complex
		Conjunctivitis/episcleritis
Laboratory	10. ANA	Lupus band test on skin biopsy
	11. Anti-dsDNA	Anticardiolipin antibody
	Anti-Sm antigen	Lupus anticoagulant
	False-positive VDRL	Hypocomplementemia
	LE preparation	

ANA, antinuclear antibody; ARA, American Rheumatism Association; AVN, avascular necrosis; dsDNA, double-stranded deoxyribonucleic acid; LE, lupus erythematosus; SLE, systemic lupus erythematosus; VDRL, venereal disease research laboratory.

- Joints commonly involved are PIPs, MCPs, carpus bones, knees, and ankle.

4. Diagnostic Studies
- Serum RF usually positive.
- Positive antinuclear antibodies (ANAs), sensitive but not specific for SLE.
- Positive antibodies to anti–double-stranded deoxyribonucleic acid (anti-dsDNA) antibody and to anti-Smith (anti-Sm), specific but not sensitive for SLE CBC, may disclose hemolytic anemia, leukopenia, lymphopenia, or thrombocytopenia.

5. Management
- Goal of treatment is to suppress disease manifestation while minimizing the cumulative toxicity of treatment.
- Supportive treatment; avoidance of, or protection from, ultraviolet light.
- Early intervention when infection occurs with acute flares of SLE.
- Avoid physical and emotional stress.
- Treatment: symptomatic, local steroids or antimalarial drugs for cutaneous manifestations and NSAIDs for arthritic symptoms.
- Immunosuppressive agents such as cyclophosphamide and azathioprine are used in cases resistant to corticosteroids.

F. Ankylosing Spondylitis

1. Etiology
- Usually affects males more than females.
- Onset: usually 15 to 30 years of age.

2. Pathology
- Chronic inflammatory disease of joints in axial skeletal and sacroiliac joints.

3. Clinical Features
- Onset: usually gradual, with intermittent periods of diffuse low back pain, and profound morning stiffness.
- Patients cannot put their head down flat while lying in supine.
- Symptoms advance in a cephalad direction, back motion becomes restricted.
- May result in fixed cervical, thoracic, or lumbar hyperkyphosis and restriction of chest expansion.
- May have painless effusions of larger joints.
- May have chin-on-chest deformity, which is defined as hyperkyphosis where an affected patient's cervicothoracic region maintains a curve >50° to create a humpback appearance.
- May present with associated findings of uveitis.
- Often associated with heart disease and pulmonary fibrosis.
- Extraskeletal manifestations: aortitis, colitis, arachnoiditis, amyloidosis, and sarcoidosis.

4. Diagnostic Studies
- Elevated ESR, histocompatibility antigen, and HLA-B27 usually positive.
- Test for RF is usually negative.
- Earliest radiographic changes are in sacroiliac joints, showing subchorial erosion of the sacroiliac joints.
- Later changes of spine show squaring and generalized demineralization of vertebral bodies and progressive ankylosis.
- The term *bamboo spine* is used to describe late radiographic findings (Figure 10–2).

5. Management
- Goal: preserve motion.
- NSAIDs, rest, and physiotherapy to maintain joint movement are helpful to control inflammation.
- For patients whose symptoms are refractory to NSAIDs, TNF inhibitors, such as etanercept, adalimumab, and infliximab, are alternatives.
- If deformity progresses quickly, assistive mobilization devices may be necessary.
- Osteotomy.

G. Bursitis

1. Etiology
- Inflammation of synovium-like cellular membrane overlying bony prominences.
- Caution for prepatellar bursitis in certain occupations where individuals work on hands and knees in tight spaces (e.g., heating, ventilation, and air conditioning [HVAC] employees or plumbers).

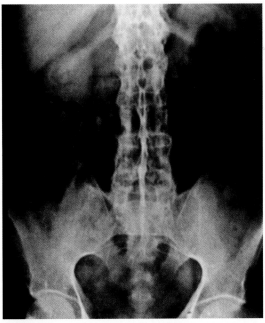

FIGURE 10–2. Radiograph of the pelvis in advanced ankylosing spondylitis. Both sacroiliac joints have undergone bony fusion, and prior sacroiliac sclerosis and erosions are now gone. Bilateral syndesmophytes bridge intervertebral disks at multiple lumbar levels, and there is marked osteopenia. (From Humes DH, ed. *Kelley's Essentials of Internal Medicine.* 2nd ed. Philadelphia, PA: Lippincott Williams & Wilkins; 2001:360, with permission.)

- Certain comorbidities can predispose individuals to olecranon bursitis, particularly patients with gout and RA.
  2. **Pathology**
     - Inflammation may be secondary to trauma, infection, or arthritic conditions (e.g., gout, RA, and osteoarthritis [OA]).
     - Normal structure allows skin, tendon, and muscle to slide over each other.
     - As a result of the trauma, infection, or inflammation, fluid accumulates in bursa.
     - Fibrinous loose bodies, adhesions, or fibrosis may occur in bursa.
  3. **Clinical Features**
     - Usually begins abruptly with focal soft-tissue swelling.
     - May be painful or painless with crepitus over a bony prominence.
     - Active and passive ROM limited.
     - Common locations include subdeltoid, olecranon, ischial, trochanteric, semimembranosus-gastrocnemius, and prepatellar bursa.
  4. **Diagnostic Studies**
     - Radiographs of affected bony prominence to disclose soft-tissue calcifications and osseous abnormalities.
     - Joint aspiration should also be considered for synovial fluid analysis.
  5. **Management**
     - Bursitis caused by trauma responds to rest, immobilization, NSAIDs, and local corticosteroid injections.
     - Avoid repetitive motions.
     - Prevent recurrence with use of protective padding and elbow and knee pads.
     - Treatment of underlying collagen vascular disease or crystalline arthritis controls bursitis.
     - Bursitis due to infection requires antibiotics based on synovial fluid analysis results.
     - Olecranon and prepatellar bursae must be drained.
     - Most common sites affected: olecranon and prepatellar bursa.
     - Most common cause of septic bursitis: *S. aureus*.

H. Adhesive Capsulitis (Frozen Shoulder)
  1. **Etiology**
     - Specific etiology is unknown.
     - There may be an inflammatory component that leads to stiffness in shoulder.
     - Has been observed in the presence of subacromial impingement as well as C-spine degenerative disease, acromioclavicular (AC) arthritis, post-traumatic bursitis, and inflammatory synovitis of shoulder.
     - Most resistant form of adhesive capsulitis can occur with certain medical conditions—most commonly, DM.
     - Has tendency to occur during fifth to sixth decades and appears to affect females more than males.
  2. **Pathology**
     - Pain and stiffness in glenohumeral joint that cannot be explained on the basis of joint incongruity.
     - Typically lasts 18 to 24 months.
  3. **Clinical Features**
     - Three clinical phases: (1) painful phase with gradual onset of diffuse pain; (2) phase of progressive stiffness with decreased ROM, affecting activities of daily living; and (3) thawing phase with gradual return of motion.
     - Usually, no precipitating cause is identified, although it is not unusual to get a history of shoulder trauma.
     - There is usually generalized aching of the shoulder, and this leads to stiffness.
     - Patient voluntarily restricts the motion of the affected shoulder, leading to more stiffness.
     - The more the stiffness, the more the pain; thus, a cycle ensues.
     - Pain: often worse at night.
     - Patient progressively becomes disabled functionally.
     - Hallmark objective finding on clinical examination is that of restriction of passive ROM in comparison with unaffected side.
  4. **Diagnostic Studies**
     - No studies are diagnostic of adhesive capsulitis, although plain film radiographs should be completed to assess for underlying pathology (i.e., subacromial impingement, rotator cuff tear, calcific tendinitis, and malignancy).
  5. **Management**
     - Mainstay of treatment: rehabilitation program designed to improve ROM in shoulder, decrease stiffness, and increase strength, which includes passive as well as active stretching of restricted planes of motion.
     - Exercises should be performed in therapy office and at home.
     - Anti-inflammatory and pain medications.
     - Refractory patients may benefit from closed manipulation of shoulder under general anesthesia and arthroscopic release.
     - If high risk of fracture to humerus exists, such as would be the case in osteopenic patient, rare consideration may be given for open release of adhesions to restore motion to shoulder.

I. Rotator Cuff Tendinitis
  1. **Etiology**
     - Usually develops between adolescence and 40 years of age.
     - Common in athletes and laborers with repeated overhead motions.

2. **Pathology**
   - Tendons of rotator cuff are supraspinatus, infraspinatus, teres minor, subscapularis (SITS).
   - Supraspinatus tendon is the most commonly affected site for rotator cuff tendinitis.
   - Rotator cuff tendinitis results from impingement syndrome and is characterized by pain with overhead activity.

3. **Clinical Features**
   - Reproducible pain by abduction and internal rotation of upper extremity.
   - Pain over deltoid.
   - Positive *Empty Can* or supraspinatus test: pain in affected extremity with abduction against resistance.
   - Positive *Neer* impingement test: pain elicited by passively moving patient's arm in forward flexion in the scapular plane.

4. **Diagnostic Studies**
   - Usually normal radiographs.

5. **Management**
   - Ice for the first 24 to 48 hours.
   - Shoulder pendulum and wall-climbing exercise.
   - Discontinue aggravating activity, especially overhead use of upper extremities.
   - NSAIDs and physical therapy.
   - Chronic tendinitis: local corticosteroid injections.

J. de Quervain Tenosynovitis

1. **Etiology**
   - Repetitive motion disorder caused by pinch, wrist/thumb flexion and can occur with racket sports and golfers; there is a history of no direct trauma.
   - Most common in 30- to 50-year-old women engaged in repetitive actions.

2. **Pathology**
   - Stenosing tenosynovitis affects abductor pollicis longus (APL) and extensor pollicis brevis (EPB).

3. **Clinical Features**
   - Pain (APL and EPB) at site; increased with gripping and extending thumb.
   - Tenderness of first dorsal compartment and radial styloid.
   - Positive Finkelstein test: fist with thumb across palmar surface of hand as ulnar deviated by the examiner.
   - Pain distal to styloid process of radius indicative of de Quervain disease.

4. **Diagnostic Studies**
   - Usually normal radiographs.

5. **Management**
   - Immobilization (i.e., splinting) of thumb, keeping the interphalangeal (IP) joint free.
   - NSAID, phonophoresis, and activity modification.
   - If symptoms persist, additional therapy of local corticosteroid injections warranted and, occasionally, surgical release of first compartment.

- Surgery complications include injury to the sensory branch of the radial nerve or failure to decompress the EPB.

K. Flexor Tenosynovitis (FT)

1. **Etiology**
   - Inflammation of a tendon and its corresponding sheath within the hand.
   - Can be infectious if secondary to a skin wound or via hematogenous spread as seen in gonococcal tenosynovitis.
   - Can be inflammatory if secondary to comorbidities such as DM type II, SLE, RA, psoriatic arthritis, or sarcoidosis. Can also occur from overuse (e.g., trigger finger).
   - Caution in IV drug users, immunocompromised patients, or those with animal bites, most commonly cats.

2. **Pathology**
   - Infectious: a closed-space infection of the tendon and tendon sheath layers (inner visceral and outer parietal) that can spread to adjacent bony structures and/or the synovial space.
   - As infectious fluid accumulates within the flexor tendon sheath, pressure increases within the compartment. This affects movement of the affected digit and can result in tendon necrosis and/or ischemia.
   - Most common infectious organisms: *S. aureus* and *Streptococcus*.
   - Inflammatory: secondary to an overgrowth of fibrous tissue. This results in a constriction of the tendon within the tendon sheath and produces pain, swelling, and tenderness.
   - Overuse syndromes occur in three stages as a result of microtrauma: inflammatory, proliferative, and maturation.

3. **Clinical Features**
   - Most important for infectious causes is Kanavel's four signs:
     - Finger held in slight flexion.
     - Fusiform swelling.
     - Tenderness along tendon sheath.
     - Pain with resisted finger flexion.
   - In overuse conditions, can expect to feel a palpable cord along the tendon sheath, tenderness at the proximal aspect of the tendon sheath, and a "catching-sensation" as the finger is flexed.

4. **Diagnostic Studies**
   - Infectious: CBC and ESR/CRP may be elevated and can also order plain radiographs to rule out bony involvement. (MRI can aid in diagnosis, but not required if diagnosis is clinically apparent.)
   - If infection is suspected, synovial fluid culture must be obtained to guide antibiotic therapy; may also aid in determination of noninfectious etiologies.

5. **Management**
   - Infectious FT: orthopedic emergency, surgical intervention is usually required if no improvement within 12 to 24 hours of empiric IV antibiotics (e.g., penicillin with first-generation cephalosporin).
   - Noninfectious FT: nonoperative conservative management is mainstay of treatment with judicious long-term monitoring. If no symptomatic improvement in 3 to 6 months, patients are considered for flexor tenosynovectomy.

L. Lateral Epicondylitis (Tennis Elbow)
   1. **Etiology**
      - Can be the result of overuse injuries, poor technique in racket sports, or wrist weakness, resulting in forced extension of wrist (e.g., tennis players making backhand strokes and people knitting).
   2. **Pathology**
      - Degeneration or inflammation at extensor muscle group origin, principally in extensor carpi radialis brevis; rubs and rolls over lateral epicondyle and radial head.
      - Pulling of extensor origin, resulting in micro-tears at the peristernal insertion.
   3. **Clinical Features**
      - Localized tenderness of lateral epicondyle, exacerbated by resisted wrist extension, pronation of forearm, and gripping activities.
   4. **Diagnostic Studies**
      - Usually normal radiographs.
   5. **Management**
      - Avoidance of painful activity.
      - Rest, ice applications, and NSAIDs.
      - Physical therapy: for example, stretching, strengthening, U/S, and electrical stimulation—is helpful in reducing symptoms and permitting return to function.
      - Lateral epicondylitis: tennis elbow strap designed to decentralize the area of stress.
      - Equipment modifications may be helpful (flexible racket and larger grip).
      - Neutral wrist position is maintained by wrist brace.
      - Corticosteroid injections may be added if conservative measures are unsuccessful.
      - Surgical (release of the common extensor origin and/or debridement of the pathologic tissue) options are reserved for severe refractory patients.

M. Medial Epicondylitis (Golfer's Elbow)
   1. **Etiology**
      - Less common and more difficult to treat than lateral epicondylitis.
      - Overuse of flexor forearm muscles stresses and inflames tendinous insertion at medial epicondyle.
      - Seen in certain manual activities, household activities, and golfers.

2. **Pathology**
   - Inflammation of affected area at pronator teres–flexor carpi radialis interface.
3. **Clinical Features**
   - Tenderness is localized to the region of medial epicondyle.
   - Reproduced by forcefully extending elbow against resistance with forearm supinated and wrist dorsiflexed.
   - Medical epicondyle pain is worse with pulling activities and elbow flexion.
4. **Diagnostic Studies**
   - Usually normal radiographs.
5. **Management**
   - See section II.K.5.

N. Lumbosacral Sprain and Strain
   1. **Etiology**
      - Cause: acute or chronic muscle tendon or ligamentous strain, lumbar disk herniation, degenerative changes of spine, or osteoporosis.
      - History of twisting or lifting.
      - Predisposing factors include repetitive movements of lifting, pushing, pulling, or bending; sedentary lifestyle; obesity; poor posture; stress; and loss of flexibility.
   2. **Pathology**
      - Tearing of muscle fibers or distal ligamentous attachments of the paraspinal muscles.
      - Most often at iliac crest or lower lumbar/upper sacral region.
   3. **Clinical Features**
      - Discloses tense, hard, paraspinal, paravertebral muscle spasms of the lumbosacral spine.
      - Possible absence of normal lordotic curve or presence of a list or both.
      - Decreased ROM of the lumbosacral spine.
      - Absence of neurologic involvement (pain radiating below the knee and ankle reflex changes).
   4. **Diagnostic Studies**
      - Baseline radiographs are not indicated; if obtained, may be normal or show degenerative joint or reverse lordotic curve.
      - The Agency for Healthcare Research and Quality guidelines for obtaining radiographs are summarized in Table 10–4.
      - MRI and CT scan not necessary for initial evaluation—indicated when symptoms persist with neurologic involvement.
   5. **Management**
      - Brief bed rest; more than a day or 2 in bed is usually counterproductive.
      - Begin walking as soon as possible; do as much normal activity as possible.
      - Ice massage to muscle spasm for the first 48 hours, followed by moist heat the following day.
      - Analgesics or NSAIDs; muscle relaxers for the first several days may be helpful.

TABLE 10–4.   AHRQ Criteria for Lumbar Radiographs in Patients with Acute Low Back Pain

Possible fracture: major trauma (any age), minor trauma in patients >50 y of age, long-term corticosteroid use, osteoporosis, >70 y

Possible tumor or infection: history of cancer, constitutional symptoms, recent bacterial infection, injection drug use, immunosuppression, supine pain, nocturnal pain

From the Agency for Healthcare Research and Quality. http://www.ahrq.gov/.

- Strengthening of paravertebral muscles with William McKenzie flexion extension exercises.
- Education regarding proper lifting technique, proper body mechanics, and weight loss if patient is obese.

O. Cervical Sprain and Strain

1. Etiology
- Overuse of musculature of posterior neck and shoulders as a result of unbalanced force exerted on area.
- Commonly seen after sudden turning of neck.
- Acceleration or "whiplash": acceleration flexion-extension neck injury—result of sudden, abrupt movement of head such as motor vehicle accident (MVA), sporting activity, assaults, and accidental fall.
- Torticollis (stiff neck) occurs predominantly after excessive exposure to cold or activities requiring unusual or prolonged rotation or twisting of neck musculature.

2. Pathology
- Result of tearing of musculature and supporting structures of neck.
- Neck muscles respond to overuse by tightening into protective spasm to prevent further disruption.

3. Clinical Features
- May include pain increased with movement, discomfort, and tightness in posterior neck; visual symptoms, dizziness, tinnitus, and headache; and tension-like, beginning in occiput region.
- Referred pain to interscapular area and shoulder.
- Palpable muscle spasms, unilateral or bilateral of the sternocleidomastoid, trapezium, or paraspinal muscles; muscle trigger points can be localized.
- Decreased ROM of the neck.
- Neurologic examination is often normal.

4. Diagnostic Studies
- C-spine radiographs: not needed for uncomplicated diagnosis; indicated if persistent symptoms; or to rule out acute fracture at the time of injury, joint subluxation, congenital anomalies, or OA.
- Most common radiographic findings: straightening of normal lordotic curve indicating acute muscle spasm.
- MRI: indicated for disk herniation and detection of cord abnormalities.

- Bone scan: indicated for osseous involvement.
- CT scan: indicated for spinal stenosis and nerve root compression.

5. Management
- NSAIDs, analgesics, and muscle relaxants.
- Ice for 24 hours, then alternate with heat.
- Use of collar may be helpful in acute phase of injury; long-term use is not recommended.
- Decreased activity for 24 to 48 hours; then, as tolerated, begin physical therapy (i.e., ROM exercises, ultrasonography, and deep massage) 48 to 72 hours after initial examination.
- Patients with paresthesia, muscle weakness, loss of reflexes, sensory loss, or evidence of bony injury require immediate stabilization with rigid cervical collar; additional studies include MRI and neurologic consult.

P. Fibromyalgia

1. Definition
- A clinical syndrome characterized by diffuse pain, extreme fatigue, stiffness, painful tender points, and sleep disturbance.
- The American College of Rheumatology defined two criteria for diagnosing fibromyalgia in 1990: (1) history of widespread pain and (2) pain in at least 11 of 18 tender point sites on digital palpation with force of 4 kg.

2. Etiology
- Thought to be a disorder in restorative stage 4 sleep.
- Commonly affects middle-aged females, but can also affect either gender of any age.
- The third most common rheumatic disorder, after OA and RA.

3. Pathology
- Muscle biopsy may show type II muscle fiber atrophy, moth-eaten appearance of type I fibers, or ragged red fibers, all of which suggest subclinical injury to muscle, thought to be caused by chronic muscle tension or chronic hypoxia.
- Muscles at tender points show decreased oxygenation and evidence of abnormal energy metabolism.
- As yet, none of these findings occur consistently enough to be useful as diagnostic test.

4. Clinical Features
- Patients frequently are unable to localize their pain.
- Patients feel worst in the morning; fatigue is a major component of disorder.

- Symptoms are worsened by physical and psychological factors (e.g., cold, noise, and stress).
- There may be complaints of numbness and tingling, often mistaken for nerve entrapment syndrome.
- No physical findings suggest inflammation (e.g., painful, swollen joints).
- Upon careful questioning, patients almost uniformly report frequently waking at night; detailed sleep pattern history is important in the diagnosis of fibromyalgia.
- There may be symptoms of depression and hypochondriasis, although no evidence exists that fibromyalgia patients as a group are different psychologically from those with chronic pain.

5. **Diagnostic Studies**
   - No radiographic findings.
   - Laboratory studies: normal except in disclosing diseases such as hypothyroidism and DM, which can mimic fibromyalgia.

6. **Management**
   - Goals of therapy: provide education as to how sleep deprivation can decrease pain threshold and lead to more sleep deprivation.
   - Pharmacotherapy is used to help patients reestablish normal sleep pattern.
   - Tricyclics: for sleep.
   - Fibromyalgia involves serotonin deficiency; serotonin reuptake inhibitors may benefit patients.
   - Analgesics may be used for nighttime pain.
   - Physical therapy should be geared toward conditioning exercise program.
   - Aerobic exercises are aimed at increasing cardiovascular work, which improves stage 4 sleep.
   - Swimming: exercise of choice because of relaxing effect of water on muscles.
   - Biofeedback may be helpful in controlling stress.

III. Inherited or Developmental Disorders

A. Scoliosis

1. **Definition**
   - Lateral curvature of spine of >10°, usually thoracic or lumbar, associated with rotation of vertebrae.
   - Curve may be convex to right or left.
   - Rotation of vertebral column around its axis occurs and may cause rib-cage deformity.
   - May be associated with kyphosis (humpback) or lordosis (swayback).
   - Most common type: idiopathic (80% of patients), usually begins between ages 8 and 10 years; more common in girls than in boys (4:1–5:1); classically asymptomatic.
   - Most patients have a family history.

2. **Etiology**
   a. **Structural Scoliosis**
      - Idiopathic.
      - Congenital defects of spine.
      - Paralytic or musculoskeletal (due to polio, cerebral palsy, or muscular dystrophy).
      - May be related to hormonal factors (melatonin), brainstem, or proprioception disorder.
   b. **Functional Scoliosis**
      - Poor posture.
      - Uneven leg length.
   c. **Classification of Scoliosis by Cause (Table 10–5)**

3. **Clinical Features**
   - Patients are often referred from school screening.
   - Forward bending test: most sensitive clinical test for scoliosis because it brings into profile rotation of ribs and vertebrae.
   - While standing behind the patient, ask the patient to bend forward with arms hanging free, feet together, and knees straight.
   - Examine for the elevation of rib cage on one side and the depression on the other.
   - In the lumbar spine, examine for the elevation of paravertebral muscle mass on one side.
   - There may be visible pelvic obliquity with patient standing erect.
   - Presence of café au lait spots, skin tags, or axillary freckles is suggestive of neurofibromatosis.
   - Presence of hairy patches or dimples over the spine is suggestive of a spinal dysraphism; this term refers to a group of neurologic disorders that cause spinal malformations.

TABLE 10–5.	Classification of Scoliosis by Cause

- Idiopathic scoliosis: infantile (younger than 3 y), juvenile (from 3 to 10 y of age), adolescent (from 10 y of age to skeletal maturity)
- Neuromuscular scoliosis: neuropathic (e.g., cerebral palsy, spinal cord trauma, poliomyelitis, and muscular dystrophy)
- Congenital scoliosis: failure of formation, failure of segmentation
- Neurofibromatosis
- Connective tissue scoliosis: Marfan syndrome, Ehlers–Danlos syndrome
- Osteochondrodystrophy: diastrophic dwarfism
- Metabolic scoliosis: secondary to nerve root irritation, postural

Data from Hu SS, Tribus CB, Tay BK, et al. Disorders, diseases, and injuries of the spine. In: Skinner HB, ed. *Current Diagnosis and Treatment in Orthopedics.* 4th ed. New York, NY: McGraw-Hill; 2006:chap 4. Available at: https://accessmedicine.mhmedical.com/content.aspx?bookid=675&sectionid=45451710.

4. **Diagnostic Studies**
   - Obtain anteroposterior (AP), lateral radiographs to measure curve.
   - Preferable to use film size at least 14 in × 17 in.
   - The magnitude of scoliosis curves is determined using the Cobb angle; measured using the upper and lower most vertebrae affected by the curve and determining the angulation between these vertebrae.
   - MRI or myelograms with CT scanning indicated for noted structural abnormalities on plain films, excessive kyphosis, juvenile onset, rapid curve progression, neurologic signs/symptoms, and left thoracic/thoracolumbar curves.

5. **Management**
   - Most idiopathic curves do not progress to the point of requiring treatment.
   - Treatment options include observation, bracing, and surgery.
   - Exercise and electrical stimulation have shown little effect on the normal history of curve progression.
   - Curve observation: indicated while child is growing.
   - Bracing: reserved for children and some adolescent patients with progressive curves in the 20° to 40° range; however, bracing is not always effective, even with a well-made brace and good compliance.
   - Surgery to fuse involved vertebrae: appropriate for progressive curves of more than 50°.
   - Pseudoarthrosis of fusion or paralysis can occur following surgery.
   - Surgery complication is a neurologic deficit not present preoperatively.

B. **Kyphosis**
   1. **Definition**
      - An excessive (>45°) outward curvature of the thoracic vertebrae, resulting in a rounded or *hunchback* appearance of the upper back.
      - Can affect patients of any age but most commonly seen in adolescence because of periods of rapid bone growth.
      - Most common type affecting children or adolescents is postural; other types are Scheuermann and congenital.
   2. **Etiology**
      a. **Postural Kyphosis**
         - Idiopathic and affects females more than males.
         - Noted as poor posture without significant vertebral abnormalities; often able to be corrected by encouraging patient to "stand up straight."
         - Painless and rarely leads to functional disability in adulthood.

   b. **Scheuermann Kyphosis**
      - More common in adolescent males than females and progression ceases when growth is complete.
      - Caused by a spinal structural abnormality where several spinal vertebrae have a triangular-type appearance; most commonly appreciated at thoracic level.
      - Can be painful and unable to be corrected if patient stands straight.
   c. **Congenital Kyphosis**
      - Present at birth caused by incomplete development or abnormal fusion of vertebrae in utero.
      - Often requires surgical intervention at young age to prevent progression.
      - Can be associated with other congenital defects (e.g., cardiac, pulmonary, or renal).

3. **Clinical Features**
   - Varies based on the type of kyphosis and degree of curve.
   - Can present with back pain, fatigue, stiffness, or tight hamstring muscles.
   - If curves are severe, neurologic symptoms or cardiopulmonary compromise can occur.

4. **Diagnostic Studies**
   - Obtain AP, lateral radiographs to measure curve.
   - MRI indicated for noted structural abnormalities on plain films, neurologic or cardiopulmonary symptoms, or rapidly progressing curves.

5. **Management**
   - Conservative management is recommended for postural kyphosis and Scheuermann's curves <75°, including physical therapy, NSAIDs, and observation.
   - Bracing is sometimes recommended for patients with Scheuermann kyphosis who are still growing.
   - Surgical intervention via spinal fusion is recommended for patients with neurologic or cardiopulmonary complications, those with Scheuermann's curves >75°, and patients who fail conservative management.
   - Individuals with congenital kyphosis will often undergo surgery without initial conservative measures.

C. **Spinal Stenosis**
   1. **Etiology**
      - Narrowing of spinal canal or neural foramina produces nerve root compression, root ischemia, variable back, and leg pain.
      - Central stenosis produces compression of the thecal sac.
      - Usually affects men twice as often as women.
      - More common in late middle age.
      - Lateral stenosis produces compression of the individual nerve roots.

- Impingement of nerve roots lateral to the thecal sac as they pass through the lateral recess and into the neural foramen.
- Nerve root compression can occur at more than one level.
- Seen more frequently in combination with central stenosis.
- Can appear as an isolated entity involving middle-aged or young adults with symptoms of radicular pain unrelieved by rest and without tension signs.

2. **Pathology**
- Acquired stenosis: most common type; usually degenerative, resulting in the loss of disk volume; increased pressure on apophyseal joints; and hypertrophy of soft tissue and bony structures, resulting in decrease in the diameter of spinal canal.
- Can be congenital, idiopathic, or developmental.

3. **Clinical Features**
- Insidious back pain that increases with time and extremity paresthesia with ambulation and extension, relieved by lying supine or with flexion of spine.
- Complaints of lower extremity pain, numbness, "giving way."
- Possible pain and sensitivity loss over one or more dermatomes.
- ROM of spine discloses pain with extension.
- Normal pulses.
- May have neurologic findings.

4. **Diagnostic Studies**
- Radiographs disclose disk degeneration, facet hypertrophy, flattening of lordotic curve, and subluxation.
- Plain CT scan, post-myelogram CT scan, and MRI: standard imaging modalities to assess nerve root entrapment.
- Bone scan or MRI may be helpful to rule out malignancy.
- Electromyogram (EMG) may be used to assess nerve root involvement, but sensitivity is variable and depends on examiner.

5. **Management**
- Majority of patients can be treated conservatively.
- Discourage activities that cause pain.
- Rest, physical therapy (i.e., flexion-based exercises), NSAIDs, weight reduction, back exercises, exercise program.
- Spinal or facet joint corticosteroid injection for refractory pain.
- Surgery is indicated for patients with positive studies, persistent pain, and alteration in activities of daily living.

D. Developmental Dysplasia of the Hip
- Previously called congenital hip dysplasia.
- "Screening for DDH: the U.S. Preventive Task Force concluded that there is insufficient evidence to recommend routine screening for developmental dysplasia of the hip in infants as a means to prevent adverse outcomes."
- Potential harms from screening include examiner-induced hip pathology caused by vigorous provocative testing, elevated risk for certain cancers from increased radiation exposure from follow-up radiographic tests, parental psychosocial issues from the diagnosis and therapy, and false-positives results, leading to unnecessary and potentially harmful follow-up and intervention.

1. **Etiology**
- Unknown.
- Ethnic, genetic factors have a role.
- Increased incidence in North American Indians and firstborn Caucasian children.
- Almost nonexistent in Chinese and African American infants.
- About 60% of children with developmental dysplasia of the hip (DDH) are firstborn.
- Eighty percent of DDH occurs in girls.
- Left hip is more commonly affected than the right hip.
- Positive family history.
- Other predisposing factors include conditions that limit fetal movement in uterus (e.g., oligohydramnios, intrauterine torticollis, and breech fetal positioning).

2. **Pathology**
- Any hip in which normal relation between acetabulum and femoral head is altered.
- By 11 weeks of gestation, hip joint is fully formed.
- At birth, femoral head is firmly seated within acetabulum and held there by surface tension of synovial fluid.
- In hips with dysplasia, fit is lost and head can be displaced easily from acetabulum.
- Pathologic specimens show varying degrees of hip joint malformation from mild capsular laxity to severe acetabular, femoral head, and neck malformations.
- Congenital hip dysplasia: refers to hip that may be provoked to sublux or dislocate (regarding degree of contact between acetabulum and femoral head) but can be reduced into acetabulum.
- Congenital hip dislocation: condition where no contact exists between the femoral head and acetabulum and femoral head is not reducible.

3. **Clinical Features**
- Most patients are detectable at birth.
- Despite screening examinations, some patients are missed.
- Diagnostic test for DDH: caused by femoral head gliding in and out of acetabulum over a ridge of abnormal acetabular cartilage.
- Common maneuvers performed during physical examinations are the Ortolani (decreases markedly after 1–2 months of age) and Barlow tests.

- Three phases are recognized commonly: (1) dislocated (Ortolani-positive, early, Ortolani-negative, late, when femoral head cannot be reduced); (2) dislocatable (Barlow-positive); and (3) capable of being subluxed (Barlow-suggestive).
- In older children, secondary adaptive changes may be evident to include waddling gait and asymmetry of the gluteal, thigh, and labial folds.
- May also appreciate shortening of affected leg.

4. **Diagnostic Studies**
   - Radiographs and U/S are not needed when clinical examination is negative.
   - U/S: good adjunct in infants before femoral heads start to ossify.
   - Normal radiographs do not rule out the possibility of DDH.

5. **Management**
   - Goal: contains femoral head within acetabulum, thereby stimulating growth and deepening of acetabulum and development of joint stability.
   - An abduction brace: usually sufficient for newborns and infants; should be continued until acetabular development and joint stability have occurred.
   - Closed manipulation of joint under general anesthesia may be necessary in refractory patients, and open reduction is reserved for patients who fail to maintain closed reduction.
   - Physical examination discloses mild-to-moderate restriction of hip motion.
   - Abduction can be particularly limited, easily noticeable if both legs are spread at the same time; this maneuver prevents pelvis from tilting.

E. **Legg–Calvé–Perthes Disease**
   1. **Etiology**
      - Idiopathic osteonecrosis of femoral head in children.
      - Thought to be related to interruption of blood flow to femoral epiphysis; femoral head has tentative blood flow.
      - Typically affects children between ages 4 and 10 years.
      - Four times more common in boys than in girls.
      - Unilateral in 90% of patients.
      - Increased incidence with a positive family history, low birth weight, and abnormal birth presentation.
      - Uncommon in African Americans.
   2. **Pathology**
      - After bone dies and loses structural integrity, articular surface of femoral head may collapse, leading to deformity and arthritis.
      - Self-limiting disease with revascularization usually occurs within 2 years.
      - Patients presenting with a bone age of 6 years have a poor prognosis.

3. **Clinical Features**
   - Presenting complaint: limping for several weeks.
   - Pain, often knee pain, effusion from synovitis, remember that hip pain is often referred to the knee.
   - Limp worsens by day's end, related to activity.
   - Complaints of pain usually involve aching into groin or proximal thigh.

4. **Diagnostic Studies**
   - AP, frog-leg lateral radiographs of pelvis show increased density of femoral head as an early sign; gross deformity in patients with advanced disease.
   - Radiographs may be negative at first, because of initial softening of the femoral head that is sufficient to cause symptoms, but insufficient to change the radiographic appearance of the femoral head.
   - In the initial stage of the disease (1–3 months), the capital femoral epiphysis fails to grow because of the lack of the blood supply. The hip radiograph demonstrates widening of the cartilage space of the affected hip and a small size ossific nucleus of the femoral head, followed by a subchondral stress fracture line in the femoral head. As the disease progresses, the femoral head becomes more radiopaque and calcification of the necrotic marrow occurs, resulting in crushing of the avascular trabeculae in the dome of the epiphysis.
   - If plain radiographs are normal, MRI (very sensitive) or bone scan is an excellent diagnostic tool.

5. **Management**
   - No current interventions accelerate the process of revascularization.
   - Observation: typically indicated for children younger than 6 years who do not exhibit significant subluxation and maintain at least 40° to 45° of abduction.
   - NSAIDs help decrease pain and inflammation in patients without allergy or sensitivity to these medications.
   - More significant treatment includes bracing with bed rest to "contain" femoral head within acetabulum and minimize flattening.
   - Before initiating treatment, motion must be regained; bed rest and traction are commonly required.
   - Osteotomy and other surgery are reserved for older children; best performed by pediatric orthopedic surgeon.

F. **Slipped Capital Femoral Epiphysis (SCFE)**
   1. **Etiology**
      - Most common hip pathology in adolescence with slightly higher occurrence in males than in females.
      - Highest risk factor is obesity.
      - Increased incidence in children with a history of radiation to the affected hip.

- Common in African Americans and Asian Pacific Islanders.
- High association with certain endocrine disorders (e.g., hypothyroidism, acromegaly, hyperparathyroidism) and osteodystrophy of chronic renal failure.
- Left hip is more common.

2. **Pathology**
   - Increased hormonal and biomechanical forces act upon a weakened area of the physis.
   - The slippage occurs at the vulnerable hypertrophic layer of the physis relative to the femoral neck.
   - The epiphysis remains in the acetabulum, whereas the femoral neck moves anteriorly and rotates externally.
   - This movement is commonly referred to as "a scoop of ice cream falling off its cone."

3. **Clinical Features**
   - Presenting complaint: groin and thigh pain for several weeks to months, but can present with knee pain (usually referred from the hip).
   - On physical examination, will note decreased hip flexion and internal rotation.

4. **Diagnostic Studies**
   - AP and frog-leg lateral radiographs of bilateral hips are required.
   - Key findings on AP radiograph are Klein's line and epiphysiolysis (early indication of SCFE) via evidence of growth plate widening.
   - If plain radiographs are normal, MRI can be used.

5. **Management**
   - Goal of treatment is stabilize the hip to prevent progression of the slippage and promote closure of the femoral physis.
   - Surgical repair is almost always surgical.
   - Various forms of operative repair can be used, such as in situ stabilization with contralateral prophylactic in situ pinning, epiphyseal reduction and pinning, or proximal femoral osteotomy.

6. **Complications**
   - Avascular necrosis (AVN) is one of the most significant complications.
   - Can also see chondrolysis, limb length discrepancy, progression of slippage, or contralateral SCFE if prophylactic pinning not performed initially.

G. Pes Planus (Flatfoot)

1. **Etiology**
   - May be acquired (congenital), result of trauma, tendon degeneration, or arthritis.
   - Between ages 3 and 5 years, normal longitudinal arch develops in most children.
   - Estimated that by age 10, only 4% of population has pes planus.
   - Always bilateral.

2. **Pathology**
   - Loss of support for arch and subsequent acquired flatfoot deformity.
   - Characterized as either flexible or rigid (tarsal coalition).
   - Flexible: most common form in children.

3. **Clinical Features**
   - Loss of longitudinal arch on weight bearing.
   - Heel becomes more valgus and forefoot abducted.
   - When child is not weight bearing or is standing on tiptoes, arch is recreated.
   - ROM is usually normal, but secondary contracture of Achilles tendon may develop in older children or adults.
   - Flexible flatfoot: usually painless.
   - If pain is present, it does not usually develop until patient is adolescent or adult.
   - Aching occurs along plantar aspect of midfoot.
   - There may be some aching into leg.

4. **Diagnostic Studies**
   - Radiographs are not usually necessary in asymptomatic children.
   - Standing lateral radiographs of foot show loss of longitudinal arch.
   - On standing AP view, there may be lateral shift (subluxation) of navicular on the head of talus.

5. **Management**
   - Conservative management for congenital flatfoot deformities.
   - Modifications to shoe and orthotic devices have not been proved to alter natural development of longitudinal arch.
   - A longitudinal arch support may benefit the patient, not necessary for the asymptomatic flexible flatfoot.
   - For symptomatic flexible flatfoot, a semi-rigid longitudinal arch support and Achilles stretching exercise may be of some benefit.
   - In symptomatic patients, acetaminophen, local heat, and massage may be used.
   - If fatigue symptoms or activity-related discomfort persists, shoe modifications provide support.

H. Osgood–Schlatter Disease

1. **Etiology**
   - 5:1 incidence in active adolescents (11–15 years of age) versus more sedentary; 2:1 to 3:1 greater incidence in boys.
   - Onset of the disease during early adolescence coincides with the development of the secondary ossification.

2. **Pathology**
   - Osteochondritis of the tibial tuberosity.
   - Results from repetitive injury or small avulsion injuries at the bone-tendon junction where the patellar tendon inserts into the secondary ossification center of the tibial tuberosity.
   - Can occur unilaterally or bilaterally.

3. **Clinical Features**
   - Pain exacerbated by running, jumping, and kneeling activities.
   - Some report pain after prolonged sitting with knees flexed.
   - Tenderness and swelling at insertion of the patellar tendon into the tibial tubercle.
   - Motion is typically unrestricted.
   - Patellofemoral joint is stable.

4. **Diagnostic Studies**
   - In acute phase of initial episode, radiographs usually show soft-tissue swelling.
   - In more chronic patients, small spicules of heterotopic ossification may be seen anterior to the tibial tuberosity, with local prominence.

5. **Management**
   - Ice after sports, NSAIDs, quadriceps stretching, and use of a protective knee pad for those who have pain with kneeling.
   - Temporary cessation of provocative activity and, occasionally, immobilization are indicated for more recalcitrant symptoms.
   - Return to full training for athletes can average 6 to 7 months.
   - Surgery is considered for patients symptomatic after growth is completed.

IV. Degenerative Disorders

A. Osteoarthritis (Degenerative Joint Disease, DJD)

1. **Etiology**
   - Most common form of arthritis.
   - Eighty percent of adults aged 65 years and older demonstrate radiographic changes of OA.
   - Younger than 45 years, the disease is more prevalent in men.
   - Older than 55 years, the disease is more prevalent in women.

2. **Pathology**
   - Joints undergo degenerative changes, including subchondral bony sclerosis and loss of articular cartilage.
   - OA is the result of failed attempt of chondrocytes to repair damaged cartilage; characterized by increased water content, alterations in proteoglycans, collagen abnormalities, and binding of proteoglycans to hyaluronic acid.
   - OA can be primary from an intrinsic defect or secondary from a trauma, infection, or congenital disorders.

3. **Clinical Features**
   - Common sites involved are hand: DIP and PIP.
   - Other sites involved are wrist, hip, knee (most common joint affected), and cervical/lumbar spine.
   - Onset: insidious, usually pain and stiffness after exercise or use of joint.
   - Pattern of involvement: multiple joints; however, often initially with single joint involvement.

- Slowly progressive disease.
- Classic hand deformities: Heberden's nodes, hard and painless nodules of dorsolateral aspects of DIP joint secondary to bony overgrowth; Bouchard's nodes, hard and painless nodules on PIP.

4. **Diagnostic Studies**
   - Radiographic characteristic: osteophytes and "joint space" narrowing, subchondral cysts from microfractures/bone repair.
   - Hand: DIP, PIP, MCP, and carpometacarpal joints of the thumb.
   - Foot: evidence of hallux valgus at first metatarsophalangeal (MTP).
   - Hip: superolateral involvement (Figure 10–3).
   - Knee: asymmetric involvement.
   - MRI: reserved for preoperative evaluation and management.

5. **Management**
   - Treatment begins with supportive measures (i.e., activity modification and cane), NSAIDs, glucosamine chondroitin, capsaicin topical skin cream, and application of heat.
   - Modalities may include physical therapy or acupuncture.
   - Intra-articular corticosteroid injection.
   - Intra-articular viscosupplement injection.
   - Surgical procedures ranging from arthroscopic debridement to arthroscopic total joint arthroplasties may be useful and advance patients resistant to nonoperative treatment.

6. **Comparison of OA and RA (Table 10–6).**

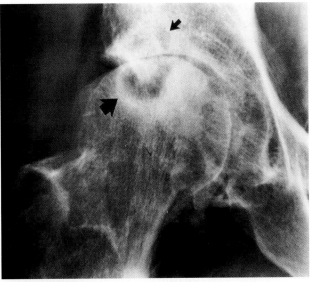

FIGURE 10–3. Osteoarthritis of the hip. There is narrowing of the hip joint, particularly superiorly. Large degenerative synovial cysts (geodes) are present in both the femoral head (*large arrow*) and the acetabulum (*small arrow*). Note the osteophyte formation in both the acetabulum and the femoral head. (From Daffner RH, ed. *Clinical Radiology: The Essentials.* 2nd ed. Baltimore, MD: Lippincott Williams & Wilkins; 1999:438, with permission.)

TABLE 10–6.   Comparing Osteoarthritis and Rheumatoid Arthritis

	Osteoarthritis	Rheumatoid Arthritis
Average age of onset	Usually after fourth decade of life	Usually between third and fifth decades of life
Pathophysiology	Generalized joint wear and tear	Autoimmune process affecting synovial membranes → joint destruction
Associated symptoms	No systemic symptoms	(+) fatigue, malaise, weight loss
Duration of morning stiffness	<30 min	>1 h
Joints involved	Weight bearing (hip, knee), DIP and PIP (spares MCP except first MCP)	Symmetrical involvement of small joints (spares DIP)
Joint characteristics	Hard/bony, mild enlargement	Soft, tender, warm, and erythematous
Joint abnormalities	Heberden's nodes (DIP) Bouchard's nodes (PIP)	Ulnar deviation, swan-neck, and boutonniere deformities
Laboratory findings	(−) ESR/CRP, RF, and anti-CCP	(+) ESR/CRP, RF, and anti-CCP
Radiologic findings	Joint space narrowing, subchondral sclerosis, osteophytes	Periarticular swelling, fusiform appearance, synovial hypertrophy, and pannus formation
Hallmark pharmacologic interventions	Acetaminophen, NSAIDs	DMARDs and immunomodulators

Anti-CCP, anti-cyclic citrullinated protein; CRP, C-reactive protein; DIP, distal interphalangeal; DMARDs, disease-modifying antirheumatic drugs; ESR, erythrocyte sedimentation rate; MCP, metacarpophalangeal; NSAIDs, nonsteroidal anti-inflammatory drugs; PIP, proximal interphalangeal; RF, rheumatoid factor.

B. Disk Herniation/Herniated Nucleus Pulposus

1. **Etiology**
   - Usually a disease of young and middle-aged adults because disk nucleus desiccates and is less likely to herniate in older patients.

2. **Pathology**
   - Disk degeneration with aging includes loss of water content and annular tears.
   - Molecular changes in disk with aging alter structural properties of disk and annulus fibrosis that contains the disk.
   - Most often involves L4–L5 disk, followed closely by L5–S1 in the lumbar spine.
   - Lumbar central prolapse may precipitate cauda equina compression syndrome—a medical emergency presenting with bowel and bladder dysfunction, saddle anesthesia, and lower extremity motor sensory dysfunction. This diagnosis requires emergent MRI and surgical decompression to prevent permanent dysfunction.

3. **Clinical Features (Table 10–7)**
   - May present with low back pain with radiation below knee and sciatica involving lower nerve root at that level (leg pain more than back pain). In the cervical spine, presentation may be neck pain with radicular paresthesia from nerve root involvement.
   - Self-protected gait; localized tenderness, spasm of affected area; decreased spine flexion; increased pain with Valsalva maneuvers (i.e., coughing, sneezing, and bowel movements); diminished or absent reflexes; diminished sensation in dermatome pattern; with positive tension signs.
   - Lumbar: positive straight leg raising and sitting nerve root test, positive contralateral straight leg raising test specific herniated nucleus pulposus (HNP).
   - Occupational risks such as jobs that require lifting, prolonged standing, or repetitive lifting need to be assessed.
   - Note Waddell and nonorganic physical signs for inappropriate symptoms.

4. **Diagnostic Studies**
   - Radiography may demonstrate disk space narrowing and rule out other pathologic evidence and should be deferred for 6 weeks.
   - CT myelography demonstrates cord and nerve root compression.
   - MRI is superior for identifying cord pathology and neural tumors.
   - EMG demonstrates findings 3 weeks after nerve root pressure, although it rarely provides more information than good physical examination. This may be used for preoperative evaluation and management.

5. **Management**
   - Limited activity, short-term bed rest (2 days) with support underneath knees and neck, NSAIDs, ice, progressive ambulation, and mobilization with back rehabilitation successful in returning most patients to normal function.
   - Early intervention with physical therapy may be helpful for symptomatic relief.

TABLE 10–7.   Neurologic Syndromes Produced by Lumbar Disk Protrusion

	L5	S1	L4 (Less Common)
Disk protrusion	Lateral protrusion at L4–L5	Lateral protrusion at L5–S1; central protrusion at L4–L5	L3–L4
Sensory disturbances	Pain and paresthesia in the region of the hip, groin, posterolateral thigh, and dorsal surface of foot, especially between first and second toes	Pain and paresthesia in midgluteal region, posterior part of thigh, calf, outer plantar surface of foot to fourth and fifth toes	Pain in anterior thigh
Weakness	Dorsiflexors of foot or extensor of big toe; walking on heels is more difficult than walking on toes	Flexor muscles of toes and foot, abductors of toes, hamstring muscles; walking on toes is more difficult than on heels	
Reflex loss	Usually none, although ankle jerk may be diminished	Loss or decrease of ankle jerk	Loss of knee jerk
Methods for diagnosis	CT; MRI; myelography; EMG of paraspinal muscles (wait 3 wk after initial injury)	See L5 syndrome; MRI especially good; loss of asymmetry of H-reflex	See L5 syndrome

CT, computed tomography; EMG, electromyogram; MRI, magnetic resonance imaging.
From Paty DW, Beall SS. Neurology. In: Kelley WN, ed. *Essentials of Internal Medicine.* 1st ed. Philadelphia, PA: JB Lippincott Company; 1994:724, with permission.

- Aerobic conditioning, proper lifting education, and body mechanics are important factors in avoiding missed work days and returning patients to work.
- If patients fail to improve with 6 weeks of conservative treatment, further diagnostic studies are indicated (e.g., bone scan to rule out spinal tumors or infection).
- Lumbar epidural steroids may be helpful in patients with predominantly sciatica.
- Patients with positive studies, neurologic findings, tension signs, without mitigating psychosocial factors are the best candidates for surgical discectomy.

C. Cervical Radiculopathy

1. **Definition**
   - Cervical disk abnormality that results in nerve root irritation, most commonly at C6 and C7.
2. **Etiology**
   - In younger patients, often secondary to acute cervical disk herniation.
   - In older adults, this occurs most commonly because of cervical disk degeneration, osteophyte production, and foraminal narrowing.
   - Increased prevalence in patients with manual labor occupations and smokers.
3. **Pathology**
   - Most commonly focuses on C3 to C7 vertebrae and corresponding nerve roots.
   - As disk degeneration occurs, the foramina narrow and compress the corresponding nerve root.
   - This increased pressure on the exiting nerve is responsible for the patient's radicular symptoms.

4. **Clinical Features**
   - Decreased active ROM in extension, rotation, and lateral bending (either toward or away from affected side).
   - Cervical paraspinal tenderness is common and usually more pronounced ipsilaterally.
   - Muscle spasms may also be present.
   - Muscle strength, reflexes, and sensory tests should be performed: results will vary depending on the affected vertebrae and degree of severity.
   - Test of choice is the Spurling maneuver: patient's head is rotated and extended and provider applies downward pressure to the head.
   - The test is positive if patient reports pain that radiates to upper extremity on side that head is rotated toward.
   - Lhermitte sign, a lightening sensation down the spine upon neck flexion, should be negative in cervical radiculopathy.
5. **Diagnostic Studies**
   - Plain film radiography should be the initial test for cervical disk abnormalities.
   - The American College of Radiology recommends MRI for patients with chronic neck pain with neurologic symptoms and normal plain films.
   - MRI is very useful for detection of soft-tissue abnormalities such as disk herniations.
6. **Management**
   - Treatment begins with conservative measures such as, NSAIDs, activity modification, epidural corticosteroids, or a cervical collar for comfort.
   - Modalities may also include physical and occupational therapy.

TABLE 10–8.		Cervical Radiculopathy Patterns			
Nerve Root	Interspace	Pain Distribution	Motor	Sensory	Reflex
C4	C3–C4	Lower neck, trapezius	–	Lower neck, upper shoulder	–
C5	C4–C5	Lateral arm	Deltoid, elbow flexion	Lateral forearm	Biceps
C6	C5–C6	Lateral arm, thumb	Biceps, wrist extension	Lateral forearm, thumb	Brachioradialis
C7	C6–C7	Lateral forearm, middle finger	Triceps, wrist flexion	Dorsal forearm, middle finger	Triceps
C8	C7–C8	Medial forearm, ulnar digits	Finger flexors	Medial forearm, ulnar digits	–
T1	C8–T1	Ulnar forearm	Finger intrinsics	Ulnar forearm	–

- Surgical interventions are considered for patients who fail conservative management after several months or present with severe neurologic compromise.

7. **Cervical Radiculopathy Patterns (Table 10–8)**

V. Trauma

A. Fractures

1. **Classification Considerations**
   - Direction of fracture line: oblique, transverse, and spiral.
   - Condition of bone: comminuted, impacted, segmented, pathologic, stress, avulsion, and incomplete.
   - Condition of soft tissue: open/closed fracture.
   - Deformity: displacement, angulation, rotation, and shortening.

2. **Clavicle Fractures**
   a. **Etiology**
      - Most common fracture in children, with majority in middle one-third of the clavicle.
      - Twice as common in males as in females.
      - Clavicle fractures of adolescents and adults result from moderate- or high-energy traumatic impacts (i.e., MVA and sports injury).
      - Clavicle fractures in children younger than 2 years: suspect abuse.
   b. **Mechanism of Injury**
      - Fall on outstretched hand and shoulder or direct trauma to clavicle.
   c. **Clinical Features**
      - Pain with ROM, deformity, tenderness, and swelling of shoulder.
      - Patient may hold arm against chest to protect against motion.
      - Crepitus at fracture site.
      - Evaluate carefully for neurovascular (NV) injury, pneumothorax, and hemothorax.
      - Most common NV sequelae are subclavian vessel or brachial plexus injuries—check for clavicle hematoma, bruit, diminished extremity pulses, and weakness.

- Fractures at the lateral one-third may be associated with disruption of the coracoclavicular ligament.
- Fractures at the medial one-third need to be evaluated for chest injury.
   d. **Diagnostic Studies**
      - AP and 45° cephalic tilt view.
      - Ultrasonography may be substituted for plain radiography in an urgent/emergent setting.
   e. **Management**
      - Middle third clavicle fractures: arm sling for 4 to 6 weeks for adults.
      - Indications for orthopedic consult include NV compromise, distal and proximal clavicle fractures.
      - Indications for acute operative management include displaced fractures with compromise of skin, open fractures, and vascular injuries.
   f. **Complications**
      - Rare.
      - Must closely evaluate for other associated injuries.

3. **Humerus: Midshaft Humerus Fractures**
   a. **Etiology**
      - Most humeral shaft fractures occur as a result of direct injuries, including falls, direct blow to arm, MVAs, and gunshot wounds.
      - Common site of pathologic fracture from metastatic breast cancer.
   b. **Mechanism of Injury**
      - Direct blow or bending force applied to midhumerus.
      - Caused by fall onto arm or elbow or violent muscle contraction; suspect physical abuse in children with long spiral fractures.
   c. **Clinical Features**
      - Cardinal signs of fracture: pain, swelling, deformity, and crepitation.
      - Shortening of upper extremity.
      - Careful NV evaluation.

- Weak or absent dorsiflexion of wrist or decreased sensation on dorsum of hand suggests radial nerve injury.
- Evaluate for compartment syndrome.
  d. **Diagnostic Studies**
  - Two radiographs of humerus taken at 90° to each other.
  - Include radiographs of shoulder and elbow.
  e. **Management**
  - Uncomplicated fractures: coaptation splints, upper arm sling and swathe, orthopedic referral 3 to 5 days. Surgical reduction depends on the type of fracture, displacement, and patient compliance, which may include plating or intramedullary rods.
  - Emergent referral with NV deficit, open fractures, or spiral fractures; radial nerve injury, nonunion, brachial artery and vein.
  f. **Complications**
  - Radial nerve injury can occur.
4. **Humerus: Humeral Head Fractures**
  a. **Etiology**
  - Humeral head fractures can occur from low-energy (e.g., falls) or high-velocity (e.g., MVAs and penetrating trauma) injuries.
  - Third most common fracture in the elderly.
  b. **Mechanism of Injury**
  - Direct blow to humeral head.
  c. **Clinical Features**
  - Cardinal signs of pain, swelling, decreased ROM, and ecchymosis of chest, humerus, and forearm.
  - Careful NV evaluation because humeral head fractures can have associated axial nerve injury with decreased sensation of shoulder and deltoid weakness.
  d. **Diagnostic Studies**
  - Radiographs of humerus using AP, scapular Y, and axillary views.
  e. **Management**
  - Uncomplicated fractures: upper arm sling with orthopedic referral and eventual physical therapy.
  - Surgical intervention with NV deficit, open fractures, or significantly comminuted injuries.
  f. **Complications**
  - Nonunion or malunion, AVN, axillary nerve injury, and adhesive capsulitis.
5. **Elbow: Radial Head and Neck Fractures**
  a. **Etiology**
  - Relatively common injury; present in nearly 20% of all elbow injuries. Radial head fracture is most common in adults, whereas radial neck fracture is most common in children.
  b. **Mechanism of Injury**
  - Commonly occurs as a result of direct fall on outstretched arm, with arm in pronation that forces radial head into capitellum.

  c. **Clinical Features**
  - Swelling of lateral elbow.
  - Limited ROM, especially with forearm rotation and elbow extension.
  - Pain increased with passive supination and pronation ROM.
  - Point tenderness of radial head.
  - Careful NV evaluation is imperative, with attention to brachial artery and median nerve function.
  d. **Diagnostic Studies**
  - AP, lateral, and oblique radiographs of elbow.
  - Radiographs may be normal.
  - Positive fat pad sign (sail sign): sail-shaped lucency in front of joint, indicative of intra-articular hemarthrosis, may be only clue to nondisplaced radial head fracture (Figure 10–4).
  e. **Management**
  - Acute treatment: long arm splint, elbow at 90°, follow-up with orthopedist.
  - Definitive treatment, nondisplaced fractures: casting with sling for comfort, active ROM exercises, and analgesics.
  - Immediate orthopedic consult for open or closed reduction for fracture dislocations, restricted ROM, and severe comminution. Closed reduction can result in long-term stiffness and decreased ROM.
  f. **Complications**
  - Minimal limitation of elbow extension and forearm rotation; chronic pain.
6. **Forearm: Fractures of Shaft of Radius (Galeazzi Fractures)**
  a. **Etiology**
  - Radial shaft fracture at the junction of middle and distal thirds of radius.
  - Complicated by subluxation or dislocation at distal radioulnar joint (DRUJ).
  b. **Mechanism of Injury**
  - Fall on extended, pronated wrist or direct blow to dorsolateral aspect of wrist.
  c. **Clinical Features**
  - Pain, swelling, and deformity of wrist.
  - Tenderness of wrist and DRUJ.
  - Distal ulna head displaced posteriorly.
  - Anterior interosseous nerve palsy may occur, which results in loss of pinch.
  d. **Diagnostic Studies**
  - Radiographs to include entire length of radius and ulna, wrist, and elbow.
  - AP and lateral radiographs.
  - Findings suggestive of DRUJ disruption: widening of DRUJ on AP view, fracture of base ulnar styloid, dislocation of radius, shortening of radius beyond 5 mm relative to distal ulna.

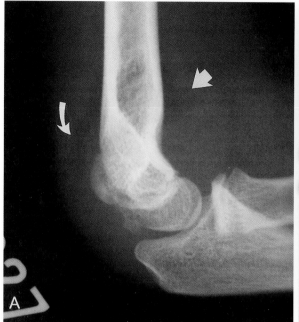 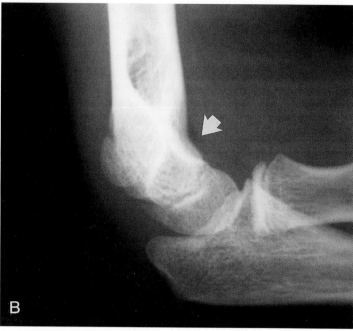

FIGURE 10–4. Elbow fat pad. **A:** Lateral radiograph shows elevation of the anterior (*large arrow*) and posterior (*curved arrow*) fat pads in patient with a subtle fracture of the distal humerus. **B:** Lateral radiograph of the opposite shows the normal position and appearance of the anterior fat pad (*arrow*). The posterior fat pad is never visible under normal circumstances. (From Daffner RH, ed. *Clinical Radiology: The Essentials*. 2nd ed. Baltimore, MD: Lippincott Williams & Wilkins; 1999:459, with permission.)

- CT scanning is indicated to evaluate the DRUJ disruption for preoperative evaluation and management.

e. **Management**
- Well-molded sugar-tong splint, referral to orthopedic surgeon for next day.
- ORIF.

f. **Complications**
- Dorsal angulation of radial fracture.
- Subluxation of DRUJ.
- Compartment syndrome.

7. **Nightstick Fractures: Isolated Fracture of the Ulna**

a. **Etiology**
- Results from direct trauma, common in MVAs, block a punch or blow.

b. **Mechanism of Injury**
- Direct blow to the shaft of the ulna by hard object such as bat, stick, and golf ball.
- Occasionally caused by fall with direct contact to the ulna shaft.

c. **Clinical Features**
- Point tenderness/pain, specific swelling at fracture site.
- Pain at fracture site with elbow or wrist ROM.
- Detectable deformity if displacement has occurred.
- With displacement of >50% or angulation of >10°, can suspect associated wrist or elbow injury.

d. **Diagnostic Studies**
- AP, lateral, and oblique views of the shaft of the ulna.
- Consider additional studies of elbow and wrist if angulation or displacement has occurred.

e. **Management**
- Nondisplaced fracture acute phase: long arm cast or functional bracing.
- Displaced/angulated: long arm splint with orthopedic surgical referral for ORIF.

8. **Forearm: Monteggia Fracture**

a. **Etiology**
- Fracture of proximal third of ulna with anterior dislocation of radial head.

b. **Mechanism of Injury**
- Fall on outstretched, extended, pronated elbow.
- Direct blow to posterior aspect of the proximal ulna.

c. **Clinical Features**
- Pain at elbow.
- Radial head is palpated in antecubital fossa; forearm is shortened.
- Radial nerve neurapraxia is common.
- Patients may demonstrate loss of thumb extension, or paresthesias to dorsum of thumb, second and third fingers.

d. **Diagnostic Studies**
- AP and lateral radiographs to include entire length of radius and ulna, wrist, and elbow.

e. **Management**
- Double sugar-tong splint, promptly referred to orthopedic surgeon.
- ORIF; pediatric patients may only require closed reduction and immobilization.

f. **Complications**
- Neurapraxia of radial nerve.
- Compartment syndrome.
- Nonunion.

9. **Wrist: Colles Fracture**
  a. **Etiology**
  - Sixty to 70% of Colles fractures occur among postmenopausal women.
  - Ten to 15% occur in younger patients from violent injuries.
  - Fracture of lower end of radius with posterior displacement of distal fragment.
  - Smith fracture: fracture of lower radius with anterior displacement.
  - Occurs in younger adults from accidents on bicycles, motorcycles.

  b. **Mechanism of Injury**
  - Fall on outstretched hand with wrist in extension.

  c. **Clinical Features**
  - Pain, swelling, tenderness, and ecchymosis dorsum of wrist.
  - "Dinner fork deformity" as a result of displacement.
  - Limited ROM.
  - Palmar paresthesias caused by tension or pressure on the median nerve.
  - Evaluate median nerve function and capillary refill.

  d. **Diagnostic Studies**
  - AP, lateral, and oblique radiographs of wrist.
  - CT scanning may be used preoperatively for evaluation and management planning.
  - Examine radiographs for associated fractures (i.e., ulnar styloid, scaphoid, and lunate), scapholunate dissociation.

  e. **Management**
  - Acute treatment: double sugar-tong or volar splint, wrist 15° in palmar flexion and ulnar deviation, forearm neutral position, elbow 90°.
  - Referral to orthopedic follow-up.
  - Indications for orthopedic consult: intra-articular extension, severe comminution, inability to maintain reduction, progressive symptoms of median nerve injury and open fractures.

  f. **Complications**
  - Malunion.
  - Joint stiffness.
  - Median nerve compression.
  - Extensor pollicis longus tendon rupture.

10. **Wrist: Scaphoid Fractures**
  a. **Etiology**
  - Commonly occurs because of fall during athletic activities.

  b. **Mechanism of Injury**
  - Fall on an extended wrist, outstretched hand.

  c. **Clinical Features**
  - Radial side wrist pain, classically in anatomic snuffbox.
  - Anatomic snuffbox tenderness positive or negative *must be written* on all charts of patients with hand injuries.
  - Concavity of snuffbox may be obscured because of slight swelling.
  - High index of suspicion is necessary to avoid complications that would delay recognition and treatment.

  d. **Diagnostic Studies**
  - Posteroanterior (PA), lateral, and right and left obliques; PA views of clenched fist in radial and ulnar deviation.
  - Negative radiographs do not exclude scaphoid fracture.
  - Examine radiographs for signs of ligament disruption and scapholunate dissociation.
  - Repeat radiographs in 2 weeks may disclose fracture.
  - If radiographs remain negative, CT or MRI is indicated.

  e. **Management**
  - Thumb spica splint for suspected, nondisplaced scaphoid fractures or for navicular tenderness even with negative radiography.
  - Orthopedic consult for displaced fractures and nondisplaced proximal scaphoid fractures because of increased incidence of poor healing, nonunion, and early signs of AVN.

  f. **Complications**
  - Fractures of middle and proximal portion of scaphoid prone to AVN and nonunion, because of vascular anatomy.

11. **Hand: Metacarpal Neck Fractures**
  a. **Etiology**
  - Fracture of fifth metacarpal, most commonly known as boxer's fracture, followed by fourth and second metacarpal.
  - Least common in first metacarpal.

  b. **Mechanism of Injury**
  - Direct impact on metacarpal head with hand in clenched fist position.
  - Palmar displacement of metacarpal head.

  c. **Clinical Features**
  - Careful inspection of skin over MCP joint for laceration caused by a tooth, especially if a history of striking a person in the mouth.
  - Ensure no rotational deformity is present.

- MCP joint depressed.
- MCP joint tender, swollen, decreased ROM.
  d. **Diagnostic Studies**
  - Lateral radiograph to measure angle of displacement in conjunction with AP and oblique views.
  e. **Management**
  - Lacerations over MCP joint; treat similarly to a human bite using antibiotics such as oral amoxicillin/clavulanic acid.
  - Fourth and fifth metacarpal neck fractures with 20° to 40° angulation, without rotational deformity—ulnar gutter splint (wrist, 15°–30° extension; MCP, 70°–90°; PIP/DIP, 5°–10°).
  - Second and third metacarpal neck fractures usually require open reduction and fixation.
  - Rotational malalignment, multiple fractures, and open fractures require orthopedic consultation.
  f. **Complications**
  - Prominent metacarpal head in palm (affects grip).
  - Loss of reduction and rotational malunion.
12. **Hand: Mallet Finger Fractures (Avulsion Fractures)**
  a. **Etiology**
  - Forced flexion of fingertip against actively extended digit.
  - Occurs in sports (e.g., catching a ball) and minor incidents (e.g., putting on socks, washing laundry, and making beds).
  b. **Mechanism of Injury**
  - Avulsion of extensor tendon from base of distal phalanx.
  c. **Clinical Features**
  - Pain, swelling, and tenderness of DIP joint.
  - Inability to extend distal phalanx.
  d. **Diagnostic Studies**
  - AP, lateral, and oblique radiographic views of digit.
  e. **Management**
  - Extension splinting of DIP joint for 6+ weeks.
  - Indications for pinning include displaced (>2 mm) fragment or avulsions involving >30% of articular surface of distal phalanx.
  f. **Complications**
  - Mallet finger deformity.
13. **Gamekeeper/Skier's Thumb**
  a. **Etiology**
  - Injury to the ulnar collateral ligament (UCL) of the thumb, causing instability of the MCP joint.
  b. **Mechanism of Injury**
  - Forced abduction of the thumb usually from a fall.
  - Most often associated with skiing injuries secondary to falling with ski pole in affected hand.

  c. **Clinical Features**
  - Pain, swelling, and point tenderness at the ulnar aspect of the MCP joint.
  - Valgus stress may reveal unstable MCP joint.
  - Weakness in pinch strength.
  d. **Diagnostic Studies**
  - Plain radiograph (AP and lateral) and stress X-rays may be used for preoperative evaluation and management.
  e. **Management**
  - Partial UCL tears should be immobilized in a thumb spica splint or cast for up to 4 weeks.
  - Complete rupture requires surgical repair and bracing.
14. **Subungual Hematoma**
  a. **Etiology**
  - Bleeding and increased pressure under nail.
  b. **Mechanism of Injury**
  - Direct trauma to nail.
  c. **Clinical Features**
  - Evidence of bleeding under the nail.
  - Increasing pain that increases with dependency.
  d. **Diagnostic Studies**
  - Plain radiograph to rule out fracture to be done before evacuation of hematoma.
  e. **Management**
  - Mild hematoma may be treated conservatively with ice and elevation.
  - Moderate-to-severe symptoms require evacuation of nail bed.
15. **Hip Fractures: Femoral Neck Fractures**
  a. **Etiology**
  - Common in elderly persons, who have decreased bone mass and increased frequency of falls.
  - More common in women than in men.
  b. **Mechanism of Injury**
  - Minor or indirect trauma in elderly patients, especially those with osteoporosis.
  - Younger patients' femoral neck fractures caused by high impact major trauma (i.e., MVA).
  c. **Clinical Features**
  - Hip pain; leg may be slightly shortened and externally rotated.
  - Evaluate NV status.
  d. **Diagnostic Studies**
  - AP with hip maximally internally rotated and lateral view of hip.
  e. **Management**
  - Orthopedic consult.
  - Operative treatment most often needed.
  f. **Complications**
  - Incidence of AVN of femoral head and nonunion increased because of compromise of blood supply to femoral head after fracture, infection, emboli, and nonunion.

16. **Intertrochanteric Fractures**
    a. **Etiology**
       • Fracture between the greater and the lesser trochanters of the femur.
       • Common in elderly with osteoporosis.
    b. **Mechanism of Injury**
       • Associated with fall, MVA, or direct impact.
       • May have twisting mechanism of the lower extremity.
    c. **Clinical Features**
       • Pain and inability to weight bear on affected side.
       • Extremity usually held in external rotation.
    d. **Diagnostic Studies**
       • Plain radiograph with AP and cross-table lateral view of the hip and full-length view of the femur.
    e. **Management**
       • Orthopedic consult with ORIF is required unless medically unstable.
    f. **Complications**
       • Nonunion.
       • Medical instability because of prolonged bed rest and immobility.

17. **Subtrochanteric Fracture**
    a. **Etiology**
       • Common in elderly with osteoporosis.
       • Occurs in younger patients with high-energy impact trauma (MVA).
       • Femur fracture just inferior to the lesser trochanter.
    b. **Mechanism of Injury**
       • Falls, trauma, MVA, and gunshot wounds.
    c. **Clinical Features**
       • Pain, swelling, and deformity present.
       • Lower extremity shortening may be present.
       • ROM is extremely limited.
    d. **Diagnostic Studies**
       • AP radiographs of the femur with cross-table lateral.
    e. **Management**
       • Orthopedic evaluation for ORIF.
    f. **Complications**
       • Nonunion.
       • Shortening of extremity.

18. **Pelvis Fracture: Acetabulum**
    a. **Etiology**
       • Commonly occurs in younger patients from high impact trauma (MVA).
    b. **Mechanism of Injury**
       • High impact trauma such as MVA or fall/jump from height.
       • Fractures are identified and classified by the exact location of the fracture line(s).
    c. **Clinical Features**
       • Acetabular fractures most often occur with associated injuries to lower extremity and abdominal and neurologic injury.
       • Lower extremity may be positioned as to the position of the hip joint.
    d. **Diagnostic Studies**
       • AP radiographs of the pelvis, with lateral and oblique.
       • CT scanning may be necessary to identify associated injuries and preoperative evaluation and management planning.
    e. **Management**
       • Medical stabilization and preoperative preparation.
       • Orthopedic referral for ORIF.
    f. **Complications**
       • Infection, deep vein thrombosis (DVT), sciatic nerve damage, and vascular injury.

19. **Pathologic Fractures**
    a. **Etiology**
       • Fracture from minimal infarct to weakened bone from medical condition.
       • May be a result of tumor, infection, and genetic disorder.
    b. **Mechanism of Injury**
       • Minor fall, trauma, or axial load.
       • Occurs at the area of cortex weakness.
    c. **Clinical Features**
       • Pain, swelling, and deformity at fracture site.
       • Sudden loss of use where fracture has occurred.
    d. **Diagnostic Studies**
       • Plain radiography may identify the fracture site.
       • CT/MRI scanning may be required for preoperative evaluation and management planning.
    e. **Management**
       • Medical evaluation and stabilization.
       • Orthopedic consult for the evaluation of healing potential and recovery.
    f. **Complications**
       • Nonunion.
       • Recurrence.

20. **Patellar Fracture**
    a. **Etiology**
       • Commonly occurs in younger patients from direct blow or trauma.
       • More common in women than in men.
    b. **Mechanism of Injury**
       • Fall with direct trauma, impact with dashboard in MVA.
    c. **Clinical Features**
       • Pain, swelling, and deformity.
       • Limited knee extension with pain.
    d. **Diagnostic Studies**
       • AP, lateral, and Merchant views of the knee.
    e. **Management**
       • Immobilization for nondisplaced fractures 4 to 6 weeks.
       • ORIF for displaced fractures.

f. **Complications**
- Infection if skin abrasion is present.
- Nonunion.
- Loss of ROM secondary to prolonged immobilization.

21. **Pilon Fracture (Also Called Tibial Plafond Fracture)**
    a. **Etiology**
    - Fracture of the distal tibia from impact with the talus.
    - Interrupts the joint space of the ankle joint.
    b. **Mechanism of Action**
    - Injury occurs from forceful axial load to high impact trauma such as MVA.
    c. **Clinical Features**
    - Severe pain, rapid swelling, and deformity.
    d. **Diagnostic Studies**
    - Plain radiographs with AP, lateral, and mortise views.
    - CT scanning for preoperative evaluation and management planning.
    e. **Management**
    - Medical stabilization.
    - Surgical stabilization is required. Technique varies with associated injuries.
    f. **Complications**
    - Soft-tissue injuries.
    - Infection and osteomyelitis.
    - AVN.

22. **Tibia/Fibula Fractures**
    a. **Etiology**
    - Occurs from impact direct trauma.
    - Tibia fracture is the most common long bone fracture.
    - Tibia fractures may occur in shaft, plateau, and distal malleolus.
    - Fibula fractures may occur in shaft, head, and distal malleolus.
    b. **Mechanism of Injury**
    - Occur from fall, athletic trauma.
    - High impact: MVA and gunshot wounds.
    c. **Clinical Features**
    - Pain, deformity, unable to weight bear if tibial fracture.
    - Isolated fibula fracture may allow weight bearing.
    - Plateau fractures may have effusion at the knee.
    d. **Diagnostic Studies**
    - Plain radiographs include AP and lateral views of entire shaft.
    - CT scanning in tibial plateau fractures because they are easy to miss.
    e. **Management**
    - Medical stabilization.
    - Antibiotic prophylaxis if open fracture.
    - Orthopedic referral.

- Immobilization with variable weight-bearing status for nondisplaced fractures.
- Displaced fractures may require open reduction and fixation.

f. **Complications**
- Nonunion distal tibia is a common area for a nonunion.
- Infection, osteomyelitis.
- Loss of ROM secondary to prolonged immobilization.

23. **Pediatric Fractures**
- Distal radius fractures: occur from fall on outstretched hand; see fracture management and Salter–Harris classification of pediatric fractures.
- Supracondylar fractures of the humerus: occur from fall on outstretched hand, very common, usually extra-articular.
- Tillaux fractures: fracture of the tibial epiphysis from fall or athletic injury.
- Torus fractures: fracture of one side of the cortex causing "buckle" in the bone shaft.
- Triplane fractures: fracture that occurs through physis, epiphysis, and metaphysis, resulting in closure and failure of growth plate.

24. **Salter–Harris Classification Fractures**
    a. **Etiology**
    - Fractures involving the physis: the cartilaginous epiphyseal plate near the ends of the long bones of growing children.
    b. **Pathology**
    - Five types:
      - Type I: fracture of growth plate.
      - Type II: fracture of growth plate with fracture of metaphysis.
      - Type III: fracture of growth plate and portion of epiphysis.
      - Type IV: single fracture through growth plate, metaphysis, and epiphysis.
      - Type V: nothing fractured, crushing injury to growth plate.
    c. **Clinical Features**
    - Potential for growth disturbances is least for type I and increases with each type; the worst prognosis is associated with type V fractures.
    - Swelling and tenderness in the region of the physis.
    d. **Diagnostic Studies**
    - Plain film radiographs.
    e. **Management**
    - Immobilization.
    - Refer to orthopedist for follow-up.
    - Gentle reduction attempted initially for type I and II fractures usually requiring general anesthesia.
    - Type III and IV fractures usually require open reduction to align the growth plate correctly.

- Type V fractures have a high complication rate because they are not identified early.

25. Spinal Fractures
  - Important to use risk stratification and medical decision-making tools to determine whether patients require C-spine radiographs in the setting of trauma.
  - Several methodologies exist for adults, including the NEXUS Criteria and Canadian C-spine Rule (separate pediatric algorithms have also been designed).

26. Jefferson Fracture
  a. Etiology
    - Described as a four-part burst fracture of the Atlas combined with posterior and anterior arch fractures.
    - Low risk of neurologic compromise because the C1 foraminal opening is wide.
    - One-third is associated with an axis (C2) fracture, 50% will have additional spinal injuries, and transverse spinal ligament involvement is possible.
  b. Mechanism of Injury
    - Associated with axial compression, lateral compression, or hyperextension.
  c. Clinical Features
    - Pain and point tenderness at level of fracture.
    - May develop neurologic symptoms (Wallenberg syndrome) if vertebral artery injury occurs.
  d. Diagnostic Studies
    - Radiographs: open mouth odontoid and lateral C-spine should be obtained.
    - CT scan is study of choice to delineate fracture line and rule out additional spinal injuries. May also be necessary for complete visualization of fracture.
    - MRI should be ordered if neurologic symptoms develop and sensitive for detecting transverse ligament involvement.
  e. Management
    - Orthopedic consult and neurosurgical consult if neurologic symptoms occur.
    - Nonoperative: hard collar or halo immobilization.
    - Operative: C1-C2 fusion if neurologic involvement or unstable fracture.

27. Hangman Fracture
  a. Etiology
    - Defined as a traumatic anterior spondylolisthesis caused by bilateral fractures of the pars interarticularis.
    - Low risk of neurologic comprise.
    - Thirty percent are associated with concomitant spinal injuries.
  b. Mechanism of Injury
    - Associated with hyperextension (leads to pars fracture) or secondary flexion (disrupts

posterior longitudinal ligament and causes cervical disk subluxation).
  c. Clinical Features
    - Pain and point tenderness at level of fracture.
    - Patients are usually neurologically intact.
  d. Diagnostic Studies
    - Radiographs: flexion and extension C-spine films should be ordered.
    - On plain film, will appreciate prevertebral soft-tissue swelling, bilateral fractures of the pars interarticularis, and anterior subluxation of C2.
    - CT scan is study of choice to delineate fracture line and rule out additional spinal injuries. May also be necessary for complete visualization of fracture.
    - MRI should be ordered if neurologic symptoms develop or there is concern for vertebral artery injury.
  e. Management
    - Orthopedic consult and neurosurgical consult if neurologic symptoms occur.
    - Nonoperative: hard collar or closed reduction/halo immobilization for several months.
    - Operative: cervical reduction with stabilization if neurologic involvement or significant displacement.

28. Clay Shoveler Fracture
  a. Etiology
    - Defined as an avulsion fracture of the spinous process.
    - Most commonly affects C7 but can occur between C6-T3.
    - Very low risk of neurologic comprise and usually occurs in isolation.
    - Can occur because of direct or indirect trauma (e.g., sudden ligamentous flexion or extension).
    - Commonly seen in MVAs or as a result of strenuous manual labor (e.g., shoveling soil).
  b. Mechanism of Injury
    - High-velocity direct trauma to the spinous process to cause fracture.
    - Sudden flexion or extension movement to cause ligamentous disruption with associated avulsion fracture.
  c. Clinical Features
    - Sudden onset of "knife-like" pain between the scapula and at the base of the neck.
    - Decreased flexion and extension of head and neck.
    - Associated with crepitus, point tenderness at fracture level, and localized swelling.
    - Neurologic examination should be unremarkable.
  d. Diagnostic Studies
    - Radiographs: AP and lateral C-spine and thoracic views are imperative.

- CT scan is study of choice in high-velocity trauma.
- MRI is not required for isolated injury.
  e. **Management**
  - Orthopedic consult.
  - Most commonly, patients require only conservative management, including NSAIDs, rest, and collar for comfort.
  - Surgical intervention is only used if patients fail conservative treatment or have persistent pain or malunion.

29. **Spinal Compression Fractures**
  a. **Etiology**
  - Burst fracture: occurs in young people usually from jump/fall from height.
  - Lumbar compression fractures: occur in the elderly from osteoporosis, tumor, or systemic illness.
  - Pathologic fracture: compression fracture secondary to tumor, malignancy.
  b. **Mechanism of Injury**
  - Burst: axial load in fall from height transferred through the spine.
  - Compression: soft cortex fails with time and degeneration.
  c. **Clinical Features**
  - Pain and point tenderness at level of fracture.
  - May develop neurologic symptoms if nerve compression occurs.
  d. **Diagnostic Studies**
  - AP and lateral plain radiographs.
  - CT scanning may be necessary for complete visualization of fracture.
  - MRI should be ordered if neurologic symptoms develop.
  - CT-guided biopsy if malignancy is suspected.
  e. **Management**
  - Orthopedic consult.
  - Neurosurgical consult if neurologic symptoms and signs occur.
  - Kyphoplasty/vertebroplasty may be attempted.
  - Analgesics for pain control.
  - Bracing and rehabilitation services.

30. **Stress Fractures**
  a. **Etiology**
  - Consistent overloading of bone that eventually weakens the periosteum to failure.
  - Common in athletes such as runners and gymnasts.
  - Also occurs in the military because of excessive marching.
  b. **Mechanism of Injury**
  - Pattern of overuse, without single traumatic injury.
  - Sudden onset of vigorous activity without appropriate training or preparation.

  c. **Clinical Features**
  - Tenderness of affected area at the end of activity early on, then advancing to pain during entire activity and at rest.
  - History may include change of sport, surface used in training, change of shoes, and sudden onset of repetitive activity.
  - Areas most common: metatarsals, midshaft of the tibia, midshaft of the femur, and humerus.
  - Adolescents are predisposed because of weaker bone, increase in formal activities, and ignoring of pain symptoms.
  d. **Diagnostic Studies**
  - AP/lateral X-ray may disclose cortical fracture line.
  - If negative, repeat in 2 weeks, looking for a periosteal reaction of bone healing.
  - Bone scanning with technetium will disclose stress fractures and stress reactions within 10 days of the injury.
  - MR testing can be done, but is not cost-effective unless suspicious of tumor.
  e. **Management**
  - Discontinue the causative activity and adjust training regimen.
  - Rest phase should be 4 to 6 weeks.
  - Occasionally, a splinting device is necessary for comfort, such as a Reece-orthopedic shoe or removable walking cast.
  - Exercise may continue using non–weight-bearing activity such as swimming, which may promote healing if fracture is of a weight-bearing bone.
  - Prevention of reoccurrence should include proper footwear, gait analysis, appropriate rehabilitation, and consistent training surface.
  f. **Complications**
  - Surgical intervention is rarely required.
  - Recurrence is common.

B. Dislocations
1. **Elbow**
  a. **Etiology**
  - Disassociation of ulna to humerus and then to elbow.
  - Most common dislocation in children.
  b. **Mechanism of Injury**
  - Fall on outstretched hand.
  - Usually, hyperextension injury.
  c. **Clinical Features**
  - Moderate-to-severe pain, with obvious deformity.
  - NV compromise may occur (brachial artery, median, ulnar, and radial nerve).
  - Associated with supracondylar and radial head fractures.

d. **Diagnostic Studies**
- X-ray AP/lateral.
- CT scanning may be required to determine occult fracture.

e. **Management**
- Reduction should be accomplished as soon as possible: usually under sedation.
- X-ray prereduction and postreduction.
- Document NV status prereduction and postreduction.
- Stable reduction can be splinted in 90° of flexion for 7 to 10 days, followed by progressive ROM.
- Open treatment is indicated for persistent instability, intra-articular fragments, medial epicondylar fractures, and coronoid process fractures.

f. **Complications**
- NV injury.
- Associated fractures.

2. **Glenohumeral Dislocation**

a. **Etiology**
- Most common dislocated joint in adults.
- Anterior (majority) or posterior displacement of the humeral head from the glenoid fossa. Inferior, superior, and intrathoracic dislocations are rare and are associated with significant trauma.

b. **Mechanism of Injury**
- Anterior: forced external rotation and abduction of arm, most common shoulder dislocation (e.g., direct blow to arm while throwing).
- Posterior: rare (<5%), humeral head drops below glenoid fossa (e.g., occurs with severe muscle constriction such as seizure and electrocution).

c. **Clinical Features**
- Acute pain, deformity, and loss of arm movement.
- First-time dislocation traumatic to soft tissue.
- Recurrence is common.
- Check NV status: axillary nerve injury may occur.

d. **Diagnostic Studies**
- Plain radiographs with AP/lateral/Y (scapular) views prereduction and postreduction.

e. **Management**
- Reduction with sedation.
- Document NV status prereduction and postreduction.
- Sling plus swathe for 4 weeks in young patients and 2 weeks in elderly persons, then rehabilitation.
- Recurrent dislocations can require surgical correction.

f. **Complications**
- NV injury: axillary nerve.
- Recurring injury.
- Associated soft-tissue injury.

3. **Hip Dislocation**

a. **Etiology**
- Uncommon injury occurring with high impact trauma, such as MVA football injury and skiing injury.
- Most hip dislocations are posterior.

b. **Mechanism of Injury**
- Direct trauma forces femoral head from acetabulum.

c. **Clinical Features**
- Severe lower extremity pain with loss of ROM and weight bearing.
- Posterior dislocation: lower extremity shortened, internally rotated, and adducted.
- Anterior dislocation: externally rotated, but may be extended or flexed.

d. **Diagnostic Studies**
- AP, cross-table lateral, and oblique radiographs of the pelvis prior to reduction.
- CT or MRI indicates postreduction for associated injury.

e. **Management**
- Orthopedic consultation.
- Urgent closed reduction with sedation.
- Open reduction may be required if closed reduction is unsuccessful.

f. **Complications**
- AVN, associated injuries, and OA.

4. **Patellar Dislocation**

a. **Etiology**
- Displacement of patella from the femoral condyles.

b. **Mechanism of Injury**
- Usually occurs from a twisting injury to the extended knee.
- More common in women.
- Occurs with strong muscle contraction of quadriceps in full extension.

c. **Clinical Features**
- Pain associated with obvious deformity and knee effusion.
- NV compromise is rare.

d. **Diagnostic Studies**
- AP/lateral plain radiographs with sunrise view—pre- and post-reduction.

e. **Management**
- Reduction with sedation.
- Immobilization in extension for 3 weeks.
- Rehabilitation referral.

5. **Knee Dislocation**

a. **Etiology**
- Uncommon injury, associated with direct trauma.

b. **Mechanism of Injury**
- Direct impact to knee joint with associated injury.
- Occurs from MVA, fall, and athletic injuries.

c. **Clinical Features**
- Severe pain and deformity.
- Weight bearing not possible.
- NV status should be carefully examined.

d. **Diagnostic Studies**
- Plain radiograph pre- and post-reduction.
- Ultrasonography to evaluate vascular status.
- CT angiography to evaluate arterial status, even if there is spontaneous reduction.

e. **Management**
- Orthopedic referral.
- Urgent reduction and splinting.
- Evaluation and monitoring of NV status.

6. **Ankle Dislocation**

a. **Etiology**
- Occurs with major trauma or injury.
- Rarely includes fracture because of complex ankle anatomy.

b. **Mechanism of Injury**
- Major trauma such as MVA or high-velocity athletic injury.

c. **Clinical Features**
- Pain, edema, deformity, and non–weight bearing.
- Dislocation may be anterior, posterior (most common), lateral, or superior.
- NV status must be evaluated.

d. **Diagnostic Studies**
- Plain radiographs AP and lateral.
- Pre- and postreduction films.
- CT scanning may be used for preoperative evaluation and management planning.

e. **Management**
- Orthopedic referral.
- Urgent reduction.
- Surgical repair likely requires ORIF.

7. **Foot Dislocation**

a. **Etiology**
- Uncommon and occurs from trauma or athletic injury.
- More common in men than in women.
- Usually occurs in the Lisfranc (between the midfoot and the forefoot) joint.

b. **Mechanism of Injury**
- High impact trauma, athletic injuries.

c. **Diagnostic Studies**
- Plain radiographs including AP, lateral, and oblique; pathognomonic sign for Lisfranc injury is the Fleck sign (bony fragment between first and second metatarsal representing an avulsion fracture).

- CT scanning for the evaluation of associated fractures.
- MRI for tendinous/ligamentous-associated injuries.

d. **Clinical Features**
- Pain, edema, and deformity.
- Can also appreciate plantar ecchymoses with Lisfranc fractures.
- NV status must be evaluated.

e. **Management**
- Orthopedic referral.
- Urgent reduction with pre- and post-radiographs.
- Commonly requires surgical reduction.

C. **AC Subluxation (Shoulder Separation)**

1. **Etiology**
- Typically due to fall onto the tip of the shoulder with arm tucked into side or onto the outstretched hand.

2. **Pathology**
- **Six types**: regarding the degree of AC displacement:
  - Type I: sprain of AC ligaments.
  - Type II: AC joint disruption.
  - Type III: disruption of coracoclavicular ligament with 25% to 100% increase in coracoclavicular space compared with normal side.
  - Type IV: posterior displacement of distal clavicle into or through trapezius.
  - Type V: detachment of deltoid and trapezius muscle from distal half of clavicle; coracoacromial space 100% to 300% greater than in normal shoulder.
  - Type VI: decrease in coracoclavicular space with clavicle inferior to acromion and coracoid.

3. **Clinical Features**
- Pain over the joint.
- Lifting arm: painful if not impossible.
- Obvious deformity with type III and higher, examining patient with shirt removed.
- Patient has difficulty or inability to raise arm at shoulder.

4. **Diagnostic Studies**
- AP radiograph of both shoulders with and without 10-lb weights placed in patient's hands, which tend to increase the degree of separation in affected shoulder, such that it is more apparent in comparison with uninjured side, as well as ipsilateral views without weights.
- Attention must be given to ruling out differential pathology (e.g., fracture of acromion and clavicle, as well as rotator cuff tear).

5. **Management**
- Types I, II, and III may be treated with the use of sling for 1 to 3 weeks.
- As pain diminishes, initiate protected ROM protocol, with the use of ice and NSAIDs.

- Progress to strengthening and rehabilitation over time.
- In types IV and V, closed reduction may be attempted; however, types V and VI typically require open surgical reduction with repair of disrupted ligaments.

D. Rotator Cuff Tear

1. Etiology
- Multifactorial to include fatigue failure of cuff tissue (e.g., repetitive overhead use); mechanical failure associated with subacromial impingement, normal aging, and intrinsic etiology such as hypovascularity and tendinopathy.
- Most tears begin at supraspinatus tendon on greater humeral tuberosity.
- As tears enlarge, they extend posteriorly to involve infraspinatus and teres minor or anteriorly to involve subscapularis.
- Most common cause of shoulder pain in patients older than 40 years.
- Traumatic event initiates symptoms in half of patients.
- Appears to affect men and women equally and involves both dominant and nondominant arms.

2. Pathology
- Investigation of vascular anatomy of rotator cuff has demonstrated dearth of vascularity involving insertion of supraspinatus at greater tuberosity.
- Critical area because most cuff tears originate here.
- Also suggested that hypovascularity of tendon may contribute to poor repair potential after tear has occurred.
- Tear may spread because of increased tension on remaining intact fibers, with resulting sequential failure.

3. Clinical Features
- Most common symptom: pain, usually associated with mild-to-moderate dysfunction and some limitation of ROM.
- Night pain is common because of the inability to sleep on involved side.
- More significant tears of supraspinatus involve pain and loss of motion with respect to abduction, forward elevation, and internal rotation.
- There is usually weakness (because of both reduction of intact muscle fibers and painful inhibition), particularly involving abduction.
- There may be visible muscle atrophy of infraspinatus and supraspinatus fossae.
- Orthopedic physical examination test of choice is the *Drop Arm* sign (patient unable to hold affected arm in 90° of abduction), where a positive test indicates a supraspinatus tear.

4. Diagnostic Studies
- MRI can be sensitive and specific for partial- and full-thickness tears.
- Sonography can evaluate a tear and biceps tendon.
- Plain film radiography is not specific or sensitive for full-thickness tears, although stress views may accentuate humeral head migration.
- Greater tuberosity sclerosis, spurring, and cyst formation, along with subacromial spurring, are associated with chronic rotator cuff disease and may be evident on plain film radiography.

5. Management
- Based on the level of pain, dysfunction, and anatomy of the tear.
- Conservative: rehabilitation, NSAIDs, corticosteroid intra-articular injection, and ROM preservation.
- Surgical intervention: patients who remain symptomatic can benefit from arthroscopic debridement, bursectomy, and acromioplasty, with or without distal clavicle resection.

E. Subacromial Impingement Syndrome

1. Etiology
- Any pathologic process that decreases space between the rather rigid coracoacromial arch and greater tuberosity of supraspinatus insertion may result in mechanical squeezing of rotator cuff and bursa between these two hard surfaces.
- Patients are typically older than 40 years.

2. Pathology
- Morphologic alterations in anterior acromion (e.g., spurring) or changes in rigidity of coracoacromial ligament may result in decreased pliability of these structures, which may begin to compress rotator cuff as arm is brought up into forward elevation.
- Theorists have questioned whether the presence of subacromial impingement is primary or contributing factor in the formation of rotator cuff tears.

3. Clinical Features
- Patients usually have history of pain, particularly with use of arm above chest or shoulder level.
- In early stages, pain occurs with activity and resolves at rest.
- With disease progression, patients attempt to rest affected arm at their side with resulting stiffness, possibly leading to adhesive capsulitis.
- Pain eventually occurs even at rest.
- In all stages, pain may be reported to radiate into the deltoid, as well as back into the scapula and lateral to the base of the neck.
- A positive impingement sign can be demonstrated in early stages of impingement, in which pain is reproduced as arm is brought into full forward elevation, thereby causing coracoacromial arch to contact greater tuberosity.
- Pain with abduction and internal rotation of affected arm.
- Diffuse tenderness to palpation as well as painful inhibition to strength testing may also be present.

- Relief of pain with subacromial space injection of Xylocaine diagnostic of subacromial impingement syndrome.

4. **Diagnostic Studies**
   - Plain radiographs often demonstrate signs of mechanical impingement (e.g., sclerosis, spur formation, and cystic changes) in area of supraspinatus insertion of greater tuberosity.
   - These changes are usually demonstrable on AP view.
   - Lateral view may show encroachment of subacromial spur.
   - MRI demonstrates bone changes, as well as any associated rotator cuff deterioration, cuff tears, and changes in subacromial bursa.

5. **Management**
   - Goals of therapy: restore and maintain ROM, reduce inflammation of soft tissues, and strengthen supporting musculature.
   - Subacromial injection of corticosteroid plays a role in patients who do not experience relief with oral anti-inflammatory medications.
   - Patients who fail conservative therapy may be candidates for surgical treatment of impingement lesions.
   - Surgical options include resection of coracoacromial ligament, anterior acromioplasty, distal clavicle excision, and bursectomy.

F. Thoracic Outlet Syndrome

1. **Etiology**
   - Idiopathic etiology, but is associated with heavy loading of brachial plexus and overuse injuries.
   - Has occurred in the presence of congenital abnormalities (e.g., a cervical rib, abnormally long transverse process of seventh cervical vertebra, and anomalous fibromuscular band in thoracic outlet).
   - Post-traumatic fibrosis of scalene muscles has also been implicated.
   - Poor posture with slumping shoulders may contribute.
   - Women 20 to 50 years old are most commonly affected.

2. **Pathology**
   - Compression of structures (e.g., brachial plexus and subclavian artery or vein) because they exit a narrow space between superior shoulder girdle and first rib.
   - These structures may be affected either individually or in combination.

3. **Clinical Features**
   - Symptoms consistent with nerve compression are most common, including paresthesias of arm, forearm, and ulnar side of hand.
   - There can be pain involving upper arm, shoulder, and neck.
   - Other complaints include headaches, weakness, and loss of coordination.

- Symptoms of vascular compression can include swelling and discoloration of arm.
- The Adson sign and the Wright's test are useful in assessing vascular compression.
- Occasionally, there can be emboli of arteries and thrombosis of subclavian vein.

4. **Diagnostic Studies**
   - AP and lateral radiographs of C-spine identify cervical rib or abnormally long transverse process.
   - Views of lung help rule out an apical lung tumor or infection.
   - Ultimately, no gold-standard diagnostic tool for the presence of thoracic outlet syndrome; however, MRI, electrodiagnostic evaluation with evoked potentials, and U/S can be helpful in ruling out alternative diagnoses.
   - Color-flow duplex scanning for vascular evaluation.
   - Arteriography is useful in assessing compression of the axillary artery.

5. **Management**
   - Because diagnosis is both clinical and controversial, most patients are treated conservatively.
   - Physical therapy programs stress muscle strengthening and postural education.
   - Avoidance of strenuous physical activity, heavy load to area (backpack), and prolonged overhead tasks.
   - Function must be optimized because possible sequelae include frozen shoulder, complex regional pain syndrome (reflex sympathetic dystrophy [RSD]), and brachial plexus injury.
   - NSAIDs, muscle relaxants, and transcutaneous electrical nerve stimulation (TENS) units can help decrease the severity of symptoms.
   - Surgical resection of cervical rib may be considered in refractory patients; however, complication rate is high and success rate variable.

G. Subluxation of the Radial Head (Nursemaid's Elbow)

1. **Etiology**
   - Most common elbow injury in young children.
   - Parent or older sibling lifts, swings, or pulls a child when forearm is pronated and elbow extended.

2. **Pathology**
   - Radial head pulled in distal direction and becomes loaded or wedged in annular ligament.

3. **Clinical Features**
   - Immediately after injury, child cries, but initial pain subsides quickly.
   - Thereafter, child is reluctant to use arm, but otherwise does not appear in great distress.
   - There is typically tenderness over radial head as well as resistance of attempted supination; however, there is no swelling at the elbow.

4. Diagnostic Studies
- Radiographs are usually normal; used to rule out other injuries, if history is uncertain or examination is equivocal.

5. Management
- Closed manipulation to reduce injury; should only be performed by providers familiar with the treatment of this type.
- Immobilization: unnecessary unless delay occurs from time of injury until radial head has been reduced or unless the child does not move the arm after a couple attempts of reduction; in this patient, sling may be used with expectation that normal function of arm returns in a few days.

H. Apophysitis of the Hip and Pelvis

1. Etiology
- Overuse injury to the growth plate in adolescent patients.
- Occurs from tendinous attachment at apophysis, causing irritation at the site of attachment.

2. Mechanism of Injury
- Overactivity/overuse of muscles surrounding the pelvis and hip.

3. Clinical Features
- Dull pain at the site of inflammation.
- May be slight swelling, no deformity.

4. Diagnostic Studies
- Plain radiograph is only indicated if symptoms persist.

5. Management
- Rest, ice, and flexibility exercises.
- Avoidance of overuse activities.
- Physical therapy for flexibility routine for return to athletics.

I. Osteochondritis Dissecans

1. Definition
- Condition in which segment of articulating and underlying subchondral bone becomes separated from surrounding bone.
- Typically involves the knee.

2. Etiology
- Trauma: possibly result of focal insufficiency in end-arterial blood supply, leading to necrosis.
- Primarily affects children younger than 12 years and young adults.
- Male:female ratio, 3:1.

3. Pathology
- Primary change in bone.
- Loss of subchondral bone support leads to degenerative cartilage changes: softening, fibromatous, and fissuring.

4. Clinical Features
- Intermittent joint pain, clicking, swelling, locking, and stiffness.
- May be asymptomatic until fragment detaches, then experience locking or giving way in the knee.

- Focal tenderness over involved part of joint.
- May have effusion, atrophy of supporting musculature, crepitus, and decreased ROM.

5. Diagnostic Studies
- **Imaging**
  - Plain radiographs, AP, lateral, and "tunnel" view; first study to confirm diagnosis.
  - Appears as well-demarcated fragment of bone surrounded by radiolucent zone.
  - If separated, fragment may be seen elsewhere in joint and defect is present in articular surface.
- **MRI**
  - Useful to delineate bony lesion.
  - Difficult to assess and identify the status of overlying articular cartilage.
  - Healing progression is difficult to follow.
- **CT scan**
  - Provides architectural description of lesion.
  - Essentially replaced by MRI.
- **Arthroscopy**
  - Definitive procedure to assess underlying cartilage and for definitive treatment.

6. Management
- Non–weight-bearing immobilization with intermittent maintenance of ROM.
- Follow closely 12 weeks for healing; fragment displacement may occur, for which arthroscopy is indicated.
- Should be followed initially every 6 to 8 weeks with serial radiographs to check for healing and possible displacement.
- Expect healing in 3 months.
- In 1 year, radiographs usually show no residual abnormality.
- NSAIDs can help with discomfort and inflammation.
- Most lesions heal without surgical intervention.
- On occasion, early surgical intervention is needed.
- Orthopedic consultation is recommended.

J. Chondromalacia (Patellofemoral Syndrome)

1. Etiology
- Typically idiopathic, although other causes include cumulative trauma, patellar instability, patellar malalignment, synovitis, increased patellar compression, and primary OA.
- May result from weakness of quadriceps mechanism, particularly involving vastus medialis obliquus (VMO).
- Affects women more than men.
- In the absence of trauma, condition is often bilateral.

2. Pathology
- Refers to softening or fissuring of articular surface of patellofemoral joint.
- Outcome: OA of patellofemoral joint.

3. **Clinical Features**
   - Usually anterior knee pain in area where patellar articulation is worse.
   - Increased pain with prolonged sitting as well as jumping, climbing, and squatting.
   - There may be history of knee giving way.
   - Positive apprehension test: whereby patient becomes apprehensive if examiner attempts to move patella medially or laterally with knee extended.
   - Pain is also increased with hyperflexion of knee.
   - Comparative thigh circumference may show atrophy of affected side involving VMO.

4. **Diagnostic Studies**
   - Plain radiograph evaluation includes AP, lateral, patellar (Merchant) views; last view is helpful in ruling out malalignment and arthritis of patella.

5. **Management**
   - Begin strengthening using a vastus medialis rehabilitation (VMO) flexibility program; assists in stabilizing the patella and improving its ability to track within the patellar groove.
   - Weight loss is recommended to decrease stress on the patellofemoral joint.
   - Short-term NSAID use.
   - Use of elastic knee sleeve for patellar stabilization.
   - Sleeve may incorporate doughnut for purposes of improving tracking of patella within femoral sulcus.

K. Iliotibial Band Syndrome

1. **Etiology**
   - Lateral knee pain from inflammation of iliotibial band (ITB) bursa.
   - Occurs with continuous running/movement.
   - Most common cause of knee pain in runners.

2. **Mechanism of Injury**
   - Occurs from lack of flexibility of the ITB.

3. **Features**
   - Pain during onset of running, then resolves.
   - Point tender over lateral condyle.
   - Pain occurs with stair climbing and running downhill.
   - Ober test causes pain and resistance to adduction.

4. **Diagnostic Studies**
   - No imaging is necessary.

5. **Management**
   - Physical therapy for flexibility regime.
   - NSAIDs for anti-inflammatory effect.
   - Resistant symptoms may respond to corticosteroid injection.

L. Posterior Cruciate Ligament (PCL) Injury

1. **Etiology**
   - Patient reports fall onto flexed knee or sustained an anterior force to bent knee (dashboard injury).
   - Can occur alone, but typically occurs in association with tear(s) of anterior cruciate ligament (ACL), collateral ligament, or meniscus.

2. **Pathology**
   - Believed to be the most important of knee ligaments because it provides 95% of total resistance to posterior translation at all angles of flexion.

3. **Clinical Features**
   - Bruising anteriorly, especially on anteromedial aspect of proximal tibia; should alert to possible posterior soft-tissue injury.
   - Large effusion is commonly present and persists for several days following injury.
   - Tests classically indicative of PCL tear include posterior drawer and posterior pivot shift tests.
   - There may be visible posterior sag (subluxation) of tibia.

4. **Diagnostic Studies**
   - Arthrocentesis can be performed in acute phase to relieve pressure and generally returns blood; if fat globules are present, associated fracture is likely.
   - AP, lateral, and Merchant (patellar) radiographs are usually negative; however, "tunnel" view is best to view intercondylar notch to identify occasional bony avulsion.
   - MRI will demonstrate acute and chronic injury, as well as combination injury to ACL and meniscus.

5. **Management**
   - Depends on patient age, degree and age of injury, as well as involvement of other structures.
   - Initial treatment includes rest, ice, compression, and elevation (RICE), along with knee immobilizer, crutches, and short-term NSAIDs.
   - Additional treatment includes physical therapy to regain ROM and establish quadriceps dominance because it helps to compensate for lost function of PCL.
   - Need for surgical reconstruction of PCL based on response to conservative treatment.

M. Anterior Cruciate Ligament (ACL) Injury

1. **Etiology**
   - Seventy percent of ACL injuries occur during sporting events.
   - Decelerating, twisting, cutting, or jumping injury associated with a "pop" or giving-away episode.

2. **Pathology**
   - Three bands of ACL: primary restraint of anterior translation of tibia regarding the femur.
   - Most commonly, tear is interstitial, irreparable.

3. **Clinical Features**
   - Large effusion is commonly present.
   - Anterior drawer test is often positive (knee flexed to 90°); however, the Lachman test (knee flexed 15°–20°) is more sensitive and is easier to perform immediately after injury.
   - Pivot shift test is also helpful.
   - These tests show laxity in ACL such that tibia displaces anteriorly.

4. Diagnostic Studies
- Arthrocentesis can be performed in acute phase to relieve pressure and generally returns blood; if fat globules are present, associated fracture is likely.
- AP, lateral, and Merchant (patellar) radiographs: usually negative, although they may show avulsion of either tibial attachment of ACL or lateral capsular margin of tibia (Segond fracture).
- MRI will demonstrate and diagnose acute and chronic injury, as well as combination injury to ACL and meniscus.

5. Management
- Depends on patient age, degree and age of injury, as well as involvement of other structures.
- Initial treatment includes RICE, knee immobilizer, crutches, and NSAIDs.
- Additional treatment can range from physical therapy and bracing to surgical reconstruction of ligament and repair of associated tissues.
- Despite treatment, some patients have residual ACL laxity, necessitating bracing to stabilize knee for the performance of certain activities.
- Chronic ACL laxity may predispose traumatic extension of injury, as well as injury to associated structures.

N. Collateral Ligament Injury
1. Etiology
- Typically traumatic.
- Medial collateral ligament (MCL) tears commonly result from valgus force without rotation.
- Less common lateral collateral ligament (LCL) injury: result of pure varus producing force to knee.
- These injuries can occur alone or in combination with meniscal, ACL, or PCL tear.

2. Pathology
- Partial or complete tear of primary, medial, or lateral stabilizer of knee.
- Examination disclosing joint space opening of <5 mm considered a grade I tear of involved ligament, whereas opening of <10 mm considered a grade III (complete) tear.
- Grade II tear falls between these two extremes.

3. Clinical Features
- Localized swelling, pain, ecchymosis, and stiffness of involved side (medial or lateral).
- May develop difficulty with continued ambulation and participation with athletics following acute injury.
- MCL may be tender anywhere between medial femoral condyle insertion and its tibial insertion.
- LCL may be tender anywhere from lateral femoral condyle insertion to fibular head insertion.
- Knee examined in 25° of flexion to relax posterior capsule, whereas varus and then valgus force is applied by palm of examining hand to involved knee.

4. Diagnostic Studies
- Plain film X-rays, although typically negative, may show avulsion from femoral origin of MCL or fibular insertion of LCL.
- MRI may be used for preoperative evaluation and management planning.

5. Management
- Treatment of all grades of MCL tears is usually conservative because potential for MCL healing is great.
- RICE, coupled with crutches and short-term NSAIDs, is usually adequate for MCL tears, as well as grades I and II LCL tears.
- Grade III LCL tears invariably involve tear to posterolateral capsular complex; best treated surgically to avoid late healing instability.
- For grades II and III MCL injuries, use of hinged knee brace with gradual return to full weight bearing over a 4-week period.
- Rehabilitation includes early ROM and quadriceps strengthening exercises.

O. Meniscal Tear
1. Etiology
- Results from trauma or degenerative change; however, may report history of minimal or no trauma.
- Ligamentous instability can predispose meniscal tears.

2. Pathology
- Meniscus fibrocartilage serves to increase knee stability and joint congruency and to improve nutrition and lubrication of articular cartilage.
- Tears can be partial thickness or complex.

3. Clinical Features
- Patient complains of joint line pain, catching, popping, and locking.
- There may be effusion evident as well as thigh wasting.
- Compression testing (e.g., Apley and McMurray) may elicit pain (Table 10–9).

TABLE 10–9.	Summary of Selected Special Orthopedic Tests for Patellar Injuries
Affected Anatomy	**Orthopedic Test**
Anterior cruciate ligament	Anterior drawer test or Lachman's test
Posterior cruciate ligament	Posterior drawer test
Lateral collateral ligament	Varus stress test
Medial collateral ligament	Valgus stress test
Meniscus	McMurray's test or Apley's grind test

4. **Diagnostic Studies**
   - Obtain AP, lateral, notch, patellar views to provide overall assessment of joint congruity, degree of joint space narrowing, or DJD.
   - MRI is the diagnostic procedure of choice in determining both the presence and the degree of tear.
5. **Management**
   - Conservative care consists of activity modification, NSAIDs, and rehabilitation.
   - Failure of conservative care arthroscopy is indicated.
   - Partial-thickness tears, as well as stable vertical or oblique tears <5 mm long, can be left alone.

P. **Ankle Sprains**
  1. **Etiology**
     - Falls, twisting injuries, and MVAs.
     - May be classified as grade I, II, or III.
     - Grades I and II: incomplete tears and differ in severity; grade III: complete dissolution of ligamentous connection.
     - Sprains (ligament tears) must be differentiated from strains (muscle-tendon unit tears), although often difficult.
     - Patients may report that they felt a "pop," followed by immediate pain, swelling, and inability to walk.
  2. **Pathology**
     - Collateral ligaments (anterior talofibular and calcaneofibular) are injured 85% of the time, as would be consistent with inversion injury.
     - Differential diagnosis includes peroneal tendon tear or subluxation, neurapraxia of superficial and deep peroneal nerve, sprain of subtalar joint, fracture of base of fifth metatarsal or talar dome, avulsion fracture of calcaneus or talus, or injury to calcaneocuboid joint.
     - Injury to syndesmosis, thick ligaments connecting distal fibula and tibia, occurs in 5% of ankle sprains.
     - Less common eversion injuries involve deltoid ligaments.
  3. **Clinical Features**
     - Pain on palpation of injured ligaments helps determine specific structures involved, although tenderness may be more diffuse, to include side opposite area of subjective complaint.
     - There may also be swelling and ecchymosis.
     - There may be reduction in joint mobility from swelling and painful inhibition.
     - *Drawer* testing may disclose joint instability or laxity.
     - Gait may be antalgic, favoring affected side.
  4. **Diagnostic Studies**
     - Radiographs of ankle are indicated according to Ottawa Ankle rules.

- MRI, CT scan, and CT arthrography are helpful in ruling out ligamentous disruption, occult fracture in refractory patients.
5. **Management**
   - Three phases of treatment that can last 2 weeks for minor injuries and up to 8 weeks or longer for more complicated injuries.
   - **Phase 1**
     - Consists of NSAIDs, ice compression, and elevation.
     - Brace or air stirrup can provide limitation of inversion/eversion, as well as promote soft-tissue healing.
   - **Phase 2**
     - Begins when patient can bear weight without increased pain.
     - Continue use of stirrup or brace.
     - Begin exercise to increase ROM and strength.
   - **Phase 3**
     - Usually begins 4 to 6 weeks after injury.
     - Begin functional conditioning with proprioceptive, endurance, agility training.

Q. **Achilles Tendon Rupture**
  1. **Etiology**
     - Most common of the Achilles tendon disorders.
     - Seventy-five percent of ruptures occur during sports-related activities (i.e., basketball, racket sports, soccer, and softball).
     - Common in patients between ages 30 and 50 years.
  2. **Pathology**
     - Mechanism of injury is mechanical overload from an eccentric contraction of the gastrocsoleus.
  3. **Clinical Features**
     - History of sudden, sharp pain in calf.
     - Sudden pain in the heel after attempting pushing-off movement.
     - Accompanied by an audible pop.
     - Ankle plantar flexion is markedly weak or absent.
     - Positive Thompson test (patient prone and affected knee bent 90°, squeezing the calf causes plantar flexion of the foot if the Achilles tendon is intact or partially torn, but not in the presence of a complete rupture).
  4. **Diagnostic Studies**
     - MRI will demonstrate full-thickness tear and location of fragment.
     - Plain film of tibia and fibula indicated to rule out associated bony abnormality.
     - Can also consider the use of bedside U/S to detect evidence of Achilles rupture.
  5. **Management**
     - Initial emergency department management requires posterior splinting and non–weight-bearing instructions.
     - Surgical repair allows for early ROM.

- Closed management usually consists of long leg casting in slight plantar flexion with gradual dorsiflexion.

R. Plantar Fasciitis

1. **Etiology**
   - Most common cause of heel pain.
   - Inflammation and/or irritation of the plantar fascia from repetitive strain injury.
   - Risk factors: tighter calf muscles that make it difficult to flex foot, obesity, high.
2. **Mechanism of Injury**
   - Running injury, poor footwear, hard surface with prolonged activity.
   - May have history of increase in activity.
3. **Clinical Features**
   - Heel pain most severe with the first few steps upon awakening, then decreases.
   - Pain, then increases after prolonged use.
   - Greater pain after (not during) exercise or activity.
4. **Diagnostic Studies**
   - Plain radiograph may reveal calcaneal spur.
5. **Management**
   - Physical therapy for stretching of the plantar fascia.
   - Night splint, orthotics, taping arch support for athletic events.
   - Surgery considered only after 12 months of aggressive nonsurgical treatment.

S. Spondylolysis

1. **Etiology**
   - Defect in pars interarticularis.
   - Most common form of low back pain in children and adolescents.
2. **Pathology**
   - Defect in pars caused by fatigue fracture from repetitive hyperextension (i.e., gymnasts and football lineman), in which there is a hereditary predisposition, congenital, and trauma or is associated with disk degeneration.
   - Usually affects L5 on S1 or L4 on L5.

3. **Clinical Features**
   - Appears late in childhood or early adult life with low back pain, often with sciatica and occasionally with neurologic loss in lower extremity.
   - Palpation of lumbar spine may disclose definite step in line of spinous process.
   - Pain worse with activity and improve with rest.
4. **Diagnostic Studies**
   - Plain lateral and oblique radiographs of spine show defect in the "neck" of "Scottie dog," in which "Scottie dog" becomes decapitated; the "head" of the dog is formed by articular process, and the "eye" is the pedicle.
   - Bone scan shows increased uptake at the pars interarticularis.
5. **Management**
   - Treatment aimed at symptomatic relief to include activity restriction, flexion exercise, strengthening exercises (i.e., back and abdomen), and bracing.
   - Bracing or casting advocated for acute lesions.
   - Surgery is indicated if conservative measures are not effectively severe or high-grade slippage that is progressively worse.

T. Spondylolisthesis (Table 10–10)

1. **Etiology**
   - Forward slippage of one vertebra on another.
   - Isthmic spondylolisthesis is most common.
   - Presents during the preadolescent growth, between ages 7 and 10 years.
   - The increased physical activities in adolescence and adulthood, along with wear and tear of daily, result in spondylolisthesis.
   - Males are more likely than females to develop symptoms from this disorder, primarily because of engaging in more physical activity, such as weightlifting, gymnastics, or football.
2. **Pathology**
   - Spondylolisthesis can be classified into five types (see Table 10–10).

TABLE 10–10.	Classification of Spondylolisthesis		
Class	**Type**	**Age**	**Pathology/Other**
I	Congenital	Child	Congenital dysplasia of S1 superior facet
II	Isthmic	5–50	Predisposition leading to elongation/fracture of pars (L5–S1)
III	Degenerative	Older	Facet arthrosis leading to subluxation (L4–L5)
IV	Traumatic	Young	Acute fracture/other than pars
V	Pathologic	Any	Incompetence of bony elements
VI	Postsurgical	Adult	Excessive restriction of neural arches/facets

3. **Clinical Features**
   - May be asymptomatic or may present with back and leg pain.
   - Rarely present with radicular pain or bowel or bladder dysfunction.
   - Young patients may have Phalen–Dickson sign: tight hamstrings and a knee-bent, hips-flexed gait.
   - Palpation may disclose a step-off secondary to a prominent spinous process.

4. **Diagnostic Studies**
   - Radiographic examination will show a defect on the lateral view; percent of slippage is measured on this view.
   - Oblique radiographs will demonstrate the "broken neck" on the "Scottie dog."
   - MRI is useful for identifying damage to the intervertebral disks.
   - Bone scans are useful for identifying stress fractures.

5. **Spondylolisthesis Grading System**
   - A method of grading spondylolisthesis is the Meyerding classification, based on the ratio of overhanging part of the superior vertebral body and AP length of the adjacent inferior vertebral body.
     - Grade I: 0% to 25% of the vertebral body has slipped forward.
     - Grade II: 26% to 50%.
     - Grade III: 51% to 75%.
     - Grade V (spondyloptosis) >100%, vertebral body complete fallen off.

6. **Management**
   - Low-grade spondylolisthesis (grade I or II) can be managed with conservative measures, such as restriction of aggravating activity, bracing, NSIADs, and physical therapy.
   - Surgical intervention (spinal fusion) is reserved for patients who fail to respond to conservative measure or if there is a progression in the slippage.
   - The goals of spinal fusion are to prevent further progression of the spine, stabilize the spine, and alleviate significant back pain.

VI. Other Disorders

A. Scleroderma (Systemic Sclerosis)

1. **Etiology**
   - Immunologic mechanisms and heredity (certain HLA subtypes) play a role in the etiology; autoimmunity, fibroblast dysregulation, and occupational exposure (i.e., trichloroethylene, silica dust, bleomycin, pentazocine, epoxy, and polyvinyl chloride) have been implicated.
   - Systemic sclerosis occurs in between 4 and 12 patients per million population per year.
   - Four times more common in women than in men.
   - Present in all racial groups and geographic areas.
   - Disease onset is highest between 25 and 50 years of age; rare in children.
   - Raynaud phenomenon: initial complaint in 60% to 70% of patients.

2. **Pathology**
   - Involves vascular damage and activation of fibroblasts; collagen and other extracellular proteins in various tissues are overproduced.
   - Characterized by thickening and fibrosis of skin (scleroderma) and internal organs (heart, lungs, kidneys, and GI tract).
   - Skin thickening caused by accumulation of collagen in lower dermis.
   - Fixation and immobility of skin caused by replacement of subcutaneous tissue with fibrous band.

3. **Clinical Features**
   - Variable in extent and progression.
   - Two principal syndromes of prognostic and therapeutic importance (Table 10–11):
     - Diffuse scleroderma: at risk for rapidly progressing, widespread skin involvement, and early development of complement of internal organ abnormalities.
     - Limited scleroderma, slowly progressive skin changes: restricted to fingers, hands, and face and may have extended course of illness before visceral abnormalities. This group has CREST syndrome variant of scleroderma (subcutaneous calcinosis, Raynaud phenomenon, esophageal dysmotility, sclerodactyly, telangiectasia).
   - Common findings include subcutaneous edema, fever, and malaise. Skin becomes thickened and hidebound, with loss of normal folds, telangiectasia, pigmentation, and depigmentation.
   - Dysphagia, hypomotility of GI tract, pulmonary fibrosis, pericarditis, and myocardial fibrosis.

4. **Diagnostic Studies**
   - Nonspecific serologic abnormalities are common.
   - Usually, ANA, Scl-70 (topoisomerase I), and anti-centromere antibodies positive.
   - RF positive.
   - Moderate elevations of ESR; hypergammaglobulinemia, proteinuria, and cylindruria appear with renal involvement.
   - In lung involvement pulmonary function, chest CT and echocardiography will be able to define severity; acute alveolitis used to detected by high-resolution chest CT.

5. **Management**
   - Treatment: symptomatic and supportive.
   - Goal: reduction of tissue fibrosis; interferon-γ, photoactivated methoxypsoralen, experimental anti-mast cell drugs, methotrexate, carboprostacyclin, and D-penicillamine are the agents tried or under investigation.

TABLE 10–11.   An Approach to Classification of Systemic Sclerosis

Characteristics of Disease	Diffuse Scleroderma	Limited Scleroderma
Onset of Raynaud phenomenon	<2 y before other symptoms	>2 y before other symptoms
Initial symptoms	Finger edema	Raynaud phenomenon (>90%)
	Arthralgia	
	Raynaud phenomenon	
	Visceral complaint	
Tendon friction rubs	60%	<1%
Extent of skin involvement	Acral and trunk	Acral only
Pace of skin involvement	Rapid in first 2 y	Minimal
Visceral involvement[a]		
GI	90% early	70% early
Lung	70% early	60% late
Heart	50% early	50% late
Kidney	25% early	Rare
Anticentromere antibody	<50%	60%–70%
Antitopoisomerase 1 antibody	30%–40%	<5%

[a]Type of visceral involvement, total percentage risk, and peak incidence of onset (early = first 3 years; late = after 3 years).
From Hume HD, ed. *Kelley's Essentials of Internal Medicine.* 2nd ed. Philadelphia, PA: Lippincott Williams & Wilkins; 2001:373.

- Glucocorticoids are useful in inflammatory muscle disease and active interstitial lung inflammation.
- Occupational and vocational therapy to maintain hand function.

B. Complex Regional Pain Syndrome (CRPS)
- Formerly called RSD.
- Other synonyms for RSD are still in use: sympathetically maintained pain, shoulder-hand syndrome, Sudeck atrophy, minor dystrophy.
1. Etiology
- Unknown.
- Bone or soft-tissue injury commonly precipitates RSD.
- Nerve-injured patients are particularly susceptible.
- Injury may be trivial in nature.
- Thirty percent of patients have no injury.
2. Pathology
- Autonomic nervous system (ANS) dysfunction; chronic neuropathic pain that follows soft-tissue or bone (type I) or nerve injury (type II) and lasts longer and is more severe than expected.
3. Clinical Features
- More commonly affects upper extremity, but can occur in lower extremity.
- Three stages
  - Stage 1: can last up to 3 months. Hallmark is pain out of proportion to original injury. ANS symptoms can include swelling of affected extremity, increased sweating, change in skin color from red to cyanotic, temperature changes, increased hair growth, and nail growth.
  - Stage 2: occurs after 3 to 4 months and marked by loss of skin lines, change in skin appearance to pale and waxy, joint stiffness, brittle nails, muscle spasms, and persistent pain.
  - Stage 3: occurs after 8 to 9 months, when irreversible changes occur. Extremity becomes atrophic with loss of muscle and skin, permanent joint contractures, loss of motion, and persistent pain that becomes severe.
- Serious consequences include loss of function of affected extremity.
- Psychiatric problems include anxiety, depression, and potential for suicide.
4. Diagnostic Studies
- Plain film radiographs, obtained in any stage, may show spotty areas of osteoporosis or demineralization in bones of affected extremity.
- Bone scans may show increased uptake in the limb, usually distal to the point of injury.
5. Management
- Treat as early as possible using multiple modalities (drugs used for neuropathic pain, physical therapy, sympathetic blockade, psychological treatments, neuromodulation, and mirror therapy).
- Sympathetic anesthetic blocks can be diagnostic or therapeutic.

- If block results in pain relief, series of three to six blocks over a 2- to 3-week period is indicated.
- Immediately after each block, ROM and stress-loading programs are begun, usually under direction of physical or occupational therapist.
- Physical and/or occupational therapy is helpful in maintaining motion and decreasing pain.
- Oral steroids, NSAIDs, and tricyclic antidepressants can decrease pain and allow patient to sleep, but do not alter the course of disease.
- TENS is a useful adjunct in control of pain and may obviate need for stronger narcotic pain medication.
- Biofeedback may assist patient in controlling autonomic functions of body that regulate sweating, skin temperature, and blood flow.

C. Pronator Teres Syndrome (PTS; Also Called Pronator Syndrome)

1. **Etiology**
   - Source of compression includes fascial bands, tumors, ganglions, the anconeus epitrochlearis, cubitus valgus, bony spurs, and a medial epicondyle nonunion.
   - PTS is rare entrapment syndrome, most common in women.
2. **Pathology**
   - Median nerve compressed in the proximal forearm by one or more of the following structures: ligament of Struthers, lacertus fibrosus, pronator teres muscle, or proximal fibrous arch on the undersurface of the flexor digitorum superficialis muscle.
3. **Clinical Features**
   - More severe pain in the volar forearm than in the wrist or hand.
   - Pain increases with activity.
   - Paresthesias may resemble carpal tunnel syndrome.
   - Sensory and motor deficits similar to carpal tunnel syndrome.
   - Dysesthesia may include distribution of the palmar cutaneous nerve.
   - Tinel sign is positive at the forearm, not at the wrist.
   - Phalen maneuver will not provoke symptoms, usually no night pain.
   - Resisted forearm pronation with elbow extended reproduces pain.
4. **Diagnostic Studies**
   - EMG and a nerve conduction velocity study are helpful to confirm diagnosis.
   - U/S and MRI are helpful to investigate entrapment syndromes.
5. **Management**
   - Splinting for 3 to 6 months.
   - NSAIDs, corticosteroids.
   - Corticosteroids have been used.

- Surgical treatment for global decompression of all potential sites of compression yields a variable treatment.

D. Ulnar Neuropathy (Cubital Tunnel Syndrome)

1. **Etiology**
   - Source of compression includes fascial bands, tumors, ganglions, the anconeus epitrochlearis, cubitus valgus, bony spurs, and a medial epicondyle nonunion.
   - Most often caused by leaning on the elbow or prolonged and excessive flexion.
2. **Pathology**
   - The region that the ulnar nerve is most commonly compressed is at the cubital tunnel along the medial elbow.
3. **Clinical Features**
   - Paresthesia and numbness involving the ring and little fingers.
   - Symptoms may be aggravated by full flexion of the elbow and may awaken the person from sleeping with the elbows flexed.
   - Patients may have clumsiness and lack of dexterity.
   - Positive Tinel sign at the elbow.
   - Positive Froment sign: as the patient tries to hold a piece of paper placed between the thumb and the index finger, the IP joint flexes in an attempt to substitute flexor pollicis longus activity for lost adductor pollicis strength.
   - An ulnar claw hand is MCP joint extension and IP joint flexion of the small and ring fingers caused by an imbalance between intrinsic and extrinsic hand muscles.
4. **Diagnostic Studies**
   - EMG.
5. **Management**
   - Conservative treatment: elbow pads to protect the ulnar nerve from trauma.
   - Splint holding the elbow at 45° of flexion.
   - Surgical decompression of the ulnar nerve.

E. Carpal Tunnel Syndrome

1. **Etiology**
   - Disorder is often seen with a history of repetitive use of hands, prolonged use of vibratory tools.
   - May also occur in pregnancy, amyloidosis, FT, endocrine disorders (DM and hypothyroidism), and tumors within the carpal tunnel and may follow injuries of wrists.
   - Most common in women aged 30 to 50 years.
2. **Pathology**
   - Compression of median nerve within carpal canal that rests under transverse carpal ligament (nerve entrapment).
3. **Clinical Features**
   - Onset is usually insidious and decreased hand strength.

- History of weakness, clumsiness in the hand, paresthesia in the median nerve distribution.
- Paresthesia in the median nerve distribution increased with use and awakes patient from sleep.
- Positive Tinel and/or Phalen tests signifying reproduction of pain and paresthesias in the median nerve distribution.
- Positive compression test: compress carpal canal for 30 seconds, paresthesia of median nerve distribution. Decreased sensation and two-point discrimination of median nerve. Muscle weakness or atrophy of thenar eminence is late finding.

4. **Diagnostic Studies**
   - Nerve conduction studies (EMG) are useful in locating lesion of median nerve.

5. **Management**
   - Immobilization of wrist (i.e., splinting, worn by patient to hold wrist in neutral position), particularly while sleeping.
   - Treat underlying disorders (i.e., diabetes, RA, hypothyroidism) can help relieve symptoms.
   - Modify activity to reduce repetitive use, NSAIDs.
   - Persistent symptoms require additional therapy of local corticosteroid injections.
   - Relative indication for surgery: constant sensory loss, failure of nonoperative treatment, and thenar atrophy.

F. Radial Tunnel Syndrome (Posterior Interosseous Nerve Syndrome)
1. **Etiology**
   - Compression of the radial nerve throughout the arm in the extensor/supinator muscle mass.
   - Compression at the elbow can result from trauma, ganglia, lipomas, bone tumors, or radiocapitellar (elbow) synovitis.
   - Paresthesias in the radial nerve distribution may occur.
2. **Mechanism of Injury**
   - May be history of humeral fracture and overuse.
3. **Clinical Features**
   - Paresthesia in the radial nerve distribution.
   - Pain in the dorsum of the forearm and lateral elbow; pain is precipitated by attempted extension of the wrist and fingers and forearm supination.
   - May be weakness associated with grip.
   - Disorder sometimes confused with lateral epicondylitis.
4. **Diagnostic Studies**
   - Radiograph and MRI may be necessary to identify fracture or lesion-causing compression.
   - EMG study will determine location and severity of compression.
5. **Management**
   - Conservative care including immobilization and NSAIDs.

- Surgical decompression is indicated if conservative care fails after 3 months, if wrist drop or weakened digital extension develops.

G. Tarsal Tunnel Syndrome (Posterior Tibial Nerve Neuralgia)
1. **Etiology**
   - Compression of the tibial nerve in the medial aspect of the ankle.
   - At the level of the ankle, the posterior tibial nerve passes through a fibro-osseous canal and divides into the medial and lateral plantar nerves. Tarsal tunnel syndrome refers to compression of the nerve within this canal, but the term has been loosely applied to neuralgia of the posterior tibial nerve resulting from any cause.
2. **Mechanism of Injury**
   - May occur with a history of prior ankle or foot trauma, body mechanics dysfunction.
   - Occasionally, nerve is compressed by tumor or growth.
3. **Clinical Features**
   - Pain, paresthesia at the medial aspect of the ankle, which increases with eversion.
   - Pain is worse with standing or walking; pain at rest may occur as the disorder progresses.
   - Positive Tinel sign at the medial ankle.
   - Abnormal sensory examination.
4. **Diagnostic Studies**
   - EMG study will confirm location and severity of compression.
   - MRI may be indicated to evaluate for tumor or growth-causing compression.
5. **Management**
   - Corticosteroid examination into the tunnel.
   - Night splint may improve symptoms.
   - Foot inversions with braces or orthoses.
   - Surgical excision of tumor or growth, or decompression of nerve, may be indicated if conservative care fails.

H. Ganglion Cyst
1. **Etiology**
   - Most common soft-tissue tumor of the hand, occurring in the hand and wrist.
   - Usually dorsal carpal ganglion and located over scapholunate ligament, but can be volar.
   - Usually develop spontaneously in adults aged 20 to 50 years, with a female:male preponderance of 3:1.
2. **Pathology**
   - Thought to be the result of outpouching of wrist capsule and contains fluid similar to joint fluid.
   - Origin (stalk) from wrist joint.
3. **Clinical Features**
   - Lesions: soft, mobile, and nontender.
   - Cyst may transilluminate.

4. **Management**
- Reassure patient.
- Most ganglia require no treatment.
- Aspiration with large-bore (16G or 19G) needle is helpful to confirm diagnosis; surgical excision if it recurs and is symptomatic or if concern is present regarding exact nature of mass.

I. Popliteal (Baker) Cyst
1. **Etiology**
   - A cyst in the posterior aspect of the knee owing to intra-articular pathology in the knee.
2. **Mechanism of Injury**
   - Most popliteal cysts are a result of a meniscal tear that causes an irritant to the posterior joint capsule that causes the cyst.
3. **Clinical Features**
   - Patients may identify a fullness and palpate the cyst in the popliteal space.
   - Cyst is generally painless.
   - Cystic fluid may leak into the calf, causing calf tightness and/or pain.
4. **Diagnostic Studies**
   - Sonography will confirm popliteal cyst and rule out DVT.
   - MRI testing may be necessary to determine intra-articular pathology.
5. **Management**
   - Aspiration and intra-articular corticosteroid injection.
   - Immobilization, rest, and compression for a brief period may contribute to the success of the steroid injection.
   - Surgical excision may be required if conservative treatment fails.

J. Dupuytren Contracture (Palmar Fibromatosis)
1. **Etiology**
   - Usually seen in men between ages 40 and 60 years.
   - Is autosomal dominant condition with variable penetrance.
   - May occur more commonly among patients with diabetes, alcoholism, or epilepsy. However, the specific factors that cause the palmar fascia to thicken and contract are unknown.
   - Associated with epilepsy, alcoholism, diabetes, cirrhosis, and tuberculosis.
2. **Pathology**
   - Disease represents pathologic change in preexisting normal fascia.
   - Proliferative fibrodysplasia of subcutaneous palmar connective tissue can lead to contractures because of nodules and cords that develop progressively.
3. **Clinical Features**
   - Nodules are often painful when first noticed.
   - Ring and little finger are most often involved.
   - Thumb web space can also be involved.

- Pathognomonic sign: nodule located at distal palmar crease or over proximal phalanx of finger.
- Flexion contracture: most frequently an MCP joint; can affect PIP joint; rarely, DIP joint.
- Other areas involved include dorsum of PIP joints, dorsum of penis (Peyronie disease), and plantar fascia (Ledderhose disease).

4. **Management**
   - Corticosteroid injection (before contracture develops).
   - Injection of clostridial collagenase for certain contractures.
   - If the hand cannot be placed flat on a table or, especially, when significant contracture develops at the PIP joints, surgery is usually indicated.

K. Charcot Joint (Diabetic Foot, Neuropathic Foot, Neurogenic Arthropathy)
1. **Etiology**
   - Peripheral neuropathy resulting from DM, peripheral vascular disease, amyloid neuropathy (secondary amyloidosis), Arnold–Chiari malformation, degenerative spinal disease with nerve root compression, or other disease states.
   - Because of lack of sensation and impaired tissue nutrition, repetitive intrinsic/extrinsic trauma leads to fractures of surrounding bony anatomy.
2. **Pathology**
   - Impaired deep pain sensation or proprioception affects the joint's normal protective reflexes, often allowing trauma (especially repeated minor episodes) and small periarticular fractures to go unrecognized.
   - Increased blood flow to bone from reflex vasodilation, resulting in active bone reabsorption and contributing to bone and joint damage.
   - Joints damaged and ultimately disintegrated by multiple nonhealing fractures.
   - Usually occurs in midfoot, although other joints can be involved, from ankle to MTP joints.
3. **Clinical Features**
   - Advanced changes typically alert patient; include swelling, pain, redness, and alteration in the shape of the foot.
   - Associated changes may include skin breakdown and discharge, leading to the formation of painless ulcer.
   - Joint destruction out of proportion to pain is often with rapid progression to joint disorganization in advanced stages.
4. **Diagnostic Studies**
   - Plain film radiographs disclose evidence of fracture and associated changes, although they may be read as normal with early Charcot's patients with swelling and pain.
   - Difficult to differentiate Charcot's changes with osteomyelitis, although as a rule, osteomyelitis

develops in an adult patient with diabetes only if overlying skin has been violated.

5. **Management**
   - Relative rest to include non–weight bearing and stabilization (e.g., bracing and casting).
   - In advanced patients, surgical resection of bony prominences or arthrodesis may be necessary.
   - Multidisciplinary consult is often necessary to treat associated disease entity involvement.

L. **Gout**
   1. **Etiology**
      - Ninety percent of patients with primary gout are men older than 30 years.
      - Onset is usually postmenopausal for women; runs in families.
      - Patients with the metabolic syndrome are at risk of gout.
      - May be precipitated by rapid fluctuations in serum urate levels from food and alcohol excess, surgery, diuretics, or uricosuric drugs.
   2. **Pathology**
      - Disorder of metabolism, causing hyperuricemia, leading to monosodium urate (MSU) crystal deposition in joints.
      - Urate levels can be elevated because of decreased excretion (most common) and increased production.
   3. **Clinical Features**
      - Sudden onset, frequently nocturnal pain.
      - Involved joint swollen, exquisitely tender; overlying skin tense, warm, and dusky red.
      - MTP joint of great toe is most susceptible.
      - Feet, ankles, and knees are commonly affected.
      - Distribution of the arthritis is usually asymmetric.
      - Tophi (crystal deposition) present in ear helix, eyelid, olecranon, and Achilles are usually in chronic form.
   4. **Diagnostic Studies**
      - Radiographs disclose "punched-out" periarticular effusions, radiolucent urate tophi, and soft-tissue tophus.
      - Elevated serum acid level (>7.5 mg per dL).
      - During attack, ESR and WBC count are frequently elevated.
      - Joint fluid analysis shows MSU crystals (thin, tapered intracellular crystals), strongly negative birefringence.
   5. **Management**
      - Termination of an acute attack with NSAIDs, corticosteroids, or colchicine.
      - Prevention of recurrent acute attacks with daily colchicine or an NSAID.
      - Prevention of further deposition of MSU crystals, reduction in flare incidence, and resolution of existing tophi by lowering the serum urate level (by decreasing urate production with allopurinol,

febuxostat, or uricase, or increasing urate excretion with probenecid or sulfinpyrazone).
      - Restrict diets high in purine (e.g., kidney, liver, and sweet breads).
      - Avoid food or alcohol that precipitates attack.

M. **Pseudogout (Chondrocalcinosis)**
   1. **Etiology**
      - Often seen in persons older than 60 years.
      - May be familial.
      - May be associated with metabolic disorders (e.g., hyperparathyroidism, Wilson disease, DM, hyperthyroidism, and gout).
   2. **Pathology**
      - Deposition of calcium phosphate crystals in articular cartilage.
      - Crystals are shed into the joint, and this leads to phagocytosis and enzyme release by leukocytes.
   3. **Clinical Features**
      - Acute or recurrent and rarely chronic arthritis.
      - Usually involves large joints (e.g., knees and wrists).
   4. **Diagnostic Studies**
      - Radiographs disclose calcification of cartilaginous structures and signs of DJD.
      - Normal serum urate levels.
      - Identification of calcium pyrophosphate crystals in joint aspirates is diagnostic of pseudogout.
   5. **Management**
      - Treat primary disease.
      - NSAIDs.
      - Colchicine oral (PO) is effective for prophylaxis.
      - Joint aspiration.
      - Intra-articular injection of triamcinolone.
      - Significant joint destruction: surgical treatment indicated.

N. **Bunion—Hallux Valgus**
   1. **Etiology**
      - Bunion is a bursa over an unduly prominent first metatarsal.
      - Exostosis (excess bone) on the metatarsal.
      - Intrinsic factors include pes planus, metatarsus primus varus, RA, and connective tissue disease.
      - Most common cause is poorly fitting or high-heel shoes, thus more commonly appreciated in females than males.
   2. **Pathology**
      - Hallux valgus deformity consists of the great toe in a valgus position.
   3. **Clinical Features**
      - Medial eminence pain of the first metatarsal.
      - Medial head deviation of the head of the first metatarsal.
      - Bursa thickening.
   4. **Diagnostic Studies**
      - Radiographs, weight-bearing AP, lateral, and oblique.

5. **Management**
   - Soft felt pad, allows toes to spread in the forefront, provides arch support to help support stress on feet.
   - Comfortable, wide-laced shoes that provide sufficient width and depth in the toe box, so are not pushed inward.
   - Medications; acetaminophen, anti-inflammatory, and cortisone injections.
   - Surgical management is recommended for painful deformity.

O. **Hammer Toe**
1. **Etiology**
   - Flexion deformity of the PIP joint of the toe with hyperextension of the MTP and DIP.
2. **Mechanism of Injury**
   - Idiopathic, but associated with second toe longer than first, poor footwear, a traumatic toe injury, arthritis, unusually high foot arch, tightened ligaments, or tendons in the foot.
3. **Clinical Features**
   - Obvious deformity with pain at PIP from constant contact with shoe.
   - Callous formation may occur at PIP.
4. **Diagnostic Studies**
   - Weight-bearing AP and lateral radiographs of the foot.
5. **Management**
   - Conservative care includes bracing or strapping.
   - Surgical correction of the deformity is based on flexible or fixed deformity, may include surgical procedures such as tendon transfer, joint resection and fusion, and performed to improve balance and mobility while reducing pain.

P. **Interdigital Neuroma (Morton Neuroma)**
1. **Etiology**
   - Compression of the common digital nerve; perineural fibrosis and entrapment of the interdigital nerve.
   - Most common site between the third and fourth metatarsal heads, can occur between the second and third metatarsal heads.
   - Common in middle-aged females.
2. **Mechanism of Injury**
   - Compression occurs from overuse, poor-fitting shoes, and degenerative disease.
3. **Clinical Features**
   - Pain and point tenderness in the area of the neuroma.
   - Pain is sharp and burning typical of nerve pain, most commonly plantar surface of the web space.
   - Positive web-space compression test.
   - Mulder's click: a bursal click may be elicited by squeezing metatarsal.
4. **Diagnostic Studies**
   - MRI is the only study that can isolate the neuroma, but is used in preoperative evaluation and planning.

5. **Management**
   - Nonoperative; wide shoe box with firm sole and metatarsal pad, corticosteroid injections.
   - Operative: neurectomy—indications are failure of nonoperative management.

REVIEW QUESTIONS

1. Which of the following is most consistently seen in Osgood–Schlatter disease?
   a) Greater incidence in females.
   b) Age of onset >18 years of age.
   c) Positive McMurray sign.
   d) Exacerbated by kneeling and jumping.
   e) Positive RF.

2. A 54-year-old man with insulin-dependent DM has developed flexion contractures of the MCP and PIP joints in the long and ring fingers of his dominant hand. Which of the following is the most likely diagnosis?
   a) Peyronie disease.
   b) Volkmann's contracture.
   c) Ledderhose disease.
   d) Carpal tunnel syndrome.
   e) Dupuytren contracture.

3. A patient arrives at the office with an acute onset of low back pain after picking up a 50-lb box. Physical examination discloses a decreased left ankle reflex, decreased sensation of the foot, and positive straight leg raise. Which of the following is the most likely diagnosis?
   a) HNP L2–L3.
   b) HNP L3–L4.
   c) HNP L4–L5.
   d) HNP L5–S1.
   e) Cauda equina syndrome.

4. Which of the following is not a characteristic of carpal tunnel syndrome?
   a) Positive Tinel sign.
   b) May occur in pregnancy.
   c) Atrophy of the hypothenar eminence.
   d) Symptoms increase while sleeping.
   e) Positive carpal compression.

5. A 23-year-old man developed a sudden onset of right knee pain. Examination discloses redness and swelling of the conjunctiva, knee tenderness, and dysuria. Which of the following is the most likely diagnosis?
   a) Chondromalacia patellae.
   b) Reactive arthritis.
   c) Charcot's joint.
   d) Pes anserine bursitis.
   e) Rheumatoid arthritis.

6. A 3-year-old boy complains of elbow pain after wrestling with his brother. The father states his son cried initially and is currently reluctant to use his right elbow. On examination, tenderness of the radial head increased with supination is noted. His NV status is normal. Radiographs show subluxation of the radial head. Which of the following is the standard treatment of choice?

   a) Open reduction: percutaneous pinning.
   b) Sugar-tong splint.
   c) Closed reduction.
   d) Observation.
   e) Application of an above elbow cast.

7. A 13-year-old teenager complains of a loss of the longitudinal arch while standing, minimal valgus of the heels and fore feet abducted, full ROM of the ankle, and no tenderness. Which of the following is the treatment of choice?

   a) Custom-molded foot orthoses.
   b) Observation.
   c) Local heat.
   d) Surgery.
   e) Acetaminophen.

8. A 10-year-old boy arrives at the emergency department after twisting his ankle while playing baseball. Radiographs of the ankle show a fracture of the growth plate and portion of the epiphysis. Which of the following is the most likely diagnosis?

   a) Salter type I.
   b) Salter type II.
   c) Salter type III.
   d) Salter type IV.
   e) Salter type V.

ANSWERS TO REVIEW QUESTIONS

1. **Answer: D**. Osgood–Schlatter disease results from repetitive injury or small avulsion injuries at the bone–tendon junction where the patellar tendon inserts into the secondary ossification center of the tibial tuberosity. Greater incidence is seen in males and active adolescents. Pain is exacerbated by running, jumping, and kneeling activities. (Osgood–Schlatter disease, clinical characteristics)

2. **Answer: E**. Dupuytren contracture is usually seen in men between ages 40 and 60 years; associated with epilepsy, alcoholism, DM, cirrhosis, and tuberculosis. Flexion contracture of the penis is Peyronie disease, and plantar fascia is Ledderhose disease. See Chapter 10, Section VI.J. (Dupuytren contracture, clinical presentation)

3. **Answer: D**. An HNP L5–S1 discloses motor deficits with eversion of the foot, decreased ankle reflex, sensory deficit of the lateral foot, and positive straight leg raise. (Disk herniation, physical examination)

4. **Answer: C**. Muscle atrophy or weakness on the thenar eminence is present in carpal tunnel syndrome. Clinical features of carpal tunnel syndrome include positive Tinel sign, positive Phalen sign, and positive compression tests. (Carpal tunnel syndrome, clinical characteristics)

5. **Answer: B**. Reactive arthritis is characterized by a triad of features including, arthritis, conjunctivitis, and urethritis or cervicitis. Most patients' symptoms develop within days or weeks of a sexually transmitted infection (i.e., *C. trachomatis*). The arthritis is most commonly asymmetric and frequently involves the large weight-bearing joints (i.e., knee, ankle). Charcot's joint is a peripheral neuropathy resulting from DM, peripheral vascular disease, and other disease states. The joint is damaged and ultimately disintegrated by multiple nonhealing fractures. Pes anserine bursitis (knee) is associated with overuse syndrome (i.e., running, walking). (Reactive arthritis, clinical presentation)

6. **Answer: C**. Subluxation of the radial head (nursemaid's elbow) is caused a parent or sibling lifting, swinging, or pulling a child. The arm of the child is pronated, and elbow devices have not proven effective. Symptomatic patients may require acetaminophen, local heat, massage, and orthosis. (Subluxation of the radial head (nursemaid's elbow), management)

7. **Answer: B**. Pes planus (flatfoot) is a loss of support for the arch and subsequent acquired flatfoot deformity. In an asymptomatic patient, no treatment is required. Orthotic devices have not proven effective. Symptomatic patients may require acetaminophen, local heat, massage, and orthosis. (Pes planus (flatfeet), management)

8. **Answer: C**. In the Salter–Harris classification fractures, a Salter type III is a fracture of the growth plate and a portion of the epiphysis. (Salter fractures, classifications)

SELECTED REFERENCES

Browner BD, Levine AM, Jupiter JB, Trafton PG, Krettek C, eds. *Skeletal Trauma*. Vols 1 and 2. 3rd ed. Philadelphia, PA: WB Saunders; 2009.

Bucholz RW, Berrey BH, Birch JG, et al. *Orthopaedic Decision Making*. 2nd ed. St Louis, MO: Mosby; 1996.

Clark DC. Common acute hand infections. *Am Fam Physician*. 2003;68(11):2167–2176.

Coleman R, Reiland A. Orthopedic emergencies. In: Humphries RL, Stone C, eds. *Current Diagnosis and Treatment Emergency Medicine*. 7th ed. New York, NY: McGraw-Hill; 2011:chap 28. Available at: http://www.accessmedicine.com/content.aspx?aID=55750959.

Daffner RH, ed. *Clinical Radiology: The Essentials*. 2nd ed. Baltimore, MD: Lippincott Williams & Wilkins; 1999:405–493.

Dambro MR, ed. *Griffith's 5-Minute Clinical Consult*. 20th ed. Baltimore, MD: Lippincott Williams & Wilkins; 2012.

Dandy DH, Edwards DJ, eds. *Essential Orthopedics and Trauma*. 5th ed. Philadelphia, PA: Elsevier Science; 2009.

Eiff PM, Hath RL, Calmbach WL, eds. *Fracture Management for Primary Care*. 1st ed. Philadelphia, PA: WB Saunders; 1998.

Engstrom JW, Deyo RA. Back and neck pain. In: Kasper D, Fauci A, Hauser S, Longo D, Jameson J, Loscalzo J, eds. *Harrison's Principles of Internal Medicine*. 19th ed. New York, NY: McGraw-Hill; 2014. Available at: http://accessmedicine.mhmedical.com/content.aspx?bookid=1130&sectionid=79724373

Feliciano DV, Moore EE, Mattox KL, eds. *Trauma*. 6th ed. Stamford, CT: Appleton & Lange; 2008.

Goljan EF, ed. *Pathology*. 1st ed. Philadelphia, PA: WB Saunders; 1998.

Goroll AH, May LA, Mulley AG, eds. *Primary Care Medicine Office Evaluation and Management of the Adult Patient*. 3rd ed. Philadelphia, PA: Lippincott-Raven; 1995.

Hahn BH. Systemic lupus erythematosus. In: Longo DL, Fauci AS, Kasper DL, Hauser, SL, Jameson, JL, Loscalzo J, eds. *Harrison's Principles of Internal Medicine*. 18th ed. New York, NY: McGraw-Hill; 2012:chap 319. Available at: http://www.accessmedicine.com/content.aspx?aID = 9136499.

Halpern CH, Grady M. Neurosurgery. In: Brunicardi F, Andersen DK, Billiar TR, et al., eds. *Schwartz's Principles of Surgery*. 10th ed. New York, NY: McGraw-Hill; 2015. Available at: http://accessmedicine.mhmedical.com/content.aspx?bookid=980&sectionid=59610884

Hughes SPF, Porter RW. *Textbook of Orthopaedics and Fractures*. 1st ed. New York, NY: Oxford University Press; 1997.

Keenan ME, Mehta S, McMahon PJ. Rehabilitation. In: Skinner HB, McMahon PJ. eds. *Current Diagnosis & Treatment in Orthopedics*. 5th ed. New York, NY: McGraw-Hill; 2014:chap 12. Available at: http://accessmedicine.mhmedical.com/content.aspx?bookid=675&sectionid=45451718

Kelley WN, ed. *Textbook of Internal Medicine*. 3rd ed. Philadelphia, PA: Lippincott-Raven; 1998.

Kimberly RP. Lupus erythematosus: systemic and local forms. In: Kelley WN, ed. *Textbook of Internal Medicine*. 1st ed. Philadelphia, PA: JB Lippincott; 1989:286–290.

Korn JH. Musculoskelatal and connective tissue disease: approach to the patient with rheumatic disease. In: Andreoli TE, Carpenter, CCJ, Griggs, RC, Loscalzo L, eds. *Cecil Essentials of Medicine*. 6th ed. Philadelphia, PA: Elsevier; 2004:731–734.

Langford CA, Gilliland BC. Periarticular disorders of the extremities. In: Longo DL, Fauci AS, Kasper DL, Hauser, SL, Jameson, JL, Loscalzo J, eds. *Harrison's Principles of Internal Medicine*. 18th ed. New York, NY: McGraw-Hill; 2012:chap 337. Available at: http://www.accessmedicine.com/content.aspx?aID = 9139675.

Mengel MB, Schweinfurt LP, eds. *Ambulatory Medicine*. 5th ed. Stamford, CT: Appleton & Lange; 2005.

Menkes JS. Initial evaluation and management of orthopedic injuries. In: Tintinalli JE, Stapczynski JS, Ma, OJ, Cline DM, Cydulka, R, Meckler, GD, eds. *Tintinalli's Emergency Medicine: A Comprehensive Study Guide*. 7th ed. New York, NY: McGraw-Hill; 2011:chap 264. Available at: http://www.accessmedicine.com/content.aspx?aID=6390597.

Miller MD, ed. *Review of Orthopaedics*. 5th ed. Philadelphia, PA: WB Saunders; 2008.

Newell KA. Common fractures and dislocations. In: Moser RL, ed. *Primary Care for Physician Assistants*. 1st ed. New York, NY: McGraw-Hill; 1998:353–357.

Paty DW, Beall SS. Neurology. In: Kelly WN, ed. *Essentials of Internal Medicine*. 1st ed. Philadelphia, PA: JB Lippincott; 1994:673–750.

Puffer JC. *Sports Medicine*. New York, NY: McGraw-Hill; 2003.

Rab GT. Pediatric Orthopedic Surgery. In: Skinner HB, McMahon PJ. eds. *Current Diagnosis & Treatment in Orthopedics*. 5th ed.

New York, NY: McGraw-Hill; 2014:chap 10. Available at: http://accessmedicine.mhmedical.com/content.aspx?bookid=675&sectionid=45451716

Rempel DM, Amirtharajah M, Descatha A. Shoulder, elbow, & hand injuries. In: LaDou J, Harrison RJ. eds. *Current Diagnosis & Treatment: Occupational & Environmental Medicine*. 5th ed. New York, NY: McGraw-Hill; 2013. Available at: http://accessmedicine.mhmedical.com/content.aspx?bookid=1186&sectionid=66478559.

Shah A, Clair EW. Rheumatoid arthritis. In: Longo DL, Fauci AS, Kasper DL, Hauser, SL, Jameson, JL, Loscalzo J, eds. *Harrison's Principles of Internal Medicine*. 18th ed. New York, NY: McGraw-Hill; 2012:chap 321. Available at: http://www.accessmedicine.com/content.aspx?aID = 9136970.

Simms RW. Musculoskeletal and connective tissue disease: nonarticular soft tissue disorders. In Andreoli TE, Carpenter CCJ, Griggs RC, Loscalzo J, eds. *Cecil Essentials of Medicine*. 6th ed. Philadelphia, PA: Elsevier; 2004:783–788.

Skihhner HB. *Current Diagnosis and Treatment in Orthopedics*. 4th ed. New York, NY: Lange Medical Books/McGraw-Hill; 2006.

Snider RK, Greene WB, Johnson TR, et al. *Essentials of Musculoskeletal Care*. 2nd ed. Rosemont, IL: American Academy of Orthopaedic Surgeons; 2006.

Tay BB, Freedman BA, Rhee JM, Boden SD, Skinner HB. Disorders, diseases, and injuries of the spine. In: Skinner HB, McMahon PJ. eds. *Current Diagnosis & Treatment in Orthopedics*. 5th ed. New York, NY: McGraw-Hill; 2014:chap 4. Available at: http://accessmedicine.mhmedical.com/content.aspx?bookid=675&sectionid=45451710.

Thomas BJ, Fu FH, Muller B, et al. Orthopedic surgery. In: Brunicardi F, Andersen DK, Billiar TR, et al., eds. *Schwartz's Principles of Surgery*. 10th ed. New York, NY: McGraw-Hill; 2015. Available at: http://accessmedicine.mhmedical.com/content.aspx?bookid=980&sectionid=59610885.

Tierney LM Jr, McPhee SJ, Papadakis MA, eds. *Current Medical Diagnosis and Treatment*. 51st ed. Norwalk, CT: Appleton & Lange; 2012.

Tintinalli JE, Ruiz E, Krome RL, eds. *Emergency Medicine: A Comprehensive Study Guide*. 5th ed. New York, NY: McGraw-Hill; 2010.

Vanderhave K. Orthopedic surgery. In: Doherty GM, ed. *Current Diagnosis & Treatment: Surgery*. 14th ed. New York, NY: McGraw-Hill; 2014. Available at: http://accessmedicine.mhmedical.com/content.aspx?bookid=1202&sectionid=71527086.

Wasserman AM. Diagnosis and management of rheumatoid arthritis. *Am Fam Physician*. 2011;84(11):1245–1252.

Weinstein SL, Buckwalter JA, eds. *Turek's Orthopaedics Principles and Their Application*. 5th ed. Philadelphia, PA: JB Lippincott; 1994.

Wilson SC, Skinner HB. Orthopedic infections. In: Skinner HB, ed. *Current Diagnosis and Treatment in Orthopedics* . 4th ed. New York, NY: Mcgraw-Hill; 2006: chap 7. https://accessmedicine.mhmedical.com/content.aspx?bookid=675&sectionid=45451713.

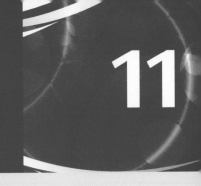

11

Head, Ears, Eyes, Nose, and Throat Disorders

Michelle L. Heinan

I. Eye

THE EYELIDS/CONJUNCTIVA/LACRIMAL GLAND

A. Hordeolum (Figure 11–1)

1. **Definition**
   - Acute localized swelling of upper or lower eyelid.
2. **Etiology**
   - Caused by staphylococcal organism.
   - Internal hordeolum is a Meibomian gland abscess.
   - External hordeolum is smaller and on the margin of the lid (sty) in the tear gland or a follicle of an eyelash.
3. **Clinical Features**
   - May occur on the upper or lower eyelid.
   - Tender to touch, painful.
   - Red, swollen.
   - Vision acuity is normal.
4. **Diagnostic Studies**
   - None.
5. **Management**
   - May resolve spontaneously.
   - Topical antibiotic solution or ointment may assist in the acute phase.
   - Warm compresses for 15 minutes three to four times per day.
   - May need incision and curettage if no improvement within 48 hours.
   - Refer to ophthalmologist if no improvement in 1 to 2 weeks.

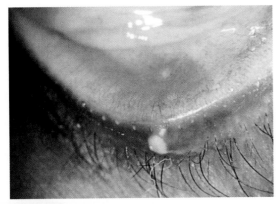

FIGURE 11–1. Hordeolum (sty). (From Weber J, Kelley J. *Health Assessment in Nursing*. 2nd ed. Philadelphia, PA: Lippincott Williams & Wilkins; 2003, with permission.)

B. Entropion

1. **Definition**
   - Inward turning of the lower eyelid.
2. **Etiology/Pathology**
   - Older population.
   - Extensive scarring of the conjunctiva and tarsus.
   - Scarring, infection, or spastic conditions.
   - May be congenital.
   - Caused by weakness of the muscle surrounding the lower part of the eye.
3. **Clinical Features**
   - Redness.
   - Light sensitivity.
   - Dryness.
   - Increased lacrimation.
   - Foreign-body sensation.
   - Scratching of the cornea by lashes.
   - Eye irritation.
   - Decreased vision.
   - Eyelid crusting.
   - Mucous type discharge.
4. **Diagnostic Studies**
   - None.
5. **Management**
   - Artificial tears; ocular ointment at bedtime for lubrication.
   - Surgical tightening of muscles if lashes rub against cornea.
   - Cool compresses to decrease swelling.
   - Epilation of the eyelashes.
   - Botox.
   - Skin tape.

C. Ectropion

1. **Definition**
   - Outward turning of the eyelid exposing palpebral conjunctiva.
2. **Etiology**
   - Common in elderly individuals.
   - Following a seventh nerve palsy.
   - Orbicularis oculi muscle relaxation.
   - Can be congenital or have cicatricial causes.
   - Eyelid growths.
3. **Clinical Features**
   - Excessive lacrimation.
   - Drooping of the eyelid.
   - Exposure keratitis.

- Cosmetic deformity.
- Redness.
- Light sensitivity.
- Dryness.
- Foreign-body sensation.
4. **Diagnostic Studies**
    - None.
5. **Management**
    - Artificial tears.
    - Surgery (lid tightening).

D. Blepharitis (Figure 11–2)

1. **Definition**
    - Bilateral eyelid margin inflammation.
    - Anterior or posterior; can coexist.
    - Anterior: *Staphylococcus* or seborrheic.
    - Posterior: Meibomian gland dysfunction (MGD).
2. **Etiology**
    - May be caused by a *Staphylococcus aureus* infection (usually ulcerative).
    - May be caused by *Staphylococcus epidermidis* or coagulase-negative staphylococci.
    - Seborrhea is associated with brows, ears, and/or scalp seborrhea and is nonulcerative. Pityrosporum ovale is involved but is not a causative agent. Seborrhea has no ulcers, scales are greasy, and lid margins are less red than the ulcerative.
    - Possibly caused by type IV hypersensitivity reaction.
    - Associated with dry eye syndrome.
    - More common in women than in men.
    - Caused by excessive secretions from eyelid glands, poor eyelid hygiene, bacterial infection, viral or fungal infection, gram-negative organisms, *Streptococcus*, herpes simplex, herpes zoster, or mites.
3. **Clinical Features**
    - Anterior blepharitis: granulations or scales are attached to the eyelashes; eyes are red and swollen (red rimmed).

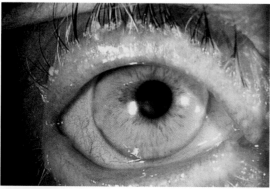

FIGURE 11–2. **Blepharitis.** (From Weber J, Kelley J. *Health Assessment in Nursing.* 2nd ed. Philadelphia, PA: Lippincott Williams & Wilkins; 2003, with permission.)

- Posterior blepharitis: MGD that causes inflammation of the eyelid; bacterial infection.
- With *Staphylococcus*, a primary glandular dysfunction with a strong association to acne rosacea; telangiectasia.
- Orifices are plugged; glands are dilated; abnormal secretions (cheesy secretions).
- Epithelial keratitis.
- Cornea develops peripheral vascularization and thinning.
- Meibomian glands are inflamed.
- Mild entropion with tears of an abnormal greasy or frothy consistency.
- Burning, itching, and irritation of eyes.
- Dry eye.
- Difficulty wearing contacts.
- Blurred vision.
- Light sensitivity.
- Complications include chalazion, hordeolum, recurrent conjunctivitis, epithelial keratitis, corneal infiltrates, abnormal lid or lash positioning, and inferior corneal thinning.
4. **Diagnostic Studies**
    - Cultures in severe cases.
5. **Management**
    - Anterior: keep scalp, eyelids, and eyebrows clean.
    - Warm compresses followed by scrubbing the lids.
    - Remove scales with damp cotton applicator and baby shampoo; rinse with clean water.
    - Apply bacitracin or erythromycin eye ointment every day to lid margins.
    - Posterior: eyelid massage and expression of the Meibomian gland on a regular basis; management of face and scalp dermatology problem.
    - To control MGD, need to add an oral antibiotic (tetracyclines, doxycycline, minocycline, or erythromycin). Prednisolone may be used.
    - Topical antibiotics to lid four times a day.
    - Artificial tears should be used on a daily basis.

E. Chalazion (Figure 11–3)

1. **Definition**
    - A localized swelling on the upper or lower eyelid.
2. **Etiology**
    - Most are caused by blockage of the Meibomian gland duct by an accumulation of secretion.
    - Other factors may be the presence of seborrhea, viral infection, immunodeficiency, or acne rosacea.
3. **Clinical Features**
    - Hard, nontender swelling of the upper or lower eyelid.
    - Conjunctiva is usually red and elevated in the area of the lesion.
    - Lesion usually points inward.
    - If large enough, may cause astigmatism or distort vision from pushing on the cornea.
    - May have a history of blepharitis.

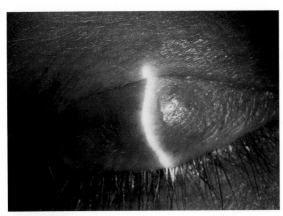

FIGURE 11–3. **Chalazion.** (From Tasman W, Jaeger E. *The Wills Eye Hospital Atlas of Clinical Ophthalmology*. 2nd ed. Philadelphia, PA: Lippincott Williams & Wilkins; 2001, with permission.)

4. **Diagnostic Studies**
   • None.
5. **Management**
   • Visual field and visual acuity testing.
   • Warm compresses 15 minutes three to four times per day.
   • Referral to ophthalmologist if no improvement on its own.
   • Injection of a corticosteroid or incision and curettage may be necessary.

F. **Conjunctivitis**
   1. **Definition**
      • Inflammation of the conjunctiva.
   2. **Etiology/Pathology**
      • Viral: usually caused by an adenovirus type 3, Herpes Simplex.
      • Bacterial: Chlamydiae, gonococci, *S. aureus*, *Streptococcus pneumoniae*, *Haemophilus* species, *Pseudomonas*, *Moraxella*, *MRSA*.
      • Allergic.
      • Chemical.
      • Direct contact via fingers, towels, or other contaminated objects or surfaces.
      • *Staphylococcus* species found more in adults.
      • Gonococcal
         • Contact from genitalia-infected secretions.
         • Consider other sexually transmitted diseases or HIV.
   3. **Clinical Features**
      a. **Bacterial**
         • Eyelashes stick together in the morning.
         • Purulent discharge.
         • Very contagious.
         • Vision does not blur.
         • Eye is infected.
      b. **Gonococcal**
         • Lid edema.
         • Purulent discharge.

         • Tender to palpation.
         • Redness.
         • Preauricular lymphadenopathy.
         • Urethritis is probably present.
         • Copious discharge from eye that appears 2 to 5 days after exposure.
         • Complication: corneal ulcer and perforation.
      c. **Viral**
         • Associated with malaise, fever, pharyngitis, and preauricular lymphadenopathy.
         • Burning, pruritic, or gritty sensation.
         • Watery discharge, injected conjunctiva.
         • Watery eyes; second eye usually becomes infected within 1 to 2 days.
         • Mild photophobia.
         • Eyelashes stick together in the morning.
      d. **Allergic**
         • Watery, stringy discharge, injected conjunctiva.
         • Eyelashes stick together in morning.
         • Both eyes are affected.
         • Scratchy, erythema.
         • Minimal photophobia.
         • Burning sensation.
   4. **Diagnostic Studies**
      • Scrapings and cultures to be done in serious cases.
   5. **Management**
      a. **In All Cases**
         • Avoid rubbing eyes.
         • Wash hands frequently; avoid using same towels as everyone else.
         • Contact lens wearers should dispose of the lens case, disinfect contact lens, and not use contacts until treatment is completed.
      b. **Viral**
         • Usually will heal within 2 weeks.
         • Cold compresses.
         • Artificial tears can be used.
      c. **Bacterial**
         • Topical antibiotic drops or ointment such as erythromycin ophthalmic ointment (mainly used for children) or sulfa ophthalmic drops for 5 to 7 days.
         • If no improvement in 48 to 72 hours despite treatment, refer to ophthalmologist.
         • Gonococci: Gram stain confirmed by gram-negative diplococci, refer immediately to ophthalmologist, hospitalization for intravenous (IV), and topical antibiotic therapy. Considered emergency caused by corneal involvement.
         • One gram intramuscular (IM) Ceftriaxone is beneficial to give initially.
         • Chlamydial treatment should be added.

d. **Allergic**
- Remove allergen if known.
- Possible treatment options are use of Iodoxamine tromethamine, cromolyn Na, olopatadine, ketorolac tromethamine, levocabastine HCl, naphazoline HCl, or pheniramine maleate.
- Systemic antihistamines.

G. Dacryocystitis (Figure 11–4)

1. **Definition**
   - Nasolacrimal system obstruction resulting in a lacrimal sac infection.
   - Reason for obstruction is unknown.

2. **Etiology/Pathology**
   - Usually present in people over 40; peaks at ages 60 to 70; postmenopausal women; and infants.
   - Congenital: both sexes are at equal risk. In acute cases, *S. aureus* and β-hemolytic strep.
   - Children: *S. epidermis* and α-hemolytic strep.
   - Usually unilateral.
   - In chronic cases, *S. epidermidis*, anaerobic strep, *Candida albicans*.
   - Results from chronic mucosal degeneration, ductile stenosis, stagnation of tears, and bacterial overgrowth.
   - *Haemophilus influenzae* in children.
   - Cause is usually unknown, but can be the result of trauma, nasal diseases, or a dacryolith.
   - Congenital, may be due to infection or an incomplete canalization of the duct.

3. **Clinical Features**
   - Sudden onset of pain, redness of tear sac region, tenderness, and swelling.
   - Purulent material may be expressed from the sac.
   - Must remove obstruction or recurrences are common.
   - In chronic cases associated with obstruction of the nasolacrimal duct, pus or mucus may be expressed in these cases.
   - In some cases, it may cause orbital cellulitis.
   - Discharge and tearing is present in chronic cases (tear film may decrease visual acuity).

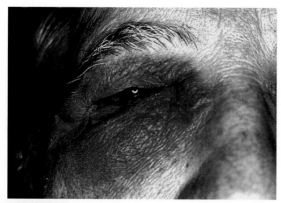

FIGURE 11–4. **Acute dacryocystitis.** (From Tasman W, Jaeger E. *The Wills Eye Hospital Atlas of Clinical Ophthalmology*. 2nd ed. Philadelphia, PA: Lippincott Williams & Wilkins; 2001, with permission.)

4. **Diagnostic Studies**
   - Usually none; consider computed tomography (CT) scan or magnetic resonance imaging (MRI) when the etiology is in question.
   - Staining of smear taken from expressed tear sac secretions.
   - Complete blood count (CBC) to check for leukocytosis.
   - Antinuclear antibody to rule out lupus.
   - Blood cultures.
   - Antineutrophil cytoplasmic antibody testing to rule out Wegener granulomatosis.

5. **Management**
   - Children: oral Augmentin, Unasyn, or Levaquin along with topical antibiotic drops/ointment, warm compresses, and acetaminophen. Aggressive treatment in children needed to avoid orbital cellulitis.
   - Severe cases in children: IV vancomycin. Referral to an ophthalmologist.
   - Adults: Augmentin, Unasyn, or Levaquin along with topical antibiotic drops/ointment, warm compresses, and ibuprofen. Rarely dacryocystorhinostomy is needed.
   - Acutely ill patients: should be hospitalized and treated with IV antibiotic (nafcillin or cloxacillin), blood and secretion cultures, warm compresses, and ibuprofen.
   - Imaging studies.
   - Removal of obstruction.
   - Probing of the nasolacrimal system.
   - Laser-assisted endoscopic dacryocystorhinostomy and balloon dilation.
   - Congenital: warm compresses, lacrimal sac massage, antibiotics (topical and/or oral). Usually resolves spontaneously. Probing of the nasolacrimal system can be done.

H. Conjunctival Foreign Bodies

1. **Etiology**
   - Results from trauma to the conjunctiva by a foreign body.

2. **Pathology**
   - Foreign body sets off inflammatory reaction.

3. **Clinical Features**
   - Acute pain.
   - Foreign-body sensation.
   - Redness.
   - Excessive tearing.
   - Visual acuity may or may not be affected.
   - May cause corneal abrasion.

4. **Diagnostic Studies**
   - Check visual acuity and visual fields.
   - Slit lamp and/or funduscopic examination.
   - Fluorescein staining.
   - Evert the eyelids to check for foreign body and abrasions.

5. **Management**
   - Instillation of a local anesthetic.
   - Normal saline flush and removal of the foreign body using a sterile cotton-tipped applicator.
   - Reassessment in 24 hours by fluorescein staining.
   - Antibiotic ophthalmic ointment.
   - Referral to ophthalmologist if corneal epithelium is not healing properly within 24 hours or if unable to remove the foreign body completely.

I. Orbital Cellulitis

1. **Definition**
   - Severe infection of the eye tissue.
   - No involvement of the globe.
   - May cause intracranial infection, vision loss, or potential death.

2. **Etiology/Pathology**
   - Occurs in children, immunocompromised and geriatric populations.
   - Bacteremia.
   - Complications from eye surgery.
   - Paranasal sinusitis (most common).
   - Dental infection.
   - Mucocele infection.
   - Dacryocystitis.
   - Orbital trauma.
   - Ear infection.
   - *S. aureus*, *Streptococcus pyogenes*, *S. pneumoniae*.
   - Fungal infection of *Mucorales* or *Aspergillus* can threaten life.
   - Erosion of the orbital bone is possible, resulting in a brain abscess or meningitis.

3. **Clinical Features**
   - Decreased vision, double vision, vision loss, proptosis, and pain and warmth around the eyes.
   - Purulent drainage may be present in case of infection.
   - Diffuse unilateral lid swelling, fever, and conjunctival hyperemia.
   - Limitation to extraocular movements.

4. **Diagnostic Studies**
   - Check visual acuity and extraocular movements
   - Cultures/smears to determine organism (nasal, blood, conjunctiva).
   - Consult otolaryngologist.
   - CT of orbit to check for foreign body, abscess, or sinusitis.

5. **Management**
   - Requires prompt treatment and hospitalization.
   - Refer to ophthalmologist.
   - Consult neurologist if suspected meningitis.
   - Consult otolaryngology if severe rhinosinusitis.
   - Immediate treatment with IV antibiotics depending on renal function.
   - Local sprays to reduce sinus decongestion, oral or nasal decongestants, or antihistamines can be administered.
   - Blood cultures.
   - Gram staining.
   - Monitor body temperature, visual acuity, degree of proptosis, and ocular motility to determine progress.
   - Examine patient on outpatient basis (after switching to oral antibiotics) every 2 to 4 days until resolved.
   - Surgical drainage may be needed if an abscess has formed.
   - Switch to oral antibiotics when the eye has improved and afebrile.

J. Pterygium

1. **Definition**
   - A thickening of the conjunctiva in the shape of a triangle usually on the nasal side growing inward toward the cornea.

2. **Etiology/Pathology**
   - Male.
   - Comes from the limbus and grows toward or onto the cornea.
   - Genetic.
   - Older age.
   - Linked to those in tropical climates, exposed to the sun, working outside, human papillomavirus (HPV) infections, tumor suppressor *gene p53* has an abnormal conjunctival expression, and abnormal human leukocyte antigen (HLA) expression.

3. **Clinical Features**
   - Eye is usually red.
   - Irritation.
   - May cause visual impairment.
   - Sight can be affected if the pterygium grows into the region of the cornea.
   - Causes difficulty for those who want to wear contacts because of irritation.
   - Most of the time bilateral.

4. **Diagnostic Studies**
   - Photographs or video keratography that shows progression.

5. **Management**
   - Over-the-counter topical ointment, drops, or gels.
   - Surgery.
   - Nonsteroidal anti-inflammatory drugs (NSAIDs) and glucocorticoids.
   - Refer to ophthalmologist.

THE CORNEA

A. Corneal Abrasion (Figure 11–5)

1. **Definition**
   - An irregularity of the cornea, superficial in nature.

2. **Etiology/Pathology**
   - Results from trauma to cornea by a foreign body, contact lens, and fingernail.

3. **Clinical Features**
   - Acute pain.
   - Redness.

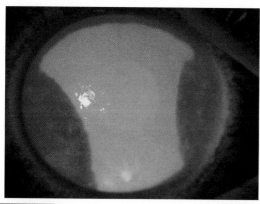

FIGURE 11–5. **Corneal abrasion.** (From Tasman W, Jaeger E. *The Wills Eye Hospital Atlas of Clinical Ophthalmology.* 2nd ed. Philadelphia, PA: Lippincott Williams & Wilkins; 2001, with permission.)

- Photophobia.
- Excessive tearing.
- Foreign-body sensation.
- Blurred vision.
- History of recent trauma.
- Usually presents with the eye closed.

4. **Diagnostic Studies**
- Check visual acuity, extraocular movements, and visual fields.
- Slit lamp and/or funduscopic examination.
- Fluorescein staining: defect will appear as a bright green area with black light.
- Evert the eyelids to check for foreign body or abrasions.

5. **Management**
- Remove foreign body, if present. Depending on how embedded the object is into the cornea, use a moistened, cotton-tipped applicator, sterile 25G needle, or Alger brush.
- Antibiotic ophthalmic ointment.
- Oral pain medication.
- Reassessment in 24 hours by fluorescein staining.
- Referral to ophthalmologist if corneal epithelium is not healing properly within 24 hours or if unable to remove the foreign body completely (if present).

B. Corneal Ulcer

1. **Definition**
- Corneal tissue necrosis.

2. **Etiology/Pathology**
- Most commonly caused by an infection of bacteria, fungi, amoeba, or virus.
- Noninfectious causes can be from inflammatory disorders, dry or allergic eyes, or neurotrophic keratitis.
- Caused most commonly by *Pseudomonas, S. pneumoniae, Staphylococcus, Chlamydia,* and *Acanthamoeba, Fusarium* species.
- Usually with corneal trauma, corneal foreign body, inadequate contact lens sterilization, or sleeping in contact lenses.

- Can occur as a result of complications from chronic blepharitis, conjunctivitis, herpes simplex keratitis, trachoma.
- Can result from a vitamin A.
- Can result from eyelid abnormalities where the cornea is exposed because of the lack of complete eyelid closure.

3. **Clinical Features**
- Photophobia, foreign-body sensation, ache, increased tearing initially (minimal).
- Begins as a gray, circumscribed opacity that eventually necrosis, forming an excavation of the cornea.
- Dendritic lesions seen in herpes simplex keratitis.
- Eye is red, injection circumcorneal.
- Corneal sensation is decreased.
- If fluorescein is applied, this area will stain green showing the defect.
- In chronic cases, corneal neovascularization and pus in the anterior chamber may be present.
- There may be purulent or watery discharge.
- Decrease in visual acuity.
- Perforation can occur, causing leakage of aqueous humor.

4. **Diagnostic Studies**
- Fluorescein staining.
- Giemsa and Gram staining.
- Culture.

5. **Management**
- Immediate referral to ophthalmologist for treatment.

C. Corneal Foreign Body (Figure 11–6)

1. **Etiology**
- Results from trauma to the cornea by a foreign body on the surface of, or embedded into, the cornea.

2. **Pathology**
- Foreign body sets off inflammatory reaction.
- If foreign body is not removed, it can cause infection, tissue necrosis, or both.

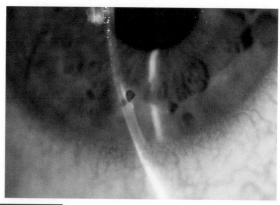

FIGURE 11–6. **Corneal foreign body.** (From Tasman W, Jaeger E. *The Wills Eye Hospital Atlas of Clinical Ophthalmology.* 2nd ed. Philadelphia, PA: Lippincott Williams & Wilkins; 2001, with permission.)

3. **Clinical Features**
   - Acute pain.
   - Redness.
   - Photophobia, excessive tearing.
   - Foreign-body sensation.
   - Blurred vision.
   - History of recent trauma.
   - Usually presents with the eye closed.
   - May see a ring infiltrate surrounding the site of the foreign body if embedded for >24 hours.
4. **Diagnostic Studies**
   - Check visual acuity.
   - Penlight exam.
   - Slit lamp.
   - Visual fields and extraocular movements.
   - Tetanus immunization status.
   - Fluorescein staining: the foreign body will be dark with an area of green surrounding it under the black light.
   - Evert the eyelids to check for foreign body or abrasions.
5. **Management**
   - Instill topical anesthetic.
   - Depending on how embedded the object is into the cornea, use a moistened cotton-tipped applicator, a sterile 25G needle, or an Alger brush.
   - Antibiotic ophthalmic drops, such as Polytrim, Sulamyd, or Tobrex, should be applied.
   - Contact lens wearers should be treated with ciprofloxacin or ofloxacin.
   - Oral pain medication, if needed.
   - Reassessment in 24 hours by fluorescein staining.
   - Referral to ophthalmologist if corneal epithelium is not healing properly within 24 hours or if unable to completely remove the foreign body.

THE GLOBE
A. Optic Neuritis
1. **Definition**
   - Inflammation of the optic nerve.
2. **Etiology/Pathology**
   - Associated with demyelinative disease (i.e., multiple sclerosis).
   - May occur in association with viral infections (mumps, measles, influenza, and those caused by the *Varicella zoster* virus).
   - Possibly genetic.
   - Women more than men.
   - People living at higher latitudes.
   - May occur with systemic lupus erythematosus.
   - Toxic substance exposure (e.g., methanol, tobacco).
   - Metabolic or nutritional issues.
   - Vascular insufficiency.
3. **Clinical Features**
   - Unilateral vision loss that develops suddenly.
   - Vision varies from 20/30 to no light perception.
   - Patient has pain particularly with any type of eye movement.

- Monocular field defects are possible.
- Color vision loss.
- Afferent pupillary defect (Marcus Gunn pupil).
- Disc margin blurring.
- More severe cases show a vitamin D deficiency.
- In acute phase, the optic nerve appears normal and then becomes swollen.
- Occasional flame-shaped peripapillary hemorrhages are present.
- Optic atrophy occurs if enough optic nerve fibers are destroyed.
- Visual acuity usually improves within 2 to 3 weeks and frequently returns to normal.

4. **Diagnostic Studies**
   - MRI can be done to determine the risk of developing multiple sclerosis.
5. **Management**
   - Referral to ophthalmologist.
   - Referral to a neurologist if demyelinating disease.

B. Retinopathy
1. **Definition**
   - Progressive damage to the eye's retina.
   - One of the leading causes of blindness.
2. **Etiology/Pathology**
   - Can be caused by long-term uncontrolled diabetes or hypertension.
   - Can result in vision loss.
   a. **Diabetic Retinopathy**
      - **Nonproliferative** (Figure 11–7A, B)
        - Capillary microaneurysms develop.
        - Tortuous and dilated veins.
        - Hard exudates.
        - Flame-shaped hemorrhages.
      - **Maculopathy**
        - Increasing ischemia.
        - Cotton-wool patches.
        - Retinal vein beading.
        - Closure of retinal capillaries.
      - **Proliferative**
        - Ischemia stimulates vessels that leak serum proteins.
        - Neovascularization can result.
        - Massive vitreous hemorrhage can result, causing sudden loss of vision.
        - Adhesions can develop.
        - Bands form and contract on the vitreous, causing retinal detachment or retinal tear.
        - Hemorrhage and swelling, leaking of fluid into the retina.
        - New growth of blood vessels within the eye.
   b. **Hypertensive Retinopathy**
      - Accumulation of the development of atherosclerosis from long-standing hypertension.
      - Acute elevation of blood pressure results in loss of autoregulation in the retinal circulation, causing vasoconstriction and ischemia.

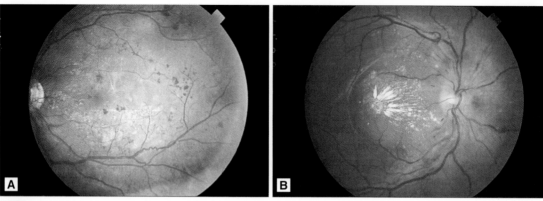

FIGURE 11–7. **A:** Fundus with diabetic retinopathy and neovascularization of the optic disc. **B:** Hypertensive retinopathy. (From Tasman W, Jaeger E. *The Wills Eye Hospital Atlas of Clinical Ophthalmology.* 2nd ed. Philadelphia, PA: Lippincott Williams & Wilkins; 2001, with permission.)

3. **Clinical Features**
   a. **Diabetic Retinopathy**
   - Decreased visual acuity and color vision.
   - Retinal hemorrhage, retinal edema, hard exudate, neovascularization, macular exudate, retinal detachment.
   b. **Hypertensive Retinopathy**
   - Decreased visual acuity.
   - Retinal hemorrhage, retinal edema, cotton-wool exudates, copper/silver wiring, arteriovenous nicking, optic disc swelling, retinal detachment.
4. **Diagnostic Studies**
   - Fluorescein angiography.
   - Optical coherence tomography (OCT) and referral to ophthalmologist.
5. **Management**
   - For patients with type 1 diabetes: referral to ophthalmologist 3 years after onset and then annually.
   - For patients with type 2 diabetes: referral to ophthalmologist at the time of diagnosis and annually.
   - Control blood glucose levels and lipid levels.
   - Women wishing to conceive should be referred to an ophthalmologist for evaluation.
   - Pregnant patients should be seen by ophthalmologist in the first trimester, then every 3 months until delivery.
   - Removal of vitreous hemorrhage.
   - Treatment may include argon laser panretinal photocoagulation, vitreoretinal surgery, and treatment of systemic disease.
   - Hypertensive retinopathy: control blood pressure, look for other end organ disease.

C. **Retinal Detachment (Figure 11–8)**
   1. **Etiology**
   - Three types
     - Rhegmatogenous retinal detachment (RRD): the most common.

   - Exudative or serous retinal detachment (ERD).
   - Tractional retinal detachment (TRD).
2. **Pathology**
   - RRD: a break in the retina allows the vitreous fluid to leak, causing the detachment. Caused by spontaneous, penetrating, or blunt trauma.
   - ERD: accumulation of subretinal fluid causes the detachment. This detachment usually results from inflammation or a tumor.
   - TRD: adhesions form, causing a traction on the retina, which forces it to separate or tear. This type of detachment occurs with sickle-cell disease, trauma, or proliferative diabetic retinopathy.
   - Bilateral detachments are possible for patients who have had bilateral cataract extractions.

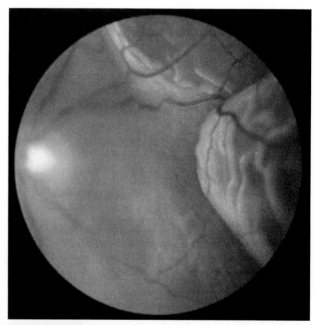

FIGURE 11–8. **Retinal detachment.** (From Moore KL, Dalley AF II. *Clinical Oriented Anatomy.* 4th ed. Baltimore, MD: Lippincott Williams & Wilkins; 1999, with permission.)

- More common in patients with myopia >6 diopters.
- Young people can sustain traumatic detachments.
- Usually occurs in patients over 50 years old.
- Cataract extraction and myopia are possible causes.
- Can result in blindness or loss of light perception.
- Leukemia, diabetes, angiomatosis, eclampsia, breast cancer, melanoma, and sickle-cell disease all increase the risk of retinal detachment.

3. **Clinical Features**
   - Photopsia.
   - Shower of floaters.
   - Decreased visual acuity.
   - Objects appear to have a wavy type of distortion.
   - Visual field defects show as a late symptom.
   - Flashing lights occur when the posterior vitreous separates.
   - Asymptomatic until the inferior detachment progresses and reaches the fovea.
   - Intraocular pressure (IOP) is >4 to 5 mm Hg in comparison with the unaffected eye.
   - On examination, multiple tears may be present.
   - Usually asymptomatic unless central vision is threatened, in which case the patient can suffer severe and abrupt vision loss.
   - Appears as a concave, smooth-surfaced detachment with marginal fibrovascular bands extending into the vitreous body.

4. **Diagnostic Studies**
   - Ocular ultrasonography may assist with the diagnosis.
   - Slit lamp.
   - No laboratory tests are usually needed unless a cause for the detachment is unknown.
   - CT or MRI is used only if a tumor or foreign body is suspected.

5. **Management**
   - Emergent referral to ophthalmologist.
   - Choice of treatment depends on the size, location, and type of detachment. In some cases, the detachment can be handled medically.
   - Possible treatment methods include surgery, laser therapy, pneumatic retinopexy, cryotherapy, scleral buckling, reattachment, and intraocular gas.

D. **Retinal Vascular Occlusion**
   1. **Definition**
      - Occlusion of the central retinal artery or vein by an embolus, causing profound vision loss.
   2. **Etiology/Pathology**
      - Artery: usually occurs in patients between the ages of 50 and 80 who often have concurrent hypertension, hyperlipidemia, cardiac arrhythmia, diabetes, or atherosclerosis.
      - Artery: may be secondary to giant cell arteritis.
      - Artery: systemic vasculitis, thrombophilia (congenital or acquired), hyperhomocysteinemia, oral contraceptives, or migraine in younger patients.
      - Vein: most common on awakening. Screen for systolic hypertension, diabetes, hyperlipidemia, and glaucoma. Smoking and oral contraceptives can be contributing factors.

   3. **Clinical Features**
      - Sudden, painless, unilateral loss of vision, visual field, or both, lasting from minutes (amaurosis fugax) to permanent.
      - Vein: retinal venous dilatation, retinal cotton-wool spots, optic disc swelling, retinal hemorrhages, and dilation and tortuosity of the retinal veins.
      - Vein: possible neovascular glaucoma can develop in the first 3 months.
      - Artery: a cherry red spot is seen at the fovea.
      - Artery: blood in the veins has a "box car" appearance.
      - Occasionally, an embolus can be visualized.
      - Artery: visual acuity is restricted to the temporal areas or by counting fingers.
      - Artery: swelling of the retina (lasts 4–6 weeks).
      - Artery: after 4 to 6 weeks, retina appears normal, but the optic nerve is pale and arterioles attenuated.
      - Artery: cotton-wool spots are limited to the region affected.
      - Artery: if head and neck pain are associated, consider internal carotid artery dissection.

   4. **Diagnostic Studies**
      - In addition, order electrocardiogram, fasting blood sugar, lipid profile, partial thromboplastin time, erythrocyte sedimentation rate, antiphospholipid antibodies, plasma homocysteine, lupus anticoagulant, and C-reactive protein in younger patients; labs to rule out associated conditions, duplex ultrasound of the carotid; echocardiogram.

   5. **Management**
      - Cause must be determined to prevent stroke.
      - Emergency referral to ophthalmologist.
      - Vein: panretinal laser photocoagulation for those at risk for neovascular glaucoma.
      - Intravitreal injections.
      - Vein: vitrectomy with radical optic neurotomy.
      - Vein: branch vein occlusion may benefit from injection of tissue plasminogen activator.
      - Artery: patient must lie flat with high levels of inhaled oxygen.
      - Artery: IV acetazolamide.
      - Thrombolysis may improve outcome.
      - Artery: if giant cell arteritis is suspected, give high dose of corticosteroids and biopsy the temporal artery.
      - Low-dose aspirin.
      - Check for sources of emboli including carotids or cardiac.

- Artery: inhaled oxygen.
- Artery: reduction of IOP and vascular resistance to flow (digital globe massage, paracentesis, and carbonic anhydrase inhibitors).
- Referral to cardiologist to rule out arrhythmia.
- Cardiac disease may need surgery or anticoagulation.

E. Cataract
1. **Definition**
   - Opacities of the lens.
2. **Etiology/Pathology**
   - Usually bilateral (but asymmetric).
   - Due to injury, age, systemic disease, congenital, or inhaled corticosteroid treatments.
   - Common loss of vision, particularly in elderly people.
   - Usually occurs at >60 years of age.
   - Cigarette smoking and alcohol increase risk.
   - Exposure to ultraviolet (UV) light.
   - Malnutrition.
   - Diabetes mellitus.
   - Metabolic syndrome.
3. **Clinical Features**
   - Can be visualized with ophthalmoscope or slit lamp.
   - Shadows or black spots in red reflex.
   - Hazy, blurred, or distorted vision.
   - Loss of color vision.
   - Difficulty night driving and reading fine print.
   - Painless decline of vision.
   - Double vision.
   - Difficulty visualizing the retina because of opaque lens; fundus reflection is absent and the pupil becomes white.
4. **Diagnostic Studies**
   - Thorough eye examination by ophthalmologist or optometrist.
5. **Management**
   - Surgery is indicated when there is visual impairment.

F. Glaucoma
1. **Definition**
   - Disease of the optic nerve related to abnormal drainage of aqueous from the trabecular meshwork, which may cause increased ocular pressure resulting in decreased peripheral fields and possible blindness.
2. **Etiology**
   - Populations at risk for open-angle glaucoma include people of African American origin and non-Hispanic white women; Asian and Inuits heritage for angle closure; people with vascular diseases such as hypertension; those with migraines, diabetes, or cardiovascular disease; older adults; those with high myopia; and people with a family history of glaucoma.

3. **Pathology**
   a. **Open-Angle Glaucoma**
      - Lack of proper drainage of the aqueous through the trabecular meshwork, causing damage to the optic nerve and resulting in vision loss.
      - May be associated with increased ocular pressure.
      - Occurs in 90% to 95% of glaucoma cases.
   b. **Acute (Angle Closure) Glaucoma**
      - Primary can occur only with the closure of a preexisting narrow anterior chamber angle.
      - Secondary to long-standing anterior uveitis or dislocation of the lens.
4. **Clinical Features**
   a. **Open-Angle Glaucoma**
      - Asymptomatic until late in the disease.
      - Chronic, slow, and progressive visual field loss.
      - Increased cup:disc ratio on funduscopic examination.
   b. **Acute Closure Glaucoma**
      - Ocular pain and decreased vision.
      - Halos around lights.
      - Conjunctiva is injected; cornea is cloudy.
      - Reduced visual acuity.
      - Treat within 24 hours.
      - Painful.
      - Pupil is mildly reactive in a mid-dilated state.
      - Nausea and abdominal pain may occur.
      - Physical examination: visual field defects.
      - Enlarged or excavated optic disc with pallor.
5. **Diagnostic Studies**
   - Thorough eye examination by ophthalmologist including tonometry.
   - Field testing.
   - Pachymetry.
6. **Management**
   a. **Open-Angle Glaucoma**
      - Prostaglandins are number one treatment.
      - α-Adrenergic blocking eye drops (timolol, levobunolol, betaxolol), β_2-agonist eye drops, prostaglandin analogs, or carbonic anhydrase inhibitors.
      - IOP >40 is emergent.
      - IOP 30 to 40 should be seen within 24 hours.
      - Laser surgery (trabeculoplasty).
   b. **Acute-Angle Closure Glaucoma**
      - Decrease of IOP by laser (argon or yttrium aluminum garnet).
      - Systemic acetazolamide or Mannitol.
      - Laser peripheral iridotomy or iridectomy.
      - Pilocarpine after IOP begins to drop.
      - Prophylactic iridotomy on uninvolved eye.
      - Refer to ophthalmologist.

G. Strabismus
1. **Etiology**
   - Basically unknown, but can be hereditary.
   - Can be the result of stroke, thyroid disease, tumor, nerve conditions, or trauma.

- Can present at birth or shortly thereafter.
- Can also develop from 6 months to 7 years of age.

2. **Pathology**
   - Poor development of one eye with decreased visual acuity, which can lead to amblyopia and blindness if not corrected.

3. **Clinical Features**
   - Most common presentation is esotropia (cross-eyed) or exotropia (wall-eyed).
   - Both eyes are not able to align simultaneously on an object.
   - Presentation at birth is a congenital esotropia.
   - Development between 6 months and 7 years has some accommodative component.
   - One eye wanders out when patient is ill, tired, or compromised in some way (intermittent exotropia).
   - Eye wanders longer and more frequently with time. Eventually leads to eye turning outward all the time (constant exotropia).

4. **Diagnostic Studies**
   - Hirschberg light reflex test.
   - Cover/uncover test.
   - Referral to ophthalmologist or optometrist.

5. **Management**
   - Check visual acuity; if amblyopia is present, patch good eye.
   - Make sure that there is no regression of the good eye during the time it is patched.
   - Surgery may be necessary to straighten eyes.
   - Late-onset cases usually cause diplopia.
   - May be treated with eyeglasses, prisms, or a vision therapy program called orthoptics.
   - Eye patch or surgery may be necessary.
   - Referral to a neurologist if underlying disease is suspected.

H. Nystagmus

1. **Definition**
   - Unilateral or bilateral oscillation of the eye that is dependent on gaze with one eye more pronounced.
   - Can be horizontal, vertical, or rotary.

2. **Etiology/Pathology**
   - May occur with ocular lesion, esotropia, or hypoplastic visual pathways.
   - Likely ocular, but may have central nervous system (CNS) or inner ear involvement.
   - May be genetic.
   - Other eye problem.
   - Caused by head injury, stroke, Ménière syndrome, alcohol or drug use, or multiple sclerosis.

3. **Clinical Features**
   - Must occur in normal fields of vision.
   - Occurs in one or more planes.
   - Photophobia.
   - Dizziness.
   - Tilted head position.

4. **Diagnostic Studies**
   - When testing eyes, material to occlude the eye should be held 12 in away from the eye not being tested. Placing the material close to the eye worsens the condition of nystagmus and does not give a good read on acuity.
   - Electroretinogram to rule out retinal pathology.
   - Referral to ophthalmologist for iris transillumination.
   - Neurologic exam.
   - Possibly MRI or CT.

5. **Management**
   - Referral to ophthalmologist.
   - Glasses or contacts can improve vision.
   - Possible surgery or treatment with prisms.

I. Macular Degeneration

1. **Definition**
   - Unilateral progressive vision loss.

2. **Etiology/Pathology**
   - Over the age of 55.
   - Family history.
   - Smoker (current or previous).
   - Light colored iris.
   - Lack of physical activity.
   - Possibly due to low intake of essential vitamins.
   - Cardiovascular disease.
   - Red or blond hair.
   - Female.
   - Caucasian.

3. **Clinical Features**
   - Hard and soft drusen on ophthalmoscopic examination.
   - Distorted images.
   - Neovascular type (wet): confluent, large soft drusen.
   - Neovascular type (dry): more rapid loss of vision.
   - Atrophic type: bilateral gradual and progressive vision loss.
   - Central vision loss, periphery remains intact.

4. **Diagnostic Studies**
   - Biomicroscopic funduscopic exam.
   - Fluorescein angiography to confirm wet age-related macular degeneration.
   - OCT to assess treatment response.

5. **Management**
   - Stop smoking and increase physical activity.
   - Eat dark green leafy vegetables and take antioxidants, zinc, copper, carotenoids.
   - Avoid excessive sunlight.
   - Consult retina specialist.

J. Papilledema

1. **Definition**
   - Increased intracranial pressure that causes swelling of the optic disc.

2. **Etiology/Pathology**
   - Causes can be meningitis, encephalitis, pseudotumor cerebri, cerebral trauma or hemorrhage, brain tumor, or abscess.

3. Clinical Features
- Most of the time is bilateral.
- No warning symptoms except for a couple of seconds of diminished vision.
- Headache, nausea, vomiting if intracranial pressure increased.
- Tortuous retinal veins, optic disc retinal hemorrhages, swollen, and hyperemic optic disc.
- Pupillary response and visual acuity are abnormal in advanced conditions.

4. Diagnostic Studies
- Thorough ophthalmoscopic examination.
- OCT
- Neuroimaging to search for cause.
- Lumbar puncture if mass lesion ruled out.

5. Management
- Determine the cause.
- Treat the underlying condition.
- Reduce intracranial pressure.

K. Blowout Fracture
1. Definition
- Fracture of the floor of the orbit, resulting in an increase in IOP.

2. Etiology/Pathology
- Blunt force trauma against the eye.

3. Clinical Features
- Intraocular muscles and fat pads may be caught in fracture.
- Eye redness.
- Epistaxis.
- Nose, teeth, and cheek numbness.
- Nausea.
- Vomiting.
- Possible fracture of facial bones.
- Skull/brain injury.
- Eye injury.
- Enophthalmos.
- Possible infraorbital rim, upper lip, and cheek anesthesia.
- Upward gaze diplopia signifying inferior rectus muscle entrapment.
- Step off of infraorbital rim.
- Look for retinal detachment, lens dislocation, ruptured globe, and hyphema.

4. Diagnostic Studies
- Orbital CT.

5. Management
- Tetanus.
- Pain control.
- Possible prophylactic antibiotics.
- Possible oral steroids.
- Possible surgery.
- Ice.
- Decongestants.
- Educate patient on avoidance of nose blowing and valsalva.

- Consult with ophthalmologist and maxillofacial surgeon.

L. Hyphema
1. Definition
- Anterior chamber bleeding.

2. Etiology/Pathology
- Usually blunt trauma.
- Nontraumatic: newborn after stressful birth, blood dyscrasias, juvenile xanthogranuloma, herpes virus infection.

3. Clinical Features
- May be associated with other ocular injury such as retinal detachment or edema, glaucoma, subluxation of the lens, or iritis. Those patients with sickle-cell trait or anemia who have an elevated intraoculation pressure.
- Pain.
- Photophobia.
- Decreased vision.
- Blood in the anterior chamber.

4. Diagnostic Studies
- Refer to ophthalmologist.
- Possible CT.

5. Management
- Refer to ophthalmologist.
- Shield over eye, head elevated.
- Bedrest.

II. Ear
THE EXTERNAL EAR
A. Otitis Externa
1. Etiology
- A bacterial infection of the external auditory canal.
- Fungal infection.
- Swimming or use of cotton-tipped applicators removes the protective layer of cerumen, resulting in maceration.
- Trauma, eczema, foreign body, otorrhea, and contact dermatitis are contributing factors.

2. Pathology
- *Pseudomonas aeruginosa.*
- *S. aureus.*
- *Streptococcus.*
- *Moraxella catarrhalis.*
- *H. influenzae.*
- *Proteus.*
- Chronic cases are fungal: *Candida, Aspergillus.*

3. Clinical Features
- Localized infection sometimes forming a boil, called furunculosis, which causes pain on pushing on the tragus.
- Generalized, painful.
- May note drainage at the opening of the external auditory canal.
- Hearing not affected, or minimal.

- Swelling of the canal.
- Discharge noted in the canal.
- Facial nerve function should be normal.
- Severe infection may show signs of auricular or postauricular cellulitis, which may resemble a mastoid abscess.
- Malignant external otitis is a separate entity caused by *P. aeruginosa* in patients with diabetes, which results in erosion of tissue and bone and needs immediate attention by an otolaryngologist.
- Discharge noted in the canal.

4. **Diagnostic Studies**
   - Cultures in cases of treatment failures or refractory.
5. **Management**
   - Cortisporin otic (if tympanic membrane [TM] is intact). Ofloxacin otic or Cipro HC Otic can be used. Ofloxacin otic is the drug of choice when a perforated TM cannot be ruled out.
   - Systemic antibiotics in case of cellulitis, or possible system involvement.
   - Refer resistant cases to an ear, nose, and throat (ENT) specialist.
   - Oral analgesics if needed for pain.
   - Educate patient on not getting water in ear.
   - Remove purulent debris.
   - No swimming until completion of antibiotics.
   - Recommend baths instead of showers.
   - Educate patient on not storing medications in the refrigerator.

B. **Foreign Body**
1. **Etiology**
   - Most often seen in children.
2. **Pathology**
   - Foreign body of metallic origin.
   - Foreign body of plant or organic matter.
3. **Clinical Features**
   - May have conductive hearing loss.
   - May have otalgia or discharge if secondarily infected.
   - Bleeding is possible if the object is sharp.
4. **Diagnostic Studies**
   - None.
5. **Management**
   - For solid material, a loop, or a hook, or an alligator forceps may be used. Be careful not to rupture TM; may irrigate if it is a rounded object, such as a bead.
   - Do not put water in the ear if the foreign body is of organic matter; it will cause the object to swell.
   - If an insect is the foreign body, lidocaine or mineral oil can be used to immobilize the insect before removal.
   - Irrigation (use room temperature sterile water or normal saline) if TM is intact.
   - After removal of foreign body, otic topical antibiotics with steroid can be prescribed.

C. **Neoplasm**
1. **Etiology**
   - Chronic irritation.
   - Sun exposure.
2. **Pathology**
   - Most common carcinomas of ear canal are squamous cell.
3. **Clinical Features**
   - Can mimic a persistent otitis externa.
   - Extremely high 5-year mortality rate.
   - The neoplasm spreads to the cranial base lymphatics rapidly.
   - May cause conductive hearing loss from buildup of debris and exudates.
   - Biopsy is warranted if otitis externa does not resolve with appropriate therapy.
4. **Diagnostic Studies**
   - Biopsy.
5. **Management**
   - Proper and timely referral to the ENT department.
   - Wide surgical resection.
   - Radiation therapy.

D. **Hearing Impairment (Table 11–1)**
1. **Etiology**
   a. **Conductive**
      - Foreign body, cerumen impaction, otitis media, perforation or immobilization of the TM, otosclerosis, ossicular discontinuity/fixation, or tumors.
      - Usually has a history of previous ear disease.
      - Onset in childhood to age 40.
   b. **Sensorineural**
      - Common causes include natural aging (presbycusis), drugs (e.g., aspirin, aminoglycosides, gentamycin), head trauma, excessive noise exposure, and acoustic neuroma.
      - Onset from middle to late years.
2. **Pathology**
   a. **Conductive Loss**
      - Disruption of the external or middle ear, impairing sound conduction to the inner ear.
      - Sound wave conduction is obstructed by canal obstruction, fluid in middle ear, or ossicular disease such as otosclerosis.
   b. **Sensorineural Loss**
      - Impaired nerve impulse transmission to the brain; inner ear or cochlear nerve disorder losses of both air and bone thresholds are diminished.
      - Seen in damage or dysfunction to cochlea/hair cells and eighth cranial nerve disease/trauma, tumors such as acoustic neuroma or CNS disease.
      - Systemic causes such as diabetes mellitus.
3. **Clinical Features**
   a. **Conductive**
      - Examination of auditory canal may disclose foreign body, cerumen impaction, otitis externa, or exostosis.

TABLE 11–1. **Patterns of Hearing Loss**

	Conductive Loss	Sensorineural Loss
Impaired understanding of words	Minor	Often troublesome
Effect of noisy environment	May help	Increases the hearing difficulty
Usual age of onset	Childhood, young adulthood	Middle and old age
Ear canal and drum	Often a visible abnormality	Problem not visible
Weber test (in unilateral hearing loss)	Lateralizes to the impaired ear	Lateralizes to the good ear
Rinne test	BC > AC or BC = AC	AC > BC
Causes	Plugged ear canal, otitis media, immobile or perforated drum, otosclerosis, foreign body	Sustained loud noise, drugs, inner ear infections, trauma, hereditary disorder, aging

AC, air conduction; BC, bone conduction.
From Bickley LS, Szilagyi PG. *Bates' Pocket Guide to Physical Examination and History Taking.* 5th ed. Philadelphia, PA: Lippincott Williams & Wilkins; 2007:114, with permission.

- Examination of TM may disclose bulging, perforation, scarring, inflammation, fluid levels, or hemotympanum.

b. **Conductive Loss**
  - Weber test: sound lateralizes to affected ear (Figure 11–9).
  - Rinne test: bone conduction (BC) > air conduction (AC) or BC = AC (negative Rinne) (Figure 11–10).

c. **Sensorineural**
  - Upper tones are lost.
  - Gradually progressive.
  - May occur suddenly and needs immediate attention by an otolaryngologist.
  - Usually bilateral and symmetric, but one side may start first or be worse than the other.
  - More difficult to hear in noisy environment.

- Patient has difficulty hearing own voice.
- May have a history of excessive noise exposure, inner ear infections, trauma, and use of medications such as salicylates, aminoglycosides, quinine derivatives, and loop diuretics.
- Nothing can be found on physical examination of the ear.

d. **Sensorineural Loss**
  - Weber test: sound lateralizes to the good ear.
  - Rinne test: AC > BC (positive Rinne).

4. **Diagnostic Studies**
  - Audiogram: establishes pattern of hearing loss. Normal hearing: 0 to 20 dB. Severe loss by a threshold of 60 to 80 dB.
  - MRI: used to rule out multiple sclerosis or acoustic neuroma in certain cases.
  - CT scans: used in middle-ear and mastoid problems.

5. **Management**
  - Conductive hearing loss can be usually resolved with medical and/or surgical measures (cerumen

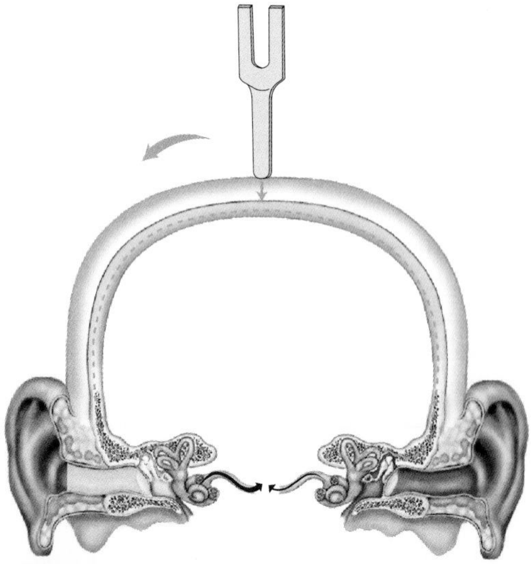

FIGURE 11–9. **Weber test.** (From Bickley LS, Szilagyi PG. *Bates' Guide to Physical Examination and History Taking.* 8th ed. Philadelphia, PA: Lippincott Williams & Wilkins; 2003, with permission.)

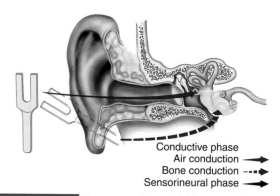

FIGURE 11–10. **Rinne test.** (From Bickley LS, Szilagyi PG. *Bates' Guide to Physical Examination and History Taking.* 8th ed. Philadelphia, PA: Lippincott Williams & Wilkins; 2003, with permission.)

or foreign-body removal, topical antibiotics for otitis externa).
- ENT referral for conditions not responsive to treatment and for sensorineural hearing losses, especially sudden hearing loss.
- Sensorineural hearing losses may be stabilized.
- Routine audiograms for those exposed to high levels of noise.
- Amplification or hearing aids.
- Cochlear implant for those with significant sensorineural hearing loss.

E. Hematoma of the External Ear
1. **Etiology**
   - Due to trauma.
   - Hematoma develops between the cartilage and the perichondrium.
2. **Clinical Features**
   - Purplish swelling of the upper part of the ear.
   - Obscured cartilage folds.
3. **Management**
   - Refer to an ENT physician.
   - Aspiration of the area with specifically applied pressure dressing.
   - Recurrent hematomas require surgical drainage.

THE MIDDLE EAR

A. Otitis Media
1. **Etiology**
   - Common in children (90% before the age of 6), although it can occur in adults.
   - Adults usually develop otitis media when they have had several infections as a child.
   - Higher risk for children with cleft palates, immune disorders, or Down syndrome.
   - Children feeding in less than an upright position are more predisposed to infections.
   - Upper respiratory infection (URI) predisposes, as well as day-care attendance.
   - Peaks in winter and spring.
   - Children with allergies (particularly those with large adenoids).
   - Exposed to smoking, including wood-burning stoves.
   - Familial.
   - Bacterial infection of middle ear.
   - Incidence decreases with age.
   - If unilateral in adult, ENT referral to rule out nasopharyngeal tumor.
2. **Pathology**
   - Eustachian tubes are narrow, more horizontal, and short.
   - Eustachian tubes can be obstructed secondary to large adenoids, causing poor drainage.
   - Most common causative organisms include *S. pneumoniae*, *H. influenzae*, and *S. pyogenes*.
   - Acute otitis media, viral in nature (respiratory syncytial virus [RSV]), can cause 25% of the cases seen.

- Eustachian tube malfunction causes a buildup of mucus and fluid, which becomes secondarily infected by bacteria.
3. **Clinical Features**
   - In younger patients, it can be associated with conductive hearing loss, resulting in cognitive learning problems and deficiency in verbal abilities.
   - URI with runny nose and congestion may be associated.
   - Conjunctival inflammation.
   - May be asymptomatic.
   - Sometimes systemic with diarrhea and/or vomiting.
   - Difficulty hearing.
   - Otalgia.
   - Check for dental problems, tonsillitis, cervical lymphadenopathy, and retropharyngeal cancer.
   - Infection may present as irritability and fever.
   - TM is often bulging and erythematous with decreased or poor light reflex.
   - Decreased visible landmarks.
   - May see cloudy, purulent fluid behind TM.
   - Possibility exists for rupture of the TM.
   - Decreased TM mobility on pneumatic insufflation.
   - Pain may precede redness.
   - Check gross hearing and whisper tests.
   - Otalgia should resolve after 24 hours.
4. **Diagnostic Studies**
   - No studies are necessary unless the child is appearing ill; refer to ENT for tympanocentesis.
   - Check for iron-deficiency anemia if the child has had multiple episodes of acute otitis media.
   - Tympanometry, if available.
   - ENTs will order a CT or MRI to check for tumors, nerve damage.
5. **Management**
   - Analgesics/antipyretics (i.e., Tylenol, codeine if necessary).
   - Auralgan every 2 hours may be used topically for ear pain.
   - Antibiotics (amoxicillin, amoxicillin/clavulanate potassium).
   - In the case of a penicillin allergy, use trimethoprim-sulfamethoxazole (TMP-SMZ) or erythromycin.
   - Reevaluate if pain and fever persist after 3 days of treatment.
   - Decongestants (e.g., oral pseudoephedrine or oxymetazoline 0.05% topical in nose) relieve URI or Eustachian tube blockage.
   - Avoid antihistamines: may cause thickened secretions.
   - Myringotomy: use in patients with increased hearing loss, poor response to medical therapy, or intractable pain.

B. Serous Otitis Media

1. **Etiology**
   - Common in children because Eustachian tube is smaller and more horizontal.
   - In adults with unilateral serous otitis media, nasopharyngeal carcinoma must be ruled out.
   - Viral.
   - Mycoplasmal.
   - May occur in adults after flying due to a barotrauma, allergens, or an URI.
2. **Pathology**
   - Serous or mucoid secretions filling middle ear and interfering with the TM movement and ossicular chain function, resulting in conductive hearing loss.
   - Often due to Eustachian tube blockage or dysfunction, resulting in negative pressure.
   - Common in adults after having viral URI or barotrauma.
3. **Clinical Features**
   - No acute symptoms. In children, usually discovered when the child first goes to school and hearing loss is suspected by the teacher.
   - Conductive hearing loss.
   - TM may be retracted, clear, or dull with bony landmarks intact.
   - May have clear fluid behind TM or air bubbles.
   - Decreased tympanic mobility.
   - Fever and pain are not present.
4. **Diagnostic Studies**
   - Tympanogram diagnostic, and should be done in all suspected cases.
5. **Management**
   - Oral/topical decongestants used in Eustachian tube blockage.
   - Some practitioners use short courses of oral steroids (prednisone) and/or antibiotics (amoxicillin, Augmentin, or TMP-SMZ).
   - Laser expansion via endoscopy in recalcitrant cases.
   - Ventilation tubes if medical treatment fails.

C. TM Rupture

1. **Etiology**
   - Usually due to acute otitis media.
2. **Clinical Features**
   - Discharge noted.
   - Possible conductive hearing loss.
3. **Diagnostics**
   - Possibly an audiogram.
4. **Management**
   - Most perforations heal within 2 weeks.
   - Wear ear plugs for bathing.
   - Surgical repair for those perforations that do not heal in 3 to 6 months or if audiogram is at or above 30 dBs.
   - Refer to ENT for surgical repair and timing.

D. Cholesteatoma

1. **Etiology**
   - Prolonged dysfunction of the Eustachian tube.
2. **Clinical Features**
   - Squamous epithelium-lined sac develops and then fills with desquamated keratin when obstructed.
   - Chronically infected.
   - Erodes bone.
   - Penetrates mastoid and ossicular chain.
   - Can cause facial paralysis if left untreated.
   - Retraction pocket of epitympanic.
   - Keratin or granulation tissue from perforated TM.
3. **Diagnostic Studies**
   - Refer to ENT.
4. **Management**
   - Refer to ENT.
   - Surgery.

E. Mastoiditis

1. **Etiology**
   - Inflammation of the mastoid.
   - Mainly in children under 2 years of age.
   - Inadequate treatment of acute otitis media.
2. **Pathology**
   - *S. pneumoniae.*
   - *S. pyogenes.*
   - *H. influenzae.*
   - Occasionally gram-negative bacilli and anaerobes.
3. **Clinical Features**
   - Preauricular pain.
   - Fever.
   - Erythema and tenderness of the mastoid process.
   - Pinna displaced outward.
   - Acute otitis media.
   - Meningitis and brain abscess are complications.
4. **Diagnostic Studies**
   - CT scan.
5. **Management**
   - IV antibiotics.
   - Myringotomy with drainage and culture.
   - Mastoidectomy if treatment fails.

THE INNER EAR

A. Labyrinthitis

1. **Etiology**
   - Mainly viral.
   - Can be caused by bacteria, although unusual.
   - Common in adolescents and young adults.
   - Familial and/or seasonal.
   - History of URI, otitis media, or sinusitis.
   - Paralysis of the vestibular nerve.
   - Trauma to head or ear.
   - Benign middle ear tumor.
   - Alcohol abuse.
2. **Pathology**
   - Vestibular neural input disrupted to the cerebral cortex and brain stem.

- Secondary to a URI that consists of infection of the labyrinth.
- Vertigo is caused by edema and inflammation.
- Viral infection that affects the cochlea and labyrinth.

3. **Clinical Features**
   - History of URI.
   - Self-limiting.
   - May last 7 to 10 days.
   - During recovery period, sudden rapid movements of head can bring on transient vertigo.
   - Vital signs: may have orthostatic changes.
   - Nausea and vomiting.
   - Subsequent episodes can occur 12 to 18 months after the initial episode. Each episode is less severe and shorter in duration.
   - Vertigo.
   - Nystagmus (rotary away from affected ear).
   - Neurologic deficits are uncommon; CNS assessment usually is normal.
   - CNS abnormality suggests a central process.
   - Detailed history to rule out psychiatric, cardiovascular, pulmonary, CNS, or metabolic disorders.
   - Comprehensive physical examination including head, ears, eyes, nose, and throat (HEENT), neuro with mental status examination, hearing and speech evaluation.

4. **Diagnostic Studies**
   - Audiologic testing.
   - Electronystagmography (ENG), depending on findings.
   - CT scan or MRI may be warranted based on the undetermined or determined neurologic findings.

5. **Management**
   - Use of methylprednisolone is possible to decrease inflammation.
   - Antibiotics if febrile.
   - Antihistamines, antiemetics, and anticholinergics.
   - If ill, may require hospitalization.
   - Epley maneuver.
   - Patient reassurance.

B. **Ménière Syndrome**
   1. **Etiology**
      - Malfunction of the endolymphatics.
      - Condition affecting the inner ear.
      - May be associated with trauma, syphilis, or may be idiopathic or autoimmune.
      - Occurs mainly in middle age.
      - Males > females.
      - Caucasians have the syndrome more frequently.
      - Inherited, history of allergies, or exposure to noise.
      - No differentiation between ears.
      - Bilateral in 20% of patients.
   2. **Pathology**
      - Imbalance in secretion and absorption of endolymphatic fluid that causes buildup of fluid in cochlea.

- Associated hair-cell damage as a result of semicircular duct swelling.
- Distention of endolymphatic compartment of inner ear.

3. **Clinical Features**
   - Vertigo is sudden, lasting 1 to 8 hours, and can be debilitating. Patient feels as if everything is moving.
   - Vestibular nystagmus.
   - Fullness or pressure in the ears.
   - Nausea and vomiting are possible.
   - Tinnitus.
   - Fluctuant sensorineural hearing loss.
   - HEENT, hearing acuity, speech discrimination, neurologic examination with reflexes, mental status examination, and gait should be checked. Also, the cardiovascular, pulmonary, endocrine, and psychological status of the patient should be evaluated.

4. **Diagnostic Studies**
   - ENG.
   - Audiometry.
   - EEG.
   - Rotational testing.
   - CT or MRI to rule out lesions.

5. **Management**
   - Decrease the endolymphatic hydrops.
   - Valium 5 mg IM or 10 mg PO.
   a. **Anticholinergics**
      - Antivert 25 to 50 mg q6h.
      - Low-sodium diet (goal of therapy is to decrease endolymphatic pressure).
      - Most cases can be corrected with the diuretic and low-sodium diet.
      - Avoid caffeine, alcohol, and smoking.
      - Advise patient to get enough sleep.
      - Manage stress.
      - ENT referral.
      - If medical therapy is not effective, surgical intervention may be considered.
   b. **Vestibular Neurectomy**
      - Labyrinthectomy is the "gold standard" if hearing is already lost.
      - Resection of the eighth cranial nerve is possible, but has complications.

C. **Tinnitus**
   1. **Etiology**
      - A symptom present in ear disease.
      - Abnormal noises are heard in the head or ears.
      - Characterized as a "ringing" in the ears.
      - Important but nonspecific and has many causes.
      - Can be caused by pathology of external ear with extension to the inner ear and CNS pathology.
      - Cause may also be psychogenic, cerebrovascular (e.g., aneurysm), or musculoskeletal (e.g., temporomandibular joint dysfunction).

2. **Pathology**
   - Condition may originate in outer, middle, or inner ear, or within the nerve supply of the ear (CN III).
   - Also consider glomus tumors, cerebral vascular disease, carotid bruit, flow impedance disorders, arteriovenous malformation, and aneurysm if pulsatile.
3. **Clinical Features**
   - May have a history of occupational exposure to noise.
   - May have a history of use of ototoxic drugs.
   - May find cerumen impaction, foreign body, otitis media, or ruptured TM.
   - Often have accompanied sensory hearing loss.
   - Occasional high-pitched ringing is normal.
   - If severe, concentration or sleep may be affected.
4. **Diagnostic Studies**
   - ENT referral.
   - Audiogram.
   - MRI.
   - Venography.
5. **Management**
   - Treat underlying cause.
   - Change ototoxic medicines.
   - Noise protection.
   - Several drugs have been tested, but a question of efficacy exists; antidepressants (e.g., nortriptyline) may be tried in severe cases.
   - May need ENT referral, especially if basic measures are not successful or if tinnitus becomes debilitating.
   - Hearing aid.
   - Antidepressants have been effective in treatment.
   - Habituation technique.

D. **Vertigo**
1. **Etiology**
   - Symptom of vestibular disease.
   - Sensation of motion, spinning, or tilting.
   - Perception of things spinning around the patient.
   - Can be due to peripheral or central lesions.
   - Peripheral causes usually have sudden onset.
2. **Pathology**
   - Pathology of inner ear (e.g., labyrinthitis, Ménière syndrome).
   - Pathology of eighth cranial nerve (i.e., acoustic neuroma, vasculitis, metastatic disease).
   - CNS pathology (i.e., occlusion of vertebral and posterior inferior cerebellar artery), cerebellar disease, brain stem lesions.
   - Triggers: high-sodium diet, fatigue, stress, bright lights.
   - Must rule out systemic disease: hypoglycemia, headache disorder (migraine), postural hypotension, seizure disorder, anemia, electrolyte abnormalities.
   - Can be part of a side effect of medications including tranquilizers, antibiotics, anticonvulsants, and analgesics.

3. **Clinical Features**
   - May be so severe that the patient cannot stand or walk.
   - May have associated nausea and vomiting.
   - May have nystagmus; in peripheral lesions, nystagmus is usually horizontal or rotational; in central lesions, nystagmus can be bidirectional or vertical.
   - Patient may have associated tinnitus with hearing loss.
   - Systemic causes may have palpitation, irregular pulse, signs consistent with congestive heart failure, and decreased cardiac volume; symptoms usually improve upon lying down.
   - Need to look at gait, conduct the Romberg test, and evaluate for nystagmus.
4. **Diagnostic Studies**
   - ENG, MRI, vestibular-evoked myogenic potentials, caloric stimulation, and audiometry.
5. **Management**
   - Diagnose underlying cause.
   - In acute situations, Meclizine, Dramamine, scopolamine; these drugs may slow down long-term recovery.
   - Vitamin D may be helpful.
   - Avoid alcohol, caffeine, and tobacco.
   - Use antibiotics if middle ear infection is present.
   - Antihistamines may be possible.
   - Antidepressants: in some cases.
   - Otolaryngologic consult.

E. **Acoustic Neuroma**
1. **Etiology**
   - Schwannoma of the eighth cranial nerve.
   - Unilateral.
   - Hereditary syndrome possibly associated.
2. **Pathology**
   - Internal auditory canal benign lesions.
3. **Clinical Features**
   - Unilateral hearing loss.
   - Deterioration of speech discrimination.
   - Vestibular dysfunction more as disequilibrium rather than vertigo.
4. **Diagnostic Studies**
   - Enhanced MRI.
5. **Management**
   - Observation.
   - Excision or stereotactic radiotherapy.
   - Vascular endothelial growth factor blocker for those with hereditary syndrome.

F. **Dysfunction of the Eustachian Tubes**
1. **Etiology**
   - URI.
   - Allergies.
   - Trapped air in the middle ear results in negative pressure.
2. **Clinical Features**
   - Ear fullness.
   - Decreased hearing.

- Retraction and decreased mobility of the TM.
- If partial block, ears will pop and crackle.
  3. **Management**
  - Systemic decongestants.
  - Intranasal decongestants.
  - Allergy patients can use intranasal corticosteroids.

G. Barotrauma
  1. **Etiology**
  - Inability to equalize pressure in the ears.
  - Attributed to flying, underwater diving, or rapid change in altitude.
  2. **Clinical Features**
  - Ear fullness.
  3. **Management**
  - Attempt to yawn, swallow, or autoinflate.
  - Decongestant or nasal spray.
  - If on-the-ground and the above treatment fails, myringotomy or insertion of tubes.
  - Avoid diving if URI or allergies.

III. Nose

INFLAMMATORY DISEASE

A. Allergic Rhinitis
  1. **Etiology**
  - Common.
  - Nasal mucosa membranes affected.
  - Affects all ages, mostly during adolescence and early adulthood.
  - Airborne particles inhaled, causing immunoglobulin E (IgE)-mediated response in the nasal mucosa.
  - Two subgroups: perennial and seasonal.
  - Most common in spring to late summer.
  - Mold spores/plant pollens.
  2. **Pathology**
  - Allergen enters through the nose, is trapped by mucosa of turbinates, eliciting IgE-mediated response; mast cells release mediators and histamines.
  - Tissue edema and eosinophil infiltration results, causing itching, increased nasal secretions, and sneezing.
  - Allergens: tree pollens, ragweed, grass.
  - Present in work or home environment: dust, animal dander, mold spores, mites, and chemical agents occasionally.
  - Antigen exposure causes degranulation of mast cells, releasing histamine as well as various other inflammatory mediators, which set off a cascade of inflammatory responses.
  - Allergens usually are small particles ($<50\ \mu$m), which enables them to be airborne easily.
  - These allergens are usually present in the environment in large amounts.
  - Ragweed is the most significant cause in the Midwestern and Eastern United States in late summer

through early fall, whereas grass pollen is most significant in late spring through early summer.
  3. **Clinical Features**
  - Clear, watery nasal discharge.
  - Sneezing: more apt to occur in early morning hours.
  - Sensation of plugged ears, postnasal drip, and nasal congestion.
  - Itching of nose, palate, and throat.
  - Nasal mucosa pale or blue in color, boggy, and edematous.
  - Conjunctival injection with tearing.
  - Alteration or loss of smell.
  4. **Diagnostic Studies**
  - Allergy skin testing.
  - Radioallergosorbent testing: usually reserved for children, patients, or both, who cannot undergo skin testing (e.g., dermatographism, eczematoid dermatitis); may be used as screening examination if skin testing is not available.
  - Nasal smear examination for eosinophils.
  5. **Management**
  - Intranasal corticosteroid sprays (fluticasone propionate, flunisolide, beclomethasone).
  - H_1 receptor antagonists (fexofenadine, cetirizine, loratadine).
  - H_1 receptor antagonist sprays can also be effective (azelastine, levocabastine), or adjunct therapy such as intranasal anticholinergic agents.
  - Attempt to maintain allergen-free environment (e.g., cover pillows and mattresses with plastic covers, avoid or get rid of household pets, avoid damp environments).
  - Air purifiers may help.
  - Keep humidity low ($<50\%$ prevents mold and dust mites).
  - Use air conditioners, especially in sleeping areas.
  - Antihistamines, topical nasal steroids.
  - Cromolyn sodium can be used as an adjunct.
  - Treat any concurrent sinusitis.
  - Immunotherapy for pharmacotherapy failures.

B. Nasal Polyposis
  1. **Etiology**
  - Associated with allergies in 40% of patients with sinus infection.
  - Associated with asthma, aspirin intolerance, and alcohol intolerance.
  - Exact cause unknown, although strangulation of the swollen mucosa as it bulges through the small ostia of the ethmoid sinuses may be the cause.
  - The mucosa will swell due to infection, viruses, allergens, and environmental conditions.
  - Genetic predisposition exists.
  - If present in children, suspect cystic fibrosis.
  - Polyps can recur postsurgical excision.

2. **Pathology**
   - Composed of edematous stroma; within this stroma, numerous eosinophils, lymphocytes, neutrophils, and plasma cells are present.
   - Recurrent episodes of rhinosinusitis can cause development of polyps.
   - Frequently polyps are a primary phenomenon and cause secondary rhinosinusitis.
3. **Clinical Features**
   - Mucosal covered, pale, edematous mass.
   - May be multiple.
   - Hyposmia/anosmia.
   - Nasal mucosa may be boggy.
   - Nasal obstruction.
   - If polyp is extremely large, the patient may be a mouth breather.
   - Occasionally, polyps become so edematous and they protrude from the nostril.
4. **Diagnostic Studies**
   - Nasal endoscopy.
   - CT scan.
   - Run sweat test if cystic fibrosis is suspected.
5. **Management**
   - Topical nasal corticosteroid sprays 1 to 3 months for small polyps.
   - Oral steroid therapy: short course.
   - Treat allergies, if present.
   - Oral doxycycline can assist in reducing the size of polyp(s).
   - Refer to otolaryngologist.
   - If patient has polyps and asthma, do not give acetylsalicylic acid (ASA) for any reason because this can cause bronchospasm.
   - If medical management fails, surgical removal may be necessary. If the patient has recurrent polyps or is at high risk, an ethmoidectomy may be indicated.

TRAUMA

A. Epistaxis
1. **Etiology**
   - Nose bleeding from infection, trauma, allergic rhinitis, foreign body, renal failure, abnormal anatomical features, coagulation problems, alcohol abuse, inhaling street drugs, some medications (e.g., nasal corticosteroid spray, NSAIDs), nasal defects, hypertension, atherosclerotic cardiovascular disease, heredity hemorrhagic telangiectasia, or tumors.
   - Use of blood thinners and anticoagulants.
2. **Pathology**
   a. **Anterior Epistaxis**
      - Originates from the anterior aspect of the nose; Kiesselbach plexus bleeding is the most common location.
   b. **Posterior Epistaxis**
      - Usual source is from a nasal branch of the sphenopalatine artery and associated with hypertension and atherosclerotic disease.

3. **Clinical Features**
   a. **Anterior Epistaxis**
      - Patient may have a history of recent URI, trauma, or allergy exacerbation.
      - May have a history of recent use of inhaled irritants (i.e., cocaine, nasal sprays).
      - Bleeding from anterior nares, usually unilateral, with no sensation of blood dripping down the back of the throat.
      - Blood is bright red.
   b. **Posterior Epistaxis**
      - An anterior site of bleeding is not visualized.
      - Patient has blood dripping down the back of the throat.
      - Patient expectorates blood.
      - Blood is dark red.
4. **Diagnostic Studies**
   - Hemoglobin and hematocrit for baseline.
   - If patient is under the age of 2 or has a family history of bleeding disorders, full workup is needed.
5. **Management**
   a. **Anterior Epistaxis**
      - Direct pressure.
      - Use of vasoconstrictive and anesthetic agents.
      - Chemical, electrical, or thermal cautery.
      - Anterior nasal packing with petroleum jelly gauze with antibiotic prophylaxis (e.g., Augmentin).
      - Short-acting topical nasal decongestant.
      - Gelfoam or Surgicel may be used.
      - Avoid NSAIDs, ASA, and nose blowing.
   b. **Posterior Epistaxis**
      - Posterior balloon with petrolatum gauze packed in the anterior nose.
      - Posterior nasal packing.
      - Epistat if no mucosal tear.
      - Opioids may be needed.
      - Immediate referral to otolaryngologist.
      - Check arterial blood gas.
      - Hospitalization for observation.
      - Continuous oxygen (O_2) saturation monitoring due to the possibility of respiratory failure leading to death.

B. Foreign Body of the Nose
1. **Etiology**
   - Usually a bead or seed is placed in the nose.
2. **Clinical Features**
   - Foul-smelling discharge from affected nostril.
   - Rhinorrhea.
   - Bleeding.
   - Halitosis.
   - Possible nasal obstruction.
3. **Management**
   - Older children can try to blow their nose to dislodge foreign body.
   - Removal of foreign body with the use of topical anesthesia, nasal decongestion, restraints, and good lighting.

- If foreign body is wedged in, refer to ENT.
- If a battery-operated foreign body is in the nose, it has to be removed within 4 hours. A battery itself is a true emergency.

IV. Sinuses
A. Rhinosinusitis
1. **Etiology**
   - Inflammation or infection of the paranasal sinuses (one or both) affecting both adults and children.
   - Viral URI is the most common cause.
   - Predisposing factors: allergic sinusitis, nonallergic sinusitis, immune deficiency, anatomical anomalies.
   - Poor draining abilities result in bacterial overgrowth secondary to mucus accumulation.
   - Maxillary sinuses are the most common site of infection, 25% of which is a result of dental causes.
   - More difficult to drain maxillary sinuses because the cilia are moving against gravity toward the upper-placed sinus ostium.
2. **Pathology**
   - The four paranasal sinuses (ethmoid, maxillary, sphenoid, and frontal) drain into the nasal cavity.
   - Partial or complete obstruction due to mucosal swelling that narrows the ostia.
   - Respiratory mucosa and cilia line the sinuses, enabling the mucous to be sent toward the ostia to drain.
   - The ostiomeatal complex is the most common site for obstruction.
   - Main pathogens are *S. pneumoniae* and *H. influenzae*.
   - Increase in β-lactamase producing *H. influenzae*.
   - *S. pneumoniae*, *M. catarrhalis*, and *H. influenzae* most common organisms in children.
   - Bacterial sinusitis can develop from a viral sinusitis.
   - *S. aureus* and respiratory anaerobes more frequently present in chronic sinusitis.
3. **Clinical Features**
   a. **Acute**
      - Headache, facial pain/pressure over sinus area, nasal congestion, cough, purulent nasal drainage or postnasal drip, pain/pressure on bending over or lying down. Halitosis and low-grade fever are possible.
      - Dental pain, ear popping, fatigue, fever (children).
      - History of recent URI or allergic rhinitis.
      - On physical examination: examination of the nose, ears, throat, lungs, and neuro is important for headache/facial pain complaints. Check dentition. Percussion for tenderness over frontal and/or maxillary sinuses. Percussion may or may not elicit pain; transillumination does not work well.

   b. **Chronic**
      - Persistent infection or inflammation; subtle, nonspecific signs and symptoms.
      - Purulent postnasal drip, headache, nasal congestion, sinus pressure, coughing, clearing of throat, sore throat, decrease or loss of smell, malaise.
      - Symptoms longer than 12 weeks.
4. **Diagnostic Studies**
   - Sinus X-rays: Caldwell (frontal), submentovertical (ethmoid), Waters (maxillary), and lateral (sphenoid); check for air–fluid levels, mucosal thickening, or opacification; films may be normal despite diagnosis of sinusitis.
   - CT scan of coronal plane can be used only in acute complicated sinusitis, recurrent or chronic sinusitis; cost is equal to that of four plain sinus X-rays.
   - If malignancy is suspected, MRI with gadolinium is recommended.
5. **Management**
   - Fourteen days of oral antibiotics for acute sinusitis; 4 to 6 weeks for chronic disease.
   - In treatment, consider the severity, duration, and frequency of the infection; age of the patient; underlying conditions; history; and response to previous treatment.
   - Amoxicillin 250 to 500 mg PO TID; macrolides for penicillin allergic individuals.
   - Bactrim or Septra 80 to 160 trimethoprim, 400 to 800 sulfamethoxazole PO BID.
   - Augmentin 250 to 500 PO TID for β-lactamase-inhibiting properties.
   - Macrolides if penicillin allergy.
   - Fluoroquinolones if treatment fails.
   - Oral or nasal decongestants.
   - Mucolytics.
   - Avoid antihistamines.
   - Acetaminophen or ibuprofen can be used for headache/facial pain.
   - Topical corticosteroids for chronic (not acute).
   - IV antibiotics if frontal sinuses infected and not responding to treatment.
   - Surgery if all other treatments fail.
   - Otolaryngologic evaluation if no response to medical regimen, disease suspected outside the sinus cavity, or for chronic disease.

V. Mouth
INFLAMMATORY LESIONS
A. Herpetic Stomatitis
1. **Etiology**
   - Common viral infection of the mouth.
   - Most often occurs in children and young adults.
   - Can occur in immunocompromised patients.

2. **Pathology**
- Caused by the herpes simplex virus (HSV-1 or HSV-2).
- HSV infects the trigeminal nerve ganglion and can remain dormant for long periods.
- Triggers: immunosuppression, trauma, fatigue, fever, cold, UV light, stress.

3. **Clinical Features**
- Widespread gingivostomatitis.
- Painful lesions.
- Burning sensation.
- Multiple vesicles that rupture to form ulcer.
- Irritability.
- Fever.
- Headache.
- Drooling.
- Difficulty swallowing.
- Arthralgias.
- Pharyngitis.
- Cervical lymphadenopathy.
- Repeated recurrences.

4. **Diagnostic Studies**
- None.

5. **Management**
- Self-limited.
- Analgesics.
- Hydration.
- Acyclovir can be used.
- Viscous lidocaine if severe pain.

B. **Herpes Simplex**

1. **Etiology**
- Viral infection.

2. **Pathology**
- HSV, type 1 or type 2.
- Occurs 2 to 20 days postexposure.

3. **Clinical Features**
- Grouped vesicles on the lips, buccal mucosa, or both, which erupt, producing flat ulcers.
- Most commonly seen at the vermillion border.
- Fever.
- Headache.
- Malaise.
- Repeated recurrences.
- May be associated with erythema multiforme

4. **Diagnostic Studies**
- Tzanck smear of lesion confirmatory.
- Smear shows multinucleated giant cells.

5. **Management**
- Self-limited.
- Can consider giving acyclovir 200 mg five times a day for 5 days, famciclovir 125 mg BID for 5 days, or valacyclovir 500 mg BID for 5 days.
- Patient education regarding prevention of transmission.

C. **Oral Candidiasis**

1. **Etiology**
- Represents an opportunistic infection in infants, leukocyte disorders, denture wearers, patients with anemia, poor oral hygiene, nutritional deficiencies, use of corticosteroids or antibiotics, and immunocompromised persons (i.e., patients with AIDS, chemotherapy or radiation therapy recipients, patients with diabetes).

2. **Pathology**
- Inflammation and edema of the underlying epithelium.

3. **Clinical Features**
- Occurs when defenses are lowered in the host.
- Difficult to tolerate hot and cold beverages and solid food.
- Tongue may be depapillated, shiny, and smooth.
- Can occur on any mucosal surface.
- Usually painful.
- White patches that leave a raw, inflamed area if rubbed off.
- Mucosa may be normal or erythematous.

4. **Diagnostic Studies**
- Potassium hydroxide prep if unsure of diagnosis.
- Prep will disclose spores.

5. **Management**
- Topical (clotrimazole troches) or systemic antifungal therapy (fluconazole by mouth, particularly if the esophagus is involved).
- Nystatin powder for denture wearers.
- If the above therapy fails or patient is immunocompromised, Amphotericin B can be given intravenously.

D. **Aphthous Ulcers (Figure 11–11)**

1. **Etiology**
- Common disorder of oral mucosa.

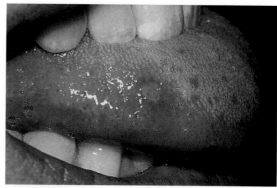

FIGURE 11–11. Aphthous stomatitis. (From Goodheart HP. *Goodheart's Photoguide of Common Skin Disorders.* 2nd ed. Philadelphia, PA: Lippincott Williams & Wilkins; 2003, with permission.)

2. **Pathology**
   - Caused by nonspecific acute inflammation, possibly herpesvirus 6.
   - Trauma.
   - Systemic disorders.
   - Nutritional deficiencies particularly B and C vitamins.
   - Hormonal fluctuations.
   - Poor oral hygiene.
3. **Clinical Features**
   - Painful, round, shallow ulcers with yellow–gray fibrinoid centers and erythematous halos.
   - Present on nonkeratinized mucosa (buccal and labial mucosa).
   - Repeated recurrences.
   - May be associated with stress.
4. **Diagnostic Studies**
   - Biopsy if no clear-cut diagnosis or if large and persistent ulcer.
5. **Management**
   - Self-limited.
   - Topical analgesics (i.e., Anbesol gel, viscous lidocaine).
   - Avoidance of spicy, hot, and citrus foods.
   - Possible use of corticosteroid gels or ointments (puts patient at risk for oral candidiasis).
   - Cimetidine can be used for maintenance if recurrent ulcers.
   - If unresponsive to treatment, laser therapy can be utilized.
   - Vitamin supplementation.
   - Biopsy if unclear diagnosis.

E. **Gingivitis**
   1. **Etiology**
      - An inflammatory periodontal disease.
   2. **Pathology**
      - Accumulation of plaque between the gingiva and teeth.
      - Misaligned teeth.
      - Trauma.
   3. **Clinical Features**
      - Bleeding gums with light contact.
      - Swollen, erythematous, and/or tender gingiva.
      - Bulbous interdental papillae.
      - Halitosis may be present.
   4. **Diagnostic Studies**
      - Dental X-rays.
      - Dental exam.
   5. **Management**
      - Referral to dentist for dental cleaning and regular follow-ups.
      - Repair of teeth or orthodontics.
      - Treat related illnesses.
      - Brush teeth at least twice daily.

   - Floss teeth nightly.
   - Use an antibacterial mouth rinse.

F. **Necrotizing Ulcerative Gingivitis (Trench Mouth)**
   1. **Etiology**
      - Occurs in young adults under stress, in malnourished persons, or underlying systemic disease.
   2. **Pathology**
      - Caused by a wide variety of spirochetes and fusiform bacilli that normally inhabit the mouth.
   3. **Clinical Features**
      - Erythema, edema, and ulceration of the gingiva.
      - Grayish membrane forms over the inflamed and ulcerated gingival margins.
      - Halitosis, fever, cervical lymphadenopathy, and malaise.
   4. **Diagnostic Studies**
      - None.
   5. **Management**
      - Correction of dietary inadequacies.
      - Alter or remove underlying factors.
      - Warm half-strength peroxide rinses.
      - Oral penicillin or tetracycline if needed.
      - Two percent viscous lidocaine.
      - Avoid irritants.
      - Dental curettage.
      - Dental follow-up.

DISEASES OF THE TEETH

A. **Dental Caries**
   1. **Etiology**
      - Decay of the tooth enamel, causing exposure of the pulp.
   2. **Pathology**
      - Caused most commonly by *Streptococcus mutans*, *Streptococcus sobrinus*, or any other acid-producing bacteria.
      - Pulp exposure if left untreated.
      - Usually fever, swelling, and pain if abscess forms from necrotic pulp.
   3. **Clinical Features**
      - Asymptomatic in early stages.
      - Toothache.
      - Sometimes tooth is decayed.
      - First visible as a chalky white deposit in the enamel surface.
      - Teeth may become brown or black and soft.
      - Percuss on tooth to pinpoint correct tooth.
      - Bone loss at advanced stages.
   4. **Diagnostic Studies**
      - X-rays.
   5. **Management**
      - Referral to dentist for repair or extraction.
      - Incision and drainage (I&D) of abscess if present.

- Root canal with crown if needed.
- Oral antibiotics.
- Oral probiotics may be useful.
- Saline rinses.
- Sealants.
- Fluoride application.
- Instruct patient on proper oral/dental hygiene.
- Modify smoking and/or intakes of foods or beverages high in sugar.
- Follow up with dentist.

B. Dental Abscess

1. Etiology
- Decay of tooth extending beyond the enamel into the dentin and finally into the tooth pulp.
- Trapped debris and plaque between gingiva and tooth.

2. Pathology
- Polymicrobial.
- Most commonly caused by *Bacteroides*, *Fusobacterium*, *Peptococcus*, *Peptostreptococcus*, and *Streptococcus viridans*.

3. Clinical Features
- Severe toothache.
- Swelling.
- Redness.
- Heat sensitivity.
- Fluctuant mass.
- Lymphadenopathy.
- Possible nausea, vomiting, chills, and fever.
- Could have respiratory difficulty.

4. Diagnostic Studies
- X-rays.
- Blood cultures may be needed.

5. Management
- Referral to dentist.
- I&D if necessary, or aspiration.
- Oral antibiotics.
- May require root canal therapy.
- NSAIDs.

C. Parotitis

1. Etiology
- Elderly who are postoperative.
- Guanethidine or iodides can cause swelling.
- Chronic cases are due to autoimmune
- processes.
- Dehydration.

2. Pathology
- Depends on the cause.
- Can be bacterial or viral.
- Polymicrobial.
- *S. aureus.*
- Mumps.

3. Clinical Features
- Pain caused by chewing.

- Progressive swelling and pain of the glands (pre- and postauricular).
- Fever.
- Viral: present bilaterally, malaise, fever, anorexia.
- Tender to palpation, erythema and swelling noted at gland on visual examination.
- Purulent saliva.

4. Diagnostic Studies
- Saliva culture and needle aspiration.
- Amylase.
- Check rheumatoid factor, anti-SS-B, and anti-SS-A.
- Sialography.
- Ultrasound.
- If suspected malignancy, CT scan and MRI with gadolinium enhancement.

5. Management
- Treat underlying condition.
- IV antibiotics.
- Possible hospitalization.
- I&D if no response in 48 hours.
- Interventional sialoendoscopy.
- Incisional biopsy.
- Surgery.
- Dental care.

D. Sialadenitis

1. Etiology
- Inflammation of the submandibular or parotid gland.
- Malnourished.
- Elderly postoperative patient.

2. Pathology
- *S. aureus.*
- Mumps.
- Influenza A.
- Epstein–Barr virus.
- Coxsackie virus A and B.

3. Clinical Features
- Swelling of the gland.
- Duct opening tenderness and erythema.
- Swelling and pain when eating.
- Usually occurs when patient in dehydrated state or has chronic illness.
- Purulent drainage.
- Chronic: low-grade fever, malaise, headache, myalgias.

4. Diagnostic Studies
- CT or ultrasound if no response to treatment.

5. Management
- Hydration.
- Gland massage.
- IV antibiotics. Less severe: oral antibiotics.
- NSAIDs for pain.
- Warm compresses.

PREMALIGNANT AND MALIGNANT LESIONS

A. Leukoplakia/Erythroplakia of Mouth and Tongue (Figure 11–12)

1. **Etiology**
   - Leukoplakia: chronic irritation of tissue (e.g., from trauma, alcohol, tobacco).
   - Leukoplakia: previous history of malignancy or premalignancy of digestive tract.
   - Erythroplakia more likely to be cancer than leukoplakia.

2. **Pathology**
   - Leukoplakia: increased thickness of the keratin layer, neovascularization.
   - Leukoplakia: if epithelial dysplasia is present, the lesion is considered precancerous.
   - Erythroplakia: usually contains squamous cell carcinoma.

3. **Clinical Features**
   - Leukoplakia is a flat or raised white lesion on the oral mucosa or tongue and cannot be removed by rubbing the surface.
   - Erythroplakia is a reddish, velvety lesion on the oral mucosa or tongue and presents with erythema.
   - Most cases of erythroplakia are precancerous or cancerous.
   - Thorough examination of the mouth.
   - Check for lymph node enlargement.
   - Fiber-optic examination.

4. **Diagnostic Studies**
   - Biopsy or exfoliative cytologic examination.

5. **Management**
   - Otolaryngologic referral.
   - Some clinical trials support the use of β-carotene, retinoids, and vitamin E.
   - Possible laser vaporization for leukoplakia.
   - Cryosurgery, laser ablation for erythroplakia.

- Avoid alcohol and tobacco (including smokeless tobacco).
- Fine-needle aspiration biopsy of enlarged lymph nodes.
- If biopsy is positive for oral squamous cell carcinoma, surgery/radiation therapy is recommended.

B. Neoplasms of the Tongue

1. **Etiology**
   - Most common carcinoma of the tongue is squamous cell carcinoma; more common in men than women, a family history of aerodigestive cancers, older age.
   - Most common on lateral tongue.

2. **Pathology**
   - Caused by carcinogenic agents such as tobacco, alcohol, environmental exposures, geographic location, and betel nuts.

3. **Clinical Features**
   - Begins as a painful, indurated plaque on the tongue that ulcerates.
   - Presents as a nonhealing ulcer or exophytic lesion.
   - Patient may also have associated lymphadenopathy.
   - May have referred ear pain.
   - Hemoptysis.
   - Dysphagia.
   - Odynophagia.
   - Feeling of a mass in the throat.
   - Mass in the neck region.
   - In advanced disease, the tongue may be fixed.

4. **Diagnostic Studies**
   - Biopsy.
   - CT with contrast.
   - Chest X-ray.
   - Liver function tests, CBC, HPV, renal tests, and BMP.
   - Bone scan if indicated.
   - Positron emission tomography scan if unclear diagnosis, primary site of cancer not located, or for pretreatment assessment.

5. **Management**
   - Surgery, radiation therapy alone or with brachytherapy, and chemotherapy.
   - Consult oncologist.
   - Follow-up imaging if nonsurgical treatment.

VI. Throat

INFLAMMATORY DISEASES

A. Laryngitis

1. **Etiology**
   - Laryngeal mucous membrane infection.

2. **Pathology**
   - Usually viral.
   - Can be caused by adenovirus or influenza.
   - Other viruses: RSV, Coxsackie virus, rhinovirus.

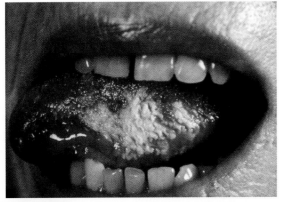

FIGURE 11–12. **Oral hairy leukoplakia.** (From Goodheart HP. *Goodheart's Photoguide of Common Skin Disorders.* 2nd ed. Philadelphia, PA: Lippincott Williams & Wilkins; 2003, with permission.)

- Bacterial causes: *H. influenzae, M. catarrhalis, S. pneumoniae.*
- Caused by URI, trauma to the throat, vocal abuse, toxic exposure, gastrointestinal or pulmonary complications, smoking, laryngopharyngeal reflux, and, occasionally, allergy.

3. **Clinical Features**
   - Hoarseness, cough, and sore throat.
   - Possible pain and difficulty swallowing.
   - Rhinorrhea.
   - Fever if infective causes.
   - Possible vesicles on the soft palate.
   - Lymphadenopathy.
   - May be associated with URI if acute.
   - If lasts >2 weeks, otolaryngologic evaluation is needed.

4. **Diagnostic Studies**
   - Laryngoscopy if suspected masses, infection, structural abnormality, and vocal cord dysfunction.

5. **Management**
   - Voice rest.
   - Do not clear throat.
   - Smoking and alcohol cessation.
   - Humidifier.
   - Hydration.
   - Treat underlying cause.
   - Surgery may be indicated in chronic cases.

B. **Bacterial Pharyngitis/Tonsillitis**

1. **Etiology**
   - Inflammation of the oropharynx.

2. **Pathology**
   - Eighty percent are viral: adenovirus, herpesvirus, rhinovirus, coronavirus.
   - Bacterial: group A β-hemolytic streptococci (GABHS), mycoplasma, Group G and C *Streptococcus, Neisseria gonorrhoeae, Chlamydia,* antibiotic-resistant *S. pneumoniae.*
   - Usually occurs in the winter/spring.
   - Spread by droplets.

3. **Clinical Features**
   - GABHS: tender cervical lymphadenopathy, fever over 38° C, no cough, pharyngotonsillar exudate.
   - Headache.
   - Acute onset of sore throat with difficulty swallowing.
   - Fever > 101° F.
   - Malaise, anorexia.
   - Arthralgias, myalgias.
   - Nausea/vomiting, abdominal pain in children.
   - Patient appears ill.
   - Tachycardic.
   - Tender, enlarged lymph nodes.
   - Erythema with or without exudate.
   - Petechiae of soft palate and strawberry tongue with strep. Scarlatiniform rash may be present.

4. **Diagnostic Studies**
   - Rapid strep-antigen testing.
   - Throat culture.
   - CBC with differential.

5. **Management**
   - Oral antibiotics (PenVK or cefuroxime axetil; erythromycin as an alternative to penicillin or for suspected mycoplasma or chlamydial bacteria).
   - Amoxicillin or Azithromycin if compliance concern.
   - Steroids may be necessary, although rarely used.
   - Decadron 10 mg IM for rapid resolution of symptoms.
   - Hydration, rest, ibuprofen for pain and decrease fever.
   - Patient not infectious after 24 hours of antibiotic therapy.
   - Otolaryngologic referral if history of recurrent symptomatic infections.

C. **Viral Pharyngitis/Tonsillitis**

1. **Etiology**
   - Inflammation of the pharynx or tonsils.

2. **Pathology**
   - Respiratory viruses are the most common cause of sore throat.
   - Adenovirus, herpesvirus, rhinovirus, and coronavirus.

3. **Clinical Features**
   - Acute onset of sore throat.
   - May be accompanied by conjunctivitis, rash, cough, sputum production, rhinitis, and systemic symptoms.
   - Pharyngeal erythema, exudates, tonsillar enlargement, and cervical adenopathy may be present.
   - Look for ulcers in the mouth.

4. **Diagnostic Studies**
   - Check liver/spleen size.
   - CBC for atypical lymphocyte.
   - Monospot.

5. **Management**
   - Hydration, gargles, and appropriate analgesics.
   - Lozenges also may be helpful.

D. **Epiglottitis**

1. **Etiology**
   - Acute inflammation of the supraglottic larynx, including epiglottitis that can progress rapidly to upper airway obstruction.
   - Occurs in children aged 2 to 7 years, but may also occur in adults.
   - More common in patients with diabetes.
   - In pediatric patients, symptoms can progress in 12 to 24 hours after onset.

2. **Pathology**
   - Usually caused by *H. influenzae* type b (this organism is rare in adults).

3. **Clinical Features**
   - Acute onset of high fever, sore throat, odynophagia, irritability, hoarseness, and restlessness.
   - Rapid development of a sore throat with subjective complaints of odynophagia that outweigh the physical findings.
   - Moderate-to-severe respiratory distress.
   - Drooling, inspiratory stridor.
   - Patient prefers sitting, leaning forward with elbows on knees.
4. **Diagnostic Studies**
   - Lateral X-ray of the upper airway shows epiglottic swelling.
   - Laryngoscopy in adults.
5. **Management**
   - Immediate otolaryngologic/pediatric evaluation.
   - Secure airway.
   - Do not instrument patient.
   - Preferred approach is nasotracheal intubation in operating room by otolaryngologist with a pediatric anesthesiologist present. Oral intubation for adults as indicated.
   - Hospitalize in ICU.
   - Oxygen saturation with pulse oximetry.
   - IV antibiotics (ceftizoxime, cefuroxime) with possible steroids (dexamethasone).

INFECTION

A. Peritonsillar Abscess

1. **Etiology**
   - Infection from the tonsil to the peritonsillar fascial planes.
2. **Pathology**
   - Complications of mononucleosis, tonsillitis, and peritonsillar cellulitis.
   - Polymicrobial.
   - Usually *Streptococcus* or *Staphylococcus*.
   - Anaerobic bacteria: *Bacteroides*.
3. **Clinical Features**
   - Symptoms usually begin when patient is on the antibiotic.
   - Young adults < 30 years.
   - Increased incidence in winter months.
   - Follows a 2- to 3-day history of a sore throat.
   - Inflammation, cellulitis, and pocket of pus in the supratonsillar space.
   - Can produce trismus.
   - Fever, odynophagia, headache, and malaise.
   - Referred pain to the ear.
   - Sore throat is more on one side.
   - Drooling.
   - Mild tachycardia.
   - Deviated uvula with peritonsillar swelling, erythema of posterior pharynx.
   - Exudate may or may not be present.
   - Ipsilateral lymph node enlargement of the anterior chain.

4. **Diagnostic Studies**
   - CT is used for diagnosis between a peritonsillar abscess and peritonsillar cellulitis.
5. **Management**
   - Pediatrics: IV hydration and antibiotics.
   - Surgery if no relief.
   - Most cases can be handled outpatient.
   - Admit patient if severe pain, dyspnea, trismus, and drooling.
   - Consult otolaryngologist.
   - I&D or aspiration of the abscess.
   - Consider immediate tonsillectomy.
   - Broad spectrum cephalosporin.
   - Before abscess formation, Clindamycin with oral amoxicillin may clear a peritonsillar cellulitis and prevent abscess formation.

REVIEW QUESTIONS

1. A patient presents with a hard, nontender swelling on the right upper eyelid. The conjunctiva is red. The lesion turns inward. What is the most likely diagnosis?
   a) Corneal ulcer
   b) Pterygium
   c) Chalazion
   d) Meibomian gland abscess

2. John Smith presents to the clinic after sustaining a foreign body to the right eye. On examination, there is a small piece of metal located at the 8 o'clock position on the cornea. He is complaining of blurred vision, excessive tearing, and pain. Which of the following would NOT be in the current treatment for this gentleman?
   a) Visual acuity
   b) Fluorescein staining
   c) Cultures from the secretions
   d) Refer to an ophthalmologist if not improving in 24 hours

3. In a retinal artery occlusion, the provider must look for a history of:
   a) Using oral contraceptives
   b) Smoking
   c) Hypertension
   d) Glaucoma

4. What diagnosis is characterized as a malfunction of the endolymphatics affecting the inner ear, can be associated with trauma, syphilis, or possibly be idiopathic, and occurs mainly in middle age? There is fullness or pressure of the ears, tinnitus, and with possible nausea and vomiting.
   a) Ménière syndrome
   b) Vertigo
   c) Labyrinthitis
   d) Acoustic neuroma

5. What condition of the mouth presents with acute inflammation, possibly from a herpesvirus 6, and painful, round, shallow ulcers on the buccal mucosa?

   a) Gingivitis
   b) Aphthous ulcers
   c) Gingivostomatitis
   d) Dental caries

6. A 50-year-old man who works in a factory presents to you complaining of hearing loss in his right ear. He states that his wife complains about him turning up the TV and not responding when she speaks to him. The patient states he wears hearing protection intermittently. On examination, you would expect to find:

   a) Weber lateralizes to the left ear and the Rinne is AC > BC.
   b) Weber lateralizes to the right ear and the Rinne is AC > BC.
   c) Weber lateralizes to the left ear and the Rinne is BC > AC.
   d) Weber lateralizes to the right ear and the Rinne is BC > AC.

ANSWERS TO REVIEW QUESTIONS

1. **Answer: C**. Chalazion is a localized swelling on the upper or lower eyelid. The most common etiology is blockage of the Meibomian gland duct by an accumulation of secretion. Other factors may be the presence of seborrhea, viral infection, immunodeficiency, or acne rosacea. Clinical features include a hard, nontender swelling of the upper or lower eyelid; the conjunctiva is red and elevated. Corneal ulcer is defined as corneal tissue necrosis. It is most commonly caused by infection of bacteria, fungi, amoeba, or virus. Corneal ulcer clinical features include photophobia, foreign-body sensation, ache, and increased tearing initially; the fluorescin applied to the area will stain green, Pterygium is a thickening of the conjunctiva in the shape of a triangle usually on the nasal side growing inward toward the cornea. Blepharitis is defined at bilateral eyelid margin inflammation. Clinical features of anterior blepharitis include granulations or scales attached to the eyelashes, and the eyes are red and swollen. Clinical feature of posterior blepharitis is defined as MGD and causes inflammation of the eyelid.

2. **Answer: C**. A corneal abrasion is defined as a superficial irregularity of the cornea. It results from trauma to the cornea by a foreign body, contact lens, or fingernail. Clinical features include acute pain, redness, photophobia, excessive tearing, foreign-body sensation, and blurred vision. Diagnostic studies include to check visual acuity and visual fields, slit lamp, and/or funduscopic examination, fluorescein staining will detect the defect as a bright green area with black light. Management includes removal of the foreign body, if present; antibiotic ophthalmic ointment, oral pain medication, reassessment in 24 hours if fluorescein staining and referral to ophthalmologist if corneal epithelium is not healing properly within 24 hours if unable to remove the foreign body completely.

3. **Answer: C**. Retinal artery occlusion usually occurs in patients between the ages of 50 and 80 who often have concurrent hypertension, hyperlipidemia, cardiac arrhythmia, diabetes or atherosclerosis, and may be secondary to giant cell arteritis. Clinical features include sudden painless, unilateral loss of vision, and/or visual field lasting from minutes (amaurosis fugax) to permanent. A cherry red spot is seen at the fovea. Visual acuity is restricted to the temporal area or by counting fingers, swelling of the retina may last 4 to 6 weeks, and cotton-wool spots are limited to the region affected.

4. **Answer: A**. Ménière syndrome is a malfunction of the endolymphatics, a condition of the inner ear. It may be associated with trauma or syphilis, occurs mainly in middle age, and effects males more than females. Clinical features include vertigo that is sudden, lasting 1 to 8 hours, and can be debilitating. The patient feels as if everything is moving; there is vestibular nystagmus; fullness or pressure of the ears; tinnitus and fluctuant sensorineural hearing loss.

5. **Answer: B**. Aphthous ulcer is a common disorder of oral mucosa caused by nonspecific acute inflammation, possibly herpesvirus 6. Clinical features are painful, round, shallow ulcers with yellow–gray fibrinoid centers and erythematous halos present on nonkeratinized mucosa (buccal and labial mucosa); repeat recurrences; it may be associated with stress. Management includes topical analgesics (i.e., Anbesol gel, viscous lidocaine) and possible use of corticosteroid gels or ointments (puts patient at risk for oral candidiasis). Cimetidine can be used for maintenance if ulcers recur; if unresponsive to treatment, laser therapy can be utilized.

6. **Answer: A**. Sensorineural loss. The Weber test sound will lateralize to the good ear; Rinne test: AC > BC (positive Rinne).

SELECTED REFERENCES

American Association for Pediatric Ophthalmology and Strabismus. *Blowout Fracture*. 2017. San Francisco, CA: American Association for Pediatric Ophthalmology & Strabismus. https://aapos.org/terms/conditions/28. Accessed July 18, 2017.

Bruch JM, Kamani, DV. Hoarseness in adults. *UpToDate*. 2017. https://www.uptodate.com/contents/hoarseness-in-adults. Accessed July 18, 2017.

Chow AW. Complications, diagnosis, and treatment of odontogenic infections. *UpToDate*. 2017. https://www.uptodate.com/contents/complications-diagnosis-and-treatment-of-odontogenic-infections. Accessed July 17, 2017.

Corey L. Herpes simplex virus infections. In: Kasper D, Fauci A. Hauser S, Longo D, Jameson JL, Loscalzo J, eds. *Harrison's Principles of Internal Medicine*. 19th ed. New York, NY: McGraw Hill; 2015.

Duncan KO, Geisse JK, Leffell DJ. Epithelial precancerous lesions In: Goldsmith LA, Katz SI, Gilchrest BA, Paller AS, Leffel DJ, Klaus W, eds. *Fitzpatrick's Dermatology in General Medicine*. 8th ed. New York, NY: McGraw Hill; 2012.

Effron D, Forcier BC, Wyszynski RE. Funduscopic findings. In: Knoop KJ, Stack LB, Storrow AB, Thurman RJ, eds. *Atlas of Emergency Medicine*. 4th ed. New York, NY: McGraw Hill-Medical; 2015.

Fazio SB, Emerick K. Salivary gland stones. *UpToDate*. 2017. https://www.uptodate.com/contents/salivary-gland-stones. Accessed July 15, 2017.

Gappy C, Archer SM, Barza M. Orbital cellulitis. *UpToDate*. 2017. https://www.uptodate.com/contents/orbital-cellulitis. Accessed July 24, 2017.

Garrity J. *Papilledema*. Kenilworth, NJ: Merck Manual Professional Version. 2017. http://www.merckmanuals.com/professional/eye-disorders/optic-nerve-disorders/papilledema#v957654. Accessed July 14, 2017.

Ghosh C, Ghosh T. Eyelid lesions. *UpToDate*. 2017. https://www.uptodate.com/contents/eyelid-lesions. Accessed July 14, 2017.

Healthwise Staff. Meniere syndrome. *eMedicine*. 2013. https://www.emedicinehealth.com/meniere_disease/article_em.htm. Accessed July 23, 2017.

Jacobs DS. Corneal abrasions and corneal foreign bodies: clinical manifestations and diagnosis. *UpToDate*. 2017. https://www.uptodate.com/contents/corneal-abrasions-and-corneal-foreign-bodies-clinical-manifestations-and-diagnosis. Accessed July 14, 2017.

Jacobs DS. Pterygium. *UpToDate*. 2017. https://www.uptodate.com/contents/pterygium. Accessed July 14, 2017.

Lee N, Romanyshyn J, Caria N, Setton J. Benign & malignant lesions of the oral cavity, oropharynx & nasopharynx. In: Lalwani AK, ed. *Current Diagnosis and Treatment of Otolaryngology-Head and Neck Surgery*. 3rd ed. New York, NY: McGraw Hill-Medical; 2011:377–386.

Lustig LR, Schindler JS. Ear, nose & throat disorders. In: Papdakis MA, McPhee SJ, eds. *Current Medical Diagnosis and Treatment*. 56th ed. New York, NY: McGraw Hill-Medical; 2016.

Mayo Clinic Staff. *Diabetic Retinopathy*. Mayo Clinic. 2015. http://www.mayoclinic.org/diseases-conditions/diabetic-retinopathy/basics/treatment/con-20023311. Accessed July 23, 2017.

Mayo Clinic Staff. *Gingivitis*. Mayo Clinic. 2017. http://www.mayoclinic.org/diseases-conditions/gingivitis/home/ovc-20305807. Accessed July 23, 2017.

Osborne B, Balcer LJ. Optic neuritis: pathophysiology, clinical features, and diagnosis. *UpToDate*. 2017. https://www.uptodate.com/contents/optic-neuritis-pathophysiology-clinical-features-and-diagnosis. Accessed July 14, 2017.

Paysse EA, Coats DK. Approach to a child with persistent tearing. *UpToDate*. 2017. https://www.uptodate.com/contents/approach-to-the-child-with-persistent-tearing. Accessed July 14, 2017.

Riordan-Eva P. Disorders of the eyes and lids. In: Papadakis MA, McPhee SJ, eds. *Current Medical Diagnosis and Treatment*. 56th ed. New York, NY: McGraw Hill-Medical; 2016.

Shtein RM. Blepharitis. *UpToDate*. 2017. https://www.uptodate.com/contents/blepharitis. Accessed July 14, 2017.

Simic PJ. Labyrinthitis. *eMedicineHealth*. 2016. http://www.emedicinehealth.com/labyrinthitis/article_em.htm. Accessed July 14, 2017.

Tubert D. *What is hyphema?* San Francisco, CA: American Academy of Ophthalmology; 2016. https://www.aao.org/eye-health/diseases/what-is-hyphema. Accessed July 14, 2017.

Usatine RP, Smith MA, Mayeaux EJ, Chumley HS. Nasal polyps. In: Usatine RP, Smith MA, Mayeaux EJ, Chumley HS. *Color Atlas of Family Medicine*. 2nd ed. New York, NY: McGraw Hill Professional; 2013. Accessed July 15, 2017.

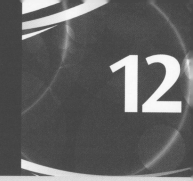

Neurologic Disorders 12

Randi Beth Cooperman • Ilaria Gadalla • Sonia V. Otte • Adrian Andrews

I. Diseases of Peripheral Nerves

A. Complex Regional Pain Syndrome (CRPS; Formerly Reflex Sympathetic Dystrophy)

1. Definition

- Rare, chronic pain disorder affecting the extremities, usually after an injury.

2. Etiology

- Several mechanisms have been identified as possible causes for CRPS, including inflammation, autoimmune processes (e.g., elevation of proinflammatory monocytes), peripheral and central sensitization, as well as alterations in sympathetic and central nervous system (CNS) function.
- Often preceded by trauma, even minor, to the area.
- Psychological stress is not considered causative.

3. Clinical Features

- Chronic musculoskeletal disorder without systemic involvement.
- Severity of the symptoms is generally out of proportion to the extent of the preceding event or injury.
- Pain is also out of proportion to the level of stimulation.
- Symptoms can begin days to weeks after the preceding incident.
- Symptoms can, but do not always, progress from the involved area being initially painful and swollen with skin changes (color and temperature) to dystrophic if left untreated.
- Symptoms are not limited to one peripheral nerve distribution area and can involve a whole limb area (e.g., lower leg) or even anatomical quadrant.
- Limited range of motion (ROM) of the area.

4. Diagnostic Studies

- Clinical diagnosis, but X-ray or bone scan may be helpful in ruling out differential diagnosis.

5. Management

- No long-term, effective treatment has been proven.
- Patient education and early treatment are paramount.
- Early mobilization after trauma or surgery lessens the likelihood of development.
- Major portion of treatment is exercise and mobilization of the area through physical therapy.
- Nonsteroidal anti-inflammatory drugs (NSAIDs) are helpful in mild cases. Oral prednisone at 30 to 60 mg per day is used for more severe cases for 2 weeks followed by a 2-week taper.
- Gabapentin has been used in treatment, as well as topical capsaicin and nortriptyline.
- Intravenous (IV) bisphosphonates (e.g., alendronate) may reduce symptoms.
- Spontaneous remission of symptoms is rare, but can occur in mild cases within several weeks to months.

B. Peripheral Neuropathies

1. Definition

- Can be divided into two categories: polyneuropathies and mononeuropathies/multiple mononeuropathies.
- Polyneuropathies cause *general* nerve dysfunction (e.g., Charcot–Marie–Tooth disease, familial amyloid neuropathies, Guillain–Barré syndrome, chronic inflammatory demyelinating polyneuropathy, diabetic neuropathy, critical illness polyneuropathy, and toxin-induced neuropathies).
- Mononeuropathies affect single or multiple peripheral nerves and cause *focal* nerve dysfunction (e.g., carpal tunnel syndrome, ulnar palsy, and peroneal neuropathy).

2. Etiology

- Polyneuropathies reflect the pathology of the underlying disease process. Some conditions/systems include endocrine, metabolic, infectious, hereditary, toxic, immune-mediated, and neoplastic.
- Underlying processes seen in mononeuropathies include inflammatory, compressive, and hereditary.
- The cause of about one-third of neuropathies is unknown.

3. Pathology

- Affects nerve axons, myelin sheath, and blood vessels–supplying nerves.
- Polyneuropathies affecting:
  - Axons have a slow degeneration of long and short nerve fibers.
  - Myelin sheath has demyelination of peripheral nerves resulting in blocked conduction.
  - Blood vessels develop ischemia and infarction of the corresponding peripheral nerves.
- Many neuropathies have both axonal degeneration and demyelination.

- In mononeuropathies, the pathologies are usually compressive (e.g., carpal tunnel syndrome), inflammatory (e.g., Bell's palsy), hereditary, or involve multiple mononeuropathies (e.g., vasculitis, leprosy, and amyloidosis).

4. Clinical Features
- General motor signs and symptoms include muscle weakness, atrophy, and decreased or absent reflexes in correlating nerve distribution.
- General sensory signs and symptoms such as numbness, tingling, pain, or sensory loss in correlating nerve distribution.

5. Diagnostic Studies
- Standard studies include complete blood count (CBC), comprehensive metabolic panel (CMP), vitamin B_{12} level, glucose tolerance test, thyroid function test, rapid plasma reagin (RPR), nerve conduction studies, electromyogram, serum protein electrophoresis, and immunofixation electrophoresis.
- Based on the suspected underlying condition or system, specific testing may be indicated such as lumbar puncture (LP), nerve biopsy, muscle biopsy, skin biopsy, and Lyme antibody.

6. Management
- Treat underlying cause.
- If underlying cause of neuropathic pain is unknown, focus management on pain control with tramadol, creams, patches, transcutaneous nerve stimulation, and alternative treatments (e.g., acupuncture).
- Consider tricyclic antidepressants (e.g., amitriptyline or venlafaxine) and anticonvulsants (e.g., gabapentin or pregabalin).

II. Headaches
A. Headache
1. Etiology
- Irritation of intracranial pain-sensitive structures, including cranial nerves, venous sinuses, cervical nerves, and large arteries.

2. General Disease and Pathology
- Headaches are classified into three groups:
  - Primary headaches that do not have an underlying pathology related to them (migraines, tension headaches, cluster headaches, etc.).
  - Secondary headaches that are related to an underlying pathology (infection, medications, vascular, nonvascular, and disordered homeostasis).
  - Cranial neuralgia syndromes that result from disorders of cranial nerves and/or cranial branches.

3. Clinical Features
- Red flags (headache warning signs that could indicate secondary headaches):
  - New-onset headaches in patients older than 50 years, those with a history of cancer or with HIV, or those with risk factors for cerebral venous sinus thrombosis.
  - A headache that reaches peak intensity in seconds to minutes ("thunderclap").
  - Any headaches accompanied by fever, neck pain, visual disturbance, or jaw claudication.
  - Any patient with neurologic symptoms (change in cognition, limb or facial weakness, extended aura, etc.) or neurologic abnormalities on physical examination.
  - Although migraine is the most common cause of morning headaches, a headache that wakes one from sleep requires further workup.
  - Headaches that are brought on by Valsalva or physical exertion or that vary with changes in posture.
  - Thunderclap headaches, those suggestive of increased intracranial pressure (ICP) or those suggestive of infection, need immediate specialist assessment.
  - All patients presenting with a headache should have a full cervical examination (inspection for posture, palpation of muscle tone and any muscle or bony prominence tenderness, and full ROM in all directions).
  - New-onset headaches or those that are different from what the patient usually experiences should be evaluated through physical examination with blood pressure (BP) and full neurologic examination (including fundoscopic examination).
  - Headache diaries or various assessment tools should be used to track headache patterns.

4. Diagnostic Studies
- Magnetic resonance imaging (MRI) should be considered in patients who have a headache that is brought on, not aggravated, by cough; those with Short-lasting Unilateral Neuralgiform headache attacks with Conjunctival injection and Tearing (SUNCT); and those who present with cluster headaches (see below) or paroxysmal hemicranias.
- Computed tomography (CT) should be considered in patients who have abnormal neurologic examinations of unexplained origin unless MRI is more appropriate.
- CT should also be used within 12 hours from onset in those with thunderclap headaches, or "worst headache of my life" headaches.
- A lumber puncture with oxyhemoglobin and bilirubin should be performed in patients with thunderclap headaches who have normal CT results or those with suspected meningitis with a normal neurologic examination.

B. Cluster Headache

1. Etiology

- Unknown, may have a positive family history of cluster headaches, associated with smoking and head trauma as well.
- More common in men than women. Onset is generally between 20 and 50 years.
- Onset later in life.
- Occurs in less than 10% of patients with headaches.

2. Pathology

- Pathophysiology thought to involve hypothalamic activation and possible vasodilatation and activation of the trigeminovascular system and autonomic features.

3. Clinical Features

- Severe, often excruciating, unilateral, periorbital or temporal sharp and piercing pain.
- The pain is deep, nonthrobbing, and may radiate to the forehead, temple, or cheek; less frequently to the ear, occiput, and neck.
- Associated unilateral lacrimation, nasal congestion, and ocular redness; rhinorrhea and Horner syndrome.
- Episodic type is more common (80%–90% of patients with cluster headaches) than chronic type (10%).
- Episodic is at least two cluster periods that can last from 7 days to 1 full year and have symptom-free periods in between clusters of at least 1 month.
- In the chronic type, symptom clusters last a year or longer and remission is less than 1 month.
- Headache duration ranges from 15 minutes to several hours with an average of 1 hour. Frequently occur near bedtime and often awaken patients from sleep.

4. Diagnostic Studies

- MRI to rule out differential diagnosis of severe headache.
- Rule out intracranial hemorrhage, tic douloureux, glaucoma, sinusitis, and dental abscess.

5. Management

- Inhalation of 6 to 10 L of 100% O_2 for 15 to 20 minutes.
- Abortive therapy first-line choice is subcutaneous sumatriptan (6 mg).
- Intranasal triptans can be used for those who cannot tolerate subcutaneous route.
- May spontaneously regress with varying period until next episode.
- Preventive therapy includes lithium, divalproex, verapamil, methysergide, and corticosteroids.
- Surgical options include trigeminal nerve sectioning or injection.
- Reduce stress through relaxation, can use biofeedback, and reduce tobacco and alcohol use.

C. Migraine Headache (with Aura and without Aura)

1. Etiology

- Cause remains unknown in the majority of cases.
- Presents in patient usually before age 40, often during adolescence.
- The lifetime prevalence of migraines is 20% to 25%. About 28 million people in the United States are estimated to have migraines (18% female and 6% male) and over 4 million have at least one attack per month.
- Migraines tend to decrease with age.
- Certain medications may cause or worsen migraines (e.g., sildenafil and analgesics).
- Obesity may increase frequency and severity, but not prevalence of migraines.
- Oral contraceptives are not associated with increased risk; however, some resources suggest that women with migraine with aura and those older than 35 years with migraine without aura should not use combined oral contraceptive pills.
- Current evidence also cannot establish a link between food triggers and migraines.

2. Pathology

- Pathophysiology includes genetic predisposition, hormonal factors, and CNS response to stimuli.
- No longer considered to be caused by vascular dilation and constriction phenomena.
- Thought to be related to primary neuronal dysfunction with activation of trigeminovascular system reflex, cortical spreading depression, and serotonins.

3. Clinical Features

- Most common cause of morning headaches.
- Severe, periodic headaches that cause disability. The headache is usually unilateral and is associated with nausea, vomiting, and photophobia.
- Typically last several hours to several days and can include unilateral pain (sometimes of pulsating nature) of moderate-to-severe intensity.
- Visual symptoms are most common.
- Sensitivity to light and sound can occur either during or in between attacks.
- Physical activity may also worsen symptoms.
- Migraine headaches can be preceded by a typical aura in 30% of patients with migraines.
- Auras are defined as a sensory, visual, or motor disturbance (manifesting singly or together) that precede the headache.
- May include scintillating scotomata, multiple small dots, homonymous visual disturbances, hemisensory disturbance, speech disturbance, and vertigo.
- Other premonitory symptoms include fatigue, diminished concentration, sensitivity to light and sound, nausea, and blurred vision.
- Patients have a normal neurologic examination.

4. Diagnostic Studies
- In patients with a clear history of migraine, without red flag signs or symptoms, and without an abnormal neurologic evaluation, neuroimaging is not indicated.

5. Management
- NSAIDs, triptans, and antiemetics are commonly used.
- Patients find comfort in lying down in a dark, quiet place.
- Stress management is recommended to reduce the number and severity of migraines.
- NSAIDs are recommended for acute treatment in patients with all severity levels of migraine.
- Paracetamol 1,000 mg can be used for acute treatment in mild-to-moderate migraines.
- If simple analgesics have not been effective, other abortive therapy includes oral triptans, and they should be taken at onset or as soon thereafter as possible. Note that triptans are contraindicated in patients with various types of heart disease.
- Oral, rectal, or IV antiemetics may be helpful in reducing nausea.
- Prophylaxis includes β-blockers. The recommended first-line therapy for migraine prophylaxis is 80 to 240 mg of propanolol. Timolol, atenolol, nadolol, and metoprolol can be used as alternatives.
- Antiepileptics may also be beneficial (e.g., sodium valproate, gabapentin, and topiramate).
- Antidepressants and botulinum toxin A can be used as prophylaxis as well.
- Aspirin is contraindicated in the third trimester of pregnancy.

D. Tension-Type Headache
1. Etiology
- May be caused by sustained craniocervical muscle contractions.
- Physical manifestation of psychosocial stresses.
- Associated with depressed state and anxiety.
- The most common form of headache.
- Usually begins in middle age and affects women more than men.

2. Clinical Features
- Recurrent and episodic in nature. No aura.
- Constricting, bilateral, "band-like distribution" tends to occur later in the day and is associated with anorexia.
- May be accompanied by pressure-like squeezing and tightening pain in the neck and shoulder; occasional nausea that occurs 15 days per month for more than 6 months.
- Tension headache should be considered when a patient has a bilateral, nondisabling headache and has a normal neurologic physical examination.
- Physical examination may show neck or head musculature contraction.
- Complete neurologic examination indicated in any new-onset headache, with imaging studies to rule out intracranial abnormalities if indicated.

3. Management
- Stress management, relaxation therapy, and physiotherapy.
- Aspirin and paracetamol for acute tension headache treatment.
- Consider tricyclics (e.g., amitriptyline at bedtime) for prophylaxis of chronic tension headaches.
- Although not first line, botulinum toxin A may be recommended as a prophylaxis of tension headaches.

III. Infectious Disorders
A. Encephalitis
1. Etiology
- May be viral, bacterial, fungal, protozoal, or helminthic.
- No pathogen identified in up to 70% of cases.
- Involves inflammatory response of the brain with neurologic dysfunction.
- Herpes simplex encephalitis (herpes simplex virus, HSV) is the most common viral encephalitis; 70% mortality rate if left untreated; type 2 causes neonatal encephalitis; and type 1 presents in older persons.
- Arboviruses (epidemic viral encephalitis):
  - Carried by mosquitoes and ticks and tend to be seasonal.
  - Include three viruses causing Western, Eastern, and Venezuelan equine encephalitis; two flaviviruses causing St. Louis and Japanese B encephalitis; and bunyaviruses causing California encephalitis.
  - Leading causes of arbovirus encephalitis in the United States—St. Louis and California encephalitis.
- Myxovirus (mumps and measles encephalitis):
  - Most common childhood encephalitis.
  - Occasionally occurs in epidemics.
  - Mumps encephalitis: usually mild, seen most in late winter.
- Measles encephalitis: 15% mortality rate. Number of cases is declining secondary to vaccinations.
- Cytomegalovirus (CMV): one of the most common causes of encephalitis in the immunosuppressed population.

2. Pathology
- Viral invasion of the brain parenchyma.
- Meningoencephalitis is seen more often than pure encephalitis.
- Primary viral invasion of CNS.
- Infection agents by age:

- Infants: consider herpes simplex type 2, CMV, rubella, *Listeria monocytogenes*, *Treponema pallidum*, and *Toxoplasma gondii*.
- Infants/children: consider influenza virus, Japanese encephalitis virus, Eastern equine encephalitis virus, and Murray Valley encephalitis virus.
- Elderly: consider St. Louis virus, *L. monocytogenes*, West Nile virus, and Eastern equine encephalitis virus.

3. Clinical Features
- Presentation is nonspecific and acute with fever, headache, and altered mental status.
- Signs and symptoms based on specific area of the brain involved and severity of infection.
- May include emesis, photophobia, nuchal rigidity, hepatitis, rash, lymphadenopathy, rash, respiratory complaints, urinary symptoms, retinitis, dementia, cranial nerve defects, cerebellar involvements, seizures, and parkinsonism.
- Ask about recent travel, exposure to animals (e.g., dogs, cats, bats, skunks, raccoons, rodents, some primates, sheep, goats, white-tailed deer, birds, horses) or insects (e.g., mosquitoes, ticks, sandflies, tsetse flies), recent illness or immunizations, immune status, recreational activities, occupational exposures, and note season of the year.
- Encephalitis is usually transient and accompanies a systemic viral illness.

4. Diagnostic Studies
- MRI is the most sensitive imaging test in the evaluation of encephalitis.
- CT is an alternative when MRI cannot be performed.
- Neuroimaging must be used.
- CBC and CMP.
- Cerebrospinal fluid (CSF) analysis is necessary, unless contraindicated, through LP and polymerase chain reaction (PCR) nucleic acid amplification testing.
- PCR testing for herpes simplex in all patients with suspected encephalitis.
- Electroencephalogram (EEG) rarely helpful in establishing etiology.
- Normal glucose shows elevated protein and lymphocytic pleocytosis.
- Elevated RBCs are seen in herpes encephalitis.
- Brain biopsy is reserved for patients with focal abnormalities on MRI, who deteriorate clinically despite antiviral therapy, and in whom PCR studies are inconclusive.

5. Management
- No definitive treatment in many cases.
- Acyclovir (10 mg per kg IV every 8 hours in children and adults who have uncompromised renal function, 20 mg per kg for neonates) should be started as soon as possible in all patients with suspected encephalitis while waiting for the results of further testing.
- Starting treatment for herpes simplex encephalitis as early as possible reduces the likelihood of serious complications or death.
- CMV: ganciclovir/foscarnet combination.
- Influenza virus: oseltamivir.
- Treat etiologic bacterial, rickettsial, fungal, or ehrlichial infections with specific agent for that organism.
- Consider high-dose steroids in suspected postinfectious encephalomyelitis.
- Supportive measures include antipyretics, analgesics, anticonvulsants, and rest.
- Watch for syndrome of inappropriate antidiuretic hormone secretion (SIADH).

B. Acute Meningitis
1. Etiology
- Noninfectious conditions such as tumors, cysts, medication, sequelae of neurologic procedures, or systemic illness.
- Viruses, bacteria, fungus, protozoa, and helminths.
- Inflammation of the meninges of the brain and spinal cord.
- Estimated 2 to 5 per 100,000 people in the Western world.
- Permanent neurologic complications in 30% to 50% of illness survivors.
- Pathogens gain entry through various routes.

2. Pathology
- Spread from contiguous sites of infection (e.g., paranasal sinusitis, mastoiditis, otitis, and osteomyelitis of the skull or vertebrae).
- Direct implantation through LP, penetrating wounds, or surgery.
- Organism enters intravascular space and choroid plexus, but no opsonization occurs due to low number of WBCs in CSF; inflammatory reaction occurs with lysis of bacteria and release of cell wall components into subarachnoid space and formation of purulent exudates. Meningeal inflammation begins with increased cytokines (interleukins and tumor necrosis factor), amino acids, and free oxygen (O_2) radicals, which then leads to increased permeability of blood–brain barrier, obstruction of CSF flow dynamics, ischemia, and necrosis.
- Bacterial: includes both gram-negative and gram-positive organisms.
- Majority of cases of acute bacterial meningitis (ABM) in immunocompetent infants over 4 weeks of age, children, and adults are caused by *Streptococcus pneumoniae* or *Neisseria meningitidis*.
- *S. pneumoniae* is the most common cause of community-acquired ABM.
- *L. monocytogenes* and staph are also common, and <10% of cases are caused by gram-negative bacilli

such as *Escherichia coli*, *Klebsiella*, *Enterobacter*, and *Pseudomonas aeruginosa*.

- The most common causative organisms in ABM in immunocompromised patients are *L. monocytogenes*, *S. pneumonia*, *P. aeruginosa*, and *N. meningitidis*.
- Nosocomial infections are caused mostly by staphylococcal strains.
- Aseptic meningitis is caused by viruses (e.g., Coxsackie viruses, echoviruses, polioviruses, and human enteroviruses 68 to 71 and, less commonly, HSV type 2, mumps, and HIV).
- Fungi occur in malnourished, debilitated, or immunosuppressed patients.
    - Most common pathogens include *Cryptococcus* and *Coccidioides*.
    - Rare pathogens include *Histoplasma*, *Candida*, and *Paracoccidioides*.
- Tuberculosis (TB), caused by *Mycobacterium tuberculosis*, is seen in malnourished, debilitated, or immunosuppressed persons.
    - More common in less-developed areas of the world.
    - Accounts for approximately 15% of extrapulmonary TB in the United States.
- Spirochetal meningitis, caused by *T. pallidum* and *Borrelia burgdorferi*, is associated with neurosyphilis and Lyme disease.

3. Clinical Features

- Most patients have some of the following four symptoms: mental status change, fever, headache, and stiff neck.
- Change in mental status can vary from confusion to coma.
- Photophobia, nausea, and emesis may also be present.
- Late: seizures, stupor, coma, cranial nerve palsies, deafness, focal neurologic signs, and papilledema.
- Positive Kernig and Brudzinski signs.
- In infants: irritability, lethargy, seizures, anorexia, and bulging fontanelles.
- May have rash of meningococcemia: diffuse, erythematous maculopapular rash on trunk/extremities/mucous membranes/conjunctiva; becomes petechial.
- Rapidly evolving rash indicates *N. meningitidis* pathogen.

4. Diagnostic Studies

- Obtain blood cultures immediately in suspected meningitis prior to initiating antibiotic therapy.
- Obtain fast-track neuroimaging, if at all possible, prior to LP if available to look for possible LP contraindications (intracranial mass lesions, midline shift, and obstructive hydrocephalus).
- LP should be done as soon as possible: CSF examination is essential to diagnosis unless

contraindication(s) like papilledema, focal neurologic sign, or coagulopathy is(are) present.
- LP is the most definitive diagnostic study for suspected ABM.
- CSF profiles differ between the various types of pathogens (Table 12-1).
- Other testing such as possible latex agglutination antigen tests detect *Haemophilus influenzae*, *S. pneumoniae*, and *N. meningitidis*.

5. Management

- Hospitalization for observation and prompt administration of appropriate IV antibiotics are essential.
- Admission to a neurologic ICU is preferable if possible.
- **Bacterial meningitis**
    - IV third-generation cephalosporins (e.g., cefotaxime or ceftriaxone) are the initial drugs of choice in the absence of antibiotic resistance and penicillin (PCN) allergy and can be started empirically.
    - Begin with an empirical broad-spectrum antibiotic, then tailor therapy when the organism is identified and its sensitivities are determined.
    - *L. monocytogenes*: third-generation cephalosporin plus amoxicillin.
    - PCN-resistant pneumococcus: vancomycin plus third-generation cephalosporin.
    - Dexamethasone with or shortly before first administration of antibiotics.
    - Suspected *N. meningitidis* due to rapidly evolving rash on physical examination: IV benzylpenicillin in the absence of PCN allergy.
    - Common initial antibiotic therapy for ages 2 months to adult:
        - Ceftriaxone, 2 g IV q12h, and vancomycin, 10 to 15 mg per kg IV q6h; if patients older than 50 years, add ampicillin 2 g IV q8h.
        - Dexamethasone 0.15 mg per kg IV q6h for 2 to 4 days. Inhibits interleukins and stabilizes the blood–brain barrier, and decreases meningeal inflammation.
    - Consider prophylaxis of household occupants, daycare workers, and teachers with rifampin, ceftriaxone, or ciprofloxacin.
    - Therapy duration: *S. pneumonia*, 10 to 14 days; *N. meningitidis*, 3 to 7 days; *H. influenza*, 7 days; *L. monocytogenes*, 14 to 21 days; and gram-negative bacilli, 21 days.
- **Viral meningitis**
    - Supportive treatment (analgesics for headache and antiemetics for nausea and vomiting).
    - Hospitalization is not required; observation at home by a responsible person is routine.
    - Prognosis is excellent; full recovery in 1 to 2 weeks.

TABLE 12–1.	Spinal Fluid Profiles in Acute Meningitis			
Variables	Pressure	White Blood Cells (cells/mm^3)	Protein	Glucose
Viral	nl or slight ↑	5–1,000	Slight ↑	nl
Bacterial	↑	1,000–10,000	↑	↓
Chronic/tuberculosis	↑	25–500	↑	↓

↑, increase; ↓, decrease; nl, normal.

- **Fungal meningitis**
  - Hospitalize for observation and appropriate IV antifungal medication: amphotericin B (lipid complex, liposomal or colloidal dispersion) for several weeks to months; addition of flucytosine may potentiate efficacy. Followed by 8 weeks of treatment with fluconazole.
  - Complications and neurologic sequelae are the same as bacterial meningitis.
  - Mortality rate is 20% to 50%.
- **TB meningitis**
  - Initial therapy: rifampin, isoniazid, pyrazinamide, and ethambutol (RIPE).
  - Adjunctive corticosteroids with dexamethasone.
  - Specific treatment regimen depends on known regional antibiotic sensitivities and culture information, but duration of therapy is 18 to 24 months.
- **Spirochetal meningitis**
  - Treatment of CNS syphilis is IV PCN G for 10 to 14 days or procaine PCN plus probenecid both for 14 days.
  - Treatment for neurologic manifestations of Lyme disease is IV ceftriaxone for 14 days.

IV. Movement Disorders

A. Essential Tremor (Familial Tremor, Benign Essential Tremor, and Senile Tremor)

1. **Etiology**
   - An uncontrollable (involuntary) rhythmic, oscillatory movement at rest involving the head, voice, or hands that worsens with intentional movement.
   - Causes may include medications, alcohol or drug withdrawal, brain lesions, or systemic diseases.
   - Can begin at any age, increasing incidence with aging.
   - Most common of all movement disorders.
2. **Pathology**
   - No associated neurologic disorder.
   - Sometimes autosomal dominant.
3. **Clinical Features**
   - Tremor at rest that increases when under emotional stress.
   - On finger-to-nose test, tremor increases as "target" is approached.
   - Typically improves with ingestion of a small amount of alcohol for a short time.

4. **Diagnostic Studies**
   - Physical examination should include evaluation of limb supported at rest, elevated versus gravity, and with goal-directed movements.
   - No CT, MRI, hematologic, or serum abnormalities.
   - Differential diagnosis to include Parkison's disease, myoclonus, ethyl alcohol (ETOH) withdrawal, drug-induced, thyroid abnormalities, and heavy-metal poisoning.
5. **Management**
   - Identify and remove any possible causative medications.
   - Treatment unnecessary unless causing disability.
   - Stress reduction.
   - Propranolol (60–240 mg per day), primidone (starting at 50 mg daily, increasing to 125 mg three times daily), alprazolam (up to 3 mg daily, divided), and gabapentin (1,800 mg daily, divided).
   - Reassure this is not associated with other conditions.
   - Surgical options for refractory cases: deep brain stimulation and unilateral thalamotomy.

B. Huntington Disease

1. **Definition**
   - Progressive, fatal hyperkinetic movement disorder with dementia and chorea (abnormal movements).
2. **Etiology**
   - Autosomal dominant inherited disorder with a prevalence of 5 per 100,000 people.
   - Onset is usually between ages 35 and 40 and death results 10 to 20 years later.
3. **Pathology**
   - Abnormal genetic repeat in the Huntington gene; length of repeat may correlate with the speed of progression of the disease.
   - Decreased activity of acetylcholine (ACh) and γ-aminobutyric acid neurons and increased activity of dopaminergic neurons.
   - Microscopic hallmark: preferential loss of medium-sized spiny neurons from striatum to external pallidum.
4. **Clinical Features**
   - Family history of Huntington disease.
   - Triad of extrapyramidal movement disorder, dementia, and behavioral disturbances.

- Most common initial symptoms are behavioral changes, such as mood changes and irritability, or antisocial behavior. Subsequent development of dementia follows.
- Cognitive/intellectual changes and abnormal or bizarre movements are hallmarks of the illness. The dyskinesia portion can begin as apparent restlessness or fidgeting but progress to full chorea-like movements, rigidity, and dystonia.

5. Diagnostic Studies
- Genetic testing.
- In diagnosed cases, neuroimaging (MRI or CT) can demonstrate cerebral atrophy and atrophy of the caudate and putamen. Decreased striatal metabolic rate is shown on positron emission tomography (PET).

6. Management
- There is no cure or treatment to slow or halt the progression of Huntington disease.
- Treatments are for symptom reduction only.
- Tetrabenazine, reserpine, or amantadine can be used for chorea symptoms (12.5 mg two to three times daily).
- Treat psychosis with atypical antipsychotics.
- Offer genetic counseling to offspring.

C. Parkinson Disease

1. Etiology
- A progressive neurodegenerative disease.
- Occurs in all ethnic groups and in men and women equally.
- Generally begins between the ages of 40 and 70 years with peak onset in the sixth decade.

2. Pathology
- Loss of dopamine in the corpus striatum; degeneration of the substantia nigra in the midbrain. Cytoplasmic inclusion bodies in neurons of substantia nigra.
- Hallmark: eosinophilic cytoplasmic neuronal inclusions (Lewy bodies).
- Loss of pigmented cells in the nigra, locus coeruleus, and dorsal motor nucleus of the vagus.

3. Clinical Features
- Resting tremor: described as "pill-rolling"—decreases with voluntary movement. Unilateral or asymmetric.
- Cogwheel rigidity: elicited by passive movement.
- Bradykinesia: slowness of voluntary movement; and difficulty turning in bed, walking, chewing food, rising from chairs, and other activities.
- Expressionless, unblinking, mask-like face.
- Postural instability: inability of the patient to keep from losing his or her balance when jostled (e.g., when in a crowd).
- Stooped posture.

- Festinating gait, shuffling steps, and reduced arm swing.
- Micrographia (small handwriting).
- Drooling secondary to failure to swallow saliva with normal frequency.
- Nonmotor clinical features: cognitive dysfunction and dementia, psychosis, hallucinations, mood disorders, fatigue, sleep disturbance, and autonomic and olfactory dysfunction.

4. Diagnostic Studies
- Clinical diagnosis based on a constellation of signs and symptoms.
- Presence of cardinal manifestations: tremor, bradykinesia, rigidity, and gait disturbance.
- Response to dopaminergic therapy.
- Dopamine transporter (DaT) SPECT (single-photon emission computed tomography) detects degeneration of nigrostriatal nerve cells. Parkinson disease will show asymmetric loss.
- Differential diagnosis: neurodegenerative disorders, dementia with Lewy bodies, corticobasal degeneration, secondary parkinsonism (drug effect), and essential tremor.

5. Management
- Consider signs and symptoms, age, stage of disease, and degree of functional disability.
- Options include nonpharmacologic, pharmacologic, and surgical.

a. Nonpharmacologic
- Education, support, exercise, and nutrition.
- Maintenance of optimal general health and neuromuscular efficiency with a planned program of exercise and rest.

b. Pharmacologic
- Symptomatic treatment:
  - Exogenous levodopa (precursor to dopamine) in combination with peripheral dopa decarboxylase inhibitor in younger patients.
  - Carbidopa/levodopa starting dose: 25 mg/100 mg three times daily.
    - Start low and titrate upward.
    - Early side effects: nausea, vomiting, and hypotension.
    - Late side effects: dyskinesias (involuntary movements including restlessness, head-wagging, grimacing, lingual–labial dyskinesia, and dystonia), psychiatric (depression, altered sleep patterns, vivid nightmares, auditory and visual hallucinations, paranoia, and frank psychosis), and fluctuations in motor performance (on–off phenomenon).
  - Due to tolerance and side effects, it is recommended that drug therapy with carbidopa/levodopa be delayed until symptoms significantly affect the patient's life.

- Dopamine agonists (e.g., bromocriptine, pramipexole, ropinirole) have direct dopaminergic effect on striatal neurons.
  - Adverse effects: unpredictable sleepiness or compulsive behaviors (gambling, shopping, or hypersexuality).
- Amantadine (100 mg twice daily): antiviral that allows release of dopamine from presynaptic storage sites.
  - Adverse effects include visual hallucinations, skin rash, and nausea.
- Anticholinergic agents (e.g., trihexyphenidyl and benztropine).
  - Useful for tremor.
  - Adverse effects include dry mouth, blurred vision, urinary retention, and confusion.
- Surgical options: deep brain stimulation, thalamotomy, and pallidotomy.

V. Vascular Disorders

A. Cerebral Aneurysm/Intracranial Aneurysm

1. Etiology

- "Berry" or saccular aneurysms.
- Multiple aneurysms present in 20% of cases.
- Typically occur anterior to the circle of Willis.
- Subarachnoid hemorrhage (SAH) is a complication, and the risk of this is increased in "nonwhite" females, those who drink 150 mg of ETOH or more per week, tobacco users, and those with hypertension (HTN) or hypercholesterolemia. Older age is also a risk factor for SAH in the presence of an intracranial aneurysm.

2. Clinical Features

- Can be asymptomatic or have nonspecific symptoms until rupture and result in SAH.
- After rupture, patient may complain of sudden onset of severe headache (i.e., "thunderclap" or "worst headache of my life") followed by neck stiffness, photophobia, nausea, and vomiting. The classic sudden onset of "worst headache of my life" is seen in SAH. Focal neurologic deficits are seen depending on the location of the bleed.
- The aneurysm itself may be asymptomatic, but resulting SAH may present with loss of consciousness, headache, nausea, and/or focal neurologic deficits.

3. Diagnostic Studies

- Angiography is definitive.
- CT or MRI may not be thorough enough for smaller lesions, especially when surgery is being considered.

4. Management

- Bed rest and reduction of strain/increased ICP.
- Prompt endovascular/surgical treatment needed for symptomatic aneurysms that have not yet ruptured.
- Monitor aneurysms smaller than 10 mm with angiograms. Consider surgery at size over 10 mm.

B. Intracranial Hemorrhage

1. Disease

- Intracranial and SAH are subclassifications of hemorrhagic stroke.

2. Etiology/Pathology

- HTN is usually the cause of a spontaneous intracerebral hemorrhage (ICH) that did not occur from trauma, if the patient does not have evidence of a vascular abnormality such as an angioma or aneurysm.
- Usually occurs in the basal ganglia, pons, thalamus, and cerebellum.
- Bleeding disorders, tumors, liver disease, alcohol abuse, and anticoagulation therapy can also be causes.
- Older age and male sex are risk factors.
- Bleeding occurs into the subarachnoid space usually when secondary to an arteriovenous malformation (AVM) or aneurysm.

3. Clinical Features

- Hemorrhages occur suddenly and are accompanied by loss of consciousness in half of patients.
- Nausea, vomiting, and headache can be present.
- There can be corresponding focal symptoms depending on the cerebral location of the bleed.
- Hypertensive etiology hemorrhage is usually accompanied by a rapidly progressive hemiplegia or hemiparesis.
- Extraocular movements may be compromised, depending on the location of the bleed as well.
- Look for changes in respiration, ataxia, change in small and reactive pupils, and facial weakness.

4. Diagnostic Studies

- Noncontrast CT is superior to MRI.
- CT angiography for smaller bleeds.
- Look for predisposing factors in lab work.
- LP if CT is negative.

5. Management

- Supportive to symptoms.
- Monitor for signs of brainstem herniation.
- Discontinue all antithrombotic agents.
- ICP alleviating techniques, including BP control (systolic < 140), may be helpful in some cases.
- Fresh-frozen plasma (FFP) and vitamin K (if vitamin K antagonist associated ICH).
- Cerebellar hemorrhage requires prompt surgery/hematoma evacuation.

C. Cerebrovascular Accident (Stroke)

1. Etiology

- Fifth leading cause of death, and leading cause of disability in the United States.
- Ischemia occurs due to reduction in cerebral blood flow with symptoms occurring within 10 seconds

due to lack of glycogen in neurons and "energy crisis."

- Eighty percent of all strokes are ischemic (due to thrombus, emboli, or systemic hypoperfusion) and 20% are hemorrhagic (i.e., ICH and SAH).
- Cerebral thrombosis includes lacunar (e.g., small vessel, penetrating arteries, atheroma, and lipohyalinosis) and large vessel thrombosis (e.g., atherosclerosis and dissection).
- Cardioembolic sources: atrial fibrillation, myocardial infarction (MI), mural thrombus, valvular lesions/prosthesis, anomalies, dilated cardiomyopathy, and bacterial endocarditis.
- Hypercoagulable disorders: venous sinus thrombosis (complication of pregnancy, postpartum, sepsis, and brain abscess/meningitis), polycythemia, factor V Leiden mutation, protein C and S deficiencies, antiphospholipid antibody syndrome, acquired antithrombin (AT) III deficiency, oral contraceptives, sickle cell disease, and homocystinemia.
- Vascular etiologies: fibromuscular dysplasia, temporal arteritis, vasculitis, and moyamoya disease.

2. Pathology
- Atherosclerotic damage to aortic arch, carotid bifurcation, or intracranial vessels occurs that produces local thrombus and distal embolism with injury to vascular endothelial cells.
- Nonmodifiable risk factors include increasing age, male, African American, family history, sickle cell disease, and hypercoagulable state.
- Modifiable risk factors include hypercholesterolemia, HTN, atrial fibrillation, diabetes mellitus (DM), asymptomatic carotid stenosis, transient ischemic attack (TIA), smoking, oral contraceptive use, obesity, alcohol consumption, and physical inactivity.

3. Clinical Features
- Ischemic and hemorrhagic stroke: symptoms determined by vascular territory of affected vessel and variable acute or subacute neurologic deficits (e.g., headache, alteration of consciousness, speech disturbance, aphasia or dysarthria, visual deficits, apraxia, agnosia, motor or sensory dysfunction).
- ICH: abrupt onset of severe headache, hemiplegia, and diminished level of consciousness; may not see these findings if hemorrhage is small.
- SAH: abrupt onset of headache (i.e., "thunderclap" or "worst headache of my life"), photophobia, nuchal rigidity, Kernig sign, and alteration of consciousness.

4. Diagnostic Studies
- CBC to rule out polycythemia; elevated WBCs are present in infective endocarditis, prothrombin time (PT), partial thromboplastin time (PTT), platelet count, consider syphilis serology, blood cultures, cholesterol profile, electrocardiography (ECG)/telemetry, chest X-ray (CXR), and cardiac echo (transthoracic or transesophageal).
- Noncontrast CT scan of head is preferable to MRI in acute stages (first 48 hours) because it is faster and detects intracranial hemorrhage better than MRI in the first 48 hours after an acute bleed. Poor detection in posterior fossa stroke, which may remain "normal" in the initial 12 to 24 hours.
- MRI/magnetic resonance angiography (MRA). Diffusion-weighted MRI is more sensitive than non–diffusion-weighted MRI for visualizing cerebral ischemia.
- EEG not routinely indicated; useful in distinguishing focal seizure activity from fluctuating symptoms of stroke or TIA.
- Carotid ultrasound (U/S) identifies occlusion or stenosis of carotid arteries.
- Cerebral angiography identifies stenosis, thrombosis, aneurysms, AVMs, and other cerebrovascular abnormalities.
- LP (if no contraindication) if suspicion for SAH and negative CT scan. Monitor for xanthochromia.

5. Management
- Thrombolytics, anticoagulation, antiplatelets, carotid endarterectomy/stent/angioplasty, surgical decompression, medical management, rehabilitation, and secondary prevention.
- Thrombolytics: recombinant tissue plasminogen activator (rtPA).
- rtPA most beneficial if within 3 hours of symptoms or no more than 4.5 hours and if no evidence of hemorrhage on CT.
- Contraindications to rtPA: head trauma or stroke in past 3 months, SAH, prior ICH, intracranial neoplasm or aneurysm, recent brain or spine surgery, active bleed, platelets <100,000, pregnancy, seizure, major surgery or trauma within 14 days, acute MI within 3 months, and BP <180/105 mm Hg.
- Anticoagulation with warfarin if chronic atrial fibrillation, cardioembolic source, recent MI, or valvular disease/prosthetics.
- Antiplatelet therapy: aspirin, clopidogrel, and dipyridamole.
- Must pass swallow study or aspirin should be given rectally.
- Surgical options: ICP monitor, decompression craniotomy with evacuation of hemorrhage, and craniectomy and expansion duraplasty if edema or increased ICP.
- Primary and secondary stroke prevention: evaluate clinical risk profile and manage modifiable risk factors, control HTN, treat hypercholesterolemia, smoking cessation, weight loss, and exercise.

- Supportive therapy: consultation with appropriate rehabilitation services; may include speech, occupational, and physical therapy, as well as social services.

D. Transient Ischemic Attack

1. Etiology

- Characterized by transient focal ischemic cerebral neurologic deficits, lasting <24 hours (usually 5 minutes to 1 hour).
- Cerebrovascular accident (CVA) following TIA most likely in the following 48 hours.
- Risk stratification scale: ABCD score (age, blood pressure, clinical presentation, duration of symptoms and diabetes mellitus). Risk increases as score increases. Hospitalize for score of 3 or more.
- Emboli are the most important cause; most common source is carotid or vertebrobasilar circulations.
- Cardiac causes of embolic TIA include atrial fibrillation, rheumatic heart disease, mitral valve disease, cardiac arrhythmia, infective endocarditis, and atrial myxoma.
- Less common causes include fibromuscular dysplasia, meningovascular syphilis, and inflammatory arterial disorders (e.g., giant cell arteritis, systemic lupus erythematosus [SLE], polyarteritis, granulomatous angiitis) and hematologic causes like sickle cell, polycythemia, and syndromes with increased viscosity.
- Crescendo TIAs: occurrence of increasing number and frequency with a high likelihood of evolving to stroke (two or more attacks within 24 hours).

2. Clinical Features

- Symptoms vary markedly among patients; however, for a given patient, symptoms tend to be constant.
- Symptoms:
  - Weakness or heaviness of the contralateral arm, leg, or face.
  - Numbness and paresthesias.
  - Slowness of movement.
  - Dysphasia.
  - Transient vision loss (amaurosis fugax) can be monocular or bilateral, lasting seconds to hours.
  - Abrupt onset without warning.
  - Rapid recovery, usually 1 to 2 hours, but can be within minutes.
  - One-third of patients with TIAs continue to have attacks without sequelae, one-third experience spontaneous remission, and one-third subsequently suffer brain infarction.

3. Diagnostic Studies

- CT scan or MRI of head: excludes small cerebral hemorrhage or tumor that may mimic TIA symptoms; carotid duplex U/S: detects stenosis of internal carotid artery, CT angiography, MRA, or conventional angiography: evaluates carotids and circle of Willis.
- Assess patient for risk factors: CBC, fasting blood glucose, serum cholesterol profile, ECG, echo (if suspect cardiac source emboli), blood cultures (if endocarditis is suspected), and Holter monitor (if transient, paroxysmal cardiac arrhythmia is suspected).

4. Management

- May warn of imminent stroke; therefore, treatment should be aggressive.
- Treat or modify controllable risk factors.
- Antiplatelet therapy, such as aspirin 81 to 325 mg daily or clopidogrel 75 mg daily.
- If atrial fibrillation or cardioembolism, treat with anticoagulants: heparin, follow with warfarin.
- Depending on angiographic findings, consider carotid endarterectomy, angioplasty, or stenting.

VI. Other Neurologic Disorders

A. Cerebral Palsy

1. Definition

- State of impaired muscle tone, movement, and coordination, which varies in severity from patient to patient. The condition is nonprogressive, but does not resolve.

2. Etiology

- Caused by brain injury or insult that occurred either prenatally, during birth, or in the perinatal phase. Intrauterine hypoxia is a common cause of insult.

3. Clinical Features

- Limb spasticity is common (75% of cases) and various limbs and combinations can be affected.
- Fine movement deficits and decreased coordination, as well as involuntary movements, may be associated.
- Seizure disorders are also possible.
- Intellectual disabilities are seen in a majority of cases. Behavioral disorders, vision impairment, hearing loss, and speech difficulties are also common.
- Physical examination may reveal limb spasticity, hyperreflexia, scissor gait, and microcephaly.

4. Diagnostic Studies

- U/S (in infants) or MRI (in older children) may reveal the etiology or the extent of the involved cerebral area. However, etiology is not found in 20% to 30% of cases.
- Definitive diagnosis should only be made after the first year of life due to rapid development until age 1.

5. Management

- Supportive care.
- Occupational, physical, and speech therapy are essential.

- Pharmacologic therapy for seizure control or muscle spasticity (e.g., diazepam or baclofen) may be needed.
- Patients with mild forms may improve over time. In some cases, intellectual capacity is normal, and those children can lead productive lives of normal span.

B. Concussion

1. Definition
- A mild traumatic brain injury (TBI) with or without a loss of consciousness, causing a change in mental status.

2. Etiology
- Secondary to a blunt or acceleration–deceleration injury to the head.

3. Clinical Features
- Signs and symptoms are often very subtle.
- Diagnosis depends on any alteration in mental processes following a head trauma.
- May include any of the following physical, cognitive, or behavioral changes or deficits: short- and long-term memory impairment, altered cognition, dizziness, vertigo, confusion, nausea/vomiting, headache, photophobia, blurred vision, brief loss of consciousness, change in concentration, balance disturbance, fatigue, seizure, anxiety, depressed mood, or tinnitus.
- Depression or changes in social participation or quality of participation can be common.

4. Diagnostic Studies
- Thorough initial neurologic evaluation is critical, including testing cognition, memory, and cerebellar function.
- Indications for head CT include: age over 65 years, seizure, focal neurologic findings or indication of a basilar skull fracture on examination, Glasgow Coma Scale (GCS) <15, two or more episodes of postinjury vomiting, moderate-to-severe headache, history of fall of >4 ft, past medical history of coagulopathy, and retrograde amnesia for greater than 30 minutes.
- Head CT is usually negative, even in mild TBI, but can be used to look for other results of trauma that may require surgical intervention.
- CT is not required of all patients. If CT is not indicated, patients can be carefully monitored at home by a caregiver every hour for 24 hours.
- Spine injury may also result from the traumatic event, so cervical spine X-rays should be considered for concussion patients with neck pain or neurologic deficit resembling cord compression.

5. Management
- No pharmacologic management. Supportive care.
- "ABCs" (airway, breathing, and circulation) and cervical spine should be addressed.

- Patient and a caregiver must be carefully educated about warning signs and why and when to return to the emergency department (ED) or for further care including, but not limited to, a persistent change in memory or cognition, headache, vomiting, or irritability.
- Patients should be admitted if GCS <15, coagulopathy, seizure episode, or no proper caregiver at home.
- Athletes may downplay symptoms to avoid being removed from practice or a game, so consultation with providers trained in concussion evaluation may be helpful.
- A graded return to activity program should be utilized, which involves a patient being asymptomatic for at least 24 hours prior to progressing to the next stage. In general, patients will progress from light to moderate to normal exercise/activity. Symptoms remaining after 3 weeks require consultation.
- There is no set amount of time for monitoring after a mild TBI.
- Symptoms generally resolve for a majority of patients within the first 4 weeks, but can remain in some patients until 3 months. Up to 10% to 15% of patients may still experience lingering symptoms at 1 year.
- A second concussion occurring while a patient continues to have symptoms from the initial trauma may lead to long-term sequelae or death (second impact syndrome).

C. Postconcussion Syndrome

1. Etiology
- Results when symptoms of mild TBI, such as headache, judgment, memory or concentration problems, dizziness, irritability, depression, anxiety, sleep disturbance, and fatigue, remain unresolved for months to years after the initial injury.
- Postconcussion *symptoms* include those lasting for 4 weeks or less after an injury.
- Postconcussion *syndrome*, on the other hand, can be used to indicate symptoms remaining 1 month to a year or more after an initial TBI.

2. Clinical Features
- Persistence of common symptoms of concussion, such as headache, insomnia, and alterations in concentration.
- No relationship to severity of symptoms or findings on initial evaluation.
- Symptoms can be vague and overlap with other pathologies.

3. Diagnosis
- Standardized tools, such as the Post-Concussion Symptom Scale (PCSS) and Graded Symptom Checklist (GCS), are used to assist with diagnosis.

4. Management
- Primarily supportive and rehabilitative in nature.
- Treat symptomatically with NSAIDs or triptans for headache.
- Consider selective serotonin reuptake inhibitors (SSRIs) and tricyclic antidepressants for headache and mood disorders.
- Consultation with concussive specialist for further neuropsychological testing.

D. Dementia

1. Definition
- Persistent, progressive decline of cognitive abilities that results in the loss of function in work or social situations. In contrast to delirium, patients are usually alert and have a stable level of consciousness (Table 12–2).

2. Etiology
- May be acquired, a primary neurodegenerative disorder, or secondary to another disease process (e.g., CVA in vascular dementia).
- Common causes include Alzheimer disease (50%–70% of cases), vascular dementia (20%–30% of cases), Lewy body disease, Parkinson disease, frontotemporal dementia, thyroid disease, vitamin deficiencies (e.g., vitamins D and B_{12}), chronic alcoholism, metastatic or primary brain tumor, normal pressure hydrocephalus, and medications.
- Risk factors include advanced age, family history of dementia, prior severe head injury, and vascular risk factors (e.g., HTN, cardiovascular disease, obesity, and DM).
- Patients with mild cognitive impairment progress to dementia at an annual rate of 10% to 15%.

3. Clinical Features
- Presenting symptoms vary depending on the portion of the brain affected.
- Most common features include memory loss, aphasia (word-finding difficulty), visuospatial dysfunction (poor recognition of previously familiar places), apathy, and apraxia (inability to perform learned motor behaviors).
- Executive function is also impaired, which affects judgment, organization, attention, and processing speed.
- Impairment in cognitive factors would be greater than would be expected for the patient's educational level and age.
- Parkinsonian movements or other motor abnormalities may be seen on physical examination and may help reveal the underlying neurologic etiology.

4. Diagnostic Studies
- Potentially treatable causes of dementia should be ruled out through laboratory testing, which includes vitamin B_{12}, folate, serum electrolytes, liver function, renal function, and a thyroid panel. If suspected, testing for HIV, syphilis, and Lyme disease should also be considered.
- Head CT or brain MRI should also be performed.
- Neuropsychological testing is used to document the patient's level of cognitive impairment. The Montreal Cognitive Assessment (MoCA) and Mini-Mental Status Examination (MMSE) are a few of many tests currently available.

TABLE 12–2. Dementia versus Delirium: Clinical Differences

Clinical Feature	Delirium	Dementia
Onset	Acute, over days to weeks	Insidious, over months to years
Course	Fluctuating symptoms	Stable but with progressive decline
Duration	Days to weeks or months	Years until inevitable death
Awareness	Reduced	Clear
Attention	Impaired—distractible	Usually normal for discrete tasks
Alertness	Fluctuates, often lethargic or hypervigilant	Usually normal
Orientation	Impaired	Impaired
Memory	Immediate and recent memories impaired	Recent and remote memories impaired
Perception	Hallucinations common	Intact
Thinking	Fragmented and disorganized with transient delusions	Impaired abstract thinking, vague content, agnosia
Language	Speech slow or rapid, often incoherent	Word-finding difficulty, aphasia
Psychomotor	Variable; hyperkinetic or hypokinetic	Apraxia as dementia progresses
Sleep–wake cycle	Disrupted or reversed	Reversed or fragmented

From Agronin ME. *Alzheimer Disease and Other Dementias.* 2nd ed. Philadelphia, PA: Lippincott Williams & Wilkins; a Wolters Kluwer business; 2008.

5. Management
- Treat any underlying causative pathology.
- Cholinesterase inhibitors (CEIs) (e.g., donepezil and rivastigmine) are considered first line. These medications may help delay (but not prevent) disease progression.
- SSRIs may be helpful in treating associated depression and anxiety.
- Encourage physically and mentally stimulating activities.
- Predictable daily routine with environmental cues helps with reorientation.
- Strong family and caregiver involvement is critical.

E. Alzheimer Disease
1. Etiology
- Most common type of dementia.
- Worldwide prevalence of Alzheimer disease is expected to increase from 44 million in 2014 to 135 million in 2050.
- Risk factors include genetic presence of APOE e4 allele (chromosome 19), prior head injury, and depression later in life.

2. Pathology
- Extracellular deposition of amyloid-β protein, intracellular neurofibrillary tangles (composed of hyperphosphorylated tau protein), and loss of neurons are hallmark features.
- Initially, the disease affects the hippocampus and then spreads to the parietal, temporal, and frontal lobes.
- The level of ACh deficit (secondary to the loss of choline acetyltransferase) corresponds well with the disease presentation.

3. Clinical Features
- Most common initial symptom is progressive memory impairment for newly acquired information, while memory for remote events remains unimpaired.
- Visuospatial dysfunction (getting lost in previously known places), emotional changes (e.g., depression and agitation), language impairment (e.g., difficulty in word-finding), and apraxia are common early symptoms.
- Patients may also note trouble with activities of daily living (ADLs) such as toileting, feeding, and dressing, as well as independent ADLs such as balancing a checkbook, using a cell phone, and shopping.

4. Diagnostic Studies
- Clinical diagnosis of exclusion because definitive diagnosis is only possible with biopsy (rarely performed) or autopsy.
- As with all dementia patients, important to rule out other possible underlying etiologies through CBC, electrolytes, thyroid panel, vitamin B_{12}, folate, glucose, lipid profile, renal studies, and liver function tests. If appropriate, consider HIV, Lyme titers, and neurosyphilis testing as well.
- Biomarker testing (e.g., T-tau, P-tau, and β-amyloid) is discouraged due to the financial burden and lack of specific disease-modifying treatment.
- Routine APOE genotyping is not recommended due to the absence of preventative therapy.
- PET scan with radiolabeled ligand for β-amyloid protein may assist in the diagnosis of a patient with cognitive impairment.
- EEG, CT scan, or MRI is performed to rule out vascular disease, subdural hematoma, mass lesions, hydrocephalus, demyelinating disease, and leukodystrophies.
- Neuropsychological testing with the MoCA or MMSE may detect subtle cognitive impairment.

5. Management
- CEIs (e.g., rivastigmine, galantamine, and donepezil) may provide modest improvement in mild-to-moderate disease, but they will not affect the overall disease process.
- N-Methyl-D-aspartate (NMDA) receptor antagonists (e.g., memantine) are considered second-line therapies and have shown some effectiveness in prolonging daily function for moderate-to-severe disease.
- Antipsychotics are not recommended for aggression/psychosis in dementia.
- *Ginkgo biloba* is not shown to prevent or treat cognitive decline in Alzheimer disease.
- Evaluation of a patient's ability to make decisions (e.g., financial planning) and a driving assessment are recommended.
- Assist caregivers in simplifying communication with the patient and in creating a daily structure.
- Patients and caregivers should be directed to community and online resources, such as through the Alzheimer's Association.
- After initial diagnosis, life expectancy is 3 to 15 years.

F. Delirium
1. Definition
- Acute alteration in consciousness associated with cognitive abnormalities, memory impairment, and perceptual disturbances. Delirium can be distinguished from dementia due to its transient, fluctuating course, which is often reversible.

2. Etiology
- Variable: may be secondary to infection, medications, hypoxemia, alterations in electrolytes, alcohol withdrawal, and coronary ischemia.
- May coexist with dementia.
- Common risk factors include advanced age, cognitive impairment, polypharmacy, severe illness, visual and auditory impairment, and depression.

3. Clinical Features
- Most common initial symptom is an abrupt behavioral or mental status change.

- Sudden onset of the inability to maintain attention and concentration is also common.
- Short-term memory and recall are also decreased or absent.
- Patients have decreased orientation and may experience hallucinations or other disturbances in perception.

4. Diagnostic Studies

- Thorough investigation of all medications, as well as physical and neurologic examinations, is critical.
- Assessment instruments, such as the Confusion Assessment Method (CAM), can be used to validate diagnosis.
- In order to determine underlying cause, perform ECG, urinalysis, and select laboratory tests, including CBC, serum electrolytes, serum glucose, blood urea nitrogen (BUN), creatinine, and liver function tests.
- Urine toxicology and head CT may be required in some cases as well.

5. Management

- Supportive care with focus on the treatment of underlying pathology.
- Extensive review and reconciliation of all medications.
- Provide environment for the patient to become reoriented, which includes having family members or a caregiver at bedside.
- Avoid use of physical restraints because they have been found to increase morbidity and mortality.
- If nonpharmacologic management is not successful, antipsychotics are considered the drugs of choice. Oral haloperidol and quetiapine are often used.

G. Guillain–Barré Syndrome (Acute Idiopathic Polyneuropathy)

1. Definition

- Acute, immune-mediated demyelinating disorder with progressive weakness and sensory deficits.

2. Etiology

- May follow recent immunizations (such as influenza), surgery, or recent infections.
- Commonly associated with *Campylobacter jejuni* infection, as well as CMV and infectious mononucleosis.
- May also be immunologically related, but the exact pathology is unclear.

3. Pathology

- Demyelination (most common) or axonal degeneration.

4. Clinical Features

- Initial symptoms often include paresthesias of the feet.
- Shortly after onset, weakness generally occurs distally (commonly in the legs) and progresses in an ascending, symmetrical manner.

- Dysesthesia, radicular pain, and neuropathic pain may also occur. However, symptoms of sensory decline are typically less prominent than weakness.
- Deep tendon reflexes are generally decreased or absent.
- Autonomic processes can also be affected and may be life-threatening in some cases due to arrhythmias, respiratory complications, and hypertension/hypotension.
- Facial weakness and ophthalmoplegia may be present as well.
- Symptoms typically peak within 4 weeks of onset.
- Asymmetric deficits should lead one to consider spinal cord origins.

5. Diagnostic Studies

- After 2 to 3 weeks, CSF analysis will show markedly increased protein, otherwise normal cell content (albuminocytologic dissociation).
- Electromyography (EMG) may reveal axonal degeneration.
- Forced vital capacity (FVC) should be monitored for respiratory decline.
- Rule out other causes of neuropathies. Heavy-metal toxicity, tick-caused paralysis, polio, and botulism can also cause weakness/paralysis.

6. Management

- Hospitalize until stable and able to confirm no signs of respiratory compromise.
- IV immunoglobulin (400 mg per kg daily for 5 days) and plasmapheresis are both considered therapies of choice. No benefit is known for using both in combination.
- Prednisone is not effective and not indicated.
- Patients with decreasing FVC should be admitted to ICU. If FVC is below 15 mL per kg, intubation should be performed.
- Measures should be taken to avoid atelectasis and thrombosis.
- With proper care, 80% to 90% of patients are able to recover without significant long-term disability. Recovery may take several months to a year. Mortality may occur in 5% to 10% of patients secondary to respiratory failure, arrhythmias, or thromboembolism.

H. Multiple Sclerosis

1. Etiology

- Common neurologic disorder in temperate regions.
- More common presentation in younger adults (<55 years) and of Western European descent.
- Genetic association and possibly autoimmune.
- Female predominance.

2. Pathology

- Demyelination in white matter of the CNS and optic nerves with axonal damage possible.

3. Clinical Features

- Most common initial symptoms include pares-thesias, weakness or numbness of a limb, optic neuritis (retrobulbar), ophthalmoplegia, urinary symptoms (sphincter problems), visual concerns, diplopia, or equilibrium disturbances.
- Forms include relapsing–remitting, primary progressive, and secondary progressive.
- Diagnosis must involve various parts of the nervous system being affected at various times.

4. Diagnostic Studies

- No one key definitive diagnostic study.
- MRI more helpful than CT.
- T1 and T2 MRI are helpful for demonstrating multiple lesions (Dawson fingers) and in identifying various progressions of the disease.
- MRI shows reduced or permanent demyelination.
- CSF analysis shows oligoclonal bands or increased immunoglobulin G (IgG).

5. Management

- High-dose steroids may reduce duration of acute exacerbations.
- Plasma exchange for patients unresponsive to steroids.
- There is no method to prevent progression.
- Support groups and antidepressant therapy are helpful.
- Treat symptoms: spasticity with baclofen, inability to urinate with cholinergics, and paresthesia with carbamazepine.
- β-Interferon, subcutaneous glatiramer acetate, and other disease-modifying therapies are also helpful in relapsing–remitting or secondary progressive disease.

I. Myasthenia Gravis

1. Etiology

- Autoimmune disorder.
- Most common disorder of neuromuscular transmission.
- Involves fluctuating weakness in ocular, bulbar, limb, and respiratory muscle.
- Associated with fatigue; weakness increases with exercise of affected muscles and improves with rest.
- Peak age of incidence in women is 20 to 30 years.
- Male incidence peaks over the fifth decade.

2. Pathology

- Interference of neuromuscular transmission at the postsynaptic site.
- Caused by antibodies to the ACh receptor protein.
- Abnormal hyperplasia or neoplasms of the thymus gland or hypothyroid/hyperthyroid disease are present in the majority of these patients.

3. Clinical Features

- Usually insidious onset.
- Course of the illness is extremely variable; danger of death is greatest in the first year after diagnosis.
- Fluctuating weakness may worsen as the day progresses; repeated or persistent activity of a muscle group (typically proximal muscles) exhausts its contractile power; rest partially restores strength.
- Common presenting features are diplopia, ptosis, weakness of eye closure (present in 90% of cases), bulbar involvement (seen in 80% of patients), difficulty chewing, regurgitation of fluids, dysphagia, low voice volume, and nasal speech.
- Disease progresses until muscle weakness is noted in the limbs, neck, and respiratory muscles (results in diminished vital capacity).
- Deep tendon reflexes are seldom altered.
- Smooth and cardiac muscles are not involved.
- Pupils respond normally to light and accommodation.
- Associated disorders include SLE, rheumatoid arthritis, thymic tumors (in ~ 10% of patients with myasthenia—predominately older males), and thyrotoxicosis (in about 5% of patients with myasthenia).

4. Diagnostic Studies

- Clinical diagnosis: sustained activity that results in weakness and contractility that improves with rest are virtually diagnostic (e.g., increasing droop of eyelid while looking at the ceiling or diplopia when fixating in lateral or vertical gaze for 2–3 minutes).
- Thyroid function studies.
- CXR and CT of mediastinum: rule out thymoma.
- Serum anticholinergic (anti-ACh) receptor antibody levels for binding, blocking, or modulating types (radioimmunoassay method most accurate and most widely used); 15% of patients with myasthenia gravis may be seronegative.
- May also test for muscle-specific receptor tyrosine kinase antibodies.
- Electrodiagnostic studies: repetitive nerve stimulation studies and single fiber EMG.
- Tensilon (edrophonium anticholinesterase inhibitor) test may help establish diagnosis. Initially 2 mg IV is given (dosage is repeated to 10 mg); if objective abatement of muscle weakness is determined within 1 to 2 minutes, myasthenia gravis is highly likely.
- Neostigmine 1.5 mg IM should improve myasthenic weakness in 10 to 15 minutes.
- Ice pack test in patients with ptosis: place ice pack on eyelids to cool muscles for 1 minute, then test for ptosis.

5. Management

- Anticholinesterase agents: pyridostigmine 30 to 60 mg every 4 hours.
- Neostigmine 15 mg every 4 hours.

- Observe for cholinergic crisis: nausea, vomiting, pallor, sweating, salivation, colic, diarrhea, meiosis, and bradycardia.
- Intermittent eye patching to eliminate diplopia.
- Rapid immunomodulating agents.
- Plasmapheresis, intravenous immunoglobulin (IVIG): temporary measure, used for managing acute exacerbations or in preparation for thymectomy.
- Chronic immunomodulating and immunosuppressive agents.
- Immunosuppressants: azathioprine 2 to 3 mg/kg/day or cyclosporine 5 mg/kg/day in patients with severe generalized weakness.
- Corticosteroids for moderate-to-severe symptoms refractory to CEIs. Hospitalization and careful observation for respiratory difficulty is advisable.
- Surgical thymectomy: improvement in 75% to 80% of patients. Recommended in patients aged 18 (postpubertal) to 59 years, especially in those not responding to other therapy.
- Myasthenic crisis: rapid and severe deterioration with respiratory failure and quadriparesis. Requires plasma exchange and ventilator management.

J. Seizure Disorders

- Seizure: a paroxysmal event due to abnormal, excessive hypersynchronous discharges from an aggregate of cortical neurons.
- Epilepsy: recurrent, unpredictable, and unprovoked seizures due to a chronic, underlying process.

1. Etiology

- May result from primary CNS dysfunction, underlying metabolic derangement, or systemic disease.
- Febrile seizures of childhood, idiopathic (most common), head trauma, stroke, vascular malformations, SAH, mass lesions, meningitis, brain abscess, encephalitis, cardiac arrest, and eclampsia.
- Hypoglycemia, hyponatremia, hypocalcemia, hyperosmolar state, uremia, hepatic encephalopathy, drug overdose, drug withdrawal (alcohol most common), and hyperthermia.

2. Pathophysiology

- Sudden, excessive, and disorderly electrical discharge of CNS neurons.
- Initiation phase: high-frequency action potentials lead to longer depolarization of neuronal membrane, influx of extracellular calcium, and opening of sodium channels.
- Propagation phase: nearby excitatory neurons are recruited with loss of inhibitory neurons and changes in the amount and conductance of neurotransmitters and ion channels.

3. Clinical Features

a. Partial (Focal) Seizures

- Simple partial seizures: consciousness is preserved; common auras include an epigastric rising sensation, nausea, feelings of fear, detachment, déjà vu, and involuntary movement.

b. Simple Partial Seizures

- Motor: focal twitching of extremity.
- Somatosensory: hallucinations, flashing lights, and paresthesias.
- Autonomic: pallor, flushing, sweating, piloerection, rising epigastric sensation, and vomiting.
- Dysphasia, distortion of memory, forced thinking, fear, hallucinations, and feelings of déjà vu.
- Complex partial seizures: focal seizure activity with transient impairment of consciousness (e.g., illusions, hallucinations, and dyscognitive states).

c. Complex Partial Seizures

- Most common type of adult seizures; formerly known as psychomotor or temporal lobe seizures.
- Usually begin with aura and patient's eyes indicate an awake state during the seizure.
- Typical behaviors are automatisms (e.g., lip-smacking, chewing, and repeated swallowing).
- Motor: focal rhythmic twitching of extremity; the involved area may enlarge through the recruitment of more neurons and result in "Jacksonian march" (increased motor deficit).
- In postictal state, a focal deficit such as hemiparesis (Todd paralysis) may persist (up to 36 hours) or complaints of headache, confusion, and fatigue.
- Partial seizures with secondary generalization:
  - Activity spreads to involve both hemispheres and usually involves tonic–clonic activity (also called generalized tonic–clonic seizure activity).
  - Crying with onset, halted respirations, cyanosis, foaming at the mouth, tongue biting and oral trauma, aspiration, and bladder and fecal incontinence.
  - Postictal lethargy and deep stupor.

d. Generalized Seizures

- Generalized seizures: all are characterized by abrupt loss of consciousness with no detectable focal onset.
  - Absence seizures (petit mal): sudden, brief loss of consciousness without loss of postural control; typically begin in childhood with episodes of staring or "daydreaming"; minimal motor manifestations (e.g., eyelid twitching); 60% spontaneously remit.

- Myoclonic seizures: brief jerks involving part or all of the body.
- Clonic: rhythmic jerking of the body.
- Tonic: brief attacks of stiffness (usually extensor spasms) in part or all of the body.
- Atonic: losses of postural tone (i.e., drop attacks) resulting in falls.
- Tonic–clonic (grand mal): bilateral tonic extension of trunk and limbs (tonic phase), followed by loud vocalization (cry) and synchronous muscle jerking (clonic phase); urinary incontinence, cyanosis, and tongue biting are common.

4. Differential Diagnosis
- Includes syncope, psychological disorders (e.g., pseudoseizures), migraine, TIA, cardiac arrhythmia, vascular disease, sleep disorders, movement disorders, and metabolic disturbance.

5. Diagnostic Studies
- EEG is the most important laboratory test for diagnosis, although it may be normal or nonspecific.
- MRI is the study of choice for detection of epileptogenic lesions and supports EEG.

6. Management
- Treat underlying condition that causes or contributes to seizure activity: correct metabolic disturbance (hyponatremia, hypoxemia, and hypokalemia/hyperkalemia), resect tumor, manage AVMs, and treat infection (brain abscess).
- Avoid precipitating factors such as sleep deprivation, alcohol intake, and stress.
- Antiepileptic drugs (AEDs):
  - Therapeutic drug monitoring should be used to determine compliance and minimize toxicity.
  - Follow serum drug levels, liver function tests, and CBC.
  - Start low and titrate dose upward until seizures are controlled or dose-related side effects occur (abnormal liver functions, nausea, emesis, vertigo, neutropenia, sedation, polycystic ovarian syndrome [valproate], rash [lamotrigine], and gingival hyperplasia [phenytoin]).
- If poorly controlled, add second agent and while weaning first agent.
- Patient education is crucial.
- Psychosocial issues to consider with AED therapy:
  - Noncompliance (50%).
  - Social implications include loss of independence (driving restrictions dependent on state law), unemployment, restricted alcohol intake, risk of seizure-related injury, and sudden death.
- Generalized tonic–clonic seizures: valproic acid, lamotrigine, carbamazepine, levetiracetam, phenytoin, phenobarbital, and primidone.
- Partial seizures (with/without secondary generalization): carbamazepine, oxcarbazepine, topiramate, levetiracetam, lamotrigine, zonisamide, valproic acid, phenobarbital, primidone, and gabapentin.
- Absence seizures: ethosuximide, valproic acid, clonazepam, and lamotrigine.
- Myoclonic seizures: valproic acid, clonazepam, phenytoin, lamotrigine, and topiramate.
- Phenobarbital first-line for children.
- Moderation in diet (ketogenic diet, modified Atkins diet, and low glycemic-index diet), alcohol intake, and exercise.
- Surgical treatment options if medically refractory: cortical resection, hemispherectomy, corpus callosotomy, lesionectomy, deep brain stimulation, responsive neurostimulator, and vagal nerve stimulator.

K. Status Epilepticus
- True medical emergency.
- Most common neurologic emergency.
- Continuous seizure activity or frequent seizures without interictal return to baseline clinical state of greater than 15 to 20 minutes duration.

1. Etiology
- AED withdrawal or noncompliance, metabolic disturbance, drug toxicity, CNS infection, tumors, head trauma, SAH, and withdrawal of alcohol, baclofen, benzodiazepines, or barbiturates.

2. Treatment
- Airway and oxygen; consider intubation.
- Rapid neurologic assessment.
- Draw chemistry profile and toxicology screen while establishing venous access.
- Give thiamine, ampule of D50, and naloxone.
- Lorazepam 0.02 to 0.03 mg per kg, diazepam 0.1 to 0.3 mg per kg, or midazolam 0.2 mg per kg.
- Close monitoring of hemodynamics.
- Load with fosphenytoin or phenytoin (rate not to exceed 50 mg per minute); risk of arrhythmias and hypotension.
- Continuous ECG and monitoring BP, oxygenation/ventilation.
- If persistent activity at 30 to 60 minutes, add phenytoin 5 to 10 mg per kg, and phenobarbital 50 to 100 mg per minute to maximum of 25 mg per kg.
- If persistent activity >60 minutes, give midazolam, propofol, or pentobarbital (5–15 mg per kg) load.

L. Syncope
1. Etiology
- Abrupt transient loss of consciousness and postural tone followed by rapid and complete recovery.
- Lightheadedness, loss of strength, and other symptoms that characterize an impending or incomplete fainting spell (presyncope).

- Cardiac structural defects such as aortic stenosis, hypertrophic obstructive cardiomyopathy, and tetralogy of Fallot.
- Reduction in cerebral blood flow (the most common type of syncope); includes vasodepressor syncope (rapid drop in BP and slowing of heartbeat often precipitated by fear, pain, and anxiety).
- Impaired cerebral metabolism (e.g., anoxia, hypoglycemia, acidosis, drug intoxication, acute alcoholism, hyperventilation, and associated respiratory alkalosis).
- Other causes include reduced blood volume secondary to obstruction, cardiac arrhythmias, pulmonary embolism, and orthostatic hypotension.

2. Pathology
- A small number of patients have a primary neurologic or cerebrovascular cause that includes transient brainstem ischemia (e.g., vertebrobasilar migraine or ischemia) or subclavian steal.
- Decreased cardiac output due to second- or third-degree conduction blocks can be exhibited in these patients.

3. Clinical Features
- Sensations of lightheadedness; sudden, brief loss of consciousness and decreased muscle tone, dizziness, weakness, diaphoresis, pallor, nausea, temperature change, or decreased motor power may be a prelude to the full episode.
- Can be present immediately before or after the syncopal episode.
- More apt to occur in standing position.
- Focal neurologic symptoms associated with syncope suggest an underlying disorder such as TIA or epilepsy.
- Exertional syncope is associated with obstructive cardiac etiologies.

4. Diagnostic Studies
- Complete history: number of episodes, associated symptoms, prodrome, position, preceding events, duration, recovery, age, medications, comorbidities, and temporal relationship to eating.
- Physical examination: orthostatic BP, Valsalva maneuvers, carotid sinus massage, and complete neurologic examination.
- ECG, ambulatory electrocardiograph 24 to 48 hours, cardiac echo, EEG, CT, carotid U/S, loop recorder, cardiac enzymes, brain natriuretic peptide, and exercise test.
- In more extreme cases, tilt table or electrophysiologic study (EPS).
- EEG or ambulatory ECG is diagnostic in 5% to 10% of cases. If symptoms develop while being monitored and no ECG changes occur, rhythm disturbance is eliminated as possibility.
- Ambulatory EEG if seizure disorder is suspected.

5. Management
- Dependent on etiology.

M. Gilles de la Tourette Syndrome (Tourette Disorder)
- Series of motor or phonetic tics or repetitious behaviors.

1. Etiology
- Onset usually in childhood between the ages of 2 and 15.
- Commonly diagnosed as psychiatric disorders initially.
- Can be a presentation of Wilson disease.

2. Pathology
- Autosomal dominant features with variable penetration.

3. Clinical Features
- Patients have tic-like movements of the face, head, and shoulders, including blinking, shrugging, head thrusting, and sniffling. Verbal or phonetic tics can include grunts, barks, throat-clearing, obscene words, coughs, hisses, repeating others' speech, repeating words or phrases, or imitating others.
- Tics can include self-harmful behaviors such as pulling hair and biting lips or tongue.
- Often associated with obsessive–compulsive symptoms as well.
- Diagnosis can be clinical and is often missed initially.

4. Management
- Behavioral therapy such as habit reversal is helpful to avoid social embarrassment and other social implications.
- Symptomatic: α-adrenergic agonists such as clonidine and guanfacine, haloperidol or other antipsychotics, dopamine-blocking medicines, or botulinum toxin are used.
- Deep brain stimulation is used for severe cases.
- Refer all patients with suspected Tourette syndrome to appropriate specialists.

N. Altered Level of Consciousness
- Unresponsive state, coma, and unarousable.

1. Etiology
- Toxic: drugs, medications, alcohol, and chemicals.
- Metabolic disorders: hypoglycemia/hyperglycemia, hypoxia, ammonia, thyroid, and hyponatremia/hypernatremia.
- Toxic–metabolic: organ-system failure (e.g., carbon dioxide narcosis, renal and hepatic failure, sepsis, and Wernicke encephalopathy).
- CNS: seizures, brainstem hemorrhage, tumor, stroke, trauma, herniation syndrome, and increased ICP (Cushing triad: bradycardia, HTN, irregular respiration).
- Other: hypothermia/hyperthermia, conversion disorder, malingering, thrombotic thrombocytopenic purpura, and fat emboli.

2. **Pathology**
   - Impaired reticular activity in the brainstem and innervated regions.
3. **Clinical Features**
   - Variable based upon etiology.
   - Fixed, dilated pupils with atropine overdose; pinpoint pupils with opioid overdose; and pupils smaller but responsive to light with metabolic encephalopathy.
   - Cheyne–Stokes respiration with metabolic etiologies.
   - Decorticate posture with central herniation.
   - Extensor posturing with cerebellar hemorrhage.
4. **Diagnostic Studies**
   - CT without contrast of the head to rule out neurosurgical emergency.
   - Labs: glucose, electrolytes, calcium, arterial blood gases (ABG), renal and liver function, and toxicology.
   - LP and EEG may be helpful.
5. **Management**
   - Supportive to symptoms.
   - Treat underlying cause.
   - Glucose, thiamine, and naloxone as indicated.
   - Hypertonic saline or mannitol for increased ICP.

REVIEW QUESTIONS

1. A 45-year-old man presents to the emergency room after having three witnessed seizures with bilateral tonic extension of limbs and synchronous muscle jerking in the past 24 hours. He has a past medical history of seizures previously associated with alcohol withdrawal and a history of end-stage liver disease secondary to alcoholic cirrhosis. He is currently on a liver transplant list and sober for 2 years. His current medications include furosemide, spironolactone, nadolol, and multivitamins. On physical examination, he is awake and alert, afebrile, and has a heart rate of 82 beats per minute with a BP of 116/78 mm Hg. He appears jaundiced, and his belly is hard and distended with a positive fluid wave. His legs show 2 to 3+ pitting edema. Lab studies show a normal serum creatinine and no blood ethanol. Serum electrolytes are normal. MRI of the brain shows chronic left frontotemporal encephalomalacia consistent with old trauma. An EEG indicates left temporal sharp waves. Which of the following is the best treatment for this patient?

   a) Valproic acid
   b) Phenytoin
   c) Levetiracetam
   d) Oxcarbazepine

2. A 30-year-old man presents after experiencing a 4-day history of worsening right eye pain and a 2-day history of visual disturbance in the right eye. The pain is aggravated by eye movement. Three years ago, the patient experienced a transient neurologic event without seeking medical attention. He stated he had arm clumsiness and a mildly unsteady gait, which resolved within a week. He has no other medical history and is not on medications. On physical examination, temperature is 97.2° F, BP is 125/56 mm Hg, pulse rate is 80 bpm, and respiratory rate is 16 breaths per minute. Pupillary reactivity is normal individually, but when a light is rapidly moved from the left to the right eye, the right pupil dilates by 2 mm. Visual acuity is 20/100 in the right eye and 20/20 in the left. Other findings from the physical examination are normal. Which of the following diagnostic tests is most appropriate to perform?

   a) LP
   b) MRI of the brain
   c) EEG
   d) CT of the head

3. A 20-year-old man presents with persistent headaches for 1 week following a head injury. He admits that he fell on his head during an amateur football game 1 week ago. He states that he never lost consciousness, but he felt very confused for about half an hour after the injury. No significant findings were noted on the sideline. He was removed from the game and recommended to follow up with his primary care. The day after the injury, he woke up with a mild headache with dizziness, which persisted for 4 days. He states that the dizziness has largely dissipated; however, he continues to have a slight headache, which is well-controlled with acetaminophen. He denies any cognitive deficits, but states that he has still not returned to his college classes or to physical activities. Physical examination—including neurologic examination—is unremarkable, and vital signs are all within normal limits. What is the most appropriate management plan for this patient at this time?

   a) Obtain head CT
   b) Obtain cervical spine X-rays
   c) Recommend sumatriptan for persistent headaches
   d) Prohibit participation in contact sports until patient is asymptomatic

4. A 90-year-old woman with a history of Alzheimer disease and HTN presents with a sudden increase in confusion and behavioral changes for the past 5 days. Her husband states that she has been on donepezil since her diagnosis 2 years ago, and he has only noticed a slow progression of her symptoms. However, 5 days ago, he noted that she was unable to locate the kitchen in their home, easily lost focus in conversations, became severely agitated in the evening, and noted hearing strange noises at night. Her

only medications are donepezil and lisinopril, which she has been on for years. Vitals signs are temperature of 99.3° F, BP of 115/70 mm Hg, pulse rate of 82 bpm (regular), and respiration rate of 12 breaths per minute. On physical examination, the patient appears drowsy and is not oriented to time or place. She is unable to stay focused or follow basic commands. No other significant findings were noted on physical examination. What is the most appropriate next step in this patient's management?

a) Discontinue donepezil
b) Obtain brain MRI
c) Start on haloperidol
d) Thorough evaluation for possible concurrent illness

5. A 57-year-old woman presents to the ED with sudden onset of severe headache and right-sided weakness followed by a temporary loss of consciousness. Her husband states this occurred 30 minutes ago. She has a history of HTN and takes amlodipine. She has a 25 pack-year smoking history. Physical examination shows a BP of 146/72 mm Hg, pulse rate of 88 bpm (regular), and a respiration rate of 14 breaths per minute. The patient does not follow commands. Pupils are equal and reactive to light bilaterally. An ECG shows normal sinus rhythm with no ST elevation. Which of the following is the most appropriate next step?

a) LP
b) CT of the head without contrast
c) MRI of the brain without contrast
d) Administration of rtPA

6. A 62-year-old man is evaluated for a 1-year history of tremor, which is more prominent on his left side. He reports increasing issue with balance and numerous falls. He has no cognitive symptoms, but has a history of acting out dreams during sleep. Physical examination shows a BP of 118/82 mm Hg and a pulse rate of 60 bpm sitting, and 86/62 mm Hg with pulse of 76 bpm standing. Respiration rate is 20 breaths per minute. Multiple bruises are noted on both upper and lower extremities secondary to falls. The patient has decreased facial expression and a tremor at rest that is more prominent on the right side. His gait is ataxic with a wide base, and he has decreased arm swing. Which of the following is the most likely diagnosis?

a) Essential tremor
b) Stroke
c) Parkinson disease
d) Huntington disease

7. A 36-year-old man with a 10 pack-year history of smoking presents with persistent, severe, right-sided periorbital headaches for the past week. His headaches occur once to twice daily and can last for 1 to 2 hours. He also experiences right-sided tearing, rhinorrhea, and nausea without vomiting. He notes that he typically has about

3 months of similar symptoms every spring for the past few years. He states that resting, NSAIDs, and prednisone do not provide relief. He notes that subcutaneous sumatriptan can quickly relieve symptoms, but his headaches are occurring too frequently to safely take sumatriptan each time. Vital signs are temperature of 98.7° F, BP of 128/80 mm Hg, pulse rate of 84 bpm (regular), and respiratory rate of 14 breaths per minute. Physical examination—including neurologic examination—was unremarkable. What is the most appropriate next step in this patient's management?

a) Start on 100% O_2 immediately
b) Add verapamil
c) Add propranolol
d) Add amitriptyline

ANSWERS TO REVIEW QUESTIONS

1. **Answer: C.** Levetiracetam is the preferred medical management for patients with liver disease due to the minimal hepatic metabolism. Valproic acid, phenytoin, and oxcarbazepine should be avoided because of their influence on the enzymatic metabolism in the liver and subsequent hepatotoxicity. Levetiracetam, gabapentin, and pregabalin are the most appropriate choices for antiepileptic management due to their renal excretion; they are least likely to interact with other medications and cause hepatotoxicity.

2. **Answer: B.** The MRI of the brain allows the provider to determine prognostic information in the risk of developing multiple sclerosis. Optic neuritis is suggestive of inflammatory demyelination in the CNS. An LP, EEG, and CT of the head will not provide the necessary information (white matter lesions of the brain on MRI) to confirm the diagnosis of multiple sclerosis.

3. **Answer: D.** The headache and dizziness that this patient is experiencing are considered postconcussion symptoms. Postconcussion symptoms occur within 4 weeks of a TBI and may include headache, concentration problems, dizziness, anxiety, sleep disturbance, and fatigue. Since this patient is an athlete, a graded return to activity program should be implemented. The patient should be asymptomatic for at least 24 hours before progressing to an increased level of activity. Head CT and cervical spine X-rays are not required at this time because the patient is not exhibiting any of the indications for further imaging. No additional medication is required because the patient states that his headaches are well-controlled with acetaminophen.

4. **Answer: D.** The patient is exhibiting the classic presentation of delirium—a sudden alteration in consciousness with perceptual changes and impairment in memory, attention, and concentration. Delirium is most commonly secondary to infection, medications, hypoxemia, electrolyte abnormalities, and coronary

ischemia. Therefore, to determine an etiology, the patient's history should be thoroughly evaluated for a possible concurrent illness. To narrow in on a cause, diagnostic tests and studies should be ordered, such as ECG, urinalysis, and select laboratory tests. Brain MRI is not required for this patient. The patient is only on two medications, which she has been on for several years. Therefore, medications are not the likely cause of her sudden delirium. Antipsychotics (e.g., haloperidol) should only be considered if nonpharmacologic management is unsuccessful.

5. **Answer: B**. A sudden-onset severe headache that is associated with focal weakness or altered consciousness is often associated with SAH or other intracranial bleed or, less frequently, cervical artery dissection or ischemic stroke. The patient's vital signs are stable, so the first step to diagnose the cause will be a CT of the head without contrast. If the CT brain does not reveal the cause or a bleed, then an MRI or LP can be considered. Administration of rtPA should never occur as a first step until a bleed and other risk factors are ruled out. The risk of hemorrhage is too high.

6. **Answer: C**. Parkinson disease remains a clinical diagnosis. The typical features are bradykinesia, resting tremor (often unilateral), and postural instability. Physical features can include craniofacial hypomimia (masked facial expression). The multiple falls and bruises allude to postural instability. An essential tremor is more noticeable in action, not at rest. A stroke should show motor or sensory deficits, not a tremor or masked facial expression. Huntington disease is characterized by choreiform movements, psychiatric problems, and dementia.

7. **Answer: B**. Severe unilateral headaches with ipsilateral rhinorrhea and lacrimation are characteristic symptoms of cluster headaches. This patient is exhibiting the episodic form of cluster headaches based on his symptom-free periods. Based on the frequency of his symptoms, abortive therapy with 100% O_2 or sumatriptan is not appropriate for long-term management. Therefore, this patient will require effective preventative therapy using a medication such as verapamil.

SELECTED REFERENCES

Agronin ME. *Alzheimer Disease and Other Dementias: A Practical Guide.* 2nd ed. Philadelphia, PA: Wolters Kluwer; 2008.

Alguire PC, Dodick DW, Ende J, eds. *MKSAP 15 Medical Knowledge Self-Assessment Program: Neurology.* 15th ed. Philadelphia, PA: American College of Physicians; 2009.

Biller J. *Practical Neurology.* 5th ed. Philadelphia, PA: Wolters Kluwer; 2017.

Griggs RC, Wing EJ, Fitz JG. *Andreoli and Carpenter's Cecil Essentials of Medicine.* 9th ed. Philadelphia, PA: Elsevier Inc; 2016.

Hammer GD, McPhee SJ. *Pathophysiology of Disease: An Introduction to Clinical Medicine.* 7th ed. New York, NY: McGraw Hill Companies Inc; 2014.

Le T, Bhushan V, Chen V, King M. *First Aid for the USMLE Step 2 CK Clinical Knowledge.* 9th ed. New York, NY: McGraw Hill Companies, Inc; 2016.

Masters PA, Kaniecki R, Ende J, eds. *MKSAP 17 Medical Knowledge Self-Assessment Program: Neurology.* 17th ed. Philadelphia, PA: American College of Physicians; 2015.

Papadakis MA, McPhee SJ, Rabow MW, eds. *Current Medical Diagnosis and Treatment.* 56th ed. New York, NY: McGraw Hill Companies Inc; 2017.

Sloane PD, Slatt LM, Ebell MH, Smith MA, Power D, Viera AJ. *Essentials of Family Medicine.* 6th ed. Philadelphia, PA: Wolters Kluwer; 2012.

Skin Disorders

Megan Schneider • Diana Smith

I. Eczematous Eruptions
A. Seborrheic Dermatitis
1. Etiology
- Not clearly defined.

2. Pathology
- Precise pathology not known, but skin rash occurs in areas of high sebaceous gland concentration and activity such as the scalp, face, and body folds.
- Histopathologic studies show a nonspecific inflammatory reaction in the dermis, spongiosis, and dilated follicular openings with neutrophils.
- The role of *Pityrosporum ovale*, a skin commensal, in the pathogenesis of seborrhea is not clear, although some patients show improvement with antifungal preparations.

3. Clinical Features
- Seborrhea (Figure 13–1) occurs in infants and adults; adult men are more affected than women.
- Pattern of involvement in infants includes scalp (cradle cap), flexural areas, and perioral region with erythematous plaques with fine, white scales to thick, yellow-brown, waxy plates of scales.
- Areas of involvement in adults are scalp, eyebrows, eyelashes, beard, and mustache, as well as nasolabial folds, postauricular sulci, trunk, and intertriginous regions of groin.
- Pruritus, itching, and burning sensations may occur in adults.

4. Diagnostic Studies
- Not typically performed; diagnosis based on clinical findings.

5. Management
- Selenium sulfide shampoos, 2% ketoconazole shampoo, or ketoconazole cream.
- Sodium sulfacetamide 10% sulfur 5% lotion/cream.
- Ciclopirox 1% shampoo.
- Severe cases may require oral antifungal therapy. (Patients with serum and crust are treated with oral antistaphylococcal antibiotics.)
- Corticosteroid (CS) preparations for inflammation may be used with close monitoring for skin atrophy.

B. Atopic Dermatitis
1. Etiology
- Typically, disorder begins in childhood.
- Hereditary predisposition to atopic dermatitis (Figure 13–2) with slight predominance in males.
- Trigger factors for the development of atopic dermatitis include allergens and contact irritants such as wool, nickel, fragrances, and latex; cold, dry climate; stress; and foods.

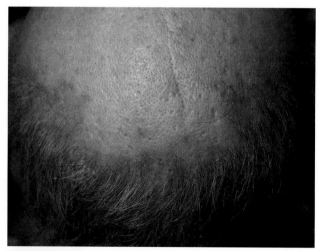

FIGURE 13–1. Seborrheic dermatitis. (Image provided by Stedman's.)

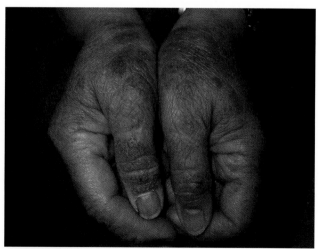

FIGURE 13–2. Atopic dermatitis. (Image provided by Stedman's.)

2. **Pathology**
- Altered immune reactions occur in genetically predisposed persons when exposed to trigger factor(s):
  - Increased T-cell activation.
  - Abnormal cell–mediated immunity.
  - Overproduction of immunoglobulin E (IgE).

3. **Clinical Features**
- Pruritus is a hallmark of atopic dermatitis causing "itch–scratch cycle."
- Acute lesions are erythematous, edematous papules/plaques with poorly defined borders; scaling may or may not be present. Oozing and crusting of lesions and secondary bacterial infection occur. Excoriations are common.
- Chronic lesions are characterized by lichenification and painful fissures, or nummular configuration (Figure 13–3).
- Other manifestations of atopy may be present: conjunctival and pharyngeal irritation/itching, rhinorrhea, edema, and discoloration of nasal mucosa, Dennie–Morgan sign.

4. **Diagnostic Studies**
- Serum IgE levels are increased.
- Radioallergosorbent test may be performed, but is of limited value in the management of patients.
- Viral culture for herpes simplex virus (HSV) to differentiate HSV infection from crusting atopic dermatitis.

5. **Management**
- Avoidance of triggers and elimination of scratching are essential to management.
- Application of topical, nonsteroidal immunomodulators such as pimecrolimus or tacrolimus.
- Use of leukotriene inhibitors and/or cyclosporine to interrupt/suppress aberrant T-cell activity.
- Acute lesions require wet dressings; topical or systemic antibiotics (e.g., cephalexin, dicloxacillin) for *Staphylococcus aureus* infection; topical CSs for inflammation; and oral antihistamines for pruritus.
- Chronic lesions necessitate daily hydration of skin with unscented bath oils and application of unscented emollients or mentholated lotions; oral antihistamines for pruritus; topical CSs or tar-based ointments for inflammation; and cyclic administration of erythromycin or other anti-staphylococcal regimen to control staphylococcal colonization.

C. **Lichen Simplex Chronicus**

1. **Etiology**
- Pruritic lichenified skin plaques, worsened by repetitive scratching, often located on the neck, extensor surfaces of the upper extremity, inner thighs, anterior lower extremities, and anogenital region.
- More common in women with a history of atopy.

2. **Pathology**
- Repetitive excessive scratching of the skin leads to an "itch–scratch cycle" that damages the skin and promotes hypertrophy and lichenification. Lichenification exacerbates pruritus. Initial source of pruritus may include mechanical or chemical irritation, excessive moisture, dermatitis, psoriasis, candidiasis, or other nondermatologic causes of pruritus.

3. **Clinical Features**
- May occur as a solitary lesion or with multiple lesions. Lichenified plaques present as thickened skin that may be red, hyperpigmented, or hypopigmented with excoriations, fissures, or scaling.
- Intense pruritus of lichenified skin occurs paroxysmally. Pruritus may be worse at night, and patients may scratch in their sleep.

4. **Diagnostic Studies**
- Clinical diagnosis based on history and physical examination.
- Histopathology can confirm diagnosis.

5. **Management**
- Goal of treatment is to control "itch–scratch cycle." Manage cause of pruritus by removing possible triggers and treating underlying pruritic condition.
- Control pruritus
  - Cool compresses, over-the-counter (OTC) anti-itch products.
  - Topical CSs used as first-line medication. May consider intralesional triamcinolone injection with severe symptoms that do not resolve with conservative measures.
  - Sedating oral antihistamine at bedtime to reduce scratching during sleep.
  - Consider counseling to address habitual scratching that may result from anxiety or depression.

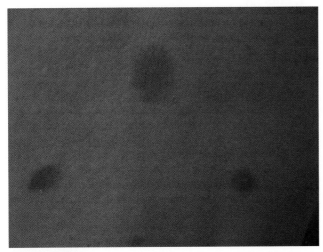

FIGURE 13–3. Nummular eczema. (Image provided by Stedman's.)

II. Papulosquamous Diseases

A. Psoriasis

1. Etiology

- Hereditary disorder affecting men and women equally and triggered by factors such as stress, physical trauma, medications (including systemic and class I topical CSs), and, occasionally, acute streptococcal infections.

2. Pathology

- Epidermal cells are produced at an accelerated rate due to a T-cell–mediated alteration in the cellular kinetics of keratinocytes causing the cell cycle to be significantly shortened (10 times faster than normal) and their maturation to be abnormal.
- T-cell activation and proliferation lead to production of cytokines interleukin-2, tumor necrosis factor-α (TNF-α), and interferon-γ. Under the influence of cytokines, inflammation and hyperproliferation of the epidermal keratinocytes occur.

3. Clinical Features

- Lesions of psoriasis are variable in distribution, arrangement, shape, and type.
- Five variants are plaque, pustular, guttate, inverse, and erythrodermoid.
- Plaque lesions (Figure 13–4) are the most common type of lesions—oval to round, erythematous plaques with distinct borders, and covered with silvery-white, thick scale on scalp, elbows, forearms, hands, knees, feet, and lumbosacral region. Auspitz phenomenon occurs with removal of scale.
- Nails are pitted in about 25% of patients with psoriasis; oil spots—yellow-to-brown discolorations under nail bed are pathognomonic for psoriasis.

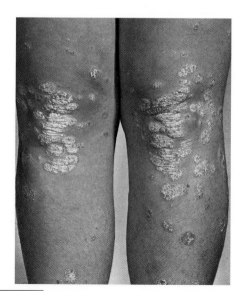

FIGURE 13–4. **Psoriasis.** (From Hall JC, ed. *Sauer's Manual of Skin Diseases.* 10th ed. Philadelphia, PA: Lippincott Williams & Wilkins; 2010, with permission.)

- Less common lesions of psoriasis:
  - Pustular: deep, sterile, yellow pustules that evolve into red macules on palms and soles occurring as exacerbations and remissions for years.
  - Guttate: small, erythematous papules with fine scale occurring as discrete lesions and confluent plaques; can occur after streptococcal infection.
  - Inverse: occur in axillary or inguinal regions and lack characteristic scale.
  - Erythrodermoid: generalized, involving most of the skin; patient is acutely ill in a hypermetabolic state typically requiring hospitalization.

4. Diagnostic Studies

- Skin biopsy demonstrates pathophysiology of increased mitosis in keratinocytes and endothelial cells, and inflammatory cells in the dermis and epidermis.

5. Management

- **Categories of therapeutics used to treat psoriasis:**
  - Topical preparations: tar-based medications, anthralin, and high-potency CSs are first-line therapy for plaque-type psoriasis; vitamin D analogs (calcipotriene) and retinoids (vitamin A analogs; tazarotene) are alternatives to topical CSs without risks of skin atrophy.
  - Phototherapy with ultraviolet B (UVB) light or photochemotherapy with psoralen UVA-range light treatment.
  - Antimetabolites: methotrexate (MTX).
  - Immunosuppressives: cyclosporin A.
  - Biologics: immunomodulators, such as alefacept, that interfere with T-cell activation and block costimulatory molecules, and efalizumab, a monoclonal IgG antibody that blocks T-cell binding.

B. Pityriasis Rosea

1. Etiology

- Unknown etiology; possibly related to viral syndrome occurring before the onset of skin lesions as reported by about 20% of patients.

2. Pathology

- Unknown mechanism causes eruption of solitary erythematous plaque followed by generalized erythematous rash within 1 to 2 weeks of original lesion; typically, all lesions resolve spontaneously within 6 to 12 weeks.
- Disorder occurs more frequently in spring and fall seasons.

3. Clinical Features

- Single, oval, pink-red plaque with a collarette scale on the advancing border, measuring 2 to 5 cm, usually erupts on trunk; "herald patch."
- Multiple, smaller oval lesions appear on the trunk, upper arms, and thighs with their long axes along

FIGURE 13–5. **Pityriasis rosea.** (Courtesy of Syntex Laboratories, Inc.)

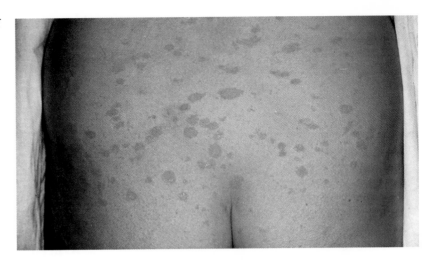

the lines of cleavage producing a classic "Christmas tree" pattern (Figure 13–5).
- Pruritus accompanies lesions in most patients.

4. Diagnostic Studies
- Not typically required.
- Diagnosis based on clinical findings.

5. Management
- Lesions of pityriasis rosea resolve spontaneously without therapy.
- Pruritus may necessitate therapy for patient comfort—oral antihistamines, emollients, and low-potency CSs are sufficient for most patients.
- Oral erythromycin stearate 250 mg four times daily (for adults) for 2 weeks effectively controls eruption.
- Rarely, severe pruritus occurs, requiring either systemic CSs or UVB therapy.

C. Cutaneous Drug Reaction

1. Etiology
- Medications administered topically, enterally, or parenterally induce changes in skin and mucous membranes.
- Most cutaneous drug reactions are hypersensitivity-immune responses (types I–IV); nonimmunologic drug reactions can also occur.
- Most cutaneous drug reactions are self-limiting if the offending medication is discontinued; life-threatening reactions can be unpredictable.

2. Pathology
- **Immune response to drug causes hypersensitivity reactions I to IV:**
  - Type I: IgE-mediated urticaria and angioedema.
  - Type II: cytotoxic reactions (drug, in combination with cytotoxic antibodies, causes lysis of cells).
  - Type III: drug-induced vasculitis and serum sickness (deposition of immune complexes in small vessels).
  - Type IV: morbilliform reactions (cell-mediated immune reaction, Figure 13–6).

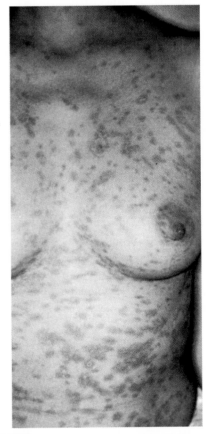

FIGURE 13–6. **Cutaneous drug reaction.** (From Hall JC, ed. *Sauer's Manual of Skin Diseases.* 10th ed. Philadelphia, PA: Lippincott Williams & Wilkins; 2010, with permission.)

- Nonimmunologic, cutaneous drug reaction: genetic inability to detoxify or acetylate certain medications, particularly anticonvulsants and sulfonamides.

3. Clinical Features
- Exanthematous or morbilliform rashes are the most common skin eruption from drug reaction characterized by generalized distribution of bright

red macules and papules that coalesce to form plaques; rash typically begins 2 to 3 days from the onset of medication use. Antibiotics, nonsteroidal anti-inflammatory drugs (NSAIDs), allopurinol, and thiazide diuretics are frequently the cause of the skin eruption.

- Urticarial (IgE-mediated) lesions are the second most common form of cutaneous drug reactions, occurring usually within minutes to hours of drug administration. Urticarial lesions are edematous, erythematous wheals and plaques that blanch and disappear within 24 hours after offending medication is stopped. Antibiotics, NSAIDs, opiates, and radiocontrast media are the most common offending agents.
- Erythema multiforme (EM) is the third most common cutaneous drug rash depicted as discrete, erythematous iris or target lesions. For more details on EM, see section III.
- Less common forms of drug reactions are acneiform, eczematous, exfoliative, fixed, photosensitive, and vasculitic.
- Fever and abdominal and joint pains may accompany cutaneous drug reactions.

4. Diagnostic Studies
- Diagnosis is usually based on clinical findings.

5. Management
- Discontinuation of causative medication.
- Oral antihistamine for exanthematous drug eruption.
- Drug-induced urticaria/angioedema, use systemic CSs, and antihistamines.
- EM minor drug reactions require symptomatic therapy.

D. Lichen Planus

1. Etiology
- T-cell–mediated autoimmune disorder that may affect the skin, scalp, nails, oral mucosa, or genital mucosa. Occurs equally in men and women and may be triggered by drugs (e.g., NSAIDS or ACE-inhibitors), stress, or infectious causes. Exact etiology unknown.

2. Pathology
- Lymphocytes attack skin or mucosal cells causing apoptosis and triggering inflammatory response.

3. Clinical Features
- *Pruritic purple planar* (flat-topped) *polygonal papules* that coalesce into *plaques* most commonly on the flexor extremities, genitalia, and oral mucosa (referred to as the "six Ps").
- In addition to the six Ps, cutaneous lesions may also present with Wickham striae (covering of lacy reticular white lines). May occur along lines of trauma (Koebner phenomenon).

4. Diagnostic Studies
- Clinical diagnosis based on history and physical examination.
- Histopathology can confirm diagnosis.

5. Management
- Potent topical CSs are the first-line medication for cutaneous lesions. Topical CSs, such as clobetasol propionate ointment, are also first-line medication for oral lesions. Oral prednisone for 4 to 6 weeks reserved for severe lesions refractory to topical steroids.
- Control pruritus with oral antihistamine.

III. Desquamation Diseases
A. Erythema Multiforme

1. Etiology
- Acute mucocutaneous eruption usually secondary to drugs or infection.
- The majority of cases are precipitated by infection, especially HSV and mycoplasma pneumoniae, which may precede the eruption by a week. Other infectious causes include cytomegalovirus (CMV), human immunodeficiency virus (HIV), hepatitis C, and varicella zoster virus (VZV). Infectious causes are usually associated with EM minor, which is defined as cutaneous lesions on <10% of the body surface area (BSA) and mucosal lesions on no more than one surface.
- NSAIDs, sulfonamides, and anticonvulsants are common causes of medication-associated eruptions. Drug causes are usually associated with EM major, which is defined as cutaneous lesions on <10% of the BSA and mucosal lesions on two or more surfaces.
- Other reported triggers may include food additives, vaccines, and idiopathic causes.
- Prevalence is greatest in adults younger than 30 years.
- EM is considered a distinct clinical syndrome from Steven–Johnson syndrome/toxic epidermal necrolysis (SJS/TEN), but they share similar features.

2. Pathology
- Cell-mediated hypersensitivity reaction triggers inflammatory cascade.
- Medication-associated EM may have alternative mechanism from infectious cause.

3. Clinical Features
- Lesions are often described as typical target lesions or atypical target lesions. Early lesions appear as round erythematous and edematous papules that may have a hypopigmented surrounding halo. As lesions enlarge, concentric circles develop producing the typical target lesion. Commonly located on extensor surfaces, but lesions may also occur on palms and soles.

- Atypical lesions are usually flat and round, but may contain a central blister.
- Lesions are fixed for >1 week, which can help differentiate the lesions from urticarial.
- Mucosal lesions most commonly occur on the oral mucosa, but may also involve the ocular, genital, respiratory, or pharyngeal mucosa.
- Prodromal symptoms of fever, malaise, or myalgia more often precipitate EM major.
- The eruption of EM minor is often self-limited in duration to 1 to 3 weeks.

4. **Diagnostic Studies**
- Clinical diagnosis.
- EM minor defined as:
  - Cutaneous involvement <10% of the BSA.
  - Minimal mucosal involvement (≤1 mucosal surface).
  - Lack of, or only mild, prodromal symptoms.
  - Self-limiting course of duration 1 to 3 weeks, and lesions that heal without scarring or recurrence.
- EM major defined as:
  - Involvement of ≥2 mucosal surfaces.
  - Cutaneous involvement <10% of the BSA, but more extensive skin involvement than with EM minor.
  - Systemic prodromal symptoms of fever, malaise, or myalgias common, occurring up to 1 week prior to skin lesions.
  - Variable course that may be self-limiting, episodic, or recurrent.

5. **Management**
- Mild EM may not require any therapy and EM minor is often self-limited.
- Discontinue any suspected drug causes.
- Treat any suspected infectious causes, such as antivirals for HSV.
- Supportive treatment may include:
  - Oral antihistamines for pruritus.
  - Topical CSs for pruritus or pain.
  - Anesthetic mouthwash for oral lesions.
- For recurrent EM, antivirals (acyclovir 400 mg PO BID) are commonly given to reduce recurrences.

B. **Steven–Johnson Syndrome/ Toxic Epidermal Necrolysis**
1. **Etiology**
- SJS is considered to be less severe than TEN, but is likely part of same disease spectrum.
- Characterized as a severe mucocutaneous reaction involving epidermal necrolysis and sloughing.
- Medications are the most common precipitating cause, especially antibiotics (sulfonamides, penicillins, cephalosporins, quinolones, and tetracyclines), antifungals, anticonvulsants, allopurinol, and NSAIDs. The reaction usually occurs 7 to 10 days after the initiation of the causative drug or within 2 days of reexposure to a drug that previously caused SJS or TEN. Symptoms related to anticonvulsants often occur within the first 8 weeks of initiation of new anticonvulsant therapy.
- Immunocompromised patients are at increased risk.

2. **Pathology**
- Pathogenesis is uncertain but appears to have an immune response mechanism and an association with genetic susceptibility.

3. **Clinical Features**
- Constitutional symptoms, such as fever, malaise, anorexia, or pharyngitis, are associated with more severe eruptions.
- Painful erythematous dusky red or purpuric macules have a tendency to coalesce. Necrotic epidermis detaches from the dermis and fills with fluid to form flaccid bullae with full-thickness necrosis. Lesions often begin on the trunk and extend to the face and extremities. Demonstrates positive Nikolsky sign (rubbing the skin with lateral traction induces blister formation).
- Painful mucosal lesions involve two or more mucus membranes. Oral and ocular mucosae are most commonly affected. Erythema and erosions of the buccal, ocular, and genital mucosa are present in more than 90% of patients. The epithelium of the respiratory tract is involved in 25% of cases of TEN, and gastrointestinal (GI) lesions can also occur.
- Lesion classification:
  - SJS:
    - Detachment <10% of the BSA.
    - Usually presents with systemic symptoms.
  - Overlap SJS/TEN:
    - Detachment between 10% and 30% of the BSA.
    - Always presents with systemic symptoms.
    - More necrolysis than SJS.
  - TEN:
    - Detachment >30% of the BSA.
    - Poorly delineated plaques with confluence of lesions.

4. **Diagnostic Studies**
- Suspect SJS or TEN based on characteristic history and physical examination, especially if after the initiation of a common causative drug.
- Biopsy can help distinguish between TEN and staphylococcal scalded skin syndrome. Biopsy will show full-thickness epidermal necrosis.
- Associated anemia and leukopenia are common.
- Monitor renal and liver function tests and electrolytes. Acute renal failure may occur.

5. Management
- Discontinue suspected causative drug. Early withdrawal of causative agent is associated with lower mortality.
- Patients should be admitted to the ICU or burn unit for supportive care. Supportive care includes resuscitation, hydration, and maintenance of electrolytes; ocular lubrication and topical antibiotics; and maintaining skin barrier with nonadherent dressings.
- Prophylactic antibiotics are not recommended.
- Complications include sepsis, interstitial pneumonitis, organ failure, and death.

IV. Acneiform Lesions
A. Acne Vulgaris
1. Etiology
- Most common chronic skin disease of adolescents and young adults.
- Tends to be more severe in males than in females.
- Stress, environmental, and genetic factors contribute to the development of acne.

2. Pathology
- Complex process of hormonal influence on pilosebaceous units interacting with bacteria *Propionibacterium acnes*.
- Androgens stimulate sebaceous glands to produce increased quantities of sebum, and bacteria secrete lipase to convert lipids to fatty acids; both the sebum and fatty acids cause inflammatory response in the pilosebaceous unit.
- Hyperkeratinization occurs in the lining of follicle causing follicular plugging.
- Comedones (whiteheads and blackheads) are formed.
- Papules, pustules, nodules, and scarring develop as a result of follicular rupture and complement activation inducing an inflammatory response.

3. Clinical Features
- Lesions of acne vulgaris are noninflammatory (comedones) and inflammatory (papules, pustules, and fluctuant nodules) classically on the face, neck, thorax, buttocks, and upper arms.
- Severe forms of acne have inflammatory cysts, and sinus tracts, abscesses, and scarring.

4. Diagnostic Studies
- Diagnostic studies are not necessary to diagnose acne vulgaris.
- Hormone studies: dehydroepiandrosterone sulfate, free testosterone, follicle-stimulating hormone, and luteinizing hormone levels—may be useful to rule out polycystic ovary syndrome as an underlying cause of severe, persistent acne in a hirsute female.

5. Management
- Comedolytics: topical tretinoin.
- Sebum suppressive medications: antiandrogens such as spironolactone, oral contraceptives; systemic isotretinoin. Potential side effects and teratogenic risks from systemic isotretinoin require additional monitoring of liver function, triglyceride levels, and prevention of pregnancy throughout therapy.
- Anti-inflammatories, including benzoyl peroxide; topical and systemic antibiotics (i.e., topical erythromycin or clindamycin, oral tetracycline or erythromycin); and intralesional triamcinolone acetonide.
- Therapies for disfigurement caused by acne lesions include dermabrasion, chemical peels, carbon dioxide (CO_2) laser resurfacing, scar revision, injection with collagen or fat, and soft-tissue augmentation.

B. Rosacea
1. Etiology
- Unclear etiology; persistent vasomotor instability may be an underlying factor leading to permanent vasodilation and lesion formation.
- Predominantly affects women of Celtic origins between the ages of 30 and 50.
- History of facial flushing in the presence of increased temperature or with alcohol consumption.

2. Pathology
- Increased reactivity of facial capillaries to heat and other stimuli causes flushing and, later, development of telangiectases.
- Perifollicular inflammation and dilated capillaries give rise to papule, pustule, and nodule formation.
- Demodex mite presents in increased numbers in facial skin of persons with rosacea, but a direct cause and effect has not been demonstrated in pathogenesis of rosacea.

3. Clinical Features
- Symmetric erythema of face, telangiectases, papules, small pustules, and central facial edema characterize rosacea (Figure 13–7).
- Comedones are absent in rosacea.
- Rhinophyma and metophyma occur.
- Chronic conjunctivitis, blepharitis, and episcleritis cause characteristic red eyes.
- Rosacea keratitis can lead to corneal ulceration.

4. Diagnostic Studies
- Skin biopsy may be helpful for staging of rosacea.

5. Management
- Topical metronidazole, sulfacetamide plus sulfur lotion, clindamycin, or erythromycin.

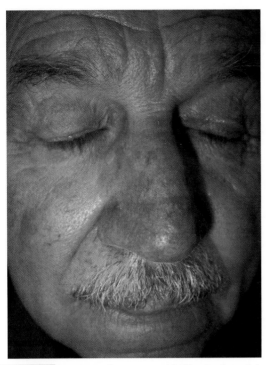

FIGURE 13-7. **Rosacea.** (Image provided by Stedman's.)

- Systemic tetracycline, doxycycline, erythromycin, or minocycline.
- Bactrim DS or metronidazole used for resistance cases. (Resistant cases can be treated with 100-200 mg per day of minocycline or with 200 mg of metronidazole twice daily.)
- Isotretinoin is useful for severe and/or granulomatous rosacea.
- Clonidine to reduce facial flushing.
- Avoidance of factors provocative of facial flushing: hot beverages, alcohol, sunlight, and spicy foods.
- Avert paradoxical exacerbations of existing telangiectasias, papules, and pustules by abstaining from use of potent topical fluorinated steroids on the face.

V. Neoplasms

- Neoplasms of the skin are classified by tissue type and as benign—not causing harm—or malignant—harmful; characterized by anaplasia, invasion, and metastasis.
- Common benign and malignant skin tumors are summarized in Table 13-1 and pictured in Figures 13-8 to 13-11.

TABLE 13–1.	Neoplasms			
Tumor	**Etiology**	**Characteristics**	**Location**	**Management**
Benign				
Hemangioma	Proliferation of endothelial cells that develop at birth	Red to purple vascular nodule or plaque	Primarily head and neck	Resolve spontaneously by age 5
Lipoma	Composed of fat cells; some contain connective tissue	Soft, mobile, round or lobulated subcutaneous tumors	Neck, trunk, extremities	Excision
Epidermal cyst (sebaceous cyst)	Invagination of epidermis into dermis with subsequent detachment from epidermis	Soft, mobile dermal to subcutaneous nodule; not tender until rupture occurs	Face, neck, ears, scalp, upper trunk	Spontaneous rupture is common
Seborrheic keratosis	Hereditary; lesions appear after age 30	Tan to brown or black macules, papules, nodules with a waxy and "warty" look	Face, trunk, upper extremities	Cryotherapy for irritated lesions only
Skin tag (acrochordon)	Lesions occur in obese persons and in pregnancy	Pedunculated, soft, fleshy, skin colored, round to oval tumors	Neck, axillae, groin	Electrodesiccation
Actinic keratosis	Considered premalignant neoplasm, may develop into SCC; chronic cumulative UV exposure	Erythematous macules or papules with coarse sandpaper scale and yellow-brown hyperkeratosis without underlying induration	UV-exposed areas at highest risk, including face and scalp	Biopsy to exclude malignancy; topical chemotherapy such as 5-fluorouracil or imiquimod; cryosurgery or Mohs for those who cannot adhere to or fail topical regimen

(continued)

Table 13–1.	Neoplasms (continued)			
Tumor	**Etiology**	**Characteristics**	**Location**	**Management**
Malignant				
BCC (most common skin cancer in the United States)	UV exposure is the greatest risk factor, but unlike SCC, BCC can occur in relatively non–sun-exposed areas	Shiny, pink to red nodule, may have "rodent" ulceration with rolled border, telangiectasia Translucent pearly appearance, overlying telangiectasias and rolled borders, +/− central crusting or ulceration, +/− flesh-colored, brown, black, or blue	Any skin or mucous membrane surface can be affected	Mohs or surgical excision, monitor for new lesions
Melanoma	Genetic predisposition, sunlight exposure	"ABCDEFG" (asymmetry, irregular borders, multicolored, diameter >6 mm, elevated surface, firm, growing)	All areas of skin containing melanocytes	High potential for metastasis; surgical excision with wide margins up to 2 cm; sentinel node biopsy, chemotherapy or radiation therapy
SCC (second most common skin cancer in the United States)	UV exposure, immunosuppression	Nonhealing, expanding, firm tender, keratotic, or eroded nodule with easy bleeding, indurated ill-defined base, may be umbilicated or ulcerated, may have thick adherent scale	UV-exposed areas at highest risk	Mohs or surgical excision, monitor for new lesions Potential for metastasis via hematogenous and lymphatic channels exists
Kaposi sarcoma	Vascular neoplasm affecting skin and mucosal surfaces HIV+ patients and immunosuppressed populations at greatest risk	Painless purple to brown vascular macules, nodules, or plaques on skin tension lines, purpuric oral lesions, lymphadenopathy	Along skin tension lines and in oral mucosa	Highly active antiretroviral therapies for HIV+ patients with or without chemotherapy, surgical excision, or radiation

BCC, basal cell carcinoma; SCC, squamous cell carcinoma.

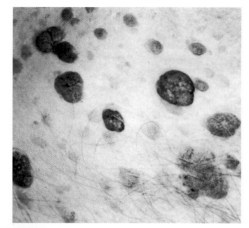

FIGURE 13–8. Seborrheic keratoses. (From Hall JC, ed. *Sauer's Manual of Skin Diseases*. 10th ed. Philadelphia, PA: Lippincott Williams & Wilkins; 2010, with permission.)

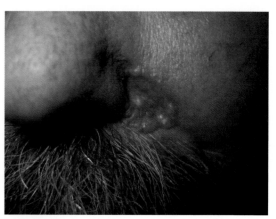

FIGURE 13–9. Basal cell carcinoma. (Image provided by Stedman's.)

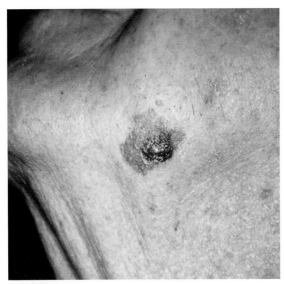

FIGURE 13–10. **Malignant melanoma.** (Courtesy of Syntex Laboratories, Inc.)

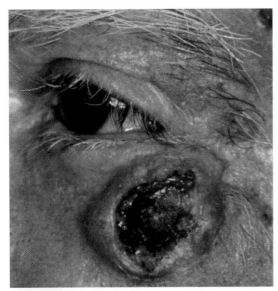

FIGURE 13–11. **Squamous cell carcinoma.** (From Chern KC, Saidel MA: Ophthalmology Review Manual, 2nd ed. Lippincott Williams & Wilkins, a Wolters Kluwer business, 2012, Fig. 7-17.)

VI. Viral Diseases

A. Herpes Simplex Infections

1. Etiology
- HSV type 1 (HSV-1, primary agent of nongenital infections) and HSV type 2.
- Extragenital types: labialis, gingivostomatitis, whitlow, gladiatorum, and eczema herpeticum.
- Urogenital and neonatal infections.

2. Pathology
- Transmission by way of direct skin-to-skin or skin-to-mucosa contact.

- Virus penetrates epidermal cells, reproduces, lyses infected cells, and causes intraepidermal lesions and local inflammation.
- Virus migrates to autonomic and/or sensory ganglia and lies dormant awaiting reactivation.
- Neonatal transmission from HSV-infected mother to infant during vaginal delivery.

3. Clinical Features
- Primary infection has incubation period of 2 to 20 days; symptomatic primary infection with fever, headache, malaise, myalgia, and regional lymphadenopathy is relatively uncommon. Children with primary HSV infection tend to present with gingivostomatitis, whereas young women with primary HSV infection tend to present with herpetic vulvovaginitis.
- Recurrent HSV classically displays a prodrome (in 24 hours preceding lesion outbreak) of burning, itching, and tingling; systemic symptoms are not usually present.
- Characteristic skin lesions (Figure 13–12) are painful vesicles on erythematous base, evolving into pustules and, finally, erosions that may be moist or crusted. Mucosal vesicles quickly become painful erosions; gingiva involved with edema, tenderness, and purplish discoloration.
- Recurrent HSV infections tend to have fewer lesions than primary outbreak. Recurrences of genital herpes are more frequent than herpes labialis and are precipitated by body stressors, UVB exposure.
- Immunocompromised patients are at high risk for HSV reactivation and may require antiviral prophylaxis.

4. Diagnostic Studies
- HSV viral culture, antigen detection tests, and HSV antibody titers.
- Tzanck smear of vesicle fluid positive for herpesvirus (not specific to simplex or zoster) when multinucleated giant cells are observed.

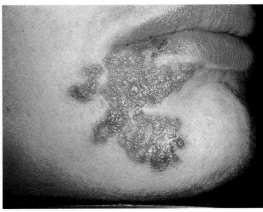

FIGURE 13–12. **Herpes simplex.** (Courtesy of Dermik Laboratories, Inc.)

5. Management

- Skin-to-skin contact should be avoided during outbreak of cutaneous HSV infection.
- Acyclovir 5% ointment. Apply six times daily for 7 days. Approved for initial genital herpes and limited mucocutaneous HSV infections in immunocompromised individuals.
- Penciclovir 1% cream. Apply every 2 hours while awake for recurrent orolabial infection in immunocompetent individuals.
- For severe disease caused by proven or suspected acyclovir-resistant strains, hospitalization should be considered. Foscarnet, 40 mg per kg of body weight, every 8 hours until clinical resolution is attained. Appears to be the best available treatment.
- Childbearing-aged women who have genital herpes should inform health care providers who care for them during pregnancy about HSV infection.
- Episodic antiviral therapy during recurrent episodes might shorten the duration of lesions.
- Suppressive antiviral therapy can ameliorate or prevent recurrent outbreaks and asymptomatic transmission.
- The safety of systemic acyclovir and valacyclovir therapy in pregnant women has not been established. Current findings do not indicate an increased risk for major birth defects after acyclovir treatment. The first clinical episode of genital herpes during pregnancy may be treated with oral acyclovir. Acyclovir treatment near term might reduce the rate of abdominal deliveries among women who have frequently recurring or newly acquired genital herpes by decreasing the incidence of active lesions. Routine administration of acyclovir to pregnant women who have a history of recurrent genital herpes is not recommended by most clinicians.
- Analgesic use is dependent on the extent and severity of a patient.
- Cool compresses. Extensive erosions on the vulva and penis may be treated with cool water, silver nitrate 0.5%, or Burrow's compresses applied for 20 minutes several times daily. This effective local therapy reduces edema and inflammation, macerates and debrides crust and purulent material, and relieves pain. The legs may be supported with pillows under the knees to expose the inflamed tissues and promote drying.
- Herpetic facial paralysis: reactivation of geniculate ganglion infection implicated in pathogenesis of idiopathic facial palsy (Bell palsy). HSV-1 shedding detected in 40% of cases. Inflammation plays a major role in pathogenesis; glucocorticoids may be effective.

- Condom use is suggested for all sexual encounters because sexual transmission of HSV has been documented during periods without obvious lesions (asymptomatic viral shedding).
- Consider testing for HIV and syphilis in patients with primary HSV genital infection.

B. Herpes Zoster Infection

1. Etiology

- VZV reactivation from latency in sensory and autonomic ganglia of patients with prior primary VZV infection.

2. Pathology

- Replication of VZV occurs in ganglia when cellular and humoral immunity wane with increasing age; immunosuppression from chemotherapy, HIV disease; malignancy; and after radiotherapy (5% of all VZV reactivation occurs in children <15 years of age). Reactivated VZV travels down the sensory nerve causing itching, burning, and pain in area where lesions appear.

3. Clinical Features

- Prodrome of neuralgia and paresthesia in the area of involved dermatome before eruption of lesions. Few patients have constitutional symptoms of headache, malaise, and fever.
- Active-stage lesions (Figure 13–13) appear as erythematous papules evolving into grouped and/or confluent vesicles filled with clear fluid, changing to pustules, and finally red-brown crusting lesions occurring in unilateral, dermatomal pattern. Thorax affected most frequently (>50%), followed by trigeminal, lumbosacral, and cervical areas (10%–20% each). Multidermatomal (contiguous

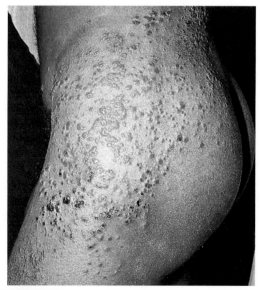

FIGURE 13–13. **Herpes zoster.** (Courtesy of Dr. J. Rico and Dr. N. Prose, Owen/Galderma.)

or noncontiguous) and recurrent eruptions occur in HIV-infected persons. Ophthalmic zoster may cause serious complications—ophthalmologist should always be consulted.
- Chronic stage of postherpetic neuralgia (PHN) persists for weeks to years. Nerve damage from inflammation and scarring may cause nerves to misfire resulting in burning, lancinating, and shooting pain after lesions resolve.

4. Diagnostic Studies
- Diagnostic testing is generally not necessary. Viral culture to rule out HSV may be useful in select patients.
- Tzanck smears are nonspecific and do not differentiate herpes zoster from herpes simplex.

5. Management
- Prevention: VZV vaccine can increase immunity, and oral antiviral agents can reduce the incidence of VZV reactivation.
- Immunization: VZV vaccine may boost humoral and cell-mediated immunity and decrease the incidence of zoster in populations with declining VZV-specific immunity.
- **Active herpes zoster requires the following:**
  - Antiviral agents (acyclovir, valacyclovir, and famciclovir as first-line agents; foscarnet for resistant VZV, and combination of acyclovir with recombinant α-2-interferon for the prevention of disseminated zoster in immunosuppressed patients).
  - Pain management with narcotic analgesics, if necessary.
  - Moist dressing application to affected area(s).
  - Chronic PHN requires pain management by way of topicals (lidocaine gel, capsaicin cream), transcutaneous electrical nerve stimulation, nerve block; oral tricyclic antidepressants; and/or analgesics.

C. Molluscum Contagiosum
1. Etiology
- Caused by poxvirus, molluscum contagiosum virus (MCV-1 and MCV-2), transmitted by skin-to-skin contact. Occurs primarily in children, sexually active adults, and HIV-infected persons.

2. Pathology
- Self-limited viral infection of epidermis in which infected keratinocytes have increased turnover rate as they migrate toward the superficial epidermis.
- The incubation period for the virus is 3 weeks to 3 months from initial exposure to virus.

3. Clinical Features
- Lesions are small, discrete, umbilicated, dome-shaped papules, and range in color from pearly white to skin tone (Figure 13–14).

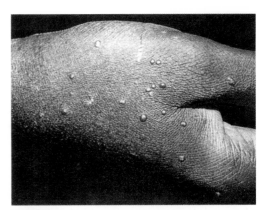

FIGURE 13–14. Molluscum contagiosum. (Courtesy of Dr. J. Rico and Dr. N. Prose, Owen/Galderma.)

- There may be a single lesion or multiple lesions present on the face, trunk, extremities, and/or genital region. (HIV-infected patients tend to have larger lesions occurring over wider body distribution; lesions in immunocompromised patients tend to be resistant even to aggressive therapy.)
- Lesions typically resolve spontaneously in 3 to 6 months without scarring.
- Autoinoculation occurs frequently causing the lesions to occur for 6 months to 3 years from the onset of initial lesions.

4. Diagnostic Studies
- Molluscum bodies (inclusion bodies) are visible on the examination of lesion biopsy.
- Diagnostic studies are not necessary to make diagnosis.

5. Management
- Avoid skin-to-skin contact with individuals who have mollusca. HIV-infected patients with mollusca in the beard area should be advised to minimize shaving facial hair or grow a beard.
- Immunocompetent patients do not require therapy unless lesions are in the area of frequent irritation/trauma or autoinoculation is persistent.
- Therapeutic interventions include curettage, cryosurgery, electrodesiccation, and topical retinoic acid.

D. Human Papillomavirus Infections
1. Etiology
- Human papillomavirus (HPV) is a papovavirus causing cutaneous and mucosal infections in humans.
- Common cutaneous HPV infections are common warts, plantar warts (Figure 13–15), and flat warts (verruca vulgaris/plantaris/plana, respectively).
- Cutaneous transmission occurs by way of direct contact of virus at point of small epidermal defect.
- Mucosal HPV infections cause genital warts (condylomata acuminata), cervical dysplasia/carcinoma, and intraepithelial neoplasia of anogenital region.

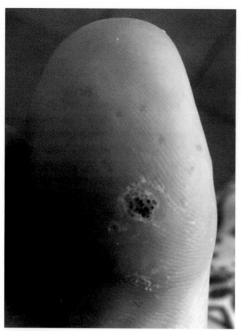

FIGURE 13–15. **Plantar warts.** (From Gru AA: Pediatric Dermatopathology and Dermatology. Wolters Kluwer, 2019, Fig. 19-14.)

2. Pathology

- Several HPV types infect keratinized skin causing slow-growing, benign epithelial hyperplasia.
- The HPV replicates within the differentiated cells of the epidermis causing excessive proliferation and retention of the stratum corneum. This process, in turn, causes papule formation.

3. Clinical Features

- Clinical presentation: varies with the type of HPV causing infection, in addition to the location and size of the lesion(s). Viral warts tend to be asymptomatic, but may cause discomfort or tenderness depending on the location and size of the lesion.
- Verruca vulgaris and plantaris: firm, hyperkeratotic papules measuring between 1 and 10 mm with red-to-brown punctations (thrombosed capillary loops are pathognomonic for warts). Borders may be rounded to irregular with vegetations and clefts.
- Verruca plana: numerous, discrete, small, flat, flesh-colored papules measuring 1 to 5 mm in diameter and 1 to 2 mm in height, typically on the face, hands, and shins.
- Condylomata acuminata: tiny papules evolve into soft, fleshy, cauliflower-like lesions, skin colored to pink or red, occurring in clusters in the genital regions and oropharynx. Lesions persist for months to years; may resolve spontaneously, remain unchanged, or grow if not treated. Increased risk of cervical dysplasia/carcinoma.

4. Diagnostic Studies

- Cutaneous HPV lesions are diagnosed based on clinical characteristics.
- Mucosal HPV lesions are also diagnosed clinically, but they may require acetic acid testing for whitening (nonspecific finding), or biopsy.
- Testing for sexually transmitted infections (HIV and syphilis) should be considered for patients with genital HPV lesions; anoscopy or proctoscopy may be necessary. Periodic Papanicolaou (Pap) smear testing of women for cervical carcinoma is essential after detection of HPV infection.

5. Management

- Prevention:
  - Avoidance of contact with infectious lesions.
  - Barrier methods of contraception may be helpful in preventing transmission of condyloma acuminatum and other anogenital HPV-associated diseases. Condom use to prevent HPV transmission and Pap smears to screen for cervical dysplasia are essential adjunctive therapies in the management of condylomata acuminata.
  - Vaccines consisting of virus-like particles (VLPs) against certain HPV types (including 6, 11, 16, and 18) can help prevent anogenital papillomavirus disease. The 9-valent HPV vaccine is the only HPV vaccine currently used in the United States; however, bivalent and quadrivalent vaccines were used in the past.
  - Change to the above sentence.v All HPV vaccines have minimal side effects. The main adverse effects of the vaccines are pain, swelling, and erythema at the injection site. A small number of subjects may experience a low-grade fever. The current Centers for Disease Control and Prevention (CDC) recommendations include administration of any HPV vaccine to both girls and boys ages 11 to 12 (can be administered as young as 9 years old), with a second dose 6 to 12 months later. Vaccine schedules are also recommended for males and females ages 13 to 26, gay, bisexual, transgender, or immunocompromised individuals who have not been previously vaccinated.
- **Verruca vulgaris and plantaris therapies include the following:**
  - Topicals: OTC salicylic acid preparations and plasters.
  - Cryotherapy, electrocautery, CO_2 laser surgery, hyperthermic immersion, and intralesional bleomycin.
  - Verruca plana: tretinoin cream; topical 5-fluorouracil for recalcitrant flat warts.

- Condylomata acuminata: therapies are similar to those used for common warts.
- Patient applied topicals:
  - External genital warts: podofilox 0.5% solution or gel, twice daily for 3 days, followed by 4 days with no therapy, for a total of 4 weeks.
  - Imiquimod 5% cream: once daily at bedtime, three times weekly for up to 16 weeks.
- Cryotherapy, electrocautery; CO_2 laser, interferon, and topical 5-fluorouracil are reserved for use on recalcitrant condylomata acuminata.

E. Viral Exanthems

- Exanthems: cutaneous expression of a primary systemic infection caused by viruses, bacteria (including *Rickettsia*), and parasites.
- A summary of common viral exanthems is shown in Table 13–2.

TABLE 13–2. Viral Exanthems

Exanthem	Rash Characteristics	Pattern/ Progression	Incubation, Season, and Transmission	Etiologic Agent	Therapies	Complications
Rubeola (measles)	Erythematous maculopapular rash; often slightly hemorrhagic; as rash fades in same pattern it appeared, desquamation and tan yellow discoloration occur; these resolve within 7–10 d	Rash begins faintly at hairline, lateral upper neck, rapidly spreading across face, neck, arms, and upper chest in the first 24 h; spreads next to back, abdomen, thighs in the second 24 h; feet involved by third day	9-to-12-d incubation Spring Transmission via inhalation of aerosolized respiratory droplets Prodromal phase with fever, coryza, and Koplik spots	Measles virus (paramyxovirus)	Prevention by immunization with live attenuated measles vaccine; antipyretics for high fever, adequate fluids, bed rest for acute infection; treatment of complications as appropriate	Encephalitis, pneumonia, otitis media, thrombocytopenia; disseminated intravascular coagulation in rare cases
Rubella (German measles)	Pink macular, popular rash; confluent on trunk; no scaling or residual pigmentary changes	Rash begins on forehead/ face and moves interiorly to trunk and extremities on first day; rash fades within 3 d	14-to-21-d incubation Spring Transmission via inhalation of airborne respiratory droplets	Rubella virus (togavirus)	Prevention by immunization with attenuated live rubella virus	Congenital rubella syndrome if exposure occurs in first trimester of pregnancy without adequate maternal immunization

(continued)

TABLE 13–2.   **Viral Exanthems (*continued*)**

Exanthem	Rash Characteristics	Pattern/ Progression	Incubation, Season, and Transmission	Etiologic Agent	Therapies	Complications
Varicella zoster (chicken pox)	Intensely pruritic, erythematous papules evolve rapidly into vesicles (dewdrops on rose petal); vesicles umbilicate and form pustules with creamy white exudate; redbrown crusts form; crusts resolve in 1–3 wk	Within 8-to-12-h period first crop of lesions appear and evolve; lesions first occur on face/scalp; next lesions appear on extremities and trunk with all stages (papules to crusts) of lesions present at same time	10-to-21-d incubation Winter and spring Transmission via airborne droplets and from direct contact with uncrusted lesions	VZV (herpesvirus)	Immunization available; acute infection treat pruritus with lotions and antihistamines; oral acyclovir decreases severity of infection; bacterial superinfections treat with antibiotics	Bacterial superinfection of lesions with *Staphylococcus aureus and Streptococcus pyogenes* group A may be the most common complication in children <5 y; varicella encephalitis, Reye syndrome, and pneumonia complicate varicella in older patients
Roseola infantum (exanthema subitum)	Small, blanchable, pink macules and papules that may be discrete or confluent	Rash appears on neck and trunk suddenly after 3–4 d of high fever in otherwise healthy child	5-to-15-d incubation	Herpesvirus type 6 and type 7	Supportive therapy	Rare sequelae
Erythema infectiosum (fifth disease)	Slapped cheeks: edematous, erythematous confluent plaques of malar region; reticulated, lacy erythematous macules on neck, trunk, and extensor surfaces of extremities	Facial plaques occur first, fading over 1–4 d; rash appears on neck, trunk, and extensor extremities lasting 5–9 d; lesions may recur for weeks to months	4–14 d Late winter and early spring Transmission via droplet aerosol	Parvovirus B19	Supportive therapy	Unusual
Hand-foot-mouth disease	Multiple small pink to red, linear, discrete macules on hands, feet, buccal mucosa, hard palate, and tongue; vesicles have clear fluid	Macules evolve into vesicles rapidly; oral vesicles become painful erosions causing refusal to eat in young children	3–6 d Warm months in temperate climates Transmission via oral–oral or oral–fecal routes	Coxsackievirus A16	Lidocaine solution for oral lesions; supportive therapy	Sequelae rare; Coxsackievirus infection implicated in aseptic meningitis, myocarditis, and spontaneous abortion

VII. Bacterial Infections

A. Impetigo

1. Etiology

- *Staphylococcus aureus* and/or group A α-hemolytic *Streptococcus pyogenes* (GABHS) cause epidermal infection.
- Age of onset:
  - Primary infections more common in children. Secondary infections, any age. Bullous impetigo: neonates, especially; children <5 years of age.

2. Pathology

- Minor tears in skin act as a portal of entry for common skin flora, or skin flora secondarily infect skin traumatized by other dermatoses.

3. Clinical Features

- **a. Nonbullous**
  - Small vesicles/pustules form erosions covered by honey-colored crusts.
  - Occurs on the face, neck, arms, legs, and buttocks.
- **b. Bullous**
  - Vesicles and bullae with clear-to-turbid fluid rupture to form shallow erosions with gray-to-hemorrhagic crusts.
  - Lesions develop on the face, hands, trunk, and intertriginous areas.

4. Diagnostic Studies

- Not performed routinely.
- Culture grows *Staphylococcus aureus* and/or *Streptococcus pyogenes* group A.
- Gram stain of lesion: gram-positive cocci in clusters or tetrads (*Staphylococcus*) or in chains (*Streptococcus*) with polymorphonuclear neutrophils.

5. Management

- Daily bath with benzoyl peroxide wash (bar).
- Check family members for signs of impetigo. Use ethanol or isopropyl gel for hands and/or involved sites.
- Two percent mupirocin ointment TID for 10 days has been shown to be as effective as oral antibiotics.
- Amoxicillin with clavulanate, dicloxacillin, clarithromycin, and azithromycin for *S. aureus* or mixed infections.
- Penicillin VK, erythromycin, and cephalexin for GABHS.

B. Cellulitis and Necrotizing Cellulitis

1. Etiology

- *Staphylococcus aureus* and GABHS most common in adults.
- *Haemophilus influenzae*, GABHS, and *S. aureus* are most common in children.
- Multiple other gram-positive and gram-negative organisms, as well as fungi, may be the causative organism.

2. Pathology

- Organisms enter the skin through small breaks in the epidermis, infecting the dermal and subcutaneous tissues.
- Virulent organisms may disseminate by way of blood or lymphatics.

3. Clinical Features

- Erythematous, edematous, tender area of variable size, with increased temperature and irregular but distinct borders (Figure 13–16).
- Commonly occurs on lower extremities of adults, whereas lesions caused by *H. influenzae* in children occur most frequently on face and neck. Extremital lesions in children tend to be caused by *S. aureus*.
- Lesions of necrotizing cellulitis/fasciitis change rapidly from tender induration to necrotic tissue.
- **Risk factors for development of cellulitis include the following:**
  - Immunosuppression from diabetes, HIV, malignancy, and cirrhosis.
  - Trauma to skin from injection drug use, bites, burns, lacerations, abrasions, and surgical incisions.
  - Skin disorders/dermatoses, lymphedema, and peripheral vascular disease.

4. Diagnostic Studies

- Common forms of cellulitis may not require extensive diagnostic testing.
- Cultures for bacteria or fungi from lesion, exudates, or biopsy specimen for atypical cases of cellulitis.
- Gram stain; potassium hydroxide (KOH) preparation for fungi.
- Skin biopsy may be useful to differentiate noninfectious causes of tender, erythematous, edematous skin lesions from infectious causes.
- Skin biopsy necessary to confirm the diagnosis of necrotizing cellulitis/fasciitis.

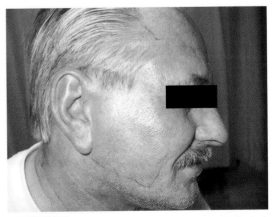

FIGURE 13–16. **Streptococcal cellulitis (erysipelas).** (Image provided by Stedman's.)

5. Management
- Amoxicillin with clavulanate, dicloxacillin, clarithromycin, and azithromycin for penicillinase-producing organisms.
- Penicillin VK, erythromycin, and cephalexin if organism is not penicillinase producing.
- Cephalosporin recommended for *H. influenzae* infections.
- Treatment of necrotizing cellulitis/fasciitis caused by *S. aureus* and GABHS organisms requires nafcillin, oxacillin, or cefazolin intravenous (IV).
- Surgical exploration and debridement, and histopathologic examination of tissues required for necrotizing infections of soft tissues.

C. Folliculitis, Furuncle, and Carbuncle

1. Etiology
- Bacterial causes: *S. aureus*, most common cause; *Pseudomonas aeruginosa*, "hot tub folliculitis."
- Fungal causes: *Candida*, dermatophytes.
- Others: syphilis, herpes simplex.

2. Pathology
- Occlusion of skin with hair follicles, from clothing, prosthetic devices, and natural skin folds predisposes to infectious folliculitis.
- Shaving, plucking, and waxing of hair are additional means of inciting folliculitis.
- Infections of the upper portions of the hair follicle can progress to deeper infections such as furuncles (deep nodule or abscess) or a carbuncle (confluent, interconnecting abscesses involving several hair follicles).

3. Clinical Features
- Bacterial folliculitis: lesions are singular or clustered, small papules, or pustules with surrounding erythema.
- Bacterial furuncle: a tender nodule (1–2 cm) with a central plug of necrotic material above a fluctuant abscess, and the surrounding area of cellulitis.
- Bacterial carbuncle (Figure 13–17): larger and more painful than furuncle, involving many interlocking furuncles/abscesses and openings draining pus. Cellulitis surrounds the carbuncle as evidenced by erythema and induration of the area.
- Hematogenous spread of the localized infection is possible causing bacteremia and distant metastatic foci of infection.

4. Diagnostic Studies
- Folliculitis may require Gram stain and culture for bacteria; KOH preparation or culture for fungi.
- Gram stain and culture of exudate from furuncle and carbuncle.
- Blood cultures may be necessary in febrile patients.

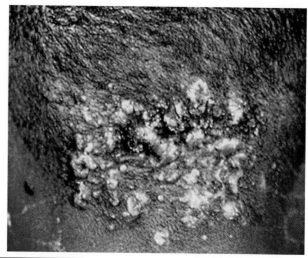

FIGURE 13–17. **Carbuncle.** (From Engleberg NC, DiRita V, Dermody TS: Schaechter's Mechanisms of Microbial Disease, 5th ed. Lippincott Williams & Wilkins, a Wolters Kluwer business, 2013, Fig. 64-4.)

5. Management
- Bacterial folliculitis: treatment, mupirocin ointment or systemic therapy with dicloxacillin, and cephalexin for *S. aureus*.
- Hot tub folliculitis: no therapy necessary; lesions resolve spontaneously in most patients. Recalcitrant lesions may be treated with ciprofloxacin.
- Furuncle/carbuncle: treatment includes heat to the affected area to promote drainage.
- Incision and drainage are the therapy of choice in healthy persons.
- Systemic antibiotics should be given to immunocompromised patients.
- Prevention of recurrent lesions by decreasing carrier state of *S. aureus* with nasal application of mupirocin ointment and use of antibiotic soaps.

D. Erysipelas

1. Etiology
- Most often caused by group A β-hemolytic streptococci (*Streptococcus pyogenes*).
- Less frequently by groups C or G streptococci.
- Rarely group B streptococcus or *Staphylococcus aureus*.

2. Pathology
- Erysipelas is a superficial form of cellulitis involving the epidermis with dermal lymphatic involvement. Organisms enter the skin through breaks in the epidermis. Surgical incision, venous insufficiency, stasis ulcers, insect bites, dermatologic conditions may all act as entry points of infection. Bacteria from nasopharynx may be the source of facial erysipelas as recent history of strep pharyngitis often precedes diagnosis; however, the exact mode of transmission is unknown.

3. Clinical Features
- Localized area of erythema and swelling with sharply demarcated borders, with or without vesicles/bullae. Areas of erythema are shiny and smooth with warmth to palpation. Rapid advancement of erythematous border is often noted.
- Constitutional symptoms include intense pain, fever/chills, and malaise.
- Areas involved are most often the central face or lower extremities.
- Most often diagnosed in children and the elderly.

4. Diagnostic Studies
- Leukocytosis.
- May have positive blood cultures.

5. Management
- Prompt diagnosis and treatment is essential due to the rapid progression and possible spread to deeper tissue.
- Parenteral or oral penicillin (depending on severity) is the drug of choice: Penicillin VK and dicloxacillin.
- First-generation cephalosporin, erythromycin, and clindamycin for penicillin-allergic patients.
- Vancomycin for facial erysipelas or suspected methicillin-resistant *S. aureus*.
- Supportive measures include hydration, analgesics, and cold compresses to affected areas.

E. Skin Manifestations of Systemic Bacterial Infections (Table 13–3; Figures 13–18 to 13–20)

VIII. Fungal Infections
A. Dermatophytoses
1. Etiology
- *Microsporum*, *Trichophyton*, and *Epidermophyton* species commonly transmitted as fomites from other people; from contact with pets such as dogs and cats; and autoinfection from one area of dermatophyte infection to another body region.

2. Pathology
- Dermatophytes infect the keratinized tissues: stratum corneum, hair, and nails by digesting keratin.
- Factors facilitating dermatophyte infection include increased skin moisture from humidity, occlusive clothing/gear, and sweating; chronic dermatoses such as atopy; altered immunity from CS use, chemotherapeutics, HIV, and diabetes mellitus (DM); and decreased circulation to distal extremities as in chronic arterial insufficiency.

3. Clinical Features
- Areas affected by dermatophytes and classic lesions:

a. Hair
- Tinea capitis findings range from annular, scaling lesions, and broken hair shafts to inflammatory pustules and scarring alopecia.
- Tinea barbae lesions are papules and pustules of the hair follicles and are easily confused with *Staphylococcus* folliculitis and acne vulgaris.

b. Nails
- Onychomycosis: inclusive term for nail infections caused by all forms of fungi—dermatophytes (tinea unguium), molds, and yeasts; occurs most commonly on great toe with findings ranging from opaque, thickened, and cracked nails to subungual hyperkeratosis and onycholysis. Progresses to other nails if not treated with systemic antifungals.

c. Epidermis (Figure 13–21)
- Tinea faciale/manuum/corporis/cruris/pedis lesions are erythematous plaques with clearly defined borders, scaling, cracking, and vesicles. Bullae and erosions occur on the hands and feet as well.

4. Diagnostic Studies
- Direct microscopy of skin/nail/hair scrapings with KOH preparation for fungal elements.
- Wood's lamp examination for green fluorescence of *Microsporum* species.
- Fungal cultures may be obtained, but require 4 to 6 weeks for the growth of organisms.

5. Management
a. Prevention
- Apply powder containing imidazoles or tolnaftate to areas prone to fungal infection after bathing.

b. Hair and Nails
- For infections of keratinized skin: use if lesions are extensive or if infection has failed to respond to topical preparations, such as griseofulvin for hair infections; itraconazole or terbinafine for nail infections.
- Be aware of drug–drug interactions and hepatotoxicities with systemic antifungal therapies.
- Extensive fungal infections of the hair and scalp may require surgical drainage of pus, antibiotic therapy, or both for secondary bacterial infections.

c. Epidermis
- Topical antifungals are adequate for superficial epidermal dermatophyte infections.
- Systemic therapies should be considered for recalcitrant infections.

TABLE 13–3. Skin Manifestations of Systemic Bacterial Infections

Disease	Causative Organism	Pathophysiology	Skin Rash	Management	Sequelae/Prognosis
Rocky Mountain spotted fever	*Rickettsia rickettsii* **Rickettsia**	*Dermacentor variabilis* (dog) and *Dermacentor andersoni* (wood tick) transmit *R. rickettsii* to human through bite	Characteristic rash of small blanching, pinking macules begins on wrist and ankles spreading to the palms and soles; within a day, rash spreads proximally on the extremities, the trunk, and face; lesions become hemorrhagic within 4–5 d	Doxycycline Tetracycline (alternative: chloramphenicol)	DIC can occur as does death from delayed/ incorrect diagnosis; sequelae include multiple types of neurologic deficits
Meningococcemia	*Neisseria meningitidis* **Gram- negative diplococci**	Bacterial invasion (meningococcal) of endothelial cells and neutrophils causes damage and necrosis of vessel walls; skin infarction, edema, and RBC leakage cause skin lesions; endotoxin from meningococci causes hypotension	Small, irregular pink to purple macules, papules, and petechiae over entire body; purpura, ecchymoses, and areas of black-gray necrosis appear in fulminant meningococcemia	Empiric antibiotics: vancomycin IV and ceftriaxone IV, add ampicillin IV for older adults and immunocompromised patients; contact prophylaxis: rifampin, ceftriaxone, ciprofloxacin for adults	Acute infection fatal if not treated Early treatment in acute infection has >90% recovery rate Cranial nerve deficits can persist Adrenal hemorrhage (Friderichsen– Waterhouse) and purpura fulminans at presentation have high mortality
Gonococcemia	*Neisseria gonorrhoeae* **Gram-negative diplococci**	Immune complex formation and deposition from hematogenous dissemination of untreated mucosal *N. gonorrhoeae* infection cause hemorrhagic and painful skin lesions	Erythematous macules become painful pustules with central hemorrhage and/or necrosis in the acral areas—primarily on fingers, small joints of hands; may be in web spaces, on feet	Ceftriaxone IM Cefixime Quinolones (not approved for use in pregnancy, lactation, or for persons ≦17 y age)	Dissemination of gonococcus to joints, tendons, liver, and endocardium can occur; untreated endocarditis can be fatal; skin/joint lesions typically resolve gradually

Scarlet fever	*Streptococcus pyogenes* group A **Gram-positive cocci** (GABHS)	Exotoxin produced by GABHS from infection of pharynx, tonsils, or skin causes exanthem, petechiae	Fine, erythematous rash on trunk; punctate lesions evolve into confluent scarlatiniform rash; Pastia lines; desquamation occurs after 4–5 d as exanthem disappears	Penicillin Erythromycin Azithromycin Cephalosporins	*Nonsuppurative:* acute glomerulonephritis, rheumatic fever, erythema nodosum *Suppurative:* local extension of infection—peritonsillar abscess, acute sinusitis, suppurative cervical lymphadenopathy
Toxic shock syndrome	*Staphylococcus aureus* **Gram-positive cocci** MTSS: tampon use associated NMTSS: deep abscesses, surgical wound, postpartum infections, osteomyelitis	Toxin (TSST-1) from *S. aureus* absorbed through mucous membranes or wound causing systemic illness of fever, erythroderma, hypotension, and multiorgan failure	Sunburn type rash of diffuse macular erythema, and erythema of mucous membranes (conjunctival, oral, vaginal); ulcerations may occur on mucosal surfaces; palmar and plantar epidermal desquamation occurs 7–14 d after onset of skin rash	Critical care admission for organ failure Antistaphylococcal therapy: IV nafcillin, oxacillin, and cefazolin Find and treat source of local *S. aureus* if NMTSS	NMTSS has higher mortality than MTSS, has high incidence of recurrence in untreated cases; risk can be greatly reduced with judicious use of tampons (lowest absorbency left in place for short time frames—4–6 h) and antibiotic therapy
Lyme disease	*Borrelia burgdorferi* **Spirochete**	*Ixodid scapularis* and *Ixodid pacifica* (deer) ticks transmit *B. burgdorferi* after biting and feeding on human (>18-h contact)	Erythema migrans lesion occurs at bite site in 75% of patients with Lyme disease; lesion is erythematous macule or papule, which enlarges to plaque with central clearing over several days	Doxycycline PO for adults and children >8 y Amoxicillin PO for children <8 y Ceftriaxone IM Avoid ticks and rapid removal of ticks	Neurologic manifestations of meningoencephalitis, cranial nerve palsies, sensory/motor deficits, mental status changes occur Cardiac abnormalities of AV block, left ventricular dysfunction, and pericarditis are transient Arthritis of single or multiple joints—most commonly the knee—occur in 60% of untreated cases

(continued)

TABLE 13–3. Skin Manifestations of Systemic Bacterial Infections (*continued*)

Disease	Causative Organism	Pathophysiology	Skin Rash	Management	Sequelae/Prognosis
				After a recognized tick bite, the risk of infection with *B. burgdorferi* is low. Option to use single dose of doxycycline 200 mg for adults to prevent Lyme disease in the following circumstances: Attached tick identified as *Ixodes* nymph or adult, tick appears engorged or is estimated to be attached for >36 h, prophylaxis given within 72 h of tick removal, in a endemic area, without contraindications for doxycycline; amoxicillin should not be substituted for doxycycline	
Syphilis	*Treponema pallidum* **spirochete** Positive fluorescent treponemal antibodies (**FTA**) on dark-field microscopy	Sexually transmitted bacterial infection; primary lesion occurs at site of inoculation; infection becomes systemic shortly after inoculation; organism may remain latent for decades	*Primary:* chancre (small papule becomes painless ulceration with raised border) *Secondary:* erythematous maculopapular rash diffusely over body; condylomata lata; patchy hair loss *Tertiary:* gumma; annular nodules	*Primary and secondary syphilis:* benzathine penicillin 2.4 million units IM *Late latent syphilis:* benzathine penicillin 2.4 million units IM/wk for 3 consecutive weeks *Neurosyphilis:* penicillin G IV or procaine penicillin IM with probenecid of 10–14 d	Untreated primary syphilis may progress to secondary syphilis, and eventually to tertiary syphilis; late complications include endocarditis and neurosyphilis; syphilis can be transmitted to the fetus in utero; fetal outcomes vary from mild congenital syphilis infection to stillbirth depending on factors ranging from duration of infection to host resistance

AV, atrioventricular; DIC, disseminated intravascular coagulation; IM, intramuscular; IV, intravenous; MTSS, menstrual toxic shock syndrome; NMTSS, nonmenstrual toxic shock syndrome; RBC, red blood cell.

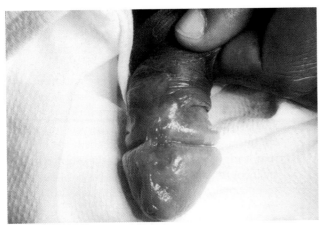

FIGURE 13–18. **Primary syphilis.** (Courtesy of the Centers for Disease Control and Prevention Public Health Image Library.)

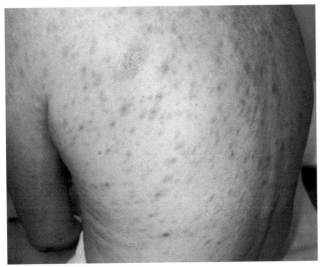

FIGURE 13–19. Secondary syphilis. (Image provided by Stedman's.)

B. Tinea Versicolor (Figure 13–22)
1. Etiology
- *Malassezia furfur* (previously known as *P. ovale, Pityrosporum orbiculare*).
- Lipophilic yeast that normally resides in the keratin of skin and hair follicles of individuals at puberty and beyond.
- An opportunistic organism, causing pityriasis versicolor and *Malassezia* folliculitis; it is implicated in the pathogenesis of seborrheic dermatitis.
- *Malassezia* infections are not contagious.
- Overgrowth of resident cutaneous flora occurs under certain favorable conditions.
2. Pathology
- Lipophilic yeast (normal skin flora) present in bodily areas with increased sebaceous activity.
- Infection occurs more frequently in summer with excess heat and humidity.

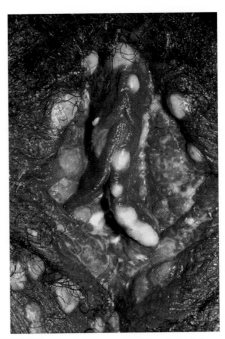

FIGURE 13–20. **Secondary syphilis (condylomata lata).** (From Edwards L, Lynch PJ: Genital Dermatology Atlas and Manual, 3rd ed. Wolters Kluwer, 2018, Fig. 5-17.)

- Risk of overproliferation of resident flora increased in Cushing disease, CS therapy, immunosuppression, oral contraceptives, pregnancy, malnutrition, and burns.
3. Clinical Features
- Multiple, well-delineated round to oval macules of various colors (white to hues of brown) and size (1–30 cm) distributed over the upper trunk, neck, upper arms, axillae, abdomen, groin, and thighs with fine scale visible on scraping.
- Lesions are typically asymptomatic; they may be hypopigmented or hyperpigmented.

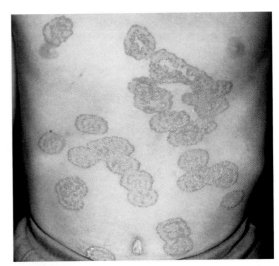

FIGURE 13–21. **Tinea corporis.** (From Hall JC, ed. *Sauer's Manual of Skin Diseases.* 10th ed. Philadelphia, PA: Lippincott Williams & Wilkins; 2010, with permission.)

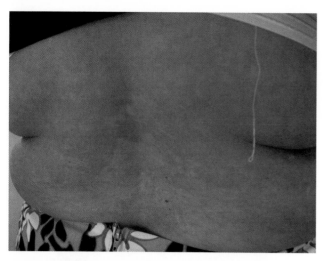

FIGURE 13–22. Tinea versicolor. (Image provided by Stedman's.)

4. **Diagnostic Studies**
- Direct microscopy of scale mixed with KOH shows classic "spaghetti and meatball" configuration of fungal hyphae and spores.
- Wood's lamp examination for yellow-green fluorescence of scales.

5. **Management**
- Once-weekly application of ketoconazole 2% shampoo (Nizoral), applied as a lotion to the neck, trunk, and proximal extremities 5 to 10 minutes before showering, may help prevent recurrences.
- Selenium sulfide suspension 2.5%. When applied for 10 minutes every day for 7 consecutive days, the suspension (available as Selsun or in generic forms) resulted in an 87% cure rate at a 2-week follow-up evaluation. Blood and urine levels determined during this study showed that no significant absorption of selenium took place. The suspension is applied to the entire skin surface from the lower posterior scalp area to the thighs. Another commonly recommended schedule is to apply the lotion and wash it off within 24 hours. This is repeated once each week for a total of 4 weeks. There are many suggested variations of this treatment schedule. Wash the scalp with the lotion at the same time.
- Terbinafine solution (Lamisil solution 1% spray bottle). Application of the spray to the affected areas twice a day for 1 week is effective. Lamisil spray is available as an OTC product.
- Miconazole, ketoconazole, clotrimazole, econazole, or ciclopirox olamine is applied to the entire affected area once or twice a day for 2 to 4 weeks. The creams are odorless and nongreasy but expensive.

C. **Mucosal Candida**
1. **Etiology**
- *Candida albicans* and other *Candida* species.
2. **Pathology**
- Suppression of immunity, systemic antibiotic therapy, or both cause the overgrowth of *Candida* organisms of the normal flora, resulting in oral and/or vulvovaginal candidiasis. Severe immunocompromise of HIV disease and chemotherapy may lead to deep candidiasis of the esophagus and tracheobronchial tree, as well as invasive candidiasis and fungemia.
3. **Clinical Features**
- Candidal lesions are white plaques on an erythematous surface that bleeds when the lesions are gently dislodged.
- Vaginal discharge is white, thick, curd-like, typically occurring in the week before the onset of menses.
- Mucosal and deep candidal infections are clinical markers and defining criteria in HIV disease.
4. **Diagnostic Studies**
- KOH preparation visualized by direct microscopy for pseudohyphae and budding yeasts.
5. **Management**
- Topical antifungal therapy with itraconazole solution, clotrimazole troche for oropharyngeal candidiasis; HIV patients respond to topical therapy, but they tend to have recurrences and eventually require systemic prophylactic therapy.
- Uncomplicated candidal vulvovaginitis may be treated with a single-dose oral fluconazole, or 3 to 7 days of therapy with imidazoles (e.g., terconazole and miconazole).

D. **Cutaneous Candida**
1. **Etiology**
- *Candida albicans*.
2. **Pathology**
- *Candida albicans* superficially infects moist, warm skin, macerated and occluded, such as intertriginous areas, genital regions, and web spaces (Figure 13–23).
- Risk factors for developing cutaneous candidiasis include occupations requiring frequent hand-wetting or immersing in water, use of occlusive clothing/diapers, obese stature, immobility, and CS therapy.
3. **Clinical Features**
- Erythematous papules and pustules coalesce forming plaque of erythema with fine scale at visually distinct margin of lesion; erosions and edema of affected area are common.
- Satellite lesions are characteristic of cutaneous candidiasis.

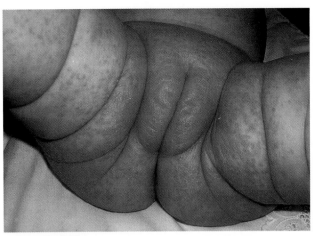

FIGURE 13–23. **Candidiasis.** (From Gru AA: Pediatric Dermatopathology and Dermatology. Wolters Kluwer, 2019, Fig. 2-26A.)

4. Diagnostic Studies
- KOH preparation of lesion scraping visualized under direct microscopy for budding yeasts and pseudohyphae.

5. Management
- Topical nystatin cream or imidazole creams.
- Prevention of lesions by keeping skin dry, frequent diaper changes, and use of cotton undergarments and nonocclusive clothing; using powder with antifungal such as miconazole; decreasing *C. albicans* colonization by washing with benzoyl peroxide soap.
- Castellani paint brings almost immediate relief of symptoms (i.e., candidal paronychia).

IX. Insects/Parasites
A. Scabies
1. Etiology
- *Sarcoptes scabiei*, an ectoparasite, is the etiologic agent of scabies.
- Transmission: usually spread by skin-to-skin contact; fomites.

2. Pathology
- The scabies mite, *Sarcoptes scabiei*, is transmitted by skin-to-skin contact, or from clothing or bedding infested with the mite. (The mite is able to survive more than 2 days while off human skin where it normally feeds and multiplies.) The female mite burrows into the skin to lay eggs, feed, and defecate leaving scybala (fecal particles) to incite a hypersensitivity reaction in the host; the mites can exist for months to years.
- Pruritus and dermatitis develop from sensitization to *Sarcoptes scabiei* within 1 month of initial infestation. Subsequent infestations cause immediate pruritus.

- Persons living in institutionalized facilities are at higher risk for scabies infestation.

3. Clinical Features
- Intense pruritus with minimal skin findings is a classic presentation of scabies.
- Mite burrows (5 mm to several centimeters in length) occur in areas where stratum corneum is thin, such as finger webs, wrists, genital region, inframammary ridge, and buttocks (Figure 13–24).
- Crusted lesions containing high concentrations of mites are more likely to occur in immunocompromised patients.
- Smooth nodules measuring 5 to 20 mm may be part of the clinical picture in a small minority of patients (<10%).
- Secondary lesions from scratching and rubbing, and bacterial infection, are common, as are urticaria and eczematous dermatitis at sites of infestation.

4. Diagnostic Studies
- Direct visualization of mite, eggs, and scybala under microscope from a skin scraping of burrow, flexor aspects of wrists, and penis. A drop of mineral oil is placed over a burrow, and the burrow is scraped off with a No. 15 scalpel blade and placed on a microscope slide.

5. Management
- Choice of scabicide is based on effectiveness, potential toxicity, cost, extent of secondary eczematization, and age of patient.
- Permethrin is effective and safe but costs more than lindane.
- Lindane is effective in most areas of the world, but resistance has been reported. Seizures have occurred when lindane was applied after a bath or used by patients with extensive dermatitis. Aplastic anemia after lindane use was also reported. No controlled studies have confirmed that two applications are better than one. Clean clothing

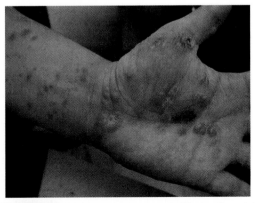

FIGURE 13–24. **Scabies.** (Image provided by Stedman's.)

should be put on afterward. Clothing and bedding are decontaminated by machine washing at 60° C. Pruritus can persist for up to 1 to 2 weeks after the end of effective therapy. After that time, cause of persistent itching should be investigated.

- **Recommended regimens:**
  - Permethrin 5% cream applied to all areas of the body from the neck down. Wash off 8 to 12 hours after application. Adverse events are very low. Permethrin (Elimite cream, Acticin cream) is a synthetic pyrethrin that demonstrates extremely low mammalian toxicity. It is the drug of choice for the treatment of scabies in children and adults of all ages. Several studies show that it is more effective than lindane.

    A diminished sensitivity to permethrin has been documented. One application is said to be effective, but a second treatment 1 week after the first application is now a standard practice. The OTC permethrin preparation (Nix) is lower in strength (1%) and ineffective against scabies. Unlike lindane, permethrin undergoes insignificant absorption (2%), after which it is rapidly degraded.
  - Lindane (γ-benzene hexachloride) 1% lotion or cream applied thinly to all areas of the body from the neck down; wash off thoroughly after 8 hours. **NOTE:** Lindane should not be used after a bath or shower, and it should not be used by persons with extensive dermatitis, pregnant or lactating women, and children younger than 2 years. Mite resistance to lindane has developed in North, Central, and South America and Asia. Low cost makes lindane a key alternative in many countries.
  - Lindane is available as a cream, shampoo, and lotion. Lotion dispensed from bulk containers may not be agitated; therefore, the concentration of lindane may be inadequate. Reports of lindane resistance have appeared. A second treatment 1 week after the first application is standard practice. A follow-up examination at 2 to 4 weeks is recommended. Approximately 10% of lindane is absorbed through intact skin. Lindane accumulates in fat and binds to brain tissue. Pruritus may persist for weeks. Additional, unprescribed applications, without documented evidence of persistent infestation, may be dangerous. Lindane should be avoided in children younger than 2 years, pregnant or nursing women, and patients with HIV or AIDS. Children with severe, underlying, cutaneous disease may be at greater risk for toxicity. This is also true for premature, emaciated, or malnourished children and those with a history of seizure disorders.

- **Alternative regimens**
  - Crotamiton 10% cream applied thinly to the entire body from the neck down, nightly for two consecutive nights. Wash off 24 hours after second application.
  - Crotamiton (Eurax lotion). A study of children with scabies showed an 89% cure rate after 4 weeks with permethrin 5% cream (Elimite) and a 60% cure rate with crotamiton cream. The toxicity of crotamiton is unknown. Reported cure rates for once-a-day application for 5 days range from 50% to 100%.
  - Sulfur 2% to 10% in petrolatum applied to skin for 2 to 3 days. Sulfur has been used to treat scabies for more than 150 years. The pharmacist mixes 6% (5%–10% range) precipitated sulfur in petrolatum or a cold cream base. The compound is applied to the entire body below the neck once each day for 3 days. The patient is instructed to bathe 24 hours after each application. Sulfur applied in this manner is highly effective, but these preparations are messy, have an unpleasant odor, stain, and cause dryness. Sulfur in petrolatum was thought to be safer than lindane for treating infants, but the safety of topical sulfur has never been established.
  - Benzyl benzoate 10% and 25% lotions. Several regimens are recommended. Swabbing only once; two applications separated by 10 minutes, or two applications within a 24-hour or 1-week interval. Twenty-four hours after application, preparation should be washed off and clothes and bedding changed. The compound is an irritant and can induce pruritic irritant dermatitis, especially on face and genitalia.
  - Benzyl benzoate with sulfiram. Several regimens are recommended, swabbing only once.
  - Esdepallethrine 0.63%.
  - Malathion 0.5% lotion.
  - Sulfiram 25% lotion. Can mimic effect of disulfiram. No alcoholic drinks should be consumed for at least 48 hours.
  - Ivermectin 0.8% lotion.
  - Systemic ivermectin.
  - Ivermectin 200 μg per kg PO. Single dose reported to be very effective for common as well as crusted scabies. To be repeated in 15 to 30 days. Average adult dose is 15 mg. Two to three doses, separated by 1 to 2 weeks, usually required for heavy infestation or in immunocompromised individuals. May effectively eradicate epidemic or endemic scabies in institutions such as nursing homes, hospitals, and refugee camps. Not approved by the U.S. Food and Drug Administration or European Drug Agency.

- For infants, young children, and pregnant/lactating women, permethrin or crotamiton regimens or precipitated sulfur ointment should be used with application to all body areas. Lindane and ivermectin should not be used.
- All clothing, bedding, and towels must be washed and/or dried using heat and should have no contact with body for minimum of 72 hours.
- Fingernails should be trimmed and scabicidal lotion left under nails to eradicate mites—reapply lotion after hand-washing.
- Sexual partners within last month should be examined and treated.

B. Pediculosis Capitis, Corporis, and Pubis

1. Etiology
- Lice infestations in humans are caused by ectoparasites.
  - Head lice: *Pediculus humanus* var. *capitis*.
  - Body lice: *P. humanus corporis*.
  - Pubic lice: *Phthirus pubis* (Figure 13–25).

2. Pathology
- All three lice are transmitted by person-to-person contact or by fomites such as hats, headsets, clothing, and bedding. Body and pubic lice require direct physical contact, whereas head lice are transmitted more frequently by way of fomites.

3. Clinical Features
- Pruritus in affected area is the most common presenting symptom.
- Lice and nits (small, white, oval-shaped capsules firmly attached to hair shaft at exit point of hair follicle) are visible on gross examination.
- Excoriations, secondary bacterial infections, or both may be present.
- Papular urticaria at site of lice bites may be present.
- Eyelashes may be infested with *Phthirus pubis* in prepubertal patient, or infrequently, *Pediculus humanus capitis*.
- Body lice live in clothing (near seams) and bedding; they infest human host only for feeding.

4. Diagnostic Studies
- Diagnostic studies are not necessary for the diagnosis of lice infestation; the diagnosis is clinical based on observation of lice/nits.

5. Management
- Topically applied insecticides. Ideally, should have 100% activity against louse and egg. Malathion kills all lice after 5 minutes of exposure, and >95% of eggs fail to hatch after 10 minutes of exposure. Synthetic pyrethroids, synergized pyrethrins, and Malathion are the most efficacious and safe. Lotion preparations are preferred. Creams, foams, and gels are also available.

- **Recommended regimen**
  - Permethrin: synthetic pyrethroid. OTC 1% products—Nix 5% product—Elimite is prescription. Product applied to infested area(s) and washed off after 10 minutes. Not totally ovicidal. Has residual activity in that the incubation period of louse eggs is 6 to 10 days. Should be reapplied in 7 to 14 days.
  - Pyrethrin and piperonyl butoxide: pyrethrins derived from extract of chrysanthemums. Products include RID mousse, RID shampoo, A-200, R and C, Pronta, and Clear Lice System.
  - Malathion 0.5% in 78% isopropyl alcohol (Ovide): applied to involved site for 8 to 12 hours; binds to hair providing residual protection. Indicated in lindane-resistant cases. Should not be used in children younger than 6 months.
- **Alternative regimen**
  - Pyrethrins with piperonyl butoxide applied to scalp and washed off after 10 minutes.
  - Lindane 1% shampoo applied for 4 minutes and then thoroughly washed off. Not recommended for pregnant or lactating women. Not totally ovicidal and lacks residual activity in that the incubation period of louse eggs is 6 to 10 days. The agents should be reapplied in 7 to 14 days. Retreatment may be necessary if live lice are found or eggs are observed at the hair–skin junction.
  - Ivermectin 0.8% lotion or shampoo.
- **Systemic therapy**
- Oral ivermectin 200 μg per kg. Repeat on day 10 to kill emerging nymphs.

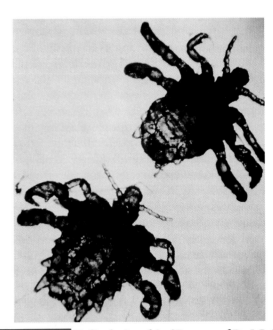

FIGURE 13–25. **Pediculosis pubis.** (Courtesy of Dr. J. Boley.)

- Acquired resistance to insecticides occurs worldwide mainly to pyrethrins and pyrethroids, but also to Malathion. If resistance is suspected, an alternative agent should be used. Other alternatives include newer insecticides and oral ivermectin in cases of resistance to both pyrethroids and Malathion.
- Head lice: comb hair with fine-toothed comb to remove nits after lotion application.
- Body lice: discard infested clothing or treat with 1% Malathion powder or 10% dichlorodiphenyl-trichloroethane powder (nits viable in clothing for 1 month).
- Pubic lice: treat sexual partner(s); bedding and clothing need to be decontaminated by washing, drying, or both, with heat and removal from body contact for at least 72 hours; eyelashes should be coated with petroleum jelly or occlusive ophthalmic ointment two or three times per day for 10 days.

X. Other
A. Hidradenitis Suppurativa
1. Etiology
- Etiology unknown but can be associated with severe acne and pilonidal sinuses.
- Predisposing factors include obesity, apocrine duct obstruction, and a family history of acne, hidradenitis suppurativa.

2. Pathology
- Previous theory of duct obstruction, dilation, and resultant inflammatory changes is questionable in the presence of histopathologic findings of multiple sinuses of follicular origin and epithelium-lined cysts.
- Initial occlusion of the follicle with keratinous material may be followed by cystic alteration of the hair follicle and involvement of the apocrine gland.
- Bacterial infection facilitates extension of the disease with sinus tract formation and scarring.

3. Clinical Features
- Commonly affects the axillary, inguinal, and perianal regions.
- Women have higher incidence of axillary involvement; men prone to anogenital involvement.
- Lesions include double blackheads; tender, inflammatory nodules/abscesses; sinus tracts; and scarring in the form of band or bridge fibrosis, keloids, and contractures.
- Purulent drainage from abscesses, sinus tracts, or both.

4. Diagnostic Studies
- No specific studies necessary for diagnosis of hidradenitis suppurativa.
- Bacterial cultures of exudate from lesions may guide antibiotic therapy.

5. Management
- Weight loss helps to reduce activity.
- Smoking cessation.

- **Abscesses should be managed aggressively—incision and drainage of fluctuant masses and intralesional injection of all nodules/abscesses with triamcinolone acetonide.**
- Systemic antibiotic therapy (tetracycline derivative, cephalosporin, clindamycin, ciprofloxacin, doxycycline, and minocycline) based on culture and sensitivity report.
- Isotretinoin may be useful early in the disease.
- Surgical management of recurrent hidradenitis with fibrosis and sinus tract formation.
- Antiandrogens (oral contraceptives and spironolactone), oral CSs, cyclosporine, and CO_2 laser vaporization are other therapeutic options.
- TNF-α blockers.

B. Urticaria/Angioedema
1. Etiology
- IgE or complement-mediated edema of the dermis and/or subcutaneous tissues.
- Urticaria may be caused by antigens from foods, drugs, insect bites; physical or environmental stimuli such as exposure to sunlight or cold, pressure/vibrations, exercise; and infectious etiology such as viral hepatitis and infectious mononucleosis.
- Idiopathic (40% of all patients) and hereditary causes of urticaria also exist.

2. Pathology
- Mast cells are stimulated to degranulate by IgE or complement activation.
- Histamines cause vasodilation of venules and resultant edema of dermis and subcutaneous tissues.

3. Clinical Features
- Typical urticarial lesions are blanchable, pink, edematous papules or plaques that may be oval, linear, or bizarre in pattern—the lesions may coalesce.
- Acute lesions of urticaria typically resolve within 24 hours.
- Angioedema is a painless, deeper form of urticaria classically affecting the eyelids, lips, tongue, hands, feet, and genitals; the larynx and GI tracts are affected less commonly—anaphylaxis can occur with IgE-mediated reactions.

4. Diagnostic Studies
- Urticaria and angioedema are diagnosed on clinical findings.
- Persistent urticaria and hereditary angioedema may require diagnostic studies.

5. Management
- Identify and eliminate causative factors when possible.
- Oral antihistamines are the mainstay of therapy for acute episodes of urticaria.

C. Pressure Ulcers

1. Etiology

- Skin ulceration that occurs when skin is compressed between a bony prominence and a hard surface such as a bed or wheelchair.
- Risk factors include impaired mobility (prolonged hospitalization, impaired cognition, sedation, and neurologic impairment), exposure to moisture (bladder or bowel incontinence, sweat), impaired wound healing (immunosuppressed, poor nutrition, and impaired circulation), and age >65.

2. Pathology

- Focal ischemia of skin and subcutaneous tissue occurs when external pressures compress an area and prevent proper circulatory perfusion. This most often occurs over bony prominences such as the hip, sacrum, or heel—but can occur anywhere depending on the positioning of the patient. Local friction and sheer forces may generate epidermis and superficial dermis erosion. Maceration of area secondary to incontinence or sweat may facilitate or worsen the breakdown of the skin tissue.
- Skin quality also plays a role in the development of pressure ulcers. Skin atrophy with aging, dehydration, malnutrition, and hypoproteinemia may all increase skin vulnerability.

3. Clinical Features

- Pressure ulcers are staged according to a standardized scale. The most popular scale used has been developed by the National Pressure Ulcer Advisory Panel (NPUAP):
  - Stage 1: intact skin with an area of nonblanchable erythema, usually over a bony prominence.
  - Stage 2: partial-thickness loss of dermis with or without ulceration; may have open/ruptured serum-filled blister.
  - Stage 3: full-thickness skin loss exposing subcutaneous fat. Bone, tendon, or muscle is not visible.
  - Stage 4: full-thickness skin loss with visible bone, tendon, or muscle. Slough or eschar may be present.
  - Unstageable: full-thickness skin loss but covered with slough or eschar, therefore preventing the full assessment of the ulcer.
  - Suspected deep tissue injury: pressure ulcers do not necessarily move from Stages 1 to 4. Sometimes pressure ulcers present with signs indicative of a deeper tissue injury (Stage 3 or 4) with the overlying skin intact. Findings in this category suggest underlying tissue damage or necrosis and include purple or maroon discoloration of intact skin with or without blistering, bogginess of surrounding area, and/or temperature changes (warmth or coolness). Individuals with darker skin tones may be more difficult to assess.

- Complications may include infection, osteomyelitis, cellulitis, and sepsis.

4. Diagnostic Studies

- Clinical evaluation.
- Nutritional assessment.
- Routine wound culture is not recommended; however, if signs or symptoms of infection are present, further diagnostic evaluations may be helpful. If osteomyelitis is suspected, complete blood count, blood cultures, erythrocyte sedimentation rate or C-reactive protein, and bone biopsy should be performed. Magnetic resonance imaging may be helpful in some cases to evaluate the extent of infection.

5. Management

- Risk assessment and prevention: assess risk for pressure ulcer development using standardized scale (Norton scale, Braden scale, etc.). For patients at high risk for developing pressure ulcers, efforts for ulcer prevention should be employed. Prevention efforts include:
  - Frequent turning and repositioning of patient.
  - Use of protective padding in pressure point areas.
  - Use of support surfaces: (1) static surfaces such as foam mattresses, or gel/liquid/air devices to help distribute weight over larger surface areas; (2) dynamic surfaces are electric-powered devices that either inflate/deflate air surfaces thereby shifting contact surfaces, or help reduce moisture.
- Appropriate wound care including cleaning, debridement, and dressings. Constant monitoring, reevaluation, and restaging of the pressure ulcer should be conducted on an ongoing basis.
- Pain management: NSAIDS or acetaminophen may be used for moderate pain. Opioids should be avoided because they may lead to sedation and further immobility. Topical opioid/non-opioid/anesthetic preparations may be used during dressing changes or debridement.
- Monitor for infection.
- Monitor nutritional status.
- Manage any fecal or urinary incontinence.
- Surgical therapy: most patients can be managed without surgery; however, skin grafts, musculocutaneous flaps, and free flaps may be appropriate when immediate wound coverage is required or would improve the patient's quality of life.

D. Bullous Pemphigoid

1. Etiology

- Idiopathic, chronic autoimmune skin disorder. Genetic and environmental factors may play a role.
- Possible triggers may include certain drugs (furosemide, penicillin, spironolactone, and antipsychotics), physical trauma or radiation, other dermatologic conditions, or other chronic medical disorders (rheumatoid arthritis, multiple sclerosis, and DM).

2. Pathology

- IgG autoantibodies bind to the subepidermal basement membrane activating complement and inflammatory mediators. Inflammatory cells, in turn, release proteases that interfere with the hemidesmosomes causing a loss of cohesion between epidermal cells and the extracellular matrix creating blistering or bullae.

3. Clinical Features

- Often initially present with pruritic urticarial lesions. Most patients develop tense bullae—with or without erythematous bases. Bullae can occur on any part of the body, but are typically found on the lower abdomen, groin, and intertriginous/flexural surfaces of joints. Oral mucosal lesions are rare. Negative Nikolsky sign.
- Other forms of manifestation include vesicular, vegetative, nodular, and acral forms.
- Primarily diagnosed in adults >60 years old. Males are diagnosed at twice the frequency of females.
- Bullae that erupt produce ulcers, but nontraumatized lesions typically heal well.
- Bullous pemphigoid may have cycles of exacerbation and remission that can last for years.

4. Diagnostic Studies

- Skin biopsy is performed for histology and direct immunofluorescence testing.
  - Histology: from edge of lesion, skin is biopsied and histologic examination reveals subepidermal blisters with inflammatory infiltrates that are typically polymorphous with eosinophilic predominance; early in the disease mast cells and basophils may be prevalent.
  - **Direct immunofluorescence testing** is performed on normal looking skin (~3 mm from edge of lesion). Results of direct immunofluorescence microscopy reveal linear deposits of IgG and/or C3 in the epidural basement membrane in patients with bullous pemphigoid.
- Serum IgG titers are performed using enzyme-linked immunosorbent assay (ELISA) and tested for IgG antibodies to BPAg1 and BPAg2. Titer tests are positive in ~75% of patients with bullous pemphigoid.

5. Management

- High-potency topical CSs or oral steroids depending on severity.
- Combination of tetracycline, nicotinamide, and minocycline may be effective.
- Dapsone may be used and is particularly effective in treating oral mucosal lesions.
- In recalcitrant cases, IV immune globulins, methotrexate, rituximab, and omalizumab have been used with success.

E. Skin Manifestations of Internal Diseases

- Many systemic diseases manifest through the skin.
- Several lesions with their characteristics, locations, and disease associations are described in Table 13–4.

TABLE 13–4.   Skin Manifestations of Internal Diseases

Lesion	Characteristics	Location	Associated Disease/Medication Use or Exposure
Acanthosis nigricans	Diffuse velvety, thickening, and hyperpigmentation	Axillae and body folds	Adenocarcinoma of GI or GU tract, endocrine disorders
Erythema nodosum	Tender, indurated nodules in subcutaneous fat	Lower legs most frequent location; knees, arms	Poststreptococcal infection, oral contraceptives, sulfonamides
Heliotrope	Reddish-purple hue with edema	Eyelids and periorbital region	Dermatomyositis
Livedo reticularis	Mottled blue discoloration of skin in net-like pattern	Arms, legs, buttocks	Vascular disorders, SLE
Myxedema	Edematous, doughy induration of skin	Generalized	Hypothyroidism
Necrobiosis lipoidica	Distinct, waxy, multicolored (pink, yellow, tan) plaque, late ulceration with pain	Shin	DM
Periungual telangiectasia	Erythema and telangiectases, thrombosis of capillary loops	Periungual	Dermatomyositis, SLE
Vitiligo	White macules or plaques caused by destruction of melanocytes	Around eyes, mouth, elbows, digits, knees, low back, genital region	Thyroid disease, Addison disease, DM, pernicious anemia

DM, diabetes mellitus; GU, genitourinary; SLE, systemic lupus erythematosus.

REVIEW QUESTIONS

1. Which of the following findings may be present in lichen planus?

   a) Wickham striae
   b) Koplik spots
   c) Bull's-eye lesion
   d) Lesions with central clearing
   e) Pastia lines

2. A 5-year-old patient presents with pruritic papules with a honey-colored exudate on his bilateral cheeks. His parents report that they noted insect bites at that location previously. Which of the following is the most likely etiology?

   a) HSV
   b) Varicella zoster virus
   c) Human papillomavirus
   d) *Staphylococcus aureus*
   e) *Sarcoptes scabiei*

3. A 38-year-old woman presents with "a new mole." The lesion is a single-round tan 3-mm papule with a waxy and warty appearance on her trunk. She denies pain or pruritis. Which of the following is the most likely diagnosis?

   a) Seborrheic keratosis
   b) Actinic keratosis
   c) Seborrheic dermatitis
   d) Melanoma

4. A 20-year-old man who recently returned from 4 weeks of hiking presents with a faint red rash that started on his wrists and ankles 2 days ago and now has extended to his palms and soles and proximal extremities. He is febrile and ill appearing. Which of the following is the most important treatment to initiate at this time?

   a) Benzathine penicillin 2.4 million units IM once (secondary syphilis)
   b) Doxycycline 100 mg PO BID
   c) Ketoconazole 2% topically (tinea)
   d) Supportive therapy only (HFMD)

5. Which of the following increases a patient's risk of developing cellulitis?

   a) Diabetes
   b) Overuse of COs
   c) Cutaneous HPV lesions
   d) Occlusive clothing
   e) UV exposure

ANSWERS TO REVIEW QUESTIONS

1. **Answer: A**. Wickham striae are lacy reticular lines that may overlay the purple pruritic polygonal planar papules and plaques (six Ps) of lichen planus. Koplik spots are white grain of sand lesions on an erythematous base that occur on the oral mucosa in measles. The erythema migrans lesions of Lyme disease are often described as bull's-eye lesions. Often the lesions of tinea are described as having a central clearing. Pastia lines are red or hyperpigmented lines in skin creases that occur in scarlet fever.

2. **Answer: D**. Impetigo can be clinically diagnosed in this patient based on the papules with honey-colored crusts. Impetigo often occurs at sites of minor skin tears, such as excoriations from insect bites. *Staphylococcus aureus* and *Streptococcus pyogenes* most commonly grow from cultures of the lesions. HSV causes painful vesicles that ulcerate. Varicella zoster virus (chicken pox) causes pruritic lesions in multiple stages of development (papules, vesicles, umbilicated ulcers, and pustules). Red-brown crusts may develop. HPV causes warty growth. *Sarcoptes scabiei* is the mite that causes scabies, which often presents as pruritic burrows.

3. **Answer: A**. This is the classic description of seborrheic keratosis, which often occurs after age 30. Seborrheic keratosis is a benign neoplasm and only requires removal for cosmetic appearance or if lesions are irritated. Actinic keratosis (AK) is a premalignant neoplasm that may progress into squamous cell carcinoma. AK is often described as erythematous macules or papules with a sandpaper scale and typically appears on sun-exposed locations such as the face. Seborrheic dermatitis can occur in both adults and children ("cradle cap"). In adults, it often occurs on the scalp, eyebrows, nasolabial folds, and trunk and is described as red plaques with flaky white to yellow-brown scales. Lesions of melanoma will often be asymmetrical with irregular borders and multicolored. An enlarging diameter over 6 mm is also more likely to be melanoma.

4. **Answer: B**. The lesions of Rocky Mountain spotted fever (RMSF) typically start on wrists and ankles and spread centrally and to the palms and soles. Patients usually also present with high fever, chills, myalgias, headache, and nausea/vomiting. Rapid diagnosis of RMSF is critical because mortality is high if left untreated. Treatment with doxycycline is similar to other tick-borne and Rickettsial diseases. Benzathine penicillin is used for the treatment of secondary syphilis (doxycycline is also a treatment option). Secondary syphilis lesions may also occur on the palms and soles, but the rash distribution is often generalized. Ketoconazole is an antifungal that can be used in the treatment of tinea, which may present in a number of different ways, including erythematous plaques; however, tinea usually does not occur with systemic symptoms. Supportive treatment is a reasonable choice for many viral exanthems, including hand-foot-mouth disease (HFMD). HFMD often presents with nonrupturing vesicles on the palms and soles, along with painful oral lesions.

5. **Answer: A**. Risk factors for the development of cellulitis include immunosuppression (DM, HIV, and malignancy),

skin trauma (IV drug use, bites, burns, and lacerations), and skin disorders (lymphedema and peripheral vascular disease). Use of COs is a risk factor for cutaneous candidiasis along with moist occlusive clothing. The lesions of HPV, especially condylomata acuminata, are associated with increased risk of cervical dysplasia. UV exposure is a risk factor for malignant skin neoplasms, such as basal cell, squamous cell, and melanoma.

SELECTED REFERENCES

Behrman RE, Kliegman RM, Jenson HB, eds. *Nelson's Textbook of Pediatrics*. 19th ed. Philadelphia, PA: WB Saunders; 2011.

Braunwald E, Fauci AS, Kasper DL, Hauser SL, Longo DL, Jameson JL, eds. *Harrison's Principles of Internal Medicine*. 17th ed. New York, NY: McGraw-Hill; 2008.

Fitzpatrick TB, Johnson RA, Wolff K, Suurmond D, eds. *Color Atlas and Synopsis of Clinical Dermatology: Common and Serious Diseases*. 6th ed. New York, NY: McGraw-Hill; 2009.

Gilbert DN, Sande MA, Moellering RC, eds. *The Sanford Guide to Antimicrobial Therapy 2003*. 41st ed. Dallas, TX: Antimicrobial Therapy; 2011.

Habif TP, ed. *Clinical Dermatology: A Color Guide to Diagnosis and Therapy*. 4th ed. St. Louis, MO: Mosby; 2004.

Hall JC, ed. *Sauer's Manual of Skin Diseases*. 10th ed. Philadelphia, PA: Lippincott Williams & Wilkins; 2010.

Leonardi CL, Papp KA, Pariser DM. Recent developments in t-cell specific biological therapy for the treatment of psoriasis *Dermatology Times*. Iselin: UBM Americas; 2003;24:S1.

Male Reproductive Disorders

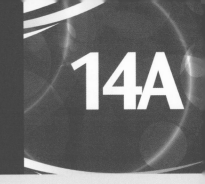

Janina Iwaszko

I. Disorders of the Testes

A. Testicular Torsion

1. Definition
- Rotation of the testicle and spermatic cord with its blood vessels causes obstruction of blood flow.
- It is a urologic emergency.

2. Etiology
- Unknown.
- Most common in teenage boys (average age 16–17.5); also occurs in neonates (extravaginal); however, it may occur at any age.
- Incidence decreases with age.
- Often difficult to differentiate from epididymitis.
- The differential diagnosis of acute scrotal pain includes testicular torsion, torsion of the appendix testis, appendix epididymis, and epididymitis.

3. Pathology
- Incomplete fixation of the testis to the tunica vaginalis.
- The most common abnormality linked with testicular torsion is the 'bell clapper' abnormality, where the testis lies transverse within the scrotum due to inadequate fixation to the tunica vaginalis.

4. Clinical Features
- Acute onset of severe testicular, scrotal, inguinal, or lower abdominal pain. Possibly nausea and vomiting.
- Recent history of trauma, an athletic event, strenuous physical activity; however, it may occur during sleep.
- There is an increased number of young boys presenting to the emergency department with non-specific abdominal pain, initially diagnosed with viral syndrome or gastroenteritis, only to return in 1 to 2 days with a testicular torsion.
- On examination, reveals a swollen, tender, often retracted testicle that may lie in the horizontal plane (bell clapper deformity).
- Cremasteric reflex absent on the affected side.
- "Blue dot sign" at the upper pole of the testicle—can be a sign of testicular appendix torsion.

5. Diagnostic Studies
- Gold standard: radionucleotide study used to detect blood flow to the testes, but may take time and can delay surgical intervention.
- Ultrasound (U/S) demonstrates diminished blood flow to the affected testicle with up to 98% accuracy.
- Emergency surgical exploration is necessary for diagnosis.
- Urine is usually clear with a normal urinalysis; in one-third of cases, there is a peripheral leukocytosis.

6. Management
- A surgical emergency.
- While awaiting surgical intervention, manual detorsion of the affected testis may be attempted.
- Ancillary studies should not delay operative intervention, should occur within 4-6 hours since testicular infarction will occur within 6 to 12 hours of torsion.
- Acute torsion must be differentiated from hernia, orchitis, epididymitis, urolithiasis.
- Urgent urologic consultation and urgent surgery: detorsion, orchidectomy may be warranted, if gonad infarcted.
- Ischemia of the testicle may result in irreversible damage.

B. Acute Epididymitis

1. Definition
- Acute inflammation, infection of epididymis.
- Must rule out testicular torsion.

2. Etiology/Pathology

a. Bacterial
- In younger age group (men >40 years), it is usually sexually transmitted and associated with urethritis. The causative organisms are *Chlamydia trachomatis*, *Neisseria gonorrhoeae*, and *Ureaplasma*.
- In older men (men 40 years of age and older), underlying structural urologic abnormalities, bacterial prostatitis, or a history of recent genitourinary tract manipulation is present. Gram-negative urinary pathogens (e.g., *Escherichia coli*, *Klebsiella*) are typically causative agents. Amiodarone has been associated with self-limited epididymitis, which is a dose-dependent phenomenon.

b. Viral
- Patients with HIV infection, cytomegalovirus, and *Cryptococcus* can also get epididymitis.

c. Traumatic or Chemical
- Seen in young men; sterile urine reflux causes a "chemical" inflammation, leading to the more chronic form of epididymitis.

3. Clinical Features
- This may be an acute (<6 weeks) or chronic (>6 weeks) condition.
- Gradual onset of pain in the testicle, scrotum, inguinal canal, lower abdomen.
- Symptoms may follow acute physical strain (heavy lifting), trauma, or sexual activity.
- The onset of pain in the epididymitis is most often more gradual (1–2 days) than that of testicular torsion.
- Younger patients may have concurrent symptoms of dysuria and penile discharge consistent with urethritis.
- Older patients may have symptoms consistent with prostatitis.
- On examination, a firm, tender mass along the testicle may be palpable and can progress to a more diffuse mass with swelling of the scrotum.
- A urethral discharge should be sought because asymptomatic urethritis may be present, especially in patients >40 years.

4. Diagnostic Studies
- Often based on physical examination findings.
- Urinalysis often shows pus, bacteria; however, absence of both does not rule out diagnosis.
- In the sexually transmitted variety, Gram staining the urethral discharge may be diagnostic of gram-negative intracellular diplococcic (*N. gonorrhoeae*). White cells without visible organisms on urethral smear represent nongonococcal urethritis, and *C. trachomatis* is the most likely pathogen.
- Culture of epididymal aspirates in patients for whom medical therapy fails, or in those who develop recurrences without a diagnosis of cause.
- U/S often helpful in differentiating epididymitis from testicular torsion or other causes of scrotal masses.

5. Management
- Bed rest, scrotal elevation, ice to the affected area.
- Nonsteroidal anti-inflammatory drugs (NSAIDs), analgesics for pain and swelling.
- Antibiotics based on suspected etiology (i.e., chemical: tetracycline, NSAID; gonococcal: ceftriaxone, doxycycline, NSAID; *Chlamydia*: ceftriaxone, ofloxacin, NSAID; *E. coli*: trimethoprim/sulfamethoxazole, NSAID; *Klebsiella*: trimethoprim/sulfamethoxazole, NSAID).

C. Orchitis
1. Definition
- Rare condition consisting of infection of the testicle.
2. Pathology
- Most common presentation as a sequelae to mumps in postpubertal males (seen in 25% of adult males with mumps); presents within 1 to 2 weeks of primary infection.
- Syphilis and other viral infections also have been implicated.
- Untreated epididymitis can progress to the testicle, resulting in epididymo-orchitis.
- Bacteria typical cause in this setting.

3. Clinical Features
- Unilateral or, rarely, bilateral swelling of testicle.
- Fever.
- Malaise.
- History of recent mumps, preceding or concurrent parotid swelling supports mumps orchitis.

4. Diagnostic Studies
- U/S is helpful in differentiating orchitis from other testicular and scrotal pathology.

5. Management
- Symptomatic; bed rest, anti-inflammatory agents, scrotal elevation.
- Treat underlying illness and consider urology referral.

D. Hydrocele, Spermatocele, and Varicocele
1. Definition
- Hydrocele: cystic fluid-containing scrotal mass should be differentiated from.
- Spermatocele: cystic fluid- and sperm-containing mass of the epididymis, palpable separately from the testis.
- Varicoceles: cystic vein containing mass of testicle.

2. Pathology
- Idiopathic fluid accumulation between layers of the tunica vaginalis.
- May be due to trauma, tumor, fluid overload, infection.
- Inadequate venous return due to obstruction of pampiniform plexus. Left spermatic vein drains into left renal vein, whereas the right drains directly into the inferior vena cava, explaining the preponderance of left varicoceles.

3. Clinical Features
- Slow-growing, painless masses.
- On examination, swelling with standing and transillumination typically present.
- Swelling can make palpation of testicle and epididymis difficult.
- Varicoceles often have "bag of worms" appearance, which represents twisting and dilation of pampiniform plexus.
- Rule out testicular tumor because swelling may obscure mass.

4. Diagnostic Studies
- U/S useful in differentiating cystic from solid masses, testicular from extratesticular masses.
- Complete blood cell count may be helpful to rule out infections such as epididymitis.

5. Management
- Most often, no treatment is necessary unless for infertility (decreased sperm count secondary to increased temperature).
- Then, surgical treatment may be of benefit.

E. Undescended Testicle

1. Etiology
* Cryptorchidism: one of the most common congenital disorders.
* Incidence approximately 2% to 5% at birth.
* Reason unclear, but may result from chromosomal disorders.
* Incidence greater in premature and low-birth-weight infants.

2. Pathology
* Testes located outside scrotum, typically in inguinal canal, but also in abdominal cavity or other ectopic places.

3. Clinical Features
* On examination, one or both testes are absent from external scrotal sac.
* May be palpated in inguinal canals.
* Must assess for testes that is descended, but retracted due to a strong cremasteric reflex.

4. Diagnostic Studies
* U/S may assist in locating testes.

5. Management
* Most cryptorchid testes will descend spontaneously during first 6 months of life.
* Orchiopexy is the treatment of choice as soon as possible after 4 months of age and completed before the child is 2 years old.
* If discovered after puberty, orchiectomy typically performed because the undescended testicle is a cancer risk.
* Human chorionic gonadotropin (hCG) injections may stimulate descent in some instances.

6. Complications
* Testicle cancer: men with a history of cryptorchidism have a higher likelihood of developing a testicular germ cell tumor.
* Infertility: low sperm counts, poor sperm quality, and decreased fertility are more likely to occur among men who have has an undescended testicle.

F. Male Infertility

1. Etiology/Pathology
* Males contribute to couple's infertility in >25% of instances.
* Thirty to 40% of male infertility is idiopathic.
* One to 2% is due to hypothalamic pituitary disease.
* Ten to 20% is due to testicular disease.
* Ten to 20% is due to genetic disorders of spermatogenesis.
* Ten to 20% is due to post-testicular defects of sperm transport.

2. Clinical Features
* Inability to conceive after 1 year of trying under a physician's guidance/fertility consultation.

3. Diagnostic Studies
* Evaluate external sexual organs, especially testes for varicocele and cryptorchidism.
* Semen analysis after 3 to 5 days' abstinence, evaluated for number, shape, motility of sperm.
* Hormone studies: luteinizing hormone (LH), follicle-stimulating hormone (FSH), testosterone levels are checked (Table 14A–1).
* Testicular biopsy, vasography may be used in some patients with azoospermatism.

4. Management
* The treatment of male infertility is outlined in Table 14A–2.

G. Primary Tumors of the Testes

1. Etiology/Pathology
* Most common solid malignancy in men of age 20 to 35.
* More often involves the right testicle.
* Approximately 10% of testicular cancer develops in patients with a history of cryptorchidism.
* Ninety-five percent are germ cell tumors (evenly distributed between seminomas and nonseminomas), the remaining are mainly sex cord–stromal tumors.
* These diseases can be divided into two categories: seminoma and nonseminomatous.
* Seminoma is defined by its general lack of marker production and excellent therapeutic response to radiation therapy.
* Nonseminomatous germ cell tumors may be pure histologic type or composed of a mixture of two or more types—that is, embryonal carcinoma, teratocarcinoma, endodermal sinus (yolk sac) tumors, and choriocarcinoma.

2. Clinical Features
* Painless enlargement of the testis.
* Testicular mass.
* Rarely: secondary hydroceles, gynecomastia.
* Stage I, confined to testis; Stage II, retroperitoneal nodal involvement; and Stage III, involvement elsewhere (usually lung).

TABLE 14A–1.	Evaluation of the Infertile Male
Abnormality	**Etiology**
↑FSH, ↑LH, ↓testosterone	Primary testicular failure
↓FSH, ↓LH, ↓testosterone	Hypothalamic pituitary disease
NI to ↓FSH, ↑LH, ↑testosterone	Azoospermia/severe oligospermia Partial androgen resistance
NI FSH, LH, testosterone	Obstruction of epididymis or vas deferens
↑FSH, NI LH, nl testosterone	

FSH, follicle-stimulating hormone; LH, luteinizing hormone; NI, normal.
From Hume HD, ed. *Kelley's Essentials of Internal Medicine.* 2nd ed. Philadelphia, PA: Lippincott Williams & Wilkins; 2001:733, with permission.

TABLE 14A–2. Treatment of Male Infertility

Category	Cause	Treatment
No treatment	Primary testicular failure	AID or adoption; androgen replacement if necessary
Specific treatment	Hypogonadotropic hypogonadism	Gonadotropins/GnRH
	Hyperprolactinemia	Bromocriptine
Potentially helpful treatment	Sexual dysfunction	Counseling
	Obstructive azoospermia	AIH
		Vasovasostomy or epididymovasostomy, microsurgical retrieval of spermatozoa followed by IVF
Value of treatment controversial	Varicocele	Varicocele ligation
	Sperm autoimmunity	High-dose glucocorticoids, IVF
	Genital tract infection	Antibiotics
	Idiopathic oligospermia, asthenospermia, or teratozoospermia	IVF, tubal embryo or zygote transfer; micromanipulation

AID, artificial insemination with donor sperm; AIH, artificial insemination with husband sperm; GnRH, gonadotropin-releasing hormone; IVF, in vitro fertilization.

From Hume HD, ed. *Kelley's Essentials of Internal Medicine.* 2nd ed. Philadelphia, PA: Lippincott Williams & Wilkins; 2001:733, with permission.

3. **Diagnostic Studies**
   - Evaluate hCG, α-fetoprotein, and LDH.
4. **Management**
   - Orchiectomy and retroperitoneal irradiation.

II. Disorders of the Penis
A. Male Sexual Dysfunction
1. **Definition**
   - Consistent inability to generate or maintain an erection.
   - May also include lack of libido and ejaculatory disorders.
2. **Etiology/Pathology**
   - Neurologic, vascular, endocrine, local disorders, as well as trauma/surgery, drugs, and psychogenic causes contribute.
   - Based on underlying cause.
   - Lack of neurologic intervention, blood supply, and circulating hormones are some predisposing factors (i.e., erectile dysfunction [ED]).
3. **Clinical Features**
   - Thorough sexual history taking should disclose duration, nature of onset of sexual dysfunction.
   - Abrupt onset more likely suggests psychogenic causes, especially if morning erections persist.
   - Gradual worsening of symptoms indicates systemic cause.
4. **Diagnostic Studies**
   - Thorough medical history and physical examination to assess signs and symptoms of systemic diseases.
   - Examination of genitals, auscultation for bruits; perineal pinprick sensation; rectal tone; prostate examination; penis for plaques or deformities; and testes for size, shape, position.
   - Evaluation of sexual dysfunction not standardized.

- Initial history and physical and basic laboratory work including testosterone level.
- Additional hormonal testing should be done if testosterone level is low.
- Clinical suspicion should be used to evaluate other possible etiologies.
- Nocturnal penile tumescence used to evaluate sleep erections (differentiates organic from psychogenic causes).
- Duplex U/S scanning used most frequently to determine penile blood flow.
- Angiography used for patients who may be surgical candidates.

5. **Management**
   - Testosterone injections used if levels are low.
   - Drugs such as yohimbine and trazodone have been tried.
   - Intracorporeal injection therapy with prostaglandin (PGE_1), combination of papaverine and phentolamine, Caverject also used.
   - Vacuum pumps, penile revascularization, penile prosthesis provide relief.
   - Psychotherapy also may be of benefit in treating psychogenic sexual dysfunction.
   - Sildenafil (Viagra) has been approved for use in select patients. Its use is contraindicated in patients using other forms of nitrates; potential hypotensive effects of nitrates with its use.

B. Priapism
1. **Definition**
   - Disorder consisting of prolonged erections without sexual excitation.
   - Pathologic erection in which both corpora cavernosa are engorged with stagnant blood.

- Infection and impotence are common complications.

2. Etiology/Pathology
- Idiopathic: 40% to 50%.
- Sickle-cell disease: 11%.
- Drugs and alcohol: 20%.
- Injection of erectile-aiding agent: 30%.
- Trauma: <10%.
- Divided into high-flow (arterial) or low-flow (venous) status (latter most common).
- Main causes of infertility: varicocele, 30% to 40% of patients.
- Others: hormonal, chromosomal, idiopathic, duct obstruction, cryptorchidism, torsion, infections.

3. Clinical Features
- Erection, with glans penis and corpus spongiosum typically not engorged.
- Low flow: very painful.
- High flow: little or no pain, usually secondary to trauma.
- End result: ischemia with necrosis, infarction, infection, urinary retention, impotence.

4. Diagnostic Studies
- Magnetic resonance imaging used to detect thrombosis associated with priapism.
- Cavernous aspiration with blood gas or Doppler ultrasound.

5. Management
- Goal of treatment: detumescence and preserving potency. Terbutaline given orally or subcutaneously occasionally reverses priapism.
- In low-flow cases, injections directly into the corpora with α-adrenergic agents, phenylephrine unless contraindicated (patients with cardiac or cerebrovascular history).
- Needle aspiration of corpora.
- Recurrent or prolonged episodes require surgical treatment.
- Attempt to treat underlying disease process; sickle-cell patients often benefit from hydration, ±transfusions.
- Ice packs, pressure dressings, cold and hot enemas, nitrates, hypotensive agents have been tried.

C. Paraphimosis
1. Definition
- Entrapment of a retracted foreskin that cannot be reduced behind the coronal sulcus.
- If the paraphimosis is not promptly reduced, initial venous engorgement of the glans penis leads to swelling and eventually the arterial blood supply becomes compromised, and the glans may necrose.

2. Clinical Features
- Pain, swelling, and erythema of the foreskin.
- Dysuria, decreased urinary stream, and possible urinary obstruction.

- If severe, the constriction causes edema and venous engorgement of the glans, which can lead to arterial compromise with subsequent tissue necrosis.

3. Management
- If no necrosis is present: apply methods to reduce swelling with pain control: ice, compression bandages and/or osmotic agents.
- Squeezing the glans firmly for 5 minutes to reduce the swelling can lead to successful reduction of the foreskin.
- Using the index fingers to pull the prepuce distally while pushing the glans into the prepuce.
- Local infiltration of anesthesia with vertical incision of the constricting band can be performed by the urologist if manual reduction fails.

III. Disorders of the Prostate
A. Prostatitis
1. Definition
- Acute or chronic bacterial infection.
- Inflammation of the prostate gland.
- Nearly half of all men experience symptoms of prostatitis in their lives.

2. Etiology/Pathology
- Causative agents for acute bacterial prostatitis include gram-negative bacilli (most often *E. coli*) and *Pseudomonas* species and less commonly by gram-positive organisms (e.g., enterococci); however, *Chlamydia* and *Trichomonas* are noted in the younger age groups. Chronic bacterial prostatitis may evolve from acute bacterial prostatitis; many men have no history of acute infection. Gram-negative rods are the most common etiologic agents, but only one gram-positive organism (*Enterococcus*) is associated with chronic infection.
- Some patients have complaints consistent with prostatitis, but no organism can be identified.

3. Clinical Features
a. Acute
- Patients are typically acutely ill.
- Symptoms include dysuria, fever, chills, perineal discomfort/pain.
- Irritative urinary symptoms such as frequency, urgency, and urge incontinence.
- Obstructive voiding symptoms such as urinary dribbling, hesitancy, and possibly acute urinary retention and associated with low back and perineal discomfort.
- Pain at the tip of the penis.
- Perineal or suprapubic pain; exquisite tenderness is common on rectal examination.
- Prostatic massage should not be performed because of the risk of bacteremia.
- Rectal examination shows tender, "boggy" prostate.

b. **Chronic**
- Symptoms typically milder than those in acute form.
- Chronic prostatitis is a cause of relapsing urinary tract infection (UTI) in men.
- Perineal or suprapubic discomfort, often dull and poorly localized.
- Fever uncommon.
- Rectal examination can be normal.

4. **Diagnostic Studies**
- Gentle prostate (PR) examination reveals a warm, firm, edematous and exquisitely tender prostate.
- Complete blood count reveals leukocytosis and, often, raised C-reactive protein (CRP) or raised prostate-specific antigen (PSA).
- Urinalysis, expressed prostatic massage secretions; postmassage urine should be analyzed for leukocytes and bacteria.
- Vigorous prostatic massage should be avoided in acute setting to avoid bacteremia.

5. **Management**
- For acute prostatitis, antibiotics should be chosen on likely etiology.
- Some patients with acute prostatitis require intravenous antibiotics, hospitalization.
- Supportive therapy with sitz baths, analgesics, and stool softeners.
- Helpful, but nonspecific, is a 4- to 6-week course of antibiotic, regardless of etiology.
- Treatment for chronic prostatitis is usually unsatisfactory because of the inability of antimicrobial agents to diffuse into prostatic fluid.
- Trimethoprim–sulfamethoxazole has resulted in moderately high cure rates, treatment must be prolonged (8–12 weeks), and relapse is frequent.
- Also consider a fluoroquinolone.

B. **Benign Prostatic Hyperplasia**
1. **Definition**
- Benign enlargement of prostatic gland.
2. **Etiology/Pathology**
- Etiology unclear, but androgens (testosterone) are a factor, as demonstrated by the lack of this condition in castrated men.
- Hyperplasia of stromal and glandular elements of prostate.
- Gland enlargement creates urethral narrowing that affects bladder emptying, which can lead to bladder wall hypertrophy distension.
- In severe hypertrophy, ureters dilate, hydronephrosis and renal impairment ensue.
- Increases in frequency progressively with age in men >50 years.
- Twenty percent in men aged 41 to 50, 50% in men aged 51 to 60, and >90% in men aged 80 and older.

- Symptoms are also age related.
- At age 55, approximately 25% of men report obstructive voiding symptoms, at age 75, 50% of men report a decrease in the force and caliber of the urinary stream.

3. **Clinical Features**
- Obstructive symptoms: hesitance, decreased force and caliber of stream, sensation of incomplete bladder emptying, double voiding (urinating a second time within 2 hours), straining to urinate, and postvoid dribbling.
- Irritative symptoms: urgency, frequency, and nocturia.
- Rectal examination discloses enlarged uniform prostate, nontender and free of nodules.
- Size does not always correlate with degree of symptoms.

4. **Diagnostic Studies**
- Careful history with attention to medication use, particularly anticholinergic agents that can cause difficulty urinating.
- Abdominal examination may disclose distended bladder.
- Rectal examination should be performed, gently palpating contour of prostate, note size and consistency of the prostate.
- Urinalysis, serum prostate-specific antigen (PSA), blood urea nitrogen, and creatinine levels should be ordered.

5. **Management**
- Patient education regarding the condition is essential.
- Avoidance of drugs that can worsen symptoms.
- Observation versus medical versus surgical treatments should be based on the degree of symptoms and whether renal impairment is present.
- Exclude urethral stricture, bladder calculi, UTI, and carcinoma of the prostate or bladder.
- Selective α_1-blockers such as prazosin (Minipress), terazosin (Hytrin), and doxazosin (Cardura) often provide improvement of symptoms.
- Hormonal therapy with finasteride (Proscar), a 5α-reductase inhibitor, reduces prostate size and symptoms.
- Combination therapy: α-blocker and 5α-reductase inhibitor (e.g., long-term combination therapy with doxazosin and finasteride) is safe and overall clinical progression of benign prostatic hyperplasia (BPH) significantly more than either drug alone.
- Transurethral resection of prostate removes the zone of the prostate around the urethra leaving the peripheral portion of the prostate and prostate capsule, useful in eliminating symptoms, but

carries a slight risk of anesthesia, postoperative sexual dysfunction.

- Consider open simple prostatectomy when the prostate is too large to remove endoscopically.
- Transurethral laser-induced prostatectomy under transrectal U/S guidance is a minimally invasive procedure; advantages of laser surgery include outpatient surgery, minimal blood loss, and rare occurrence of transurethral resection syndrome; disadvantages of laser surgery include lack of tissue for pathologic examination, longer postoperative catheterization time, and more frequent irritative voiding complaints.

IV. Disorders of Testosterone Secretion

A. Male Hypogonadism

1. **Etiology/Pathology**
   - Primary hypogonadism: caused by insufficient testosterone secretion by the testes themselves (more common), or due to decreased gonadotropin secretion of the pituitary gland.
   - Secondary hypogonadism: alcohol, chronic illness, Cushing syndrome, hemochromatosis.
   - The deficiency of testosterone contributes to reduced sperm count, ED, and can produce osteoporosis.

2. **Clinical Features**
   - Decreased libido, ED, fatigue, depression.
   - Physical signs: diminished sexual hair growth, decrease of testicular mass, loss of muscle mass with increase in weight.

3. **Diagnostic Studies**
   - Decreased morning serum testosterone level.
   - LH and FSH should be measured; they are elevated in patients with testicular dysfunction and low in patients with pituitary (secondary hypogonadism) disorders.

4. **Management**
   - Testosterone replacement therapy should be started only after evaluation for prostate cancer.
   - Forms of replacement: oral preparations, intramuscular, and transdermal (skin patches).

REVIEW QUESTIONS

1. Which of the following is the most common age range for testicular torsion to occur?
   a) 13 to 14.5 years old
   b) 14 to 15.5 years old
   c) 15 to 16.5 years old
   d) 16 to 17.5 years old

2. Which of the following bacteria is the most common pathogen for acute epididymitis in men 40 years of age or older?
   a) *Escherichia coli*
   b) *C. trachomatis*
   c) *N. gonorrhoeae*
   d) *Streptococcus mitis*

3. Which of the following is the most likely complication in a patient with a past medical history of undescended testicle?
   a) Epididymitis
   b) Infertility
   c) Testicular torsion
   d) Inguinal hernia

ANSWERS TO REVIEW QUESTIONS

1. **Answer: D.** Testicular torsion is defined as a rotation of the testicle and spermatic cord with its blood vessels causing obstruction of blood flow. It is an urologic emergency. Most common in teenage boys (average age 16–17.5 years); also occurs in neonates (extravaginal); however, it may occur at any age. Incidence decreases with age. Often difficult to differentiate from epididymitis. The differential diagnosis of acute scrotal pain includes testicular torsion, torsion of the appendix testis, appendix epididymis, and epididymitis. (Testicular torsion, epidemiology)

2. **Answer: A.** Acute epididymitis is an acute inflammation, infection of epididymis. In younger age-group (men younger than 40 years), it is usually sexually transmitted and associate with urethritis. The causative organisms are *C. trachomatis*, *N. gonorrhoeae*, and *Ureaplasma*. In older men (men 40 years of age and older), underlying structural urologic abnormalities, bacterial prostatitis, or a history of recent genitourinary tract manipulation is present. Gram-negative urinary pathogens (e.g., *E. coli*, *Klebsiella*) are typically causative agents. Amiodarone has been associated with self-limited epididymitis, which is a dose-dependent phenomenon. (Acute epididymitis, clinical features)

3. **Answer: B.** Undescended testicle, cryptorchidism is one of the most common congenital disorders. The incidence approximately 1% to 3% at birth and is greater in premature and low-birth-weight infants. Clinical features include examination, one or both testes are absent from external scrotal sac, may be palpated in inguinal canals and must assess for testes descended, but retracted due to a strong cremasteric reflex. The diagnostic study is an U/S, which may assist in locating the testes. The management of most cryptorchid testes will descend spontaneously during first year 6 months of life. Orchiopexy is the treatment of choice

as soon as possible after 4 months of after age and completed before the age of 2 years. If discovered after puberty, orchiectomy typically performed because the undescended testicle is a cancer risk. hCG injections may stimulate descent in some instances. Complications of include testicular cancer and infertility. Low sperm counts, poor sperm quality, and decreased fertility are more likely to occur among men who've had an undescended testicle. This can be due to abnormal development of the testicle and might get worse if the condition goes untreated for an extended period. (Undescended testicle, clinical features)

SELECTED REFERENCES

Bates B, ed. *A Guide to Physical Examination and History Taking.* 10th ed. Philadelphia, PA: JB Lippincott; 2008.

Bennett JC, Plum F, eds. *Cecil Textbook of Medicine.* 22nd ed. Philadelphia, PA: WB Saunders; 2004.

Bondesson JD. Urologic conditions. In: Knoop KJ, Stack LB, Storrow AB, et al, eds. *The Atlas of Emergency Medicine.* 3rd ed. New York, NY: McGraw-Hill; 2010:chap 8. Also available at: http://www.accessmedicine.com/content.aspx?aID=6002004. Accessed January 7, 2012.

David AK, Johnson TA Jr, Phillips DM, et al, eds. *Family Medicine: Principles and Practice.* 6th ed. New York, NY: Springer-Verlag; 2003.

DeCherney AH, Nathan L, eds. *Current Obstetric and Gynecologic Diagnosis and Treatment.* 11th ed. New York, NY: McGraw-Hill; 2011.

DeGowin RL, ed. *Degowin and Degowin's Diagnostic Examination.* 9th ed. New York, NY: McGraw-Hill; 2009.

Doherty GM, ed. *Current Surgical Diagnosis and Treatment.* 13th ed. Norwalk, CT: McGraw-Hill Companies; 2010.

Geisler WM, Krieger JN. Epididymitis and the acute scrotum syndrome. In: Klausner JD, Hook EW III, eds. *Current Diagnosis and Treatment of Sexually Transmitted Diseases.* New York, NY: McGraw-Hill; 2007:chap 6. http://www.accessmedicine.com/content.aspx?aID=3027157. Accessed January 7, 2012.

Gillenwater JY, Grayhack JT, Howards SS, et al, eds. *Adult and Pediatric Urology.* 4th ed. St Louis, MO: Mosby; 2002.

Goroll AH, May LA, Mulley AG, eds. *Primary Care Medicine, Office Evaluation and Management of the Adult Patient.* 6th ed. Philadelphia, PA: Lippincott-Raven; 2009.

Greenfield LJ, Mullholland MW, Oldham KT, et al, eds. *Essentials of Surgery, Scientific Principles in Practice.* Philadelphia, PA: Lippincott-Raven; 2010.

Hatcher RA, Trussell J, Stewart F, et al, eds. *Contraceptive Technology.* 17th ed. New York, NY: Ardent Medica; 1998.

Isselbacher KJ, ed. *Harrison's Principles of Internal Medicine.* 18th ed. New York, NY: McGraw-Hill; 2011.

Kavoussir LR, ed. *Campbell-Walsh Urology.* 7th ed. Philadelphia, PA: WB Saunders; 2007.

La Rochelle J, Shuch B, Belldegrun A. Urology. In: Brunicardi FC, Andersen DK, Billiar TR, et al, eds. *Schwartz's Principles of Surgery.* 9th ed. New York, NY: McGraw-Hill; 2010:chap 40. http://www.accessmedicine.com/content.aspx?aID=5025145. Accessed January 7, 2012.

Mackett CW III, Nusbaum MR. Adult sexual dysfunction. In: South-Paul JE, Matheny SC, Lewis EL, eds. *Current Diagnosis and Treatment in Family Medicine.* New York, NY: McGraw Hill; 2010.

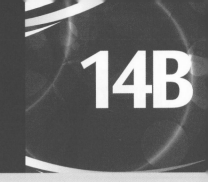

Female Reproductive Disorders

Janina Iwaszko

Note: Carcinomas are addressed in Chapter 17

I. Infections (Table 14B–1)
A. Diseases Characterized by Vaginal Discharge
1. **Bacterial Vaginosis (BV)**
   a. **Etiology/Pathology**
      - Most common cause of vaginitis and vaginosis (the latter is the term used in the absence of inflammation).
      - Complex change in the composition of normal vaginal flora (*Gardnerella vaginalis*, *Mobiluncus* species, anaerobic gram-negative rods, and *Peptostreptococcus* species).
      - Marked decrease in the lactobacilli acidophilus that maintains vaginal pH.
      - Overall prevalence of 29.2%; 45.2% among women who reported having sex with another women.
   b. **Clinical Features**
      - Copious watery, foul-smelling (fishy, rotten smell), gray-white discharge.
      - May be associated with pruritus.
      - BV alone does not cause dysuria, dyspareunia, pruritis, or vaginal inflammation.
      - The presence of these symptoms suggests mixed vaginitis.
      - No associated lesions.
      - May be asymptomatic (>50%).
   c. **Diagnostic Studies**
      - Saline wet mount: clue cells (>20% of epithelial cells) and marked decrease in lactobacilli, few white blood cells (WBCs).
      - Positive "whiff-amine test" (fishy odor) with a drop of 10% potassium hydroxide (KOH).
      - pH > 4.5.
      - Can do Gram stain of discharge if unsure of diagnosis (large number of small gram-negative bacilli and a relative absence of lactobacilli).
   d. **Complications**
      - Associated with preterm labor, premature rupture of membranes, chorioamnionitis, postpartum endometritis, posthysterectomy vaginal cuff cellulitis, postabortion infection, and pelvic inflammatory disease (PID).
      - May experience recurrence despite treatment.
   e. **Management**
      - Consider not treating asymptomatic women (U.S. Centers for Disease Control and Prevention [CDC] recommendation).
      - Treatment should be considered for relief of symptoms or prevention of postoperative infection.
      - Resolves spontaneously in <30% nonpregnant women or approximately 50% pregnant women.
   f. **Treatment**
      - Treatment is recommended for women with symptoms. The established benefits of therapy in nonpregnant women are to relieve vaginal symptoms and signs of infection.
      - **Metronidazole**
        - Five hundred milligrams orally twice a day for 7 days; or
        - 0.75% gel, one full applicator (5 g) intravaginally, once a day for 5 days; or
      - **Clindamycin**
        - Two percent cream, one full applicator (5 g) intravaginally at bedtime for 7 days; or
        - Three hundred milligrams PO twice a day for 7 days; or
        - One hundred milligram ovules intravaginally once at bedtime for 3 days; or
        - Clindesse vaginal cream: one full applicator (5 g) intravaginally one-time dose.
        - Tinidazole 1 g orally once daily for 5 days.
      - Chronic or recurrent infection: 0.75% metronidazole gel, one full applicator (5 g) intravaginally two times a week for 4 to 6 months.
      - Avoid douching: promotes loss of vaginal lactobacilli.
      - Unclear if sexually transmitted; currently, treating partners is not necessary, further studies are needed.
        - Use of condoms by male partners associated with a reduced risk of recurrence.
        - Consider screening female partners because BV is frequently found in both members of monogamous lesbian couples.
      - Pregnant women with BV.
        - Treatment is highly recommended to avoid any chance of preterm labor.

TABLE 14B–1.   Comparisons of Infections

	Etiology/ Pathology	Clinical Features	Diagnostic Studies	Complications	Management
Diseases characterized by vaginal discharge					
Bacterial vaginosis	Overgrowth of normal vaginal flora Marked decrease in the lactobacilli acidophilus that maintains vaginal pH. Most common cause of vaginitis	Copious watery, foul-smelling, gray-white discharge May be associated with pruritus; no associated lesions May be asymptomatic (>50%)	Wet mount: clue cells, few WBCs, decrease in lactobacilli Positive "whiff test" pH > 4.5	Recurrence common; unclear if sexually transmitted; treating partners is not necessary but consider screening female partners May be associated with preterm labor, premature rupture of the fetal membrane, chorioamnionitis, postpartum endometritis, posthysterectomy, vaginal cuff cellulitis, postabortion infection, and PID	Metronidazole orally or intravaginally Clindamycin orally or intravaginally Avoid douching: promotes loss of vaginal lactobacilli Use condoms with male partners
Trichomoniasis	*Trichomonas vaginalis*, sexually transmitted	Malodorous, frothy, yellow-green vaginal discharge Pruritus or pain Vaginal erythema Cervical petechiae Male partners may develop urethritis or balanitis, but usually asymptomatic	Wet mount: WBCs, motile trichomonads, pH > 4.5 Rapid tests available	Associated with perinatal complications Increased incidence in the transmission of HIV	Metronidazole Tinidazole Treat partner Spermicidal agents decrease transmission Evaluate for other STIs
Vulvovaginal candidiasis	Overgrowth of *Candida albicans*	Vaginal discharge, pruritus, dysuria, ±dyspareunia Erythematous, edematous vulva, ±excoriations Thick, cottage cheese-like discharge	KOH: budding hyphae and spores. pH ≤ 4.5	May be unrefractory in pregnancy, HIV infection, and diabetes mellitus	Intravaginal options: Butoconazole Clotrimazole Miconazole Nystatin Terconazole Oral: Fluconazole Prevention
Cytolytic vaginitis	Overgrowth of lactobacilli	Nonodorous white to opaque vaginal discharge, vaginal and/or vulvar itching, vaginal or vulvar burning	Saline wet preparation: copious amounts of lactobacilli and a large number of epithelial cells pH between 3.5 and 4.5	None documented	Discontinue tampon use; sitz bath with sodium bicarbonate or sodium bicarbonate douche

TABLE 14B–1.	Comparisons of Infections (*continued*)				
	Etiology/ Pathology	Clinical Features	Diagnostic Studies	Complications	Management
Gonorrhea	*Neisseria gonorrhoeae* Coinfection with *Chlamydia* common	Incubation period: 3–5 d Asymptomatic or purulent vaginal discharge, urinary frequency, dysuria, chronic cervicitis	Culture Nucleic acid hybridization tests Nucleic acid amplification tests	May cause PID, infertility, increased risk of ectopic pregnancy, disseminated infection, arthritis Neonatal gonococcal conjunctivitis/ pharyngitis/ respiratory/ systemic infection	Ceftriaxone Cefixime Treat for *Chlamydia* Notify and treat partners Avoid sexual activity for 7 d following treatment
Chlamydia	*Chlamydia trachomatis* Most common cause of cervicitis Cause of LGV in tropical countries Coinfection with gonorrhea common	May be asymptomatic May cause mucopurulent cervicitis, urinary frequency, dysuria, abdominal pain, PID, and/or postcoital bleeding	Ligase chain reaction test: most sensitive/ specific Others: culture, direct fluorescent antibody, DNA probe test, enzyme immunoassay	PID, infertility, ectopic pregnancy, premature labor and delivery Postpartum infection Atypical cytologic findings on Pap smear	*Recommended*: Azithromycin Doxycycline *Alternatives*: Erythromycin Ofloxacin Levofloxacin Test for gonorrhea Treat partners LGV: doxycycline Avoid sexual activity for 7 d following treatment
		Diseases characterized by genital ulcers			
Genital HSV infections	HSV Transferred during symptomatic and asymptomatic viral shedding Sexually transmitted	Primary outbreak: 2–7 d from exposure, resolves in 2–6 wk Prodromal symptoms Multiple vesicles erode into painful ulcers Fever, malaise, inguinal lymphadenopathy, dysuria or other urinary symptoms With cervical infection: profuse watery discharge Virus remains in the sacral ganglia: recurrence in the same location Some outbreaks are asymptomatic	Viral culture for HSV Serum antibody titers Tzanck smear: multinucleated giant cells	HSV infection during pregnancy associated with congenital malformations C-section if active herpetic lesions or prodromal symptoms at time of delivery Prophylactic oral acyclovir after 36 wk	Self-limiting infection, lesions heal spontaneously Dosing varies depending on first episode, suppression therapy or episodic treatment for recurrence Acyclovir Famciclovir Valacyclovir
Syphilis	*Treponema pallidum*	*Primary*: Painless ulcer, 10–90 d after exposure	Darkfield examination for spirochete	Neurosyphilis	Benzathine penicillin G 2.4 million units intramuscular

(*continued*)

TABLE 14B–1. Comparisons of Infections (*continued*)

	Etiology/ Pathology	Clinical Features	Diagnostic Studies	Complications	Management
	Contracted by direct contact with an infectious moist lesion May be congenital	Lesions heal in 1–5 wk ± painless lymphadenopathy *Secondary:* Generalized, maculopapular rash, condyloma lata, fever, sore throat, diffuse adenopathy, patchy alopecia Develops average ~6 wk (0.5–6 mo) after initial infection, resolves in 2–6 wk Serology positive in this stage *Latent:* Infectious in the first 1–2 y of latency *Tertiary:* Occurs 4–20+ y after initial infection in one-third of untreated patients	Serologic tests: become positive 1–4 wk after the 1° lesion appears Venereal Disease Research Laboratory, rapid plasma reagin, fluorescent treponemal antibody absorption For neurosyphilis, cerebrospinal fluid finding useful for monitoring resolution following treatment	Jarisch–Herxheimer reaction Congenital syphilis	*For primary, secondary syphilis and latent (of <1 y):* 1 dose *For late latent:* weekly dose for 3 wk (7.2 million units total) Treat partners Offer HIV testing
Chancroid	*Haemophilus ducreyi* Uncommon in the U.S. sexually transmitted, lesions on the hands have occurred. Incubation period is 3–5 d	Soft, painful, shallow, genital ulcer Multiple, small papules or vesicles may develop Lesion produces heavy, foul-smelling, contagious discharge Painful inguinal adenitis common, with abscess formation	Clinical diagnosis Culture is diagnostic but positive in less than one-third of cases PCR available (not FDA-cleared)	Secondary infections, scarring	Azithromycin Ceftriaxone Erythromycin Ciprofloxacin
Others					
HPV	Virus with double-stranded DNA Five types with oncogenic potential Two types linked to genital warts	Most asymptomatic Flat, papular, or pedunculated growths May have vaginal discharge, pruritus. postcoital bleeding	Pap smear: characteristic changes when high risk oncogenic types present Nucleic acid tests Acetowhite staining of epithelium Colposcopy and biopsy	Associated with cervical dysplasia Condylomas may proliferate during pregnancy and resolve after delivery	*Office treatment:* Podophyllin Cryotherapy Trichloroacetic acid Bichloroacetic acid Surgical removal *Outpatient treatment:* Podofilox Aldara (imiquimod)
	Sexually transmitted				*Prevention:* Quadrivalent HPV vaccine (Gardasil)

TABLE 14B–1.	Comparisons of Infections (*continued*)				
	Etiology/ Pathology	**Clinical Features**	**Diagnostic Studies**	**Complications**	**Management**
PID	*N. gonorrhoeae* *C. trachomatis* Other microbes Risks: multiple partners, not using condoms	*Acute:* Appears ill May have fever, abdominal tenderness, purulent vaginal discharge, cervicitis, cervical motion tenderness, adnexal tenderness or mass, uterine tenderness *Chronic:* Less severe symptoms with a history of PID in the past	Wet mount. CBC, erythrocyte sedimentation rate, C-reactive protein (β-human chorionic gonadotropin), Gram stain Culture for gonorrhea and chlamydia Pelvic U/S Culdocentesis	Infertility Ectopic pregnancy Chronic pelvic pain	*Acute:* Antibiotics to cover gonorrhea, chlamydia, anaerobes NSAIDs *Chronic:* Antibiotics for 2–3 wk and NSAIDs Surgery screen partners for STIs and treat, if necessary
Toxic shock syndrome	Toxins produced by *Staphylococcus aureus*	Sudden onset of high fever, watery diarrhea, nausea, vomiting, sore throat, headache, diffuse macular rash, myalgias Appear acutely ill, fever $\geq 39°$ C (102.2° F) Tachycardia, dehydration, hypotension, erythematous rash, erythematous conjunctiva and pharynx, muscle and abdominal tenderness Pelvic examination should be done, remove tampon if present Multisystem involvement	CBC with differential, electrolytes, urine analysis, blood urea nitrogen, creatinine, liver function tests Culture suspected sources of the staphylococcal toxins	May progress to hypotensive shock in <48 h Death	Admission to hospital Supportive measures Search for source and treat Antistaphylococcal antibiotics
Bartholin gland cyst/ abscess	Retained secretions from duct obstruction leads to gland enlargement May be infected by gonococcus, *Escherichia coli*, *Staphylococcus*	*Not infected:* Nontender unilateral vulvar mass in the area of the Bartholin gland *Infected:* painful, unilateral vulvar mass, with associated inflammation and edema	Culture exudates	Recurrence	Simple asymptomatic cyst: no treatment Incision and drainage, may require marsupialization

CBC, complete blood count; HPV, human papillomavirus; HSV, herpes simplex virus; LGV, lymphogranuloma venereum; NSAIDs, nonsteroidal anti-inflammatory drugs; PID, pelvic inflammatory disease; STI, sexually transmitted disease; WBC, white blood cells.

- Clindamycin 300 mg or Metronidazole 500 mg twice daily for 7 days.
- Topical medications: Clindamycin 5 g or Metronidazole 500 mg twice daily for 7 days. (This treatment may give symptomatic relief, but it is insufficient in preventing pregnancy complications.)

2. **Trichomoniasis**
   a. **Etiology/Pathology**
      - Caused by infestation of *Trichomonas vaginalis*, a unicellular flagellate protozoan.
      - Sexually transmitted.
   b. **Clinical Features**
      - Maybe present in asymptomatic carrier state.
      - Up to 50% of women may be asymptomatic.
      - Copious, frothy, yellow-green vaginal discharge, usually worse after menses or during pregnancy in 10% to 30% of women.
      - Other women may have a clear or mucopurulent urethral discharge and/or dysuria.
      - May have foul odor and secondary vulvitis.
      - May have pruritus, dysuria, lower abdominal pain, or dyspareunia.
      - Generalized vaginal erythema and, in a small number of cases, cervical-petechiae "strawberry cervix."
      - Often, simultaneous infection of urinary tract.
      - Male sex partners may develop urethritis or balanitis but often are asymptomatic.
   c. **Diagnostic Studies**
      - Saline wet mount shows motile trichomonads, increased WBCs: sensitivity approximately 60% to 70%.
      - pH > 5.0.
      - OSOM *Trichomonas* rapid test (immunochromatographic capillary flow dipstick technology): sensitivity >83%, specificity >97%.
      - May be seen on Pap smear.
      - Affirm VP III (nucleic acid probe test): sensitivity >83%, specificity >97%.
      - Culture: most sensitive specific but not commonly done.
   d. **Complications**
      - Associated with perinatal complications.
      - BV.
      - Increased incidence in the transmission of HIV.
   e. **Management**
      - Metronidazole 2 g PO in a single dose or 500 mg BID for 7 days.
      - Tinidazole 2 g PO in a single dose.
      - Must treat partner also, who is usually asymptomatic.
      - Spermicidal agents (nonoxynol-9, etc.) decrease the transmission of *Trichomonas*.
      - Evaluate for other sexually transmitted infections (STIs) and BV.

3. **Vulvovaginal Candidiasis**
   a. **Etiology/Pathology**
      - Caused from overgrowth of *Candida albicans* (present in normal vaginal flora) due to a change in normal vaginal environment.
      - Consider *Candida glabrata*, if KOH is negative, but yeast is suspected clinically.
   b. **Clinical Features**
      - Ten percent to 20% of women of reproductive age with *Candida* infection are asymptomatic.
      - Vaginal discharge, pruritus of vulva and vaginal introitus, burning when urine touches the skin (secondary to inflammation and excoriation), vulva feels swollen, sore, and/or dyspareunia.
      - Erythematous, edematous vulva, possibly with excoriations from scratching.
      - Vagina may have thick, cottage cheese-like discharge.
   c. **Diagnostic Studies**
      - Yeast, pseudohyphae and budding hyphae and spores visible with 10% KOH solution.
      - Normal vaginal pH (<4.5).
      - Gram stain if suspect *C. glabrata*.
      - Yeast culture rarely indicated.
   d. **Complications**
      - Yeast infections may be unrefractory in pregnancy, HIV infection, and diabetes mellitus.
   e. **Management**
      - Treatment only indicated for relief of symptoms.
      - **Intravaginal options**
        - Butoconazole
          - Two percent cream 5 g intravaginally for 3 days.
          - Butoconazole 1–sustained release, single intravaginal application.
        - Clotrimazole
          - One percent cream 5 g intravaginally for 7 to 14 days.
          - One hundred milligram vaginal tablet for 7 days.
          - One hundred milligram vaginal tablet, two tablets for 3 days.
        - Miconazole
          - Two percent cream 5 g intravaginally for 7 days.
          - One hundred milligram vaginal suppository, one suppository for 7 days.
          - Two hundred milligram vaginal suppository, one suppository for 3 days.
          - One thousand two hundred milligram vaginal suppository, one suppository for 1 day.
          - Nystatin 100,000-unit vaginal tablet, one tablet for 14 days.

- Tioconazole 6.5% ointment 5 g intravaginally in a single application.
  - Terconazole
    - About 0.4% cream 5 g intravaginally for 7 days.
    - About 0.8% cream 5 g intravaginally for 3 days.
    - About 80 mg vaginal suppository, one suppository for 3 days.
  - Oral: Fluconazole 150 mg PO, one tablet in single dose.
  - Discuss vulvovaginal hygiene: keep vulva dry; wear 100% cotton underwear; and avoid tight-fitting clothing, feminine deodorant products, and bubble baths.

4. **Cytolytic Vaginitis**
   a. **Etiology/Pathology**
   - Caused by an overgrowth of lactobacilli.
   - Etiology remains unknown.
   - Often misdiagnosed as BV or candidiasis.
   b. **Clinical Features**
   - Symptoms may vary with menstrual cycle.
   - Variable symptoms may include white vaginal discharge, vaginal and/or vulvar pruritus, vulvar burning or vulvar dysuria, and/or dyspareunia.
   - Minimal exam findings may include white or opaque discharge, tenderness with speculum insertion, and/or slightly erythematous vulvar and vaginal tissue.
   c. **Diagnostic Studies**
   - Saline wet preparation: copious amounts of lactobacilli and a large number of epithelial cells.
   - Exclude bacterial vaginitis, trichomoniasis, and candida infections.
   - pH normal: 3.5 to 4.5.
   d. **Management**
   - Discontinue tampon use to decrease vaginal acidity.
   - Sitz bath with 2 to 4 tbsp of sodium bicarbonate.
   - Sodium bicarbonate douche with 1 tbsp of sodium bicarbonate to 1 pint of warm water.
   - Treatment may have to be repeated before relief is achieved.

5. **Gonorrhea**
   a. **Etiology/Pathology**
   - *Neisseria gonorrhoeae* contracted by sexual contact with an infected person.
   - Coinfection with *Chlamydia* common.
   b. **Clinical Features**
   - Incubation period: 3 to 5 days.
   - Usually asymptomatic.
   - If symptomatic: vaginal mucopurulent discharge, cervicitis, urinary frequency, dysuria, rectal discomfort from perineal spread.
   - Can progress to PID, disseminated infection, and arthritis.
   c. **Diagnostic Studies**
   - Nucleic acid amplification tests (NAATs): most sensitive and specific:
     - Endocervical specimen.
     - Vaginal specimen.
     - Urine.
   - Culture: endocervical specimen.
   - Nucleic acid hybridization tests: endocervical specimen.
   - Gram stain: not specific for endocervical specimens, therefore not recommended.
   d. **Complications**
   - May cause PID, infertility, increased risk of ectopic pregnancy secondary to tubal scarring, premature rupture of membranes, low birth weight, spontaneous abortion, chronic pelvic pain, and neonatal conjunctivitis.
   e. **Management**
     - **Recommended regimens: one time dose**
       - Ceftriaxone 250 mg intramuscular (IM); or
       - Cefixime 400 mg: 1 tablet or 10 mL (200 mg per 5 mL) orally.
     - **Alternative regimens: one time dose**
       - Ceftizoxime 500 mg IM; or
       - Cefoxitin 2 g IM, administered with probenecid 1 g orally; or
       - Cefotaxime 500 mg IM.
     - Also treat with Azithromycin 1 g orally × one for presumptive coinfection with chlamydia.
     - Partners within the last 60 days, or last partner if >60 days, should be notified and treated.
     - Avoid sexual activity for 7 days following treatment.
   f. **Screening: U.S. Preventive Services Task Force (USPSTF) Recommendations**
     - All sexually active women and men under the age of 26.
     - Any woman or man at increased risk for infection: positive for other STIs, new or multiple sexual partners, erratic condom use, and having sex for drugs or money.

6. *Chlamydia*
   a. **Etiology/Pathology**
   - *Chlamydia trachomatis* contracted by sexual contact with an infected person.
   - Most common cause of cervicitis.
   - Cause of lymphogranuloma venereum (LGV) in tropical countries.
   - Coinfection with gonorrhea common.
   b. **Clinical Features**
   - May be asymptomatic.
   - May cause mucopurulent cervicitis, urinary frequency, dysuria, abdominal pain, PID, and/or postcoital bleeding.

- Discharge tends to be less purulent and painful, and more watery than discharge of gonorrhea.
  c. **Diagnostic Studies**
    - NAAT of vaginal swabs.
    - Culture, direct fluorescent antibody, enzyme immunoassay, and DNA probe test.
    - Ligase chain reaction (LCR) test is the most sensitive and specific. Can be run on a urine specimen.
  d. **Complications**
    - PID, infertility, and ectopic pregnancy.
    - Premature labor and delivery.
    - Postpartum infection.
    - Atypical cytologic findings on Pap smear.
  e. **Management**
    - **Recommended regimens**
      - Azithromycin 1 g orally single dose therapy; or
      - Doxycycline 100 mg orally, twice a day × 7 days.
    - **Alternative regimens**
      - Erythromycin base 500 mg orally four times a day × 7 days; or
      - Erythromycin ethylsuccinate 800 mg orally four times a day × 7 days; or
      - Ofloxacin 300 mg orally twice a day × 7 days; or
      - Levofloxacin 500 mg orally once daily for 7 days.
    - Also test for gonorrhea.
    - Partners within the last 60 days, or last partner if >60 days, should be notified and treated.
    - Avoid sexual contact for 7 days after treatment.
    - For LGV doxycycline 100 mg twice a day × 21 days.
  f. **Screening: USPSTF Recommendations**
    - All sexually active women and men under the age of 26.
    - Any woman or man at increased risk for infection: positive for other STIs, new or multiple sexual partners, erratic condom use, and having sex for drugs or money.

B. Diseases Characterized by Genital Ulcers
  1. **Genital HSV Infections**
    a. **Etiology/Pathology**
      - Herpes simplex virus (HSV).
      - Transferred during both symptomatic and asymptomatic viral shedding.
      - Sexually transmitted (oral, anal, or vaginal intercourse) through direct contact with contaminated secretions or mucosal surfaces.
    b. **Clinical Features**
      - Primary outbreak occurs 2 to 7 days from the time of exposure.
      - Prodromal symptoms (itch/tingle) may be experienced prior to the development of multiple vesicles that erode into painful ulcers on labia and around introitus.
      - May have fever, malaise, and tender, inguinal lymphadenopathy in severe infections.
      - Dysuria or other urinary symptoms, including urinary retention, may develop.
      - Herpes outbreaks on the cervix cause a profuse watery discharge and no other symptoms.
      - Lesions are self-limited, resolving in 2 to 6 weeks.
      - The virus remains in the sacral ganglia and can recur any time with lesions.
      - Clinical recurrences of genital HSV are common.
      - Some outbreaks are asymptomatic.
    c. **Diagnostic Studies**
      - Polymerase chain reaction (PCR) on active genital lesion scrappings.
      - Viral culture for HSV.
      - Serum antibody titers.
      - Tzanck smear reveals multinucleated giant cells.
    d. **Complications**
      - If pregnant woman has active herpetic lesions or prodromal symptoms at the time of delivery, C-section is indicated to prevent neonatal transmission (60% fetal mortality rate with vaginal delivery; 40%–50% chance of transmission during active primary infection, 5% during recurrent infection). Consider prophylactic oral acyclovir after 36 weeks.
      - HSV infection during pregnancy also associated with congenital malformations.
    e. **Management**
      - Self-limiting infection, lesions heal spontaneously.
        - First episode
          - Acyclovir 400 mg orally three times a day × 7 to 10 days or 200 mg orally five times a day × 7 to 10 days.
          - Famciclovir 250 mg orally three times a day for 7 to 10 days; or
          - Valacyclovir 1 g orally twice a day for 7 to 10 days.
      - **Suppression therapy for ≥6 recurrences per year:**
        - Acyclovir 400 mg orally twice a day and valacyclovir 1.0 g orally twice a day.
      - **Episodic therapy for recurrent herpes:**
        - Acyclovir 400 mg orally three times a day for 5 days.
        - Acyclovir 800 mg orally twice a day for 5 days.
        - Acyclovir 800 mg orally three times a day for 2 days.

- Famciclovir 125 mg orally twice a day for 5 days.
- Famciclovir 1.0 g orally twice a day for 1 day.
- Valacyclovir 500 mg orally twice a day for 3 days.
- Valacyclovir 1.0 g orally once a day for 5 days.
  f. **Screening: USPSTF Recommendations**
  - Screening not recommended.
2. **Syphilis**
   a. **Etiology/Pathology**
   - *Treponema pallidum* (a spirochete).
   - Contracted by direct contact with an infectious moist lesion.
   - Site of infection may be the hand as a consequence of touching a lesion.
   - May be congenital.
   b. **Clinical Features**
   - Primary: chancre (indurated, firm, painless papule, or ulcer with raised borders) develops 10 to 90 days after exposure to infection. It can occur anywhere on skin or mucous membrane. The lesions heal in 1 to 5 weeks. May be associated with painless lymphadenopathy.
   - Secondary: caused by the spirochetes entering the bloodstream. Self-limited, generalized, maculopapular rash develops 2 weeks to 6 months (average ~6 weeks) after initial infection, resolves in 2 to 6 weeks. Skin lesions common in 80% of patients, classically affecting the palms and soles. Condyloma lata, fever, sore throat, diffuse adenopathy, and patchy alopecia may be present. Serology positive in this stage.
   - Latent: period after resolution of the lesions of primary and secondary infection, or the finding of a reactive serologic test without a history of therapy. Infectious in the first 1 to 2 years of latency.
     - Early latent stage: infection of <1 year.
     - Late latent stage: infection of >1 year.
   - Tertiary: occurs 4 to 20+ years after initial infection in one-third of untreated patients. Commonly causes granulomatous disease of the skin, cardiac, and neurologic problems and can affect any organ system.
   c. **Diagnostic Studies**
   - Serologic tests become positive 1 to 4 weeks after the primary lesion appears.
     - Nontreponemal tests: Venereal Disease Research Laboratory test (VDRL), rapid plasma reagin (RPR) test, and automated reagin test for screening procedures in the field.
     - Treponemal antibody tests: the fluorescent treponemal antibody absorption (FTA-ABS) test and microhemagglutination assay for *T. pallidum* detect antibody against *Treponema* spirochetes.

- Rapid Point-of-Care (POC) tests are becoming more widely available.
- For neurosyphilis, cerebrospinal fluid (CSF) findings are unreliable for excluding the diagnosis but are useful for monitoring resolution following treatment.
  d. **Complications**
  - Neurosyphilis may develop.
  - **Jarisch–Herxheimer reaction**
    - Febrile reaction occurring in 50% to 75% of patients with early syphilis treated with penicillin.
    - Occurs 4 to 12 hours after injection; lasts 24 hours.
    - Uncertain cause.
    - Generally benign.
  - With pregnancy in an infected woman, the baby will have congenital syphilis.
  e. **Management**
  - For primary, secondary, and latent syphilis (of <1 year): benzathine penicillin G 2.4 million units IM once.
  - For late latent, benzathine penicillin G 2.4 million units IM once weekly for 3 weeks (7.2 million units total).
  - Alternative treatments for nonpregnant penicillin-allergic patients: doxycycline (Vibramycin), 100 mg taken orally twice daily for 2 weeks, or tetracycline, 500 mg taken orally four times daily for 2 weeks; limited data support efficacy for ceftriaxone (Rocephin), 1 g once daily IM or IV for 8 to 10 days.
  - Partners should be notified and treated.
  - Offer HIV testing to all patients diagnosed with syphilis due to high rates of coinfection.
  f. **Screening: USPSTF Recommendations**
  - Persons at increased risk for syphilis infection.
  - All pregnant women.
3. **Chancroid**
   a. **Etiology/Pathology**
   - *Haemophilus ducreyi* (gram-negative bacillus).
   - Very uncommon in the United States.
   - Sexually transmitted, lesions on the hands have occurred.
   - Incubation period is 3 to 5 days.
   b. **Clinical Features**
   - Soft, painful, shallow genital ulcer, circumscribed circumscribed by a bright red zone of congestion.
   - Multiple, small papules or vesicles may develop.
   - Lesion produces heavy, foul-smelling, contagious discharge.
   - Painful inguinal adenitis common, often with abscess formation.
   c. **Diagnostic Studies**
   - Culturing is diagnostic, but positive in less than one-third of cases.

- PCR testing available, although not Food and Drug Administration (FDA)-cleared.
- Rely on clinical diagnosis; probable diagnosis made if:
  - One + painful genital ulcers.
  - Negative HSV test.
  - Clinical presentation is typical for chancroid.
  d. **Complications**
  - Secondary infections, scarring.
  e. **Management**
  - Azithromycin 1 g once; or
  - Ceftriaxone 250 mg IM once; or
  - Erythromycin 500 mg PO TID × 7 days; or
  - Ciprofloxacin 500 mg PO BID × 3 days.
4. **Lymphogranuloma Venereum**
   - Uncommon in the United States and in women.
5. **Granuloma Inguinale**
   - Uncommon in the United States.

C. Others

1. **Human Papillomavirus**
   a. **Etiology/Pathology**
   - Most commonly transmitted sexual infection.
   - Virus with double-stranded DNA.
   - More than 40 types of human papillomavirus (HPV) identified: types 16, 18, 31, 33, and 35 appear to have the most oncogenic potential and are considered "high risk."
   - Types 6 and 11 are associated with genital condyloma and considered "low risk."
   - When vulvar lesions are present, the entire lower tract is usually involved.
   - Sexually transmitted, both partners infected.
   - Condyloma lesions, also known as warts, are benign and not related to the development of cervical cancer.
   b. **Clinical Features**
   - Most types cause an asymptomatic infection.
   - Flat, papular, or pedunculated growths.
   - Warts are either external or internal.
   - With florid condylomas, may have vaginal discharge and pruritus.
   - Postcoital bleeding may occur.
   - Massive proliferation seen in immunosuppression (pregnancy, HIV infection, diabetes, renal transplant) and treatment often is difficult.
   c. **Diagnostic Studies**
   - Characteristic changes may be present on Pap smear when high-risk types of HPV are present.
   - Nucleic acid tests.
   - Acetowhite staining of epithelium with dilute acetic acid solution.
   - Colposcopy and biopsy.
   d. **Complications**
   - Associated with cervical dysplasia, regular Pap smears recommended.

- Condyloma may proliferate during pregnancy and spontaneously resolve following delivery.
  e. **Management**
  - Most lesions respond within 3 months of treatment.
  - **Office treatment**
    - Podophyllin resin 10% to 25% in a compound tincture of benzoin applied to each wart (not in pregnancy) repeated weekly. Wash off after 1 to 4 hours to reduce local irritation.
    - Cryotherapy internally.
    - Trichloroacetic acid or bichloroacetic acid (BCA) 80% to 90% applied to each wart, repeated weekly if needed.
    - Surgical removal, tangential shave excision, curettage, or electrosurgery.
  - Most lesions respond within 3 months of treatment.
  - **Outpatient treatment**
    - Not in pregnancy.
    - Podofilox (0.5% solution of gel), apply BID × 3 days, repeat weekly for up to 4 weeks.
    - Imiquimod (Aldara), applied externally overnight three times a week for up to 16 weeks.
  - **Prevention**
    - Quadrivalent HPV vaccine (Gardasil).
      - Three-dose schedule, second and third doses: 2 and 6 months after the first dose.
      - Routine vaccination of females aged 11 to 12 years; can be started as young as age 9 years. Recommended up to 26 years of age.
      - Screenings for cervical cancer and HPV DNA or HPV antibody prior to vaccination are not needed.
      - No therapeutic effect on current infection.
      - May be used in immunocompromised and lactating women, not given in pregnancy.
2. **Pelvic Inflammatory Disease**
   a. **Etiology/Pathology**
   - Infectious inflammation of upper genital tract (uterus, fallopian tubes, ovaries, pelvic peritoneum) following disruption of the endocervical mucus barrier.
   - Polymicrobial infection caused most commonly by *N. gonorrhoeae* and *C. trachomatis*.
   - Other microbes may be present.
   - Having multiple partners, not using condoms puts patients at high risk.
   b. **Clinical Features**
   - Patient is usually in reproductive years with a history of unprotected sex.
   - Onset often associated with menses.
   - **Acute**
     - Appears ill.

- May have lower abdominal tenderness that is often bilateral and associated with menses, purulent vaginal discharge, cervicitis, cervical motion tenderness, adnexal tenderness or mass, uterine tenderness.
  - **Chronic**
    - Symptoms of low-grade fever, weight loss, and abdominal pain may present with a history of PID diagnosis in the past.
- c. **Diagnostic Studies**
  - β-human chorionic gonadotropin (β-hCG) test to rule out intrauterine or ectopic pregnancy.
  - Wet mount: BV, *Trichomonas*, and/or WBCs may be present.
  - Blood work: complete blood count (CBC; increased WBCs), erythrocyte sedimentation rate (increased), β-hCG (rule out ectopic), and C-reactive protein (elevated).
  - Gram stain: gram-negative kidney-shaped diplococci in polymorphonuclear leukocytes.
  - NAAT for *C. trachomatis* and *N. gonorrhoeae*.
  - Cervical cultures for gonorrhea and chlamydia.
  - Pelvic ultrasound (U/S): most valuable for following abscess progression or regression.
- d. **Complications**
  - Salpingitis, oophoritis, peritonitis, and tubo-ovarian cyst.
  - Increases risk of infertility.
  - Ectopic pregnancy.
  - Chronic pelvic pain.
  - Occasionally patient ends up with diagnostic laparoscopy because symptoms may mimic acute appendicitis.
- e. **Management**
  - Screen partners for STIs and treat, if necessary.
  - **Acute**
    - Inpatient or outpatient treatment, depending on the severity of symptoms.
      - All pregnant or immunocompromised women with PID should be hospitalized.
    - Antibiotic therapy needs to cover gonorrhea, chlamydia, and anaerobes.
    - Pain management with nonsteroidal anti-inflammatory drugs (NSAIDs).
  - **Chronic**
    - Antibiotics for 2 to 3 weeks and NSAIDs.
    - Surgery (TAH-BSO) if associated with intractable pelvic pain and/or tubo-ovarian abscess.
3. **Toxic Shock Syndrome**
  a. **Etiology/Pathology**
    - Toxins produced by *Staphylococcus aureus*.
  b. **Clinical Features**
    - Sudden onset of high fever, watery diarrhea, nausea, vomiting, headache, myalgias, diffuse macular rash, and sore throat.

- Tachycardia, dehydration, and possibly hypotension.
- Appear acutely ill, fever $\geq$39° C (102.2° F); erythematous, sunburn-like rash is seen over the face, proximal extremities; erythematous conjunctiva and pharynx; and muscle and abdominal tenderness.
- Pelvic examination should be done, remove tampon if present.
- Mucosal lesions should be sought, and a culture for *S. aureus* performed.
- Multisystem involvement is the rule (three or more of the following involved: muscular, mucous membranes, renal, hepatic, hematologic, and CNS).
  c. **Diagnostic Studies**
    - Based on clinical presentation.
    - Assess for effects on various organ systems: CBC with differential, electrolytes, urine analysis (UA), blood urea nitrogen (BUN), creatinine, liver function tests (LFTs), blood and throat cultures, CSF culture, if indicated.
    - Culture suspected sources of the staphylococcal toxins.
  d. **Complications**
    - May progress to hypotensive shock in 48 hours.
    - Thirty percent of women who suffer from toxic shock syndrome (TSS) have recurrences (greatest risk is in the first three menstrual cycles after the original episode).
    - Mortality rate: 3% to 6%.
    - Major causes of death from TSS are adult respiratory distress syndrome, disseminated intravascular coagulation, and hypotension.
  e. **Management**
    - Admission to hospital.
    - Supportive measures (e.g., intravenous fluids, blood pressure support, analgesics).
    - Search for source and treat (e.g., removal of vaginal products, exploration of recent surgical wounds).
    - Antistaphylococcal antibiotics.
4. **Bartholin Gland Cyst/Abscess**
  a. **Etiology/Pathology**
    - Duct obstruction leads to enlargement of the greater vestibular gland in the vulva from retained secretions. Maybe complicated with infection by gonococcus, *Escherichia coli*, *Staphylococcus*, for example.
  b. **Clinical Features**
    - Nontender unilateral vulvar mass in the area of the Bartholin gland if not infected.
    - Painful, unilateral vulvar mass, with associated inflammation and edema if infected.

c. **Diagnostic Studies**
  - Physical examination of the cyst in an appropriate location.
  - Culture exudate.
d. **Complications**
  - Recurrence.
e. **Management**
  - Simple asymptomatic cyst requires no treatment.
  - Incision and drainage (I&D).
  - Biopsy to exclude carcinoma, particularly in women >60 years old.
  - May require marsupialization.
  - Recurrent infections may require excision or marsupialization of the gland for permanent drainage.

II. Disorders of the Cervix
A. Cervical Polyps
1. **Etiology/Pathology**
   - Result of focal endocervical hyperplasia of unknown etiology. May be related to hyperestrogenism.
   - May be covered with squamous, columnar, or squamocolumnar epithelium. Often attached by a long stalk.
   - Common; occur at any age but more common in multigravidas over 20.
   - Most are benign; although low risk for cancer (0.5%: dysplasia; 0.5%: malignant), all should be removed and sent for pathologic diagnosis.
2. **Clinical Features**
   - May be asymptomatic, found on examination.
   - Symptoms
     - Bleeding: intermenstrual, postcoital, heavy, and/or prolonged.
     - Vaginal discharge: leukorrhea.
   - Soft, smooth, red approximately 0.5 to 1 cm × 1 to 2 cm growth protruding from cervical opening, or seen in the endocervical canal with the use of an endocervical speculum.
   - Fragile, may bleed on contact.
3. **Diagnostic Studies**
   - Remove polyp and send for pathologic diagnosis.
   - Polyps may be seen on transvaginal pelvic U/S, hysterosalpingogram, or saline infusion sonohysterography.
   - Culture for concomitant infections if abnormal discharge is present.
4. **Complications**
   - Cause of previously unexplained infertility.
   - Cervicitis, endometritis, and parametritis.
   - Salpingitis.
5. **Management**
   - Removal, usually done in office by twisting at the pedicle with hemostat (usually curative).

B. Nabothian Cysts
1. **Etiology/Pathology**
   - Mucus-secreting columnar endocervical epithelium becomes covered by squamous cells.
   - Secretions accumulate.
2. **Clinical Features**
   - Smooth, clear, or yellow nodule visible on examination; may be palpable.
   - Several millimeters to 3 cm in diameter.
3. **Diagnostic Studies**
   - None.
4. **Complications**
   - None.
5. **Management**
   - No treatment necessary, if asymptomatic.

III. Disorders of the Uterus
A. Fibroid Tumors (Leiomyoma)
1. **Definition**
   - Benign tumors of the uterus arising from the smooth muscle cells of the myometrium.
2. **Etiology**
   - True etiology unknown.
   - Most common pelvic tumor in females.
   - More common in African American than Caucasian females.
   - Responsive to hormones; grow during reproductive years, shrink after menopause.
3. **Pathology**
   - Benign growths, primarily of smooth muscle, originating in the myometrium.
   - Usually multiple.
   - Classification based on anatomic location.
4. **Clinical Features**
   - About 50% to 65% are asymptomatic.
   - Symptoms may include heavy or prolonged menstrual bleeding (most common), pelvic pain or heaviness, dysmenorrhea, anemia, back pain, and premature labor.
   - Uncommon symptoms due to the pressure of a large fibroid: increased urinary frequency, hydronephrosis, stress incontinence, dyspareunia, constipation, and lower extremity edema.
   - Enlarged, irregularly contoured uterus on bimanual examination.
   - May be palpable during abdominal examination.
5. **Diagnostic Studies**
   - β-hCG: rule out pregnancy.
   - Pelvic U/S: document size and position of fibroids.
   - CBC count: anemia common, leukocytosis with acute degeneration or infection.
   - Sedimentation rate may be elevated with acute degeneration or infection.
   - Intravenous pyelogram: rule out hydronephrosis.
   - Consider endometrial biopsy to rule out endometrial cancer as a cause of bleeding.

6. **Complications**
   - Anemia secondary to menorrhagia.
   - Degeneration: caused by ischemia when a fibroid outgrows its blood supply; a painful condition that may present as an acute abdomen; sarcomatous (malignant) degeneration is rare.
   - Pregnancy (rapid growth can occur due to hormones): degeneration leading to pain, premature labor, obstruction requiring C-section, and postpartum hemorrhage.
   - Possible link to fertility: myomectomy for endocavitary fibroids.
   - Spontaneous abortion.
7. **Management**
   a. **Nonpregnant, Asymptomatic Patient**
      - Follow with bimanual examination every 6 months or serial pelvic U/S to follow growth. Fibroids may shrink after menopause; consequently, postmenopausal fibroid growth considered malignancy until proven otherwise.
   b. **Symptomatic**
      - **Conservative treatment**
        - Progestin therapy for abnormal bleeding. Gonadotropin-releasing hormone (GnRH) agonists create temporary menopause and are used frequently preoperatively (fibroid tumors shrink in the absence of estrogen stimulation).
        - Mirena (levonorgestrel-releasing intrauterine device [IUD or IUC]) to treat menorrhagia.
      - **Surgical treatment**
        - Myomectomy: removes fibroids and preserves the uterus (and fertility). Depending on the location of tumors may be able to be done by laparoscope or hysteroscope.
        - Hysterectomy: performed when fertility is not an issue. Curative.
        - Embolization: embolizing agent infused into the uterine artery supplying the fibroid.

IV. Disorders of the Ovaries
A. Ovarian Cysts
1. **Definition**
   - Cystic enlargement of any of the normal ovarian structures.
   - Fluid-filled sacs often related to ovulation.
   - Common in reproductive years, usually unilateral.
2. **Etiology/Pathology**
   - Follicular cysts represent a mature follicle that fails to rupture.
   - Corpus luteum cysts develop as a result of bleeding into center of corpus luteum.
   - Theca lutein cysts are associated with elevated levels of chorionic gonadotropin. They can be associated with hydatidiform mole, choriocarcinoma,

and chorionic gonadotropin or clomiphene therapy and, rarely, with normal pregnancy.

3. **Clinical Features**
   - May be asymptomatic and an incidental finding on pelvic examination.
   - May cause a change in menstrual cycle, aching pelvic pain, dyspareunia, and abnormal uterine bleeding.
   - Palpable adnexal mass on bimanual examination.
   - Ruptured cyst can present as an acute abdomen.
4. **Diagnostic Studies**
   - β-hCG to rule out pregnancy.
   - Pelvic U/S to confirm diagnosis.
5. **Complications**
   - Bleeding, ovarian torsion (surgical emergency), rupture causing symptoms of an acute abdomen.
6. **Management**
   - Cysts usually resolve spontaneously over the next few menstrual cycles.
   - Oral contraceptives have been used in the past to aid in resolution. Data do not support increased rate of resolution.
   - If no resolution occurs, or if demonstrated continued growth is present, laparoscopic cystectomy to rule out malignancy.

B. Polycystic Ovarian Syndrome
1. **Definition**
   - Endocrine/metabolic syndrome characterized by ovulatory irregularity, obesity, hirsutism, bilaterally enlarged polycystic ovaries, menstrual irregularity, insulin resistance, and subfertility and infertility.
2. **Etiology/Pathology**
   - Etiology unknown.
   - Abnormal gonadotropin secretion with excessive androgen production with pituitary suppression.
   - Condition not always fully expressed.
3. **Clinical and Associated Features**
   - Anovulatory cycles.
   - Menstrual abnormalities, including oligomenorrhea and amenorrhea.
   - Hirsutism (50%), obesity (80%), amenorrhea (50%), abnormal uterine bleeding (30%), enlarged ovaries on bimanual examination.
   - Metabolic syndrome.
4. **Diagnostic Studies**
   - Transvaginal U/S.
   - Luteinizing hormone (LH) and follicle-stimulating hormone (FSH): rule out premature ovarian failure.
   - Thyroid-stimulating hormone (TSH): rule out thyroid disorder.
   - Prolactin level: rule out pituitary adenoma.
   - Lipid panel to evaluate for dyslipidemia.
   - Glucose tolerance test to evaluate for insulin resistance.

- Testosterone (elevated), dehydroepiandrosterone-sulfate (DHEA-S) (elevated in 50% of patients), and 17-hydroxyprogesterone.

5. Complications
- Infertility, hirsutism, and endometrial hyperplasia.
- Increased risk of early onset type 2 diabetes mellitus, cardiovascular disease, and endometrial and breast cancer.

6. Management
- Treat patient symptoms.
- Oral contraceptives regulate menstrual cycle and prevent endometrial hyperplasia; cyclic progestin can also be used.
- Metformin can restore menstrual cyclicity and insulin resistance.
- Hirsutism: spironolactone (decreases androgenic action in target organs), antiandrogens (flutamide or finasteride), low-dose oral contraceptive pill (OCP) (results after 6–12 months), depilation, and electrolysis.
- Dexamethasone for high DHEA-S levels.
- Obesity: weight reduction may help to restore ovulation.
- Infertility: induce ovulation with drugs: clomiphene (stimulates ovaries); oral hypoglycemics (reduce hyperandrogenemia and hyperinsulinemia). Refer if needed.
- Monitor lipids, glucose; consider screening carotids starting at 30 and coronary calcium starting at 45.

V. Disorders of the Breasts
- See also Chapter 17, section III.

A. Mastitis
1. Etiology/Pathology
- Congestive: bilateral breast engorgement occurring 2 to 3 days postpartum.
- Infectious: uncommon complication of breast feeding; usually unilateral: due to nipple trauma; infection with *S. aureus* or *Candida*.
- More common in first-time nursing mothers.

2. Clinical Features
- Congestive: bilateral breast pain and swelling, low-grade fever, may have axillary lymphadenopathy.
- Infectious: presents 1-week postpartum; usually unilateral breast pain; fever, chills; findings confined to one quadrant of the breast with tenderness, swelling, erythema and warmth; ± nipple discharge; and ± abscess formation (edema and fluctuation).

3. Diagnostic Studies
- Culture of abscess if draining.
- CBC, although not necessary.

4. Complications
- Abscess.

5. Management
- Congestive: if woman does not want to breast-feed—tight-fitting bra, ice packs, avoiding breast

stimulation, analgesics. If she does want to breastfeed, supportive therapy only—manually emptying breasts completely after baby is done breastfeeding, analgesics, local heat, and continuing to nurse.
- Infectious: supportive measures as above, with antibiotic therapy (antistaphylococcal) or fluconazole 200 mg orally daily.
- Abscess: surgical I&D, discontinue breastfeeding, and suppress lactation.

VI. Other Disorders
A. Pelvic Organ Prolapse
1. Definition
- Herniation of one of the pelvic organs, classified by their location.
  - Anterior vaginal wall: cystocele.
  - Apical: uterine prolapse.
  - Posterior vaginal wall: rectocele.

2. Etiology/Pathology
- Relaxation, injury, congenital or developmental weakness of pelvic support structures.
- Risk factors: age, obesity, activities that increase pressure on the pelvic floor—multiparity, chronic coughing, repetitive heavy lifting, Ehlers–Danlos syndromes.
- Staging is based on position of the prolapse to the hymen, graded 0 (no prolapse) to IV (complete prolapse).

3. Clinical Features
- Condition may affect quality of life.
- Symptoms include pressure or discomfort in the vagina or pelvis, low back pain, urinary symptoms including stress incontinence and urinary tract infection (UTI) symptoms without dysuria, sensation of something protruding from the vagina (somewhat relieved by lying down), dyspareunia, difficulty with defecation, and sexual dysfunction due to a feeling of laxity.
- Examination: bulging mass, more prominent with increased intraabdominal pressure.
- Also evaluate for urinary incontinence.

4. Diagnostic Studies
- Usually not needed.
- Pelvic U/S if questionable pelvic mass is present.
- Voiding cystourethrography (VCUG): for evaluation of bladder and bladder support.

5. Complications
- Not common.
- Ulceration of the protruding vaginal tissue, which can lead to cellulitis.
- UTI or urinary obstruction.
- Urinary or fecal incontinence.

6. Management
- Kegel exercises: strengthen pelvic floor.
- Pessary: provides symptomatic relief.

- Hormone replacement therapy (HRT): to improve symptoms due to atrophy.
- Surgery: only curative treatment; procedure-dependent on the type of prolapse.

B. Endometriosis

1. **Etiology/Pathology**
   - Cause is unknown, may be due to retrograde menstruation.
   - Endometrial tissue is found outside of the uterus eliciting an inflammatory response.
   - Occurs in women of reproductive age.
2. **Clinical Features**
   - Asymptomatic or infertility.
   - Dysmenorrhea and dyspareunia, premenstrual low back, pelvic, or rectal pain that can continue through menses and for several days afterwards.
   - Pelvic examination: usually normal; may find a tender mass or nodules in the adnexa, posterior fornix or rectovaginal septum; fixed uterus and cervical motion tenderness.
3. **Diagnostic Studies**
   - Presumptive clinical diagnosis.
   - None of value. Diagnosed with direct visualization at laparotomy or laparoscopy.
   - Histologic evaluation of a lesion biopsied during laparoscopy.
4. **Complications**
   - Infertility.
   - Otherwise rare: symptoms due to adhesions, obstruction of ureters or bowel, and ovarian torsion.
5. **Management**
   - Conservative treatment
     - Premenstrual/menstrual pain: NSAIDs; analgesics with or without narcotics.
     - Prevention of ovulation with decrease in hormone levels: continuous use of oral contraceptive pills, patch, or ring for 6 to 12 months; danazol for 4 to 6 months; GnRH analogs for 6 months; and progestins.
   - Surgical treatment
     - Laparoscopic ablation of lesions.
     - Hysterectomy with bilateral oophorectomy for women no longer interested in childbearing.

C. Stress Incontinence

- Urinary incontinence is addressed in Chapter 1.

1. **Etiology/Pathology**
   - Involuntary urinary leakage that occurs with increased intraabdominal pressure (coughing, sneezing, laughing, exertion).
   - Due to pelvic floor muscle laxity and insufficiency of the urethral sphincter.
   - Risk factors include vaginal delivery, obesity, chronic cough, heavy lifting, straining, and strenuous exercise.

2. **Clinical Features**
   - Patient leaks urine with coughing, sneezing, laughing, exercising, and straining.
   - Examination: evaluate pelvic support structures, evaluate for estrogen effect (atrophy) and anal wink reflex for neurologic defects.
   - Observe for urine leakage with Valsalva.
   - Cotton-tipped applicator test: checks for bladder neck hypermobility—positive if $>30°$ rotation is present.
3. **Diagnostic Studies**
   - UA with culture and sensitivity to rule out UTI.
   - Cystoscopy and urodynamic testing to evaluate function and rule out abnormal pathology.
4. **Complications**
   - Social and psychological effects.
   - Side effects of various treatment modalities.
   - Chafing.
5. **Management**
   - Establish bladder capacity through voiding diary. Prevent bladder filling to this capacity through fluid restriction, avoiding/decreasing alcohol, and caffeine consumption.
   - Strengthen pelvic floor muscles: Kegel exercises or electrical stimulation.
   - Biofeedback.
   - Prescription: α-adrenergic agonists (oxybutynin and ephedrine), local estrogen replacement therapy, pessary use if cystocele or urethrocele is present.
   - Collagen injection.
   - Surgery to restore bladder neck position.

D. Osteoporosis

- Addressed in Chapter 9.

VII. Menstrual Disorders

A. Disorders of Menstruation

1. **Definition**
   - Normal menstrual cycle: 24 to 38 days, lasting 4.5 to 8 days; average blood loss of 30 mL (range: spotting to 80 mL).
   - Amenorrhea: absence of menstrual periods.
   - Cryptomenorrhea (hypomenorrhea): unusually light flow, may be only spotting.
   - Menopause: cessation of menses for 6 months, not due to pregnancy.
   - Menorrhagia: normal intervals of heavy or prolonged flow.
   - Metrorrhagia: bleeding between menstrual cycles.
   - Menometrorrhagia: irregular intervals, varying amounts and duration of flow.
   - Oligomenorrhea: interval >36 days.
   - Polymenorrhea: interval <21 days.
2. **General Approach**
   - History including family history, a menstrual and reproductive history, and a general medical history including medications used, and nutritional, exercise, and emotional assessments.

- Physical examination looking for abnormal genital anatomy (including imperforate hymen, enlarged fibroid uterus), signs of androgen excess, estrogen deficiency, or an endocrinopathy.

3. **Diagnostic Studies**
- Blood: β-hCG; CBC with differential (thrombocytopenia, anemia); thyroid studies.
- Pap smear: screen for cervical cancer.
- Wet mount: cervical or vaginal infection, for example, *Trichomonas*.
- Endometrial biopsy: rule out endometrial hyperplasia.
- Pelvic U/S: confirm fibroids, detect polyps, masses.
- Hysteroscopy: allows for direct visualization of the uterine cavity with removal or biopsy of lesions.

4. **Management**
- Treat according to cause.

B. Amenorrhea

1. **Definition**
- Primary: no menarche by age 13 (girls without development of secondary sexual characteristics) or by age 15 (those with secondary sexual characteristics).
- Secondary: cessation of menses after the onset of menarche, lasting 3 or more months. This may, however, be transient, intermittent, or permanent depending on causal factors.

2. **Pathology**
- Amenorrhea is a symptom not a disease. Most common cause is pregnancy.
- Primary amenorrhea: causes include developmental anomalies or absence of reproductive organs, ovarian failure, hypogonadotropic hypogonadism, androgen insensitivity, and chronic anovulation.
- Secondary amenorrhea: causes include functional hypothalamic GnRH deficiency, CNS, pituitary gland, thyroid gland, adrenal gland, ovarian, or uterine dysfunction; prolonged, continuous, strenuous exercise, PCOS, pregnancy.

3. **Diagnostic Studies**
- Document abnormal growth and development, secondary sex characteristics, evidence of endocrine disorders, normal reproductive tract.
- Genetic karyotyping may be indicated in primary amenorrhea.
- Depends on history and physical exam findings: β-hCG, TSH, serum prolactin, testosterone, DHEA-S, FSH, LH, and estradiol level.

4. **Complications**
- Abnormal development, infertility, endometrial hyperplasia, and osteoporosis.

5. **Management**
- Depends on etiology and patient's wishes regarding fertility.
- Underlying medical problems should be corrected, often menses then resumes.

C. Menopause

1. **Definition**
- Permanent cessation of menses due to loss of ovarian function.
- Premature menopause: ovarian failure before age 40.

2. **Etiology/Pathology**
- Average age of onset in the United States, 51.3 years (range 45–55).
- May occur naturally, surgically, or secondary to medical therapy (chemotherapy, radiation).
- Occurs sooner in smokers than in nonsmokers, type 1 diabetics, women who live at high altitudes, vegetarians, and women who are undernourished.
- Climacteric (perimenopausal period) is a result of oocyte depletion.
- FSH raises and estrogen levels decline, causing characteristic signs and symptoms.

3. **Clinical Features**
- Menstrual cycle irregularities until menstruation has ceased for 1 year.
- Hot flushes and night sweats.
- Mood swings, trouble sleeping.
- Atrophic changes of vulva and vagina, causing vaginal dryness, which leads to dyspareunia.
- Pelvic relaxation and bladder problems.
- Hair and skin thinning, with growth of facial and body hair.

4. **Diagnostic Studies**
- Clinical diagnosis with 12 months of amenorrhea in the absence of other biologic or physiologic causes.
- Serum FSH and LH levels are elevated and plasma estradiol.

5. **Complications**
- Osteoporosis and fractures.
- Increased risk of cardiovascular disease.
- Psychosexual changes.
- Increased risk of endometrial cancer.

6. **Management**
- Vaginal atrophy: transdermal, intravaginal estrogen.
- Hot flushes: estrogens, progestins, clonidine, selective serotonin reuptake inhibitors (SSRIs), gabapentin.
- Osteoporosis prevention/treatment: calcium, vitamin D, regular exercise, bisphosphonates, calcitonin, estrogens (with or without progestins), selective estrogen receptor modulators (raloxifene).
- Mood lability/depression: antidepressant SSRI.
- Risk/benefit of HRT must be carefully considered.

D. Postmenopausal Bleeding

1. **Definition**
- Vaginal/uterine bleeding after menopause.

2. **Etiology/Pathology**
- Uterine causes: fibroids, endometrial problems (hyperplasia, polyp, and carcinoma).

- Cervical causes: cancer, polyp, and erosion.
- Also atrophic vaginitis and HRT.
- *Any* report of vaginal bleeding from a postmenopausal woman not on HRT, or from a woman on HRT with abnormal bleeding, is suspicious for cancer.

3. **Clinical Features**
   - Examine for friability of vaginal mucosa and cervix, evidence of cervical polyp, uterine or ovarian masses.
4. **Diagnostic Studies**
   - Pelvic examination.
   - Pap smear.
   - Pelvic U/S.
   - Endometrial biopsy.
   - Hysteroscopy with D&C (often diagnostic and therapeutic).
5. **Complications**
   - Anemia.
   - Surgery often necessary.
6. **Management**
   - Depends on etiology.

E. **Dysmenorrhea**
1. **Etiology/Pathology**
   a. **Primary dysmenorrhea**
      - Painful menstruation associated with uterine contractions mediated by elevated levels of prostaglandins.
      - No associated pelvic pathology.
      - Pain usually begins 1 to 2 years after the onset of menarche; may become more severe with time.
   b. **Secondary dysmenorrhea**
      - Pain caused by pelvic pathology (e.g., endometriosis, fibroids, PID, IUD).
      - Onset generally after the age of 25.
2. **Clinical Features**
   - Pelvic pain with the onset of menses that may radiate to the back of the legs, low back.
   - May be accompanied by nausea, vomiting, diarrhea, and headache.
   - Usually lasts 1 to 3 days.
   - Exam normal or may have uterine tenderness in the primary dysmenorrhea. In the secondary dysmenorrhea, may have findings related to the cause.
3. **Diagnostic Studies**
   - β-hCG to rule out pregnancy.
   - Secondary dysmenorrhea: depends on suspected cause (e.g., laparoscopy, MRI).
4. **Complications**
   - May be so severe, woman is unable to function adequately at home or work.
5. **Management**
   - Symptomatic treatment: heat, rest, vitamin E.
   - Antiprostaglandin (NSAID): works best when started before the onset of severe symptoms.

- Oral contraceptives/Depo-Provera/contraceptive vaginal ring: suppress ovulation and significantly reduce symptoms.
- If above treatment fails: laparoscopy to rule out causes of secondary dysmenorrhea.

F. **Premenstrual Syndrome**
1. **Etiology/Pathology**
   - Multifactorial, poorly understood; disease versus constellation of symptoms.
   - Occurs during reproductive years.
   - True etiology unknown: may include serotonin dysfunction or be related to ovarian function.
   - Premenstrual dysphoric disorder (PMDD): more severe form of premenstrual syndrome (PMS).
2. **Clinical Features**
   - Symptoms include a feeling of weight gain, mood swings, anxiety, lower extremity edema, abdominal bloating, breast pain, depression, food cravings, headache, inability to concentrate, irritability, lethargy, libido change, skin disorders, and hot flashes.
   - Symptoms occur during the luteal phase (7–14 days before the onset of menses) are relieved within 2 to 3 days of the onset of menses, and there are at least 7 symptom-free days in the follicular phase of the cycle.
   - Symptoms must be documented in at least three consecutive cycles.
   - Psychiatric history important.
   - Essentially normal physical examination.
3. **Diagnostic Studies**
   - Full menstrual cycle history.
   - Rule out thyroid disorder and anemia.
4. **Complications**
   - Underlying psychiatric illness may be present.
5. **Management**
   - Treat patient's symptoms, for example:
     - Breast pain: bromocriptine, danazol.
     - Bloating: spironolactone, calcium carbonate.
     - Mood disorders, especially for PMDD: SSRIs either daily or on symptomatic days; monophasic OCP (20 μg ethinyl estradiol and 3 mg drospirenone).
     - Water retention: spironolactone.
   - Aerobic exercise, decrease or eliminate caffeine and alcohol, low salt complex carbohydrates diet, and calcium supplementation.
   - Psychiatric referral may be necessary for underlying psychiatric disease.

VIII. Infertility
A. **Definition**
   - One year of unprotected intercourse without resulting pregnancy in women aged <35 years.
   - Six months of unprotected intercourse without resulting pregnancy in women >35 years.

B. Etiology/Pathology
- Male partner contributes to approximately 40% of cases of infertility; a combination of factors is common.
- Female: ovulatory disorders 25%, endometriosis 15%, and pelvic adhesions 12%. Also anovulatory cycles; congenital or acquired problems in fallopian tubes, cervix, or uterus.
- Sixty percent of couples will achieve a pregnancy within 3 years, in the absence of identifiable causes of infertility.

C. Clinical Features
- May have a history of menstrual irregularity, hirsutism, galactorrhea, dyspareunia, pelvic pain, IUD use, PID, and diethylstilbestrol (DES) exposure.
- Sexual history is important: frequency of penis in vaginal intercourse, ejaculation, use of lubricants, and prior contraceptive use.
- Speculum and bimanual examination, breast examination (galactorrhea), and skin examination (hirsutism).

D. Diagnostic Studies
- Postcoital microscopy on ovulatory day looking at number of motile sperm in the cervical mucus and their survival rate.
- Verification of ovulation:
  - Measure the serum progesterone level at the midpoint of the secretory phase (21st day) to evaluate for adequate luteal function.
  - Basal body temperature elevation during the luteal phase.
  - Endometrial biopsy.
  - Change in cervical mucus.
- Hysterosalpingogram for tubal patency and uterine cavity structure.
- Laparoscopy with instillation of dye: diagnostic for tubal dysfunction; able to identify and treat endometriosis, other pelvic pathology, PID; and lysis of adhesions.

E. Complications
- Risks associated with surgical procedures.
- Emotional and physical stress.

F. Management
- Best handled by an infertility specialist.
- Treatment based on etiology:
  - Nonpatent tubes: repair surgically.
  - **Anovulation or oligoovulation (treatment depends on cause)**
    - Rule out underlying endocrine disorders. Women start ovulating after endocrine problems have been corrected.
    - Polycystic ovary: induce ovulation with clomiphene citrate.
    - Exercise-induced anovulation: reduce exercise level and weight gain; hCG therapy.
    - Hyperprolactinemia: bromocriptine therapy.
- Antisperm antibodies: condom usage for 6 months.

IX. Contraceptive Counseling (Table 14B–2)
- Women should be advised of their contraceptive options and choose the method appropriate for themselves based on personal preference, health risks, and cost. Predicted pregnancy rate of 85% in a year without use of contraception.

A. Natural Family Planning (Fertility Awareness Methods)
- Requires a regular menstrual cycle and specific determination of ovulation, using basal body temperature charting, cervical mucus evaluation, and/or urine tests and patient motivation.
- Can be used with a barrier method during most fertile phase of cycle, increasing effectiveness.
- Abstaining from intercourse during fertile days, leaves few days of the month for intercourse.
- Failure rate dependent on the method used and the patient.
- No protection from STIs.

B. Coitus Interruptus
- Male withdraws penis from vagina before ejaculation.
- Failure rate due to sperm in the pre-ejaculatory fluid, premature ejaculation, and/or the deposition of semen on the vulva.
- No protection from STIs.

C. Spermicide: Nonoxynol-9
- Mechanical barrier and toxic to sperm.
- Comes in vaginal jelly, cream, gel, suppository, film, and foam.
- Available without a prescription.
- Most effective when used with other forms of birth control.
- Nonoxynol-9 can cause microabrasions to the vaginal mucosa, therefore increasing the risk of HIV transmission; sex workers and women with multiple partners should be discouraged from using methods that contain nonoxynol-9.

D. Barrier Methods
- Physical barrier between ejaculate and vagina.
  1. **Condoms**
     - Male (latex, polyurethane, lambskin) and female (polyurethane), both of which offer protection from STIs.
     - Available without a prescription.
     - Highly effective in preventing pregnancy, especially when used in combination with a spermicidal jelly, foam, or insert.
     - May decrease sensitivity for partners.
     - Female condom is awkward to use for some women; external ring may cause irritation.
     - Female condom: only female-controlled birth control with STI and pregnancy protection.

TABLE 14B–2.   Comparisons of Birth Control Methods (Predicted Pregnancy Rate of 85% in a Year without Use of Contraception)

	Description	OTC/RX	Typical Failure Rate during First Year of Use	STI Protection	Others
	Barrier methods: physical barrier between ejaculate and vagina				
Condoms: male	Latex, polyurethane, lambskin sheath	OTC	18%	Yes	Some contain nonoxynol-9 More effective if used with spermicide
Condoms: female	Polyurethane sheath with two rings to stabilize it in the vagina	OTC	21%	Yes	Only female-controlled birth control with STI and pregnancy protection More effective if used with spermicide
Diaphragm	Rubber cup-like device that holds spermicide against the cervix	RX	12%	±	
FemCap	Smaller rubber cup-like device that fits over the cervix, holding spermicide	RX	14%	±	
Contraceptive sponge	Onetime use sponge with nonoxynol-9	OTC	Nulliparous: 12% Parous: 24%	±	
	Hormonal methods				
Combination oral contraceptive pills	Contain estrogen and progestin—type varies	RX	9%	No	Contraindications for use Many noncontraceptive benefits Not for smokers >35
Progestin-only pills "Mini-pill"	Oral contraceptive pill without estrogen	RX	9%	No	May be used by women who cannot use estrogens, including lactating women Menstrual irregularities Must take at consistent time
Plan B	Two tablets of 0.75mglevonorgestrel ingested 12 h apart, or both tablets at once; initiated within 5 d of unprotected intercourse	OTC ≥ 18 RX < 18	1% when taken within 72 h	No	
Implanon	Single rod implant, releases 68 pg of etonogestrel daily	RX	0.05%	No	Office visit for insertion Lasts for 3 y
Depo-Provera	Depo medroxyprogesterone acetate intramuscular	RX	6%	No	Office visit every 3 mo for injection
Ortho Evra	Transdermal patch that delivers 150 pg norelgestromin and 20 pg ethinyl estradiol daily	RX	9%	No	Applied once a week for 3 consecutive weeks followed by 1 wk off May be less effective in women ≥198 lb

(continued)

TABLE 14B–2.   **Comparisons of Birth Control Methods (Predicted Pregnancy Rate of 85% in a Year without Use of Contraception) (continued)**

	Description	OTC/RX	Typical Failure Rate during First Year of Use	STI Protection	Others
NuvaRing	Flexible plastic ring that releases 120 pg of the etonogestrel and 15 pg of ethinyl estradiol	RX	9%	No	Inserted intravaginally for a 3-wk period, then removed for 1 wk, during which withdrawal bleeding is expected
Natural family planning Cervical mucus Symptothermal Calendar (rhythm) Standard days	Avoid intercourse or use contraception during fertile times	N/A	Up to 24%	No	Classes available
Coitus interruptus	Withdrawal of penis from vagina before ejaculation	N/A	22%	No	
Spermicide nonoxynol-9	Mechanical barrier and toxic to sperm	OTC	28%	Slight, not HIV	Vaginal jelly, cream, gel, suppository, film, foam
Intrauterine device Mirena (levo-norgestrel) ParaGard (Copper T 380A)	Intravaginal device	RX	Mirena 0.2% ParaGard 0.8	No	Mirena: 5 y ParaGard: 10 y History of pelvic inflammatory disease—absolute contraindication
Sterilization	Permanent blocking of the fallopian tubes by either mechanical or chemical means		0.5%	No	Surgical procedure Considered permanent; reversal difficult

STI, sexually transmitted disease; OTC, over the counter; RX, prescription.

- Latex allergy may deter use of male condoms; lambskin condoms do not prevent STIs.
2. **Diaphragm**
   - Requires pelvic examination and fitting by a trained health care professional.
   - Should be used with spermicidal jelly in the cup for maximum effectiveness.
   - Can be inserted several hours before intercourse, and must remain in place for 6 to 24 hours after intercourse.
   - Small risk of TSS if left in place too long.
   - Additional spermicidal jelly must be inserted into vagina with an applicator between each act of intercourse.
   - Device requires a prescription.
   - Can be messy and difficult to insert and remove.
   - Effective when used properly.

3. **FemCap**
   - Silicone rubber cap with brim and strap for removal; acts as a barrier by completely covering the cervix.
   - Used with spermicidal jelly.
   - Can be inserted several hours prior to intercourse and must remain in place for at least 8 hours; however, can remain in place for up to 48 hours.
   - Risk of toxic shock if left in place too long.
   - No additional jelly needed between acts of intercourse.
   - Requires a prescription, but no fitting required; size is determined by obstetrical history.
   - Can be messy and difficult to insert and remove.
   - Effective when used properly.
4. **Contraceptive Sponge**
   - Polyurethane sponge containing nonoxynol-9 for single use only.

- Moistened with tap water prior to insertion.
  - May be inserted a few hours prior to intercourse but must be left in place for at least 6 hours after the last act of intercourse; should not be left in place for more than 24 hours.
  - Risk of toxic shock if left in place too long.
  - No prescription needed.
  - Check for current availability; method available as of fall 2011.

E. Hormonal Methods

- Prevent pregnancy by inhibiting ovulation, thickening cervical mucus, and altering the quality of the endometrium.
- Women who smoke have a higher risk of death from cardiovascular disease and should stop combined hormonal methods at age 35 if they continue to smoke.
- Use cautiously in women with diabetes, HTN, hyperlipidemia, and history of biliary tract disease.

1. **Oral Contraceptives**
   a. **Combination (Containing an Estrogen and a Progestin)**
      - Requires an office visit and prescription.
      - Woman must remember to take a pill every day, consistently.
      - Many side effects and contraindications; however, when used correctly, are more than 99% effective against preventing pregnancy.
      - Most side effects are tolerable.
      - Offers no protection against STIs.
      - Noncontraceptive benefits include improving dysmenorrhea, controlling menstrual cycle and flow, protection against ovarian cysts, ovarian and endometrial cancer; improvement of acne; and positive effect on bone mass.
      - Women who smoke have a higher risk of death from cardiovascular disease and should stop the pill at age 35 if they continue to smoke.
      - Use cautiously in women with diabetes, HTN, hyperlipidemia, and history of biliary tract disease.
   b. **Combination Oral Contraceptives Containing Progestin Drospirenone**
      - Diuretic effect may be beneficial for women who experience water retention and bloating during menses.
      - Only combined oral contraceptive approved by the FDA for treatment of PMDD.
      - Should not be used by women with kidney, liver, or adrenal disease.
      - May increase potassium levels.
   c. **Progestin-Only Pills (No Estrogen)**
      - Requires office visit and prescription.
      - Fewer contraindications.
      - May be used by breastfeeding women.

- Slightly less effective in preventing pregnancy than combination pills.
- No protection from STIs.
- Menstrual irregularity from amenorrhea to menometrorrhagia.
- Woman must remember to take a pill every day, consistently.

   d. **Emergency Contraception: Multiple Formulas, Plan B Is Most Commonly Used**
      - Consists of two tablets of 0.75 mg levonorgestrel ingested 12 hours apart, initiated within 72 hours of unprotected intercourse.
      - Evidence-based medicine: taking both 0.75 mg tablets at once has shown to have greater efficacy at preventing pregnancy.
      - In addition, studies have shown that Plan B may be effective for up to 5 days following unprotected intercourse.
      - Over-the-counter for women over 18, by prescription for 17 and under.
      - Patients are advised to seek medical attention if menses have not begun within 21 days after treatment.
      - ParaGard (Copper IUD or IUC) can also be used as emergency contraception if inserted within 5 days of unprotected intercourse.

2. **Implantable/Injectable/Long-Acting Progestins**
   a. **Implanon**
      - Single-rod implant, releases 68 μg of etonogestrel daily.
      - Prevents ovulation in most women for 3 years.
      - Similar side effects as with other progesterone-only methods.
      - Menstrual irregularity from amenorrhea to menometrorrhagia.
      - Requires prescription and office visit for placement.
      - No protection from STIs.
      - Highly effective.
   b. **Norplant Implants**
      - Wyeth Pharmaceuticals voluntarily removed Norplant from the U.S. market on July 26, 2002, due to limitations in product component supplies. Wyeth does not plan to reintroduce it.
      - Patients need to switch to other forms of birth control after the removal at the 5-year expiration date.
   c. **Depo-Provera (Depo Medroxyprogesterone Acetate)**
      - Injectable progesterone; prevents pregnancy for 3 months at a time.
      - Similar menstrual disturbances as with other progesterone-only methods.
      - Requires prescription.

- No protection from STIs.
- Highly effective.
- Weight gain and irregular bleeding are common complaints.

3. Other Hormonal Options

a. Ortho Evra

- Transdermal patch that delivers 150 mg norelgestromin and 20 mg ethinyl estradiol daily into the circulation.
- Applied once a week for 3 consecutive weeks followed by 1 week off.
- Efficacy similar to that of oral contraceptives, but compliance may be better.
- May be less effective in women ≥198 lb.
- Requires prescription and office visit.
- No protection from STIs.

b. NuvaRing

- Flexible plastic ring that releases 120 μg of the etonogestrel and 15 μg of ethinyl estradiol daily into the circulation.
- Inserted intravaginally for a 3-week period, then removed for 1 week, during which withdrawal bleeding is expected.
- Efficacy is comparable with that of combination oral contraceptives.
- Requires prescription and office visit.
- May be removed for intercourse but must be replaced within 3 hours to maintain continued efficacy.
- No protection from STIs.

F. Intrauterine Device

- Exact mechanism of action is not currently known; may inhibit sperm transport or disrupt the uterine lining.
- Progesterone IUC has additional mechanism of cervical mucus thickening.
- Device placement (and removal) in the uterus must be done by a trained health care professional.
- Two types available:
  - Mirena (releases levonorgestrel): 5 years.
    - Similar menstrual disturbances as with other progesterone-only methods.
  - ParaGard (Copper T 380A): 12 years.
    - May cause menorrhagia in some women.
- No protection against STIs.
- Highly effective.

G. Continuous Cycling

- All combined contraceptive methods may be prescribed for continuous use by skipping the placebo or off week.
- Good option for women with menstrual migraines, dysmenorrhea, menorrhagia, endometriosis, recurrent ovarian cysts, anemia, or PMS.
- Will require additional prescriptions to cover year's supply, which may not be covered under insurance or funding.

H. Irreversible Methods: Voluntary Female Sterilization

- Women should choose this method only if they are absolutely sure that they are finished with childbearing.

1. Tubal Ligation

- A permanent mechanical blocking of the fallopian tubes achieved through a surgical procedure in which the lumen of the tube is interrupted.
- Requires surgery.

2. Transcervical Approach: Essure

- Chemical or coils are used to scar the proximal portion of the tubes or cornua.
- Can be done in office or clinic and requires local anesthesia only.

3. For All Forms of Sterilization

- Reversal is difficult and rarely successful.
- If failure occurs, it is often an ectopic pregnancy.
- No protection from STIs.
- No alteration of menstrual pattern.
- Highly effective.
- No long-term side effects.

X. General Guidelines for Women's Health Maintenance

A. Health Maintenance

- Women should have gynecologic examinations annually from age 18, or when sexually active. Risk factors such as smoking, alcohol intake, drug use, sexual promiscuity, obesity, sedentary lifestyle, and abuse should be discussed.

- **Cervical cancer screening**
  - Pap smear screening should be initiated at the age of 21.
  - Screening is recommended every 2 years between the ages of 21 and 29 as long as cytology results are negative.
  - Screening may be decreased to every 2 to 3 years in women aged 30 and older who have had three or more negative cytology results in a row and no history of cervical intraepithelial neoplasia (CIN 2) or CIN 3.
  - For women over the age of 30, screening should be done no more than every 3 years if combined with HPV DNA testing.
  - Screening may be discontinued in women between the ages of 65 and 70 years who have had three or more negative cytology test results in a row and no history of abnormal results in the past 10 years.
  - Women who have a history of DES exposure in utero require annual Pap smears.
  - HIV-positive women should have annual screening, regardless of the cytology results.
  - Discontinue routine screening in any woman who has had a total hysterectomy for benign reasons and negative history for high-grade CIN.

- **Breast cancer screening: breast self-examination**
  - Value of breast self-examination (BSE) debated; for women who choose to do BSE, review proper technique; must be done monthly by woman age ≥20, immediately after menstruation or on days 5 to 7 of cycle.
  - Clinical breast examination should be performed at least every 3 years in women between the ages of 20 and 39, then annually after the age of 40.
  - Mammogram guidelines currently are conflicting.
    - USPSTF recommends baseline mammogram at age 50, then every other year until the age of 74. Mammogram screening should be performed every other year beginning at age 40 only in women with risk factors.
    - American Cancer Society (ACS) continues to recommend baseline screening beginning at age 40 and continuing annually.
  - The decision to continue with screening mammograms after the age of 65 should be based on the patient's comorbidities, expected life span, and patient's preference. It is generally not recommended to continue routine screening after the age of 65 to 75.
  - If there is a family history of breast cancer in a first-degree relative, baseline mammogram should be done 10 years before the age at which the family member was diagnosed.
- **Colon cancer screening: done starting at age 50**
  - Annual fecal occult blood test.
  - Sigmoidoscopy every 5 years or colonoscopy every 10 years.
  - Cholesterol screening: every 5 years.

B. Wellness Promotion

- Smoking cessation; smoking specifically increases the risk of developing cervical cancer.
- Cease substance use/abuse.
- Regular exercise.
- Proper nutrition/weight management.
- Stress reduction/management.
- Immunization updates.

XI. Management of Pap Smear Results

- See also Chapter 17.

A. Normal Pap Smear Result

- Repeat in 2 years for women between the ages of 21 and 29; repeat every 2 to 3 years in women over the age of 30, but no more than every 3 years if HPV DNA testing is also done.
- Women with HIV, and those with a history of DES exposure in utero, should be screened annually.

B. Abnormal Pap Smear Result

1. **Infection**
   - Treat the specified infection.
   - If normal cytology, follow-up in 2 to 3 years.

2. **Reactive and Reparative Changes**
   - Rule out infection.
   - If cytology is negative, follow up in 2 to 3 years.
3. **Squamous Cell Abnormalities**
   - Atypical squamous cells of undetermined significance.
     - If HPV negative, repeat in 1 year.
     - If HPV positive, colposcopy needed.
     - Low-grade squamous intraepithelial lesion (SIL): colposcopy, biopsy, and treatment. Repeat Pap smear at 6 and 12 months, or have HPV testing in 1 year.
     - High-grade SIL: colposcopy, biopsy, and treat. Close follow-up for 2 years.
     - Squamous cell cancer: refer to gynecologist for colposcopy and treatment.

REVIEW QUESTIONS

1. Which of the following is recommend management for a first episode of genital HSV?
   a) Valacyclovir 1.0 g orally twice a day
   b) Acyclovir 800 mg orally twice a day for 5 days
   c) Famciclovir 1.0 g orally twice a day for 1 day.
   d) Acyclovir 400 mg orally three times a day × 7 to 10 days or 200 mg PO orally five times a day × 7 to 10 days

2. Which of the following is the most common cause of amenorrhea in a 30-year-old woman?
   a) Hypogonadotropic
   b) Uterine dysfunction
   c) Pregnancy
   d) Ovarian failure

ANSWERS TO REVIEW QUESTIONS

1. **Answer: D.** Genital HSV infections management is as follows:

   First episode:
   - Acyclovir 400 mg orally three times a day × 7 to 10 days or 200 mg PO orally five times a day × 7 to 10 days
   - Famciclovir 250 mg orally three times a day for 7 to 10 days
   - Valacyclovir 1 g orally twice a day for 7 to 10 days

   Suppression therapy for ≥6 recurrences per year:
   - Acyclovir 400 mg orally twice a day
   - Valacyclovir 1.0 g orally twice a day

   Episodic therapy for recurrent herpes:
   - Acyclovir 400 mg orally three times a day for 5 days
   - Acyclovir 800 mg orally twice a day for 5 days
   - Acyclovir 800 mg orally three times a day for 2 days
   - Famciclovir 125 mg orally twice a day for 5 days

- Famciclovir 1,000 mg 1.0 g orally twice a day for 1 day
- Valacyclovir 500 mg orally twice a day for 3 days
- Valacyclovir 1.0 g PO orally once a day for 5 days

(Genital HSV, clinical intervention)

2. **Answer: C**. Amenorrhea is a symptom, not a disease. The most common cause is pregnancy. Primary amenorrhea: causes include developmental anomalies or absence of reproductive organs, ovarian failure, hypogonadotropic hypogonadism, androgen insensitivity, chronic anovulation. Secondary amenorrhea: causes include functional hypothalamic GnRH deficiency, CNS, pituitary gland, thyroid gland, adrenal gland, ovarian, or uterine dysfunction; prolonged, continuous, strenuous exercise, PCOS, pregnancy. (Amenorrhea, clinical features)

SELECTED REFERENCES

Center for Disease Control and Prevention. Sexually transmitted diseases treatment guidelines, 2010. *MMWR Recomm Rep.* 2010;59(RR-12):1–110.

DeCherney AH, Nathan L, Goodwing TM, eds. *Current Obstetric and Gynecologic Diagnosis and Treatment*. 10th ed. New York, NY: McGraw-Hill; 2006.

Gibbs R, Karlan B, Haney A, et al. *Danforth's Obstetrics and Gynecology*. 10th ed. Philadelphia, PA: Lippincott Williams & Wilkins; 2008.

Hatcher RA, Trussell J, Nelson AL, et al, eds. *Contraceptive Technology*. 20th revised ed. New York, NY: Ardent Media; 2011.

McPhee SJ, Papadakis MA, Rabow MW, eds. *Current Medical Diagnosis and Treatment*. New York, NY: McGraw-Hill; 2012.

Zieman M, Hatcher R, Cwiak C, et al. *Managing Contraception for Your Pocket*. 2010–2012 Edition. Atlanta, GA: Bridging the Gap Foundation; 2010.

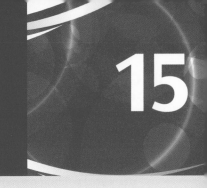

Complicated Pregnancies

Catherine Nowak • Juanita Gardner • Nina Multak

I. Rh Alloimmunization

A. Definition
- Maternal antibodies develop against fetal red blood cells (RBCs) following fetomaternal hemorrhage when fetal blood components enter maternal circulation. Untreated alloimmunization can result in hemolytic disease of the newborn (hydrops fetalis).

B. Etiology
- Rhesus factor (Rh) alloimmunization (also isoimmunization or erythroblastosis fetalis) is caused by incompatibility between fetal and maternal blood, such as the mother being Rh-negative and fetus being Rh-positive (mother Rh-negative, father Rh-positive). Rh alloimmunization typically refers to formation of antibodies to the Rh D antigen.

C. Pathology
- Rh antigens are lipoproteins located on the red cell membrane. Patients who lack a specific red cell antigen produce an antibody if exposed to the antigen.
- Rh sensitization occurs when an immune response occurs following exposure of an Rh-negative woman to Rh D antigen.
- This antibody may be harmful following an incompatible blood transfusion or a hemorrhage between a mother and an Rh-incompatible fetus. Invasive procedures during pregnancy, such as amniocentesis and chorionic villus sampling, can precipitate fetal–maternal hemorrhage.
- Rh-negative women who delivered or will deliver an Rh-positive fetus will become immunized and must be treated to prevent subsequent erythroblastosis.
- Infection, hemorrhage at delivery, threatened abortion, placenta previa, abruption, and C-section can transfer fetal blood to mother.
- Maternal antibody is transferred to fetus. The fetus' red cells get damaged. Hemolysis responds with erythropoiesis and further hemolysis.

D. Clinical Features
- Hemolytic disease in the newborn.
  - Hemolysis, bilirubin release, anemia.
- Fetal hepatosplenomegaly.
- Fetal icterus (kernicterus).
- Fetal heart failure.
- Fetal hydrops: fluid accumulation in at least two of the following extravascular areas.

- Pericardial effusion, pleural effusion, ascites, subcutaneous edema.
- Fetal death.

E. Diagnostic Studies
- **Pregnant woman**
  - ABO blood group.
  - Rh-D type.
  - Indirect erythrocyte antibody screen (titers of 1:8–1:32 are associated with fetal hemolysis).
  - Kleihauer–Betke test used to detect the presence of fetal RBCs in maternal circulation.
  - Indirect Coombs test to determine sufficient antibody.
- **Fetus: monitor for fetal anemia in second trimester**
  - Amniotic fluid assessment: increasing bilirubin levels positive sign.
  - Ultrasound (U/S) of middle cerebral artery for peak velocity: increase in flow secondary to decrease in viscosity of blood in fetal anemia.
  - Percutaneous umbilical blood sampling (PUBS) for direct measurement of fetal hematocrit.
  - Paternal blood type and Rh status is helpful.

F. Management
- **Prevention: mother**
  - Rh screening should be completed at the first prenatal visit.
  - Three hundred microgram Rh immune globulin (RhIG, RhoGAM) intramuscularly (IM) for Rh-negative mother and Rh-positive or Rh-unknown father; additional dosing may be required to ensure adequate immunoglobulin coverage.
    - Administered at 28 weeks' gestation.
    - With procedures or conditions with possibility of fetal-to-maternal bleeding.
    - With ectopic pregnancy.
    - After spontaneous, threatened, or induced abortions or vaginal bleeding.
    - Within 72 hours of delivery of Rh-D–positive infant.
- **Prevention: baby**
  - After delivery, the mother and baby are both screened.
  - Moderate–severe anemia requires transfusion of antigen-negative RBCs through U/S-guided transfusion into umbilical vein.

II. Genitourinary Infections

A. Definition
- Infection of the genitourinary tract caused by various organisms.

B. Etiology
- Bladder and ureters under pressure from uterus, with decreased voiding patterns and smooth muscle relaxation from elevated progesterone levels, may contribute to increased risk for genitourinary infections.

C. Lower Urinary Tract Infections and Asymptomatic Bacteriuria
1. **Pathology**
   - *Escherichia coli.*
2. **Clinical Features**
   - Asymptomatic.
   - Dysuria, frequency, urgency.
3. **Diagnostic Studies**
   - Urine analysis (U/A) and culture and sensitivity at onset of prenatal care or symptomatology.
4. **Management**
   - Seven to 10 days of treatment with cephalosporin, nitrofurantoin, or sulfonamide.
   - Repeat cultures following treatment.

D. Upper Urinary Tract Infections (Pyelonephritis)
1. **Pathology**
   - *E. coli* and gram-negative aerobes; bacterial invasion of renal parenchyma.
2. **Clinical Features**
   - Fever, malaise, dehydration.
   - Costovertebral tenderness or back pain.
   - Premature labor.
   - Maternal sepsis with high morbidity.
3. **Diagnostic Studies**
   - U/A with culture and sensitivity.
   - Computed tomography (CT) scan, magnetic resonance imaging (MRI).
4. **Management**
   - Admit for inpatient treatment.
   - IV hydration, antipyretics.
   - IV antibiotics with cephalosporin or penicillin and aminoglycosides.
   - Tocolytic therapy to halt contractions if preterm labor (PTL) develops.
   - Repeat cultures following treatment.

E. Vaginitis
1. **Pathology**
   - Bacterial vaginosis (previously termed *Gardnerella* vaginitis or *Haemophilus vaginalis* vaginitis).
   - Candidiasis: *Candida albicans.*
   - Trichomoniasis: protozoan parasite *Trichomonas vaginalis.*
2. **Clinical Features**
   - Bacterial vaginosis: abnormal, odorous vaginal discharge.
   - Candidiasis: white, curd-like discharge, vaginal or vulvar pruritus, dysuria.
   - Trichomoniasis: vaginal pruritis and discharge with or without odor, occasionally foamlike discharge with cervical erosion.
3. **Diagnostic Studies**
   - Bacterial vaginosis: wet mount for clue cells.
   - Candidiasis: potassium hydroxide smear for budding yeast.
   - Trichomoniasis: wet mount for *T. vaginalis* and white cells.
4. **Management**
   - Bacterial vaginosis: metronidazole or clindamycin.
   - Candidiasis: course of vaginal azoles.
   - Trichomoniasis: metronidazole.

F. Sexually Transmitted Infection
- Sexually transmitted infection (STI) is a more current term and replaces sexually transmitted disease (STD).
1. **Pathology**
   - *Chlamydia: Chlamydia trachomatis.*
   - Herpes simplex infection: Herpes simplex virus types 1 and 2.
   - *Neisseria gonorrhoeae.*
2. **Clinical Features**
   - *Chlamydia.*
     - Asymptomatic, urethritis, mucopurulent cervicitis.
   - Herpes simplex infection.
     - Tender vesicles.
     - Ulcerated tender vesicles with crusting represent older lesions.
   - *N. gonorrhoeae.*
     - Asymptomatic or nonspecific symptoms.
     - Purulent discharge from urethra, cervix, or vagina; may be greenish or yellow.
3. **Diagnostic Studies**
   - *Chlamydia.*
     - Culture.
     - Direct fluorescent antibody staining, enzyme immunoassay.
     - Nucleic acid hybridization and amplification tests (NAATs).
   - Herpes simplex.
     - Culture of vesicles for the identification of HSV.
     - Polymerase chain reaction (PCR) testing.
     - Serologic testing for HSV-1 and HSV-2 immunoglobulin.
   - *N. gonorrhoeae.*
     - Culture.
     - PCR for at-risk women.
4. **Management**
   - *Chlamydia.*
     - Azithromycin 1 g dose once **or** 7-day course of amoxicillin.
     - Retest 3 months after treatment.
   - Herpes simplex.

- Acyclovir if symptoms are severe or for suppression starting at 36 weeks to reduce viral shedding.
- Cesarean delivery only if active lesions on vulva, in vagina, or on cervix at the time of labor or rupture of membranes.
  - *N. gonorrhoeae.*
    - Ceftriaxone 125 mg IM or ciprofloxacin 500 mg orally in a single dose.
    - All neonates receive routine prophylactic ophthalmic ointment (erythromycin or tetracycline) for the prevention of gonococcal ophthalmia.

G. Group Streptococcus
1. **Pathology**
   - *Streptococcus agalactiae.*
2. **Clinical Features**
   - Asymptomatic in pregnant woman.
   - Manifestations in newborn can include septicemia, pneumonia, or meningitis.
3. **Diagnostic Studies**
   - Rectovaginal culture for group B streptococci (GBS) in all women between 35 and 37 weeks' gestation.
4. **Management**
   - Penicillin, ampicillin, cefazolin, clindamycin, or vancomycin prophylaxis for positive culture, and with PTL, premature rupture of membranes, maternal fever in women with unknown status, ideally within 4 hours of labor.

H. Syphilis
1. **Pathology**
   - *Treponema pallidum.*
2. **Clinical Features**
   - Painless ulcer at site initially.
   - Skin rash in 1 to 3 months.
   - Condyloma lata lesions in women.
   - Newborn symptoms develop up to 14 days after delivery and include maculopapular rash, hepatosplenomegaly, jaundice.
3. **Diagnostic Studies**
   - Serologic screening of all women with Venereal Disease Research Laboratory.
   - Rapid plasma reagin (RPR).
   - Sometimes treponemal-specific tests (FTA-ABS and TP-PA).
4. **Management**
   - Benzathine penicillin G 2.4 million units IM as a single dose.
   - Patient should receive a follow-up RPR test for syphilis 1 month after treatment to document decreasing titer.
   - If patients are sensitive to penicillin, they usually require desensitization.

I. HIV/AIDS
1. **Pathology**
   - Human immunodeficiency virus (HIV) is an RNA virus that belongs to the retrovirus family.

2. **Clinical Features**
   - Wide range of presentations common with HIV/AIDS diagnosis.
   - Candidiasis, bacterial vaginosis, genital herpes, and syphilis may be common in pregnancy.
   - Decline in absolute $CD4^+$ counts.
3. **Diagnostic Studies**
   - Enzyme-linked immunosorbent assay (ELISA).
   - Western blot if positive ELISA.
   - Rapid HIV testing is an alternative for at-risk women of unknown infection status presenting in labor.
   - Monthly viral load and $CD4^+$ counts in HIV-positive pregnant women.
4. **Management**
   - Antiretroviral therapy.
     - Zidovudine (AZT) 100 mg orally five times daily has been shown to reduce viral transmission to the fetus.
   - Vaccinations.
   - Should be followed at a high-risk clinic, internist specializing in treating HIV-positive persons, or a maternal–fetal medicine specialist.
   - Planned cesarean at 38 weeks for women with viral load >1,000 copies per mL.

J. Chorioamnionitis, Inflammation of Fetal Membrane
1. **Pathology**
   - Ascending genital tract infection most commonly caused by *Bacteroides* and *Prevotella* species, *E. coli*, anaerobic streptococci, and GBS.
2. **Clinical Features**
   - Maternal fever.
   - Maternal tachycardia.
   - Uterine or abdominal tenderness.
   - Fetal tachycardia, distress.
3. **Diagnostic Studies**
   - Transabdominal amniocentesis for culture.
4. **Management**
   - Parenteral antibiotic.
     - Ampicillin (2 g every 6 hours) or penicillin (5 million units every 6 hours) plus gentamicin (1.5 mg per kg every 8 hours).
   - C-section for fetal distress and poor biophysical profile (BPP).

III. Genetic/Chromosomal Disorders
A. Definition
- Congenital abnormality in fetus.

B. Etiology
- Chromosomal abnormalities.
- Single gene (Mendelian) disorders.
- Polygenic or multifactorial disorders.
- Teratogenic disorders.

Risk factors
- Advanced maternal age (>35 years).
- Previous pregnancy affected by abnormality.
- History of early pregnancy loss.
- Advanced paternal age (>50 years).
- Ethnicity.

C. Pathology
- Chromosomal and gene replication errors within the cell's DNA.

D. Clinical Features
- It is estimated that 50% of early spontaneous abortions and 5% of stillborns are due to an abnormal chromosomal number.
- Clinical traits or features of newborn will vary depending on specific genetic disorder.
  - Chromosomal: trisomy 21 (Down syndrome).
    - Mental retardation.
    - Cardiac abnormalities.
    - Respiratory infections.
    - Leukemia.
    - Polygenic disorders.
    - Hydrocephaly.
    - Neural tube defects.
    - Cleft lip and palate.
    - Pyloric stenosis.
- In instances where the patient has not begun prenatal care until later in her pregnancy, a pelvic U/S may detect physical deformities such as neck webbing, neural tube disorders, anencephaly, cardiac malformations, growth restrictions, or dwarfism.

E. Diagnostic Studies
- Serum triple screen at 15 to 18 weeks to assess risk for Down syndrome, trisomy 18, and trisomy 13.
  - α-Fetoprotein (AFP).
  - Human chorionic gonadotropin (hCG).
  - Pregnancy-associated plasma protein A.
- U/S for nuchal transparency.
- Amniocentesis for karyotyping (Down syndrome) between 15 and 20 weeks' gestation.
- Chorionic villus sampling for DNA evaluation.
- PUBS or cordocentesis after 20 weeks' gestation for fetal blood analysis and DNA analysis.
- Fetal blood sampling and fetal biopsy for DNA sampling.

F. Management
- Genetic counseling for couples at increased risk for genetic abnormalities.
- Introduction to maternal–fetal medicine specialist.
- Treating pregnancy as high risk.
- Depends on genetic abnormality and severity.
- Option for termination of pregnancy.
- Postpartum support groups in instances of fetal demise or termination.
- Postpartum genetic counseling.
- Folic acid supplementation may prevent occurrence and recurrence of neural tube defects.

IV. Abortions
A. Definition
- Expulsion of all or part of the products of conception (POCs) before the completed 20th week of conception. Incidence is estimated to be 50% of all pregnancies, most occurring during the first 7 weeks.

B. Etiology
- Fetal chromosomal abnormalities (50% of all cases).
- Maternal infections.
- Uterine defects.
- Endocrine abnormalities.
- Malnutrition.
- Immunologic factors.
- Physical trauma.

C. Pathology
- Death of embryo.
- Hemorrhage, inflammation, and necrosis at the site of implantation.
- Detachment of gestational sac with uterine contractions for expulsion of the POCs.

D. Spontaneous Abortion
1. **Definition**
   - Expulsion of all or part of POCs before the completed 20th week of conception; miscarriage. Incidence is estimated to be 50% of all pregnancies.
2. **Clinical Features**
   - Passage of POCs.
   - Maybe associated bleeding, cramping, contractions, and cervical changes.
3. **Management**
   - Emotional support to family.
   - Administer Rh immunoglobulin, if needed.
   - Submit any POC, if present, to pathology.

E. Complete Abortion
1. **Definition**
   - Expulsion of all the POCs before the 20th completed week of gestation.
2. **Clinical Features**
   - Passing of entire conceptus.
   - Pain and bleeding cease after passage of tissue.
   - Cervical os closed.
   - Uterus small and nontender.
3. **Management**
   - Emotional support to family.
   - Administer Rh immunoglobulin, if needed.
   - Submit any POC, if present, to pathology.

F. Incomplete Abortion
1. **Definition**
   - Expulsion of part of POCs before the 20th completed week of gestation. Typically no viable conceptus.

2. **Clinical Features**
   - Passage of part of POC.
   - Retained tissue.
   - Continuous bleeding that can be profuse.
   - Boggy uterus with dilated os.
   - Cramps.
3. **Management**
   - Dilation and evacuation (D&E).
   - Pitocin.
   - Rh immunoglobulin, if needed.
   - Submit any POC to pathology.
   - Emotional support.

G. Inevitable Abortion

1. **Definition**
   - Bleeding or cramping before the 20th completed week with continuous and progressive dilation of the cervix and rupture of membranes; no expulsion of the POCs.
2. **Clinical Features**
   - Moderate effacement of the cervix.
   - Cervical dilation > 3 cm.
   - Rupture of the membranes.
   - Bleeding for >7 days.
   - Persistence of cramps.
3. **Management**
   - D&E for retained tissue.
   - Emotional support to family.
   - Administer Rh immunoglobulin.
   - Submit POC to pathology.

H. Threatened Abortion

1. **Definition**
   - Bloody vaginal discharge before the 20th completed week with or without uterine contraction.
2. **Clinical Features**
   - Vaginal bleeding ranges from spotting to profuse, brown to bright red, precedes uterine contraction or back pain.
   - Blood in vaginal vault.
   - Bleeding from cervical opening.
   - Cervix is closed and uneffaced.
   - No evidence of passage of tissue.
3. **Diagnostic Studies**
   - Serial β-hCG levels.
     - Decreasing β-hCG levels suggest probable loss of pregnancy.
   - Pelvic U/S to determine gestational age and viability.
     - Abnormal gestational sac, small embryo with slow heart rate suggests probable loss of pregnancy.
4. **Management**
   - No treatment modalities are available other than time.
   - Rest at home; instruct patient to call if symptoms persist or increase.
   - Reassure patient that it is not her fault.

- Symptoms remain mild or cease. Follow β-hCG every 3 days until the pattern of increasing levels and uterine growth are proven.

I. Missed Abortion

1. **Definition**
   - Death of fetus before the 20th complete week of gestation; POCs remain in utero.
2. **Clinical Features**
   - Loss of symptoms of pregnancy.
   - Decrease in uterine size.
   - Embryo has succumbed; no passage of tissue.
   - Maybe brownish vaginal discharge.
   - Cervix is firm and closed.
3. **Diagnostic Studies**
   - β-hCG decreased.
   - U/S to evaluate suspected missed abortion.
   - Pregnancy test may be negative.
4. **Management**
   - First trimester: suction curettage.
   - Second trimester: D&E or induction of labor with prostaglandin E_2 (PGE_2) suppositories 20 mg vaginally every 4 hours or misoprostol 200 mg tablets vaginally every 4 hours.
   - Emotional support to family.

J. Septic Abortion

1. **Definition**
   - Retained POCs have become infected, including uterine and adjacent organ infection.
2. **Clinical Features**
   - Severe abdominal pain.
   - Fever/chills.
   - Uterine tenderness.
   - Normal to decreased bowel sounds.
   - Brown to bloody, foul-smelling vaginal discharge.
   - Cervix may be nondilated with motion tenderness.
   - Shock.
   - Hemorrhage.
   - Possible renal failure.
3. **Diagnostic Studies**
   - Complete blood count (CBC), white blood cell (WBC) count, urinalysis, electrolytes, blood urea nitrogen (BUN) and creatine, type and screen, coagulation studies.
   - Anaerobic and aerobic cultures from blood, cervix, POC.
   - Cervical cultures for gonorrhea and *Chlamydia*.
   - Abdominal radiographs to evaluate for free air or foreign bodies, rule out perforation.
   - Chest X-ray.
4. **Management**
   - Admission to hospital.
   - Broad-spectrum antibiotics.
   - Removal of POC, D&E.
   - Hysterectomy may be needed if treatment does not resolve infection.

K. Recurrent Miscarriage

1. Definition
- Three or more consecutive spontaneous pregnancy losses.

2. Clinical Features
- Clinical features reflective of type of spontaneous miscarriage.

3. Diagnostic Studies for Etiologic Evaluation
- Radiographic or direct visualization of uterus for structural defects.
- Endometrial biopsy or luteal-phase serum progesterone levels to investigate possible luteal-phase defect (LPD).
- Evaluation for polycystic ovarian syndrome (PCOS).
- Genetic testing.
- Antiphospholipid autoantibodies for evaluation of antiphospholipid syndrome (APS).

4. Management
- LPD: 25 mg progesterone vaginal suppository twice daily.
- PCOS: metformin.
- APS: anticoagulation therapies.

L. Induced Abortion

1. Definition
- Voluntary termination of pregnancy surgically or pharmaceutically.

2. Clinical Features
- Surgical abortion.
  - Dilation and curettage (D&C) procedure for 5 to 13 weeks' gestation.
  - D&E procedure for >12 weeks' gestation.
- Pharmaceutical (medication) abortion for gestations up to 49 days.
  - Mifepristone 200 to 600 mg PO on Day 1.
  - Misoprostol 400 to 800 μg PO or p.v. on Day 3 if abortion has not occurred after mifepristone.
  - Methotrexate 50 mg per m^2 IM or 25 to 50 mg PO; has not been FDA approved for early medication abortion.

3. Diagnostic Studies
- Screening for cervical gonorrhea and *Chlamydia*.
- U/S for accurate estimation of gestational age.
- Rh(D) typing.

4. Management
- Preprocedure counseling.
- Administration of RhIG if indicated.

V. Ectopic Pregnancy

A. Definition
- Implantation of a fertilized ovum outside the uterine cavity; leading cause of maternal death in the first trimester due to hemorrhagic complications.

B. Etiology
- High risk.
  - History of ectopic pregnancy.
  - Tubal damage secondary to ligation, surgery, pathology, or infection.
  - Intrauterine contraceptive devices.
  - Assisted reproductive technology is associated with 5% increased risk for ectopic pregnancies.
- Moderate risk.
  - Infertility.
  - History of genital infections.
  - Multiple sexual partners.
- Low risk.
  - History of pelvic infections.
  - Cigarette smoking.
  - Previous abdominal or pelvic surgery.

C. Pathology
- Implantation of a fertilized ovum outside the uterine cavity, incidence by location:
  - Fallopian tube, 98.3%.
  - Abdominal, 1.4%.
  - Ovarian and cervical, 0.15% each.

D. Clinical Features
- Classic: pelvic or abdominal pain, bleeding, cervical motion tenderness, adnexal mass in a pregnant woman.
- Others: amenorrhea or irregular periods with abdominal pain.
- **Rupturing or ruptured ectopic pregnancy**
  - Severe abdominal pain, dizziness, nausea, vomiting, weakness, shock.
  - Syncope or dizziness may be present.
  - Adnexal or cervical motion tenderness.
  - Constitutes a true medical emergency.

E. Diagnostic Studies
- Serial serum β-hCG: can indicate ectopic pregnancy if levels rise <66% over 2 days, plateau or decrease.
- Transvaginal U/S: 98.9% sensitivity and 84.4% specificity.
  - Absence of intrauterine POCs.
- Presence of noncystic, extraovarian adnexal mass.
- Uterine evacuation with histologic evaluation when β-hCG and U/S are indeterminate.
- Laparoscopy: infrequently necessary for diagnosis when serial β-hCG, U/S, and uterine sampling is utilized.
  - Allows direct visualization and possible removal of ectopic pregnancy before rupture.
- Exploratory laparotomy: when ruptured ectopic is suspected or proven.

F. Management
- Expectant management for falling β-hCG levels under 1,000 mIU per mL.
  - Spontaneous resolution in 67% of ectopic pregnancies.
- Medical management for unruptured ectopic pregnancies ≤4 cm.
  - Multiple-dose methotrexate.

- Methotrexate 1 mg per kg and leucovorin 0.1 mg per kg alternating day dosing for maximum of 4 doses each.
  - β-hCG monitoring on Day 0 and then odd-numbered days, successful when 15% drop between two successive blood draws.
- Single-dose methotrexate.
  - Methotrexate 50 mg per m^2 single dose.
  - β-hCG monitoring on Days 0, 4, and 7; successful when 15% drop in levels from Day 4 to 7.
- Two-dose methotrexate.
  - Methotrexate 50 mg per m^2 on Days 0 and 4.
  - β-hCG monitoring on Days 0, 4, and 7; successful when 15% drop in levels from Days 4 to 7.
- Surgical management for ruptured ectopic pregnancy or contraindicated methotrexate therapy.
  - Laparoscopic salpingostomy: first choice "Gold standard" for unruptured tubal pregnancies <2.0 cm.
  - Explorative laparotomy and salpingectomy: alternatives.
- Administer Rh immunoglobulin if indicated.

VI. Cervical Insufficiency (Formerly Cervical Incompetence)

A. Definition
- Premature cervical dilation in the second trimester with higher risk of preterm birth.

B. Etiology
- Often no identifiable risk factors present.
- Previous procedures or trauma to cervix.
- Structural defects in uterus or cervical connective tissue.
- Diethylstilbestrol exposure in utero.
- Prior spontaneous or induced abortions.
- Multiple gestation.

C. Clinical Features
- Patient may be asymptomatic.
- Gradual and painless dilatation and effacement of the cervix.
- History of painless cervical dilation with preterm delivery.

D. Diagnostic Studies
- Serial digital examination for shortening and effacement of the cervix.
- U/S may detect cervical funneling or shortened cervix.
- Evaluate for PTL, rupture of membranes, chorioamnionitis, and fetal anomalies in women who have a short cervix.

E. Management
- Patients with a history of recurrent loss of pregnancy due to incompetent cervix should be followed early with frequent, gentle pelvic examinations and U/S.

- Weekly injections of 17α-hydroxyprogesterone caproate have shown effectiveness for nonsurgical therapy.
- Utilization of pessaries has demonstrated success in studies.
- Prophylactic, therapeutic, or emergent cerclage (surgical suture technique of the cervical os) may be necessary.
- Corticosteroids are administered to women at 24 to 34 weeks' gestation to reduce the risks of complication of preterm delivery.

VII. Preterm Labor

A. Definition
- Regular uterine contractions with progressing cervical changes (dilation, effacement) occurring before 37 weeks' gestation.
- Accounts for 75% of all neonatal morbidity and mortality.

B. Etiology
- Prior history of preterm delivery.
- Multiple gestations.
- African American race.
- Preterm, premature rupture of the fetal membranes (PPROM).
- Infections (e.g., chorioamnionitis) caused by prostaglandin endotoxin-producing bacteria (*Streptococcus, Fusobacterium, Gardnerella vaginalis*).
- Dehydration.
- Incompetent cervix.
- Uterine trauma.
- Placental abnormalities (e.g., abruptio placentae, placenta previa).

C. Clinical Features
- Low, dull backache.
- Pelvic or abdominal pressure.
- Cramps with or without diarrhea.
- Vaginal discharge increase or change (e.g., "bloody show").
- Contractions, often without pain.
- Contractions may be visible on a fetal monitor.

D. Diagnostic Studies
- Pelvic examination (sterile speculum examination); if PPROM is ruled out, a bimanual examination may be done.
  - Cervical dilation and effacement with possible premature rupture of membranes.
    - Cervical dilation $\geq$3 cm and 80% effacement = PTL.
    - Cervical dilation 2 to 3 cm and <80% effacement = PTL likely, unconfirmed.
    - Cervical dilation <2 cm and <80% effacement = PTL unlikely.
  - Mucus bloody vaginal discharge or "bloody show" may be present. If there is more significant bleeding, evaluate for placenta previa or abruption placentae.
- Nitrazine and fern test.

- Transvaginal U/S, cervical length.
  - Cervical length <20 mm with contractions = PTL.
  - Cervical length 20 to 30 mm with contractions = PTL likely.
  - Cervical length >30 mm with/without contractions = PTL likely.
- Fetal fibronectin test of cervicovaginal fluid for the presence of protein that is strongly associated with PTL if present between 20 and 34 weeks' gestation.
  - Transabdominal U/S to assess fetus (weight, position) and amniotic fluid.
  - Anovaginal GBS culture.
  - Cervical cultures for *Chlamydia* and gonorrhea.
  - Wet mount for bacterial vaginosis, *Trichomonas*, or yeast.

E. Management
- Continuous fetal monitoring.
- Tocolytic therapy: suppress uterine activity—contraindicated with intrauterine infection, severe preeclampsia, severe fetal anomaly.
  - β-Adrenergic agonists (ritodrine and terbutaline) titrate till halt of uterine contractions or development of side effects.
  - Magnesium sulfate ($MgSO_4$).
  - Calcium channel blockers (nifedipine).
  - Prostaglandin synthetase inhibitor (indomethacin).
- Antenatal corticosteroids: accelerate fetal lung maturity.
  - Single course given if between 24 and 32 weeks' gestation; maximum benefit when administered within 7 days of delivery.
  - Betamethasone 12 mg IM every 24 hours for total of two doses.
  - Dexamethasone 6 mg IM every 12 hours for a total of four doses.
- Antibiotics, GBS prophylaxis, hydration therapy, and bed rest may be beneficial.
- Delivery should occur in a hospital equipped with neonatal intensive care.
- C-section is usually done for premature breech infants who weigh under 2,000 g.

VIII. Hyperemesis Gravidarum
A. Definition
- An abnormal condition of pregnancy associated with severe nausea and vomiting, weight loss, electrolyte imbalance, and ketonuria, most often occurring in the first or second trimester.

B. Etiology/Pathology
- Unclear, thought to be multifactorial.
- May be related to rapidly rising serum levels of hormones.
- Social and psychological factors may contribute.
- Risk factors include primigravida, multiple gestations, molar pregnancy, previous hyperemesis gravidarum.

C. Clinical Features
- Morning sickness: mild nausea and vomiting, usually resolved by the 16th week of gestation.
- Hyperemesis gravidarum: severe nausea and vomiting.
- Weight loss of up to 5% of pregravid weight.
- Dehydration.
- Acidosis from starvation.
- Alkalosis from loss of hydrochloric acid in vomitus.
- Hypokalemia.

D. Diagnostic Studies
- Follow weight.
- Urinalysis for ketones.
- Electrolytes, liver function tests (LFTs), CBC and peripheral blood smear, thyroid function tests.
- Sonogram.

E. Management
- Depends on symptom severity.
- Morning sickness: usually no treatment necessary.
- Vitamin supplementation may be needed, vitamin B_6 10 to 25 mg, three times daily.
- Alternative therapies having shown benefit in research include ginger (250 mg four times daily) and acupuncture.
- Medications for antiemetic therapy doxylamine, 12.5 mg, three or four times daily and may add promethazine, 12.5 to 25 mg taken orally or rectally every 4 hours or dimenhydrinate, 50 to 100 mg taken orally or rectally every 4 to 6 hours.
- Severe hyperemesis gravidarum: admission.
- IV hydration, multivitamin and thiamin supplementation, electrolyte correction, IV antiemetic medications.
- Total parenteral nutrition for lack of response to other therapies.
- If the pregnant woman does not respond to medical treatment, a psychiatric consult is advised.

IX. Gestational Diabetes Mellitus
A. Definition
- Glucose intolerance with onset of pregnancy or first recognition during pregnancy resulting in maternal hyperglycemia. Resolves after delivery.

B. Etiology
- Risk factors:
  - History of diabetes type 1, type 2, or gestational diabetes.
  - Family history of diabetes.
  - Ethnicity: African American, Asian, Hispanic, Native American.
  - Prior macrosomic, malformed, or stillborn infant.
  - In current pregnancy, presence of fetal macrosomia, polyhydramnios, multiple gestations.
  - Older maternal age (>25).
  - Obesity (BMI > 25).

C. Pathology

- Increases in serum insulin levels, sensitivity, estrogen, progestin, and cortisol for maternal fat accumulation resulting in increased insulin resistance.

D. Clinical Features

- Gestational diabetes mellitus (GDM) affects most body systems, and the woman may present with:
  - Hypoglycemia.
  - Hyperglycemia.
  - Recurrent urinary infections.
  - Vaginal infections.
  - Hypertension.
  - Hydramnios.
  - Retinopathy.
  - Stocking/glove neuropathy.
- Infant presentation:
  - Macrosomia.
  - Polyhydramnios.
  - Neonatal hypoglycemia.
  - Hypocalcemia.
  - Hyperbilirubinemia.
  - Congenital anomalies.
  - Respiratory distress.

E. Diagnostic Workup

- Determine risk at first prenatal visit through history.
- Pregnant women not considered at risk or not yet tested are screened at 24 to 28 weeks' gestation for gestational diabetes (earlier if in high-risk category).
- Fifty grams oral glucose challenge without regard to time of day or last meal; plasma sample taken at 1 hour.
  - Level of 140 mg per dL or less is considered normal.
  - If level >140 mg per dL, patient should receive a 3-hour oral glucose tolerance test (OGTT).
- Overnight fasting with a fasting blood sugar draw, followed by 100-g glucose load; plasma glucose drawn at 1, 2, and 3 hours.
  - Fasting blood glucose = ≤95 = WNL
  - Two of the four plasma glucose levels above normal is diagnostic of GDM.
  - See Table 15–1, criterion values for diagnosis of GDM.
- Pelvic U/S to evaluate fetus for growth and abnormalities, and amniotic fluid for amount.

F. Management

- Glucose control to obtain and maintain euglycemia, monitor with frequent home blood glucose checks four times daily (fasting and 1 or 2 hours following meals).
- Optimal glucose levels for fasting is <95 mg per dL, <120 mg per dL 2 hours after meals, and <140 mg per dL 1 hour after meals.
- Glycosylated hemoglobin (HbA_{1c}) drawn monthly to evaluate control.
- Nutritionist for diabetic diet counseling.

TABLE 15–1.	Criterion Values for Diagnosis of GDM from Results of OGTT	
Time since 100-g Glucose Load (h)	Modified O'Sullivan Scale	Carpenter and Coustan Scale
Fasting	105	95
1	190	180
2	165	155
3	145	140

Note: Values are plasma glucose levels in mg per dL.

GDM, gestational diabetes mellitus; OGTT, oral glucose tolerance test.

Data from Fortner KB, Szymanski LM, Fox H, Wallach EE, eds. *The Johns Hopkins Manual of Gynecology and Obstetrics*. 3rd ed. Baltimore, MD: Lippincott Williams & Wilkins; 2006:164.

- Calorie intake should be approximately 30 kcal/kg/day of ideal body weight.
  - Diet should consist of 20% protein, 40% fat, and no more than 40% complex carbohydrates.
- Exercise.
- Pharmacologic therapy initiated when diet is ineffective.
  - Insulin, therapy of choice.
  - Does not cross the placenta and will not affect the fetus directly.
  - Maternal weight and gestational age dictate insulin dosing as does the patient's record of finger stick glucose readings to suppress gluconeogenesis.
    - Total daily dose is split between morning and evening doses. Often, NPH (intermediate-acting) and regular (fast-acting) insulin combinations are used.
    - Some practitioners split the evening dose and give the regular insulin at dinner and the NPH at bedtime to decrease the risk of nocturnal hypoglycemia.
  - Glyburide, which does not cross the placenta, is an acceptable alternative to insulin in GDM. Research has shown similar glucose control as insulin but higher rate of preeclampsia and need for infant phototherapy. However, glyburide may not be appropriate for patients with more severe GDM.
    - Start at 2.5 mg in morning and titrate up to a max of 10 mg every 12 hours.
- Fetal monitoring.
  - Biweekly starting at about 32 weeks of gestational age; adjust insulin doses depending on home glucose log.
  - Daily fetal "kick counts" monitored.
  - Fetal heart rate monitoring.
  - Nonstress test (NST).
  - BPP (U/S tests fetal respiration, tone, flexion/extension, amniotic fluid levels) or contraction stress test if NST nonreactive.
  - U/S monitoring of fetus for macrosomia and shoulder dystocia.

- Early delivery: at 38 weeks, the fetus should be evaluated by pelvic U/S for weight. If macrosomic, >4,500 to 5,000 g, an elective C-section should be performed.
- Before delivery, U/S-guided amniocentesis should be performed and amniotic fluid analyzed for the level of phospholipid and phosphatidylglycerol, an indicator of fetal lung maturity.
- Fetal intrauterine demise common with noncompliant patients.
- If PTL develops in patients with diabetes, magnesium sulfate is the tocolytic agent of choice because many of the others exacerbate diabetes-related problems.
- If there is a risk of preterm delivery, corticosteroids should be given for fetal lung maturity. However, care must be taken because corticosteroids have a hyperglycemic effect.

X. Hypertensive Disorders in Pregnancy
A. Chronic Hypertension
  1. **Definition**
     - Hypertension diagnosed preconception or before the 20th week of gestation, or persistence past 12 weeks postpartum.
     - Mild-to-moderate: systolic blood pressure (BP) 140 to 159 mm Hg, diastolic 90 to 109 mm Hg, on two separate occasions at least 6 hours apart and not more than 1 week apart.
     - Severe: systolic BP ≥ 160 mm Hg, diastolic ≥ 110 mm Hg.
     - High risk of developing superimposed preeclampsia or eclampsia.
  2. **Diagnostic Studies**
     - CBC, glucose screen, electrolyte panel, BUN, serum creatinine, creatinine clearance, uric acid, calcium.
     - Liver function tests.
     - Total urinary protein, 24-hour urine, obtain urine culture.
     - Coagulation studies such as PT, PTT, fibrin split products.
     - Twenty-four hour urine calcium measurement.
     - ECG.
     - Pelvic U/S to monitor fetus.
     - Differential diagnosis: gestational hypertension, preeclampsia.
  3. **Management**
     a. **Mild Chronic Hypertension**
        - Prenatal visits every 2 to 4 weeks, weekly beginning at 34 to 36 weeks.
        - Monitor BP and urine for protein frequently.
        - Check fundal height.
        - Ask about symptoms/signs of preeclampsia.
        - Fetal monitoring begins at 32 to 34 weeks.

- Delivery by week 39 to 40.
- Most clinicians begin pharmacologic treatment at systolic BP of 150 to 160 mm Hg or diastolic BP of 100 to 110 mm Hg.
- First-line BP-lowering agents in pregnancy: labetalol, nifedipine, methyldopa.
- Additional BP-lowering agents in pregnancy: hydralazine, hydrochlorothiazide.

  b. **Severe Chronic Hypertension**
     - May need more frequent prenatal visits to monitor.
     - Consider inpatient monitoring.
     - Monitor BP, proteinuria, and fetal growth.
     - Assess for preeclampsia.
     - If there is end-organ involvement, monitor for exacerbation.
     - U/S for fetal growth every 2 to 4 weeks beginning at 32 to 34 weeks.
     - Delivery after week 38 or when fetal lungs are mature.

B. Gestational Hypertension
  1. **Definition**
     - Hypertension detected after the 20th week of pregnancy without proteinuria. Resolves or becomes chronic or transient hypertension.
     - May also occur within 48 to 72 hours after delivery.
  2. **Management**
     - Outpatient treatment; some recommend withholding antihypertensives so as not to mask severe preeclampsia.
     - If antihypertensives are used, hydralazine or labetalol are recommended.
     - Monitor BP and proteinuria at least once a week in office setting as the majority of these patients progress to preeclampsia later in pregnancy.
     - Weekly home BP monitoring advised.
     - Draw baseline CBC, BUN, creatinine. Some practitioners recommend following a uric acid level. A rise indicates progression to preeclampsia.

XI. Preeclampsia
A. Definition
  - Hypertension and proteinuria after the 20th week of gestation.
  - Edema is no longer part of the diagnostic criteria because it occurs too frequently in normal pregnancies.
  - Can occur prior to the 20th week in trophoblastic disease or multiple gestation.
  - Categorized as mild and severe.

B. Etiology
  - Largely unknown. Incidence is 2% to 7% in nulliparous women.

C. Risk Factors
  - Nulliparity.

- Previous preeclampsia/eclampsia; family history of preeclampsia.
- Multiple gestation (i.e., twins).
- Thyroid disease.
- Extremes of age.
- Preexisting hypertensive, vascular, autoimmune, or renal disease.
- Pregestational diabetes.
- Obesity.
- Fetal hydrops.
- Trisomy 13.
- Hydatidiform mole.
- African American race.

D. Clinical Features
1. Mild Preeclampsia
- Systolic BP ≥140 mm Hg and/or diastolic BP ≥90 mm Hg in a previously normotensive woman on two separate occasions at least 6 hours apart (but no >1 week apart).
  - Proteinuria >300 mg in 24-hour period (or >+1 on urine dipstick).
2. Severe Preeclampsia
- Systolic BP ≥160 mm Hg and/or diastolic BP ≥110 mm Hg on two occasions preferably during bed rest and 6 hours apart.
- Or any of the following:
  - Proteinuria: >5 g in a 24-hour period (or +3 or greater on two urine dipsticks randomly tested at least 4 hours apart).
- Oliguria <500 mL in 24 hours.
- Thrombocytopenia (<10,000 platelets per μL).
- Pulmonary edema.
- Cyanosis.
- HELLP syndrome (special entity, **H**emolysis, **E**levated **L**iver enzymes, **L**ow **P**latelets).
- Restriction of fetal growth.
- Other symptoms include:
  - Epigastric/upper-right-quadrant pain.
  - Intrauterine fetal growth restriction (IUGR).
  - Nausea, vomiting.
  - Dyspnea.
  - Lack of fetal movement.
  - Preterm labor.
  - Elevated liver function tests.
  - Headache.
  - Visual disturbances/scotomata.
  - Altered mental status.

E. Diagnostic Studies
- Recognize preeclampsia early.
- Obtain BP measurements on two occasions with patient in left lateral position.
- U/A for protein.
- CBC, coagulation factors (PT, PTT, fibrin split products), BUN and creatinine levels, LFTs, if severe form.
- Pelvic U/S to monitor fetus.

F. Management
1. Mild
- Only cure for preeclampsia is delivery.
  - Deliver if at 34 to 36 weeks' gestation or more.
  - Restrict activity; bed rest for mild preeclampsia is controversial.
  - Daily weights and urine dipstick; weekly 24-hour urine.
  - Twice weekly NSTs and/or BPPs weekly.
  - BP control.
  - Seizure prevention.
2. Severe
- Continue to monitor mother and fetus and prevent seizures.
- Patient should be hospitalized for moderate-to-severe preeclampsia.
- $MgSO_4$ IV reduces patient's BP and helps prevent seizures, but not used until diagnosis of severe preeclampsia or start of labor.
- Hydralazine is the drug of choice (other BP-lowering agents may be necessary [e.g., labetalol, nifedipine]).
- Monitor fetal well-being, continuous heart rate, U/S, BPP.
- Consider amniocentesis to evaluate fetal lung development if fetus is 30 to 37 weeks. If lungs are immature, give corticosteroids. If fetus is between 26 and 30 weeks, give corticosteroids.
- Depending on the patient's condition, delivery of a preterm infant may be delayed for steroid treatment to facilitate lung maturity. If the patient is at term, she should be delivered by induced vaginal delivery or by C-section.
- Consider delivery regardless of maturity or gestational age in severe preeclampsia.

G. Complications
- Abruptio placentae.
- Liver failure/rupture/HELLP.
  - Congestive heart failure.
- Renal failure.
- Cerebrovascular accident (CVA).
- Adult respiratory distress syndrome.
- Fetal distress/demise.

XII. Eclampsia
A. Definition
- Occurrence of convulsions, coma, or both in a woman with preeclampsia.
- Life threatening for mother and fetus.
  - Can occur antepartum (most commonly), intra-, or postpartum.

B. Etiology
- Unknown.
- Incidence is 0.05% to 0.10% in the United States, but higher in developing countries.

C. Clinical Features
- Abrupt tonic–clonic seizure of 1 to 2 minutes duration, followed by postictal state.
- May include headache, visual changes, epigastric pain.
- Cardiorespiratory arrest may follow.
- Pulmonary aspiration.
- Other neurologic symptoms may be present.

D. Diagnostic Studies
- Studies as for preeclampsia (see section XI).
- **Differential diagnosis**
  - Until proven otherwise, a seizure during pregnancy should be considered eclampsia.
  - Others include epilepsy, encephalitis, meningitis, cerebral tumor, and CVA.

E. Management
- Airway, breathing, circulation.
- Protect the patient from injury.
- Treat hypertension as in preeclampsia.
- Drugs: $MgSO_4$ to prevent recurrence of seizure.
- Deliver fetus after patient is stabilized; be prepared for emergency C-section.
- Monitor for pulmonary edema; careful attention to fluid status.
- Monitor urine output with use of indwelling Foley catheter.

XIII. Placenta Previa
A. Definition
- The presence of placental tissue in the lower uterine segment over, or adjacent to, the cervical os.
- Results in complete or partial coverage of the cervix, ahead of presenting fetal part.
- Average presentation of first bleeding episode is 29 to 30 weeks.
- Bleeding is a result of separation of placenta from lower uterine segment and cervix.
- **Total (complete) placenta previa**
  - Internal cervical opening covered completely.
- **Partial/marginal placenta previa (previously categorized separately)**
  - Placenta lies within 2 to 3 cm of the cervical os, but not covering it.

B. Etiology
- Unknown: incidence is 0.5% to 1.0% in all pregnancies.

C. Risk Factors
- Previous uterine surgery, C-section, previous placenta previa.
- Advanced age.
  - Prior endometrial trauma, D&C, D&E.
  - Abnormality of endometrial vascularity.
- Delayed ovulation.
- Multiparity.
- Cigarette smoking.
- Cocaine use.

D. Clinical Features
- Spotting during first and second trimesters.
- Sudden painless vaginal bleeding in third trimester.
- Usually soft, nontender uterus.
- Patients with no prenatal care may present with severe vaginal bleeding.
- Prenatal patients usually receive an U/S between the 12th and 20th weeks of gestation, which allows for diagnosis before the onset of bleeding.

E. Diagnostic Studies
- Transvaginal U/S to localize the placenta.
- Additional U/Ss are necessary to establish the degree of previa because the placenta may migrate.
- Abdominal examination to assess uterine tone.
- Fetal heart rate.
- Monitor mother's vital signs.
- CBC, platelet count, coagulation studies—in patients with significant bleeding.
- Amniocentesis to determine lung maturity.
- Digital examination is contraindicated if placenta previa is present.

F. Management
- Treatment depends on the extent of bleeding, gestational age, and status of the cervix.
- Hospitalization with hemodynamic stabilization.
- Maternal and fetal monitoring.
- Steroids between 24 and 34 weeks for fetal lung development.
- Rh0(D) immunoglobulin to Rh-negative mothers.
- Pelvic rest.
- Preterm patients with one to two episodes of mild bleeding are treated with bed rest and tocolysis, if needed.
- Follow closely and monitor CBC.
- Monitor BP.
- May progress to term and deliver vaginally (marginal placenta) or by C-section (total previa).
- Patients with severe hemorrhage or third bleeding episode should be resuscitated and delivered by urgent C-section.
- Usually, if a mother is hospitalized on three separate occasions, she will remain in the hospital until delivery.
- If a patient is not bleeding during the third trimester, confirm previa through U/S, allow pelvic rest, educate patient of warning signs, avoid strenuous activity, and check fetal U/S every 3 or 4 weeks.

G. Complications
- Longer hospital stay.
- C-section.
- Abruptio placentae.
- Postpartum hemorrhage (PPH).
- Malpresentation.

XIV. Abruptio Placentae

A. Definition

- Premature partial or complete separation of the placenta from its normal implantation.
  - One of the leading causes of fetal mortality.
- Classified according to clinical findings:
  - Grade 1, mild abruption; slight bleeding.
  - Grade 2, moderate or partial abruption.
  - Grade 3, large or complete abruption (least common).
    - Grade 3 and complete separation should be considered life threatening to the mother and fetus.
    - Figure 15–1 shows common features of different types of abruption.

B. Etiology

- Primary etiology is unknown.
- Occurs in approximately 1 of 120 births.
- Abruption accounts for 10% to 15% of perinatal mortality.

C. Risk Factors

- Maternal hypertension (strongly associated with grade 3).
- Blunt abdominal trauma (initially often grade 1, can progress rapidly to grade 3).

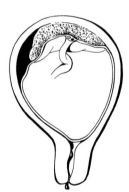
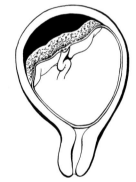

Partial separation

Complete separation with concealed hemorrhage

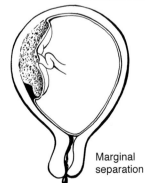

Marginal separation

FIGURE 15–1. **Various degrees of separation of a normally implanted placenta.** (From Scott JR. Placenta previa and placental abruption. In: Scott JR, DiSaia PS, Hammond GB, Spellacy WN, eds. *Danforth's Obstetrics and Gynecology*. 8th ed. Philadelphia, PA: Lippincott Williams & Wilkins; 1999:412, with permission.)

- Previous abruptio placentae.
- Chorioamnionitis.
- Multiple gestation.
- Poor nutrition (folic acid deficiency).
- Cigarette smoking; drug abuse (alcohol, cocaine).
- Advanced maternal age.
- Uterine anomalies or myomas.
- Thrombophilia defects.
- Elevated serum α-fetoprotein (AFP) during the second trimester.
- Preeclampsia.

D. Pathology

- Separation is initiated by bleeding into decidua basalis.
- Decidua splits and placenta is sheared off.
- Blood may extravasate into and through myometrium.

E. Clinical Features

- Abruption may be life threatening or, depending on grade, may be asymptomatic and only be discovered on delivery of placenta.
- Vaginal bleeding in the third trimester (80%).
- Uterine tenderness.
- Abdominal pain or back pain.
- Premature labor.
- May be fetal distress.
- Severe cases can lead to hypovolemic shock, disseminated intravascular coagulopathy (DIC), fetal distress, demise, uterine tetany.

F. Diagnostic Studies

- Pelvic U/S of fetus, placenta, and uterus.
- Clinical examination.
- Fetal heart rate monitor and tocometry may show hypertonic contractions with elevated baseline and various degrees of abnormal heart rate patterns.
- Coagulation studies: PT, PTT, fibrin, fibrin split products.
- CBC with platelet count, hematocrit, blood type and screen depending on the severity of bleeding, BUN, and creatinine.
- U/A.
- **Differential diagnosis**
  - Placenta previa (abruptio placentae has abdominal discomfort and painful contractions, whereas placenta previa does not).

G. Management

- Mild abruption: no treatment may be necessary.
- Follow closely in labor unit until fetal maturity; may be confused with premature or early labor; expect vaginal delivery.
- After abdominal trauma, patients should be observed closely for at least 24 hours.
- May place Foley catheter to measure urine output, which should be >0.5 to 1.0 mL/kg/hour.

- Administer Rh0(D) immunoglobulin to Rh-negative individuals.
- **Moderate-to-severe abruption with signs of fetal distress**, loss of fetal heart tones, or maternal signs of shock require immediate resuscitation and delivery by C-section.
- Patients should be cross-matched for 4 to 6 units of blood.
- Repeat coagulation studies and CBC to evaluate for DIC.
- **Moderate-to-severe abruption with no signs of fetal distress or maternal hypotension**: vaginal delivery may be attempted with gentle induction of labor with Pitocin, as long as no evidence of fetal distress or maternal complications is present.
- **Cesarean section** is often the form of delivery.
- Postdelivery of infant and placenta, patient may still develop complications and should be treated symptomatically.

XV. Multiple Gestations

A. Definition

- Gestation and delivery of two or more fetuses.
- One of the most common high-risk conditions.
- Twin gestation is the most common form.

B. Etiology

- Ethnic background: more common in African Americans than Caucasians or Asians.
- Maternal age: more common in women between 30 and 40 years of age.
- Infertility therapy: assisted reproductive technology.
- Hereditary: increased incidence in families.

C. Pathology

- Zygosity refers to the genetic makeup.
- Chorionicity refers to the placental composition.

- Dizygotic twins (fraternal): more common type (1 in 90 pregnancies); two separate ova are fertilized (2 eggs; 2 sperm). The placentation is always diamniotic and dichorionic.
- Monozygotic twins (identical): single ovum is fertilized and splits into distinct fetuses (1 in 250 pregnancies). May have diamniotic and dichorionic placenta; however, much more common is monoamniotic, monochorionic placenta (Figure 15–2).

D. Clinical Features

- Uterus larger than dates suggest.
- The patient may have earlier and more severe pressure in pelvis.
- Excessive maternal weight gain.
- Hydramnios (excessive amniotic fluid).
- Nausea.
- Backache.
- Varicosities.
- Constipation, hemorrhoids.
- Abdominal distension.
- Difficulty breathing.
- Multiplicity of small parts.
- Two fetal hearts detected.
- Two fetuses palpated.

E. Complications

- Higher incidence of maternal complications compared with singletons:
  - Preterm labor.
  - Preeclampsia.
  - Placental abruption.
  - Placenta previa.
  - Anemia.
  - Hydramnios.
  - Urinary tract infections (UTIs).
  - C-section.
  - Postpartum hemorrhage.

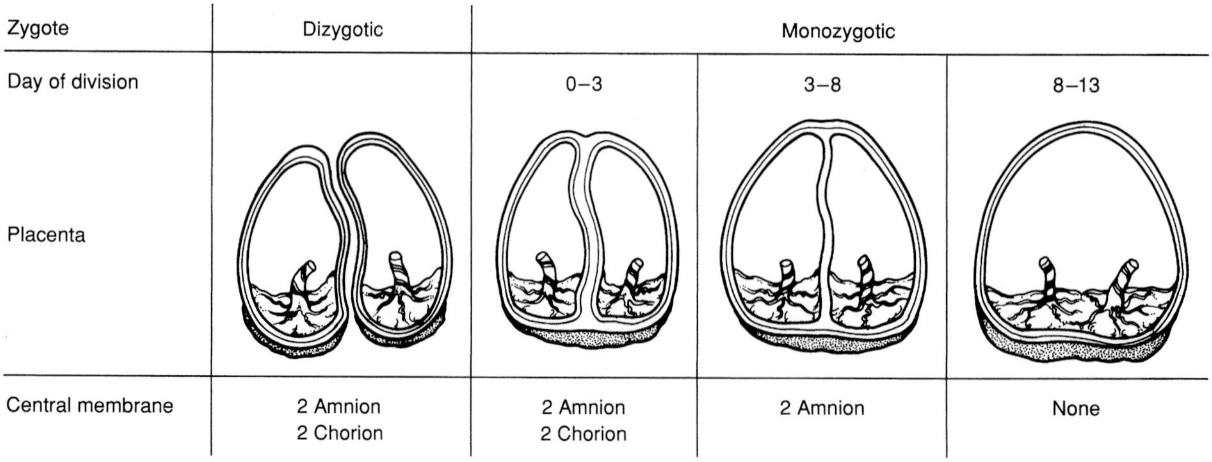

Zygote	Dizygotic	Monozygotic		
Day of division		0–3	3–8	8–13
Placenta				
Central membrane	2 Amnion 2 Chorion	2 Amnion 2 Chorion	2 Amnion	None

FIGURE 15–2. **Types of placentation in monozygotic and dizygotic twinning.** (From Spellacy WN. Multiple pregnancies. In: Scott JR, DiSaia PS, Hammond GB, Spellacy WN, eds. *Danforth's Obstetrics and Gynecology*. 8th ed. Philadelphia, PA: Lippincott Williams & Wilkins; 1999:294, with permission.)

- For the fetuses, most common problems are:
  - Low birth weight.
  - Growth restriction.
  - Premature birth.
  - Congenital abnormalities.
  - Incidence higher in monozygotic twins.
  - Cord accidents.
  - Malpresentation.
  - Vanishing twin.
  - Monoamniotic cord entanglement.
  - Twin-to-twin transfusion syndrome.
  - Molar pregnancy and fetus.
  - Delayed delivery.

F. Diagnostic Studies
- More than one heartbeat on auscultation.
- External examination: multiple heads and small parts.
- Higher levels of β-hCG, AFP, human placental lactogen, or estriol.
- Majority of multiple pregnancies are diagnosed by U/S scanning.

G. Management
- After diagnosis of multiple gestation, patient must be treated as high risk.
- Patient must be seen more frequently, as well as receive regular vaginal examination and U/S to evaluate for premature contractions, and for fetal growth and well-being.
- The role of bed rest is still being studied. Starting at approximately 24 weeks may be helpful for reducing complications and increasing fetal weight; 81% of perinatal mortality occurs before gestational week 29.
- Depending on fetal positions and gestational age, placental type, and mother's parity, vaginal delivery may be possible.
- In instances of monoamniotic monochorionic placentas or presenting twin breech, C-section is the best course.

XVI. Abnormalities of Labor
A. Definition
- Dystocia is defined as an abnormal progression of labor, or arrest of labor in either of the first two stages, that may result in modes of delivery other than spontaneous vaginal.

B. Etiology
- Protraction or arrest of active labor may be caused by:
  - Abnormalities of power (uterine contractions, cervical resistance).
  - Abnormalities of the passenger (fetal size, presentation, position).
  - Abnormalities of passage (maternal pelvimetry).

C. Clinical Features
- At first prenatal visit, especially in the case of primigravida, pelvic sizing is important.

- If noted early that the outlet may not be appropriate, patient must be watched more closely during labor.
- In instances of fetal size or presentation causing cephalopelvic disproportion, careful evaluation should be done to determine the mode of delivery.

D. Diagnostic Studies
- No laboratory studies are available that allow for prediction of abnormal labors.
- Pelvic U/S helps evaluate fetal position, presentation.
- MRI may help with some estimation of pelvimetry.
- X-ray, the original method of pelvimetry, is not commonly used today.

E. Management
- Identify the specific abnormality and determine if the problem is correctable.
- Management options vary considerably from observation to C-section.
- Augmentation with oxytocin is recommended in certain conditions.
- First stage: ambulation, positioning, hydration.
  - Latent phase: oxytocin for PROM.
  - Active phase: if inadequate progression of cervical dilation after 4 hours of favorable uterine contractions, may manage with oxytocin and/or amniotomy. If FH pattern remains reassuring, may allow labor to continue 8 hours.
- C-section delivery is usually performed in cases of cephalopelvic disproportion, fetal abnormalities such as hydrocephalus and abnormal head positions.
- Use of forceps or vacuum can sometimes accomplish a change of position or help guide and deliver the fetal head.

XVII. Malpresentations
A. Definition
- Any presentation of presenting part other than vertex: breech, transverse position, face presentation, brow presentations, compound presentation.
- Breech presentation is the most common malpresentation.

B. Etiology
- Associated with both fetal and maternal abnormalities.
- Small fetus (increased motility).
- Decreased fetal muscle strength and tone (myotonic dystrophies, chromosomal abnormalities).
- Hydrocephalus or anencephaly.
- Multiple gestations.
- Abnormally implanted placenta (obstructive normal descent).
- Multiparity (laxity of maternal abdominal and uterine musculature).
- Uterine tumor or anomalies.

C. Clinical Features

- In most instances, presenting part of the fetus can be determined before the 36th week by pelvic examination ± U/S.
- Chances of spontaneous conversion of malpresentation decreases with EGA.
- Mode of delivery depends on position.
- Risk of cord prolapse is greatest with incomplete and compound presentations.
- Risk of injury to baby increased with vaginal delivery in nonexpert hands.

D. Diagnostic Studies

- U/S: primary tool for determining fetal position.
- Vaginal/pelvic examination.
- Leopold maneuvers.

E. Management

- In cases of breech or transverse lie, external cephalic version may be attempted after 36 weeks (40% revert to original lie).
- C-section is recommended for most malpresentations.

XVIII. Shoulder Dystocia

A. Definition

- An acute obstetrical emergency, when one (usually the anterior) or both shoulders of the fetus become lodged at or behind the pubic symphysis after delivery of the head.
- Brachial plexus injury (Erb palsy) may result.
- "Turtle" sign: head retracts after each contraction.

B. Etiology

- **Risk factors**
  - Macrosomia (mother diabetic); history of macrosomic newborn.
    - Maternal obesity.
    - Multiparity.
    - Postterm gestation.
  - Bony pelvic abnormality.
  - Uterine abnormalities.
  - Abnormal contractions.

C. Clinical Features

- Rapid or precipitous descent should warn the clinician of possible shoulder dystocia.
- Condition must be recognized quickly because it could be fatal for the fetus if too much time is taken to deliver the shoulder.

D. Management

- The first-line treatment is McRoberts maneuver: maternal hyperflexion of the hips and abduction of knees and legs to increase pelvic opening. Suprapubic pressure is applied.
- A second-line choice is to perform the Wood corkscrew maneuver by rotating the posterior shoulder toward the fetal back. Rubin maneuver may be performed (hand inserted into the vagina and digital pressure applied to posterior aspect of anterior shoulder toward the fetal chest).
- It may be necessary to fracture one or both of the clavicles if none of the above are successful. Clavicles should be broken using the thumb and fracturing the bones away from the lungs.
- As a last resort, the Zavanelli maneuver involves cephalic replacement and C-section delivery.
- The longer it takes to deliver the fetus, the greater the chance for neuropsychiatric disorders and trauma to the fetus.
- After delivery, the mother may be left with the equivalent of a fourth-degree tear. The wound must be closed properly, or the mother may suffer from rectovaginal fistulae or rectal incontinence.
- The mother is given stool softeners, and wound is checked daily for evidence of hematoma or infection.

XIX. Postpartum Fever and Sepsis

A. Definition

- Infections that occur in the immediate postpartum period causing fever, sepsis, or both.
- Fever >38° C on at least two occasions (measured at least 4 hours apart) after the first 24 hours postpartum.

B. Etiology

- **Risk factors**
  - C-section.
  - Breech presentation.
  - Prolonged labor.
  - Lengthy duration of ruptured membranes.
  - Low socioeconomic status.
  - Obesity.
  - Immunosuppression/diabetes.
  - Vaginal infections, especially bacterial vaginosis.
  - Multiple vaginal examinations.

C. Clinical Features

1. **Endometritis**
   - Rare after vaginal delivery.
   - Usually presents second to seventh postpartum day.
   - Infection is usually polymicrobial in nature.
   - Patient presents with complaints of abdominal pain, high fever, chills, purulent/foul lochia.

2. **Urinary Tract Infections**
   - UTIs, especially pyelonephritis in postpartum period.
   - Usual presentation: fever, chills, frequency, and back pain.
   - Check for CVA tenderness.
   - If fever persists for more than 48 to 72 hours after antibiotic treatment, consider other problems such as wound infection, ovarian vein thrombosis, pelvic abscess, septic pelvic thrombophlebitis, and mastitis.

3. Wound Infection
- Pain, redness, and swelling in the area of incision.
- **Septic pelvic vein thrombophlebitis**
  - Persistent fever, elevated WBC, no evidence of UTI, endometritis, or abscess.

D. Diagnostic Studies
- CBC plus peripheral blood smear.
- Urinalysis.
- Blood and urine cultures; genital cultures.
- In instances of suspected phlebitis or abscesses, pelvic U/S, CT scan, or MRI may identify possible sources.

E. Management
- Patient should be admitted and started on IV antibiotics after culture and sensitivity; appropriate antibiotics may be ampicillin/sulbactam, gentamicin, clindamycin, ampicillin, or combinations thereof.
- In most instances, patients respond in 24 to 48 hours.
- If patient does not respond in 3 to 4 days, other conditions should be considered and appropriate subspecialist may be consulted.
- Prophylactic antibiotics after C-section are recommended.

XX. Postpartum Hemorrhage

A. Definition
- Emergent condition traditionally defined as bleeding in excess of 500 mL with vaginal delivery or >1,000 mL with C-section.
- Current criteria include bleeding that produces signs and symptoms and requires a blood transfusion; 10% drop in hematocrit from admission to postpartum period.
- Early PPH occurs ≤24 hours postpartum; late PPH occurs ≥24 hours, up to 6 to 12 weeks postpartum.

B. Etiology/Pathology
- The "Four Ts"
  - Tone (atony) most common cause; uterine atony (unable to contract and control bleeding).
  - Tissue: retained placenta
  - Trauma: severe vaginal or perineal tears, uterine rupture, or uterine inversion.
  - Thrombin: possible coagulopathies, congenital bleeding disorders or other coagulation defects, DIC (caused by preeclampsia, sepsis, abruptio placentae, or amniotic fluid embolus).
- Accounts for a minimum of 25% maternal deaths worldwide.
- Incidence difficult to estimate due to lack of uniform definition of PPH.

C. Clinical Features
- Hypovolemic shock: pale, clammy skin; hypotension; tachycardia; delayed capillary refill; narrowed pulse pressure.

D. Diagnostic Studies
- Vital signs.
- CBC, peripheral blood smear, PT, PTT, fibrinogen, fibrin split products.
- Type and cross-match for possible transfusion.

E. Management
- Evaluate excessive bleeding and identify/treat probable cause.
- For uterine atony: bimanual massage until fundus becomes firm and administer IV oxytocin. If unsuccessful, other agents include methylergonovine or misoprostol. Balloon catheter or packing are next-line options, whereas operative measures are a last resort.
- For retained placenta: manual removal and management of atony as above.
- If present, repair lacerations and correct coagulation defects.

XXI. Postpartum Depression (Table 15–2)

A. Definition
- Criteria for major depressive disorder are met; see clinical features below.
- Usually occurs 2 weeks to 12 months postpartum.
- Differential diagnosis includes the following:
  - Postpartum "baby" blues: common condition (affects 70%–80% of postpartum women) possibly caused by decreasing progesterone. Self-limiting and resolved within 2 weeks.
  - Postpartum psychosis: a rare (<0.2%), but serious, condition that may require hospitalization due to impairment and risk of harm to mother or baby. These patients typically have a preexisting psychotic diagnosis like bipolar disorder or schizophrenia.

B. Etiology/Pathology
- Psychosocial and/or biochemical factors such as prior history of depression, family history/genetic factors, poor social support, stressful life events, and trauma during birth.
- Incidence is between 10% and 15% of all pregnancies, including miscarriages and abortions.
- Depression occurring during pregnancy or a history of a depressive disorder before pregnancy is strong predictor of PPD.

C. Clinical Features
- The onset of PPD can vary from the immediate postpartum period to several weeks following delivery.
- Symptoms may include depressed mood, anhedonia, difficulty concentrating, guilt, suicidal ideation, anxiety, and sleep or appetite changes.
- Patients may feel lonely, isolated, unable to care for self or baby.

TABLE 15–2.	Three Categories of Postpartum Mood Disorders		
	Postpartum Psychosis	**Postpartum Depression**	**Maternity Blues**
Incidence (%)	0.1–0.2	=10	50–80
Average time	2–3 d PP	2 wk to 12 mo PP	1–5 d PP
Average duration	Variable	3–14 mo	2–3 d, resolution within 10 d
Symptoms	Similar to organic brain syndrome: confusion, attention deficit, distractibility, clouded sensorium	Irritability, labile mood, difficulty falling asleep, phobias, anxiety; symptoms worsen in the evening	Mild insomnia, tearfulness, fatigue, irritability, poor concentration, depressed affect
Treatment	A psychotic pharmacotherapy, antidepressant, 50% of patients also meet depression criteria	Antidepressant, pharmacotherapy, psychotherapy	Time, reassurance, watchful waiting; leads to PPD in 20% of patients

PP, postpartum psychosis, PPD, postpartum depression.

From Beckmann CR. *Obstetrics and Gynecology*. 5th ed. Baltimore, MD: Lippincott Williams & Wilkins; 2005:130, with permission.

- In early stages, clinicians should be attuned to patient complaints and changes in mood, affect, and appearance.

D. Diagnostic Studies

- Thyroid function should be assessed, as depression may be due to hypothyroidism.
- Order additional diagnostic studies as needed to rule out other organic causes of depression.
- PPD must be taken seriously. Patients should be screened during pregnancy and postpartum period. Evaluate mood, affect, appearance, and risks for harm to mother or baby.

E. Management

- Evaluate the severity of the condition and the potential for harm. Evaluate the need for a psychiatric evaluation. Providers must be alert for pronounced feelings of sadness or anxiety that do not improve after 10 to 14 days of delivery, particularly if the symptoms worsen.
- Antidepressant medications and/or psychotherapy are recommended for treatment for PPD. Postpartum (baby) blues does not require intervention other than support and reassurance.

REVIEW QUESTIONS

1. Your patient presents to the office for management after having had her third consecutive spontaneous abortion. She has completed genetic counseling, and an endometrial biopsy was negative for a luteal-phase defect. Labs you drew at the last visit showed elevated luteinizing and follicular-stimulating hormones (LH and FSH). Based on you suspected diagnosis, which of the following management plans should be included for this patient?

a) Twenty-five milligram progesterone vaginal suppository twice daily.
b) Metformin 1,000 mg twice daily.
c) Low-molecular-weight heparin.
d) Mifepristone 400 mg PO once daily.

2. You are treating a woman in the emergency department who just experienced a spontaneous abortion. Her medical record indicates she is Rh-negative and she tells you she is not sure what blood type the father has. When you counsel her about Rh immunoglobulin therapy, she seems hesitant and not convinced it is necessary. Which of the following should be included in educating this patient about Rh immunoglobulin?

a) "Your blood may have developed antibodies that may damage the blood cells in the circulation of your next baby."
b) "Your blood may have developed antibodies because of exposure to the baby's blood that may damage the blood cells in your circulation."
c) "Your baby's blood may have developed antibodies that may damage the blood cells in your circulation."
d) "Rh immunoglobulin therapy is not necessary now, but you will need to have it during your next pregnancy."

3. A pregnant patient presents to the emergency department complaining of urinary frequency, chills, and back pain. Your exam indicates she may be mildly dehydrated. Based on your suspected diagnosis, which of the following is the most appropriate pharmaceutical management of this patient?

a) Nitrofurantoin 100 mg PO q6h × 5 days.
b) Cephalexin 500 mg PO BID × 10 days.
c) Ceftriaxone 1 g IV OD.
d) Gentamycin 5 mg/kg/day IV.

4. A 25-year-old woman presents to the emergency department with complaints of right lower quadrant abdominal pain and nausea. Which of the following diagnostic tests must be performed urgently?

a) CT scan of the abdomen and pelvis.

b) Ultrasound of the pelvis.

c) Complete blood count.

d) Human chorionic gonadotropin.

5. Your 14-week pregnant patient calls the office because of a new onset of moderate vaginal bleeding. She denies cramping or pain. You instruct her to come to the office to be evaluated, and upon exam you find the cervix to be closed. However, you note there is some bleeding from the cervical os and blood present in the vaginal vault. Which of the following is the most appropriate management for this patient at this time?

a) Perform dilation and evacuation.

b) Perform cervical cerclage.

c) Serial β-hCG levels.

d) Transvaginal ultrasound.

ANSWERS TO REVIEW QUESTIONS

1. **Answer: B.** The most likely diagnosis in this patient is polycystic ovarian syndrome (PCOS). PCOS is the leading cause of infertility and can also cause spontaneous abortions when the couple are able to conceive. The workup for multiple spontaneous abortion should include visualization of the pelvic organs to rule out structural defects, an endometrial biopsy or luteal-phase serum progesterone levels to identify any luteal-phase defect, genetic testing for chromosomal anomalies, and evaluation for PCOS. First-line treatment for PCOS in women who desire fertility includes weight loss and metformin.

2. **Answer: A.** Maternal antibodies develop against fetal red blood cells (RBCs) following fetomaternal hemorrhage when fetal blood components enter maternal circulation. This can occur during delivery, pregnancy-related procedures such as amniocentesis, any type of abortion, and ectopic pregnancies. Put simply, women who are Rh-negative and are exposed to the blood of an Rh-positive fetus will develop antibodies to the Rh-D antigen of the fetus' blood, thus immunizing her to the Rh-D antigen. In a subsequent pregnancy, the antibodies of the mother's blood will mix with the fetal blood and attack the Rh-D antigen, causing hemolysis.

3. **Answer: C.** This patient is presenting with pyelonephritis, the most common complication of a lower urinary tract infection in pregnant women. Pyelonephritis can have serious complications such as septic shock and ARDS and must be treated aggressively with hospital admission, IV fluid hydration, and IV antibiotics. Ceftriaxone is the antibiotic of choice initially until urine cultures are reported. Gentamycin is not recommended as first line due to fetal ototoxicity.

4. **Answer: D.** All women of child-bearing age with complaints of abdominal pain must have a human chorionic gonadotropin (hCG) performed urgently to rule out pregnancy. A positive result must alert the practitioner to prove there is an intrauterine pregnancy as opposed to an ectopic pregnancy. The hallmark presentation of an ectopic pregnancy is pain, vaginal bleeding, and amenorrhea. Cervical motion tenderness and hemodynamic instability can indicate a ruptured ectopic pregnancy and must be considered a medical emergency.

5. **Answer: C.** This patient is experiencing a threatened abortion and must be treated as a viable pregnancy until proven otherwise. Serial β-hCG levels should be performed every 3 days to determine if the pregnancy remains viable. Decreasing β-hCG levels suggest that the pregnancy will likely progress to an inevitable or missed abortion. A dilation and evacuation (D&E) is performed during the second-trimester incomplete or inevitable abortions. A cervical cerclage is performed when the cervix is found to be incompetent or insufficient (shortening and opening too early in pregnancy). A pelvic ultrasound is most desirable in a patient with a threatened abortion.

SELECTED REFERENCES

Beckman CRB, Ling FW, Herbert WNP, et al, eds. *Obstetrics and Gynecology.* 7th ed. Baltimore, MD: Lippincott Williams & Wilkins; 2014.

DeCherney AH, Nathan L, Laufer N, Roman AS, eds. *Current Diagnosis and Treatment Obstetrics and Gynecology.* 11th ed. New York, NY: McGraw-Hill; 2012.

Gabbe SG, Niebyl JR, Simpson JL, eds. *Obstetrics: Normal and Problem Pregnancies.* 7th ed. Philadelphia, PA: Churchill Livingstone; 2017.

Gibbs RS, Karlan BY, Haney AF, Nygaard I, eds. *Danforth's Obstetrics and Gynecology.* 10th ed. Philadelphia, PA: Lippincott Williams & Wilkins; 2008.

Hacker NF, Gambone JC, Hobel CJ, *Hacker and Moore's Essentials of Obstetrics and Gynecology.* 6th ed. Philadelphia, PA: Elsevier; 2016.

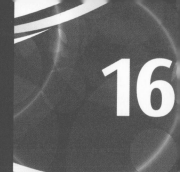

Infectious Diseases

16

William R. Short

I. Fungal (Mycotic) Infections

A. Aspergillosis

1. **Etiology**
   - *Aspergillus fumigatus*, the usual cause of aspergillosis, is a fungus capable of causing disease in healthy individuals as well as an opportunistic pathogen causing infection in immunocompromised hosts; other species also cause disease.
   - It is characterized by large septate hyphae that branch at a 45° angle.
   - *Aspergillus* is commonly found in garden and houseplant soil and compost.

2. **Pathology**
   - The immunologic status of infected hosts primarily determines the manifestations of the disease.
   - Routes of transmission include inhalation (most common), direct inoculation of the skin, or injection into the blood stream.

3. **Clinical Features**
   - Clinical features vary from a hypersensitivity reaction to life-threatening illness.
     - Allergic bronchopulmonary aspergillosis, found mainly in patients with asthma and in patients with cystic fibrosis, is characterized by thick, brown, tenacious, mucous plugs in sputum.
   - Acute invasive *Aspergillus* sinusitis may occur in persons with normal or mildly suppressed immunologic function. Symptoms include fever, headache, toothache, epistaxis, and purulent nasal discharge.
   - Aspergilloma occurs when the fungus colonizes existing cavitary pulmonary lesions; it may be an incidental finding or present with hemoptysis because of its propensity for invading blood vessels.
   - Chronic necrotizing pulmonary aspergillosis, although rare, occurs in immunocompromised patients and produces nonproductive cough, dyspnea, and pleuritic chest pain.
   - Potentially fatal invasive or disseminated aspergillosis occurs in severely immunocompromised and neutropenic patients, who may have pleuritic chest pain, cough, necrotic skin lesions, tissue infarction, wound infections, and brain abscesses.

4. **Diagnostic Studies**
   - In an immunocompetent host, isolation of organism from sputum, burn eschar, ear canal debris, or other areas usually does not indicate disease or require treatment.
   - In allergic bronchopulmonary aspergillosis, transient or migratory upper lobe pulmonary infiltrates appear; patients have eosinophilia, markedly elevated levels of total serum immunoglobulin (Ig) E, and high titers of anti-*Aspergillus* antibodies.
   - For sinusitis, diagnosis is usually based on histology following surgery.
   - Specific IgG antibody testing is not helpful in diagnosing disseminated *Aspergillus* in compromised hosts because of immunosuppression.
   - Detection of galactomannan by enzyme-linked immunosorbent assay (ELISA) or polymerase chain reaction (PCR) in serum or other body fluid samples is useful for diagnosis and treatment.
   - Computed tomography (CT) scanning of the chest may suggest invasive aspergillosis, but biopsy of lesions is the mainstay of diagnosis. Rounded nodular infiltrates are the most common finding on chest X-ray.

5. **Management**
   - Allergic bronchopulmonary aspergillosis usually responds to tapered corticosteroid therapy, postural drainage, and chest physiotherapy. Voriconazole is increasingly being used, but itraconazole is the best-studied agent.
   - Sinusitis requires a prolonged course of antifungal agents following surgical debridement in immunocompromised patients.
   - Surgical resection is the treatment of choice for symptomatic aspergilloma.
   - Chronic necrotizing pulmonary aspergillosis may require surgery in addition to antifungals.
   - Severe invasive or disseminated aspergillosis is treated with voriconazole and a lipid formulation of amphotericin B. The mortality rate for invasive disease is high, particularly in patients with refractory neutropenia.
   - Any underlying disease should be treated.

6. **Prevention**
   - Elimination of environmental exposure and prophylactic antifungal therapy is indicated in immunosuppressed and neutropenic patients.

B. **Blastomycosis**
1. **Etiology**
   - *Blastomyces dermatitidis*, a dimorphic fungus, occurs as a mold in nature and as a yeast in tissue.
   - Infection usually occurs in immunocompetent men involved in outdoor activities in proximity to waterways.
   - The fungus is endemic and limited to areas of south central and Midwestern United States and Canada.
2. **Pathology**
   - Infection is believed to occur from inhalation of fungus from rotting wood or soil.
   - Pulmonary infection is most common; hematogenous dissemination is most likely to affect bone, skin, and genitourinary system.
   - Infection rates are high in endemic areas, but symptomatic disease occurs in only about 50% of infected individuals.
3. **Clinical Features**
   - Disease may be acute or chronic.
   - Dry cough, dyspnea, headache, and fever may resemble influenza or pneumonia.
   - Symptoms may resolve or progress to productive cough, hemoptysis, pleuritic pain, weight loss, and prostration resembling a bacterial pneumonia.
   - Verrucous, crusted, or ulcerated cutaneous lesions expand and may leave a central scar with healing.
   - Ribs and vertebrae are most frequently involved in disseminated bone disease.
   - Symptoms suggesting prostatitis or epididymitis are common.
4. **Diagnostic Studies**
   - Nonspecific laboratory findings include leukocytosis and anemia.
   - Sputum, pus, cerebrospinal fluid (CSF), or tissue analysis reveals readily culture and grow thick walled cells (5–20 mcm) with single broad-based bud.
   - An available urinary antigen test has considerable cross-reactivity with *Histoplasma*, so its utility is not clear.
   - Chest X-ray findings are variable and nonspecific.
5. **Management**
   - Itraconazole is the treatment of choice for non-meningeal disease.
   - Amphotericin B is used for severe or rapidly progressing illness, treatment failures, AIDS-related, and central nervous system (CNS) disease.
6. **Prevention**
   - Patient education and awareness in endemic areas.

C. **Coccidioidomycosis**
1. **Etiology**
   - *Coccidioides immitis* or *Coccidioides posadasii*, soil molds that grow in arid regions of southwestern United States, Mexico, and Central and South America.
   - *C. immitis* is a possible agent for bioterrorism.
2. **Pathology**
   - Inhalation of highly infectious arthroconidia, the hyphae of the mold form.
   - Coccidioidomycosis is a common opportunistic infection in persons living with human immunodeficiency virus (HIV) who reside in endemic areas.
3. **Clinical Features**
   - Primary disease occurs in about 40% of infections and resembles respiratory tract infection with nasopharyngitis, bronchitis, fever, chills, cough, headache, and pleuritic pain.
   - Pain and swelling of the knees and ankles are common; erythema nodosum may also occur.
   - Persistent pulmonary cavitations, abscesses, nodules, or bronchiectasis occurs in about 5%.
4. **Diagnostic Studies**
   - The mold form is highly contagious and must be clearly labeled, so laboratory personnel do not become infected.
   - Diagnosis is established by tube precipitin test and immunodiffusion test to detect IgM antibodies.
   - Serial serologic (complement fixation) titers assess dissemination of disease and treatment; in HIV-infected patients, the false-negative rate is high.
   - Meningitis is diagnosed with CSF complement-fixing antibodies; CSF also shows lymphocytosis and reduced glucose.
   - Imaging may show pulmonary infiltrates, cavitation, hilar or mediastinal lymphadenopathy, pleural effusions, and lytic bone lesions.
5. **Management**
   - Most cases are asymptomatic and self-limited; localized lung disease is treated symptomatically.
   - Use of amphotericin B, itraconazole, fluconazole, or ketoconazole depends on the severity of disease.
   - Fluconazole is used to treat most patients with CNS disease, although intrathecal amphotericin B, voriconazole, or posaconazole may be used.
6. **Prevention**
   - Patient education and awareness in endemic areas.

D. **Cryptococcosis**
1. **Etiology**
   - *Cryptococcus neoformans*, a large, thick-walled, encapsulated budding yeast.
   - *Cryptococcus gattii* also causes disease in humans, primarily outside North America.
2. **Pathology**
   - *C. neoformans* is present in pigeon and other bird droppings and soil.

- Infection is acquired through inhalation, causing lung disease that may be localized, self-healing, or disseminated.
- Immunocompetent persons rarely develop clinical disease, but patients with hematologic malignancies, Hodgkin disease, chronic steroid use, HIV infection, or other immunodeficiency states do. It is the most common life-threatening fungal infection in AIDS patients and the third most common CNS infection in these patients.

3. **Clinical Features**
   - Disseminated cryptococcosis may affect any organ system, but the CNS is most common.
   - Onset may be acute or insidious; the more immunosuppressed the patient, the more rapid the onset.
   - In cases of CNS involvement, headache is usually the first symptom of meningoencephalitis, followed by a varying course of confusion, irritability, or dizziness appearing over weeks or months without pattern.
   - Behavioral changes, fever, seizures, cranial nerve palsies, papilledema, dementia, and decreased level of consciousness may appear later.
   - Pulmonary infections are often asymptomatic with minimum sputum production.
   - Skin and bone may be involved in disseminated disease.

4. **Diagnostic Studies**
   - Ninety-five percent of patients with HIV and solid organ transplant will show a positive result for a serum antigen test; the test is also 95% sensitive for cryptococcal meningitis in screening these patients.
   - Lumbar puncture is essential and demonstrates increased opening pressure, variable pleocytosis, increased protein, and usually decreased glucose; demonstration of *C. neoformans* by direct examination or cultural isolation from CSF or other infected sites is definitive.
   - CT or magnetic resonance imaging (MRI) of the head is indicated for papilledema or focal neurologic signs and may demonstrate cryptococcoma or hydrocephalus; MRI is more sensitive.

5. **Management**
   - Initial treatment with amphotericin B and flucytosine followed by fluconazole is the treatment of choice.
   - Hydrocephalus or high CSF pressures require ventricular shunting or repeated lumbar punctures.
   - Maintenance therapy with fluconazole prevents relapse.

6. **Prevention**
   - Immunosuppressed patients should avoid dried bird droppings.

E. **Histoplasmosis**
   1. **Etiology**
      - *Histoplasma capsulatum* is a dimorphic fungus found in soil contaminated with bat or bird droppings in many areas of the world, especially the in Ohio and Mississippi River valleys.
   2. **Pathology**
      - Infection is acquired by inhalation of spores. Spores convert to budding cells in lungs, proliferate, and spread through the bloodstream and lymphatics.
   3. **Clinical Features**
      - Most cases in immunocompetent patients are asymptomatic or mild; primary histoplasmosis typically resembles influenza.
      - Acute histoplasmosis, often epidemic, lasts 1 to 6 weeks and is characterized by fever and prostration. Findings on chest radiography may show diffuse pneumonia, but patients have few lung symptoms.
      - Progressive disseminated histoplasmosis involves all body organs and is usually fatal. Findings include fever, dyspnea, weight loss, cough, prostration, hepatosplenomegaly, oropharyngeal ulcers, and bloody diarrhea. Adrenal involvement occasionally leads to adrenal insufficiency.
      - Chronic progressive pulmonary histoplasmosis occurs primarily in older patients with chronic obstructive pulmonary disease.
      - Disseminated disease in severely immunocompromised patients may resemble septic shock.
      - Disseminated histoplasmosis is an AIDS-defining illness in persons with a positive HIV test.
   4. **Diagnostic Studies**
      - Anemia of chronic disease is common in patients with progressive lung disease.
      - Pancytopenia and elevations of alkaline phosphatase, lactate dehydrogenase (LDH), and transferrin occur in disseminated disease.
      - Sputum culture is rarely positive in acute disease; antigen testing of fluid obtained by bronchoalveolar lavage may be helpful.
      - In immunocompromised patients, bone marrow and blood culture results are usually positive.
      - In AIDS patients with disseminated disease, a urine antigen assay is >90% sensitive; a combination of screening immunodiffusion and complement fixation titers is also helpful.
   5. **Management**
      - In limited disease, spontaneous resolution may occur.
      - Itraconazole in oral solution is recommended for local or mild-to-moderate disseminated disease and for secondary prevention in those with AIDS.
      - Amphotericin B is the treatment of choice for the severely ill, immunocompromised patient and patients with life-threatening or CNS disease.

6. **Prevention**
   - Patient education and awareness in endemic areas; avoidance of areas with droppings.

II. Protozoal Diseases

A. Amebiasis

1. **Etiology**
   - *Entamoeba histolytica*: this must be distinguished from the nearly identical *Entamoeba dispar*, which produces an asymptomatic carrier state.
   - *E. histolytica* exists as cysts and motile trophozoites; cysts remain viable in soil and water for weeks to months.
   - In the United States, most cases are in immigrants from and travelers to developing nations; U.S. rates are higher in communal living facilities, day-care centers, and men who have sex with men.
   - Humans are the only hosts; person-to-person transmission can occur, and flying insects are vectors.

2. **Pathology**
   - The amoeba lives as a commensal in most infected persons, and the host serves as a carrier. Amebic dysentery is acquired by ingestion of cysts present in contaminated food or water; excystation occurs in the small intestine; trophozoites become established in the lumen of the large intestine where they encyst.
   - Trophozoites invade intestinal epithelium, causing characteristic ulcers, most commonly found in the cecum, descending colon, and rectosigmoid area, but may occur anywhere in the colon or terminal ileum.
   - The liver is the primary site of extraintestinal amebic disease, where typically a single abscess up to 15 cm diameter may form, usually in the upper right lobe; trophozoites may disseminate into lung, pleural cavity, and pericardium, and through bloodstream to brain.

3. **Clinical Features**
   - Following an incubation period of 2 to 4 weeks, some patients have acute diarrhea; however, symptoms range from none or mild to severe colitis.
   - In dysenteric colitis, early stools are watery with streaks of blood, and later with blood and necrotic tissue; patient may have high fever, abdominal cramping and tenderness, nausea and vomiting, and tenesmus.
   - Hepatic amebiasis includes development of fever, pain, and tender enlargement of the liver.
   - Other areas are rarely involved, but include skin, lungs, brain, and genitalia.

4. **Diagnostic Studies**
   - Identification of *E. histolytica* in feces microscopically and stool antigen detection is standard; serologic assays are fairly sensitive after the initial stage of disease.
   - Colonoscopy (without bowel preparation) will identify characteristic ulcers and allow collection of exudates for identification of trophozoites.
   - Ultrasonography, CT, or MRI is used to identify hepatic abscess.

5. **Management**
   - Choice of amebicides is based on location and severity of infection.
   - Metronidazole and tinidazole both eradicate amebiasis in the bowel lumen, the bowel tissue, and other tissues; diloxanide furoate, iodoquinol, and paromomycin eradicate disease in the bowel lumen.
   - Combination treatment is most effective.

6. **Prevention**
   - Adequate disposal of human feces, and water sanitation and careful handwashing are essential.
   - Travelers can minimize infection risk by drinking bottled water and by avoiding consumption of unpeeled fruits and vegetables.
   - Amebic cysts are not killed by chlorine; boiling water or treating with iodine or filtering usually ensures the absence of amoebae.

B. Giardiasis

1. **Etiology**
   - *Giardia lamblia*, a large flagellated protozoan with both trophozoite and cyst forms.
   - *Giardia* is the most common cause of epidemic waterborne diarrheal disease in the United States; is the most frequently identified intestinal protozoan in the United States and Europe.
   - It is seen frequently in daycare centers, residential facilities, and, increasingly, in food-borne outbreaks.

2. **Pathology**
   - The organism occurs in feces as a flagellated trophozoite and as a cyst.
   - Only the cyst form is infectious by the oral route through contaminated food or water, person-to-person contact, and anal–oral sexual contact. Trophozoites are destroyed by gastric acidity.
   - After the cysts are ingested, trophozoites emerge in the duodenum and jejunum, and exist as a flagellated trophozoite or cyst in the stool.

3. **Clinical Features**
   - Most infected persons are asymptomatic and clear the infection spontaneously.
   - **Three symptomatic syndromes occur:**
     - Acute diarrhea, usually mild, with copious, frothy, greasy, foul-smelling stools without blood or pus.
     - Chronic diarrhea is similar, may be daily or recurrent, and may be accompanied by weight loss; growth and cognitive development may be slowed in children. Less common symptoms include loss of appetite, nausea, vomiting, cramping, belching, flatulence, and distension.

- Malabsorption syndromes may develop with either chronic or acute diarrheal syndromes.

4. **Diagnostic Testing**
   - Obtaining three stool specimens at 2-day intervals increases the likelihood of detection of cysts and trophozoites by microscopy.
   - Antigen assays are simpler and less expensive than serial stool examinations, but will not identify other pathogens.
   - Occasionally, duodenal aspiration, endoscopic brush cytology, or duodenal biopsy is indicated.

5. **Management**
   - In adults, the treatment of choice is either tinidazole or metronidazole. Tinidazole and furazolidone are safe in pregnancy.
   - In children, furazolidone or nitazoxanide is used.

6. **Prevention**
   - Filtration of water is necessary to eliminate cysts; boiling is also effective.
   - Careful handwashing and separation of food-preparation and diaper-changing tasks in daycare centers are needed.
   - Education about safer sex practices.

C. **Malaria**
   1. **Etiology**
      - *Plasmodium falciparum*, *Plasmodium vivax*, *Plasmodium ovale*, and *Plasmodium malariae* all infect humans, with *P. falciparum* and *P. vivax* causing most disease; malaria is endemic in most tropical and subtropical areas.
      - *P. falciparum* predominates in Africa, Haiti, and the Dominican Republic; it causes most deaths.
      - Malaria is the most important tropical parasitic disease of humans with more than 1 million deaths annually.
   2. **Pathology**
      - Infected female anopheles mosquitoes transmit the disease from person to person; congenital and blood transfusion transmission also occurs.
      - **The three typical courses of disease are explained by the protozoan's life cycle:**
        - The mosquito ingests human blood containing gametocytes of the parasite, which develop into sporozoites in the mosquito's salivary glands.
        - The mosquito inoculates humans with sporozoites, which travel to the liver (exoerythrocytic stage), where they transform into merozoites in the hepatic cells.
        - The merozoites are released into the bloodstream and infect red blood cells (RBCs; erythrocytic stage).
        - In the RBCs, the merozoites undergo schizogamy, resulting in two asexual and two sexual forms; mature sexual forms infect other red blood cells, repeating the cycle.

- Recurring asexual cycles occur until host immunity stops the erythrocytic cycle.
- In *P. vivax* and *P. ovale*, dormant hepatic sporozoites may resume intrahepatic multiplication, which leads to relapses or delayed primary infection for up to 6 to 8 months.
- Recrudescent disease is recurrence due to the failure of treatment to eradicate infected RBCs.
- *P. falciparum* does not produce a dormant liver stage and does not cause late relapse. *P. malariae* has no persistent liver stage; relapse occurs because of low-level persistence in the bloodstream.
- Malaria is curable if diagnosed promptly and treated adequately.

3. **Clinical Features**
   - During an attack, a typical sequence over 4 to 6 hours includes the cold stage (shaking chills), hot stage (high fever), and sweating stage (marked diaphoresis). Patients feel well between attacks.
   - Attacks may occur every other day or every third day; following the primary attack, latent periods and recurrences are common.
   - Hepatosplenomegaly is common.
   - *P. falciparum* causes the most serious infection, with high fever, changes in level of consciousness, agitation, prostration, bleeding, and hyperventilation; complications include hypotension, shock, headache, retinal hemorrhages, convulsions, delirium, coma, mental status changes, pulmonary edema, acute tubular necrosis, renal failure, jaundice, cardiac arrhythmias, hypoglycemia, dysentery, electrolyte imbalance, and disseminated intravascular coagulation (DIC).
   - "Blackwater fever" refers to dark urine due to severe hemolysis following treatment with quinine.

4. **Diagnostic Studies**
   - Thick and thin blood films from serial finger- or earlobe-stick blood specimens obtained every 8 hours for 3 days demonstrate parasites; repeated blood films confirm success of treatment.
   - Rapid antigen detection methods are increasingly available and are nearly as sensitive and specific as blood smear analysis.
   - During attacks, leukocytosis may develop, followed by leukopenia with increased monocytes. Patients may also have thrombocytopenia, anemia, and liver function abnormalities.

5. **Management**
   - Successful treatment requires destruction of all forms of parasite.
   - Chloroquine is the mainstay of treatment for non-falciparum and for nonresistant falciparum malarias; quinine and quinidine remain effective for all malaria, but are poorly tolerated.
   - In resistant areas, treatments include artemether-lumefantrine,

artesunate-amodiaquine, artesunate-mefloquine, amodiaquine-sulfadoxine-pyrimethamine, and dihydroartemisinin-piperaquine.

- Combination therapy may slow spread of drug-resistant malaria; artemisinin derivatives are usually included.
- For *P. vivax* and *P. ovale*, primaquine prevents relapse; it eradicates dormant liver forms of all species.
- Other options include atovaquone plus proguanil (Malarone), tetracycline and doxycycline, clindamycin, azithromycin, halofantrine, and lumefantrine.

6. Prevention
- Avoid contact with mosquito vector (use protective clothing, insect repellent, and mosquito netting, besides avoiding endemic areas).
- Chemoprophylaxis depends on resistance patterns; chloroquine is preferred in nonresistant areas.
- Malarone, mefloquine, or doxycycline in resistant areas, but no prophylaxis is 100% effective.

D. Toxoplasmosis
1. Etiology
- *Toxoplasma gondii*, an obligate intracellular parasite, exists in three forms: the disease-causing trophozoite, the latent cyst, and the infective sporozoite-containing oocysts.
- Cat species, the definitive hosts, excrete oocysts in feces; these remain infective in moist soil for months to years.

2. Pathology
- Humans become infected by ingesting cysts from raw/undercooked meat, ingesting oocysts from contaminated food or water, handling cat litter carelessly, from transplacental, blood transfusion, or organ-transplantation transmission of trophozoites.
- Once ingested, bradyzoites from cysts or sporozoites from oocysts invade different types of cells, propagate as trophozoites, and cause cell death and inflammation.
- Incubation period is 7 to 14 days.

3. Clinical Features
- Initial infection is usually asymptomatic; when symptoms appear, they vary with the type of host involved.
- In a normal host, the most common manifestation is asymptomatic localized cervical lymphadenopathy; a mild infectious mononucleosis-like illness may occur.
- Manifestations of congenital toxoplasmosis vary by trimester of infection; first trimester disease is often catastrophic, resulting in abortion or stillbirth. Live-born children may demonstrate microcephaly, hydrocephaly, convulsions, psychomotor retardation, fever, hepatitis, pneumonia, and skin rash. Those infected later in pregnancy demonstrate milder disease at birth, but months later may develop epilepsy, retardation, strabismus, uveitis, or retinochoroiditis if untreated.
- In the immunocompromised host, reactivated toxoplasmosis most often affects the brain, lungs, and eye, but may affect the heart, skin, gastrointestinal (GI) tract, and the liver, or present as disseminated disease. Often, fatal encephalitis, mass lesions, and diffuse intracerebral lesions are common in patients with AIDS.
- Chronic latent infection persists in both symptomatic and asymptomatic hosts following initial infection.

4. Diagnostic Studies
- Reliable and sensitive serologic tests of blood, bone marrow, CSF, sputum, placental tissue, and others are the mainstay of diagnosis; identification of parasites in tissue or body fluids using PCR is also diagnostic.
- Chest radiographs may show interstitial pneumonia.
- In patients with HIV, CT or MRI images show multiple ring-enhancing lesions, primarily in the corticomedullary junction and basal ganglion.

5. Management
- Mild disease in immunocompetent hosts is self-limiting.
- Pyrimethamine plus sulfadiazine or clindamycin is used for severe or persistent disease; folic acid supplementation and maintenance of urinary output prevent bone marrow suppression and nephrotoxicity, respectively. Other combinations are possible.
- In immunocompromised patients, prophylaxis is indicated if serology (IgG) is positive; treatment of acute disease should be followed by continued prophylaxis.
- Pyrimethamine is teratogenic and contraindicated in first trimester of pregnancy; spiramycin is the standard therapy in pregnancy and it reduces the frequency of transmission to the fetus by about 60%.
- Spiramycin does not cross the placenta, so when fetal infection is documented or for acute infection late in pregnancy (which commonly leads to fetal transmission) treatment with combination regimens is recommended.

6. Prevention
- Careful handwashing after handling uncooked meat or working in potentially infected soil.
- Cook food to safe temperatures and clean food preparation areas and utensils thoroughly.
- Peel or wash fruits and vegetables thoroughly.

- Avoid handling cat feces, particularly changing kitty litter; scald litter pans regularly.
- Wear gloves when gardening and handling cat waste, especially if pregnant.

III. Viral Infections
A. AIDS (Tables 16–1 to 16–3)
   1. **Etiology**
      - HIV is a retrovirus. The related HIV-2 virus, found primarily in West Africans, progresses more slowly.
      - HIV is transmitted to humans by blood and less commonly body fluids (e.g., semen; cervical secretions; breast milk; CSF; and synovial, pleural, peritoneal, pericardial, and amniotic fluids); through unprotected sexual contact; blood, blood product transfusion, or organ transplantation (before routine screening); needle sharing; transplacental or perinatal infection; and occupational exposure of health care workers.
      - HIV is also present in saliva, tears, and urine, but is not transmitted through these fluids.
      - No evidence exists for spread through respiratory droplets, mosquito or other vector bites, or non-sexual contacts.

TABLE 16–1. **1993 Revised CDC HIV Classification System and Expanded AIDS Surveillance Definition for Adolescents and Adults**

CD4 Cell Category[a]	Clinical Category A	B	C	Clinical Category A	Clinical Category B	Clinical Category C
(1) ≥500/mm³	A1	B1	C1	Asymptomatic HIV infection	Symptomatic, not A or C conditions	Candidiasis: esophageal, trachea, bronchi
(2) 200–499/ mm³	A2	B2	C2	Persistent generalized lymphadenopathy	Examples include, but not limited to:	Coccidioidomycosis, extrapulmonary
(3) <200/mm³	B3	A3	C3	Acute (primary) HIV illness	Bacillary angiomatosis	Cryptococcosis, extrapulmonary
					Candidiasis, vulvovaginal: persistent >1 mo, poorly responsive to treatment	Cervical cancer, invasive
					Candidiasis, oropharyngeal	Cryptosporidiosis, chronic intestinal (>1 mo)
					Cervical dysplasia, severe or carcinoma in situ	CMV retinitis, or CMV in other than liver, spleen, nodes
					Constitutional symptoms, for example, fever (38.5° C) or diarrhea >1 mo	HIV encephalopathy
						Herpes simplex with mucocutaneous ulcer >1 mo, bronchitis, pneumonia
						Histoplasmosis, disseminated, extrapulmonary
						Isosporiasis, chronic, >1 mo
						Kaposi sarcoma
						Lymphoma, Burkitt immunoblastic primary in brain
						Mycobacterium avium or *Mycobacterium kansasii*, extrapulmonary
						Mycobacterium tuberculosis, pulmonary or extrapulmonary
						Pneumocystis carinii pneumonia
						Pneumonia, recurrent (>2 episodes in 1 y)
						Progressive multifocal leukoencephalopathy
						Salmonella bacteremia, recurrent
						Toxoplasmosis, cerebral
						Wasting syndrome due to HIV

Note: The above diseases must be attributed to HIV infection or have a clinical course or management complicated by HIV.

[a]There is a diurnal variation in CD4 counts averaging 60 per mm³ higher in the afternoon in HIV-positive patients and 500 per mm³ equivalence between CD4 counts, and CD4 percentage of total lymphocytes is ≥500 = ≥29%, 200 to 499 = 14% to 28%, and <200 = <14%.

CMV, cytomegalovirus; HIV, human immunodeficiency virus.

From Hume HD, ed. *Kelley's Essentials of Internal Medicine*. 2nd ed. Philadelphia, PA: Lippincott Williams & Wilkins; 2001:601, with permission.

TABLE 16–2.	Frequency of Symptoms and Findings Associated with Acute HIV-1 Infection in Symptomatic Patients
Symptom or Finding	**Percentage of Patients**
Fever	>80–90
Fatigue	>70–90
Rash	>40–80
Headache	32–70
Lymphadenopathy	40–70
Pharyngitis	50–70
Myalgia or arthralgia	50–70
Nausea, vomiting, or diarrhea	30–60
Night sweats	50
Aseptic meningitis	24
Oral ulcers	10–20
Genital ulcers	5–15
Thrombocytopenia	45
Leukopenia	40
Elevated hepatic-enzyme levels	21

Data from Kahn JO, Walker BD. Acute human immunodeficiency virus type 1 infection. *N Engl J Med*. 1998;339:33–39.

2. Pathology

- HIV causes immunodeficiency through viral replication within cells.
- HIV can attach to any cell with the CD4 receptor; chemokine receptors CCR5 and CXCR4 are co-receptors that are essential for viral entry.
- The CD4 (helper) cell is the primary site of infection, but HIV may also infect B lymphocytes and macrophages.
- Immunologic defects are related not only to decreasing numbers of CD4 cells but also to their inability to respond normally; autoimmunity and allergic/hypersensitivity reactions also occur.
- HIV may also cause neurologic, renal, and GI problems by direct infection of these systems.

3. Clinical Features (Figures 16–1 and 16–2)

- The mean time from exposure to HIV to development of symptoms suggesting immunodeficiency is 10 years.
- Acute HIV-1 infection presents most commonly with fever, fatigue, rash, headache, lymphadenopathy, pharyngitis, myalgias or arthralgias, nausea and vomiting or diarrhea, and night sweats; less common findings include aseptic meningitis, oral ulcers, genital ulcers, thrombocytopenia, leukopenia, and elevated hepatic enzymes.

TABLE 16–3.	Initial Evaluation of HIV-Seropositive Patients

History and physical examination

Complete blood cell count with differential and platelet counts

Serum chemistry profile

Fasting lipid profile

Urinalysis

Serologic tests

HLA-B*5701 test (if you plan on using abacavir)

Hepatitis B and C serologies

Rapid plasma reagin

Sexually transmitted disease testing

Toxoplasma gondii antibodies

Urinalysis and calculated creatinine clearance

Tuberculin skin test or interferon-γ release assay

Chest radiograph only if tuberculosis screening test is positive

Glucose-6-phosphate dehydrogenase level
The most common variant GdA⁻ is found in 10%–15% of black men and women, and Gdmed is found in men from the Mediterranean, India, and Southeast Asia.

Viral load by polymerase chain reaction

CD4⁺ lymphocyte count and percentage of total lymphocytes

HIV resistance testing

HIV, human immunodeficiency virus.
Data from Aberg JA, Gallant JE, Ghanem KG, et al. Primary care guidelines for the management of persons infected with HIV: 2013 update by the HIV medicine association of the Infectious Diseases Society of America. *Clin Infect Dis*. 2014;58(1):e1–e34.

- Findings highly specific for HIV infection include hairy leukoplakia of the tongue, disseminated Kaposi sarcoma, and cutaneous bacillary angiomatosis.
- Generalized lymphadenopathy is common in early HIV infection.
- Many HIV-positive patients have persistent fever, night sweats, and weight loss even without the presence of opportunistic infection.

4. Diagnostic Studies

- HIV ELISA screens for HIV infection; 95% of infected persons test positive within 6 weeks of infection.
- Results of HIV ELISA must be confirmed with Western blot testing; together these tests are 99.9% specific.
- ELISA and Western Blot are no longer standard of care for diagnosis.
- Fourth-generation HIV testing includes p24 antigen in addition to antibody testing and, if reactive, a follow up test to differentiate HIV-1 and HIV-2.

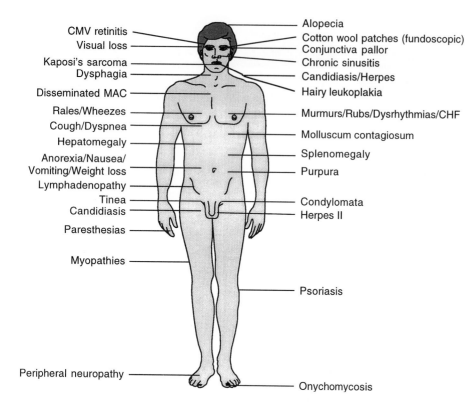

FIGURE 16–1. Spectrum of HIV (front view). CHF, congestive heart failure; CMV, cytomegalovirus; MAC, *Mycobacterium avium* complex.

- Rapid antibody testing produces results in 10 to 20 minutes.
- Anemia, neutropenia, and thrombocytopenia are common in advanced HIV infection.
- The absolute CD4 lymphocyte count is used to predict HIV progression; <200 cells per μL strongly predicts the risk of opportunistic infection or malignancy in the absence of treatment.
- CD4 lymphocyte <14% in the absence of treatment is also strongly predictive.
- HIV viral load is the best test for the diagnosis of infection before seroconversion; it is also used to monitor disease progression and response to treatment.

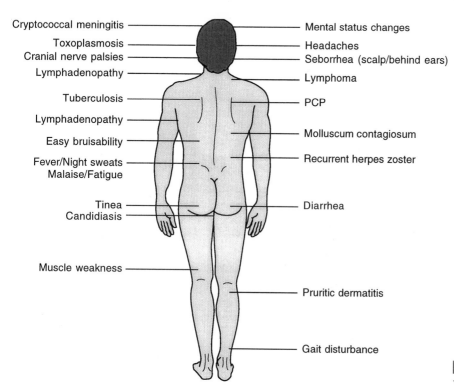

FIGURE 16–2. Spectrum of HIV (rear view). PCP, *Pneumocystis carinii* pneumonia.

5. **Management**
   - Serial viral load assessment plus CD4 counts and percentages guide therapy.
   - Management includes antiretroviral treatment, prophylaxis and treatment of opportunistic infections (INH; isoniazid for those with a positive purified protein derivative [PPD] and negative chest radiograph; flu, diphtheria tetanus [dT], pneumococcal, hepatitis A and B, human papillomavirus, haemophilus influenzae type B vaccines), and hematopoietic stimulation.
   - Initiation of antiretroviral agents is recommended for all regardless of CD4 or viral load.
   - Effective highly active antiretroviral therapies (HAARTs) are combinations of drugs from six major groups:
     - Nucleoside and nucleotide reverse transcriptase (RT) inhibitors: zidovudine, didanosine, stavudine, lamivudine, emtricitabine, abacavir, zalcitabine, and tenofovir; didanosine, zalcitabine, stavudine, and lamivudine are associated with peripheral neuropathy and emtricitabine with palmar/plantar discoloration.
     - Protease inhibitors: indinavir, nelfinavir, ritonavir, saquinavir, fosamprenavir, tipranavir, lopinavir, atazanavir, and darunavir; indinavir is associated with nephrolithiasis.
     - Nonnucleoside reverse transcriptase inhibitors: nevirapine, efavirenz, delavirdine, and etravirine.
     - Fusion inhibitors: enfuvirtide.
     - Co-receptor antagonists: maraviroc.
     - Integrase inhibitor: raltegravir, elvitegravir, and dolutegravir.
   - Adherence and drug resistance are major challenges.
   - Therapy for opportunistic infections and malignancies depends on specific problem, response to HAART, prior treatment, and the development of drug allergies.
   - For *Pneumocystis pneumonia*, options include trimethoprim-sulfa, pentamidine, atovaquone, trimethoprim with dapsone, primaquine with clindamycin, and trimetrexate. Corticosteroid therapy improves the course of moderate to severe disease in a patient who presents with PaO_2 <70 mm Hg or an AA gradient >35.
   - Cryptococcal meningitis is treated with a combination of amphotericin B and flucytosine.
   - Cytomegalovirus (CMV) infection is usually treated with ganciclovir, valganciclovir, or foscarnet.
   - Toxoplasmosis is treated with sulfadiazine or clindamycin with pyrimethamine plus folinic acid.
   - Herpes simplex infections are treated with acyclovir, famciclovir, or valacyclovir; foscarnet is used in acyclovir-resistant cases.
   - *Mycobacterium avium* complex (MAC) infection is treated with a macrolide (clarithromycin or azithromycin) plus ethambutol +/− rifabutin.
   - Lymphoma is treated with combination chemotherapy; if the CNS is involved, radiation plus dexamethasone.
   - Esophageal candidiasis is treated with fluconazole.
   - Prophylaxis for opportunistic diseases is based on CD4 count, the evidence of severe immunosuppression, and the history of prior infection.

6. **Prevention**
   - Primary prevention includes a discussion about safer sexual practices, prevention of injection drug use and needle sharing, providing perinatal HIV prophylaxis to the mother and her baby, screening of blood products, and infection control processes in the health care arena; this is recommended for health care professionals who sustain needle sticks.
   - The use of emtricitabine/tenofovir disoproxil fumarate as pre-exposure prophylaxis is an effective biomedical intervention to decrease HIV acquisition.
   - The use of antiretrovirals (emtricitabine/tenofovir disoproxil fumarate with either raltegravir or dolutegravir) for occupational exposures for 28 days.
   - The variability in the viral envelope of various HIV strains hampers vaccine development.
   - Secondary prevention includes prophylaxis of opportunistic infections, PPD testing with appropriate follow-up, screening for syphilis, vaccination for pneumonia and hepatitis B, and avoidance of pathogens such as *Toxoplasma*.

B. **Hand-Foot-Mouth Disease**
   1. **Etiology**
      - Coxsackie A16 (an enveloped RNA virus) is the enterovirus implicated most frequently.
      - Coxsackie A5 and A10 and enterovirus 71 may also cause hand-foot-mouth (HFM) disease.
   2. **Pathology**
      - Humans are the major natural host; illness may represent host immunologic response to tissue injury by virus or to persistent viral antigens.
      - Transmission is by direct contact with nose, throat, discharge, or stools of infected person.
      - Most infections are subclinical.
      - HFM usually occurs in children <5 years.
   3. **Clinical Features**
      - Mild fever, decreased appetite, rhinitis, and pharyngitis begin 3 to 5 days after exposure.
      - Vesicular lesions erupt in oral cavity (chiefly on the buccal mucosa and tongue) and on the distal extremities 1 to 2 days following initial symptoms.
      - Enterovirus 71 causes four stages of disease including HFM/herpangina, CNS disease (central hypoventilation, dysphagia, limb weakness), cardiopulmonary (pulmonary edema), and convalescence.

4. **Diagnostic Studies**
   - Diagnosis is usually made clinically.
   - In acute phase of disease, diagnosis is most readily established by isolating the virus from throat swabs and vesicles; enterovirus 71 may be isolated in the CSF.
5. **Management**
   - Primarily supportive.
6. **Prevention**
   - Careful handwashing and sanitation.

C. **Infectious Mononucleosis (Mono)**
   1. **Etiology**
      - Epstein–Barr virus (EBV), an enveloped DNA virus, found as two variants (EBV-1 and -2) of human herpesvirus 4.
      - EBV infection occurs worldwide among humans and usually occurs as a subclinical infection in early childhood; 80% of adults in the United States are seropositive for EBV. The virus persists for life.
      - Infectious mononucleosis usually occurs in young adults 15 to 25 years of age, but can occur at any age.
      - In the United States and Great Britain, seroconversion occurs in half the population before 5 years of age.
   2. **Pathology**
      - The primary mode of transmission appears to be saliva, but it may also be found in genital secretions; incubation is several weeks.
      - Saliva may be infectious for 6 or months following onset of symptoms.
      - Disease results from viral replication and host immune responses to viral antigens.
      - EBV infects epithelial cells of the oropharynx and nasopharynx and disseminates to the peripheral blood lymphocytes and plasma.
   3. **Clinical Features**
      - Most early infections are asymptomatic, but prodrome of headache, malaise, and fatigue may occur.
      - In acute disease, patient has severe sore throat, fever, malaise, myalgia, and anorexia; signs include diffuse pharyngeal inflammation, edema, tonsillar exudates, and tender lymphadenopathy particularly in the posterior cervical chain; 50% of patients have splenomegaly.
      - Petechiae on the soft palate may occur; 15% of patients have a maculopapular or petechial rash; this increases to 90% or more if ampicillin is given.
      - Fever in adults may go as high as 101° to 102° F; children may be afebrile.
      - Some patients develop hepatitis, renal failure, myocarditis, mononeuropathies, aseptic meningitis, encephalitis, dyspnea, or other manifestations.
      - Complications include bacterial pharyngitis, splenic rupture, fulminant hepatitis, pericarditis, myocarditis, and, rarely, neurologic problems.

4. **Diagnostic Studies**
   - Complete blood count initially shows granulocytopenia, followed within a week by lymphocytic leukocytosis with many atypical lymphocyte; thrombocytopenia and hemolytic anemia may rarely occur.
   - Heterophile antibody tests become positive within 4 weeks of onset.
   - During acute illness, IgM to EB virus capsid antigen (VCA) rises and falls; IgG to VCA rises and persists through life. IgG antibodies to EBV nuclear antigen appear after 4 weeks and persist. PCR analysis may help in detecting illness in children.
   - Elevated hepatic aminotransferases and bilirubin are common.
5. **Management**
   - In most cases, symptomatic treatment suffices.
   - Corticosteroids are used if lymph node enlargement threatens the airway and for hemolytic anemia and severe thrombocytopenia.
   - The value of corticosteroid therapy in impending splenic rupture, pericarditis, myocarditis, and nervous system involvement is less well established.
   - Ampicillin and amoxicillin should be avoided for the treatment of coexisting streptococcal pharyngitis; penicillin or erythromycin is preferred to avoid rash.
   - Patients must avoid contact and collision sports for at least a month to prevent splenic rupture.
6. **Prevention**
   - Avoidance of sources of infected saliva; careful dishwashing.

D. **Mumps**
   1. **Etiology**
      - Paramyxovirus, an enveloped single-stranded RNA virus, is spread by respiratory droplets.
      - Mumps occurs most often in children and the incidence is highest in the spring.
   2. **Pathology**
      - Incubation period of 14 to 21 days (average 18 days) after entry into the respiratory tract and the local lymphoid tissue, where virus replicates and then disseminates to target tissues such as salivary glands, pancreas, testes and ovaries, and CNS.
      - Tissue response is that of cell necrosis, inflammation, and mononuclear cell infiltration.
   3. **Clinical Features**
      - Tender swelling of salivary glands (particularly parotids) and facial edema are the most common findings.
      - Swelling may be unilateral or bilateral and persist 7 to 10 days; the openings of Stensen's ducts may be swollen and red.
      - Fever may be minimal in small children, but high with meningitis or orchitis.

- Orchitis, usually unilateral, is the most common extrasalivary manifestation in adults; sterility is rare. Oophoritis occurs in 5% of postpubertal women.
- Mumps is the most common cause of pancreatitis in children and is suggested by upper abdominal pain, nausea, and vomiting.
- CNS complications include encephalitis, Guillain–Barré syndrome, facial palsies, and transverse myelitis, but are rare.
- Deafness from eighth nerve neuritis develops in about 0.1%; it is typically unilateral, severe, and permanent.

4. Diagnostic Studies
- The diagnosis is usually clinical, without laboratory testing.
- Early in the illness, it is possible to isolate the virus from saliva, pharynx, CSF, or duct of the affected salivary gland for culture.
- Serum IgM elevations are diagnostic, although the rise may be delayed in persons who have been immunized.
- Serum amylase elevations are due to salivary gland involvement.
- More than half of patients have mild renal function abnormalities.

5. Management
- For most patients, symptomatic treatment, light diet, and hydration suffice.
- Infectivity occurs via saliva and urine and precedes the symptoms by about 1 day and is maximal for 3 days, although it may last a week.

6. Prevention
- The Centers for Disease Control and Prevention (CDC) recommends that children get 2 doses of measles-mumps-rubella (MMR) vaccine, starting with the first dose at 12 through 15 months of age, and the second dose at 4 through 6 years of age.

E. Rabies
1. Etiology
- Rabies encephalitis is caused by a single-stranded RNA virus of the rhabdovirus group.
- Primarily a viral infection of nonhuman carnivores; in the United States, it is most common in raccoons, skunks, bats, coyotes, and foxes; outside the United States, in dogs.
- The mortality rate exceeds 90%.

2. Pathology
- The virus gains entry into the body from saliva through a bite or an open wound; the more extensive or severe the bite/wound, and the closer to the head and neck, the higher the mortality rate.
- Incubation period is usually 3 to 7 weeks, but can be 10 days to many years.
- The virus travels through the nerves to the brain where it multiplies, and then travels back through the efferent nerves to the salivary glands.

3. Clinical Features
- The prodromal stage begins as 2 to 10 days of pain at the wound site, sore throat, low-grade fever, malaise, headache, anorexia, nausea, and vomiting; hypersensitivity to temperature changes on the skin develops.
- The CNS stage is most commonly encephalitic (delirium alternating with calm), but may be paralytic, resembling Guillain–Barré syndrome. Painful laryngospasm may occur with swallowing ("hydrophobia").
- In most cases, coma, autonomic nervous system failure, and death ensue, even with supportive treatment.

4. Diagnostic Studies
- An apparently healthy biting animal must be observed in quarantine for 10 days; sick or dead animals must be tested for rabies.
- Direct fluorescent antibody staining of biopsy or necropsy tissue is the standard for diagnosis. Skin biopsy from the back of the neck is 60% to 80% sensitive.
- Reverse transcriptase–polymerase chain reaction (RT-PCR), nucleic acid sequence-based amplification, direct rapid immunohistochemical test, and viral isolation from CSF or saliva are definitive modalities.

5. Management
- Thorough cleansing and flushing of wounds with soap and water are important; animal bites should not be sutured.
- Rabies immune globulin (preferred) or antiserum should be infiltrated around the wound.
- Inactivated rabies vaccine is given in the deltoid on 0, 3, 7 and 14 days after exposure. The fifth doses at 28 days is only given to immunosuppressed patients.
- Symptomatic treatment includes respiratory support and anticonvulsants.
- The Milwaukee protocol has been helpful in a handful of patients who survived; this includes induction of coma with ketamine, midazolam, and barbiturates, along with the administration of amantadine and ribavirin.

6. Prevention
- Vaccination of domestic and wild animals and avoidance of animal bites.
- Veterinarians, animal handlers, spelunkers, laboratory workers using rabies virus, and people planning to visit countries with a high prevalence of dog rabies should undergo preexposure prophylaxis.

F. Respiratory Syncytial Virus
1. Etiology
- Pneumovirus within paramyxovirus family; enveloped virus with a single-stranded genome; produces characteristic fusion of human cells in tissue culture (syncytial effect).

- Single most important etiologic agent in respiratory diseases of infancy (in infants, major cause of pneumonia and bronchiolitis).
- Community outbreaks of disease usually occur from late fall to early spring.

2. **Pathology**
   - Of the two subtypes identified, A is implicated in more severe clinical illness.
   - Transmission of virus to respiratory tract by way of contact with infective secretions (droplet, direct contact, and fomites). Infection is confined to respiratory epithelium with progression to middle and lower airways.
   - Mortality among infants hospitalized with respiratory syncytial virus (RSV) infection is 0.5% to 1%; it rises as high as 50% in immunocompromised children.

3. **Clinical Features**
   - Two- to 8-day incubation period (average 5 days) followed by rhinorrhea and symptoms of common viral upper respiratory tract infection such as cough, pharyngitis, and hoarseness.
   - Progression of severity peaks within 1 to 3 days; fever is variable.
   - Infants may progress to bronchiolitis and pneumonitis with cough, wheezing, and respiratory distress.
   - Tachypnea, hypoxemia, and hypercapnia occur, along with interstitial infiltrates or pulmonary collapse on chest radiography.
   - Milder illness in older children and adults includes rhinorrhea, pharyngitis, tracheobronchitis, and cough. RSV can cause acute flare-ups of chronic bronchitis and trigger asthma exacerbations.
   - Symptoms usually resolve within 5 to 7 days.
   - *Streptococcus pneumoniae* otitis media is a common complication.

4. **Diagnostic Studies**
   - Immunofluorescent antibody (IFA) or ELISA tests detect viral antigen in the cytoplasm of nasopharyngeal epithelial cells; culture remains the gold standard, but PCR is used increasingly often.

5. **Management**
   - Treatment includes hydration, humidification, and ventilatory support as needed.
   - Corticosteroids, bronchodilators, and ribavirin are used in the majority of children, but controlled studies have shown that they are of limited or no benefit; pregnant women should avoid ribavirin.
   - Palivizumab, a monoclonal RSV antibody, has replaced RSV immune globulin. Infants with high-risk conditions such as heart disease should receive palivizumab.

6. **Prevention**
   - Good handwashing, barriers to protect hands and conjunctivae in settings where high rates of transmission occur, and contact isolation are important.
   - There is no vaccination available.

G. **Severe Acute Respiratory Syndrome**
1. **Etiology**
   - Caused by the virulent severe acute respiratory syndrome–associated coronavirus (SARS-CoV).
   - The primary mode of transmission appears to be respiratory droplet and fomite contact with mucous membranes of the mouth, nose, or eyes.
   - SARS has been traced to a health care worker in China in 2002, with rapid spread to Hong Kong, Singapore, Taiwan, Vietnam, and Toronto; now seen in 30 countries, including in the United States.

2. **Pathology**
   - SARS is an atypical pneumonia that may be asymptomatic, mild, moderate, or severe, and is found in persons of all ages.
   - The incubation period is 2 to 7 days; spread to contacts of patients occurs for up to 10 days.

3. **Clinical Features**
   - Persistent fever (>100.4° F) is usually accompanied by chills, rigors, cough, shortness of breath, rales, and rhonchi. Headache, malaise, myalgia, and sore throat are common.
   - Watery diarrhea may occur late in the disease.
   - In elderly patients, the only findings may be malaise and delirium.

4. **Diagnostic Studies**
   - Chest radiographic findings may be normal or nonspecific; high-resolution computed radiography scan is likely to show ground-glass opacifications or focal consolidations.
   - RT-PCR test result for SARS-CoV in urine, stool, and nasal secretion is often negative early in the disease, but variably positive by day 14. Stool is most likely to test positive; serum serologies may not be positive for 3 weeks.
   - Leukopenia and lymphopenia are common; many patients have low-grade DIC.
   - Arterial oxygen saturation is usually <95%.

5. **Management**
   - Suspected cases should be reported to state health departments.
   - Intensive supportive treatment may be required.
   - Evidence for the use of corticosteroids, ribavirin, interferon 1, and systemic steroids is not definitive.

6. **Prevention**
   - Clinicians evaluating suspected cases should use standard respiratory precautions.
   - Family members and health care workers caring for a SARS patient should use standard infection control precautions and respiratory isolation.

H. West Nile Fever

1. **Etiology**
   - The West Nile virus (WNV) is a *flavivirus* (an arbovirus) that causes encephalitis in humans. It is the leading cause of domestically acquired arboviral disease in the United States.

2. **Pathology**
   - Infected mosquitoes are the primary vectors; birds are the main reservoir of infection.
   - Person-to-person transmission may occur through blood transfusion, organ transplantation, transplacental transmission, and, possibly, breast milk.
   - First reported in North America in 1999 in New York City area, WNV is found in the entire United States. The homeless appear to be particularly susceptible.
   - Outbreaks tend to occur in late summer and early fall.

3. **Clinical Features**
   - The incubation period is 2 to 14 days. Most infected people are asymptomatic; 20% develop a flu-like illness (fever, sore throat, headache, fatigue, malaise, nausea, and vomiting), typically lasting 3 to 6 days.
   - Less than one-third of patients develop a roseolar or maculopapular rash on the face and trunk.
   - The most common neurologic signs are stiff neck and mental status changes; 10% of patients develop flaccid paralysis, about 5% seizures. Muscle weakness reminiscent of Guillain–Barré syndrome is common.
   - Young patients tend to develop the febrile syndrome, adult's aseptic meningitis, and elderly encephalitis. Elderly patients have the greatest mortality.

4. **Diagnostic Studies**
   - IgM capture ELISA can be done on serum or CSF for diagnosis.
   - Acute and convalescent IgM antibody titers may confirm acute infection.
   - PCR testing was introduced in 2003 for blood donor screening.

5. **Management**
   - Intensive supportive measures are the only treatment. Intravenous Ig or interferon α is possibly effective.
   - West Nile meningitis and encephalitis are reportable diseases.

6. **Prevention**
   - No human arbovirus vaccine is available.
   - Mosquito control is essential, including drainage of standing water.
   - Use of insect repellent with DEET (*N, N*-diethyl-meta-toluamide); wearing long-sleeved shirts, long pants, and socks; and avoiding outdoor activities between dusk and dawn when mosquitoes are most prevalent are helpful.

IV. Bacterial Diseases

A. Anthrax

1. **Etiology**
   - *Bacillus anthracis.*
   - Spore-forming, aerobic, gram-positive rod; the spores are the infectious form of the organism.
   - Naturally occurring disease, found in sheep and goats, cattle, horses, and pigs; human disease is rare, caused by inhalation or ingestion of spores, contact with infected animals or their products, or soil inoculation.
   - Anthrax is a category A bioterrorism threat.

2. **Pathology**
   - Spores germinate into vegetative bacteria that multiply locally in the skin or GI tract or disseminate to cause systemic disease; inhaled spores are ingested by pulmonary macrophages and are carried to the regional lymph nodes before they germinate. The bacteria rapidly multiply within the lymphatics, causing a hemorrhagic lymphadenitis.
   - Invasion of the bloodstream leads to overwhelming sepsis, leading to death of the host.
   - Plasmid pXO1 encodes genes for lethal toxin, responsible for shock syndrome, and edema toxin, responsible for prominent edema in cutaneous anthrax. pXO2 encodes genes for capsule production, which protects bacteria from immune defenses.

3. **Clinical Features**
   - Cutaneous anthrax (most common) occurs within 2 weeks of exposure, beginning with a small, inflamed pruritic papule resembling an insect bite. This ulcerates and undergoes necrosis developing a black painless eschar surrounded by edema and vesicles. In severe cases of cutaneous anthrax, regional tender lymphadenopathy, fever, headache, malaise, nausea, and vomiting may occur.
   - Inhalational anthrax (<5% of cases) has a biphasic clinical pattern with an initial 1- to 3-day period of fever, malaise, dry cough, substernal pressure beginning about 10 days after exposure. The second, fulminant phase begins suddenly, typically progressing to death from sepsis in 1 to 2 days.
   - GI anthrax has not been reported in the United States; it follows ingestion of insufficiently cooked contaminated meat. Patients have oral–pharyngeal or abdominal syndromes.

4. **Diagnostic Studies**
   - Culture of skin lesion, blood, pleural fluid, or CSF reveals typical organisms (chains of "box-car" encapsulated rods).
   - Other tests are available through the CDC.
   - Mediastinal widening on chest radiography is a hallmark of inhalational disease.

5. **Management**
   - Ciprofloxacin is the drug of choice; doxycycline is also first line. Other agents include amoxicillin,

penicillin G, rifampin, clindamycin, clarithromycin, erythromycin, vancomycin, and imipenem. Combination therapy is recommended in many cases.

6. Prevention
- In case of an outbreak, prophylaxis consists of ciprofloxacin or doxycycline for 100 days or vaccination with an investigational agent and 40 days of antibiotic.
- Existing stores of an approved vaccination are reserved for military personnel and others at high risk for exposure to spores.
- Patients with draining lesions should be placed in contact isolation.

B. Botulism
1. Etiology
- *Clostridium botulinum*, a spore-forming anaerobic bacillus found in soil, produces a neurotoxin that causes paralysis by preventing the release of acetylcholine at neuromuscular junctions and autonomic synapses.
- Toxin types A, B, E, and F cause human disease.
- Botulism occurs in food-borne, infant, and wound forms; infant form is associated with ingestion of honey and wound form with injecting drug use (usually contaminated heroin).

2. Pathology
- The botulinum exotoxin binds to the synapses of motor neurons and inhibits the release of the neurotransmitter acetylcholine.

3. Clinical Features
- Symptoms begin within 72 hours of ingestion of the toxin and may progress for several days. Typically, diplopia, loss of accommodation, and other visual changes occur, followed by ptosis, cranial nerve palsies, and fixed and dilated pupils.
- Most frequent symptoms in food-borne botulism are dysphagia, dry mouth, dysarthria, fatigue, upper extremity weakness, constipation, lower extremity weakness, dyspnea, nausea and vomiting, and dizziness; respiratory dysfunction may occur from upper airway obstruction or respiratory weakness.
- Paralysis, respiratory failure, and death occur.

4. Diagnostic Studies
- The diagnosis should be thought about with the development of sudden, fluctuating, and severe weakness in a previously healthy person with a history of ingestion of home-canned food or honey.
- Demonstration of botulinum toxin in the patient's serum or feces or in the suspected food source using a mouse toxin-neutralization test confirms the diagnosis.

5. Management
- Patients should be admitted to an intensive care unit for intubation and monitoring and support of respiratory and cardiac function.

- State or federal health officials can assist in obtaining antitoxin to neutralized unabsorbed toxin.
- Prompt diagnosis decreases chance of death; full recovery may take 3 months to 1 year.

6. Prevention
- Maintenance of food at an acid pH; storage at <4° C; thorough heating before serving.
- Careful home canning.
- Infants should not eat honey.

C. Brucellosis
1. Etiology
- *Brucella* species (aerobic, slow-growing, non-motile, facultative intracellular gram-negative coccobacilli).
- The most common animal vectors are cattle, hogs, and goats.
- Rare in the United States, it is endemic in Mexico, the Mediterranean lands, Spain, and South America.
- Pulmonary forms of brucellosis are a category B (see section VIII) bioterrorist threat.

2. Pathology
- Transmission to humans is usually from handling of infected tissues or ingestion of infected unpasteurized milk and cheese.

3. Clinical Features
- Onset may be abrupt, with fever, chills, and sweats.
- Insidious onset is more common; patients experience low-grade fever, weakness, myalgia, arthralgia, headache, anorexia, weight loss, and easy exhaustion.
- Undulant fever occurs in chronic disease, with intermittent periods of normal temperature between episodes.
- Hepatosplenomegaly and lymphadenopathy are common.
- Complications include endocarditis, meningitis, encephalitis, epididymitis, orchitis, osteoarticular disease with septic arthritis, sacroiliitis, spondylitis, or osteomyelitis.

4. Diagnostic Studies
- *Brucella* species may be recovered from the culture of blood, bone marrow, CSF, urine, and other sites.
- Serum agglutination titer or rising serum titers are the usual means of diagnosis.

5. Management
- Single-drug regimens are not recommended because the relapse rates are high.
- Doxycycline plus rifampin or streptomycin or gentamicin is recommended.
- Postexposure prophylaxis is reserved for cases of febrile illness or accidental veterinary vaccine inoculation.

6. Prevention
- Eliminating livestock disease through vaccination, pasteurization of milk, and use of universal precautions are effective preventive measures.

- No human vaccine is available.
- Because brucellosis is the most common laboratory-acquired infection, laboratories should use BL-3 safety measures.

D. Campylobacter Dysentery
1. **Etiology**
   - *Campylobacter jejuni* is one of the most common causes of gastroenteritis worldwide.
   - Comma-shaped gram-negative rods commonly occur in pairs.
2. **Pathology**
   - Infection occurs with ingestion of contaminated water, raw milk, and food (especially poultry).
   - *C. jejuni* colonizes the jejunum where it elaborates an enterotoxin.
   - Three to 5 days after ingestion, overt disease occurs if organism penetrates and invades epithelial cells.
3. **Clinical Features**
   - Abrupt onset of watery diarrhea with occasional abdominal cramping relieved by defecation, plus pain, malaise, and fever.
   - Grossly bloody, loose, or watery stools occur in nearly half of patients.
   - Although frequently self-limiting, it can last more than 1 week in 10% to 20% of patients; relapse occurs in 5% to 10% of untreated patients.
4. **Diagnostic Studies**
   - Dark-field or phase contrast microscopy identifies gram-negative, S- or seagull-shaped bacteria in watery, bloody, leukocyte-filled feces.
   - Stool culture confirms the diagnosis.
5. **Management**
   - Course of disease may be shortened with treatment and is indicated in patients with high fevers, bloody stools, worsening symptoms, or unrelenting defecation.
   - Azithromycin and ciprofloxacin are both effective.
   - Fluoroquinolone resistance has been increasing, so susceptibility testing should be performed before its use.
   - Fluid and electrolyte replacement is important.
6. **Prevention**
   - Cook food, especially poultry, thoroughly and wash hands frequently.
   - Ingest only pasteurized milk; wash fruits and vegetables before use.

E. Cat-Scratch Disease
1. **Etiology**
   - *Bartonella henselae*.
2. **Pathology**
   - Cat-scratch disease is primarily found in children and young adults.
   - The major arthropod vector is the cat flea, which is responsible for cat-to-cat transmission.
   - Transmission to humans occurs through scratch, bite, or other contact with infected secretions.
3. **Clinical Features**
   - A papule or ulcer may develop within days at the inoculation site.
   - Low-grade fever, headache, and vague and generalized aches and pains follow in 1 to 3 weeks.
   - Enlarged tender regional nodes develop 1 to 7 weeks after inoculation and slowly regress within 2 to 4 months; some may suppurate.
   - In HIV-positive persons, disseminated disease (bacillary angiomatosis, peliosis hepatis) occurs.
4. **Diagnostic Studies**
   - Diagnosis is usually based on history and physical examination.
5. **Management**
   - Cat-scratch disease is usually self-limited in immunocompetent persons; macrolides or doxycyclines are used in the immunosuppressed.
6. **Prevention**
   - Avoidance of cat scratches.

F. Cholera
1. **Etiology**
   - *Vibrio cholerae* is a slightly curved gram-negative rod that elaborates an exotoxin (enterotoxin). The disease is toxin-mediated.
   - Only serogroups O1 and O139 are associated with cholera.
   - Cholera occurs in epidemics in conditions of poor sanitation and crowding in warm seasons.
2. **Pathology**
   - Organisms that survive stomach and upper intestinal acidity attach to microvilli of brush border of epithelial cells of jejunum and ileum, where they multiply and liberate cholera enterotoxin and mucinase, but do not invade the mucosa.
   - The enterotoxin produces changes leading to massive hypersecretion of water and chloride ions, resulting in up to 15 L of diarrhea daily. Death results from hypovolemia.
3. **Clinical Features**
   - Onset of symptoms is characterized by abrupt, painless, voluminous, watery diarrhea that may lead to several liters of fluid loss within a few hours; if uncontrolled, this may lead to profound shock; vomiting may follow or precede diarrhea; fever is rarely present.
   - Stools are gray and without fecal odor, blood, or pus ("rice water stool").
   - Patient may be cyanotic with sunken eyes and cheeks, scaphoid abdomen, poor skin turgor, and thready or absent peripheral pulses reflecting hypotension and dehydration.
4. **Diagnostic Studies**
   - Stool culture or agglutination studies.

5. Management
- Oral or intravenous fluid replacement is the basis of treatment.
- Antibiotic administration will shorten the course of the disease, but multiple drug-resistant strains are increasingly encountered, so susceptibility testing, if available, is advisable.

6. Prevention
- Avoidance of endemic areas.
- A vaccine is available, but provides only short-term protection, and it is not useful in managing outbreaks.
- Clean water and food and appropriate sanitation are the most effective prevention.

G. Diphtheria
1. Etiology
- *Corynebacterium diphtheriae* is a small pleomorphic gram-positive rod.
- Rare in the United States.
- Humans are the only known reservoir for *C. diphtheriae*.

2. Pathology
- The organism is spread by respiratory secretions and usually affects the respiratory tract, but may involve any mucous membrane or skin wound.
- *C. diphtheriae* produces a potent exotoxin that causes an inflammatory response and the formation of a pseudomembrane on the respiratory mucosa; it is also absorbed by the circulatory system and distributed throughout the body.
- Exotoxin also inhibits protein synthesis, which can damage the kidneys, heart, and nerves.
- Death is due to either aspiration of membrane or diphtheria's toxigenic effect on the heart.

3. Clinical Features
- Diphtheria occurs in nasal, laryngeal, pharyngeal, and cutaneous forms; pharyngeal is most common.
- After an incubation of 2 to 4 days, pharyngitis or tonsillitis, malaise, fever, and adenitis develop.
- Dense gray-white "pseudomembrane" in oropharynx may extend to larynx and trachea; scraping discloses intense underlying inflammation and edema.
- In mild cases, infection resolves and the membrane is coughed up after 5 to 10 days.
- Most common serious complications are myocarditis and neuropathies.

4. Diagnostic Studies
- Diagnosis is made clinically, but *C. diphtheriae* can be cultured on selective media from infected site.

5. Management
- Immediate administration of diphtheria antitoxin (available from the CDC) neutralizes the toxin.
- Removal of the membrane may be needed to alleviate airway obstruction.

- Hospitalization and isolation are needed until three cultures document elimination of the organism.
- Erythromycin or penicillin eliminates the organism; azithromycin and clarithromycin are options; antibiotic therapy should not be substituted for antitoxin therapy.
- Manage complications of disease by supportive measures.

6. Prevention
- The diphtheria, pertussis, and tetanus (DPT) vaccine provides active immunity. However, antitoxin levels decline slowly over time, and booster doses of toxoid should be given at 10-year intervals.
- Contacts should receive erythromycin prophylaxis for 7 days.

H. Disseminated *M. avium* Infection
1. Etiology
- *Mycobacterium avium-intracellulare* (MAI).
- This acid-fast, rod-shaped nonmotile organism is not communicable from person to person.

2. Pathology
- MAI produces a range of conditions from asymptomatic colonization to disseminated disease.
- Disseminated disease occurs in late HIV infection in patients with low CD4 counts.

3. Clinical Features
- Fever, weight loss, hepatomegaly, splenomegaly, and anemia are the most manifestations.

4. Diagnostic Studies
- Mycobacterial blood cultures have a sensitivity of 98% and are the preferred diagnostic modality.
- MAI may also be cultured from the liver, lymph nodes, and bone marrow.

5. Management
- MAC is resistant to most conventional antituberculosis drugs; it also rapidly develops secondary resistance, so combination therapy is indicated.
- The treatment of choice is a macrolide (clarithromycin or azithromycin) with ethambutol, with or without rifabutin.
- It is permissible to discontinue treatment in patients on HAART who have been treated for a year for disseminated MAC, who have no evidence of active disease, and whose CD4 counts exceed 100 cells per μL.

6. Prevention
- HIV-infected persons whose CD4 counts are <50 cells per μL should receive prophylaxis with either clarithromycin daily or azithromycin weekly.

I. Erysipeloid
1. Etiology
- *Erysipelothrix rhusiopathiae* has a worldwide distribution in a variety of animals, especially hogs.

2. **Pathology**
   - This occupational disease follows skin abrasion or puncture wound from contact with fish, shellfish, meat, and poultry.
   - Infection is usually limited to skin (mainly hands, fingers).
3. **Clinical Features**
   - Incubation period is 2 to 7 days.
   - Patients experience severe pain described as burning, itching, throbbing; nonpitting edema; purplish erythema with sharp, irregular margins extending peripherally, but clearing centrally; absent or low-grade fever.
   - Endocarditis occurs rarely.
   - Erysipeloid is self-limiting and usually resolves without treatment in 3 to 4 weeks.
4. **Diagnostic Studies**
   - Diagnosis is usually based on the typical clinical appearance in persons with occupational exposure highly suggestive of infection.
   - The organism may be cultured from biopsy material.
5. **Management**
   - The antibiotics of choice are penicillin or cephalosporins.
   - In patients allergic to penicillin, ciprofloxacin alone or erythromycin in combination with rifampin may be used.
   - The organism is resistant to vancomycin, an important consideration if the patient has endocarditis.

J. **Leprosy (Hansen Disease)**
   1. **Etiology**
      - *Mycobacterium leprae* is an acid-fast gram-variable, rod-shaped obligate intracellular bacterium.
      - It is endemic in tropical and subtropical areas of Africa, Asia, Central America, and South America, but is rare in the United States.
   2. **Pathology**
      - Leprosy is a chronic intracellular infectious disease unique to humans; its mode of transmission is thought to be respiratory.
      - Development of disease requires prolonged childhood exposure.
      - Two main types of disease occur: lepromatous and tuberculoid.
      - Lepromatous is more malignant and progressive, and occurs in persons who lack cellular resistance.
      - Tuberculoid is more benign and less likely to progress, and occurs in persons with intact immunity.
      - Borderline or intermediate cases occur.
      - Leprosy is usually not fatal and has predilection for cooler body areas (grows best at 37° C).
   3. **Clinical Features**
      - In lepromatous leprosy, patients have nodular skin lesions and slowly evolving, symmetrical nerve involvement.

- In tuberculoid leprosy, patients have macular lesions and sudden onset of sever asymmetric nerve involvement.
- Most deformity is due to trauma to, or secondary infection of, denervated tissues. Peripheral nerve damage is most common in ulnar nerve distribution (clawing of fourth and fifth fingers), posterior tibialis (clawing of toes and plantar anesthesia), and superficial peroneal (foot drop).
- Fine touch, temperature, and pain are impaired, whereas proprioception and vibratory sensation remain intact.
- Skin changes include symmetrically distributed macules, papules, plaques, nodules (lepromas); loss of eyebrows, eyelashes; rarely loss of scalp hair; leonine facies; thickened pendulous ears; spider telangiectasias; and edema of extremities.
- Eye changes include conjunctival and episcleral nodules; beading of corneal nerves; superficial punctate keratitis; interstitial keratitis with pannus formation of chronic plastic iridocyclitis.
- Upper respiratory changes include nasal stuffiness, coryza, epistaxis, and ulcers; ulcers of uvula, tonsils; loss of teeth; septal perforation, nasal collapse, hoarseness, stridor, asphyxia.
- Other organ/system changes may include hepatomegaly, splenomegaly, lymphadenopathy, testicular invasion and destruction, gynecomastia, cystic bone changes in distal phalanges, and skeletal muscle invasion. The kidneys are usually spared unless immune complex nephritis or amyloidosis occurs.
- Infection does not confer permanent immunity.

4. **Diagnostic Studies**
   - Leprosy is usually diagnosed by the presence of the characteristic peripheral nerve abnormality or the demonstration of acid-fast bacillus in the affected skin or nerve tissue.
   - Lepromin skin test, used primarily in research, usually returns a negative result in lepromatous disease, but the result is positive in tuberculoid.
   - Biologic false-positive serologic test results for syphilis, antithyroglobulin antibody, and rheumatoid factor occur.
5. **Management**
   - Combination therapy is recommended for treatment of all types of leprosy.
   - Lepromatous and borderline cases require combination therapy with dapsone, rifampin, and clofazimine for 12 months. Longer courses may be needed for patients with high burden of disease.
   - Tuberculoid leprosy is treated with dapsone and rifampin for 6 months.
   - Prevention of disability from nerve damage and management of complications are essential.

K. Salmonellosis

1. **Etiology**
   - *Salmonella enterica* is a motile gram-negative rod with many serotypes (~2,000); serotypes typhi, typhimurium, and choleraesuis cause almost all human infection.

2. **Pathology**
   - Salmonella gastroenteritis is transmitted through the fecal–oral route; it has a large animal reservoir and is transferred to humans by contaminated food (especially poultry, dairy products, meat, and eggs) or through handling of exotic pets, especially reptiles.
   - Enteric (typhoid) fever is caused by *Salmonella* species; "typhoid" is used only with serotype "typhi"; infection is transmitted by contaminated food and drink; the organisms cross the epithelium of the intestine and invade and replicate in macrophages in the mesenteric lymph nodes, spleen, and Peyer patches. The infection then localizes in the lymphoid tissues of the small intestine. Disseminated disease may occur in the lungs, gallbladder, kidneys, and CNS.

3. **Clinical Features**
   - Gastroenteritis: after incubation of 6 to 48 hours, fever, chills, nausea and vomiting, cramping, abdominal pain and diarrhea, headache, and muscle aches; diarrhea may be bloody. The disease is usually self-limiting; but in patients with sickle cell disease, bacteremia and localization to joints and bones may occur.
   - Enteric fever: the prodrome lasts 7 to 10 days with malaise, headache, cough, sore throat, abdominal pain, constipation, and stepwise fever. The patient then becomes much more ill with constipation or "pea soup" diarrhea, abdominal distension and tenderness, and possibly splenomegaly. The characteristic "rose spot" rash on the trunk appears in the second week; this is a 2- to 3-mm pink papule that fades with pressure. Improvement takes 1 to 2 weeks.
   - Complications of enteric fever include intestinal hemorrhage, which may lead to death; rarer complications include urinary retention, pneumonia, thrombophlebitis, myocarditis, psychosis, cholecystitis, nephritis, osteomyelitis, and meningitis.

4. **Diagnostic Studies**
   - Gastroenteritis: isolation of organism from stool specimen; leukocytes in stool; serotyping in outbreaks.
   - Enteric fever: blood culture is preferred.

5. **Management**
   - Fluoroquinolones are the treatment of choice for uncomplicated enteric fever and severe cases.
   - Ceftriaxone is also effective.

6. **Prevention**
   - Careful food handling, waste disposal, and water treatment.
   - For typhoid fever: immunization of household contacts, of travelers to endemic areas, and during epidemics.

L. Shigellosis/Shigella Dysentery

1. **Etiology**
   - *Shigella sonnei* in majority of cases, followed by *Shigella flexneri*; *Shigella dysenteriae* in most serious cases.
   - Invasive nonmotile gram-negative facultative rod.
   - Shigellosis is the most communicable of the bacterial diarrheas.

2. **Pathology**
   - Shigellosis is transmitted by the fecal–oral route.
   - Bacteria invade intestinal mucosa, producing local inflammation and ulceration.
   - An enterotoxin may cause watery diarrhea by inducing intestinal secretion.

3. **Clinical Features**
   - Following a 1- to 4-day incubation period, patients have abrupt onset of diarrhea mixed with blood and mucus, lower abdominal cramps, tenesmus, distension, malaise, and fever lasting an average of 7 days.
   - Sigmoidoscopy shows punctate areas of ulceration and inflamed mucosa.
   - Some patients develop disaccharidase deficiency following shigellosis; occasional reactive arthritis occurs.

4. **Diagnostic Studies**
   - Fecal smear shows leukocytes and erythrocytes.
   - Stool culture is usually positive, but blood culture is not.

5. **Management**
   - Supportive care including hydration and electrolyte replacement may be required in elderly, young, or immunocompromised patients.
   - Recommended empiric antibiotic therapy is either with a fluoroquinolone or ceftriaxone. If the isolate is susceptible, trimethoprim-sulfamethoxazole or azithromycin can be used. High rates of resistance to ampicillin make it a less effective regimen.
   - Antibiotic treatment is important in limiting course of disease and may decrease the chance of complications and transmission.

6. **Prevention**
   - Good public health and education programs; handwashing before handling food.
   - Refrigeration and proper cooking of potentially infected food.

M. Tetanus

1. **Etiology**
   - Neurotoxin tetanospasmin produced by *Clostridium tetani*.
   - Unvaccinated persons account for most cases, including newborns, elderly persons, injecting drug users, and migrant workers.

2. **Pathology**
   - Spores of *C. tetani* are found in the soil; they germinate when introduced into a wound.
   - Any wound may become colonized; puncture wounds are the most common.
   - The average incubation period is 8 to 12 days.
   - Tetanospasmin acts at the spinal of inhibitory neurons, where it cleaves a protein needed for the release of neurotransmitters.

3. **Clinical Features**
   - Diagnosis is suggested by a wound or recent history of a wound without a clear history of tetanus immunization.
   - Pain and tingling occur at the wound site, then muscle spasm of adjacent muscles.
   - Other early signs include jaw stiffness, dysphagia, stiff neck, and irritability.
   - Progression occurs usually over 2 weeks with hyperreflexia, spasms of the jaw muscles ("lockjaw" or trismus); other muscles may exhibit spasm and rigidity including facial, abdominal, neck, and back.
   - Minor stimuli precipitate painful tonic convulsions.
   - Death may occur because of spasms of the glottis and respiratory muscles.
   - Patients demonstrate clear mentation; sensory examination is normal.

4. **Diagnostic Studies**
   - This is a clinical diagnosis; however, patients will show moderate leukocytosis, normal CSF, and normal serum calcium.
   - Attempts to culture *C. tetani* from wounds are not useful in diagnosis.

5. **Management**
   - Supportive care until toxin is metabolized includes monitoring in quiet, nonstimulating environment; sedation; paralysis and mechanical ventilation as needed.
   - Intramuscular administration of tetanus immune globulin neutralizes circulating toxin; the role of intrathecal administration is under study.
   - Although the course of tetanus is not affected by debridement, appropriate wound care is essential.
   - Intravenous penicillin is the drug of choice for eradication of *C. tetani*.
   - Once well, the patient should have a full series of tetanus toxoid immunizations.

6. **Prevention**
   - DPT vaccine series in children; primary immunization in adults consists of 2 doses of tetanus toxoid 4 to 6 weeks apart and a third 6 to 12 months later.
   - Tetanus and diphtheria toxoids every 10 years throughout life or at the time of an injury if more than 5 years since the last dose.

V. Rickettsial Diseases
A. Ehrlichiosis
1. **Etiology**
   - Two forms exist in the United States: human monocytic ehrlichiosis (HME), caused by *Ehrlichia chaffeensis* and *Ehrlichia canis*; and human granulocytotropic ehrlichiosis (HGE), caused by *Anaplasma phagocytophilum* and *Ehrlichia ewingii*.
   - These are tick-borne gram-negative obligate intracellular organisms that exhibit tropism for either macrophages or granulocytes.
   - Ehrlichiosis occurs year-round in areas where ticks are active; incidence peaks in summer.

2. **Pathology**
   - The major vector of HME is the lone star tick and is endemic in the southeast, mid-Atlantic, and south central United States; vectors of HGE are deer ticks of the *Ixodes* species with the same geographic distribution as *Borrelia burgdorferi* (see section VI.A.).
   - Nonhuman hosts for HME-causing organisms include mice, dogs, and horses; for HGE-causing organisms, wood rats, deer mice, chipmunks, white-tailed deer, and white-footed mice.
   - Both types have a 7- to 10-day incubation period; the organism is present most commonly in blood, but can also be present in lymph nodes and bone marrow.

3. **Clinical Features**
   - Prodromal symptoms include rigors, malaise, and nausea, followed by abrupt onset of high fever, toxicity, myalgia, headache, and nausea.
   - Usually no rash; a few people develop maculopapular or petechial rash.
   - May progress to acute respiratory and renal failure and encephalopathy.
   - In case of HGE, fevers and malaise may occur for 2 years or more.
   - Coinfection with Lyme disease or babesiosis may occur.

4. **Diagnostic Studies**
   - Leukopenia, lymphopenia, thrombocytopenia, and elevated liver transaminases are found.
   - For HME and HGE, nucleic acid amplification by PCR is sensitive and highly specific.
   - Serologic diagnosis by IFA in acute and convalescent serum is the most widely available technique.

5. **Management**
   - Oral or intravenous doxycycline is the treatment of choice.

6. **Prevention**
   - Avoidance of tick-infested areas, protective clothing, and use of tick repellent.

B. Rocky Mountain Spotted Fever
1. **Etiology**
   - *Rickettsia rickettsii.*

- In the United States, most cases occur along the mid-Atlantic and southeastern seaboard and Mississippi River Valley.
- Most cases occur late spring and summer.

2. **Pathology**
   - The primary vector is *Dermacentor andersoni* (Rocky Mountain wood tick) in the west and *Dermacentor variabilis* (American dog tick) in the east.
   - *Rickettsia* multiplies within endothelial cells lining small blood vessels.

3. **Clinical Features**
   - Rocky Mountain spotted fever is the most serious rickettsial disease.
   - Incubation time between tick bite and onset of illness is 2 to 14 days (mean 7 days).
   - Fever, chills, headache, rash, toxicity, mental confusion, myalgias, nausea, and vomiting occur.
   - Fever rises rapidly; characteristically is high and spiking. Cough and pneumonitis may appear, as may delirium, lethargy, seizures, stupor, and coma.
   - Rash occurs between the second and sixth day of fever; initial lesions are small faint macules that blanch with pressure. Lesions rapidly become maculopapular, then petechial.
   - Rash appears first on wrists and ankles, spreading centrally but remaining more marked on extremities; palms and soles are typically involved; however, 10% have no or minimal rash.
   - Facial flushing and conjunctival injection are common.
   - Headache (beginning soon after onset) is extreme, intense, continuous, and intractable.
   - Some patients develop hepatosplenomegaly, jaundice, myocarditis, uremia, or necrotizing vasculitis.

4. **Diagnostic Studies**
   - Common findings include thrombocytopenia, elevated liver function tests, hyponatremia, and hyperbilirubinemia.
   - IFA testing of serum is most commonly used to confirm the diagnosis, but patients may not demonstrate antibody response until week 2.
   - Skin biopsy early in illness may demonstrate presence of *R. rickettsii*.

5. **Management**
   - Doxycycline is the treatment of choice; chloramphenicol in pregnant women.

6. **Prevention**
   - Avoidance of tick-infested areas, protective clothing, and the use of tick repellent.

VI. Spirochetal Diseases
A. Lyme Disease
1. **Etiology**
   - *B. burgdorferi.*
   - Lyme is the most common vector-borne infection in the United States.

- The vector is a species of the Ixodes (deer) tick; the larvae feed in late summer, nymphs in spring and early summer, and adults in fall.
- The preferred host for the larvae and nymphs is the white-footed mouse; for adults, the white-tailed deer. Most infections occur in the spring and summer.

2. **Pathology**
   - Lyme disease is transmitted through the bite of a tick that injects spirochete into the bloodstream; in most cases, the tick must be attached for at least 24 hours to transmit infection.
   - Immune complexes accumulate in joints and attract enzyme-releasing neutrophils that attack antigen–antibody complexes. Enzymes also attack joints, eroding bone and cartilage and causing arthritis-like symptoms.
   - O-antigen (lipopolysaccharide) of *Borrelia* stimulates macrophages to secrete interleukin 1, which subsequently stimulates the production of collagenase and prostaglandin. Collagenase degrades collagen, leading to the pattern of erosion seen in severe cases.
   - Prostaglandins promote pain.

3. **Clinical Features**
   - Although three stages of the disease have been described, overlap is common.
   - Early localized infection: usually about 7 days (range 3–30) after bite by an infected tick, erythema migrans rash develops typically in groin, axilla, or thigh; this expands from the site of the bite, may have central clearing or intensification, and may be up to 50 cm in diameter. About half of patients develop flu-like symptoms.
   - Early disseminated infection: if bacteremia occurs, patients progress within days to weeks to disseminated disease involving most commonly the skin, CNS, and musculoskeletal systems. Smaller skin lesions not associated with site of bite may develop; headache, stiff neck, and migratory joint, muscle, and tendon pain may occur. Persistent fatigue is common. Up to 10% of patients develop cardiac (myocarditis, pericarditis, dysrhythmias, and heart block) and up to 20% neurologic (aseptic meningitis, Bell palsy, encephalitis, personality changes, forgetfulness) symptoms. Ocular involvement may occur.
   - Late persistent infection: months to years later, patients develop variable musculoskeletal problems including joint pain without objective changes, frank arthritis of the large joints, and chronic synovitis. Neurologic involvement most commonly manifests as memory loss, mood swings, and sleep disturbance.

4. **Diagnostic Studies**
   - ELISA for serum antibodies confirmed with Western blot is the preferred methodology, but up to

half of patients will be antibody negative in the first few weeks.

- Isolation of organism in culture from biopsy of skin lesions early in the disease is readily accomplished, but culture from other sites is difficult; PCR of skin biopsy is even more sensitive.

5. **Management**
   - A tick bite is not usually treated in the absence of symptoms.
   - Early disease responds readily to doxycycline or amoxicillin, and cefuroxime for patients unable to tolerate doxycycline or amoxicillin, all for 2 to 3 weeks.
   - IV penicillin G, ceftriaxone, or cefotaxime for 2 to 4 weeks is used for CNS or cardiac disease; arthritis requires oral doxycycline or amoxicillin for up to 60 days or cefotaxime, cephotaxin, or penicillin G for up to 4 weeks.
   - "Chronic Lyme" or "post-Lyme syndrome" is treated symptomatically.

6. **Prevention**
   - LYMErix, the only licensed Lyme disease vaccine, was withdrawn from the market because of lack of demand.
   - Wearing protective clothing, avoidance of habitats of the deer tick, use of repellents and insecticides, and prompt removal of ticks prevent Lyme disease.
   - In limited circumstances, a single dose of doxycycline following tick bite may be indicated.

VII. Helminthic Infestations

A. Ascariasis

1. **Etiology**
   - *Ascaris lumbricoides* (roundworm).
   - Most common intestinal helminth worldwide.

2. **Pathology**
   - Adult ascarids inhabit the upper small intestine; females deposit eggs into intestinal lumen, which are eventually passed in the feces; eggs must mature in soil 2 to 3 weeks before becoming infective.
   - Following ingestion of contaminated food or water, eggs hatch into larvae in the small intestine, enter bloodstream, move to the right heart and then the lung, enter the alveoli, move up the bronchi, are swallowed, and return to the intestine.
   - Cycle takes 60 to 75 days.

3. **Clinical Features**
   - A small worm load is generally asymptomatic; heavier loads produce vague abdominal discomfort.
   - In higher worm loads, adults may migrate to common bile duct, pancreatic duct, appendix, or diverticula, causing symptoms associated with site of migration; very heavy disease may cause obstruction, intussusception, or other serious disease. Worms may also be coughed or vomited up.

- Nutritional disorders can occur secondary to impaired digestion or absorption of dietary proteins, particularly in children.

4. **Diagnostic Studies**
   - Recovery of characteristic egg in feces is usually sufficient for the diagnosis or identification of a large worm after it emerges from the mouth, nose, or anus.
   - Abdominal films, endoscopic retrograde cholangiopancreatography, and ultrasound may demonstrate a worm mass.
   - Pulmonary phase is diagnosed by finding larvae and eosinophils in sputum.
   - Eosinophilia occurs in the pulmonary phase; oxygen desaturation and migratory pulmonary infiltrates may occur.

5. **Management**
   - Mebendazole, albendazole, and pyrantel pamoate are the treatments of choice; in pregnant women, treatment should be delayed until after the first trimester.
   - Stools must be rechecked at 2 weeks with re-treatment as needed until all worms are removed.
   - Intestinal obstruction usually responds to conservative management while the antihelminthic agents work; surgery may be required for appendicitis.

6. **Prevention**
   - Adequate sanitation facilities, frequent handwashing, and avoidance of foods fertilized with human feces.

VIII. Pathogens with Bioterrorism Potential

- The Working Group for Civilian Biodefense compiled a list of characteristics of biologic agents that are most likely to be used as weapons of terror: high morbidity and mortality, potential for person-to-person spread, low infective dose, highly infectious when aerosolized, difficulty in making rapid diagnosis, lack of available effective vaccines, anxiety-producing potential, availability, feasibility of production, environmental stability, database of prior research and development, and potential to be "weaponized."
- **The CDC has classified potential biologic terrorism agents into three categories:**
  - Category A is the highest priority and includes anthrax, botulism, plague, smallpox, tularemia, and viral hemorrhagic fevers.
  - Category B, the second highest priority, includes brucellosis, epsilon toxin of *Clostridium perfringens*, food safety threats such as *Salmonella* species, glanders, melioidosis, psittacosis, Q fever, ricin toxin, staphylococcal enterotoxin B, typhus, viral encephalitis, and water safety threats.

- Category C bioterrorism threats are the third highest priority and include emerging infectious diseases such as Nipah and hantavirus.

A. Anthrax

- See section IV.A. for naturally occurring presentation.

1. **Etiology**
   - *B. anthracis.*

2. **Pathology**
   - Owing to availability, the agent's hardiness, ease of dispersion, and ability to cause grave illness, anthrax is considered the preferred agent of biologic terrorists.

3. **Clinical Features**
   - The form considered most likely to be used for biologic terrorism is inhalational anthrax.
   - This form is characterized by rapid progression from flu-like syndrome to lymphadenitis and hemorrhagic mediastinitis and is usually fatal within days.
   - Anthrax infection should be suspected when large numbers of patients have respiratory and flu-like symptoms outside of influenza season.

4. **Diagnostic Studies**
   - See section IV.A.
   - A 1-hour DNA test for anthrax is available from the CDC.

5. **Management**
   - Because no human-to-human cases have been found, standard precautions (routine use of gloves for skin lesions, handwashing, and use of gowns, masks, and eye protection during procedures in which splashing can occur) are sufficient for hospitalized patients.
   - Early initiation of ciprofloxacin is recommended in cases of biologic warfare because these strains may have been altered to resist standard antibiotics.
   - Burn or steam-sterilize contaminated dressings to destroy spores.
   - Notify local and state health departments, CDC, and appropriate law enforcement agencies immediately of suspected biologic terrorist attack.

6. **Prevention**
   - Vaccination is available in limited supply for those at risk (such as military personnel) and following a known exposure.
   - Chemoprophylaxis with doxycycline or ciprofloxacin may prevent the development of inhalational form if administered before disease onset.

B. Botulism

- See section IV.B. for naturally occurring presentation.

1. **Etiology**
   - *C. botulinum.*

2. **Pathology**
   - Botulinum toxin is the most poisonous substance known.

- It is a major threat because of extreme potency, degree of lethality, ease of production, and transport.

3. **Clinical Features**
   - See section IV.B.

4. **Diagnostic Studies**
   - Send samples (serum, stool, gastric aspirate, vomitus) and/or suspicious foods before treatment to CDC or special state and municipal public health laboratories for analysis.
   - Botulism is highly suspected if a large number of cases of acute flaccid paralysis with prominent bulbar palsies occur or in the presence of an outbreak of an unusual botulinum toxin type.
   - Bioterrorism is also suggested in the case of an outbreak with common geographic factor, but without a common dietary exposure or in multiple simultaneous outbreaks with no common source.

5. **Management**
   - Effectiveness of treatment based on timely diagnosis; administration of antitoxin should precede microbiologic test results.
   - Treat all those with suspected exposure and signs of illness with antitoxin and supportive measures.

6. **Prevention**
   - Investigational pentavalent (ABCDE) botulinum toxoid is available to those at high risk for exposure to botulinum toxin and the military; a recombinant vaccine is in development.

C. Glanders

1. **Etiology**
   - *Burkholderia mallei* (a small, bipolar, gram-negative, nonmotile, aerobic bacillus).
   - Although glanders is a category B agent, it is believed that attempts are being made to develop an aerosolized form of antibiotic-resistant *B. mallei* that could become a biologic weapon as potent as anthrax.
   - Eradicated in North America in 1938, glanders still occurs in Asia, Africa, and South America.

2. **Pathology**
   - Ordinarily, *B. mallei* infects horses, mules, and donkeys; pigs and cattle are resistant, but it rarely infects humans.
   - Disease is transmitted from animal-to-human by way of nasal, oral, and conjunctival mucous membranes, by inhalation into lungs, or through the lacerated or abraded skin; in humans, inoculation usually is into the skin of the hand or arm.

3. **Clinical Features**
   - After a 10- to 14-day incubation period, patients exhibit fever, rigors, night sweats, malaise, prostration, myalgia, headache, pleuritic chest pain, photophobia, lacrimation, diarrhea, and/or regional lymphadenitis.
   - The bacterium causes nodules to form in the affected area; these enlarge, forming ulcers;

crater-like ulcers on skin along course of lymph vessels of extremities commonly called *farcy*.
- Acute presentation ranges from localized suppurative infection to pulmonary infection to septicemia; patients with this form have fever, cervical adenopathy, splenomegaly, rash with generalized papular or pustular eruptions.
- Chronic indolent suppurative infection is associated with subcutaneous ulcers, lymphatic thickening, and lymphatic nodules.
- Aerosolized dissemination may lead to any of the above presentations.

4. **Diagnostic Studies**
- Serology is the preferred diagnostic modality; 16s rRNA gene sequencing is used for rapid identification.
- Chest radiography demonstrates miliary nodules, lung abscesses, and lobar or bronchopneumonia.

5. **Management**
- Long-term administration of a variety of drug combinations may be used in treatment including streptomycin and tetracycline or chloramphenicol and streptomycin.
- Abscesses need surgical drainage.

6. **Prevention**
- Standard precautions for laboratory exposures.
- No vaccine is available currently.
- Postexposure prophylaxis with Trimethoprim/ sulfamethoxazole (TMP/SMX), ceftazidime, and doxycycline.

D. **Plague**
1. **Etiology**
- *Yersinia pestis*, a nonmotile, gram-negative rod demonstrating bipolar "safety pin" staining with Wright, Giemsa, or Wayson stain.
- Optimal growth on blood or MacConkey agar at 35° C.

2. **Pathology**
- Patient is inoculated with thousands of organisms by plague-infected flea or by handling infected rodents in naturally occurring infection; person-to-person spread is through droplets.
- Aerosol dissemination leading to pneumonic plague is most likely in a bioterrorist attack.
- The incubation period is 2 to 10 days.
- Organisms spread through the lymphatic system, then to all organs through the blood.
- Plague-associated pneumonia and meningitis are often fatal.

3. **Clinical Features**
- Onset of fever, chills, weakness malaise, tachycardia, intense headache, delirium, and severe myalgias is rapid.
- Three forms of the disease exist: bubonic, septicemic, and pneumonic.
- Bubonic is the most common form (95%); it presents with an acutely swollen, extremely painful lymph node (bubo), 2 to 10 cm in diameter, in the groin, axilla, or cervical region.
- Septicemic refers to the subsequent DIC and gangrene in advanced disease. Septicemic plague denotes plague without the presence of a bubo. Patients become toxic and comatose with extensive purpura ("black death") on the distal extremities, nose, or penis.
- Pneumonic symptoms include tachypnea, productive cough, frothy blood-tinged sputum, and cyanosis. This form is usually fatal within a few hours if untreated.
- Bleeding from GI, respiratory, or genitourinary tracts is common ("red death").
- Plague is highly contagious by airborne transmission and invariably fatal if antibiotic therapy is delayed by more than 1 day after illness onset.

4. **Diagnostic Studies**
- Gram stain will demonstrate the bacillus in smears from buboes.
- Cultures from aspirate, pus, and blood are positive.
- For rapid diagnosis, direct immunofluorescence can be applied to smears of fluids or cultures.

5. **Management**
- Notify hospital, local, state, or military laboratories or, as necessary, the CDC immediately to confirm diagnosis.
- Streptomycin or gentamicin is the preferred treatment and must be begun immediately; doxycycline is an alternative.
- Patients with a cough or pneumonic plague require strict respiratory isolation for at least 48 hours after starting antibiotic therapy.

6. **Prevention**
- Doxycycline or tetracycline is used for postexposure prophylaxis.

E. **Q Fever**
1. **Etiology**
- *Coxiella burnetii* is a proteobacterium (formerly thought to be a *Rickettsia*) that is transmitted to humans primarily by inhalation of contaminated aerosols from the infected animal tissues. Ingestion of raw milk or cheese is another route.
- The animal reservoir of this zoonotic disease is primarily cattle, sheep, and goats; secondary reservoirs include cats, rabbits, pigeons, and dogs.
- *Coxiella* is resistant to heat and drying and can survive in harsh environments for weeks to months because of the formation of spore-like structures.
- Q fever is a category B bioterrorism threat.

2. **Pathology**
- Disease in animals is mild or subclinical, whereas humans may develop more serious illness.
- Person-to-person transmission is extremely rare, but maternal–fetal infection occurs.

3. **Clinical Features**
   - After a 7- to 21-day incubation period, the patient experiences fever, weight loss, severe headache, dyspnea, myalgias, nonproductive cough, and prostration.
   - More fulminant cases are associated with pneumonia, hepatitis, meningoencephalitis, or, rarely, endocarditis or osteomyelitis.
   - Culture-negative endocarditis is the most common finding in chronic disease.
   - Some patients develop chronic, relapsing disease.
   - Reactivation in pregnant women may cause spontaneous abortions, fetal death, fetal growth retardation, premature labor, and oligoamnios.
4. **Diagnostic Studies**
   - *C. burnetii* is highly infectious and must be tested in specialized laboratories.
   - The diagnostic methodology of choice is indirect immunofluorescence; ELISA and complement fixation are also appropriate.
   - Rheumatoid factor, C-reactive protein, and erythrocyte sedimentation rate levels are high; liver function test may be elevated; leukocytosis may occur.
   - Chest radiography shows patchy pulmonary infiltrates.
5. **Management**
   - Tetracycline or doxycycline is used to treat acute infection, but may not eradicate disease; newer macrolides and the quinolones are alternatives.
   - Heart valve replacement may be needed in chronic disease.
   - In case of exposure in a bioterrorist attack, doxycycline or TMP/SMX should be given for prophylaxis.
6. **Prevention**
   - Primary need is detection, prevention, and avoidance of diseased animals; milk should be pasteurized.
   - A vaccine has been used and found effective for high-risk exposures in Australia; none is available in the United States.

F. **Smallpox (Variola)**
   1. **Etiology**
      - Variola major is a DNA virus of the genus *Orthopoxvirus*, among the largest and most complex of all viruses.
      - The aerosolized form is extremely stable in cool temperatures, low humidity, and when protected from ultraviolet light.
      - Variola minor is a less severe form.
      - Smallpox is a category A bioterrorism agent.
   2. **Pathology**
      - The infectious dose is believed to be only a few virions.
      - Following implantation, the virus migrates and multiplies in the lymph nodes, spleen, and bone marrow.
      - The incubation period is about 12 days (7–17).

3. **Clinical Features**
   - The prodrome consists of abrupt onset of high fever and severe head- and backache; patients may have chills and rigors, coryza, and pharyngitis.
   - Skin eruptions begin 1 to 2 days after the development of an enanthem; these begin as macules and progress through papules, pustules, and crusting over about 2 weeks. Palmar and plantar lesions are common.
   - Skin lesions develop all at once, rather than in crops, as in varicella.
4. **Diagnostic Studies**
   - Laboratory confirmation is important; a vaccinated laboratory worker wearing gloves and a mask should collect specimens from vesicular or pustular fluid.
   - Laboratory confirmation is made by electron microscopic examination.
   - Use state or local laboratory with high-containment (BL-4) facility.
5. **Management**
   - Supportive therapy plus antibiotics in the case of secondary bacterial infection.
   - Persons in whom smallpox is suspected should be isolated and vaccinated within first few days of exposure.
   - Household and face-to-face contacts should be vaccinated, placed under surveillance, and monitored for fevers.
   - Smallpox must be treated as international health emergency (report to national officials through local and state health authorities).
6. **Prevention**
   - Vaccination is available in limited amounts for persons at risk; eczema, other dermatitides, and burns are contraindications.
   - Standard precautions include using gloves, gowns, and masks; handling laundry and waste as biohazardous; and decontaminating rooms.
   - Limited supplies of vaccinia immune globulin are available for treating severe cutaneous reactions occurring as a vaccination complication.

G. **Tularemia**
   1. **Etiology**
      - *Francisella tularensis* is one of the most infectious pathogenic bacteria.
      - Category A agent for bioterrorism due to the ease of dissemination and virulence.
      - Humans become infected because of tick or insect bite or handling animal tissues; aerosol infection is also highly likely.
   2. **Pathology**
      - The incubation period is 2 to 10 days.
      - Small, nonmotile aerobic gram-negative coccobacillus.
      - Hardy, non–spore-forming organism with thin lipopolysaccharide-containing envelope.

3. **Clinical Features**
   - Tularemia may be asymptomatic or begin with sudden onset of fever, headache, and nausea, and a papule develops at the site of inoculation with progression to ulceration.
   - Pneumonia may be primary following inhalation or the result of hematogenous spread.
   - After ingestion of infected meat or water, patients may develop GI symptoms, stupor, and delirium.
   - Tender splenomegaly is common, as are rashes, myalgias, and prostration.
4. **Diagnostic Studies**
   - Diagnosis is usually made serologically.
5. **Treatment**
   - Streptomycin is the recommended treatment; gentamicin or doxycycline is an alternative.
6. **Prevention**
   - Avoidance of ticks and deer fleas, use of insect repellents, and wearing gloves when handling animal carcasses prevent naturally occurring disease.
   - The CDC has an intradermal vaccine available.

H. Viral Hemorrhagic Fevers

1. **Etiology**
   - One of four families of viruses capable of causing febrile disease and a bleeding disorder.
   - These families pose particularly serious threats as biologic weapons, based on their infectious properties, morbidity and mortality, and transmissibility by way of aerosol dissemination: Filoviridae (Ebola and Marburg viruses), Arenaviridae (Lassa fever and the New World arenaviruses), Bunyaviridae (Rift Valley fever, Crimean–Congo hemorrhagic fever virus), and Flaviviridae (dengue, yellow fever, Omsk hemorrhagic fever, and Kyasanur Forest disease viruses).
   - None occurs naturally in the United States.
2. **Pathology**
   - Small RNA viruses with lipid envelopes act in varied ways; much is unknown.
   - Some illness results from the body's immunologic response to infection.
   - Direct and indirect cell damage leads to platelet dysfunction.
   - Filoviruses extremely virulent and cytotoxic to cells leading to necrosis of visceral organs.
   - Arenaviruses may induce secretion of inflammatory mediators from macrophages because few or absent cytopathic effects are present.
   - Infection with Rift Valley and yellow fever viruses leads to destruction of infected cells.
3. **Clinical Features**
   - Early symptoms of all these resemble influenza or gastroenteritis with headache, upper respiratory or GI symptoms, and myalgias; hepatitis is common.
   - Later manifestations are more specific to the particular virus; symptoms typically include organ failure, mental status changes, and hemorrhage.
   - Fatality rates are up to 90% with Ebola fever.
4. **Diagnostic Studies**
   - Variable clinical presentations present a major diagnostic challenge.
   - Clinical microbiology and public health laboratories are not equipped to make rapid diagnosis, so specimens must be sent to CDC or U.S. Army Medical Research Institute of Infectious Diseases.
5. **Management**
   - Early treatment with intravenous ribavirin may be useful in Lassa fever and hemorrhagic fever with renal failure.
   - No antiviral medications are currently approved, so early supportive care is essential.
   - Close and high-risk contacts must be identified and monitored for 21 days.
   - An effective vaccine is available for yellow fever, but is not useful following bioterrorist attack because of short incubation period.
   - Suspected cases must be reported to local or state health departments immediately.
6. **Prevention**
   - Avoidance of sick animals or people and arthropod bites is essential.
   - Rift Valley fever and Flaviviridae are not transmissible from person to person.
   - Airborne transmission is rare, but may be transmitted to laboratory personnel through aerosol generated during specimen processing.
   - Virus culture must occur in high-containment (BSL-4) laboratories.
   - Barrier precautions include strict hand hygiene plus double gloving, impermeable gowns, face shields, eye protection, and leg and shoe coverings.

REVIEW QUESTIONS

1. A 20-year-old man presents to the office with a fever, sore throat, and enlarged cervical, axillary, and inguinal lymph nodes. He also has a rash on his torso. Which of the following tests would be most sensitive for diagnosing acute HIV in this situation?

   a) Western Blot
   b) CD4 count and percentage
   c) Serum rapid plasma reagin (RPR)
   d) HIV viral load
   e) Skin biopsy

2. A 18-year-old woman is diagnosed with acute mononucleosis with EBV. Which of the following is not an indication for steroids?

   a) Impending splenic rupture
   b) Hemolytic anemia
   c) Severe thrombocytopenia
   d) Airway obstruction

3. A 35-year-old man noticed a rash after being out in the woods this past weekend. This manifestation is secondary to transmission of *B. burgdorferi* and is characterized by gradual expansion of erythema around the initial tick bite and is called:

   a) Erythema nodosum
   b) Erythema chronicum migrans
   c) Erysipelas
   d) Erythema multiforme
   e) Erythema marginatum

4. In the above case, what treatment would be indicated at this time?

   a) No treatment
   b) Doxycycline 100 mg bid for 14 days
   c) Doxycycline 100 mg bid for 21 days
   d) Doxycycline 100 mg bid for 28 days
   e) Doxycycline 200 mg as a single dose

5. A 52-year-old woman presents with fever, dry cough, and pleuritic chest pain after returning from a trip in the Ohio River Valley region. On physical examination, she has cervical adenopathy and decreased breath sounds at both lung bases. She admits to exploring caves and was exposed to bat droppings. What is the most likely causative organism?

   a) *A. fumigatus*
   b) *C. immitis*
   c) *H. capsulatum*
   d) *M. tuberculosis*
   e) *B. burgdorferi*

ANSWERS TO REVIEW QUESTIONS

1. **Answer: D**. An HIV viral load is the most sensitive test. It is 100% sensitive and 88% specific. A western blot is used to confirm an ELISA, but is no longer recommended. A CD4 and percentage would be checked once a diagnosis of HIV is made. The RPR would be used to check for syphilis, and a skin biopsy would not confirm the diagnosis of acute HIV.

2. **Answer: A**. The indications for steroids in mononucleosis are airway obstruction, hemolytic anemia, and severe thrombocytopenia. The value of steroids is less well established in impending splenic rupture, pericarditis, myocarditis, or nervous system involvement.

3. **Answer: B**. Erythema chronicum migrans is the initial lesion of Lyme disease and often appears at the site of the infecting tick bite. Erythema nodosum is usually secondary to a recent infection or inflammatory condition. Erysipelas is a superficial bacterial infection that extends into the lymphatics and it is usually caused by a streptococcal infection. Erythema multiforme is an acute, self-limiting, and sometimes recurrent skin condition that is a type IV hypersensitivity reaction associated with certain medications and infections. Finally, erythema marginatum is a type of erythema associated with pink rings on the torso and inner surface of the limbs that come and go for several months and can be seen in rheumatic fever.

4. **Answer: E**. Routine prophylaxis after a recognized tick bite is not recommended. A guideline from the Infectious Disease Society of America recommends prophylactic antibiotic therapy for adults and children older than 8 years, using a single 200-mg dose of doxycycline (in children, 4 mg per kg up to a maximum dose of 200 mg) only if all of the following criteria are met: The attached tick can be reliably recognized as a nymphal or adult *Ixodes scapularis*, the tick has been attached for at least 36 hours, as determined by the degree of engorgement of the tick or certainty about the time of exposure to the tick, prophylaxis can be started within 72 hours of the time the tick was removed, the local rate of infection of these ticks with *B. burgdorferi* is at least 20%, and doxycycline treatment is not contraindicated.

5. **Answer: C**. A history of pulmonary symptoms following exposure to bat droppings while in the Ohio River Valley is a classic presentation for *H. capsulatum*.

SELECTED REFERENCES

American Academy of Pediatrics Subcommittee on Diagnosis and Management of Bronchiolitis. Diagnosis and management of bronchiolitis. *Pediatrics*. 2006;118(4):1774–1793.

Anderson H, Stryjewska B, Boyanton BL, Schwartz MR. Hansen disease in the United States in the 21st century: a review of the literature. *Arch Pathol Lab Med*. 2007;131(6):982–986.

Blyth CC, Palasanthiran P, O'Brien TA. Antifungal therapy in children with invasive fungal infections: a systematic review. *Pediatrics*. 2007;119(4):772–784.

Centers for Disease Control and Prevention. Emergency preparedness and response: bioterrorism agents. https://www.nsc.org/home-safety/safety-topics/emergency-preparedness?gclid=EAIaIQobChMI1N-3tMnN3wIVhB6GCh0BRAUfEAAYASAAEgKTcvD_BwE. Accessed November-December 2011.

Franco MP, Mulder M, Gilman RH, Smits HL. Human brucellosis. *Lancet Infect Dis*. 2007;7(12):775–786.

Griffith KS, Lewis LS, Mali S, Parise ME. Treatment of malaria in the United States: a systematic review. *JAMA*. 2007;297(20):2264–2277.

Halperin JJ, Shapiro ED, Logigian E, et al; Quality Standards Subcommittee of the American Academy of Neurology. Practice parameter: treatment of nervous system Lyme disease (an evidence-based review): report of the Quality Standards Subcommittee of the American Academy of Neurology. *Neurology*. 2007;69(1):91–102.

Hankins DG, Rosekrans JA. Overview, prevention, and treatment of rabies. *Mayo Clin Proc*. 2004;79(5):671–676.

Ho W; Hong Kong Hospital Authority Working Group on SARS; Central Committee of Infection Control. Guideline on management of severe acute respiratory syndrome (SARS). *Lancet*. 2003;361(9366):1313–1315.

Hotez PJ, Molyneux DH, Fenwick A, et al. Control of neglected tropical diseases. *N Engl J Med.* 2007;357(10):1018–1027.

Hui DS, Chan PK. Clinical features, pathogenesis and immunobiology of severe acute respiratory syndrome. *Curr Opin Pulm Med.* 2008;14(3):241–247.

Jackson AC. Update on rabies diagnosis and treatment. *Curr Infect Dis Rep.* 2009;11(4):296–301.

Keiser J, Utzinger J. Efficacy of current drugs against soil-transmitted helminth infections: systematic review and meta-analysis. *JAMA.* 2008;299(16):1937–1948.

Longo D, Fauci AS, Kasper DL, Hauser SL, Jameson JL, Loscalzo J, eds. *Harrison's Principles of Internal Medicine.* 18th ed. New York, NY: McGraw-Hill; 2011.

Mandell GL, Bennett JE, Dolin R. *Principles and Practice of Infectious Disease.* Amsterdam, The Netherlands: Elsevier; 2007.

McPhee SJ, Papadakis MA, Rabow MW, eds. *Current Medical Diagnosis and Treatment.* 50th ed. Stamford, CT: Appleton & Lange; 2017.

Panel on Antiretroviral Guidelines for Adult and Adolescents. *Guidelines for the Use of Antiretroviral Agents in HIV-1-infected Adults and Adolescents.* Washington, DC: Department of Health and Human Services; 2016:1–161. http://www.aidsinfo.nih.gov/ContentFiles/AdultandAdolescentGL.pdf. Accessed May, 2017.

Patterson TF, Thompson GR, Denning DW, et al. Practice guidelines for the diagnosis and management of Aspergillosis: 2016 update by the Infectious Diseases Society of America. *Clin Infect Dis.* 2016;63(4):e1–e60.

Skalsky K, Yahav D, Bishara J, Pitlik S, Leibovici L, Paul M. Treatment of human brucellosis: systematic review and meta-analysis of randomized controlled trials. *Br Med J.* 2008;336(7646):701–704.

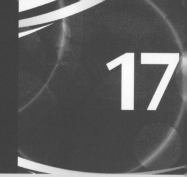

Surgery Disorders

Surgery Disorders

17

Abigail Gonnella • Randi Beth Cooperman • Justine Filippelli • Jennifer Keat-Wysocki • Tanya Konyesni • Julie Le • Scott Naples

I. Skin Disorders
A. Vascular Lesions: Hemangiomas
1. **Etiology**
   - Congenital; commonly seen in children as "birthmarks."
   - Most common benign vascular tumors of infancy.
   - Types:
     - Superficial hemangiomas are the most common of the hemangiomas; most commonly present as bright red nodules, papules, or plaque, and most of these lesions resolve spontaneously.
     - Deep, subcutaneous (SQ) hemangiomas are slightly raised, skin colored with bluish hue with or without central telangiectatic patch.
     - Cavernous hemangiomas are purely deep hemangiomas.
   - Associated syndromes:
     - Kasabach–Merritt: sudden enlargement of existing hemangioma, thrombocytopenia, and/or coagulopathy—an acute syndrome with high mortality.
2. **Pathology**
   - Increased number of blood vessels (capillary); hyperplasia of endothelial cells.
   - Proliferate after birth, grow intermittently, and commonly involute.
3. **Clinical Features**
   - Most hemangiomas are not evident at birth, but develop later in the first few days to first month of life.
   - Most hemangiomas are asymptomatic—cosmesis may be the primary concern.
   - Size and distribution are highly variable.
   - Associated syndromes must be kept in mind.
   - Complications include ulceration, bleeding, vision complications, thromboangiitis, airway, infection, and pulmonary embolism (PE); all mostly seen with large lesions.
   - History and physical examination usually suffice for diagnosis.
   - Presence at birth, size, location, rate of growth, and associated symptoms are important.
   - Raised lesions are purple, red, or pink; they have irregular borders and thinned dermis and vary in size.

4. **Diagnostic Studies**
   - Laboratory tests are indicated preoperatively to assess complications or associated illnesses. Platelet and red blood cell (RBC) count are most important.
   - Immunohistochemical marker: positive Glut-1 (glucose transporter protein) may help in the evaluation of biopsied tissue.
   - Angiography and other imaging studies (magnetic resonance imaging [MRI], computerized tomography [CT] scan) may be needed to define larger lesions, particularly when considering surgical resection or embolization.
   - Computer tomography angiography (CTA) to map lesion.
   - Ultrasound (U/S) and color Doppler imaging.
5. **Management**
   a. **Conservative Treatment**
      - Observation indicated in childhood for asymptomatic and stable lesions.
      - The majority of hemangiomas involute, leading to ulceration in a small percentage of patients.
      - In general, cosmetically acceptable hemangiomas do not need treatment.
   b. **Medical Treatment**
      - Topical corticosteroids: treat minor, recurrent ulcerations.
      - Propranolol: first-line treatment inhibits growth of severe infantile hemangiomas.
      - Vincristine: another alternative choice for lesions unresponsive to corticosteroids.
      - Interferon α-2a: no longer widely used because of complications—used only with failure of other drugs.
   c. **Surgical and Interventional Treatment**
      - Cryoablation: effective in treating small lesions; may leave scar.
        - Pulsed dye laser (PDL) is most effective for ulcerated and superficial hemangiomas.
        - Neodymium:yttrium aluminum garnet (Nd:YAG) laser: recommended for deep or rapidly growing hemangiomas.
        - Surgical resection: ample indications; may involve major amputations, reconstructions, and tissue transfer.

- Embolization: mostly used as a last resort with failure of medical therapy and palliative method for inoperable lesions.

B. Vascular Malformations

1. Etiology
- Present at birth, but may not be clinically apparent until later.
- Grow with child, never involute.
- Soft, flat, easily compressible.

2. Pathology
- Two common capillary vascular malformations are the salmon patch (nevus simplex) and port wine stain (nevus flammeus).

3. Clinical Features
- Salmon patch:
  - Most common vascular malformation of infancy.
  - Made up of superficial capillaries.
  - When located at the nape of the neck, also called "stork bite."
  - Most will fade within the first few years.
- Port wine stain:
  - Made up of superficial capillaries and deep vessels of skin and soft tissue.
  - Soft-tissue or bony hypertrophy.
  - Associated syndromes:
    - Sturge–Weber syndrome:
      - Port wine stain in ophthalmic branch of trigeminal nerve.
      - Associated with ocular (glaucoma) and neurologic (mental retardation, seizures, hemiplegia) abnormalities.
    - Klippel–Trenaunay syndrome:
      - Port wine stain over an extremity.
      - Associated bony or soft-tissue hypertrophy of extremity.
      - Termed *Parkes Weber syndrome* when arteriovenous fistula is noted.

4. Diagnostic Studies
- Immunohistochemical marker: negative Glut-1 (glucose transporter protein).
- MRI.

5. Management
- Sclerotherapy.
- Laser treatment.
- Surgery excision.
- Sturge–Weber syndrome:
  - CT or MRI.
  - Screen for eye and central nervous system (CNS) disease.
- Klippel–Trenaunay syndrome:
  - Supportive care; analgesic control, treat infection.
  - Routine measurement of extremity to detect evolving extremity hypertrophy/leg length discrepancies; may need orthopedic intervention.
  - Surgery to decrease tissue overgrowth.

C. Neurogenic Tumors (Benign)

1. Etiology
- Types:
  - Neurofibroma: benign nonencapsulated tumor of nerve fibers.
  - Schwannoma: benign, encapsulated tumor of nerve sheath (Schwann cells).
- May be solitary and sporadic or multiple and associated with neurofibromatosis (NF), a hereditary disease.
- Schwannoma or neurilemmoma is a variant arising from the perineural sheath of Schwann cells.
- NF type 1 (von Recklinghausen disease):
  - Autosomal dominant inheritance.
  - Appears to be caused by mutation of a gene on chromosome 17.
  - New mutations occasionally occur in the germ line of the unaffected parent and can be transmitted to more than one offspring.
- NF type 2.
  - Cranial nerve 8.
  - Mutation of chromosome 22.

2. Pathology
- Solitary neurofibroma: oval to elongated nuclei on fibrocollagenous background.
- Schwannoma: round, tan, yellow tumor on gross examination; spindle cells on light microscopy; entangled processes lined by continuous basal laminas on electron microscopy.
- NF: diffuse neurofibroma, café-au-lait spots, freckling, bilateral acoustic nerve schwannomas, intestinal neuromas, and arterial wall thickening.

3. Clinical Features
- Solitary neurofibroma: small (~2 to 8 mm) sessile or pedunculated skin lesions.
- Schwannoma: deep-seated tumors (retroperitoneum, mediastinum), which may reach 10 to 15 cm in diameter without causing symptoms.
- NF: seven types (NF1 through NF7) have been recognized, according to clinicopathologic characteristics:
  - Café-au-lait macules (hyperpigmentation) are noted in the first year of life.
  - Numerous neurofibromas of varying size throughout the skin.
  - Paraspinal and acoustic neuromas, and spinal cord meningiomas.
  - Axillary/inguinal freckling.
  - Rarely, adrenal or extra-adrenal pheochromocytoma is associated.
- Associated symptoms: change in vision, sensation, movement, bowel/bladder habits, hearing loss due to nerve impingement.

4. Diagnostic Studies
- Solitary neurofibroma: firm, nontender, cutaneous, or SQ nodule.

- Schwannoma: cannot be distinguished from neurofibroma clinically.
- NF: familial pattern is identifiable.
- Histopathology is essential for definitive diagnosis of any of the variants.
- MRI to assess nerve involvement.

5. **Management**
   - Most individuals with NF1 do not need treatment. Painful SQ neurofibromas can be excised. Intraspinal and -cranial tumors are typically benign and treated surgically.
   - NF is treated conservatively; lesions causing compression, pain, bleeding, or altered function may need surgical resection; select lesions may be resected for cosmetic reasons.
   - Removal of schwannomas and other tumors is often indicated for individuals with NF2, and early recognition is important for successful treatment of VIII nerve tumors.
   - Solitary neurofibromas: excisional biopsy is indicated to exclude malignancy. Surgical resection is indicated for patients with pain, neurologic deficits.
   - Genetic counseling should be provided to all patients and families.

D. Decubitus Ulcer
1. **Etiology**
   - Excessive prolonged pressure causing ischemia and eventual necrosis of skin and SQ tissues, also known as "pressure ulcer" or "pressure sore."
   - Risk factors include paraplegia, chronic illness, neuropathy, age, uremia, jaundice, diabetes, corticosteroids, cancer, chemotherapy, malnutrition, and inadequately fit casts or other means of immobilization, immunosuppression.
   - Stage I: nonblanchable erythema of intact skin, the heralding lesion of skin ulceration. In persons with darker skin, discoloration of the skin, warmth, induration, or hardness also may be indicators.
   - Stage II: partial-thickness skin loss involving epidermis, dermis, or both. The ulcer is superficial and appears clinically as an abrasion, blister, or shallow crater.
   - Stage III: full-thickness skin loss involving damage to, or necrosis of, SQ tissue that may extend down to, but not through, underlying fascia. The ulcer appears clinically as a deep crater with or without undermining of adjacent tissue.
   - Stage IV: full-thickness skin loss with extensive destruction, tissue necrosis, or damage to muscle, bone, or supporting structures (e.g., tendon and joint capsule). Undermining and sinus tracts also may be associated with Stage IV pressure ulcers.
   - Unstageable: full-thickness skin and tissue loss to unknown extent because area is covered by eschar. When eschar is removed, usually Stages III to IV.

2. **Pathology**
   - Necrosis, which may involve skin, SQ tissues, and muscles.

3. **Clinical Features**
   - Early stages: red or purple skin; late stages: necrosis (dark blue or black discoloration).
   - Size is variable; area of necrosis is usually deeper than it appears externally because SQ tissues and muscle are more sensitive to ischemia than skin.
   - Patients who are bedridden, paraplegic, or unable to sense pain should be examined frequently for damaged skin in areas of pressure, especially bony prominences.
   - Extent of necrosis is best determined by local exploration and debridement.
   - Associated illness always present.
   - Complications: cellulitis, fasciitis, osteomyelitis, abscess, sepsis, and, rarely, bleeding.

4. **Diagnostic Studies**
   - Laboratory tests and imaging may be needed (e.g., to rule out osteomyelitis, to assess nutritional status, and preoperatively).

5. **Management**
   a. **Medical Treatment**
      - When feasible, correct underlying disorders (e.g., diabetes).
      - Pain management.
      - Correct nutrition deficiencies, if present.
      - Avoid local pressure; positional changes, pressure-relieving mattress, and cushion pads.
      - Dressings, such as topical sulfadiazine (Silvadene) or adhesive colloids with hydrophilic particles (DuoDERM, Restore, J&J ulcer dressing).
   b. **Local Wound Care**
      - Stage 1: use of transparent films (prevents shearing).
      - Stage 2: keep wound moist with semiocclusive or occlusive dressings. Avoid wet to dry dressings.
      - Stages 3 and 4: drainage of any purulent collection and sharp debridement of necrotic tissue.
      - Future coverage with healthy tissue: skin grafts and rotational or advancement flaps.

II. Endocrine Disorders
A. Thyroid Carcinoma
1. **Etiology**
   - Most primary cancers of the thyroid and can be classified into *papillary, follicular, medullary,* and *anaplastic. Squamous cell carcinoma, lymphoma,* and *metastatic carcinoma* also occur, but rarely.
   - Thyroid cancer is usually a solid lesion and rarely secretes thyroid hormones.
   - Familial predisposition: medullary carcinoma is transmitted as an autosomal dominant trait—50% chance of disease in the offspring.

- Ionizing radiation—radiotherapy, atomic bomb, and nuclear accident—is a high-risk factor; thyroid cancer develops 5 to >25 years after exposure.

2. **Pathology**
   - Papillary: 50% to 80% of thyroid cancers. On histology, papillary fronds are characteristic, and laminated microcalcifications ("psammoma bodies") can be present; tumor may be multicentric; it metastasizes to regional lymph nodes.
   - Follicular: 20%; characterized by follicles containing colloid; may be encapsulated or invasive; spread is hematogenous.
   - Papillary and follicular subtypes make up approximately 90% of all thyroid cancers.
   - Medullary: <10% of all thyroid tumors; arises from C-cells that produce calcitonin; cells grow with nesting pattern; amyloid deposits can be noted.
   - Anaplastic: a most aggressive neoplasm; represents 5% to 10% of thyroid cancers; variable histologic appearance; spindle and giant cells are commonly seen.

3. **Clinical Features**
   - Papillary: appears as asymptomatic (nonfunctional) thyroid nodule; affects younger population; prognosis is generally good.
   - Follicular: slow-growing, tends to invade locally; disseminates through the bloodstream; bone metastases may cause pain. Most patients are in the fifth decade of life, and women-to-men incident ratio is 3:1.
   - Medullary: can be sporadic nonfamilial or familial. The latter form may be associated with pheochromocytoma, parathyroid adenoma, and neuroma—sipple syndrome or multiple endocrine neoplasia, type II (MEN-II).
   - Anaplastic: dismal disease; appears as painful enlargement of the thyroid; rapidly invades surrounding structures (e.g., trachea, recurrent nerves, and carotids), causing hoarseness, respiratory obstruction, dysphagia, bleeding, and other life-threatening complications.
   - Most thyroid cancers appear as a "silent" nodule; *anaplastic carcinoma* can have dramatic presentation, with pain, hoarseness, and respiratory trouble.
   - Physical examination does not distinguish between benign and malignant nodules; signs of hyperthyroidism do not exclude cancer; cervical adenopathy suggests malignancy.

4. **Diagnostic Studies**
   - Thyroid function tests are usually normal in thyroid cancer; radioimmunoassay for calcitonin is used in screening of medullary carcinoma.
   - U/S can differentiate between cystic and solid lesions.
   - Fine-needle aspiration (FNA) cytology is the most useful test to diagnose cancer; however, definitive diagnosis of thyroid follicular cancer requires histologic analysis.

5. **Management**
   a. **Medical Treatment**
      - Radioactive iodine (^{131}I) can ablate residual tumor and metastases, particularly of follicular tumors.
      - Thyroid suppressive therapy with thyroxine is given.
      - Chemotherapy (e.g., doxorubicin or multidrug regimens) can be used for metastatic disease and anaplastic carcinoma, but cure is extremely rare.
   b. **Surgical Treatment**
      - Papillary: at least thyroid lobectomy plus isthmectomy is often recommended if nodule is <1 cm. If nodule is ≥4 cm, then a total thyroidectomy is recommended.
      - Follicular: near-total thyroidectomy is favored with nodules <1 cm. If nodule is ≥4 cm, then a total thyroidectomy is recommended.
      - Medullary: total thyroidectomy should be performed (because of multicentricity).
      - Anaplastic: total thyroidectomy and radical neck dissection for resectable tumors; in most instances, surgery is palliative.
      - If there are suspicious thyroid nodules, a unilateral lobectomy can be performed. If pathology shows follicular or papillary cancer, then a complete thyroidectomy is recommended.

B. Hypercortisolism

1. **Etiology**
   - Cushing disease: hypersecretion of adrenocorticotropic hormone (ACTH) by pituitary adenoma stimulating adrenal gland to produce cortisol.
     - Hypersecretion of ACTH by a corticotropin-producing pituitary tumor much more common cause of Cushing disease than from benign or malignant adrenal tumors.
   - Cushing syndrome: constellation of signs and symptoms from excess cortisol; may be secondary to Cushing disease, adenoma of the adrenal cortex, or exogenous corticosteroids.
   - Ectopic ACTH syndrome: hypercortisolism secondary to nonpituitary tumor; usually a paraneoplastic syndrome (e.g., lung cancer secreting ACTH).
   - The most common cause of Cushing syndrome (hypercortisolism) is exogenous corticosteroid use for treatment of a variety of diseases, including asthma, autoimmune disorders, and inflammatory bowel disease.

2. **Pathology**
   - Pituitary adenoma: typically small basophilic intrasellar tumor; however, the tumor can reach large sizes and cause local compression.

- Adrenocortical adenoma: composed of lipid-rich cells arranged in clusters and cords resembling normal zona fasciculata.
- Adrenocortical hyperplasia: zona fasciculata markedly thickened by enlarged cells with abundant lipid.
- Ectopic ACTH-producing tumors: lung, thymus, and pancreas.

3. **Clinical Features**
- Truncal obesity, "moon" facies, "buffalo hump," atrophic muscles, fragile skin, ecchymoses, purple striae, supraclavicular fat pad fullness, cataracts, osteoporosis, menstrual dysfunction, hyperglycemia, hypertension, recurrent candidiasis, hirsutism, acne, poor wound healing, and psychiatric disturbances.

4. **Diagnostic Studies**
- Increased levels of cortisol in blood and urine.
- Investigate cause of hypercortisolism.
- Sellar X-rays, CT scan, and MRI to evaluate pituitary tumors.
- Abdominal imaging to evaluate adrenal tumors.

5. **Management**
   a. **Medical Treatment**
   - External radiation may be used for residual tumor after pituitary surgery.
   - Aimed at correcting the cause of hypercortisolism.
   b. **Surgical Treatment**
   - Optimal treatment is surgical resection of pituitary tumor.
   - Pituitary adenomas are preferably resected through transnasal transsphenoidal approach to the sella turcica.
   - Adrenal gland tumors can be resected by way of laparotomy, lateral or posterior (lumbar) incisions, or laparoscopy.

III. Disorders of the Breast
A. Fibrocystic Breast Changes (Fibrocystic Disease—Fibrodysplasia)
1. **Etiology**
- Most common benign condition or lesion of the breast.
- Most common cause of cyclic breast pain or mastalgia in reproductive women: affects >50% of women of reproductive age.
- Common in women between ages 30 and 50.
- Decreased incidence in postmenopausal women.

2. **Pathology**
- These lesions are benign and noted frequently in normal breasts, and therefore thought to be a "normal variant."
- Fibrous tissue and multiple cysts.
- Believed to be related to ovarian activity.
- Estrogen hormone as a causative factor.
- Gross findings reveal dense white stromal tissue admixed with variably sized cysts that may have brown or blue (blue-dome cyst) discoloration.

- Microscopic findings reveal fibrosis, cystic dilation of ducts, apocrine metaplasia, adenosis, and epithelia hyperplasia.
- Ductal and lobular hyperplasia are considered risk factors for development of cancer.

3. **Associated Factors**
- Early menarche.
- Small breast size.
- History of cyclic breast discomfort.
- Irregular menses.
- Premenopausal status.
- Late menopause.
- Normal or low body weight.
- History of spontaneous abortions.
- Possible relation to increased caffeine intake.

4. **Clinical Features**
- Cyclical breast pain or tenderness, typically bilateral breast involvement with multiple smooth lumps.
- Nipple discharge may be noted (usually green or brownish, nonbloody).
- Sudden appearance or disappearance of cysts is common.
- Symptoms are often exacerbated during premenstrual cycle.
- Fluctuations in size and breast tenderness are common.
- Physical examination demonstrates tender, nodular breast(s).

5. **Diagnostic Studies**
- Imaging:
  - U/S: pregnant women or <30 years, useful to distinguish between solid mass and cystic lesion.
  - Mammogram: women >30 and not pregnant.
- FNA of "dominant" cysts to rule out carcinoma.
- Biopsy is definitive.

6. **Management**
- Breast pain due to mammary dysplasia is treated conservatively.
- Avoidance of breast trauma; wearing a brassiere to provide support and protection.
- Nonprescription analgesics (nonsteroidal anti-inflammatory drugs [NSAIDs] or acetaminophen) for pain.
- Avoidance of caffeine and addition of vitamin E and evening primrose oil to diet may improve symptoms.
- Smoking cessation is recommended because nicotine is thought to worsen breast pain.
- Discontinuing hormone replacement and decreasing estrogen in oral contraceptive pills may improve symptoms.
- For more symptomatic women, danazol and tamoxifen have been found to be effective.

B. Intraductal Papilloma

1. **Etiology**
   - Most common cause of bloody (or blood-tinged) nipple discharge.
   - Mostly located subareolar.

2. **Pathology**
   - Polypoid epithelial tumors arise in ducts of the breast.
   - These lesions typically have a long, slender stalk and are subject to torsion.
   - Rarely, diffuse papillomas can be present; these are typically multiple, involve breasts bilaterally, have a more "serous" discharge, and are associated with increased risk of cancer.

3. **Clinical Features**
   - Appears commonly with unilateral, spontaneous bloody, serous, or cloudy nipple discharge.
   - Solitary, central papillomas located in subareolar region.
   - Peripheral papillomas are typically multiple.

4. **Diagnostic Studies**
   - Guaiac test to differentiate between bloody and brownish nipple discharge.
   - Breast imaging: U/S for all women plus mammogram for women >30 years.
   - Other imaging tests: ductography, MRI, MR ductography.
   - Biopsy results of subareolar excision for treatment of nipple discharge distinguishes between intraductal papilloma and cancer.
   - Cytology of nipple discharge rarely helpful and not cost-effective.

5. **Management**
   - Nipple duct excision over a lacrimal duct probe or terminal duct resection.

C. Fibroadenoma

1. **Etiology**
   - Most common benign breast tumor.
   - Common in adolescents and young women (<30 years).
   - Usually appears suddenly.

2. **Pathology**
   - Hallmark of lesion: presence of stromal tissue with epithelium-lined, duct-like structures, and absence of elastic tissue.
   - Typically consists of a mixture of proliferating epithelial and fibrous tissues.

3. **Clinical Features**
   - Does not change with menstrual cycle.
   - Typically painless, slow-growing mass.
   - Commonly noted on breast self-examination (BSE).
   - Palpable breast mass: round, smooth, rubbery, mobile.

4. **Diagnostic Studies**
   - Definitive diagnosis confirmed with core needle biopsy or excision.
   - U/S can distinguish between cyst and solid mass.

5. **Management**
   - Core needle biopsy or short-term (3-6 months) follow-up with repeat U/S and breast examination.

D. Breast Abscess

1. **Etiology**
   - Relatively uncommon inflammatory process; purulent collection.
   - Two types: lactational and nonlactational.
   - Infection in the nonlactating breast is rare.
   - Can develop when mastitis or cellulitis does not respond to antibiotic regimen.

2. **Pathology**
   - *Staphylococcus aureus*; *methicillin-resistant S. aureus* cases are increasing.
   - Patients with recurrent breast abscess have an increased incidence of mixed flora and anaerobic infection.

3. **Clinical Features**
   - Localized, painful, tender, erythematous, warm breast mass, breast edema.
   - Fever and chills may occur.
   - Subareolar: nipple abnormality (nipple inversion or retraction).
   - Fluctuant, tender, palpable mass.
   - Axillary lymphadenopathy.

4. **Diagnostic Studies**
   - U/S distinguishes between abscess and mastitis and may be used for guided aspiration.

5. **Management**
   - If cellulitis is discovered without a palpable mass, antibiotic treatment is usually successful.
   - No need to stop breastfeeding.
   - Drainage: FNA or open surgical drainage with adequate debridement.
   - Antibiotics based on culture and sensitivity results.
   - Recurrent or unresolved mass needs biopsy to exclude cancer.

E. Breast Carcinoma

1. **Etiology**
   - Most common cancer in women.
   - Approximately 11% of women in the United States develop breast cancer.
   - Most cancers are diagnosed through biopsy of a nodule detected on either mammogram or by palpation.
   - Caucasian women have higher incidence of breast cancer than African American women older than 40 years.
   - African American women have higher incidence when younger than 40 years and are more likely to die of breast cancer at every age compared with Caucasian women.
   - **Risk factors:**
     - Age >50.
     - Personal history of breast cancer.
     - BRCA1 and BRCA2 inherited susceptibility genes.

- Family history (first-degree relatives).
- Postmenopausal obesity.
- Alcohol consumption.
- Early menarche.
- Late menopause.
- Nulliparity or >30 years for first, full-term pregnancy.
- Dense breast tissue.

2. Pathology
- Majority of breast cancers are invasive adenocarcinomas.
- Seventy to 80% are infiltrating ductal carcinomas.
- Cords and nests of cells with varying amounts of gland formation.
- Approximately 10% are infiltrating lobular carcinomas.
  - Small cells that insidiously infiltrate mammary stroma and adipose tissue individually and in a single file pattern.
  - Have a higher frequency of bilaterality and multicentricity.
- Breast cancer spreads by both vascular and lymphatic routes.
  - Adenocarcinomas (infiltrating, intraductal) spread to bones, lungs, liver, and brain.
  - Lobular spread to meninges, peritoneum, and gastrointestinal tract.

3. Clinical Features
- Early: tumor usually painless and may be mobile.
- Most patients present due to an abnormal mammogram.
- Most common: painless breast mass.
- Most common sites: upper outer quadrant (first); beneath the nipple–areola complex (second).
- As tumor grows, it becomes more fixed to ligaments and fascia, and borders become less distinct.
- Late: skin changes ("peau d'orange") and nipple discharge occur.

4. Diagnostic Studies
- Complete history and physical examination.
- Clinical breast examination.
- Bilateral mammography.
- Mammographic findings of breast cancer include presence of soft tissue mass or density and clustered microcalcifications.
- U/S can be used to distinguish benign from malignant lesion.
  - Malignant: speculation, hypoechogenicity, microlobulation, shadowing, lesion taller than is wide, angular margins.
- MRI for high-risk patients.
- FNA or core biopsy may be used initially.
- Women presenting with signs of inflammatory breast cancer require full-thickness skin biopsies.
- Staging: removal of primary tumor and ipsilateral lymph node resection.

- Chest X-ray (CXR), bone scan, and CT for further diagnosis if there are symptoms, positive lymph nodes, or tumors >5 cm.
- Presence of estrogen and progesterone receptor assessed in the specimen.

5. Management
  a. Goals
  - Control of local disease; treatment of distant disease; improved quality of life.
  - Dependent on staging of disease and patient goals.

  b. Treatment
  - Lumpectomy and radiation therapy: standard for women with small tumors.
  - Postlumpectomy breast irradiation greatly reduces the risk of recurrence in the breast.
    - Nearly one-third of women in the United States are managed by lumpectomy.
  - Mastectomy: used for large (>5 cm) and multicentric tumors; when tumors are scattered, and suspicious microcalcifications throughout breast tissue are present; when patients are unable or unwilling to receive postoperative radiation.
  - Sentinel lymph node biopsy (SLNB) is generally the standard of care for women with localized breast cancer and clinically negative axilla.
  - Metastatic disease: treatment modified according to (1) menopausal status, (2) hormone receptor status, and (3) sites of metastases.
  - Radiation: used postlumpectomy to treat remaining breast tissue; used on axilla only for invasive disease and if no axillary dissection was performed; used if positive axillary lymph nodes were left behind during lumpectomy, and as palliative control of metastatic ulceration pain.
  - Chemotherapy: used in select patients after surgery, before resection of the primary tumor, and/or in metastatic disease.
  - Hormonal: used in metastatic cancer or adjuvant therapy in early cancer for postmenopausal women (tamoxifen); used for premenopausal women with estrogen/progesterone receptors on the surface of tumor cells.
  - Targeted therapy: used for breast cancer caused by overproduction of growth-promoting protein HER2. Trastuzumab is a monoclonal antibody that targets this protein. Lapatinib is a tyrosine kinase inhibitor that targets this protein and is used for patients who have failed treatment with trastuzumab.
  - Bisphosphonates (zoledronate or pamidronate): decrease pain associated with bone metastasis and decrease fracture risk.

IV. Vascular Disorders
A. Compartment Syndrome
1. Etiology
- Trauma of the extremity, with edema or hemorrhage in the interstitial space of a compartment (one or more muscles enveloped by fascia).
- Common causes: long bone fractures, crush injuries, rhabdomyolysis, reperfusion of ischemic tissue (revascularization of extremities), external compression (such as tight bandaging/casting), and major vein ligation.
- Occurs most commonly in lower extremity, then forearm.
- May be acute or chronic; acute compartment syndrome (ACS) is a surgical emergency.
2. Pathology
- Increase in venous pressure and inadequate venous drainage lead to increased interstitial pressure, which leads to a reduction of capillary blood flow, causing ischemia, and ultimately cellular anoxia.
- Peripheral nerve ischemia is the hallmark of the disorder.
- Anterior compartment of the tibia is the most common site of ACS.
3. Clinical Features
- Pain (early, common finding), swelling, paresthesias, paralysis, and tense compartment.
- Tingling followed by sensory loss and paralysis of distal portions of the extremity involved—Volkmann contracture in the forearm, peroneal nerve injury, and foot drop in the leg.
- Pain with passive flexion of involved extremity.
4. Diagnostic Studies
- Distal pulses are usually present, although edema may impair palpation.
- Compartment pressure can be measured by insertion of a needle connected to manometer; elevation >30 to 40 mm Hg indicates a need for decompression.
5. Management
- Main goal is to avoid permanent nerve damage.
- Fasciotomy of all compartments involved (four in the leg) should be performed, followed by wound care and delayed wound closure.

B. Arterial Disease
1. Etiology
- Narrowing of arterial lumen due to plaque formation within vessel, progressive stenosis of vessel, embolism, thrombosis, or atherosclerosis.
- Most common cause: atherosclerosis.
- Important risk factors: smoking, hyperlipidemia, diabetes.
2. Pathology
- Changes in intima, media of arterial wall due to deposits of lipids, calcium, fibrin, inflammatory cells, and hemorrhage.
- Ischemia of tissue due to imbalance in supply and demand.
3. Clinical Features
- Calf, hip, thigh claudication.
- Impotence.
- Ischemic rest pain.
- Bruits.
- Decreased/absent pulses (femoral, popliteal/pedal pulses).
- Skin changes (coloration/pigmentation/ulcerations).
4. Evaluation (5 Ps)
- Pulselessness.
- Pallor.
- Paresthesias.
- Pain.
- Paralysis.
5. Diagnostic Studies
a. Noninvasive
- Doppler U/S:
  - Ankle/brachial (blood pressure [BP] ratio) (ABI = ankle BP/brachial artery BP rest or postexercise):
    - 1.2 to 2.0 or greater: medial calcinosis or noncompressible.
    - 0.9 to 1.2: normal.
    - 0.4 to 0.9: claudication.
    - 0.2 to 0.4: rest pain.
    - 0.0 to 0.2: tissue breakdown and threat to limb loss.
b. Invasive
- Angiography gives an anatomic description of vasculature. Advanced imaging (CTA or magnetic resonance angiography [MRA]) is used only when revascularization is planned.
- Cardiopulmonary, renal assessment, necessary pre-op evaluation.
6. Management
a. Surgery
- Reserved for patients who fail medical therapy and have severe ischemia.
- Amputation for patients with gangrene/extensive infection.
- Aortoiliac occlusion: aortobifemoral or axillobifemoral bypass (last resort before amputation): percutaneous endovascular stents and laser atherectomy for high-risk patients, less invasive than bypass.
  - Synthetic material above the groin, if necessary, and autogenous vein below.
b. Medical
- Involves cardiovascular risk reduction and lifestyle modification.
- Long-term use of antiplatelet therapy (aspirin and clopidogrel).
- Heparin (acute thrombosis), but still needs surgical intervention.

7. **Carotid Artery Stenosis**
   a. **Indication**
      - May cause transient ischemic attack and neurologic deficits.
      - CVA: neurologic deficit >24 hours.
      - Cerebral angiography and carotid duplex U/S used to evaluate degree of stenosis.
      - Surgery warranted if stenosis >70%, >69% to 50% if symptomatic.
   b. **Treatment**
      - Carotid endarterectomy or angioplasty with stenting.
   c. **Contraindication**
      - Total occlusion.
      - Acute stroke.
      - Fixed severe stroke.
   d. **Outcome**
      - Stroke: 2% to 7%.
      - Transient cranial nerve injury: 10%.
      - Death: <1%.

C. **Aortic Aneurysm (AA)**
   - Weakness and dilatation of vessel wall, caused by genetic or atherosclerotic damage.
   - Most common cause is atherosclerosis—also septic emboli, vasculitis, trauma, giant cell arteritis, and Marfan syndrome.
   - Aneurysms are 85% abdominal and 15% thoracic.
   - Rupture has a mortality rate between 45% and 50%.
   - May be asymptomatic, pulsatile abdominal mass.
   - Rupture causes severe back, abdominal flank pain, and hypotension.
   - Laboratory studies: abdominal U/S, CT; aortography is *not* a diagnostic study for aneurysms.
   - Surgical treatment for ruptured AA is emergent OR with control of hemorrhage and repair of aneurysm.
   - Elective endovascular repair of abdominal AA is indicated for symptomatic patients, or patients with abdominal AA >5.5 cm, or if the aneurysm has expanded >0.5 cm in 6 months.

D. **Prevention of Thromboembolic Events**
   - Use $CHADS_2$ score = **C**ongestive heart failure, **H**ypertension, **A**ge, **D**iabetes, **S**troke to determine risk.
   - Bridging anticoagulation for high-risk patients on warfarin:
      - Stop warfarin 5 days before surgery and allow the international normalized ratio (INR) to return to near normal. If INR ≥1.5, give vitamin K.
      - Give bridging SQ low-molecular-weight heparin (LMWH) or IV unfractionated heparin (UFH). Give half of regular dose as last dose of LMWH 24 hours before surgery. Stop UFH 4 hours before surgery.
      - May need to hold heparin longer for neurosurgical and ocular cases.
   - Restart warfarin in approximately 12 to 24 hours post-op if adequate hemostasis.
   - If bridging anticoagulation is continued, restart approximately 24 hours after surgery. If high risk for post-op bleeding, restart approximately 48 to 72 hours post-op.
   - If high risk of bleeding or contraindications to antithrombotic medications, use graduated compression stockings or intermittent pneumatic compression devices.

V. Gastrointestinal Disorders
ESOPHAGUS
A. Hiatal Hernia
   1. **Etiology**
      - Portion of the stomach prolapses through diaphragmatic esophageal hiatus of the stomach into the chest.
      - Type I, sliding hernia: gastroesophageal (GE) junction above the hiatus of the diaphragm—most common type of hiatal hernia.
      - Type II, "paraesophageal" hernia: GE junction remains intra-abdominal; fundus of the stomach herniates.
   2. **Pathology**
      - Type 1, sliding hernia, does not have a hernia sac and slides into the chest because the GE junction is not fixed inside of the abdomen.
      - Type II, paraesophageal hernia, is a true hernia with a hernia sac. It is an upward dislocation of the gastric fundus through a defect in the phrenoesophageal membrane.
   3. **Clinical Features**
      - Most small, Type I sliding hernias are asymptomatic.
      - Large Type I hernias are often associated with GE reflux; symptoms include heartburn, regurgitation, and dysphagia.
      - Complications are rare with Type II hiatal hernias and are usually related to reflux.
      - Paraesophageal hernias are either asymptomatic or vague, intermittent symptoms; most commonly, epigastric or substernal pain, or postprandial fullness, nausea, retching. GE reflux symptoms are less prevalent, when compared with Type I hernias.
      - Most complications of paraesophageal hernias are due to mechanical problems caused by the hernia, such as gastric volvulus.
      - Advanced cases may result in dysphagia, bleeding from gastric ulceration, gastritis, or erosions (Cameron lesions), retrosternal pain, and respiratory symptoms from mechanical compression.
      - In a paraesophageal hernia, part of the stomach can be strangulated, leading to necrosis and perforation. This acute syndrome carries high mortality if diagnosis and treatment are delayed.

4. **Diagnostic Studies**
  - Upper endoscopy can diagnose sliding and paraesophageal hiatal hernias and allow biopsy of suspicious lesions. Small sliding hiatal hernias (<2 cm) often reduce spontaneously and can only be diagnosed with certainty during surgery.
  - High-resolution manometry (HRM) with esophageal pressure topography (EPT) can characterize a hiatal hernia by the separation of the crural diaphragm from the lower esophageal sphincter by a pressure trough.
  - Barium swallow is the most sensitive diagnostic test for paraesophageal hernias.

5. **Management**
  a. **Conservative**
    - Management of symptomatic gastroesophageal reflux disease (GERD) with postural adjustment, antacids after meals and at bedtime, histamine-2 (H_2) receptor blockers, proton-pump inhibitors, and diet modification.
    - Weight control.
  b. **Surgical**
    - Indicated for large hernias or symptomatic paraesophageal hernias, stricture, bleeding, recurrent aspiration pneumonitis, and Barrett esophagitis.
    - Emergent surgical repair for patients with gastric volvulus, uncontrolled bleeding, obstruction, strangulation, perforation, and respiratory compromise.
    - Fundoplication (Nissen-type procedure): gastric fundus is wrapped around the intra-abdominal portion of the esophagus, and the hiatus is narrowed with sutures.

B. **Esophageal Perforation**
  1. **Etiology**
    - Spontaneous or strain-induced (Boerhaave syndrome).
    - Increased intraluminal pressure at the anatomic sites of narrowing can lead to rupture of the esophagus.
    - Results in mediastinitis without prompt diagnosis and treatment.
    - Iatrogenic: endoscopy, dilation of strictures, intubation. Iatrogenic causes are the most common cause of perforation.
    - Traumatic: penetrating missile, swallowed foreign body, blunt chest or abdominal injury, surgical dissection, ingestion of caustic agents.
    - Intrinsic esophageal disease: peptic ulceration, carcinoma.
    - Anastomotic leak after esophageal surgery.
  2. **Clinical Features**
    - Usually dramatic, irreversible sepsis may ensue within 24 hours.
    - Severe retching followed by acute pain.

  - "Mackler triad"—vomiting, lower chest pain, cervical SQ emphysema—uncommon.
  - Pain (chest or epigastric—depending on location of tear); respiratory symptoms (dyspnea, cyanosis); rarely, tension pneumothorax occurs (usually following endoscopy).
  - Cervical tear: pain in the neck; crepitus; dysphagia.
  - Thoracic tear: pain in the chest or epigastric area; tachypnea, dyspnea.
  - Fever, tachycardia, tachypnea, hypotension, and shock.
  - Hamman sign: "crunching" sound heard in systole, caused by heart beating against air-filled mediastinum.
  - Mediastinal and SQ emphysema.

3. **Diagnostic Studies**
  - CXR: air in the mediastinum (the "V" sign of Naclerio), air under the diaphragm, SQ emphysema, and pneumothorax.
  - Abdominal X-ray: pneumoperitoneum.
  - Esophagogram with water-soluble contrast (Gastrografin): extraluminal leak of contrast. Use barium if negative with Gastrografin.
  - Upper endoscopy: controversial because of insufflation of air; reserve for patients in whom location of perforation is unclear from imaging.
  - CT scan of chest: if esophagography is contraindicated or results are nondiagnostic.

4. **Management**
  - Patient's oral intake is restricted.
  - Rapid resuscitation with fluids and intravenous (IV) antibiotics is paramount.
  - Perforations of the cervical esophagus may respond to broad-spectrum antibiotics, elimination of all feeding, and total parenteral nutrition.
  - A primary repair is the gold standard of care. A laparotomy is the preferred approach to repair a perforation of an intra-abdominal esophagus.
  - Drainage of the area of perforation alone should be performed only if it is a cervical perforation that cannot be visualized and there is no distal obstruction.
  - Cervical esophagostomy with gastrostomy is an alternative for a hemodynamically unstable and critically ill patient.
  - Mortality rate following operative management is dependent on location of the perforation, with cervical perforations having the lowest mortality rate (6%), thoracic perforations (27% to 34%), and intra-abdominal perforations (21% to 29%).

C. **Esophageal Carcinoma**
  1. **Etiology**
    - Peak incidence in fifth and seventh decades; male:female ratio is 3:1.
    - Squamous cell:
      - Risk factors are smoking and alcohol use.

- More common in African Americans than in Caucasians.
  - Adenocarcinoma: more common in Caucasians than in African Americans.
    - Associated with Barrett esophagus with intestinal metaplasia due to GERD; obesity and smoking are risk factors.
  - Premalignant lesions: achalasia, reflux esophagitis, radiation esophagitis, caustic burns.
2. **Pathology**
   - Squamous cell carcinoma: most common type worldwide.
   - Adenocarcinoma: arises in distal esophagus and esophagogastric junction—accounts for >60% of all esophageal cancers in the United States.
   - Rare types: anaplastic small cell carcinoma (oat cell carcinoma), adenoid cystic carcinoma, malignant melanoma, and carcinosarcoma.
   - Metastasize to lymph nodes, liver, lungs, bone, and brain.
3. **Clinical Features**
   - Dysphagia and weight loss: most common presenting symptoms.
   - Odynophagia, chest pain, and hematemesis.
   - Approximately 6% to 10% are asymptomatic at the time of diagnosis.
4. **Diagnostic Studies**
   - Endoscopic biopsy must be performed to confirm diagnosis.
   - Diagnosis requires histologic examination of tumor tissues.
   - Endoscopic resection may be feasible for small lesions (<2 cm and involve less than one-third of the circumference of the esophageal wall).
   - Brush cytology has been used for screening in some regions to increase biopsy accuracy.
   - Other studies (CT scan, bone scan) to rule out metastases.
5. **Management**
   - In the majority of patients, local tumor spread or distant metastases preclude cure.
   - Palliation (i.e., restoring the patient's ability to swallow comfortably) is important. Palliative treatment using prosthetic stents and laser can be used.
   - Major goals of palliative therapy are restoration and/or maintenance of the ability to swallow, management of pain, and prevention of bleeding.
   - Chemotherapy and radiotherapy may also be used for palliation and as adjuvants to surgical treatment.
   - Surgical resection is the treatment of choice to attempt cure and stage.
   - Preoperative chemoradiation preferred for T3 to T4, or node-positive localized cancer has demonstrated better survival when compared with local therapy alone.

- Types of surgical resections include transthoracic esophagectomy (Ivor Lewis procedure) and transhiatal esophagectomy (cervical and abdominal incisions), which allows removal of the entire esophagus without thoracotomy.

GALLBLADDER DISEASE
A. Cholelithiasis
1. **Etiology**
   - Symptomatic gallbladder stones affect 10% to 25% of the population.
   - More common in females in their forties, fertile, and obese (fat)—"the four Fs."
   - Also more common in Western Caucasian, Native American, Hispanics African Americans with sickle cell disease, patients with Crohn disease, and post-bariatric surgery patients.
2. **Pathology**
   - The gallbladder contains single or, more often, multiple stones and may have various degrees of inflammation (cholecystitis).
   - Types: cholesterol, pigmented (calcium), mixed.
   - Most common: cholesterol (>75%); pigment (15%).
3. **Clinical Features**
   - Majority of patients have no symptoms, or vague and occasional abdominal discomfort.
   - Symptoms are characterized by recurrent biliary colic attacks—right upper quadrant (RUQ) or epigastric pain, often radiating to the back, diaphoresis, nausea, and vomiting—which last 30 minutes to 6 hours, subsiding spontaneously. Biliary colic may be precipitated by fatty food and rapid weight loss in obese patients.
   - Pain of biliary colic caused by obstruction of cystic duct.
4. **Diagnostic Studies**
   - U/S is the main diagnostic tool to determine the presence of stones, inflammation of gallbladder wall, and obstruction of the extrahepatic biliary ducts.
5. **Management**
   - Avoidance of offending foods.
   a. **Medical Treatment**
      - Dissolution of gallstones through biliary lithotripsy and bile salt therapy (ursodeoxycholic acid), but has limited application and may offer only temporary relief.
   b. **Surgical Treatment**
      - Not recommended as prophylaxis in asymptomatic patients.
      - *Laparoscopic cholecystectomy* is currently the treatment of choice for symptomatic cholelithiasis.
      - ERCP (endoscopic retrograde cholangiopancreatography) for removal of common bile duct (CBD) stones in acute choledocholithiasis.

- Open cholecystectomy needed in 1% to 2% of elective procedures and 5% to 10% of acute cholecystitis.

B. Cholecystitis

1. Etiology
- Acute or chronic inflammation of the gallbladder.
- Classic syndrome: RUQ pain, fever, and leukocytosis with gallbladder inflammation.
- Gallstones are present in 95% of cases (calculous cholecystitis), presumably causing obstruction of the cystic duct (gallbladder neck).
- Less commonly: sepsis, prolonged fasting, vasculitis, and ischemia may cause acalculous cholecystitis.
- Most of these cases occur in patients hospitalized for other causes.

2. Pathology
- Acute: the gallbladder is tense and distended; may have areas of necrosis and contain purulent material. In acalculous cholecystitis, gangrene is the rule.
- Chronic: the gallbladder wall is thickened and infiltrated with chronic inflammatory cells.

3. Clinical Features
- Acute: mild-to-intense RUQ colicky/constant pain radiating to right subcapsular area, nausea and vomiting, fever, leukocytosis, RUQ tenderness, and sometimes peritonitis. (+) Murphy sign; palpation of the gallbladder.
- Pain may initially be epigastric, but rapidly advances to abdominal tenderness.
- Patients are ill appearing, febrile, tachycardiac, with RUQ guarding and positive Murphy sign.
- Chronic: ill-defined clinical picture with recurrent symptoms of biliary obstruction or vague abdominal pain and dyspeptic symptoms.

4. Diagnostic Studies
- U/S: the test of choice.
- CT/MRCP scanning: have high sensitivity and specificity for acute cholecystitis; also useful for evaluating surrounding tissues.
- Hepatobiliary scintigraphy scan (HIDA scan): for negative U/S.
- ERCP or endoscopic ultrasonography.

5. Management
a. Medical Treatment
- Sixty percent of cases resolve with antibiotics and supportive care.
- Calculous cholecystitis may be treated with antibiotics followed by surgery within a few days or, in certain cases, after 4 to 5 weeks when the inflammation is resolved.
- Antiemetics and oral analgesics.

b. Surgical Treatment
- Cholecystectomy, laparoscopic or open, carries a low morbidity and overall mortality rate of

<0.2%. Most deaths occur in elderly or severely ill patients undergoing emergency operation.
- Acalculous acute cholecystitis requires emergent surgery.
- Percutaneous cholecystostomy tube insertion for drainage of gallbladder in patients at high surgical risk until surgically stable and after antibiotic treatment.
- Removed gallbladder should be evaluated for cancer in pathology.

LIVER

A. Carcinoma

1. Etiology
- Primary hepatic carcinoma in the United States is uncommon.
- Most malignancy in the liver is metastatic versus primary (20:1); the primary is usually in the gastrointestinal (GI) tract, breast, or lung.
- Most common metastatic lesion from colorectal cancer.
- Risk factors:
  - Hepatitis B (HBV) or C (HCV) infection.
  - Aflatoxins: food contamination by *Aspergillus flavus*.
  - Cirrhosis: of any cause.
  - Parasitosis: liver fluke *Clonorchis sinensis* (Asia).
  - Genetic: deficiency in α-antitrypsin or hemochromatosis.

2. Pathology
- Hepatocellular carcinoma (HCC, hepatoma): single or multiple nodules with prominent vascularity.
- Cholangiocarcinoma: a type of adenocarcinoma arising from intrahepatic or extrahepatic bile ducts.
- Hepatoblastoma: the fetal variant of HCC with familial adenomatous polyposis; seen in infants.
- Metastatic: more commonly, multiple nodules; histology resembles that of the primary tumor; mostly GI tract adenocarcinoma.

3. Clinical Features
- Often asymptomatic early in disease, other than symptoms from chronic liver disease.
- General: anorexia, fatigue, weight loss, abdominal mass (enlarged, hard liver, or other primary tumor).
- RUQ tenderness, ascites.
- Biliary obstruction: jaundice, pruritus.
- Portal hypertension: ascites, splenomegaly, prominent abdominal veins ("caput medusae" represents periumbilical vein dilatation).

4. Diagnostic Studies
- U/S: noninvasive, inexpensive, good resolution; best for lesions, 1 cm, repeat U/S every 3 months.
- Liver function studies: α-fetoprotein (AFP) increased.

- Helical, multiphasic CT scan and MRI with contrast (CT preferred): provide precise location, extent of invasion of surrounding structures, and involvement of other organs, indicated when lesions are >1 cm.
- Percutaneous or laparoscopic needle biopsy: definitive diagnosis. Indicated when imaging is not definitive. If liver biopsy is negative, follow-up imaging in 3 to 6 months.
- PET scan for suspected metastasis to the liver.

5. **Management**
   a. **Medical Treatment**
      - Metastatic liver cancer is usually treated with chemotherapy alone; exceptions include colon cancer and neuroendocrine tumors, which may respond better to resection.
   b. **Surgical Treatment**
      - Depending on location and number of lesions, primary and metastatic tumors can be removed by local excision, right or left hepatectomy (removal of half the liver), or various types of "segmentectomies."
      - Liver transplantation for malignant tumors is evolving.
      - Cryoablation (freezing with liquid nitrogen), alcoholization, and radiotherapy are used in select patients.

B. Portal Hypertension

1. **Etiology**
   - Most common basic lesion: increased resistance to blood flow.
   - Most common cause in the United States: cirrhosis, due to chronic alcoholism (most common), posthepatitis. Elsewhere: schistosomiasis.
   - Budd–Chiari syndrome: phlebitis or web obstructing suprahepatic veins.
   - Extrinsic compression: trauma, inflammatory process, tumor.
   - Schistosomiasis: common in tropical countries.

2. **Pathology**
   - Portal pressure >12 mm Hg, with associated complications: esophageal varices, encephalopathy, hypersplenism, ascites, and spontaneous peritonitis.
   - Variceal hemorrhage is most common complication.
   - Collateral circulation develops through:
     - Coronary vein (lesser curvature of the stomach and esophageal venous plexi).
     - Superior hemorrhoidal veins (tributaries of inferior mesenteric vein).
     - Anterior abdominal wall veins (from umbilical vein).
     - Plexus of Retzius (retroperitoneal anastomoses between mesenteric veins and inferior vena cava).
   - Ascites is the result of transudation from the liver capsule.

3. **Clinical Features**
   - History, symptoms, and signs of liver disease.
   - Abdominal distension from ascites (fluid wave on examination).
   - Esophageal varices often causing massive GI bleeding.
   - Caput medusae: dilated paraumbilical veins.
   - Hemorrhoids and hemorrhoidal bleeding.
   - Other manifestations include splenomegaly, thrombocytopenia, primary peritonitis (infected ascitic fluid without visceral perforation), encephalopathy, hypersplenism (anemia, thrombocytopenia, leukopenia), and malnutrition.

4. **Diagnostic Studies**
   - Hepatic venous pressure gradient measurement.
   - Abnormal liver function tests (LFTs; bilirubin, transaminases), anemia, hypoalbuminemia.
   - U/S shows ascites, splenomegaly, and changes in liver parenchyma.
   - Duplex U/S may be useful to evaluate thrombosis of portal vein.
   - CT scan shows ascites, splenomegaly, dilated venous collaterals, associated intra-abdominal pathology (e.g., tumor), and portal vein thrombosis.
   - MRI/magnetic resonance angiography: similar result as CT scan.
   - Liver biopsy (percutaneous or laparoscopic) provides histologic diagnosis.
   - Peritoneocentesis to obtain ascitic fluid for biochemical and bacteriologic analysis.

5. **Management**
   a. **Medical Treatment**
      - Main goal is prevention and treatment of complications.
      - Mainstay of therapy for cirrhosis and portal hypertension.
      - Diuretics and nutritional measures (sodium restriction) to control ascites.
      - Endoscopic injection sclerotherapy or band ligation for bleeding esophageal varices.
      - Vasopressin with nitrates, octreotide, and propranolol to reduce portal pressure.
   b. **Surgical Treatment**
      - Control of ascites: paracentesis and peritoneovenous conduits (LeVeen and Denver shunts).
      - Decompression of the portal system:
        - Transjugular intrahepatic portosystemic shunt (TIPS).
        - Portosystemic shunts (splenorenal, mesocaval, portacaval) less commonly used but still useful in select patients.
      - Direct control of variceal bleeding via β-blockers and endoscopic ligation.
      - Devascularization procedures: splenectomy, GE devascularization (Sugiura procedure).
      - Liver transplantation.

SMALL BOWEL

A. Obstruction

1. **Etiology**
   - Adhesions from previous surgery are the most common cause.
   - Without prior surgery, incarcerated or strangulated hernias are usually the cause.
   - Other causes include tumor, radiation enteritis, inflammatory stricture (e.g., Crohn disease), intestinal torsion, peritonitis (nonmechanical obstruction or "ileus"), and ischemic disease.

2. **Pathology**
   - Adhesions are formed by fibrous tissue (bands) and may cause narrowing, kinking, twisting, or internal herniation of the bowel.
   - Inflammatory disorders such as TB and Crohn disease may cause thickening of the intestinal wall, perforation, and adhesions.
   - Adenocarcinoma is the most common tumor obstructing the small bowel or colon.

3. **Clinical Features**
   - Nausea and vomiting, obstipation, variable or crampy abdominal pain initially, followed by constant pain when necrosis or perforation is present.
   - Crampy abdominal pain has "crescendo-decrescendo" pattern.
   - Abdominal distension, increased bowel sounds or high-pitched, "tinkling" sounds on auscultation in partial obstruction, whereas muffled or absent bowel sounds in complete obstruction; no stool in the rectum unless fecal impaction is the cause.
   - Peristalsis may be visible.
   - Incarcerated (nonreducible) hernia in the groin, epigastrium, umbilicus, or at site of scar from previous operation or trauma (incisional hernia).
   - Tumor or inflammatory mass may be felt on abdominal or rectal examination.
   - Insertion of nasogastric tube (NGT) disclosing fecaloid fluid usually reflects lower small bowel obstruction or colonic obstruction.
   - Strangulated (death of tissue) results in peritoneal signs.

4. **Diagnostic Studies**
   - Obstructive series (supine and upright abdominal, and CXRs): most important test following clinical evaluation; can show intestinal distension, air–fluid levels, free air under the diaphragm in the case of perforation, and suggest underlying cause of the obstruction (e.g., large tumor, gallstone ileus).
   - CT scan may show "transition point" at obstruction or cause of obstruction such as tumor, abscess, or free air, indicating bowel perforation.
   - Blood tests may confirm dehydration, electrolyte disturbances, renal impairment, or suggest underlying cause.

5. **Management**
   a. **Medical Treatment**
      - Partial obstruction:
        - Initial treatment is IV fluids and NGT decompression.
        - Most will spontaneously resolve with decompression.
      - Complete obstruction:
        - Initial treatment is IV fluids and NGT placed on continuous suction.
        - Antibiotics may be indicated for infectious causes.
        - Serial clinical examination, electrolytes, and imaging radiographic follow-up to rule out bowel ischemia or strangulation.
   b. **Surgical Treatment**
      - Indicated for bowel perforation or when conservative management (NGT decompression and bowel rest) fails to allow bowel obstruction to resolve.
      - Exploratory laparotomy (open) or diagnostic laparoscopy may be indicated.
      - Lysis of adhesions, transection of fibrous band, tumor excision, bowel resection or diversion (colostomy, ileostomy), insertion of gastrostomy or jejunostomy tubes, and hernia repair may be needed.

B. Ileus

1. **Etiology**
   - Intestinal atony or hypotony due to nonmechanical cause; intestine is paralyzed, lacking peristaltic movements—"paralytic ileus."
   - Causes include peritonitis, electrolyte imbalance, postoperative and posttraumatic ileus, medications (narcotics), and rare dysmotility disorders.
   - Most common cause of ileus is postsurgical use of narcotic medications and spontaneously resolves over 1 to 3 days.

2. **Pathology**
   - Bowel distension, with intraluminal gas and fluid accumulation, without mechanical obstruction.
   - Nervous plexus cells may be absent in congenital dysmotility disorders.

3. **Clinical Features**
   - Distension, vomiting, and obstipation, mild-to-moderate abdominal discomfort unless peritonitis ensues.
   - Inability to tolerate a diet postoperatively.
   - Abdominal distension, hypoactive bowel sounds.

4. **Diagnostic Studies**
   - X-rays and CT scan show distension of both large and small bowel loops, no "transition zone," and air within the colon.

5. **Management**
   - The main goal is to correct any underlying pathology.

- Supportive therapy includes NPO, NGT decompression, and replacement of fluid and electrolytes.
- Consider selective opioid antagonists to prevent postoperative narcotic-induced ileus.
- Surgery is reserved for complications, such as perforation with peritonitis or abscess, for chronic and intractable patients, and rarely for diagnosis.

C. Neoplasms

1. Etiology/Pathology
- Relatively rare (2%); most common cancers are carcinoid (gastrointestinal neuroendocrine tumors) (40%) and then adenocarcinoma (30%).
- Includes sarcomas and gastrointestinal stromal tumors and lymphomas.
- Carcinoid tumors arise from neuroendocrine cells; terminal ileum is the most common site.

2. Clinical Features
- Typically asymptomatic in early stages.
- Abdominal pain and weight loss: most common presenting symptoms.
- Chronic colicky abdominal pain, chronic anemia or overt hemorrhage, small bowel obstruction, nausea, vomiting.
- Carcinoid tumors may cause bronchospasm, cutaneous flushing, diarrhea, and right-sided heart failure ("carcinoid syndrome").

3. Diagnostic Studies
- Usually, the diagnosis is established during laparotomy for intestinal obstruction.
- CT scan, enteroscopy, and laparoscopy may provide preoperative diagnosis in some patients.

4. Management
- Surgical resection is indicated for all small intestinal tumors. Survival depends on location. Carcinoid and adenoma tumors are treated with wide resection. Lymphoma is treated with abdominal radiation with or without chemotherapy.

D. Appendicitis

1. Etiology
- Obstruction of the vermiform appendix by foreign bodies, enlarged lymphatic tissue, parasites, "fecalith," or benign/malignant appendiceal tumor.
- Typically is present in second or third decade.
- Most common nonobstetric surgical disease in pregnancy.
- Perforation higher in elderly patients because of impaired blood flow (atherosclerosis) causing earlier perforation; atypical presentation.

2. Pathology
- Nonperforated (simple/uncomplicated) versus perforated (complicated).
- Early stages: vascular congestion, edema, neutrophilic infiltrates, mucosal necrosis, luminal occlusion (e.g., fecalith).
- Late stages: gangrene, perforation, abscess formation, or diffuse peritonitis.

- Cecum may be mobile; therefore, appendix may be located anywhere in the abdominal cavity, and this may cause atypical presentation.

3. Clinical Features

a. Classic Presentations
- Periumbilical discomfort, anorexia, nausea and vomiting, right lower quadrant (RLQ) pain, and fever.
- Movement of pain from periumbilical area to RLQ.
- Guarding, rigidity, + Rovsing, and + psoas signs.
- RLQ tenderness (McBurney point) with rebound, right-sided tenderness on rectal examination.

b. Less Common Presentations
- Pain in other locations than RLQ; diarrhea; diffuse peritonitis (common in children and elderly patients); chronic recurrent appendicitis (poorly defined entity; other disorders must be excluded).
- Combination of history, physical examination, complete blood count (CBC), and abdominal CT scan should provide correct diagnosis in majority of patients.

4. Diagnostic Studies
- CBC with differential demonstrates leukocytosis.
- U/S and CT scan can be helpful in doubtful cases, particularly in children and elderly and in advanced appendicitis with abscess formation.

5. Management
- Early appendicitis is best treated with urgent appendectomy and preoperative antibiotics.
- Advanced cases, with rupture and localized abscess, may be treated with IV antibiotics and U/S-guided percutaneous drainage, followed by delayed ("interval") appendectomy.
- Appendectomy can be most commonly performed through laparoscopy. Can also be performed using an oblique or transverse incision in the RLQ (McBurney and Rocky-Davis incisions).

COLON, RECTUM, AND ANUS

A. Carcinoma

1. Etiology

a. Risk Factors for Colorectal Cancer
- Smoking, heavy alcohol use, obesity, lack of fiber, overconsumption of red meat.
- Genetic: familial adenomatous polyposis, Gardner syndrome.
- Others: inflammatory bowel disease (ulcerative colitis), neoplastic polyps (usually >2 cm), age >40.

b. Risk Factors for Anal Cancer
- Human papillomavirus (HPV), prior radiation.

2. Pathology
- Colorectal: >90% adenocarcinoma.

- Anal: approximately 60% squamous cell carcinoma; approximately 20% cloacogenic.
- Most common metastasis: regional lymph nodes.
3. **Clinical Features**
   - Abdominal pain, palpable mass.
   - Colorectal: obstruction/diarrhea, bleeding, chronic anemia, perforation.
   - Rectal: hematochezia, tenesmus, discharge, obstruction.
4. **Diagnostic Studies**
   - Fecal occult blood plus rectal examination are most cost-effective screening methods (rectal examination discloses ~20% of all colorectal tumors).
   - Proctosigmoidoscopy, colonoscopy, and barium enema can provide definitive diagnosis and location.
   - Blood levels of carcinoembryonic antigen are useful to detect recurrence after surgery.
   - CT scan of abdomen/pelvis/lung to evaluate metastasis.
5. **Management**
   - Patients at increased risk should undergo periodic early screening.
   - Colon: wide surgical excision and regional lymphatics.
   - Rectal: surgery with chemoradiation.
   - Depending on location, permanent colostomy may be necessary.

B. **Anal Fissure**
   1. **Etiology**
      - Mechanical trauma, ischemia, and infection have all been postulated as causes of anal fissure.
      - Most common cause: passage of large, hard stools.
   2. **Pathology**
      - Superficial tear in the anoderm.
      - Acute: sudden tearing pain, bleeding.
      - Chronic: >6 weeks.
      - Most fissures are located on the posterior midline.
      - In the early phases, shallow ulceration with ill-defined edges; later, deeper ulcer, regular edges.
   3. **Clinical Features**
      - Painful linear or elliptic ulceration in the anal canal.
      - Rectal pain, blood stools, mucoid discharge.
   4. **Diagnostic Studies**
      - Digital examination discloses spasm of anal sphincter, and anoscopy confirms the presence of fissure—may require sedation to complete examination.
      - CBC to rule out anemia and infection.
      - Differential diagnosis: ulcerative colitis and Crohn disease, perirectal abscess, hemorrhoids, fistula-in-ano, squamous cell carcinoma, syphilis, TB, and ulcerations in immunosuppressed patients (leukemia, AIDS).

5. **Management**
   a. **Medical Treatment**
      - WASH: **w**arm water baths (sitz baths), **a**nalgesics (lidocaine jelly), **s**tool softeners, and **h**igh-fiber diet resolve 90% of cases.
      - Majority of fissures resolve spontaneously.
      - Topical nitroglycerin to relieve anal spasm and promote healing.
      - Botulinum toxin injection.
   b. **Surgical Treatment**
      - Sphincterotomy of the internal sphincter reduces spasm and allows healing; the external sphincter must be spared to preserve anal continence.
      - Anal dilatation under anesthesia can provide pain relief in 80% to 90% of cases; however, recurrence occurs in approximately 10% and sphincter dysfunction in approximately 10%.

C. **Ischemic Bowel Disease/Mesenteric Ischemia**
   1. **Etiology**
      - Thrombosis: hypercoagulable states, aortic dissection, atherosclerosis of visceral vessels (celiac trunk, superior mesenteric artery [SMA], inferior mesenteric artery [IMA] vasospasm).
      - Embolism: clot dislodged from the heart, atrial fibrillation, ventricular aneurysm.
      - Low flow: congestive heart failure (CHF), vasoconstrictive agents, shock.
   2. **Pathology**
      - SMA syndrome: extensive ischemia or necrosis of small and large intestines, from ligament of Treitz to mid-transverse colon.
      - IMA syndrome: left colon and sigmoid involvement.
      - Celiac artery is usually narrowed or occluded.
   3. **Clinical Features**
      - Acute event with rapid clinical deterioration: hypotension, shock, acidosis, renal failure, and death.
      - Manifestations more insidious in thrombosis and low flow; more abrupt in embolism.
      - Abdominal pain out of proportion with physical signs.
      - Abdominal distension, peritonitis, and bloody stools later in course.
      - Severe acidosis, with high lactic acid in the blood.
      - High degree of suspicion when risk factors are present: old age, cardiovascular disease, and low flow states.
   4. **Diagnostic Studies**
      - Plain X-rays show dilated loops with edema of the bowel wall ("thumbprinting").
      - Angiography can provide precise anatomic diagnosis and can be used for intra-arterial thrombolytic therapy in select patients.
      - CT scan can show aortic dissection, bowel distension and edema, arterial calcifications, and associated intra-abdominal pathology.

5. **Management**
    a. **Medical Treatment**
        - Rapid fluid resuscitation, intensive care, anticoagulation, and thrombolysis—urokinase, streptokinase, tissue-type plasminogen activator (tPA)—as indicated.
        - NGT placement.
    b. **Surgical Treatment**
        - Visceral thromboembolectomy and revascularization when intestines are viable.
        - Most patients require extensive bowel resection, plus enterostomy.

D. Pilonidal Cyst and Abscess
1. **Etiology**
    - Caused by hair and cellular debris finding entry into hair follicles (pit).
    - Cystic cavity containing keratin and hair in the SQ tissues of the natal cleft (between the buttocks in the sacrococcygeal area).
2. **Pathology**
    - Hyperkeratotic invagination, inflammation, granuloma, and sinus formation.
3. **Clinical Features**
    - Acute presentation: abscess; red and warm swelling, sometimes fluctuance, in the upper intergluteal fold; may be paramedian.
    - Chronic presentation: sinus felt in the natal cleft, with occasional discomfort or discharge.
4. **Diagnostic Studies**
    - Physical examination is sufficient to make the diagnosis.
    - Differential diagnosis includes hidradenitis, perirectal abscess with fistulas, and folliculitis.
5. **Management**
    - Abscess is treated with incision and drainage and removal of hair pit. Postoperative shaving and removal of hair from area have a 90% success rate.
    - Chronic noninfected, symptomatic sinuses are best excised with open packing, marsupialization, or wound flaps; only complete excision prevents recurrence.

E. Pancreatic Cancer
1. **Etiology**
    - Incidence has increased 3-fold in past 40 years.
    - In the United States, approximately 55,440 patients are diagnosed with cancer of the exocrine pancreas annually, and almost all are expected to die of the disease.
    - Second most common GI tract malignancy.
    - Fourth most common cause of cancer death.
    - Incidence increases with age and peaks in fifth and sixth decades of life.
    - Male to female incidence ratio, 1:1.
2. **Pathology**
    - Three types of tumors: (1) adenocarcinoma—arises from ductal epithelium, most common; (2) endocrine tumors; (3) cystic pancreatic neoplasms.
    - Benign neoplasms are exceedingly rare.
    - Half the lesions localized in the head; 20% in the body; <5% in the tail; 20% are multicentric.
3. **Clinical Features**
    - Most commonly, painless; jaundice is presenting symptom.
    - Severe weight loss, abdominal pain.
    - Pruritus of hands/feet.
    - Palpable nontender gallbladder (Courvoisier sign), due to neoplastic obstruction of common duct.
    - Abdominal mass or supraclavicular node (suggestive of distant metastasis).
4. **Diagnostic Studies**
    - Laboratory studies: often nonspecific, but usually support obstructive jaundice.
    - Abdominal U/S: may show dilatation of biliary ducts and, less commonly, may disclose mass at the head of pancreas.
    - CT scan: detects mass and ductal dilatation and is the test of choice for initial evaluation (helical or spiral CT).
    - ERCP (necessary if CT scan is negative): may show duodenal or ampullary lesion, "double duct sign," irregular narrowing of both intrapancreatic CBD and pancreatic duct, suggesting pancreatic cancer.
    - Laparoscopy: may be used for staging, before laparotomy.
    - Aspiration biopsy of pancreatic mass avoided for resectable tumors secondary to risk of spreading tumor cells intraperitoneally.
5. **Management**
    - Resectable tumors (<25%) in the head of pancreas treated with pancreaticoduodenectomy (Whipple procedure) or duodenal sparing procedure (modified Whipple).
    - Unresectable tumors (75%) treated with palliative biliary bypass or endoscopic stenting of the CBD.
    - Five-year survival rate after resection is <5%.
    - Chemotherapy and radiotherapy have shown some short-term benefit, but do not improve long-term survival; clinical trials continue at some large medical centers.

VI. Genitourinary Tract Disorders—Male
A. Testicular Carcinoma
1. **Etiology**
    - Most common solid tumors in male adolescents and adults (15 to 35 years).
    - Risk of testicular malignancy is 1 in 500.
    - The five-year survival rate is >95%.
    - The lifetime probability of developing testicular cancer is 0.3% for an American male.
    - Approximately 5% of testicular cancers develop in a patient with a history of cryptorchidism, seminoma being the most common.

2. **Pathology**
   - Germ cell tumors account for 95% of testicular cancer.
     - Seminomas account for 35% of all germ cell tumors.
     - Nonseminomatous germ cell tumors (NSGCTs) are all other germ cell tumors; embryonal, teratoma, choriocarcinoma, and mixed cell.
   - Non-germ cell neoplasms: Leydig cell, Sertoli cell, gonadoblastoma.
3. **Clinical Features**
   - Most commonly, single, hard, nontender mass, and painless swelling noted on testicle.
   - Other symptoms related to metastasis may be present.
   - Gynecomastia occurs in approximately 5% of men with testicular germ cell tumors.
4. **Diagnostic Studies**
   - Scrotal U/S shows a hypoechoic area in seminomas.
   - Serum tumor markers: AFP, β-subunit of human chorionic gonadotropin (β-hCG), and lactate dehydrogenase (LDH).
   - Serum AFP and/or β-hCG is elevated in 80% to 85% of NSGCTs.
   - Serum AFP is not elevated in pure seminomas.
   - CT scan of abdomen and pelvis is used to evaluate retroperitoneum for metastasis.
   - Neither scrotal U/S nor serum tumor markers are sufficiently accurate to replace radical inguinal orchiectomy.
5. **Management**
   - Inguinal orchiectomy is the mainstay of therapy and allows histologic evaluation of the primary tumor.
   - Following orchiectomy, optimal treatment depends on extension of lymph node involvement.
   - Retroperitoneal lymph node dissection (RPLND) is the only reliable method to identify nodal micrometastasis. It is the gold standard for providing accurate pathologic staging of the retroperitoneum.
   - Chemotherapy and radiotherapy may be used depending on the type of tumor and stage of disease.
   - Cisplatin-based combination chemotherapy is the standard treatment for advanced testicular germ cell tumors, seminomas, and nonseminomatous germ cell tumors.
   a. **Seminomas**
      - Low-stage disease treated with surgical orchiectomy; active surveillance is recommended.
      - High-stage disease, or those unwilling to comply with active surveillance, warrants adjuvant chemotherapy and/or radiation therapy.
   b. **Nonseminomatous Germ Cell Tumors**
      - Surgical orchiectomy if low-stage disease and normal markers.
      - RPLND if imaging evidence of >1 retroperitoneal lymph node larger than 1 cm.

c. **Renal Cell Carcinoma**
   - Most common type of renal malignancy; 5% of all adult cancers.
   - Originates in the renal cortex.
   - Classic triad: flank pain, hematuria, and a palpable abdominal renal mass.
   - Surgical radical nephrectomy is curative in majority of patients who do not have metastases.
   - There is no clear role for any type of systemic adjuvant therapy after completion of surgical resection.
d. **Wilms Tumor**
   - Most common renal malignancy in childhood.
   - Children with WAGR syndrome (chromosomal deletion of *WT1* gene) have a 50% risk of developing Wilms tumor.
   - Asymptomatic abdominal mass or abdominal swelling.
   - Hypertension, hematuria, and fever are the primary symptoms.
   - Lung is the most common metastatic site.
   - Abdominal U/S is initial study performed: detects hydronephrosis and multicystic kidney disease.
   - CT to further evaluate nature and extent of the mass.
   - Treatment: Nephrectomy. Radiation if tumor extends beyond renal capsule. Large tumors may require preoperative radiation and chemotherapy.

B. **Bladder Carcinoma**
   1. **Etiology**
      - Men affected more frequently than women.
      - More common in smokers, occupational carcinogens, schistosomiasis, chronic infection, and HPV.
   2. **Pathology**
      - Ninety percent of tumors are of transitional cell origin.
      - Squamous cell carcinoma and adenocarcinoma are less common.
      - Transitional cell carcinoma has strong link to cigarette smoking.
      - Transitional cell tumors are classified as either superficial or invasive.
   3. **Clinical Features**
      - Most common presentation is painless microscopic hematuria.
      - Other symptoms may include those of irritation (e.g., frequency and urgency).
      - Ureteral obstruction is common.
   4. **Diagnostic Studies**
      - Cystoscopy (can be diagnostic and therapeutic).
      - Small lesions can be excised or fulgurated.
      - Excretory urography for large masses used to evaluate renal pelvis and ureters because they are at risk for urothelial neoplasia.

- CT scanning of abdomen and pelvis is done to evaluate small tumors and metastasis.
5. **Management**
   - Local noninvasive disease treated with endoscopic transurethral resection and close follow-up.
   - Intravesical chemotherapeutic agents decrease recurrence.
   - Invasive disease treated with cystectomy and urinary diversion.
   - Chemotherapy and radiation reserved for invasive disease.
   - Only 50% of patients with invasive disease are rendered tumor free.
   - Radical cystectomy for recurrent cancer, diffuse transitional cell carcinoma combination chemotherapy.

C. Prostate Carcinoma
1. **Etiology**
   - Most common cancer in men worldwide.
   - Second most common cause of cancer-related mortality in men.
   - Approximately 1.6 million new cases are diagnosed each year worldwide.
   - African Americans have higher mortality rates than Caucasians.
   - Increased risk in men who have one or more relatives diagnosed before age 70.
   - Only 3% of men with prostate cancer have clinically evident disease.
   - Fifty percent of patients have advanced disease at time of diagnosis.
2. **Pathology**
   - Ninety-five percent are adenocarcinomas.
   - Five percent transitional cell carcinoma of prostatic urethra, small cell carcinoma, sarcomas.
   - Peripheral zone: area felt on digital rectal examination (DRE), most common site of origin.
   - Transitional zone or periurethral zone, next most common site (area removed by transurethral resection of prostate).
3. **Clinical Features**
   - Asymptomatic until tumor invasion of bladder or bones, or obstruction of urethra.
   - Prostate cancer rarely causes hematuria or obstruction when contained to gland.
   - Early detection relies on DRE and prostate-specific antigen (PSA) testing.
   - DRE: firm, nontender, fixed mass of prostate.
   - For men who decide to be screened, the American Cancer Society recommends PSA testing with or without DRE for average-risk men beginning at age 50. African Americans and men with a family history of prostate cancer should begin testing at age 40.
4. **Diagnostic Studies**
   - PSA level: elevated in prostate cancer.

- Men with abnormal DRE, PSA >4 ng per mL should undergo transrectal U/S (TRUS) and biopsy.
- TRUS may detect lesions in prostate, but is operator dependent; used in U/S-guided biopsy of prostate.
- PSA >10 ng per mL: radionuclide bone scan to rule out bony metastasis.
- PSA <10 ng per mL: low probability for metastatic disease.
- CT scan may not be reliable in detecting nodal involvement for prostate cancer.

5. **Management**
   a. **Organ-Confined Disease**
      - Negative bone scan, DRE not suggestive of extracapsular extension: local therapy with curative intent, radical prostatectomy, external beam radiation therapy.
      - Side effects of surgery include sexual impotence and urinary incontinence.
      - Morbidities of external beam radiation include sexual impotence, radiation cystitis, urethral stricture, and proctitis.
   b. **Advanced and Metastatic Disease**
      - Androgen ablation—either castration or medical alteration using luteinizing hormone—improved progression-free survival, but not overall survival.
      - Bone pain from metastatic disease may be treated with palliative, localized radiation therapy and analgesics.

VII. Genitourinary Tract Disorders—Female
A. Cervical Carcinoma
1. **Etiology**
   - Third most common malignancy in women in the United States.
   - Average age at diagnosis: 48, although the very young as well as the very old can be affected.
   - A bimodal distribution exists: peaks between 35 and 39 years, then again between 60 and 64 years.
   - Etiology is unknown; some risks factors include:
     - Coitus at an early age.
     - Multiple sexual partners.
     - HPV: detected in 99.7% of all cervical cancers with types 16 and 18 accounting for 70% of them.
     - Male sexual partner participating in high-risk sexual behavior.
     - Smoking.
     - Use of birth control pills.
     - Immunocompromised patients.
     - History of sexually transmitted infection (STI), vulvar or vaginal neoplasia or cancer.
     - Low socioeconomic status.

2. **Pathology**
- 69% are squamous epithelial, 25% adenocarcinoma, 6% other.
- 95% of squamous cell carcinoma occur within the transformation zone.
- Spreads by direct extension, via local lymphatics or through blood.
- Metastases: lungs, mediastinal, inguinal, axillary, and supraclavicular lymph nodes, bones, liver.

3. **Clinical Features**
- Early disease: asymptomatic and limited to the uterus; routine Papanicolaou (Pap) smear indicative.
- Irregular or heavy bleeding.
- Postcoital bleeding or spotting.
- Leukorrhea: typically sanguineous or purulent, odorous, and nonpruritic.
- Advanced disease: symptomatic, larger tumors, extension beyond the uterus, including other pelvic or retroperitoneal structures.
- Pelvic or low back pain, which can radiate to posterior lower extremities.
- Involuntary loss of urine or feces through vagina (fistula formation).
- Weight loss, anemia, weakness.
- Physical findings:
  - Enlargement; irregularity; and fixed, firm consistency of cervix.
  - Friable, bleeding, cauliflower-like lesion within vagina.
  - Ulceration may be primary manifestation of invasive disease.
  - Unilateral leg edema, sciatic pain, and ureteral obstruction indicate advanced disease.

4. **Diagnostic Studies**
- History and physical examination with Pap smear.
- Cytologic (Pap smear) studies; suspect or positive Pap smears indicate the need for further studies.
- Colposcopy and biopsy of lesions (staging of disease).
- Conization if colposcopy is nondiagnostic.
- Imagining studies such as MRI, CT scan, and/or pelvic lymphangiography may be used for staging demonstrate involvement of pelvic or periaortic lymph nodes.
- Advance disease cystoscopy, proctosigmoidoscopy.
- CXR to rule out metastatic or primary disease.

5. **Management**
- Dependent on staging and cell type, age, patient health, and attempts to include patient fertility desires.
  a. **Microinvasive Carcinoma**
  - When biopsy specimen demonstrates questionable invasion or early stromal invasion to 3 mm and no tumor or vascular space is involved, cone biopsy or simple or extended hysterectomy should be curative.

  b. **Invasive Carcinoma**
  - Radical hysterectomy.
  - With cancer staging in mind, fertility-preserving surgery preferred for young women of childbearing age or sexually active women.
  - Adjuvant radiation therapy or chemoradiation therapy is additional treatment modalities.
  c. **Palliative Care of Cervical Cancer**
  - Palliative chemotherapy and/or radiation therapy.
  - Management of ulceration, vaginal hemorrhage, and pain control.

B. **Vaginal Carcinoma**
1. **Etiology**
- 3% of primary gynecologic cancers located in the vagina.
- Secondary vaginal carcinomas are more common than primary.
- Extension from adjacent gynecologic structures is the most common cause of secondary vaginal carcinoma.
- HPV, most commonly 16 or 18 subtype infection, is a risk factor.
- Typically affects postmenopausal women.

2. **Pathology**
- 85% are squamous cell carcinoma.
- Remainder include adenocarcinomas, sarcomas, and melanomas.
- Route of metastasis is dependent on size and location of tumor within vagina:
  - Upper third:most common site (50%) of tumor metastases—similar to carcinoma of cervix.
  - Middle third:(20%) metastasize to inguinal nodes or directly to deep pelvic nodes.
  - Lower third:(30%) primarily metastasize to the inguinal lymph nodes.

3. **Clinical Features**
- Many are asymptomatic, but most common symptoms are abnormal, painless, bleeding or bloody vaginal discharge, or postcoital bleeding.
- Early: asymptomatic; typically discovered on routine vaginal cytologic examination; painless bleeding from ulcerated tumor.
- Advanced: tumor causes vaginal discharge and vulvar pruritus.
- Late: bleeding, pain, weight loss, swelling.

4. **Diagnostic Studies**
- Diagnosis of primary vaginal carcinoma cannot be made until metastases from other sources are ruled out.
- Biopsy establishes diagnosis; if positive, a search for metastatic disease is warranted.
- Staged clinically, including CXR, skeletal survey, cystoscopy, and proctoscopy.

5. **Management**
- Treatment: chemoradiation or radiotherapy with or without surgery, depending on location, size, and stage of disease.
- Prognosis: most important indicators: size and depth of tumor, and stage of disease at time of diagnosis.
- Follow-up:
  - Low risk: Every 6 months for 2 years, and then annually thereafter.
  - High risk: Every 3 months for 2 years, and then annually thereafter.
  - Advanced: as clinically indicated.

C. **Vulvar Carcinoma**
1. **Etiology**
- Fourth most common gynecologic malignancy after uterine, ovarian, and cervical.
- Occurs mostly in postmenopausal women.
- Approximately 5% of gynecologic cancers.
- More than 90% are squamous cell carcinomas.
- Typically, it is a slow-growing cancer.
- Risk factors: HPV infection, STIs, smoking, multiple sexual partners, prior history of cervical cancer, vulvar lichen sclerosis, premalignant conditions, such as vulvar intraepithelial neoplasia (VIN) and cervical intraepithelial neoplasia (CIN).
- High rate of recurrence.
- Less common types: melanoma, sarcoma, Paget disease, basal cell carcinoma, Bartholin gland adenocarcinoma.

2. **Clinical Features**
- Most common presenting complaint: vulvar pruritus.
- Patient has a long history of vulvar irritation with pruritus, local discomfort, bloody discharge, development of raised lesions.
- 20% are asymptomatic.
- Lesion may appear erythematous, ulcerative, or leukoplakic; configuration—papular or macular.
- Classic or wart-like appearance: found in younger women, associated with HPV.
- Keratinized or differentiated appearance: Found more often in older patients and associated with vulvar dystrophies.
- Lesions are generally unifocal and occur on labia majora.
- Appearance of early lesions similar to vulvar dermatitis.
- Appearance of late lesions: cauliflower or hard, ulcerated area.

3. **Diagnostic Studies**
- Colposcopic examination of vulva, vagina, cervix, perineum, perianal area.
- Anoscopy to rule out disease in the anal canal.
- Biopsy of vulvar mass or lesion.

4. **Management**
- Complete diagnostic evaluation to rule out metastases, primary or concurrent cancers.
- Treatment options include surgery, laser, and topical medications (imiquimod, topical 5-fluorouracil).
- Adjuvant radiation therapy for advanced stages.
- Chemotherapy for metastatic disease and recurrences.
- Follow-up: immediate postoperative period to detect recurrence or second primary cancer: every month for 2 years, and then every 6 months thereafter.

D. **Ovarian Carcinoma**
1. **Etiology**
- Second most common cause of gynecologic cancer in women in the United States, with 95% derived from epithelial cells.
- Each year, epithelial ovarian cancer causes more deaths of American women than all other gynecologic malignancies combined.
- Poor prognosis because 75% are diagnosed in a late stage.
- Typically occurs in postmenopausal women
- aged between 50 and 75. Risk factors:
  - Caucasian origin.
  - Breast, uterine, or colorectal cancer.
  - Nulliparity.
  - Delayed childbearing.
  - Family history of gynecologic cancer (first-degree relative).
  - Genetics: *BRACA1* or *BRACA2* mutation, Lynch syndrome.
  - Endometriosis.
  - Increase with age.
- Protective factors:
  - Oral contraceptive pills.
  - Multiparity.
  - Breastfeeding.
  - Tubal ligation.

2. **Pathology**
- Three histopathologic categories (based on cell type):
  - Epithelial neoplasms (80% to 90%).
  - Stromal cell (5% to 15%).
  - Germ cell (5%): occurs in young women and has a different course and treatment.
- Transperitoneal dissemination is the most common type of extraovarian spread.
- Most common sites of spread include omentum, peritoneum, bowel surfaces, and retroperitoneal lymph nodes.

3. **Clinical Features**
- Typically asymptomatic until disease is widely disseminated; however, symptomatic severity does not correspond to disease stage.

- History of nonspecific abdominal or pelvic complaints, such as early satiety, nausea/dyspepsia, bloating, distension, vague discomfort, change in bowel habits, and urinary urgency and frequency.
- Abdominal bloating, vague abdominal discomfort.
- Pelvic mass palpated (although masses <10 cm are often undetected by routine examination). Malignant—solid, nodular, fixed.
- Enlarging mass.
- Advance disease: large pelvic mass causing obstructive symptoms, ascites, respiratory distress secondary to pleural effusion.

4. **Diagnostic Studies**
- Complete history and physical examination with emphasis on pelvis and adnexal areas.
  a. **Radiographic Evaluation**
  - U/S (transabdominal and transvaginal examination).
  - If U/S positive, CXR to rule out lung metastasis, pleural effusion, mediastinal lymphadenopathy.
  b. **Laboratory Evaluation**
  - Serum level of CA-125 (a glycoprotein and antibody that reacts on a peritoneal cell antigen); increased or increasing levels of CA-125 indicate ovarian cancers and may be used as a monitor for known disease. *Not a screening test.*
  - Serum hCG if pregnancy is a possibility.
  - Exploratory laparotomy or laparoscopy.
  - CT or MRI as needed.
  - Barium enema or colonoscopy with patient complaints of change in bowel habits or positive guaiac stools.
  - Mammography in patients with a breast mass.

5. **Management**
- Referral to gynecologic oncology specialist.
- Surgery: mainstay of therapy (to obtain complete surgical staging of disease).
- Post-op venous thromboembolism prophylaxis.
  a. **Stages I and II**
  - Laparotomy/total abdominal hysterectomy/bilateral salpingo-oophorectomy, and chemotherapy (dependent on grade).
  - Unilateral salpingo-oophorectomy and staging biopsies if fertility is desired and determined to be Stage I/Grade 1 or of lower malignant potential.
  - Follow-up every 2 to 4 months for 2 years, then every 6 months for 3 years, and then yearly: serial serum CA-125 level to detect the presence of ovarian recurrence. Pelvic examinations, CXR, CT scans as indicated.
  - Serum CA-125 level to detect the presence of ovarian recurrence.
  b. **Stages III and IV**
  - Cytoreductive surgery and chemotherapy.
  - Chemotherapy only for patient unable to tolerate surgery.

E. **Uterine Carcinoma**
1. **Etiology**
- Endometrial carcinoma is the most common gynecologic malignancy in the United States.
- Seventy-five percent of patients presenting for initial diagnosis have disease confined to uterine corpus.
- Diagnosed primarily in postmenopausal women (mean age: 60); 30% are premenopausal or of age <40.
- Incidence higher in Caucasian women.
- Risk factors.
  - Classic triad of risk factors:
    - Obesity.
    - Diabetes mellitus.
    - Hypertension.
  - Long-term history of unopposed estrogen (either endogenously or by exogenous administration).
  - Nulliparity.
  - Uterine or ovarian cancer positive family history.
  - Tamoxifen use.
  - Lynch syndrome (hereditary nonpolyposis colorectal cancer).
2. **Pathology**
- Adenocarcinoma (Grade 1) is most common form.
- Other types: clear cell, secretory, squamous, and papillary serous endometrial carcinomas.
3. **Clinical Features**
- Seventy percent complain of abnormal vaginal discharge:
  - Seventy-five to 90% have abnormal bleeding with the amount of bleeding uncorrelated with severity.
  - Majority of abnormal uterine bleeding has benign etiology, but is of increasing concern after age 45.
- Painful or frequent urination (secondary to enlarging uterine mass).
- Premenopausal patient: prolonged (>7 days) heavy menstrual periods, intermenstrual spotting, amenorrhea >6 months.
- Advanced disease: feelings of pelvic pressure.
- Physical examination:
  - Early:
    - May have no abnormal findings.
  - Advanced:
    - Abdominal examination: ascites with palpable hepatic or omental nodules.
    - Pelvic: uterine enlargement, boggy consistency.
    - Rectovaginal examination: to determine disease infiltration.
4. **Diagnostic Studies**
- Pregnancy test.
- Transvaginal U/S.
- Hysterosonography/hysteroscope for visualizing mass or abnormality.

- Endocervical curettage, biopsy, and sampling:
  - Endocervix.
  - Entire endometrial cavity.
  - Dilation and curettage, if office sampling is inconclusive.
  - CT, MRI, or both.
5. **Management**
   - Search for metastatic disease:
     - CXR.
     - CT/MRI if a patient is staged clinically.
   - CBC, biochemical profile, including renal and LFTs, CA-125 (predicts extrauterine spread) measurement.
   - Surgery: hysterectomy with bilateral salpingo-oophorectomy and surgical staging for most patients.
     - Additional therapy depends on various factors (including staging and grade of tumor).
     - Radiation: used in bulky pelvic disease and post-op in patients with invasion in the myometrium, positive lymph nodes, or adnexa involvement.
     - Chemotherapy: for some Stage III or IV carcinomas.
     - Hormones: hydroxyprogesterone, medroxyprogesterone, or megestrol used when distant metastasis is present.

VIII. Hernia
A. Inguinal
1. **Etiology**
   - Indirect hernia: a congenital defect; persistence of the processus vaginalis.
   - Direct hernia: presumably degenerative; gradual weakening of transversalis fascia on the floor of the inguinal canal.
2. **Pathology**
   - Indirect: intraperitoneal contents protrude through the internal ring, enter the spermatic cord, and may reach the scrotum.
   - Direct: defect is medial to the internal ring and inside Hesselbach triangle (inguinal ligament, inferior epigastric vessels, and rectus muscle); protrusion usually does not reach the scrotum.
   - Contents of hernia sac may include intestine, appendix, omentum, bladder, ovary, and fallopian tubes.
3. **Clinical Features**
   - Indirect: most common in children and men and women.
   - Direct: more common in older patients; rare in women.
   - Incarceration: contents cannot be reduced back into abdominal cavity; usually painful.
   - Strangulation: incarceration associated with compromise of blood supply (ischemia or gangrene), causing pain, fever, and leukocytosis.

- Clinical evaluation should establish the presence or absence of hernia (bulge), and of incarceration or strangulation.
4. **Diagnostic Studies**
   - Groin U/S: highly sensitive and specific in the presence of a palpable mass.
   - CT scan may be necessary (e.g., in morbidly obese patients and when associated intra-abdominal pathology is suspected).
5. **Management**
   - The treatment of hernias is surgical. Occasionally, patients with prohibitive risk, or having asymptomatic hernias with a wide neck (low risk of incarceration), may be managed conservatively with a supporter (truss).
   - Incarceration requires urgent surgical reduction; strangulation is an emergency and may require resection of bowel or other strangulated structures.
   - Most elective hernia repair is conducted on an ambulatory basis, under local–regional anesthesia.
   - Open repair using synthetic mesh is the standard with fewer complications to laparoscopic repair.
   - The use of synthetic mesh has decreased the recurrence of hernias by 50% to 75%.
   - Laparoscopic repair is associated with less pain postoperatively. The rates of recurrence vary from 1% to 28% for direct and 0.6% to 3% for indirect hernias.
   - Complications of surgery include nerve entrapment, damage to spermatic cord structures, ischemic orchitis, hematoma, chronic pain, and infection.

B. Femoral
1. **Etiology**
   - Defect in the femoral canal, medial to the femoral vein (femoral anatomy—from lateral to medial: "NAV," nerve, artery, and vein).
2. **Pathology**
   - Defect is small (~0.5 to 2 cm); most common herniated structure is preperitoneal fat.
3. **Clinical Features**
   - Bulge below the inguinal ligament, usually asymptomatic.
   - The majority of cases occur in females.
   - Differential diagnosis: lymphadenopathy, varicose saphenous vein, inguinal hernia.
   - Physical examination: small bulge of the upper thigh; often nonreducible.
4. **Diagnostic Studies**
   - U/S or CT scan.
     - CT scan is useful in differentiating femoral from inguinal hernia.
   - Caution: needle aspiration or biopsy only if hernia is excluded with certainty—in view of risk of bowel perforation.
5. **Management**
   - Surgical repair is indicated because of high risk of strangulation (narrow neck).

C. Umbilical

1. **Etiology**
   - Herniation of omental or preperitoneal fat through defect in umbilicus.
2. **Pathology**
   - Children: most often congenital.
   - "Adult" umbilical hernias are usually small defects that become apparent when increased intra-abdominal pressure is present, because of obesity, ascites, or pregnancy.
3. **Clinical Features**
   - Pregnancy, intra-abdominal tumor, ascites, or bowel distension often precipitates clinical manifestation of small umbilical hernias.
   - A round defect in the aponeurosis at the level of the umbilicus can usually be felt on palpation.
   - Maneuvers to increase intra-abdominal pressure (coughing, straining) help in making the diagnosis.
4. **Management**
   - Conservative treatment: Most small umbilical hernias in children resolve spontaneously before age 5.
   - Surgical treatment: Symptomatic or large hernias are best treated by surgical closure (nonabsorbable sutures) of the defect; mesh repair may be needed for large defects.

D. Incisional

1. **Etiology**
   - Any penetrating injury to the abdomen can eventually result in hernia.
   - Physical examination; hernia is often nonreducible. Most common cause is laparotomy, particularly midline incisions.
2. **Pathology**
   - Defect in posterior fascial layers allowing passage of intra-abdominal contents.
3. **Clinical Features**
   - Bulge in the region of previous scar from surgery or penetrating trauma.
   - Incarceration and strangulation may occur except in large hernias.
4. **Diagnostic Studies**
   - History of surgery (including laparoscopy) or trauma (commonly, stab wound).
   - Physical findings consistent with fascial defect in the vicinity of a scar.
5. **Management**
   - Most incisional hernias require surgical repair; experience is growing with laparoscopic approaches; mesh is often used and has a better outcome.

IX. Disorders of Bone
A. Osteosarcoma

1. **Etiology**
   - Most common primary malignant bone tumor.
   - Account for 20% to 30% of bone tumors; of these, 70% are metastatic or hematologic in origin.
   - Five-year overall survival rate is 63%.
   - Histologic hallmark is malignant osteoid.
   - Male:female ratio is 3:2.
   - Occurs predominantly in adolescents and young adults, usually during growth spurts.
   - Eighty percent occur in patients younger than 20 years.
   - Secondary peak incidence occurs in patients aged 50 to 60, with a history of radiation therapy for other types of malignancies.
   - Risk factors:
     - Paget disease: most common condition leading to osteosarcoma development.
     - Retinoblastomas.
     - Radiation (secondary osteosarcoma).
     - Multiple exostoses.
   - Pulmonary metastases: most common spread.
     - Pulmonary metastatic disease is most common cause of death in these patients.
2. **Pathology**
   - Three common histologic subtypes:
     - Osteoblastic (most common).
     - Chondroblastic.
     - Fibroblastic.
   - Ninety percent noted in metaphyseal region of long bones; 50% of these are located around the knee area.
   - Three most common bones are distal femur, proximal tibia, and proximal humerus.
   - Always contain osteoid and callus produced by abnormal, atypical anaplastic stromal cells.
   - Malignant spindle cell produces the osteoid, deposited in thick masses between trabeculae of normal callus, which then destroys the compact bone and replaces it with abnormal callus and osteoid.
   - Periosteal reaction—occurs when tumor lifts off the periosteum and makes bizarre patterns of new bone formation—seen on plain films.
3. **Clinical Features**
   - Most common presenting symptoms: pain, swelling, palpable mass.
   - Limitation of motion if mass is present near or within joint.
   - May have tenderness, warmth, erythema, striae, or engorged veins around mass.
   - Pain: initially mild and intermittent, but rapidly progresses in severity and duration; usually worse at night or with activity.
   - May occasionally present as a pathologic fracture.
   - Systemic symptoms (fever, night sweats) are rare.
4. **Diagnostic Studies**
   - Plain radiographs should demonstrate an extensive, poorly defined destructive bony lesion, usually with extraosseous component.

- "Sunburst" appearance (extension of tumor through periosteum).
- Radionuclide bone scanning with technetium-99 (^{99}T) pyrophosphate to identify extent of primary lesion, as well as demonstrate bony metastases.
- CT scanning to assess degree of bony destruction, extent of soft-tissue involvement, relationship of tumor to neurovascular structures.
- Chest CT scan to rule out pulmonary metastases.
- MRI indicated for patients who qualify for limb-sparing surgery to assist in planning the procedure. Also delineates extent of intramedullary disease and identifies skip lesion. Single most important study for surgical staging.
- Incisional biopsy to determine type of sarcomas and plan preoperative and postoperative chemotherapy.
- Labs:
  - Elevated LDH and alkaline phosphatase (ALP) indicate poorer prognosis.
  - Elevated ALP at the time of diagnosis is more likely to indicate pulmonary metastasis.

5. Management
- Surgery is primary treatment.
- Limb-sparing resection: used for most patients with extremity sarcomas and no neurovascular involvement.
- Radical amputation for sarcomas involved with neurovascular structures.
- Preoperative chemotherapy: used to increase limb-salvaging excisions by decreasing the soft-tissue involvement.
- Serial scans (such as the thallium-201 scans) and serum ALP levels can be used to document preoperative response to chemotherapy.
- Postoperative chemotherapy: tailored to patient's response to preoperative chemotherapy and histologic determination from biopsy.

B. Osteochondroma
1. Etiology
- Most common primary benign bone tumor.
- Male:female ratio is 3:1.
- Most common sites are distal femur, proximal humerus, tibia, femur.
- Thought to be a peripheral portion of the physis herniating through the growth plate.

2. Pathology
- Aberrant cartilage growth (not neoplastic) resulting in bony mass.
- Cartilage capped bony projection on external surface of bone.
- Begins in childhood and grows until completion of skeletal maturity.
- Arises in the area of growth plates of the long bones, pelvis, spine.

3. Clinical Features
- Appears as solitary mass, typically asymptomatic (unless nerve compression, mechanical irritation, or bursa formation is present).
- Complaint of pain or growth of lesion may indicate degeneration to malignancy.
- Usually is initially found on radiographs.

4. Diagnostic Studies
- Plain films: lesion with peripheral rim of calcification and "stippled" calcification within lesion.
- Lesion grows away from growth plates.
- CT scan to distinguish benign from malignant indicators.

5. Management
  a. Prepubertal Presentation
  - May be observed, but resected immediately on growth of lesion or development of pain.
  b. Adult Presentation
  - Observation if located on extremity.
  - Resection if pelvis involved (most common site of malignant transformation).
  - Resection only if symptomatic or if growth occurs.

X. Shock
- An initially reversible abnormality of the circulatory system that results in inadequate organ perfusion and tissue oxygenation that must be recognized early and treated before progression to irreversible organ dysfunction.
- Shock can be divided into four categories: cardiogenic, obstructive, hypovolemic, and distributive, although shock may result from a combination of these categories.

A. Cardiogenic
1. Etiology
- Results from cardiac dysfunction leads to decreased cardiac output.

2. Pathology
- Cardiomyopathy (impaired myocardium secondary to myocardial infarction, CHF exacerbation, cardiac arrest, myocarditis, other sources of shock).
- Arrhythmia (brady- or tachyarrhythmias).
- Mechanical (valvular or septal defects).

B. Obstructive
1. Etiology
- An extracardiac insult resulting in poor right ventricular output, which leads to heart pump failure.

2. Pathology
- Increased external pressure on the heart or great vessels decreases heart's ability to pump.
- Common pathologies:
  - Pulmonary vascular resistance (PE, pulmonary hypertension).

- Mechanical (tension pneumothorax, pericardial tamponade, constrictive pericarditis, restrictive cardiomyopathies).

C. Hypovolemic
1. Etiology
- Loss of circulating volume reduces overall cardiac output.
- Type of loss includes blood, plasma, extracellular, extravascular, or water.
- Common causes include hemorrhagic and nonhemorrhagic (GI, skin, renal, third spacing losses).

2. Pathology
- Loss of volume: followed by increased heart rate, vasoconstriction, and maintenance of BP (compensatory response).
- BP decreases if losses are not replaced, and causes are identified and treated.
- Low cardiac output.
- High peripheral resistance.
- Low CVP.

3. Clinical Features
- Pale cool skin, slow capillary refill.
- Apprehensive, restless.
- Decreased mentation.
- Hypotension, tachycardia.
- Orthostatic hypotension.
- Oliguria, anuria.

4. Diagnostic Studies
- CBC: decreased hematocrit and hemoglobin (H&H) in hemorrhage (late sign); increased H&H in dehydration (hemoconcentration).

5. Management
- Restoration of circulating blood volume with isotonic saline.
- Transfusion with packed RBCs.
- Source of hemorrhage must be identified and controlled.
- Prevention of hypothermia.
- Aggressive treatment of coagulopathy.

D. Distributive
1. Neurogenic
a. Etiology
- Disruption or alteration of neurologic function and peripheral autonomic regulation.
- Commonly secondary to spinal cord or brain injury.

b. Pathology
- Results from blockade of peripheral autonomic regulation.
- Increase in overall vascular space without change in blood volume.

c. Clinical Features
- Hypotension.
- Paralysis, paresthesia below level of injury.

- Bradycardia or normal pulse instead of tachycardia because of autonomic dysregulation (no narrowed pulse pressure).

d. Management
- Isotonic IV fluids.
- Vasopressors.
- CVP monitoring.
- Monitoring input and output (fluids, urine).
- Electrolyte monitoring.

2. Septic and Anaphylactic
a. Etiology
- Overwhelming infection or sepsis resulting in circulatory, cellular, and metabolic abnormalities.
- Anaphylactic/allergic reaction.

b. Pathology
- Decreased peripheral vascular resistance due to:
  - Release of activated cytokines in sepsis.
  - Release of histamines in anaphylaxis.
- Presence of early, increased cardiac output.
- Capillary leak.

c. Clinical Features
- Sepsis: search for septic focus:
  - Central venous catheters.
  - Pneumonia.
  - Intra-abdominal, pelvic abscesses.
  - Urinary sepsis.
  - Physical examination findings:
    - Hypotension (decreased systolic pressure and narrow pulse pressure).
    - Warm skin/diaphoresis.
    - Rash.
    - Decreased urine output.
- Anaphylaxis etiologies:
  - Allergens (IgE dependent; foods, medications, insect bite or sting).
  - Immunologic (IgE independent).
  - Idiopathic (mast cell activation).
  - Nonimmunologic (medications, recent injection of IV contrast).
- Physical examination findings:
  - Hives.
  - Angioedema.
  - Respiratory distress.
  - Stridor.

d. Management
- Sepsis:
  - Isotonic IV fluids.
  - Vasopressors.
  - Panculture before antibiotics.
  - Treat the source if known: bacterial, fungal, viral.
- Anaphylaxis:
  - Airway management.
  - Epinephrine.
  - Antihistamines.
  - IV fluids.

XI. Trauma
A. Overview and General Management
1. Etiology
- Five million deaths per year worldwide.
- Worldwide, nine people die every minute from injuries or violence.
- Leading cause of death in people aged 1 to 44 years.
- Third leading cause of death, after cancer and atherosclerosis, in all age groups.
- The "golden hour" of care: rapid assessment and resuscitation of trauma patients improve outcomes.

a. Trimodal Distribution of Mortality
- First peak:
  - Death in seconds to minutes.
  - Usually because of apnea from brain or spinal cord injury or cardiac/aortic rupture.
- Second peak:
  - Death in minutes to hours.
  - Usually, these patients have devastating injuries, massive head trauma, or hemorrhage.
- Third peak:
  - Death in days to weeks.
  - These patients succumb to complications of their injuries, brain injury, disseminated intravascular coagulopathy, multiorgan system failure, acute respiratory distress syndrome, and sepsis.

2. Blunt versus Penetrating
a. Blunt
- Motor vehicle collisions (MVCs).
- Rapid deceleration injuries.
- Blast injuries.
- Falls.

b. Penetrating
- More common in urban settings.
- Gunshot wound (GSW).
- Stab wounds.
- Blast injuries.

B. Trauma Management
1. Primary Survey
- Aims at diagnosis *and* treatment of immediately life-threatening conditions.

a. ABCDEs of Trauma
- **A**irway (check patency; ensure passage of air) with cervical spine protection.
- **B**reathing (check ventilation; provide assistance).
- **C**irculation (check pulses, insert IVs; begin resuscitation and hemorrhage control).
- **D**isability (assess neurologic status through eye opening and pupil size, verbal and motor responses; treat brain swelling).
- **E**xposure/**E**nvironmental control (remove clothing to expose patient and examine while preventing hypothermia).

b. Airway and Breathing
- Protect or immobilize the cervical spine (C-spine).
- All traumatized patients should be presumed to have a spinal cord injury until history, physical examination, or CT scan have confirmed otherwise.
- Assessment of airway patency (exclude obstruction by tongue; foreign body [e.g., teeth]; blood; fractures; or swelling).
- Assessment of ventilatory status (cyanosis, bilateral breath sounds).
- Administration of O_2.
- Intubation if necessary.
- Surgical airway (needle or surgical cricothyroidotomy) if intubation is not feasible.
- Diagnosis of tension pneumothorax must happen early with prompt needle decompression to limit decompensation and death.
  - Immediate management: insertion of large-bore needle into pleural cavity (second intercostal space at midclavicular line).
  - Subsequent management: tube thoracotomy (placement of chest tube under water seal)—check with CXR.
  - CXR: may disclose pneumothorax/hemothorax, widened mediastinum of aortic rupture or dissection, diaphragmatic herniation of abdominal contents, and free air below the diaphragm, signifying rupture of a hollow viscus.

c. Circulation
- Assessment of circulatory status.
- Check for pulses (carotid/femoral), capillary refill (<2 seconds is normal), and BP
- Heart rate:
  - Tachycardia, noted in hypovolemic shock.
  - Bradycardia, noted in brain edema and spinal injury.
- Altered level of consciousness may indicate poor cerebral perfusion.
- Hypovolemic patients may have ashen, gray facial coloring and white extremities.
- **BP:**
  - Carotid BP >60 mm Hg.
  - Femoral BP >70 mm Hg.
  - Radial BP >80 mm Hg.
- Stop exsanguinating hemorrhage.
- Bleeding from major arteries and scalp wounds can lead to exsanguination.
- Pericardiocentesis for cardiac tamponade.
  - Signs and symptoms of pericardial tamponade: Beck triad:
    - Jugular vein distension (JVD).
    - Hypotension.
    - Muffled heart tones.
- Thoracotomy: mainly for penetrating injury of the heart or great vessels.

d. Disability
- Brief neurologic examination noting best response from patient.
- Level of consciousness: alert, responsive to verbal stimuli, responsive to painful stimuli, unresponsive.
- Pupil size/reaction.
- Unequal or nonreactive pupils are suggestive of increased intracranial pressure (ICP).
- **Glasgow Coma Scale (GCS) is used to determine the level of consciousness:**
  - Eye opening (1 to 4).
  - Verbal response (1 to 5).
  - Motor response (1 to 6).
  - GCS = (E + V + M); best possible score = 15 and worst possible score = 3.

e. Exposure
- Patients need to be fully exposed, examined, and log-rolled (most missed injuries are secondary to the practitioner's failure to inspect the entire body).
- Full assessment of vital signs is then done, evaluating heart rate, BP, respiratory rate, and temperature.
- Care is taken to keep the patient warm and avoid hypothermia.

2. History
- A brief history is obtained focusing on the following (AMPLE):
  - Allergies.
  - Medications.
  - Past medical history/pregnancy.
  - Last meal.
  - Events leading up to the injury.
  - Details surrounding incident: including speed of vehicle, caliber of bullet, seat-belt use, deformity of vehicle, height of fall, and level of injury of others involved in trauma.

3. Secondary Survey
- Complete head-to-toe physical examination performed after the primary survey, resuscitative efforts, and stabilization of vital signs.

a. Skin
- Decrease in skin color and capillary refill are signs of poor perfusion and occur early in hypovolemic shock.

b. Head
- Obvious trauma.
- Scalp lacerations and hemorrhage can lead to rapid exsanguination.
- Fractures of the skull may allow passage of pathogens into the CNS and damage to the brain itself.
- Battle sign (mastoid process ecchymosis) and raccoon eyes (periorbital ecchymosis) are seen in basilar skull fractures.

c. Eyes
- Pupillary response: compression of the third cranial nerve (oculomotor) causes pupillary dilation.
- Examine eyes early because periorbital edema may later preclude examination.
- Funduscopic examination: paying particular attention to papilledema, which often accompanies increased ICP.
- Visual acuity.
- Hemorrhage of conjunctiva or fundi, or discoloration of the lens.
- Ocular entrapment may indicate orbital fractures.

d. Ears
- Blood and cerebrospinal fluid (CSF) in the external auditory canals and hemotympanum are suggestive of basilar skull fracture.

e. Nose
- Blood flowing from the nares may represent direct trauma to the tissues of the nose, but if CSF also is present, skull fracture is suspected.
  - Halo sign: when two rings form on a gauze pad after placing a drop of blood from the ear canal or nose, represents CSF leak.
- Fracture.
- Septal hematoma may require drainage.

f. Mouth
- Lacerations.
- Dental alignment and missing or loose teeth require rapid evaluation, so emergent treatment can be undertaken. Teeth are best preserved in the patient's mouth, if no risk of aspiration is present, and reimplanted as soon as possible. Each minute the tooth is out of the mouth, tooth survival decreases by 1%.

g. Neck
- Presence of JVD is suggestive of CHF, tension pneumothorax, or pericardial tamponade.
- Evaluation of the trachea for position and alignment—the trachea shifts away from the side of a tension pneumothorax.
- Palpate posterior cervical spine to assess for point tenderness.
- Examine patient for SQ air.
- Carotid bruits may indicate carotid artery injury.
- Placement of NGT or orogastric tube can be both therapeutic and diagnostic. Traumatized patients may swallow air or have large volumes of food or liquids in their stomachs, causing decreased pulmonary function. Evacuation of gastric contents is important before any surgical procedure to minimize the risk of aspiration.
- Penetrating injuries to the neck that extend through the platysma should not be explored or probed until the patient has been taken to the operation room.

h. **Thorax**
- Equal expansion: unequal expansion in pneumothorax/hemothorax.
- Flail chest: fracture of two or more adjacent ribs in two or more places leads to paradoxical movement, and further to hypoventilation and hypoxia.
- Breath sounds: decreased or absent over pneumothorax and hemothorax.
- Heart sounds: muffled in pericardial tamponade.
- CXR to confirm the presence of pneumothorax, hemothorax, most rib fractures, or a widened mediastinum (aortic rupture).

i. **Abdomen**
- Obvious trauma: seat-belt sign, ecchymoses, or abrasion across the lower abdomen should alert the examiner to the possibility of bowel injury.
- Bowel sounds: decreased in abdominal trauma.
- Assess for distension and peritonitis.
- Upright abdominal X-ray: evaluates for free air in hollow viscus rupture.
- CT scan of abdomen and pelvis with contrast: highly sensitive in evaluating visceral, solid organ, or vascular injuries.
- Frequent reevaluation of the abdomen, because these findings often change over time.

j. **Genitalia**
- Rectal examination is performed to evaluate sphincter tone (distal neurologic function) and prostate position. A high-riding or mobile prostate, along with blood at the urethral meatus, is suggestive of urethral disruption.
- If urethral injury is not suspected, a Foley catheter is placed. Obtain urine for evaluation (U/A, urine drug screen). Foley catheter allows for accurate measuring of urine output. Adequate urine output is approximately 0.5 mL/kg/hour.
- Pelvic examination is performed to evaluate the female genitalia and bony pelvis for fracture.
- Mandatory pregnancy test for all women of childbearing age.

k. **Pelvis**
- Examination is aimed at assessment of stability of the pelvis. The pelvis is rocked and palpated, and a pelvic X-ray assessing for fracture is obtained. Massive quantities of blood can be lost into the pelvis after fracture.
- Pelvic binder is applied to patients with hemodynamic instability and open-book pelvic fractures.

l. **Extremities**
- Neurovascular examination.
- Splint obvious fractures to reduce the chance of nerve or vascular injury and blood loss. Femur

fractures may cause accumulation of several units of blood in the thigh.

m. **Neurologic**
- Serial neurologic examinations (motor, sensory, papillary response, and level of consciousness), assessing for changing neurologic status.

5. **Resuscitation**
- O_2.
- Cardiac monitoring.
- Two IVs of lactated Ringer (LR) or normal saline solution (NSS) by way of large-bore catheters are established. In any hypotensive patient, 1 to 2 L of crystalloid is infused.
- If the patient is still hypotensive after administration of 2 L of crystalloid IV fluids, begin administration of blood products.
- Blood is given as needed: "O"-negative is the *universal donor*.
- Chest tubes: placed to relieve pneumothorax or hemothorax. Blood loss of >200 mL per hour for 2 to 3 consecutive hours is suggestive of the need for thoracotomy.
- Definitive care for trauma is exploration and repair in the operating room.

C. **Head Trauma**
1. **Etiology**
- Blunt trauma is more common than penetrating.
- Injuries may be sustained from MVCs, falls, and gunshot and knife wounds.
- GCS is objective clinical measure of severity of brain injury. GCS of 8 or lower is considered severe and requires intubation.

2. **Pathology**
- Brain injury may result from axonal sheer; cerebral contusion; secondary edema; subdural, epidural, or subarachnoid hematoma.

a. **Subdural Hematoma**
- More common in elderly individuals.
- Slow, insidious onset.
- Acute subdural hematoma (SDH) is usually caused by tearing of the bridging veins.
- Arterial rupture can also result in SDH, and this source accounts for approximately 20% to 30% of SDH cases.
- Shape conforms to the contours of the brain.

b. **Epidural Hematoma**
- Typically associated with a brief period of unconsciousness followed by a lucid interval, then rapid deterioration of mental status.
- Rapid hematoma collection from middle meningeal artery rupture leads to rapid rise in ICP that causes brain herniation.
- Biconvex or lenticular in shape.

3. **Management**
- Airway maintenance with cervical spine protection, breathing and ventilation, circulation

with hemorrhage control, disability (neurologic evaluation), exposure and environmental control (ABCDEs).
- Management of hypertension and/or hypotension.
- Any patient who has had transient or persistent unconsciousness with evidence of head trauma or skull fracture should undergo CT scan of the head.
- Patients who sustain minor concussion and can be monitored at home can safely be discharged; all other patients require admission.
- Elevation of the head above the level of the heart (reverse Trendelenburg position) to reduce ICP by allowing venous outflow.
- Craniotomy and hematoma evacuation is the mainstay of surgical treatment of acute, expanding hematoma (EDH).
- Keep $PaCO_2$ at 30 mm Hg or above. Brief periods of hyperventilation are acceptable, but should be for as limited a period as possible.
- Hyperosmolar therapy using IV mannitol or hypertonic saline.
- Seizure prophylaxis with phenytoin or fosphenytoin.

D. Chest Trauma—Spontaneous Pneumothorax
1. **Etiology**
   - Young, tall, thin adults 18 to 25 years old are most commonly affected.
   - Older patients with asthma or chronic obstructive pulmonary disease are also affected.
2. **Pathology**
   - Rupture of subpleural bleb into pleural space.
   - Lung collapse results from leakage of air into pleural space.
3. **Clinical Features**
   - Chest pain, cough, and dyspnea are common.
   - Decreased breath sounds over the affected side.
   - Hyperresonance to percussion on the affected side.
4. **Diagnostic Studies**
   - CXR shows increased radiolucency over the affected side.
5. **Management**
   - Chest-tube drainage of affected pleural space.
   - Surgery for persistent pneumothorax: air leak for >7 to 10 days; incomplete lung expansion.

E. Chest Trauma—Tension Pneumothorax
1. **Etiology**
   - Usually traumatic from blunt or sharp trauma to the thorax.
2. **Pathology**
   - Air is trapped in the pleural space, causing collapse of the affected lung.
   - In the instance of tension pneumothorax, pressure in the pleural cavity increases and may cause mediastinal contents to be pushed away from the side

of the injury, resulting in decreased lung function and impediment of blood return to the heart.
3. **Clinical Features**
   - A life-threatening emergency, requiring immediate care.
   - Decreased or absent breath sounds over the affected side.
   - Hyperresonance to percussion over the affected side.
   - Increased radiolucency on the affected side.
   - JVD.
   - Tracheal shifts away from the side of the injury.
   - Diagnosis of tension pneumothorax should be made clinically, not by radiography.
4. **Management**
   - Immediate needle decompression.
   - ABCs of trauma resuscitation.
   - Pleural decompression by way of needle thoracotomy—may be lifesaving in the event of tension pneumothorax.
   - Chest-tube insertion to evacuate air and blood from the pleural cavity.

F. Chest Trauma—Hemothorax
1. **Etiology**
   - Blunt or sharp trauma to the thorax.
2. **Pathology**
   - Blood in the pleural space causing collapse of the lung.
   - Chest wall, intercostal vessels, and pulmonary vasculature are sites of hemorrhage.
3. **Clinical Features**
   - Shortness of breath, dyspnea, cough.
   - Decreased breath sounds over the affected side.
   - Dullness to percussion over the dependent areas of the affected pleural cavity.
   - Evidence of fluid within the affected pleural space with decrease in lung volume.
4. **Management**
   - Supportive care.
   - ABCs of trauma resuscitation.
   - Insertion of large-bore chest tube for evacuation of blood from the pleural cavity.
   - Surgical intervention (thoracotomy) if hemorrhage is large or continuing.

G. Chest Trauma—Atelectasis
1. **Etiology**
   - Postoperative patients: particularly thoracic and abdominal procedures.
   - Most common cause of fever in the first 24 hours after surgery.
2. **Pathology**
   - Usually due to decreased tidal volume and inability to clear secretions.
   - Bed rest and pain are the two most common predisposing factors.

- Pain causes patients to breathe more shallowly, causing decreased tidal volume; for the same reason, patients do less coughing and are less effective in clearing secretions.
- Mucus plugs create a one-way valve allowing air to escape but not enter the bronchus, causing collapse of the lung tissue.

3. **Clinical Features**
   - Shortness of breath and fever early (first 24 hours) in the postoperative course.
   - Tachypnea.

4. **Diagnostic Studies**
   - CXR shows areas of lung collapse.
   - If large areas of the lung are affected, hypoxia may be present, followed by respiratory failure.

5. **Management**
   - Management is aimed at prevention—early ambulation, use of incentive spirometry, frequent coughing and deep breathing, and aggressive pulmonary toilet.
   - Aggressive tracheal suctioning, postural drainage, and chest physiotherapy.
   - Bronchoscopy may be necessary to clear secretions.

H. Abdominal Trauma

1. **Etiology/Pathology**
   a. **Blunt Trauma**
      - Usually results in injury to the spleen and liver.
      - Knowledge of height of a fall, speed of an MVC, seat-belt use, air-bag deployment, extrication requirements, extent of damage to the vehicle, and condition of other victims are helpful in judging the potential extent of injuries. Patients who fall from a height of >15 ft have a 5% mortality rate.
   b. **Penetrating Trauma**
      - Size and length of the knife and caliber and type of gun used aid in understanding potential injuries.
      - Damage from bullet wounds is determined by speed (velocity) and size (mass) of the projectile.
      - The faster and heavier the bullet, the greater the cavitation caused; pressure, not the bullet, creates an injury tract, known as blast effect.

2. **Clinical Features**
   - Abdominal pain and tenderness are common findings.
   - Clinical index of suspicion needs to be high because many trauma patients have associated head trauma or substance abuse, and their examination may be unreliable.

3. **Diagnostic Studies**
   - Abdominal X-rays may show free air in peritoneum or retroperitoneum, fractures, and abdominal fluid collections.

- FAST: focused abdominal sonography in trauma is useful in evaluation of the heart, great vessels, kidneys, spleen, and liver. Organ disruption and fluid collections may be noted.
- CT scanning for stable patients is appropriate and highly sensitive and specific.
- Diagnostic peritoneal lavage (DPL), formerly a mainstay in diagnosis of blunt abdominal trauma, has been replaced by U/S and CT scanning.
- FAST and CT scan are helpful in patients in whom a high index of suspicion for injury exists, but who have a normal or minimally abnormal examination.

4. **Management**
   - Directed by the type and extent of injury.
   - Patients who are in shock unresolved by fluid administration, or who deteriorate, need emergent laparotomy and repair of specific damage.
   - After initial stabilization, transfer to a trauma center should be considered.

I. Burns

1. **Etiology**
   a. **First Degree: Superficial**
      - Frequently caused by excessive exposure to sunlight (sunburn).
   b. **Second Degree: Partial Thickness**
      - Frequently caused by short flash or scalding liquid exposure.
   c. **Third Degree: Full Thickness**
      - Frequently caused by high electrical current, prolonged exposure to flame, immersion in scalding liquid chemicals.

2. **Pathology**
   a. **First Degree**
      - Outer layer of the dermis.
   b. **Second Degree**
      - Superficial: upper portion of the dermis.
      - Deep: involving most, but not the entire dermis.
   c. **Third Degree**
      - Complete destruction of the dermis; may involve fat, muscle, bone.

3. **Clinical Features**
   a. **First Degree**
      - Erythema, mild discomfort.
   b. **Second Degree**
      - Blister formation, tissue edema, plasma leakage.
      - Exquisitely painful.
   c. **Third Degree**
      - Painless, leathery, charred appearance.

4. **Determining the Extent of Injury: Rule of Nines (First Degree Not Included in Calculation)**
   - Head and neck: 9%.
   - Arm (each): 9%.
   - Trunk (anterior): 18%.

- Trunk (posterior): 18%.
- Leg (each): 18%.
- Genitalia: 1%.
5. **Management**
   a. **Initial Management of All Burns**
      - Remove patient from the source of injury.
      - Stop burning.
      - ABCDEs of trauma resuscitation.
      - Administer O_2 therapy if possibility of coexisting inhalation injury exists.
      - Provide IV therapy for larger second-degree and all third-degree wounds.
      - Provide analgesia if patient hemodynamically stable.
      - Provide tetanus prophylaxis for all burn patients.
      - Systemic antibiotics not indicated in initial management.
   b. **First Degree**
      - Pain resolves in 48 to 72 hours.
      - Acetaminophen and NSAIDs usually provide adequate analgesia.
      - Local wound care and surveillance for infection; ice.
   c. **Second Degree**
      - Superficial: usually heals in 7 to 14 days:
         - Local wound care; debridement of nonviable skin.
         - Topical antibiotic.
         - Wound coverage with dressings that promote moisture retention.
         - PO analgesia (may require narcotics).
      - Deep: wound healing may be slow and unpredictable:
         - Local wound care; debridement of blisters.
         - Topical antibiotics.
         - Skin grafting as necessary.
         - Wound coverage with dressings that promote moisture retention.
         - PO narcotic analgesia.
         - May require IV analgesia with narcotics, especially for dressing changes.
   d. **Third Degree**
      - Unable to heal by reepithelialization because of the loss of epidermal appendages within the dermal layer.
      - Spontaneous healing results in burn scar contracture.
      - Early skin grafting is used to replace devitalized tissue and reduce septic complications.
      - Escharotomy is performed in patients with circumferential chest wall burns with decreased peripheral circulation and ventilatory exchange.
   e. **Therapy**
      - Parkland formula: using LR solution:

- Adults: 4 mL/kg/% total burn surface area (TBSA) burned; half given over first 8 hours and the other half over next 16 hours.
- Children: 3 mL/kg/% TBSA burned; half given over first 8 hours and the other half over next 16 hours plus maintenance.
   f. **Admission Criteria/Burn Center Transfer**
      - Age 10 to 50 with superficial partial-thickness burns of >15% TBSA or deep partial- or full-thickness burns of >5%.
      - Age <10 and >50 with superficial partial-thickness burns >10%, or deep partial- or full-thickness burns >3%.
      - Any patient with partial- or full-thickness burns to hands, feet, face, perineum, circumferential, or across major joints.
      - Chemical or electrical burns.
      - Associated inhalation injury or other trauma.
      - Coexisting medical conditions, immunocompromised.

XII. Nutrition Disorders
- Goals are to provide enough energy and nutritional reservoirs to enable the patient to maintain function, repair body, and recover from diseased or postsurgical states.
- Height and weight are most important set of vital signs in nutritional assessment.
- Calculations in caloric needs based on ideal body weight(IBW).
   - Actual body weight (ABW) or IBW should be employed in feeding calculations.
   - Percentage IBW = (ABW/IBW) ×100.
   - The following parameters should be used to determine nutritional needs:
      - If ABW < IBW, use ABW.
      - If ABW > IBW (but <120%), use IBW.
      - If ABW >120% of IBW, use adjusted/relative body weight to calculate needs: IBW+ (ABW − IBW × 0.25).
      - ABW 80% to 90% of IBW = mild malnutrition.
      - ABW 70% to 80% of IBW = moderate malnutrition.
      - ABW <70% = severe malnutrition.

A. Carbohydrates
- The primary fuel source for the body; metabolized to the form of glucose and stored as glycogen.
- RBCs, CNS, and renal medulla metabolize only glucose.
- Glucose and glycogen stores from the muscle and liver are depleted within 24 to 36 hours of fasting.
- Fat and protein are then used for fuel.

B. Fats
- Fatty acids are the basic unit of fat.
- Linoleic and linolenic acids are the essential fatty acids.

- Fat metabolism yields fatty acids, glycerol, and ketone bodies.
- Ketone bodies are used as fuel during starvation.

C. Protein (Amino Acids)

- Primary function is to maintain cellular structure and function.
- Used as fuel during starvation.

D. Caloric Requirements

- Nonprotein calories (NPC): estimated to provide enough nonprotein energy to maintain function without breaking down protein and restore lost weight.
- 500 kcal per day above estimated needs 1 lb per week weight gain; 60% of NPC should come from carbohydrates; 40% of NPC should come from fats.

1. NPC Estimation

- Harris–Benedict equation.
  - Standard for calculating energy requirements in ill and hospitalized patients.
  - Basal energy expenditure (BEE) × activity factor × injury factor.
  - Estimates BEE in kilocalories per day of a healthy, resting adult. Standard: 25 to 35 kcal/kg/day.
    - Males: BEE = $66.5 + [13.8 \text{ (weight in kg)}] + [5 \text{ (height in cm)}] - [6.8 \text{ (age in years)}]$.
    - Females: BEE = $655.1 + [9.6 \text{ (weight in kg)}] + [1.8 \text{ (height in cm)}] - [4.7 \text{ (age in years)}]$.
- Activity factor:
  - Ambulatory: 1.3.
  - Bed-bound: 1.2.
- Injury factor:
  - Fever: 1.1 (for each ° C above normal body temperature).
  - Major surgery: 1.6.
  - Elective surgery: 1.0 to 1.1.
  - Severely stressed patients: 1.6.
  - Burn patients: 2.3.
  - Multiple long bone fractures: 1.1 to 1.3.
- Indirect calorimetry.
  - The body uses O_2 and produces CO_2 in metabolism; therefore, BEE can be calculated on the basis of these measurements. These measurements are taken by "metabolic carts," which either hook into a ventilator or isolate a patient within a tent. Not useful because of its expense, unavailability in general settings, and inaccuracy for nonventilating patients or patients inspiring $>50\%$ O_2.

2. Protein Requirements

- Needs:
  - Protein is used constantly and metabolized, therefore not typically stored.
  - Minimal requirement: 0.54 g/kg/day.

- Standard healthy adult: 0.8 g/kg/day.
- Stressed patients: 1.0 to 1.5 g/kg/day.
- Losses:
  - Reflected in urine as nitrogen.
  - Standard healthy adult: 0.05 to 0.08 g/kg/day.
  - Stressed patients: 5-fold increase from normal.

3. Protein Estimation

- Laboratory values
  - Plasma proteins (e.g., albumin, prealbumin, and transferrin).
    - Albumin: reflects relationship between synthesis, degradation, and distribution of protein.
    - Transferrin: better marker of visceral protein status.
    - Prealbumin: best nutritional marker.
  - Typically decrease with decreased protein balance.
  - Not an exact measurement of protein balance.
- Nitrogen balance
  - Because nitrogen is 16% protein and excreted primarily through urine, it is reflective of protein balance. Therefore, measurement of nitrogen in urine can be used to calculate protein balance with the following formula: N balance (g) 5 [(protein intake in g/6.25)]/[(urinary N + 4)]. (**NOTE:** 4 reflects nonurinary nitrogen losses, and it increases to 6 in critically ill patients.)
- Measure of nitrogen balance can be obtained with urinary urea nitrogen.
- Nitrogen balance <0 (starvation, trauma/surgery, inadequate nutrition).

E. Method of Delivery

1. Oral

- Ideal and preferred route.
- 55% calories from carbohydrates, 15% from protein, and 30% from fat (regular diet).
  - Fat-restricted diet (cholecystitis, Crohn disease, abdominal pain) <50 g fat per day.
  - High-fiber diet (constipation, irritable bowel, colon CA) 20 to 35 g fiber per day.
  - High protein diet (cancer, malnutrition).
  - Sodium-restricted (CHF, hypertension, cardiovascular disease) 500 mg to 4 g per day.
  - Nutritional supplements.

2. Enteral Nutrition

- Used for patients with functional GI tract, but cannot or will not take nutrition orally.

a. Benefits

- Relatively inexpensive.
- Maintains mucosal structure and function.
- Protects against infection by maintaining the integrity of the mucosal lining of the small bowel.

b. **Modes**
- NGT used for short-term support; risks: aspiration, diarrhea, bronchial intubation.
  - Requires intact gag reflex.
- Gastrostomy tube: used for chronic nutritional support; allows for bolus feeding because stomach is used; good prophylaxis against gastritis; risks: aspiration and diarrhea.
  - Normally requires normal gastric function and no reflux.
  - Surgically placed.
- Jejunostomy tube: used for chronic support, patient with high aspiration risk, or both; must give continuous feedings; risk: diarrhea.
  - Surgically placed.

3. **Parenteral Nutrition**
- Used preoperatively for severely malnourished patients.
- Used, for instances, when patient's stomach or gut cannot be used (e.g., short-bowel syndrome, hepatic failure, enterocutaneous fistulas, major thermal injury, acute renal failure, and prolonged ileus).
- Requires primarily a central venous access.
- Types:
  - Peripheral parenteral nutrition (PPN): short-term intervention, use for 14 days or less, patient's oral intake improving but not sufficient.
  - Total parenteral nutrition (TPN): for full nutritional support, minimum of 7 days, more long-term usage.
- Risks:
  - Mechanical: due to line placement, pneumothorax, pleural laceration.
  - Metabolic: due to nutritional deficits, resultant metabolic disorders, dehydration.
  - Sepsis: line placement contaminants.

XIII. Wounds
A. Stages of Wound Healing
1. Physiology
- Surgical or traumatic tissue disruption causing intact skin to break down.
- Classified as acute or chronic.
2. Inflammation
- Initially, vasoconstriction to reduce blood loss after injury.
- Hemostasis (clot formation), vasodilatation follows.
- Vasodilatation allows inflow of neutrophils and monocytes.
- Phagocytosis by macrophages occurs at wound.
- Chemotactic factors stimulate migration of fibroblasts to wound.

3. Epithelialization (Migration)
- Restores denuded epithelial surface.
- Occurs 12 to 24 hours after injury.
- At 48 hours, waterproof covering achieved, preventing migration of bacteria into wound.
- Wound dressings can be removed safely after 48 hours (uncomplicated surgical wounds).
4. Proliferation Phase
- Fibroblastic synthesis (2 to 21 days): fibroblasts responsible for collagen synthesis.
- Collagen synthesis (2 to 21 days): primarily regulated by macrophages by way of cellular mediators.
- Angiogenesis (2 to 7 days): formation of new vessels, increasing vascular supply to wound.
- Contraction (2 to 20 days): gradual reduction in wound size secondary to retraction of granulation tissue.
5. Maturation Phase
- At 21 days, collagen deposition reduced.
- Wound tensile strength continues to increase.
- Prewound strength never achieved.
- Patients advised to protect wound and avoid strenuous activity for at least 6 weeks after injury.

B. Wound Closure
1. Primary Intention
- Wound edges are brought together using suture, tapes, or surgical staples.
- Used for clean wounds <6 hours old.
- Wound may be debrided and converted to clean wound if minimally contaminated.
2. Secondary Intention
- Wound left open to close by contraction and epithelialization.
3. Delayed Primary Closure (Tertiary Closure)
- Wound is closed (skin, SQ tissue) 4 to 5 days after injury.
- Delaying closure decreases risk of potentially infected wounds.
4. Contraindications to Wound Closure (Primarily Centered Around Risk of Infection)
- Wound older than 6 hours.
- Wound older than 24 hours on face.
- Wound infection present.
- Heavily contaminated wound.
- Excessive tension of wound.
- Retained foreign bodies.
5. Classification of Wounds
   a. **Clean Wounds**
   - Incision made during operative procedure.
   - Skin has been prepared adequately with appropriate disinfectant.
   - No contamination from GI, respiratory, or genitourinary (GU) tracts.
   - Infection rates <2%.

b. **Clean-Contaminated Wounds**
- Similar to clean wounds, exception being entrance into GI, GU, or respiratory tract.
- GI tract prepped to minimize amounts of bacteria.
- GU, respiratory tracts assumed to have no active infection.
- Examples: routine cholecystectomy, bladder surgery, surgery of colon after preparation.
- Infection rates of 3% expected.

c. **Contaminated Wounds**
- Major contamination of wound.
- All traumatic wounds.
- Examples: intestinal obstruction with enterotomy and spillage of contents, surgery for acute cholecystitis with spillage of pus.
- Although contamination is high, infection rates are approximately 5%.

d. **Dirty Wounds**
- Old traumatic wounds with retained devitalized tissue, foreign bodies, or fecal contamination, or wounds that involve existing clinical infection.
- Examples: skin laceration with active infection present, appendiceal abscess, perirectal abscess.
- Infection rates as high as 50% expected.

6. **Wound Infection**
  a. **Signs and Symptoms**
  - Erythema (redness, rubor).
  - Calor (heat).
  - Tenderness (dolor).
  - Discharge for >24 hours after injury.
  - Purulent discharge.
  - Lymphangitis (red streaking).
  - Pain at injury site.
  - Fluctuance, induration.

  b. **Treatment**
  - Open suture lines to allow drainage.
  - Incise and drain closed areas.
  - Oral antibiotics used for mild infection.
  - Parenteral antibiotics used for moderate-to-severe infections.
  - Agent of choice should be guided by possible contaminates.
  - Example: Augmentin (amoxicillin, clavulanic acid) for human bite wounds and first-generation cephalosporin for skin flora.

7. **Tetanus**
  a. **History**
  - Tetanus immunization status.
  b. **Following Patients Must Be Considered to Have Incomplete Immunization**
  - Age >50.
  - Foreign-born patients.
  - Unavailable or unreliable history.

8. **Anesthesia for Wound Care**
- Direct infiltration: placement of anesthesia into wound edges.
- Field block: placement of anesthetic agent parallel to the wound edge.
- Regional block: anesthetic agent in injected adjacent nerve proximal to the wound.

9. **Anesthetic Agents**
- Amides: lidocaine, mepivacaine, bupivacaine.
- Esters: procaine, tetracaine, benzocaine, and cocaine.
- Epinephrine: used to increase the time of anesthesia and reduce bleeding. Its use should be avoided in areas of terminal circulation, ears, fingers, toes, nose, and tip of the nose.
- Dosage of lidocaine is limited to 5 mg per kg without epinephrine and 7 mg per kg with epinephrine.
- Suture size and removal schedule.
  - Eyelid: remove on day 3.
  - Neck: remove on days 3 to 4.
  - Face: remove on day 5.
  - Trunk, upper and lower extremities: remove on days 7 to 10.

REVIEW QUESTIONS

1. A patient is postoperative day 4 with an ileus. What would be the best option for nutritional support?
   a) Add nutritional supplements
   b) Nasogastric tube
   c) Gastrostomy tube
   d) Parenteral nutrition

2. A 70-year-old patient with colon cancer is admitted to the hospital for fatigue and weakness. He is undergoing a nutritional assessment. What is the best laboratory test to determine protein status?
   a) Hemoglobin
   b) Transferrin
   c) Prealbumin
   d) Albumin

3. Which of the following is the most common complication of nasogastric feeding tubes?
   a) Diarrhea
   b) Aspiration
   c) Infection
   d) Intolerance

4. A 13-year-old girl presents to the office with pain in her right knee. She is a soccer player but denies any known injury or trauma. X-rays obtained show no acute fracture

or dislocation, but do show a lesion in the distal femur with a sunburst appearance. What is the most likely diagnosis?

a) Osteosarcoma
b) Chondrosarcoma
c) Osteochondroma
d) Ewing sarcoma

5. A malignant osteosarcoma has been discovered in a 19-year-old man's proximal tibia. What area are you most concerned with in regard to metastasis?

a) Lungs
b) Brain
c) Spine
d) Kidney

6. A 32-year-old man presents after being involved in a motor vehicle collision, and he appears in visible respiratory distress. Physical examination reveals decreased breath sounds on the left side, tracheal deviation to the right side, and right-sided JVD. What is your initial management of this patient?

a) Needle decompression
b) Chest X-ray
c) Chest CT with contrast
d) Emergently transfer to the operating room

ANSWERS TO REVIEW QUESTIONS

1. **Answer: D.** The etiology of an ileus is an intestinal atony or hypotony resulting from nonmechanical cause; the intestine is paralyzed, lacking peristaltic movements ("paralytic ileus"). Common causes include peritonitis, electrolyte imbalance, and postoperative and posttraumatic ileus medications (narcotics). Most common cause of ileus medications (narcotics) is postsurgical procedures that spontaneously resolve in 1 to 3 days. The clinical features include distension, vomiting, and obstipation; mild-to-moderate abdominal discomfort unless peritonitis ensues; and abdominal distension and hypoactive bowel sounds. Diagnostic studies in abdominal radiographs and CT scan show distension of both large and small bowel loops and no "transition zone." The main goal of management is to correct the underlying pathology; parenteral nutrition is the best option. Supportive therapy includes NPO and NGT decompression and replacement of fluid and electrolytes.

2. **Answer: C.** The prealbumin, a hepatic protein, is a cost-effective and sensitive method of assessing the severity of illness resulting from malnutrition in patients who are critically ill or have a chronic disease. Prealbumin levels are shown to correlate with morbidity and mortality. Serum hepatic protein levels are helpful to identify the most critical patients that may most likely develop malnutrition.

3. **Answer: B.** Complications of malpositioned feeding tubes are most often due to inadvertent placement in the

respiratory tract; a tube with feeding ports in the esophagus significantly increases the risk of aspiration.

4. **Answer: A.** Osteosarcoma is the most primary malignant bone tumor; occurs predominantly in adolescents and young adults; plain radiographs demonstrate an extensive, poorly defined destructive lesion, usually with extraosseous component; and the tumor is solid, hard, and irregular ("fir-tree," "moth-eaten," or "sunburst" appearance on radiograph) because of the tumor spicules of calcified bone radiating at right angles. Chondrosarcoma is a rare type of sarcoma; it typically affects adults between the ages of 20 and 60 and is more common in men and affects the cartilage cells of the femur, arm, pelvis, or knee; less often, it may affect the ribs. Osteochondroma is the most common benign bone tumor; most common sites are distal femur, proximal humerus, tibia, and femur. Radiographs demonstrate a lesion with peripheral rim of calcification and "stippled" calcification within lesion. Ewing sarcoma is the second most common malignant bone tumor, occurring in children and young adults; common sites are the lower extremity (femur most frequently affected), pelvis, upper extremity, axial skeleton, ribs, and face.

5. **Answer: A.** Osteosarcoma is the most common primary malignant tumor, accounting for 20% to 30% of bone tumors. Of these, 70% are metastatic or hematologic in origin. This occurs predominantly in adolescents and young adults, with 80% in patients younger than 20. Pulmonary metastases are the most common spread.

6. **Answer: A.** A tension pneumothorax is usually traumatic from blunt or sharp trauma to the thorax. Air is trapped in the pleural space, causing collapse of the affected lung. In the instance of the tension pneumothorax, pressure in the pleural cavity increases and may cause mediastinal contents to be pushed away from the side of the injury, resulting in decreased lung function. This is a life-threatening emergency requiring immediate care—immediate decompression and pleural decompression by way of a needle thoracotomy. Clinical features include decreased or absent breath sounds over the affected side; hyperresonance to percussion over the affected side; and JVD and tracheal shift away from the side of the injury.

SELECTED REFERENCES

Albanese CT, Sylvester KG. Pediatric surgery. In: Doherty GM, Way LW, eds. *Current Surgical Diagnosis and Treatment.* 12th ed. New York, NY: McGraw-Hill; 2006:1322–1323.

American College of Surgeons Committee on Trauma. *Advanced Trauma Life Support for Doctors (ATLS) Student Course Manual.* 8th ed. Chicago, IL: American College of Surgeons; 2008.

Andreoli TE, Benjamin I, Griggs RC, et al, eds. *Andreoli and Carpenter's Cecil Essentials of Medicine.* 8th ed. Philadelphia, PA: Elsevier; 2011.

Boelaert K. Revised guidelines for the management of thyroid cancer. *Nat Rev Endocrinol.* 2010;6(4):185–186.

Cooper CS, Williams RD. Urology. In: Doherty GM, Way LW, eds. *Current Surgical Diagnosis and Treatment.* 12th ed. New York, NY: McGraw-Hill; 2006:1033–1051.

Glasgow SC, Herrmann VM. Surgical metabolism and nutrition. In: Doherty GM, Way LW, eds. *Current Surgical Diagnosis and Treatment.* 12th ed. New York, NY: McGraw-Hill; 2006:140–164.

Hunt TK. Wound healing. In: Doherty GM, Way LW, eds. *Current Surgical Diagnosis and Treatment.* 12th ed. New York, NY: McGraw-Hill; 2006:75–80.

Kasper DL, Braunwald E, Fauci A, et al, eds. *Harrison's Principles of Internal Medicine.* 17th ed. New York, NY: McGraw-Hill Professional; 2008.

Kinder BK, Burrow GN. The thyroid: nodules and neoplasia. In: Felig P, Frohman LA, eds. *Endocrinology and Metabolism.* 4th ed. New York, NY: McGraw-Hill; 2001:349–383.

Schwartz LR, Balakrishnan C. Thermal burns. In: Tintinalli JE, Kelen GD, Stapczynski JS, eds. *Emergency Medicine: A Comprehensive Study Guide.* 6th ed. New York, NY: McGraw-Hill; 2004:1220–1226.

Stewart PM. Treatment of Cushing's syndrome. In: Kronenberg HM, Melmed S, Polonsky KS, et al, eds. *Williams Textbook of Endocrinology.* 11th ed. Philadelphia, PA: Saunders Elsevier; 2008:475–477.

Preventive Medicine

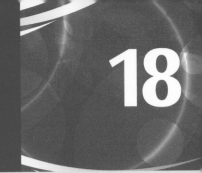

18

Parmjeet S. Saini • Patrick C. Auth

I. Primary Prevention

A. Family Violence or Domestic Violence

1. **Definition**
   - Willful intimidation, battery, sexual assault, or abusive behavior perpetrated by a family or household member or intimate partner against another with the goal of establishing and maintaining power and control.

2. **Epidemiology**
   - Approximately 1 million children are identified as physically abused in the United States each year.
   - In the United States, approximately 1 to 4 million women are physically, sexually, or emotionally abused by their intimate partners each year.
   - Women are 7 to 14 times more likely to suffer severe physical injuries from an assault by an intimate partner.
   - In 90% of abuse cases, the perpetrator is a family member, usually an adult child or spouse.

3. **Screening**
   - Family Violence Prevention Funds and Health and Human Services (HHS) recommend routine screening as opposed to indicator-based screening for all female patients older than 14 at primary care settings, emergency departments, pediatrics, and mental health clinics.
   - Confidential documentation will increase outcomes and opportunities for identification and intervention and document and report abuse and/or neglect, such as burns, bruises, and repeated suspicious traumatic injury.
   - Screening for child abuse in the primary care setting can include physical examination as well as screening questionnaires.
   - Consider using *Hawaii Risk Indicators Screening Tool* followed by the *Kempe Family Stress Inventory*.
   - The Domestic Violence Survivor Assessment tool can help health care providers and abused women identify issues and feelings created by domestic violence and helps guide counseling.
   - More research is needed to develop screening tools that are effective in the general population.

4. **Recommendation**
   - Reporting child and elder abuse to protective services is mandatory in most states, and several states have laws requiring mandatory reporting of intimate partner violence.
   - The American Academy of Pediatrics (AAP) and the American Medical Association (AMA) recommend that physicians remain alert for the signs and symptoms of children's physical and sexual abuse in the routine examination.
   - The AMA encourages physicians to inquire routinely about their patients' domestic violence histories and refer those patients with violence-related problems for medical and/or community-based services.
   - The Centers for Disease Control (CDC) and U.S. Preventive Services Task Force (USPSTF) on Community Preventive Services found that home visitation programs aimed at children with a high risk of maltreatment (e.g., single or young mothers, low-income households, families with low birth-weight infants) were effective in decreasing maltreatment episodes.
   - The American College of Obstetricians and Gynecologists (ACOG) guidelines on domestic violence recommend that physicians routinely ask women direct, specific questions about abuse.
   - The American Academy of Family Physicians (AAFP) notes that family physicians can provide early intervention in family violence through routine screening and the identification of abuse, and recommends that physicians be alert to the presence of family violence in virtually every patient encounter.
   - Screening: Agency for Healthcare Research and Quality (AHRQ) recommends Delphi Instrument for Hospital-Based Domestic Violence Program https://archive.ahrq.gov/research/domesticviol/dvtool.htm.

B. Unintentional Household Injuries among Persons 0 to 19 Years Old

1. **Definition**
   - Public health–related unintentional accidental injury.
   - Unintentional injuries are the leading cause of morbidity and mortality among children in the United States.

2. **Epidemiology**
   - Each year, among those aged 0 to 19 years, more than 12,000 people die from unintentional

injuries and more than 9.2 million are treated in emergency departments for nonfatal injuries.
- *Injuries due to transportation were the leading cause of death for children.* Combining all unintentional injury deaths among those aged between 0 and 19 years, motor vehicle traffic-related deaths were the leading cause.
- *The leading causes of injury death differed by age-group.* For children younger than 1 year, two-thirds of injury deaths were due to suffocation. Drowning was the leading cause of injury death for those aged 1 to 4 years. For children and adolescents (5–19 years), the most injury-related deaths were due to being an occupant in a motor vehicle traffic crash.
- Poisoning death rate for those older than 15 years is at least five times the rate for the younger age-group.
- *Risk of injury death varied by race.* An injury death rate was highest for American Indians and Alaska Natives and was lowest for Asian or Pacific Islanders. Overall death rates for Whites and African Americans were approximately the same.
- *Injury death rates varied by state, depending on the cause of death.* Overall, Northeast (NE) states have the lowest injury-related death rates. Fire, burn, and transportation-related injuries death rates were highest in some of the Southeast (SE) states.
- Approximately 21.8 million persons aged ≥15 years sustained nonfatal, unintentional injuries, resulting in approximately $67.3 billion in lifetime medical costs (2008).

3. **Screening**
- Injury Center suggests screening for child maltreatment prevention, motor vehicle safety, and older adult falls. Screening should be an ongoing process at primary care and community-based settings.

4. **Recommendation**
- The CDC's Community Guide "recommends child safety seat use laws, community-wide information and enhanced enforcement campaigns, and distribution or incentive programs plus education, enforcement programs to increase safety seat use in infants and children."
- The CDC recommends 0.08 blood alcohol concentration laws, lower blood alcohol concentration laws for young drivers, minimum legal drinking age laws, sobriety checkpoints, mass media campaigns, school-based programs, and alcohol server intervention training programs.
- AAFP, AAP, and AMA support primary enforcement of occupant-restraint system legislation and counseling of all parents and patients older than 2 years about accidental injury prevention, and document the use of occupant-restraint systems. In addition, providers should provide up-to-date, appropriate information for parents on car

safety seat choices and proper use. Motor vehicle occupant injuries (MVOIs) between physicians and their patients and the use of active, approved restraints for both adults and children should also be discussed.
- The ACOG recommends that clinicians counsel all women on the use of seat belts and that pregnant women be counseled on proper seat belt use during pregnancy and driving while intoxicated (DWI) alert for riding with the DWI drivers.

C. Prevention of Falls in Older Adults: Fall and Gait Disorders (Also See Chapter 6, Section IV.C.).
1. **Definition**
- An unexpected event in which the participant falls and comes to rest on the ground, floor, or lower level.

2. **Epidemiology**
- Each year, one in every three adults aged 65 and older falls, which can lead to moderate to severe injuries, such as hip fractures and head traumas, and can even increase the risk of early death.
- Falls are the leading cause of fatal and nonfatal injuries among adults aged ≥65 years (older adults). During 2014, approximately 27,000 older adults died because of falls; 2.8 million were treated in emergency departments for fall-related injuries, and approximately 800,000 of these patients were subsequently hospitalized.
- Falls are the leading cause of injury-related visits to emergency departments in the United States and the primary etiology of accidental deaths in persons over the age of 65 years.
- Most common cause of nonfatal injuries and hospital admissions for trauma.
- Annual Medicare costs for older adult falls have been estimated at $31.3 billion and that for the older adult population is expected to increase 55% by 2030.
- The highest rates were for injuries that occurred in or around the tub or shower (65.8 per 100,000) and injuries that happened on or near the toilet (22.5 per 100,000).
- Hip fracture is common after fall; over 90% of hip fractures are caused by falling; women sustain three-quarters of all hip fractures.
- The most common are fractures of the spine, hip, forearm, leg, ankle, pelvis, upper arm, and hand.
- White women are much more likely to sustain hip fractures than are African American or Asian women; people aged 85 years and older are 10 to 15 times more likely to sustain hip fractures than are those aged 60 to 65.
- Falls are the leading cause of fatal and nonfatal injuries among adults aged ≥65 years (older adults). During 2014, approximately 27,000 older adults

died because of falls; 2.8 million were treated in emergency departments for fall-related injuries, and approximately 800,000 of these patients were subsequently hospitalized.

3. **Screening**
   - During routine visits, a provider should ask elderly patients about history of falls; observe any change in mental status, change in vision, and difficulty in transferring from bed to chair/bathroom; and observe patients' gait.
   - *Tinetti Tool for Fall Screening*, designed for the adult population and elderly residents, is a simple, easily administered test that measures a resident's gait and balance. The Tinetti Assessment Tool is a task-performed examination that can be completed in 10 to 15 minutes. Scoring is based on the resident's ability to perform specific tasks and is done on a three-point ordinal scale with a range of 0 to 2. A score of 0 represents the most impairment, whereas a score of 2 represents independence. The individual scores are then combined to form three measures: an overall gait assessment score, an overall balance assessment score, and a combined gait and balance score.
   - Interpretation: the maximum score for the gait component is 12 points. The maximum score for the balance component is 16 points. The maximum total score is 28 points. In general, residents who score below 19 are at a high risk for falls. Residents who score in the range of 19 to 24 points indicate that the resident has a risk for falls (see http://fallpreventiontaskforce.org/wp-content/uploads/2014/10/Tinettitool.pdf).

4. **Recommendation**
   - The USPSTF recommends exercise or physical therapy and vitamin D supplementation to prevent falls in community-dwelling adults aged 65 years or older who are at increased risk for falls.
   - No single recommended tool or brief approach can reliably identify older adults at increased risk for falls, but several reasonable and feasible approaches are available for primary care clinicians. See the Clinical Consideration section for additional information on risk assessment.
   - The USPSTF recommends counseling older patients on measures to reduce the risk of falling. These measures include exercise (particularly training to improve balance), safety-related skills and behaviors, environmental hazard reduction, and monitoring and adjusting medications. This recommendation is based on fair evidence that these four measures reduce the likelihood of falling. The USPSTF also recommends an intensive individualized home-based multifactorial intervention for high-risk older patients in settings where adequate resources are available to deliver

such services. Several studies have examined single risk-factor modification and multifactorial interventions and have found that both can prevent falls in older patients.
   - Exercising regularly, focus on increasing leg strength and improving balance. As a result, Tai Chi programs are effective.
   - Reviewing medicines: both prescription and over-the-counter—to reduce side effects and interactions that may cause dizziness or drowsiness.
   - Eye examination/vision check once a year.
   - Making home safety improvements by reducing tripping hazards, adding grab bars and railings, and improving lighting.
   - Getting adequate calcium and vitamin D in your diet, undertaking a program of weight-bearing exercise, and getting screened and treated for osteoporosis.

D. **Motor Vehicle Occupant Restraints**
1. **Definition**
   - MVOIs are related to motor vehicle accidents (MVAs) when the seat belt and *child safety seats* are not used by the motor vehicle occupants (passengers).
2. **Epidemiology**
   - In 2013, the U.S. crash death rate was more than twice the average of other high-income countries. In the United States, front seat belt use was lower than in most other comparison countries. One in three crash deaths in the United States involved drunk driving, and almost one in three involved speeding.
   - About 90 people die each day in the United States from crashes, resulting in the highest death rate among comparison countries.
   - There were more than 32,000 crash deaths in the United States in 2013. These deaths cost more than $380 million in direct medical costs.
   - Each year, MVAs take the lives of more than 40,000 people in the United States and result in 2.7 million emergency department visits.
   - Leading cause of death among individuals aged between 3 and 33 years of age in the United States and cause morbidity for the nearly 3 million people who sustain nonfatal injuries annually.
   - Proper use of seat belt or motor vehicle occupant restraints (child safety seats, booster seats, and lap-and-shoulder belts) is associated with a 45% to 70% reduction in fatality risk. Improper use reduces the efficacy of restraints substantially.
   - All 50 states currently have laws requiring child safety seats for infants and children, and 49 states and the District of Columbia have adult seat belt laws.
   - All 50 states, the District of Columbia and Puerto Rico have laws that make it illegal to drive with a

blood alcohol concentration of 0.08 g per dL or higher, and rates of alcohol involvement among fatal crashes have decreased during the past two decades.
- Despite widespread regulation and overall increases in safer motor vehicle-related behaviors, recent crash data show that more than 50% of fatalities were among unrestrained occupants and nearly 40% involved alcohol.

3. **Screening**
- Increasing the correct use of occupant-restraint devices and decreasing alcohol-related driving (i.e., driving while under the influence of alcohol or riding with drivers who are under the influence of alcohol) are among the most important strategies to effectively reduce MVA-related fatalities.

4. **Recommendation**
- The USPSTF recommends that clinicians screen adults aged 18 years or older for alcohol misuse and provide persons engaged in risky or hazardous drinking with brief behavioral counseling interventions to reduce alcohol misuse.
- Proper seat belt recommendations can be found at https://www.cdc.gov/safechild/road_traffic_injuries/index.html.
- Counseling in primary care setting to increase the proper use of child safety seats, increase the use of safety belts, and reduce alcohol-impaired driving.

E. Pertussis (Also See Chapter 21, Section III.)

1. **Definition**
- A cough illness lasting at least 2 weeks with one of the following: paroxysms of coughing, inspiratory "whoop," or posttussive vomiting, without any other apparent cause (as reported by a health professional).

2. **Epidemiology**
- During 2014, 32,971 cases of pertussis were reported to CDC. This represents a 15% increase compared to the 28,639 cases reported during 2013.
- Age-incidence trends observed during 2014 were similar to those in 2013 and 2012. Increased rates were again observed in adolescents aged 13 through 15 years, as well as in the 16-year-olds. Most deaths occurred among babies younger than 3 months old. The incidence rate of pertussis among babies exceeded that of all other age-groups.
- Overall reporting of pertussis declined during 2013 after a peak year in 2012. During 2012, 48,277 cases of pertussis were reported to CDC, including 20 pertussis-related deaths. This was the most reported cases since 1955. In 2012, second highest rates of disease after babies were observed in children aged 7 through 10 years old. Rates increased in teens aged 13 and 14 years.

- Pertussis is an endemic (common) disease in the United States, with periodic epidemics every 3 to 5 years and frequent outbreaks.
- Since the 1980s, there has been an increase in the number of reported cases of pertussis in the United States, especially among 10- to 19-year-olds and infants younger than 6 months.
- The primary goal of pertussis outbreak control efforts is to decrease morbidity (amount of disease) and mortality (death) among infants; a secondary goal is to decrease morbidity among persons of all ages.
- Polymerase chain reaction (PCR) tests vary in specificity, so obtaining culture confirmation of pertussis for at least one suspicious case is recommended any time there is suspicion of a pertussis outbreak.
- Institutional outbreaks of pertussis are common. Outbreaks at middle and high schools can occur when protection from childhood vaccines fades. In school outbreaks, prophylaxis is recommended for close classroom and team contacts—and the pertussis booster vaccine (Tdap), depending on age. Pertussis outbreaks in hospitals and other clinical settings can put infants and other patients at risk (Figure 18–1).

3. **Screening**
- Infants younger than 6 months, who are at greatest risk of severe disease and death, continue to have the highest reported rate of pertussis, with a 60% increase in incidence observed between 2008 and 2009.
- PCR tests of nasopharyngeal swabs or aspirates can be a rapid, sensitive, and specific test for pertussis. Preferably, it should be used in addition to bacterial cultures, not as a replacement for culture tests.
- Clinical case and positive PCR tests are considered confirmed cases by the health department.

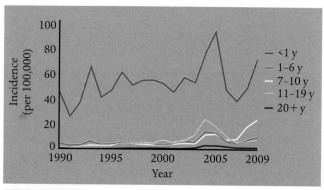

FIGURE 18–1. Reported pertussis incidence of age-group, **1990 to 2009.** (Courtesy of the CDC, National Notifiable Diseases Surveillance System, 2009.)

Patients who have not been coughing for at least 14 days are considered probable cases unless the cough continues for 14 days.

- Isolation of *Bordetella pertussis* by culture is considered to be definitive for pertussis. The *B. pertussis* bacteria are fastidious; therefore, culturing may be difficult.

4. **Recommendation**
   - Since 2005, the Advisory Committee on Immunization Practices has recommended that health care personnel receive a single dose of Tdap; after receipt of Tdap, a dose of Td is recommended every 10 years. Currently, both Tdap products are Food and Drug Administration approved for single use.
   - Persons aged 65 years and older (e.g., grandparents, child-care providers, and health care practitioners) who have or who anticipate having close contact with an infant aged less than 12 months and who previously have not received Tdap should receive a single dose of Tdap to protect against pertussis and reduce the likelihood of transmission.
   - Vaccination of susceptible persons is the most important preventive strategy against pertussis. Universal childhood pertussis vaccine recommendations have been implemented since the mid-1940s.
   - Postexposure prophylaxis. A macrolide can be administered as prophylaxis for close contacts of a person with pertussis if the person has no contraindication to its use: azithromycin, erythromycin, clarithromycin, alternate agent (TMP-SMZ).

F. **Obesity (Adult)**
   1. **Definition**
      - Obesity ranges are determined using weight and height to calculate the body mass index (BMI).
      - An adult who has a BMI between 25 and 29.9 is considered overweight.
      - An adult who has a BMI of 30 or higher is considered obese.
   2. **Epidemiology**
      - More than one-third (36.5%) of U.S. adults have obesity. Obesity-related conditions include heart disease, stroke, type 2 diabetes mellitus (DM), and certain types of cancer, some of the leading causes of preventable death.
      - Non-Hispanic blacks have the highest age-adjusted rates of obesity (48.1%) followed by Hispanics (42.5%), non-Hispanic whites (34.5%), and non-Hispanic Asians (11.7%). Obesity is higher among middle age adults aged 40 to 59 years (40.2%) and older adults aged 60 and over (37.0%) than among younger adults aged 20 to 39 (32.3%).
      - According to AMA, childhood obesity is an increasingly serious problem; 13.9% of children aged 2 to 5 years, 18.8% of children aged 6 to 11 years of age, and 17.4% of adolescents aged 12 to 19 years of age in America are obese.

- It is estimated that more than 34% of adults aged 20 and older in the United States are obese (defined as having a BMI of 30 or higher) and therefore at increased risk for cancer, diabetes, and coronary heart disease (CHD).
- Approximately 65% of obese adults aged 20 and older reported being told by their health care provider that they were overweight.
- Poor, near-poor, and middle-income obese adults were less likely than high-income obese adults to report being told by their health care provider that they were overweight.
- Obese adults with less than a high school education and those with a high school education were less likely than obese with at least some college to report being told by their health care that they were overweight.
- Obese women aged 20 and older were more likely than men to report being told by a doctor or health professional that they were overweight.

3. **Screening**
   - The USPSTF recommends screening all adults for obesity. Clinician should offer or refer patients with a BMI of 30 kg/m^2 or higher to intensive, multicomponent behavioral interventions.
   - The USPSTF recommends that clinicians screen for obesity in children and adolescents aged 6 years and older and offer or refer them to comprehensive, intensive behavioral interventions to promote improvements in weight status.
   - The USPSTF recommends that clinicians screen all adult patients for obesity and offer intensive counseling and behavioral interventions to promote sustained weight loss for obese adults.
   - The AAFP recommends that intensive counseling involve more than one session per month for at least 3 months (2003).

4. **Recommendation**
   - USPSTF recommends that high waist circumference is associated with an increased risk of type 2 DM, dyslipidemia, hypertension (HTN), CVD in patient with BMI in a range between 25 and 34.9 kg per m^2. Men having waist circumference >102 cm (40 in) and women >88 cm (>35 in) are at high risk.
   - The CDC recommends counting calories and not eating more calories than the body is using, reducing time spent watching television and other sedentary behaviors, building physical activity into regular routines, and creating opportunities for physical activity at work sites and in communities.
   - The AHRQ recommends physician-based exercise and diet counseling as an effective strategy for a weight loss intervention and regular exercise and a health aid in maintaining normal blood cholesterol levels, weight, and blood pressure, reducing the risk of heart disease, stroke, and diabetes.

G. Physical Activity

1. Definition

The CDC defines physical activity as follows:

- Recommend physical activity: moderate-intensity activities in a usual week (i.e., brisk walking, vacuuming, or anything that results in small increases in breathing or heart rate) for ≥30 minutes per day, ≥5 days per week; or vigorous-intensity activities in usual week (i.e., running, heavy hard work, or anything else that causes large increases in breathing or heart rate) for ≥20 minutes per day, ≥3 days per week, or both.
- Insufficient physical activity: doing more than 10 minutes per week of moderate or vigorous-intensity lifestyle activities (i.e., household, transportation, or lifestyle activities), but less than the recommended level of activity.
- Inactivity: less than 10 minutes per week of moderate or vigorous-intensity lifestyle activities (i.e., household, transportation, or leisure-time activity).
- Leisure-time inactivity: no reported physical activities (i.e., any physical activities or exercise such as running, calisthenics, golf, gardening, or walking) in the previous month.

2. Epidemiology

- According to Healthy People 2020 (HP2020): more than 80% of adults do not meet the guidelines for both aerobic and muscle-strengthening activities. Similarly, more than 80% of adolescents do not do enough aerobic physical activity to meet the guidelines for youth.

3. Screening

- The AAFP recognizes that regular physical activity is imperative.

4. Recommendation

- The USDHHS (HP2020), CDC, AAFP, AAP, The American Heart of Association, and ACOG recommend that health care providers counsel individuals physical activity based on the health benefits of physical activity.
- HP2020 reflects a multidisciplinary approach to promoting physical activity. This approach brings about traditional partnerships, such as that of education and health care, with nontraditional partnerships representing transportation, urban planning, recreation, environmental health, and other fields. (For more information, see http://www.physicalactivityplan.org/theplan.html.)
- According to CDC and USPSTF, 36 States reported (2008) that 25% of their population reported no leisure-time physical activity.
- According to the 2007 Youth Risk Behavior Surveillance System, 17% of high school youths are physically active.

- The *2008 Physical Activity Guidelines for Activity* recommends adults should do at least 150 minutes of moderate intensity (e.g., brisk walking) or 75 minutes of vigorous-intensity physical activity (e.g., jogging, running) per week or an equivalent combination of the two.
- For additional health benefits, adults should do more than 300 minutes of moderate intensity or 150 minutes of vigorous-intensity activity per week or an equivalent combination of the two.
- Older adults should engage in muscle-strengthening activities on at least 2 days of the week to improve.

H. Hormone Replacement Therapy

1. Definition

- There is controversy around the risks and benefits of using hormone replacement therapy (HRT) in women going through menopause and having decrease in estrogen levels.

2. Epidemiology

- White women are more likely to receive HRT counseling than black or Hispanic women with the same level of education; women with higher levels of education were more likely to receive counseling than women with less education, regardless of race or ethnicity.
- Women who had received recent preventive health services such as mammograms, Pap smears, and general examinations were much more likely to have received HRT counseling than those who had not. The more recent the services, the greater the likelihood the women had received HRT counseling.

3. Screening

- The American College of Physicians recommended that health care providers discuss HRT with all women around the time of menopause (40–60 years of age, the years when menopause is most likely to occur).

4. Recommendation

- The USPSTF recommends against the routine use of combined estrogen and progestin for the prevention of chronic conditions in postmenopausal women.
  - Postmenopausal women: the USPSTF recommends against the use of combined estrogen and progestin for the prevention of chronic conditions in postmenopausal women.
  - Postmenopausal women who have had a hysterectomy: the USPSTF recommends against the use of estrogen for the prevention of chronic conditions in postmenopausal women who have had a hysterectomy.
- The USPSTF found evidence that the use of combined estrogen and progestin results in the reduced the risk of fracture and colorectal cancer (CRC).

- The USPSTF found that combined estrogen and progestin has no beneficial effect on CHD and may even pose an increased risk. Other harms included an increased risk for breast cancer, venous thromboembolism, stroke, cholecystitis, dementia, and lower global cognitive function.
- The USPSTF could not assess the effects of combined estrogen and progestin on the incidence of ovarian cancer, mortality from breast cancer or CHD, or all-cause mortality. The USPSTF concluded that the harmful effects of combined estrogen and progestin are likely to exceed the chronic disease prevention benefits in most women.
- The USPSTF recommends against the routine use of unopposed estrogen for the prevention of chronic conditions in postmenopausal women who have had a hysterectomy.

II. Children and Adolescents

A. Dental Caries in Preschool Children (Also See Chapter 11, Section V. Diseases of the Teeth, A)

1. **Definition**
   - Dental caries (i.e., tooth decay) is an infectious, multifactorial, communicable disease caused by demineralization of tooth enamel in the presence of a sugar substrate and cariogenic bacteria found in plaque.
   - *Streptococcus mutans* is considered to be the primary strain of bacteria causing tooth decay.
   - When plaque is not regularly removed, it may calcify to form calculus (tartar) and dental caries.
   - Fluoride reduces the incidence of dental caries and slows or prevents cavities.

2. **Screening**
   - Health care providers are encouraged to screen for dental caries and identify risk factors for childhood dental caries during routine visits: frequent consumption of foods and beverages containing sugars and sticky foods, frequent bottle- and breast-feeding on demand, maternal or sibling caries, repetitive use of "sippy cup," poor oral hygiene, inadequate fluoridation, and lack of dental visits.

3. **Epidemiology**
   - According to the CDC, dental caries affects more than one-fourth of U.S. children aged 2 to 5 years, and half of those aged 12 to 15 years, half of all children and two-thirds of adolescents aged 12 to 19 years from lower-income families have decay.
   - Less than one of three children enrolled in Medicaid received at least one preventive dental screening.
   - Children and adolescents from some racial and ethnic groups have more untreated tooth decay—40% of Mexican American children aged 6 to 8 years have untreated decay, compared with 25% of non-Hispanic white.

4. **Recommendation: Dental Caries Screening from Birth through Age 5 Years**
   - The USPSTF recommends that primary care clinicians prescribe oral fluoride supplementation starting at age 6 months for children whose water supply is deficient in fluoride.
   - The USPSTF recommends that primary care clinicians apply fluoride varnish to the primary teeth of all infants and children starting at the age of primary tooth eruption.
   - The USPSTF concludes that the current evidence is insufficient to assess the balance of benefits and harms of routine screening examinations for dental caries performed by primary care clinicians in children from birth to age 5 years.
   - The USPSTF and AAFP recommend that health care providers prescribe oral fluoride supplementation to prevent dental caries based on age and fluoride concentration of patient's water supply for infants and children aged 6 months through 16 years residing in areas with inadequate fluoride in the water supply (<0.6 ppm).

B. Exercise (Physical Activity)

1. **Definition**
   - Physical activity is any bodily movement that results in the expenditure of energy and includes aerobic, muscle-strengthening, and bone-strengthening activities.
   - According to the CDC, physical activity for children and adolescents is measured on a scale of 0 to 10, where sitting is a 0 and the highest level of activity is a 10, moderate-intensity activity is a 5 or 6 and vigorous-intensity activity is a level 7 to 8.
   - Aerobic activity moderate-intensity includes brisk walking, and vigorous-intensity includes running; muscle strengthening includes gymnastics or push-ups; and bone-strengthening activities include jumping rope or running.

2. **Epidemiology**
   - According to HP2020, the following factors have a positive association with physical activity:
     - Children aged 4 to 12, gender (boys), belief in the ability to be active (self-efficacy), and parental support.
     - Adolescents aged 13 to 18 years; parental education, gender (boys) and personal goals, physical education/school sports, belief in the ability to be active (self-efficacy and support of friends and family).
     - Environmental influences positively associated with physical activity among children and adolescents include presence of sidewalks, having a destination/walking to a particular place, access to public transportation, low traffic density, access to neighborhood or school play area and/or recreational equipment.

3. **Screening**
   - The AAFP *recognizes that regular physical activity is desirable.* The effectiveness of physician's advice and counseling in this area is uncertain (2002).

4. **Recommendation**
   - The *2008 Physical Activity Guidelines for Activity* recommends that children should be active at least 60 minutes daily and that most of this time should be spent in either moderate (i.e., brisk walking) or vigorous-intensity physical activity (i.e., running) on at least 3 days per week, to include aerobic, muscle-strengthening, and bone-strengthening activities.
   - The AAFP recommends that prolonged periods of physical inactivity should be discouraged in both the home and the school.
   - Adults should do at least 150 minutes a week of moderate intensity (e.g., brisk walking) or 75 minutes a week of vigorous-intensity aerobic physical activity. Aerobic activity should be performed in episodes of at least 10 minutes and should be spread throughout the week.
   - The AAFP recommends that parents encourage their children to be physically active as part of their daily routine. The benefits of physical activity include increased cardiovascular endurance, improved large muscle strength and endurance, increased flexibility, maintenance of proper body weight, and reduction of stress.

C. **Healthy Diet (Nutrition)**
   1. **Definition**
      - The *Dietary Guidelines for Americans, 2010* emphasizes the following goals for a healthy diet:
        - Balance calories with physical activity to manage weight.
        - Consume more of certain foods and nutrients such as fruits, vegetables, whole grains, fat-free and low-fat dairy products, and seafood.
        - Consume fewer foods with sodium (salt), saturated fats, *trans* fats, cholesterol, added sugars, and refined grains.
      - **HP2020 Nutrition guideline includes the following five steps:**
        - Follow a healthy eating pattern across the life span. All food and beverage choices matter. Choose a healthy eating pattern at an appropriate calorie level to help achieve and maintain a healthy body weight, support nutrient adequacy, and reduce risk for chronic disease.
        - Focus on variety, nutrient density, and amount. To meet nutrient needs within calorie limits, choose a variety of nutrient-dense foods across and within all food groups in recommended amounts.
        - Limit calories from added sugars and saturated fats and reduce sodium intake. Consume an eating pattern low in added sugars, saturated fats, and sodium. Cut back on foods and beverages higher in these components to amounts that fit within healthy eating patterns.
        - Shift to healthier food and beverage choices. Choose nutrient-dense foods and beverages across and within all food groups in place of less healthy choices. Consider cultural and personal preferences to make these shifts easier to accomplish and maintain.
        - Support healthy eating patterns for all.

   2. **Epidemiology**
      - According to the CDC, most youths in the United States do not meet the recommendations for eating fruits and vegetables and whole grains each day, and exceed the recommended maximum daily intake of sodium (1,500–2,300 mg each day).
      - Children and adolescents between the ages of 2 and 18 years consume 40% of their daily calories from empty calories from soda, fruit drinks, dairy desserts, grain desserts, pizza, and whole milk.
      - Adolescents drink more full-calorie soda per day than milk. Males aged 12 to 19 years drink an average of 22 oz of full-calorie soda per day, more than twice their intake of fluid milk (10 oz), and females drink an average of 14 oz of full-calorie soda and only 6 oz of fluid milk.

   3. **Screening**
      - Health care providers are encouraged to screen for healthy eating to reduce the risk of heart disease, cancer, stroke, and diabetes in children and adolescents; in addition, it is important for proper growth and development and can prevent health problems such as obesity, dental caries, and iron deficiency.

   4. **Recommendation**
      - The Dietary Guidelines for Americans recommends a diet rich in fruits and vegetables, whole grains, and fat-free and low-fat dairy products for persons aged 2 years and older.
      - Key recommendations that are quantitative are provided for several components of the diet that should be limited. These components are of particular public health concern, and the specified limits can help individuals achieve healthy eating patterns within calorie limits:
        - Consume less than 10% of calories per day from added sugars.
        - Consume less than 10% of calories per day from saturated fats.
        - Consume less than 2,300 milligrams (mg) per day of sodium.
        - If alcohol is consumed, it should be consumed in moderation—up to one drink per day for

women and up to two drinks per day for men—and only by adults of legal drinking age.

- The guidelines also recommend that children, adolescents, and adults limit the intake of solid fats (major sources of saturated and trans fatty acids), cholesterol, sodium, added sugars, and refined grains.

D. Lead Levels in Children and Adolescents (Also See Chapter 2, Section I.C.)

1. Definition

- Lead is an element found in flaking lead paint, artist's paints, fruit tree sprays, solder, brass alloys, home-glazed pottery, and fumes from burning batteries.
- Repetitive ingestion of small amounts of lead is more serious than a single massive exposure.
- Toxic effects are more likely to occur if more than 0.5 mg of lead per day is absorbed.
- Lead poison causes symptoms including weakness, irritability, weight loss, vomiting, ataxia, headache, colicky abdominal pain, decreased growth in height, delayed sexual maturation, increased dental caries, and impaired neurologic development (e.g., behavioral changes, mental impairment, seizures, and coma).

2. Epidemiology

- The incidence and prevalence of lead poisoning in children has decreased since the removal of lead from paint and gasoline in the 1970s; however, there are approximately 310,000 U.S. children younger than 5 years that have elevated blood lead levels.

3. Screening

- Health care providers are encouraged to identify children at risk, eliminate exposure to known sources, and ensure adequate nutrition, including preventing and correcting iron deficiency, as key strategies in the care of all children.
- Health care providers should perform targeted screening for lead poisoning in children who are Medicaid-enrolled or Medicaid-eligible, foreign-born, or identified as high risk by the CDC.

4. Recommendation

- The CDC recommends a blood lead level of 10 μg per dL (0.48 μmol per L) or higher as abnormal and requiring follow-up and intervention; lead levels lower than 10 μg per dL can affect cognitive development.
- Recommendations for treatment of elevated blood levels include a thorough environmental investigation, laboratory testing when appropriate, iron supplementation for iron-deficient children, and chelation therapy for blood lead levels of 45 μg per dL or more. Prevention consists of education and avoidance of lead-contaminated products.

III. Cancer

A. Breast Cancer (Also See Chapter Chapter 17, Section III.E.)

1. Definition

- Cancer that forms in tissues of the breast, usually the ducts and lobules.

2. Epidemiology

- Most common cancer in pregnant and postpartum women, occurring in about 1 in 3,000 pregnant women.
- Average patient is between 32 and 38 years of age, many women choosing to delay childbearing; it is likely that the incidence of breast cancer during pregnancy will increase.
- Estimated new cases and deaths from breast cancer in the United States (2011): new cases—230,480 (females), 2,140 (males); and deaths—39,520 (females), 450 (males).
- Decline in cancer deaths among white women in this country, but survival has decreased among black women, with 28% more likely to die from the disease.

3. Screening

- The USPSTF recommends screening mammography (Grade B), with or without clinical breast examination, every 1 to 2 years for women aged 40 and older. Grade B net benefit is moderate to substantial.

4. Recommendations

- CDC makes the following recommendations: have a regular breast examination, control weight and exercise, know your family history, find out the risks and benefits of HRT, and limit the amount of alcoholic drinks.

B. Colorectal Cancer (Also See Chapter 17, Section VI.E.)

1. Definition

- Most common type is adenocarcinomas.

2. Epidemiology

- Estimated new cases and deaths from colon cancer in the United States (2011): new cases—101,340 (colon), 39,870 (rectal); and deaths—49,380 (colon and rectal combined).
- Third most common type of cancer and the second leading cause of cancer death in the United States.
- Prevention of CRC includes modifying risk factors such as weight, physical activity, smoking, and alcohol use, as well as screening for early disease.

3. Screening

- Screening is important because early stages of CRC may not present any symptoms, and also because abnormal growths can be detected before they develop into cancer.
- Early detection increases treatment options and the chances for survival. The USPSTF recommends CRC screening for men and women aged 50 years and continuation until age 75.

- The screening tests include fecal occult blood test (FOBT), flexible sigmoidoscopy, colonoscopy, proctoscopy, and barium enema.
- Insufficient evidence to assess the benefits and harms of computerized tomography (CT) colonography and fecal DNA testing as screening modalities for CRC.

4. **Recommendations**
   - High-sensitivity FOBT or fecal immunochemical testing annually, flexible sigmoidoscopy every 5 years, double-contrast barium enema every 5 years.
   - CT colonography (virtual colonoscopy) every 5 years, colonoscopy every 10 years, fecal DNA at an unspecified interval.
   - Adults aged 50 to 75 years: screen with high-sensitivity FOBT, sigmoidoscopy, or colonoscopy.

C. Lung Cancer
1. **Definition**
   - Cancer of air passages, small-cell lung cancer (SCLC) and non–small-cell lung cancer (NSCLC).
2. **Epidemiology**
   - In the United States, the estimated cases of lung cancer (SCLC and NSCLC)—new cases: 221,130 and deaths: 156,940 (2011).
   - The most common types of NSCLC are squamous and that of SCLC are adenocarcinomas.
   - Leading cause of death accounting for one in every four deaths both in men and in women.
   - NSCLCs are associated with cigarette smoke, whereas adenocarcinomas may be found in patients who have never smoked.
   - As a class, NSCLCs are relatively insensitive to chemotherapy and radiation therapy compared with SCLCs.
   - SCLC accounts for approximately 15% of bronchogenic carcinomas; at the time of diagnosis, approximately 30% of patients will have tumors confined to the hemithorax of origin, the mediastinum, or the supraclavicular lymph nodes.
   - Five-year survival rates were higher for whites (52.7%) than for blacks (47.5%) with stage I or II disease. For stages III and IV disease, 5-year survival rates were 17.7% for whites and 19.6% for blacks.
3. **Screening**
   - In patients considered to be at high risk of developing lung cancer, no screening modality for early detection has been shown to alter mortality.
   - The USPSTF recommends annual screening for lung cancer with low-dose computed tomography in adults aged 55 to 80 years who have a 30 pack-year smoking history and currently smoke or have quit within the past 15 years. Screening should be discontinued once a person has not smoked for 15 years or develops a health problem that substantially limits life expectancy or the ability or willingness to have curative lung surgery.

4. **Recommendations**
   - The USPSTF concludes that the evidence is insufficient to recommend for or against screening asymptomatic persons for lung cancer with either low-dose CT(LDCT), chest X-ray, sputum cytology, or a combination of these tests.
   - CDC makes the following recommendations: stop smoking, control weight and exercise, know your family history, and limit the amount of alcohol drinks.

D. Oral Cancer
1. **Definition**
   - Cancer of oral cavity.
2. **Epidemiology**
   - In the United States, new cases were estimated to be 39,400 and deaths to be 7,900 (2011).
   - Tobacco (cigarettes, cigars, pipes, betel, or mixed tobacco and smokeless tobacco) users or alcohol users are at elevated risk for oral cancer; and they are at particularly high risk if they use both tobacco and alcohol.
   - Persistent oral infection by carcinogenic strains of human papillomavirus and chronic sun exposure of lips are also at increased risk.
3. **Screening**
   - USPSTF concludes insufficient evidence to recommend routine screening of adults for oral cancer. Recommend oral examination during routine health care visits.
4. **Recommendations**
   - Encouraged not to use tobacco and to limit alcohol use to decrease their risk of oral cancer as well as heart disease, stroke, lung cancer, and cirrhosis.

E. Ovarian Cancer
1. **Definition**
   - Mostly epithelial carcinomas.
2. **Epidemiology**
   - Estimated new cases and deaths from ovarian cancer in the United States in 2011—new cases, 21,990; and deaths, 15,460.
3. **Screening**
   - Two tests used most often to screen for ovarian cancer are transvaginal ultrasound (U/S) and the CA-125 (cancer antigen 125) blood test, in addition to pelvic examinations.
4. **Recommendations**
   - Genetic testing for *BRCA1/2* mutation that can increase chances for breast/ovarian cancer.
   - Most breast and ovarian cancers are *not* caused by mutations in these genes; *BRCA1/2* genetic testing will be helpful only for a small number of women.
   - CDC recommends general cancer prevention, such as control weight; more fruit and vegetables; exercise; know your family history; and limit the amount of alcohol drinks.

F. Prostate Cancer (Also See Chapter 17, Section VI.C.)

1. **Definition**
   - Cancer of prostate common in older men.
2. **Epidemiology**
   - The American Cancer Society estimates about 240,890 new cases and 33,720 deaths in the United States (2011).
3. **Screening**
   - The USPSTF recommends against prostate-specific antigen–based screening for prostate cancer.
4. **Recommendations**
   - CDC recommends general cancer prevention, such as control weight; more fruit and vegetables; exercise; know your family history; and limit the amount of alcohol drinks.

G. Skin Cancer

1. **Definition**
   - Skin cancer; it could be melanoma, basal cell, squamous cell, and neuroendocrine carcinoma of skin.
2. **Epidemiology**
   - The American Cancer Society estimates that in 2011, there were 1,000,000 new cases and fewer than 1,000 deaths.
3. **Screening**
   - The only widely proposed screening procedure for skin cancer is visual examination of the skin, including both self-examination and clinical examination.
4. **Recommendations**
   - The USPSTF concludes that the current evidence is insufficient to assess the balance of the risk and benefits of using a whole-body skin examination by a primary care clinician or patient skin self-examination for the early detection of cutaneous melanoma, basal cell cancer, or squamous cell skin cancer in the adult general population.
   - The USPSTF concludes that the evidence is insufficient to recommend for or against routine counseling by primary care clinicians to prevent skin cancer.

H. Testicular Cancer (Also See Chapter 17, Section VI.A.)

1. **Definition**
   - Testicular cancer common in young or middle-aged men or germ cell cancer.
2. **Epidemiology**
   - The American Cancer Society estimates 8,290 new cases and 350 deaths (2011).
3. **Screening**
   - α-Fetoprotein, β-human chronic gonadotropin, and lactase dehydrogenase should be measured before removing the involved testicle.
4. **Recommendations**
   - The USPSTF, AAFP, and AAP recommend against screening for testicular cancer in adolescent or adult males. The American Cancer Society does not recommend testicular self-examination. Most testicular cancers are discovered accidentally by the patient or their partner. Potential harm associated with screening testicular cancer includes false-positives, anxiety, and harms from diagnostic tests or procedures.

I. Tobacco Cessation

1. **Epidemiology**
   - Tobacco use is the leading preventable cause of death, disease, and disability in the United States. Each year, around 443,000 people die from smoking or exposure to secondhand smoke, and another 8.6 million suffer from a serious illness from smoking.
   - CDC reports about 46.6 million adults in the United States smoke, and 88 million nonsmokers are exposed to secondhand smoke.
   - Adult smoking rates vary across the United States, but the states with the most smokers are in the Midwest and Southeast regions.
   - Smokers are two to four times more likely to develop heart disease, double the risk for stroke.
2. **Screening and Recommendations**
   - To increase tobacco use cessation, the United States Public Health States (USPHS) on Community Preventive Services recommends increasing the unit price of tobacco products, conducting mass media education campaigns with community interventions, and providing telephone-based cessation counseling.
   - USPHS recommends that brief advice by medical providers to quit smoking is an effective intervention.
   - HHS provides single toll-free number 1-800-QUIT NOW.
   - All 50 states offer some degree of telephone-based tobacco cessation services.

IV. Cardiovascular Disorders

A. Abdominal Aortic Aneurysm (AAA)

1. **Epidemiology**
   - AAA is more common in men and in individuals aged 65 years and older. AAA is less common in women and with black race/ethnicity.
   - AAA (from 2.9 to 4.9 cm diameter) are present in 1.3% of men (0% of women) aged 45 to 54 years and 2.5% (5.2% of women) of men aged 75 to 84 years.
2. **Screening**
   - USPSTF recommends onetime screening for AAA by U/S in men aged 65 to 75 years who have ever smoked and do not recommend U/S for those who have never smoked.
3. **Recommendations**
   - Men aged 65 to 75 years who have ever smoked: the USPSTF recommends onetime screening for

AAA with ultrasonography in men ages 65 to 75 years who have ever smoked.

- Men aged 65 to 75 years who have never smoked: the USPSTF recommends that clinicians selectively offer screening for AAA in men aged 65 to 75 years who have never smoked rather than routinely screening all men in this group.
- Women aged 65 to 75 years who have ever smoked: the USPSTF concludes that the current evidence is insufficient to assess the balance of benefits and harms of screening for AAA in women aged 65 to 75 years who have ever smoked.
- Women who have never smoked: the USPSTF recommends against routine screening for AAA in women who have never smoked.
- Less than 3.0 cm, no further screening; 3.0 to 3.9 cm, periodic rescreening with abdominal U/S until age 75 and expert opinion.
- 4.0 to 5.4 cm, rescreening with U/S and one expert opinion, at 6 months following first screening; every year until age 75.
- Greater than or equal to 5.5 cm, refer to vascular surgery for AAA repair 2. Grade A periodic surveillance offers comparable mortality benefit to routine elective surgery.

B. Hypertension

1. Definition
- The definition of HTN according to American College of Cardiology/American Heart Association Task Force on Clinical Practice Guidelines is given in Table 18–1.

2. Epidemiology
- About 75 million American adults (29%) have high blood pressure—that's one in every three adults.
- Only about half (54%) of people with high blood pressure have their condition under control.
- High blood pressure costs the nation $46 billion each year. This total includes the cost of health care services, medications to treat high blood pressure, and missed days of work.

TABLE 18–1.	Blood Pressure Levels	
Normal	Systolic: <120 mm Hg	
	Diastolic: <80 mm Hg	
Elevated	Systolic: 120–129 mm Hg	
	Diastolic: <80 mm Hg	
Stage 1 hypertension	Systolic: 130–139 mm Hg	
	Diastolic: 80–89 mm Hg	
Stage 2 hypertension	Systolic: >140 mm Hg	
	Diastolic: >90 mm Hg	

- About one of three U.S. adults—31.3%—has high blood pressure (nearly 68 million), a major risk factor for heart disease, stroke, congestive heart failure, and kidney disease.
- In 2010, high blood pressure will cost the United States $76.6 billion in health care services, medications, and missed days of work.
- About 70% of those with high blood pressure and who took medication had their high blood pressure controlled. The control rate was 46.6% among all hypertensive patients.
- Twenty-five percent of American adults have prehypertension: blood pressure numbers that are higher than normal, but not yet in the high blood pressure range. Prehypertension raises your risk of high blood pressure.
- High blood pressure increases the risk of heart disease and stroke, the first and third leading causes of death.

3. Screening
- The USPSTF recommends screening for high blood pressure in adults aged 18 years and older.

4. Recommendations
- In the general population, pharmacologic treatment should be initiated when blood pressure is 150/90 mm Hg or higher in adults aged 60 years and older, or 140/90 mm Hg or higher in adults younger than 60 years.
- In patients with hypertension and diabetes, pharmacologic treatment should be initiated when blood pressure is 140/90 mm Hg or higher, regardless of age.
- Initial antihypertensive treatment should include a thiazide diuretic, calcium channel blocker, angiotensin-converting enzyme inhibitor, or Angiotensin II Receptor Blocker (ARB) in the general nonblack population or a thiazide diuretic or calcium channel blocker in the general black population.
- If the target blood pressure is not reached within 1 month after initiating therapy, the dosage of the initial medication should be increased or a second medication should be added.
- The National Guideline Clearinghouse and the American Dietetic Association recommend dietary interventions, including dietary approaches to stop hypertension, dietary pattern and weight management, physical activity interventions, behavioral interventions, and pharmacotherapy.

C. Coronary Heart Disease

1. Epidemiology
- Leading cause of death in most Northern European, North American, and other industrialized Caucasian societies.
- Leading cause of death among African Americans, Native Americans, or Alaska Natives, Hispanics, and Whites. One-third of all deaths over age 35 are related to CHD.

- By the age of 60, 1 in 5 men and 1 in 17 women have some form of CHD. One in 15 men and women will eventually have a stroke.
- Every year about 785,000 Americans have a first heart attack. Another 470,000 who have already had one or more heart attack have another attack.
- In 2011, heart disease will cost the United States $444 billion (in health care services, medications, and lost productivity).
- About 610,000 people die of heart disease in the United States every year.
- Heart disease is the leading cause of death for both men and women. More than half of the deaths due to heart disease in 2009 were in men.
- Every year about 735,000 Americans have a heart attack. Of these, 525,000 are a first heart attack and 210,000 happen in people who have already had a heart attack.

2. **Screening and Recommendations**
- The USPSTF found insufficient evidence to recommend for or against routine screening with electrocardiogram (ECG), exercise treadmill, or electron-beam CT (EBCT) scanning for coronary calcium for either the presence of severe coronary artery stenosis or the prediction of CHD events in adults at low or high risk for CHD events.
- Recommendation for use of Aspirin:
  - Adults younger than 50 years: the current evidence is insufficient to assess the balance of benefits and harms of initiating aspirin use for the primary prevention of CVD and CRC in adults younger than 50 years.
  - Adults aged 50 to 59 years with a ≥10% 10-year CVD risk: the USPSTF recommends initiating low-dose aspirin use for the primary prevention of cardiovascular disease (CVD) and CRC in adults aged 50 to 59 years who have a 10% or greater 10-year CVD risk, are not at increased risk for bleeding, have a life expectancy of at least 10 years, and are willing to take low-dose aspirin daily for at least 10 years.
  - Adults aged 60 to 69 years with a ≥10% 10-year CVD risk: the decision to initiate low-dose aspirin use for the primary prevention of CVD and CRC in adults aged 60 to 69 years who have a 10% or greater 10-year CVD risk should be an individual one. Persons who are not at increased risk for bleeding, have a life expectancy of at least 10 years, and are willing to take low-dose aspirin daily for at least 10 years are more likely to benefit. Persons who place a higher value on the potential benefits than the potential harms may choose to initiate low-dose aspirin.
  - Adults aged 70 years or older: the current evidence is insufficient to assess the balance of benefits and harms of initiating aspirin use for the primary prevention of CVD and CRC in adults aged 70 years or older.
- The nontraditional risk factors include in this recommendation are high-sensitivity C-reactive protein, ankle brachial index, leukocyte count, fasting blood glucose level, periodontal disease, carotid intima-media thickness, coronary artery calcification score on EBCT, homocysteine level, and lipoprotein level.
  - Adults at low risk: the USPSTF recommends against screening with resting or exercise electrocardiography (ECG) for the prediction of CHD events in asymptomatic adults at low risk for CHD events.
  - Adults at intermediate or high risk: the USPSTF concludes that the current evidence is insufficient to assess the balance of benefits and harms of screening with resting or exercise ECG for the prediction of CHD events in asymptomatic adults at intermediate or high risk for CHD events.

V. EYE
A. Glaucoma (Also See Chapter 11, Section I. The Globe, F.)
1. Definition
- There are four major types of glaucoma: open-angle (chronic) glaucoma, angle-closure (acute) glaucoma, congenital glaucoma, and secondary glaucoma. In the United States, it is the second most common cause of blindness, and it is a leading cause of blindness worldwide.

2. Epidemiology
- Glaucoma is one of the leading causes of blindness in the United States, affecting an estimated 2.7 million Americans.
- Because of the asymptomatic nature of the disease, only 50% of people with glaucoma even don't know they have the condition.
- Glaucoma disproportionately affects African Americans, at six to eight times more common among African Americans than whites. Additionally, less than 40% of Hispanics with glaucoma are aware of their diagnosis. Moreover, people older than 60 years, people with diabetes, and those with a family history of glaucoma are also at high risk.
- An estimated 2.2 million Americans have glaucoma, and a similar number may have the disease without knowing it. As a result of glaucoma, 120,000 are blind.
- Risk factors include African Americans older than 40 years, everyone older than 60 years, Mexican Americans, and those with a family history of glaucoma.
- Primary open-angle glaucoma is the most common type of glaucoma.

3. **Screening**
   - The USPSTF found insufficient evidence to recommend for or against screening adults for glaucoma.
4. **Recommendation**
   - Complete eye examination before age 40 or sooner if you have the above-mentioned risk factors for glaucoma or other eye problems.
   - Laser eye surgery for high risk of acute glaucoma.

B. **Cataract**
   1. **Definition**
      - Clouding eye lens.
   2. **Epidemiology**
      - An estimated 20.5 million Americans aged 40 or older have cataract in either eye.
      - One of the leading treatable causes of blindness in the world.
      - By age 80, more than half of all people in the United States either have a cataract or have had cataract surgery.
   3. **Screening**
      - Visual acuity, dilated eye examination test, and tonometry.
   4. **Recommendation**
      - Complete eye examination before age 40 or sooner if you have above-mentioned risk factors for cataract or other eye problems.

C. **Age-Related Macular Degeneration**
   1. **Definition**
      - Associated with aging, which gradually destroys sharp, central vision.
   2. **Epidemiology**
      - More than 1.6 million Americans older than 60 years have advanced age-related macular degeneration (AMD).
      - Common among people aged 50 and older.
      - Most common cause of blindness and vision impairment in Americans aged 60 and older.
   3. **Screening and Recommendation**
      - Recommendations for prevention and screening of AMD include the following: do not smoke; prevent overexposure to the sunlight by wearing sunglasses and a hat; eat a variety and nutritious diet that includes leafy green vegetables, fruit, fish, and foods containing vitamins D, E, and C and ω-3 fatty acids; maintain a healthy weight; keep blood pressure at a normal level; follow a regular exercise routine; regularly visit an eye doctor for comprehensive eye examinations; and perform Amsler grid tests at home.

VI. Musculoskeletal Disorders
A. **Osteoporosis (Also See Chapter 9, Section IV.A.)**
   1. **Definition**
      - A condition characterized by decreased bone strength and microarchitectural deterioration of bone tissue that increases bone fragility and risk of fractures.

2. **Epidemiology**
   - In the United States, 8 million women and 2 million men have osteoporosis; it is estimated that 50% of Americans older than 50 years will be at risk of osteoporotic fractures during their lifetime.
   - Percentage of men aged 65 years and over with osteoporosis of the femur neck or lumbar spine: 5.1%.
   - Percentage of women aged 65 years and over with osteoporosis of the femur neck or lumbar spine: 24.5%.
   - Occurs more frequently with increasing age because bone tissue is progressively lost.
   - Prevalence rates are higher in women than in men; rates vary by race, with the highest in whites; and rates for all demographic groups increase with age.
   - In women, the loss of ovarian function (typically at about age 50) precipitates rapid bone loss; occurs in men and women with underlying conditions (see Chapter 9, section IV.A) or major risk factors associated with bone demineralization.
   - Causes approximately 1.5 million fractures annually in the United States, mainly of the spine and hip.
3. **Screening**
   - The dual energy X-ray absorptiometry (DXA) is used to predict fractures, to diagnose osteoporosis, and to select patients for treatment.
   - Recommendation summary. The USPSTF recommends screening for osteoporosis in women aged 65 years and older and in younger women whose fracture risk is equal to or greater than that of a 65-year-old white woman who has no additional risk factors.
   - DXA of the hip is the strongest predictor of hip fracture, and most DXA testing includes measurements of the hip and lumbar spine (central DXA).
   - The most commonly used non-DXA test in the United States is quantitative ultrasound (QUS) of the calcaneus.
   - QUS avoids ionizing radiation and is inexpensive, portable, and feasible for primary care settings.
4. **Recommendation**
   - The USPSTF recommends screening for osteoporosis in women aged 65 years or older and in younger women whose fracture risk is equal to that of a 65-year-old woman who has no additional risk factors.
   - The USPSTF concludes that the current evidence is insufficient to assess the balance of benefits and harms of screening for osteoporosis in men.
   - Osteoporosis screening recommendations of other organizations (Table 18–2).

TABLE 18–2.   Osteoporosis Screening Recommendations of Other Organizations

Organization	Recommendations	
	Women	Men
National Osteoporosis Foundation	BMD testing for all women ≥65 y and postmenopausal women <65 y, based on risk factor profile	BMD testing for all men ≥70 y and men aged 50–69 y, based on risk factor profile
World Health Organization	Indirect evidence supports screening women ≥65 y, but no direct evidence supports widespread screening programs using BMD testing	–
American College of Physicians	–	Clinicians should assess older men for osteoporosis risk factors and use DXA to screen men at increased risk who are candidates for drug therapy for osteoporosis
American Congress of Obstetricians and Gynecologists	BMD testing for all women ≥65 y and postmenopausal women <65 y who have one or more risk factors	–

BMD, bone mineral density; DXA, dual energy X-ray absorptiometry.

VII. Tertiary Prevention and Disease Management

A. Antimicrobial Resistance (Also See Chapter 16, Sections IV and VI)

1. **Definition**
   - According to the World Health Organization, antimicrobial resistance (AMR) is the resistance of a microorganism to an antimicrobial medicine to which it was previously sensitive. AMR is a consequence of the use, particularly the misuse, of antimicrobial medicines and develops when a microorganism mutates or acquires a resistance gene.

2. **Epidemiology**
   - According to the CDC, there are 440,000 new cases of multidrug-resistant tuberculosis emerging annually, resulting in at least 150,000 deaths.
   - A high percentage of hospital-acquired infections are caused by highly resistant bacteria such as methicillin-resistant *Staphylococcus aureus* (MRSA).
   - Each year in the United States, at least 2 million people become infected with bacteria that are resistant to antibiotics, and at least 23,000 people die each year as a direct result of these infections. Many more people die from other conditions that were complicated by an antibiotic-resistant infection.
   - Antibiotic-resistant infections can happen anywhere. Data show that most happen in the general community; however, most deaths related to antibiotic resistance happen in health care settings such as hospitals and nursing homes.

3. **Screening**
   - Health care providers can prevent the spread of antibiotic resistance by prescribing antibiotic therapy when it will most likely be beneficial to the patient, using antibiotics that target likely pathogens and using antibiotics for the appropriate dose and duration.

4. **Recommendations**
   - View the CDC's adult and pediatric academic detail sheets for recommended prescribing guidelines for providers: http://www.cdc.gov/getsmart/campaign-materials/info-sheets/adult-approp-summary.html and http://www.cdc.gov/getsmart/campaign-materials/info-sheets/child-practice-tips.html.
   - Pediatric treatment guidelines for upper respiratory infections: http://www.cdc.gov/getsmart/campaign-materials/pediatric-treatment.html.

REVIEW QUESTIONS

1. Which of the following is the leading cause of unintentional injuries for children aged 0 to 19 years?
   a) Drowning
   b) MVAs
   c) Poisoning
   d) Fall

2. Which race has the highest injury death rate for unintentional household injuries among persons aged 0 to 19 years?
   a) Asian
   b) White
   c) African Americans
   d) American Indians

3. Which of the following is the leading cause of fatal and nonfatal injuries among adults aged ≥65 years?

a) Poisoning
b) Fires
c) Drowning
d) Falls

4. Which of the following is recommended by the USPSTF for older patients to reduce the risk of falling?

a) Vitamin E
b) New rugs
c) Ceiling fans
d) Training to improve balance

5. Which of the following bacteria is the cause of the highest percentage of hospital-acquired infections?

a) MRSA
b) *Escherichia coli*
c) *Klebsiella pneumoniae*
d) *Clostridium difficile*

ANSWERS TO REVIEW QUESTIONS

1. **Answer: B**. Unintentional injuries are the leading cause of morbidity and mortality among children in the United States. Each year, among those 0 to 19 years of age, more than 12,000 people die from unintentional injuries and more than 9.2 million are treated in emergency departments for nonfatal injuries. Injuries caused by transportation were the leading cause of death for children. Combining all unintentional injury deaths among those between 0 and 19 years, motor vehicle traffic-related deaths were the leading cause.

2. **Answer: D**. Risk of injury death varied by race for unintentional household injuries among persons aged 0 to 19 years. An injury death rate was highest for American Indians and Alaska Natives and was lowest for Asian or Pacific Islanders. Overall death rates for Whites and African Americans were approximately the same.

3. **Answer: D**. Each year, one in every three adults aged 65 and older falls, which can lead to moderate to severe injuries, such as hip fractures and head traumas, and can even increase the risk of early death. Falls are the leading cause of fatal and nonfatal injuries among adults aged ≥65 years (older adults). During 2014, approximately 27,000 older adults died because of falls; 2.8 million were treated in emergency departments for fall-related injuries, and approximately 800,000 of these patients were subsequently hospitalized.

4. **Answer: D**. The USPSTF recommends counseling older patients on measures to reduce the risk of falling. These measures include exercise (particularly training to improve balance), safety-related skills and behaviors, environmental hazard reduction, and monitoring and adjusting medications. This recommendation is based on fair evidence that these measures reduce the likelihood of falling. The USPSTF also recommends an intensive individualized home-based multifactorial intervention for high-risk older patients in settings where adequate resources are available to deliver such services.

5. **Answer: A**. Each year in the United States, at least 2 million people become infected with bacteria that are resistant to antibiotics and at least 23,000 people die each year as a direct result of these infections. Many more people die from other conditions that were complicated by an antibiotic-resistant infection. A high percentage of hospital-acquired infections are caused by highly resistant bacteria such as MRSA.

SELECTED REFERENCES

Agency for Healthcare Research and Quality. Clinical guidelines and recommendations. 2012. http://www.ahrq.gov/CLINIC/uspstfix.htm. Last reviewed July 2018.
Agency for Healthcare Research and Quality. Preventive medicine recommendations, screening and counseling by topic. http://epss.ahrq.gov/ePSS/Topics.do?ttid=1.
Agency for Healthcare Research and Quality. Screening for and management of obesity. 2015. https://www.ahrq.gov/professionals/prevention-chronic-care/healthier-pregnancy/preventive/obesity.html. Last reviewed May 2015.
American Academy of Family Physicians. https://www.aafp.org/afp/2008/0415/p1138.html.
Centers for Disease Control and Prevention. CDC A-Z index. http://www.cdc.gov/az/.
Centers for Disease Control and Prevention. CDC childhood injury report. 2008. https://www.cdc.gov/safechild/child_injury_data.html. Updated December 23, 2015.
Centers for Disease Control and Prevention. *CDC Childhood Injury Report: Patterns of Unintentional Injuries among 0–19 Year Olds in the United States, 2000–2006.* Atlanta, GA: Centers for Disease Control and Prevention; 2008. https://www.cdc.gov/safechild/images/CDC-childhoodinjury.pdf.
Centers for Disease Control and Prevention. Fall prevention brochure and literature. https://www.cdc.gov/steadi/pdf/STEADI-PocketGuide-508.pdf.
Centers for Disease Control and Prevention. Fatalities and injuries from falls among older adults—United States, 1993–2003 and 2001–2005. *Morbidity and Mortality Weekly Report.* http://www.cdc.gov/mmwr/preview/mmwrhtml/mm5545a1.htm.
Centers for Disease Control and Prevention. Heart disease facts. https://www.cdc.gov/injury/index.html. Last reviewed November 28, 2017
Centers for Disease Control and Prevention. Injury prevention and control. https://www.cdc.gov/physicalactivity/resources/reports.html.
Centers for Disease Control and Prevention. State indicator report on physical activity, 2010 national action guide. https://www.cdc.gov/injury/researchpriorities/index.html
Centers for Disease Control and Prevention. Three priority areas for prevention. https://www.cdc.gov/mmwr/preview/mmwrhtml/mm6115a5.htm.
Centers for Disease Control and Prevention. Vital signs: unintentional injury deaths among persons aged 0–19 years—United States, 2000–2009. Atlanta, GA: Centers for Disease Control and Prevention; 2012. https://www.cdc.gov/mmwr/preview/mmwrhtml/mm6115a5.htm.
ChooseMyPlate.gov, United States Department of Agriculture. http://www.choosemyplate.gov. Accessed July 2018.
Clinical Preventive Services resources for PA (AAPA). https://cme.aapa.org/prevention.aspx.
The Community Guide. Motor vehicle injury (Multiple interventions in these areas have been recommended). http://www.thecommunityguide.org/mvoi/.

HealthyPeople.gov. Physical activity. 2008. https://www
.healthypeople.gov/2020/topics-objectives/topic/physical-activity.

National Cancer Institute. Colorectal cancer—patient version. http://
www.cancer.gov/cancertopics/types/colon-and-rectal.

National Center for Victim of Crime. https://www.legalmomentum
.org/referral-directory/national-center-victims-crime?gclid=
EAIaIQobChMI-p-_0dyz3wIVyuDICh1L7wdmEAAYASAAEgKu
xvD_BwE.

The National Highway Traffic Safety Administration. http://www
.nhtsa.gov. Accessed July 2018.

National Institute on Aging. https://www.nia.nih.gov/.

Other resources for Preventive Medicine. https://
www.uspreventiveservicestaskforce.org/Page/Name/
task-force-resources.

Recommendations for Adults. http://www
.uspreventiveservicestaskforce.org/adultrec.htm.

U.S. Preventive Services Task Force. Evidence review literature
review for fall prevention. 2012. https://jamanetwork.com/
journals/jama/fullarticle/2678103. Accessed July 2018.

U.S. Preventive Services Task Force. Menopausal hormone therapy:
preventive medication. 2012. https://www.uspreventiveservices
taskforce.org/Page/Document/UpdateSummaryFinal/
menopausal-hormone-therapy-preventive-medication. Accessed
July 2018.

U.S. Preventive Services Task Force. Dental caries in children
from birth through age 5 years screening. 2014. https://www
.uspreventiveservicestaskforce.org/Page/Document/
UpdateSummaryFinal/dental-caries-in-children-from-birth-
through-age-5-years-screening. Accessed July 2018.

U.S. Preventive Services Task Force. Grading for recommendations.
https://www.uspreventiveservicestaskforce.org/Page/Name/grade-
definitions. Accessed July 2018.

U.S. Preventive Services Task Force. Published recommendations
(A-Z topics). http://www.uspreventiveservicestaskforce.org/
uspstopics.htm. Accessed July 2018.

U.S. Preventive Services Task Force. Recommendations for Children. https://www.uspreventiveservicestaskforce.org/BrowseRec/
Index?age=Pediatric,Adolescent. Accessed July 2018.

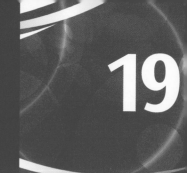

Study and Test-Taking Strategies

19

Rebecca Signore • Lindsay Matias • Valerie Damon-Leduc

How to Study

This chapter details some study and test preparation techniques that can help you plan your study time, retain relevant material, and feel more confident when you take the Physician Assistant National Certification Examination/Physician Assistant Recertification Examination (PANCE/PANRE). Although there is no single "right" way to study, identifying and utilizing the techniques that work for you are critical to your success.

Time Management

No study technique can replace managing your time well. Inevitably, studying will be only one of several competing priorities on your to-do list. It is important to remember that time management includes both creating schedules and prioritizing tasks appropriately. Creating daily, weekly, and monthly schedules, if done systematically, can give you both an immediate- and long-term visual of deadlines and obligations. This information will then allow you to arrange tasks in a way that makes sense for you. When prioritizing, keep in mind that you should consider both the urgency and the importance of a task. Responsibilities for which a deadline is quickly approaching and that have significant consequences should take precedence, followed by anything that might be due soon but has less significance or a later deadline. Create and keep these schedules and to-do lists in the way that feels most comfortable for you—electronically or on paper. There are apps and other software available for phones, tablets, and computers, and a quick internet search will reveal many free templates for a variety of scheduling options.

Although there is no magic equation to identify just how many hours of studying are needed to be successful on the exam, there are general principles of managing study time that you should know. First, studying over a sustained period is ideal, as opposed to cramming. It is best to begin preparing several months in advance rather than several days in advance. Insert study time into your daily and weekly schedule as though it is an appointment that you *must* keep. Second, try shorter but more frequent study sessions. Shorter study sessions (45 minutes to 1 hour) over several weeks allow you (and your brain) time to make connections to different material and practice recalling information. Finally, as the test date gets closer, you can lengthen the sessions, but review more material in shorter "chunks" of time. For example, in a 3-hour study session, you might decide to review six topics for 25 minutes each, allotting 5 minutes between topics for a break. Remember, as the exam nears, you should have prepared a solid foundation of the material in the previous weeks of study, so you can comfortably shift your focus to reviewing. Both preparation and review study sessions should be active because being actively engaged with the material is a fundamental characteristic of the best study techniques.

The Structure of a Study Session

When the time comes to study, it is important to find ways to make your sessions efficient and effective. Most of us have experienced how challenging it can be to reach the end of the time we have set aside, only to realize that we have not accomplished as much as we had expected. This is a common problem, but intentionally structuring your study sessions can maximize efficiency. A good formula for building a study session centers around the questions *when*, *where*, *what*, and *how*. As mentioned earlier, it is important to build study time into your schedule. It is also important to be strategic about *when* and *where* you schedule that time. Have you ever noticed that you tend to be particularly unproductive at certain times (e.g., right after lunch) or that there are times when you feel more motivated (maybe after the gym)? Noticing when you are more productive and studying during those peak times will help you to be more efficient. In the same way that you are programmed to find certain times more productive, you also associate certain locations with productivity. For most people, studying in places they associate with sleep, recreation, or other distractions can be counterproductive. Identify somewhere that you associate with focus and academics that is free from distractions. Libraries, study lounges, coffee shops, and a designated workspace at home are common examples of where many people are conditioned to stay focused.

The *what* of studying are the specific goals you set for your session. The idea of "studying" can be vague, with no clear end or measure unless you make an effort to be intentional. First, break your task into more manageable pieces. For example, when studying for the PANCE/PANRE, organize your study sessions around chapters, sections, or systems of the body to help you stay focused. This process reduces procrastination and makes the workload less intimidating. The process, or *how*, of studying is arguably the most important part of the equation. For many students, the act of studying consists of reading, writing, or memorizing. However, this passive approach to learning is ineffective for long-term retention and comprehension. The most effective techniques involve intentional interaction with the material. This kind of studying applies the principles of critical thinking and encourages you to organize, analyze, categorize, and otherwise manipulate the material. Techniques such as creating charts, tables, concept maps, diagrams, and self-testing are discussed later in the chapter.

In sum, your study sessions should aim to answer the questions *when*, *where*, *what*, and *how* as specifically as possible. For example, *I will go to the library between classes and create a flowchart of the circulatory system over the next hour and then do practice case vignettes on circulatory issues for 30 minutes*. This kind of session mapping sets you up to accomplish as much as possible in the time that you have and reinforces long-term retention.

Resource Utilization

When preparing for an exam, you have access to a wide array of resources—choosing the right ones and using them productively can make your study sessions more impactful and efficient. The materials you received and created while learning (textbooks, class notes, lecture materials, study guides, etc.) are resources that you can use to study, refresh your memory, or test yourself. There is also a wide array of reputable resources available online that can help you learn and recall information. Do not be afraid to think creatively about what study resources are and where you can find them. This text itself is a resource. You can take a complete PANCE/PANRE or a shorter practice exam and use the results to identify some of your strengths and weaknesses. That information can then guide your studying. As you review your answers to practice exams or other questions, think about what you got right and wrong, but also about how confident you were in your answers. If you got an answer right but guessed to do so, you should take some time to review related material so that when you see a similar question in the future, you can answer it confidently.

Class and review materials are not the only tools to which you have access. You should think holistically—consider any health and wellness resources you might need to help you achieve balance as you prepare for the PANCE/PANRE. It is also important to think about people as resources: instructors, people you know who work in the field, and colleagues. In addition to your individual study sessions, you can come together with your peers to form study groups or for informal conversations about material and your approaches to preparing for the exam. Working with others can provide you with new perspective, answers to questions you may have, and opportunities to demonstrate your mastery over material by teaching to others. Your peers are a good resource for accountability. If you are not sure how to study, or are having trouble sticking with a study schedule, seek their help.

Study Techniques

There are a number of study techniques you may find useful (discussed in the subsequent sections). These suggestions

have a dual benefit; you are learning as you create them and as you revisit them throughout your study sessions.

Active Reading and Annotation

Doing well on the PANCE/PANRE is not simply a matter of memorizing information. As with all studying, it is important to be active while reading. One way to encourage active reading is to annotate your text. Annotation helps you reflect and check your comprehension. As you are reading, ask yourself, "Do I *know* this information, or do I just understand it while I'm reading it?" You might create a shorthand system that visually identifies information with which you are struggling (e.g., indicated by a question mark in the margins) and information in which you feel confident (e.g., indicated by an asterisk). You could also signify how well you comprehend the information with different color highlighters (for instance, blue for information you feel good about and yellow for that which you want to review further).

Flashcards

Flashcards, although sometimes time-consuming to create, can be a helpful tool for retention and recall of information. One benefit of flashcards is that they are small and easily transportable. Carry them with you, and review a few when you have short periods of free time. Keep in mind that not all information can or should be placed on a flashcard. Flashcards should have a cue phrase on one side of the card and everything you need to know about that topic on the other side. The cue phrase is a visual indicator, and when you look at the flashcard, you should attempt to recall the information listed on the other side. Although you are not likely to remember every detail on the back of the card, your effort to remember followed by reviewing what is on the back will strengthen your retention.

Diagrams

Diagrams are visual representations that show relationships between information. They are useful when you need to know the parts of a whole and the relationships between them, like an image of the chambers and valves of the heart. You can create a diagram of your own, or take a diagram from a textbook or other source, cover the labels and related information, and relabel it to test your recall.

Tables

Organizing information into tables can help you consolidate important facts and learn the differences between items in an overarching category. For example, you could make a chart that lists different cell types and the relevant features of each cell type.

Flowcharts

Flowcharts highlight a chain of events or processes. You start with the impetus for the process and then draw where it could go from there. You map out each path that the process could take, including forks where it could go in different directions and cycles back to previous steps. You could use this to map processes of the body or even the steps involved in clinical patient care.

Concept Maps

Concept maps help to synthesize large amounts of information and identify relationships between topics. Start by choosing a complex concept or idea—a specific disease or pathology, for example. Then, proceed to branch off related information from that first idea. In the case of a disease, you may create a branch for populations, treatment options, symptoms, or diagnosis tools. Next, draw any connections between your branches. For example, if certain treatment methods are best for certain age groups, you may make a connection showing that. Continue creating branches until you have mapped out all of the connections.

Study Guides

Study guides distill information into an organized, cohesive whole. They allow you to learn and practice by putting material in your own words and in a format that works for you. Study guides are most helpful when you have many resources and want to bring together information from all of them (i.e., a textbook, lecture notes, handouts, etc.). It is important to make your own study guide, rather than using one created by a peer or one that is commercially available. Deciding what to include and what to leave out helps you think critically about the material, and putting things into your own words is a way to double-check your understanding of concepts.

Self-testing

One way to ensure that you are ready to put the information you are studying into practice is to imagine you are treating a real patient and ask yourself, "What would I see?" and "What would I do?" Asking yourself these two questions can help make the information you are studying more real. Some people like to visualize situations. Others prefer to verbalize them. Choose a method that works for you, and it will be easier to remember and apply the information later. The act of self-testing can be done either alone or with a partner. It is also beneficial to set aside time to take practice exams. Simulating the act of taking the test has multiple benefits, including checking for comprehension, identifying topics that you need to study further, and lessening test anxiety.

The Day of the Test

Just like there are best practices to preparing for an exam, there are tips to help you succeed while taking one. For each block of the exam, you should preview the list of questions and identify the ones in which you feel most confident.

Answer those questions first to ensure that you earn those points and then go back and answer the questions that are more challenging. If you run out of time for any reason, this method maximizes your points earned in that section. When you read each individual question, it is important to understand what it is asking. Identify keywords, irrelevant data, and directives (like "all," "none," or "except"), or put the question into your own words. Then try to answer the question *before* looking at the answer options. When you are unsure of an answer, use process of elimination to reduce your options. You can also use context clues. For example, the grammar or construction of the question may tell you that the answer needs to be plural. If you still cannot figure out an answer, skip it and focus on the other questions. If you have time when you finish with the block, go back and check your answers. You should only change an answer, however, if you have a valid reason. Your first instinct is more likely to be right than if you doubt yourself and change answers on a whim.

When taking your exam, it is completely normal to feel a certain amount of anxiety or stress. In fact, as long as this feeling does not overwhelm you, the adrenaline that it summons can actually help your performance, keeping you alert and focused. If anxiety around tests is something that inhibits your performance, however, keep the following in mind. First, good preparation is the best way to limit stress, so all of the hard work you do in the weeks leading up is essential. Additionally, deep breathing and positive self-talk are good techniques to help manage stress. In many cases, anxiety comes from unrealistic expectations about how you or others are doing. Minimizing these thoughts by having a positive mantra and then refocusing on the exam will help you stay calm. If you feel that your anxiety reaches a level that is unmanageable, seek out resources that offer assistance.

If you start with a well-thought-out schedule for your overall test preparation and for each individual study session, you will be on the path to success. Remember to use your resources and to study actively, incorporating some of the strategies and tools outlined in this chapter. It is important that you think beyond studying, however. Keeping a regular sleep schedule, eating healthy meals, and allowing yourself time for exercise, socialization, and relaxation in the time before the exam will help you maintain a healthy work–life balance and reduce your stress levels. All of this will lay the groundwork for good preparation leading up to the PANCE/PANRE.

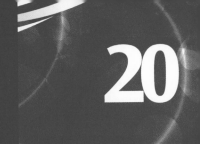

Pharmacology

20

Lawrence P. Carey • Michael C. Barros • Michael A. Mancano • Jacqueline A. Theodorou

I. Pharmacokinetics

A. Absorption

1. **Definition**
   - Ability of a drug to cross biologic membranes and enter blood.

2. **Mechanisms**
   - Passive diffusion (requires no energy): primary method for most drugs.
   - Active transport (requires energy): carrier-mediated, energy-dependent; competition is possible.
   - Facilitated diffusion: carrier-mediated, but does not require energy.

3. **Factors Affecting Absorption**
   - Route of administration (oral, intramuscular, rectal, inhalation, topical, etc.).
   - Concentration of drug.
   - Chemical properties of the agent (e.g., pKa and lipophilicity).
   - Physiologic factors (e.g., blood flow and surface area of the site of administration).
   - Metabolism before reaching the systemic circulation; oral administration occurs in intestines and liver (first-pass effect)—examples of agents with high first-pass metabolism: verapamil, morphine, propranolol, and nitroglycerin.

4. **Quantification**
   - Bioavailability (F): quantifies the amount of administered drug reaching the circulation.
   - Bioequivalence.

B. Distribution

1. **Definition**
   - Estimation of the extent of spread of total drugs throughout the body.

2. **Factors**
   - Physiologic (e.g., blood flow to organs and disease states).
   - Protein binding: movement in plasma (free drug) and binding to proteins (e.g., albumin).
   - Tissue binding: drugs can be sequestered in tissues (e.g., lipid-soluble drugs in adipose tissue).

3. **Quantification**
   - Volume of distribution (Vd): relates the amount (ratio) of drug in the body to plasma concentration; large Vd drug is widely distributed into tissue and small Vd drug is primarily in plasma.
   - Examples of agents with high Vd: meperidine, morphine, verapamil, propranolol, and quinidine.
   - Examples of agents with low Vd: nifedipine, sulfamethoxazole, theophylline, tobramycin, and warfarin.

C. Metabolism (Biotransformation)

1. **Definition**
   - Process of chemical alteration of drug molecules; primary purpose is to inactivate drugs and increase water solubility to enhance renal elimination.

2. **Major Sites**
   - Liver: primarily by way of cytochrome P450 system.
   - Lungs.
   - Gastrointestinal (GI) tract.

3. **Types**
   - Phase I: primarily cytochrome P450 system–mediated reactions such as oxidation, reduction, and hydrolysis; products are more polar.
   - Phase II: conjugation with endogenous substances such as glucuronide; products are highly polar and totally inactivate drug.

D. Excretion

1. **Definition**
   - Removal of a drug and its metabolites from the body.

2. **Sites**
   - Kidney: primary site.
   - Lungs.
   - Sweat, breast milk.

3. **Mechanism (Kidney)**
   - Glomerular filtration: drugs moved from blood to tubular fluid.
   - Tubular reabsorption: lipid-soluble drugs reabsorbed from tubular fluid into the blood vessels supplying the nephrons.
   - Tubular secretion: pumps in the tubules actively pump drugs from blood into the tubules.

4. **Factors**
   - Chemical properties: pKa, polarity.
   - Physiologic factors: renal blood flow, glomerular filtration rate (GFR), plasma protein binding.
   - Drug interactions: active transport process at tubules can be subject to competition with other drugs (e.g., probenecid).

5. **Quantification**
   - Clearance: measures rate of elimination of a drug from the body as it relates to drug concentration, including all sites of elimination.
   - Half-life ($t_{1/2}$): time required to decrease the amount of drug in the body by 50%; useful in determining dosage regimens.
   - Example $t_{1/2}$ values: morphine = 1.9 hours, warfarin = 37 hours.

II. Pharmacodynamics "What the Drug Does to the Body?"

A. Dose–Response Relationships
1. **Definition**
   - Relationship between administered dose of a drug and the resultant effect, generally expressed as a log-dose response that results in an S-shaped curve. Drug responses are graded, quantal, and time action.
2. **Features**
   - Maximum response (E_{max}): maximum possible response.
   - Effective concentration 50 (EF_{50}): concentration of the drug producing 50% of maximal response.

B. Targets of Drug Action
1. **Receptors**
   - Agonists: drugs that bind to a receptor and mimic the effect of the endogenous neurotransmitter (e.g., opioids).
   - Antagonists: drugs that block receptors and prevent binding of endogenous neurotransmitter (e.g., β-blockers).
2. **Enzymes**
   - Inhibitors: drugs that inhibit the activity of enzymes (e.g., angiotensin-converting enzyme inhibitors [ACEIs]—inhibit angiotensin-converting enzyme).
   - Activators: drugs that enhance the activity of enzymes (e.g., tissue plasminogen activator activates the enzyme plasminogen in the presence of fibrin).
3. **Channels**
   - Blockers: drugs can prevent channels from opening (e.g., calcium channel blockers).

III. Principles of Drug–Drug Interactions

A. Pharmacodynamics
1. **Physiologic: Two Drugs Taken Simultaneously That Have Effects on the Same Organ System**
   - Antagonism: agents with opposite effects (e.g., central nervous system [CNS] stimulation of pseudoephedrine and CNS depression of diphenhydramine—used to offset the adverse effects).
   - Synergism: agents with similar effects (e.g., CNS depression caused by benzodiazepines and alcohol can be fatal).

2. **Pharmacologic: Two Drugs Taken Simultaneously That Have Opposing Effects on a Receptor**
   - Receptor agonist and antagonist administered together will antagonize each other (e.g., nonselective β-receptor antagonist and a β_2-receptor agonist).

B. Pharmacokinetics
1. **Altered Absorption**
   - Changes in GI pH, motility, or blood flow to the site of administration can affect absorption.
2. **Altered Distribution**
   - Main mechanism is by way of competition for plasma protein-binding sites (primarily albumin).
3. **Altered Metabolism: Cytochrome P450 Isozymes (e.g., CYP1A2, CYP2C9, CYP2C19, CYP2D6, and CYP3A4)**
   - Inducers: promote the synthesis of P450 enzymes and thereby increase the metabolism of many drugs; may result in a lack of therapeutic effect (e.g., phenobarbital, phenytoin, and rifampin).
   - Inhibitors: prevent the metabolism of other agents; can lead to toxicity (e.g., ketoconazole, cimetidine, erythromycin, and grapefruit juice).
4. **Altered Renal Excretion**
   - Alteration in renal blood flow can affect GFR, that is, agents that decrease the renal blood flow such as vasodilators.
   - Alteration in urinary pH can affect ionization and the degree of reabsorption.
   - Drugs can compete for the tubular active transporters.

IV. Autonomic Agents

A. Muscarinic Agents
1. **Direct Agonists**
   - Work directly on muscarinic receptors sites:
     - Mechanism of action: mimic the effects of the parasympathetic nervous system (PNS) by way of direct stimulation of muscarinic receptors in autonomic nervous system (ANS) innervated by PNS.
     - Effects: eye—decrease intraocular pressure by way of enhanced outflow, pupil constriction; CVS—decrease heart rate, pulmonary, and bronchoconstriction; smooth muscle—enhance tone of GI causing increased bowel movements and urinary smooth muscle causing increased urination and stimulation of salivary secretions.
     - Therapeutic uses: wide-angle glaucoma (pilocarpine), postoperative ileus (bethanechol), postoperative or postpartum urinary retention (bethanechol), dry mouth (cevimeline, pilocarpine, echothiophate).
     - Common adverse effects: bradycardia, diarrhea, nausea and vomiting (N/V), incontinence, blurred vision.

- Contraindications/cautions: patients with asthma and cardiovascular diseases.
- Example agents: bethanechol (Urecholine), pilocarpine (Isopto Carpine), cevimeline (Evoxac), echothiophate (Phospholine Iodide).

2. **Indirect Agonists**
- Mechanism of action: mimic the effects of acetylcholine (ACH) by way of inhibition of plasma acetylcholinesterase (ACHE); increasing ACH at effector organs and effects occur at both nicotinic and muscarinic receptors.
- Primary effects are stimulation of skeletal muscle; CNS, especially learning and memory; effects similar to muscarinic agonists also occur.
- Therapeutic uses: myasthenia gravis (pyridostigmine), Alzheimer disease (donepezil, rivastigmine, galantamine), glaucoma (echothiophate), reverse effects of neuromuscular blocking agents (edrophonium, neostigmine), antidote atropine poisoning (physostigmine).
- Common adverse effects: shortness of breath, muscle fasciculations, bradycardia, and delirium.
- Contraindications/cautions: sarin is an ACHE inhibitor that is a nerve gas; many insecticides are ACHE inhibitors; poisoning is common.
- Example agents: pyridostigmine (Mestinon), edrophonium (Tensilon), donepezil (Aricept), rivastigmine (Exelon), galantamine (Reminyl), echothiophate (Phospholine), neostigmine (Prostigmin).

3. **Muscarinic Antagonists (Blockers)**
- Mechanism of action: inhibit muscarinic receptors of PNS.
- Effects: bronchodilation, relief of atrioventricular (AV) block or vagus-induced bradycardia, antitremor effects, vestibular effects, mydriasis (dilated pupil), decreased contraction (constipation) of GI and genitourinary smooth muscle (anuresis).
- Therapeutic uses: chronic obstructive pulmonary disease (COPD; ipratropium), bradycardia (atropine), motion sickness (scopolamine), Parkinson disease (benztropine, trihexyphenidyl), incontinence (tolterodine, oxybutynin).
- Common adverse effects: dry mouth, dilated pupils, blurred vision, dry skin, flushing, tachycardia, urinary retention, constipation, fever, delirium, hallucinations (overdose).
- Contraindications/cautions: glaucoma (especially narrow angle), geriatric patients (especially elderly male, risk of urinary retention).
- Example agents: ipratropium (Atrovent), atropine, scopolamine, benztropine (Cogentin), trihexyphenidyl (Artane), tolterodine (Detrol), oxybutynin (Ditropan).

B. **Adrenergic Agents**
1. **Catecholamines**
- Norepinephrine (Levophed): effects mediated primarily through activation of α-receptors; can be used mainly to elevate blood pressure.
- Epinephrine (Adrenalin): activates α_1-, α_2-, β_1-, and β_2-receptors.
- Dopamine (Intropin): low dose produces renal vasodilation by way of stimulation of D1 receptors and high dose produces cardiac stimulation by way of β_1-receptor stimulation and α_1 vasoconstriction; used in emergency management of shock and heart failure.

2. **α_1-Receptor Agonists**
- Mechanism of action: stimulate α-receptors blood vessels, cause vasoconstriction that results in increased blood pressure, decreased bleeding, relief of nasal congestion, and mydriasis.
- Therapeutic uses: emergency treatment of hypotension to preserve cerebral and coronary blood flow, decongestants, and production of mydriasis during eye examinations; midodrine is used to treat chronic orthostatic hypotension.
- Common adverse effects: hypertension leading to vascular accident (e.g., stroke), reflex bradycardia, syncope, and stress reactions.
- Contraindications/cautions: if extravasation occurs, local tissue damage is possible; overuse as a topical nasal decongestant leads to rebound hyperemia (inverse quantity of blood flow).
- Example agents: phenylephrine, midodrine (Amatine), epinephrine.

3. **α_2-Receptor Agonists**
- Mechanism of action: stimulate central α_2-receptors that cause a decrease of adrenergic activity in the CNS and result in a decrease in blood pressure and heart rate.
- Therapeutic use: hypertension.
- Common adverse effects: dry mouth, sedation, postural hypotension, inhibition of sexual function, autoimmune hemolytic anemia (methyldopa only).
- Contraindications/cautions: do not discontinue rapidly, rebound hypertension can occur.
- Example agents: clonidine (Catapres), methyldopa (Aldomet).

4. **Miscellaneous α-Agonists**
- Oxymetazoline (Afrin) and xylometazoline (Neo-Synephrine): used topically (nasally) for decongestant effect, activate α_1- and α_2-receptors.
- Pseudoephedrine (Sudafed): used as decongestant in over-the-counter (OTC) cold preparations, CNS effects may produce anorexia, used in OTC weight-loss products, activates α_1- and α_2-receptors.

- Methylphenidate (Ritalin): similar to amphetamine, promotes release and stimulation of α-receptors of norepinephrine and epinephrine used for attention-deficit/hyperactivity disorder (ADHD).
- Amphetamine and derivatives: used as an antiobesity drug and for narcolepsy.

5. **α_1-Receptor Antagonists**
- Mechanism of action: block α_1-receptors, effects are primarily on blood vasodilation, also relax the prostate and bladder neck.
- Therapeutic uses: hypertension, benign prostatic hyperplasia (BPH).
- Common adverse effects: postural hypotension resulting in syncope, dizziness, and possibly fainting, reflex tachycardia, nasal congestion, inhibition of sexual function.
- Contraindications/cautions: hypotensive effects are more prominent with the first dose; patients should be warned to rise slowly.
- Example agents: prazosin (Minipress), terazosin (Hytrin), doxazosin (Cardura), tamsulosin (Flomax).

6. **β_1-Receptor Agonists**
- Mechanism of action: stimulate β_1-receptors in the heart and kidney, resulting in positive inotropic effect and release of renin.
- Therapeutic use: emergency management of heart failure.
- Common adverse effect: tachycardia.
- Contraindications/cautions: α-receptors stimulated at a high dose, increase blood pressure.
- Example agent: dopamine, dobutamine.

7. **β_2-Receptor Agonists**
- Mechanism of action: stimulate β_2-receptors; main effects are bronchodilation and relaxation of the uterus.
- Therapeutic uses: asthma, COPD, delay premature labor (terbutaline).
- Common adverse effects: muscle tremor, heart palpitations, nervousness.
- Contraindications/cautions: blood glucose levels can rise in diabetic patients; for acute treatment of asthma, sustained release agents should not be used (e.g., salmeterol).
- Example agents: albuterol (Proventil), terbutaline, salmeterol xinafoate (Serevent), metaproterenol (Alupent).

8. **Miscellaneous β-Agonists**
- Isoproterenol (Isuprel): stimulates β_1- and β_2-receptors, used in the emergency treatment of bradyarrhythmias and cardiac shock.

9. **β-Receptor Antagonists: Selective β_1; Nonselective β_1- and β_2-Blockers**
- Mechanism of action: block β-receptors, resulting in cardiovascular effects including decreased cardiac output, decreased heart rate, decreased contractility, decreased renin secretion, reflex vasoconstriction, increased sodium and water retention, and decreased postmyocardial infarction (MI) cardiac remodeling.
- Therapeutic uses: hypertension, tachyarrhythmias, heart failure, angina, acute MI, migraine prophylaxis, essential tremor, performance anxiety, thyrotoxicosis, wide-angle glaucoma.
- Common adverse effects: bradycardia, heart block, bronchoconstriction, depression, hypotension, insomnia.
- Contraindications/cautions: can mask signs of hypoglycemia in diabetics, should not be stopped abruptly; use with caution in patients with asthma/COPD, heart block.
- Example agents: *nonselective* (block β_1 and β_2): propranolol (Inderal), timolol (Timoptic); *selective* (block β_1): metoprolol (Lopressor), atenolol (Tenormin), esmolol (Brevibloc—IV only for arrhythmias); *nonselective β-blocker and α-blocker*: labetalol (Normodyne), carvedilol (Coreg).

C. **Neuromuscular Blocking Agents (Depolarizing)**
- Mechanism of action: block nicotinic receptors in skeletal muscle and produce paralysis by producing persistent depolarization.
- Therapeutic uses: produce muscle relaxation during surgery, intubation, or other procedures.
- Common adverse effects: hypotension, respiratory arrest.
- Contraindications/cautions: drug interaction occurs with general anesthetics, resulting in enhanced effects.
- Example agents: pancuronium (Pavulon), vecuronium (Norcuron), atracurium (Tracrium), succinylcholine (Anectine).
- **NOTE:** Succinylcholine is a depolarizing neuromuscular blocking agent used as a paralytic. It produces stimulation of nicotinic receptors leading to depolarization and paralysis. Short acting, associated with risk of malignant hyperthermia.

V. Cardiovascular Agents and Antihypertensive Agents

A. **Antihypertensive Agents**
1. **Diuretics**
   a. **Thiazide Diuretics**
   - Mechanism of action: increase the urinary excretion of sodium and chloride in approximately equivalent amounts at distal renal tubule.
   - Therapeutic uses: hypertension (preferred diuretic class), edema.

- Monitor: weight, blood pressure, serum electrolytes, blood urea nitrogen (BUN), creatinine.
- Common adverse effects: hypokalemia, hyponatremia, hypomagnesemia, hypercalcemia, hyperuricemia, muscle cramps, glucose intolerance, dyslipidemia (usually transient and at high doses).
- Contraindications/cautions: anuria, lupus erythematosus, hypersensitivity to sulfonamides, photosensitivity; use with caution in patients with impaired renal function (increased risk of toxicity or azotemia, decreased diuretic effectiveness).
- Example agents: hydrochlorothiazide (Microzide), metolazone (Zaroxolyn), chlorthalidone (Hygroton).

b. **Loop Diuretics**
- Mechanism of action: primarily inhibit absorption of sodium and chloride in the renal tubules (ascending loop of Henle, proximal and distal).
- Therapeutic uses: hypertension (preferred in patients with chronic kidney disease), edema.
- Monitor: weight, blood pressure, serum electrolytes, BUN, creatinine.
- Common adverse effects: hyperuricemia, hypokalemia, hyponatremia, hypomagnesemia, hypocalcemia, muscle cramps, bladder spasm, loss of appetite.
- Contraindications/cautions: anuria, liver disease, photosensitivity, ototoxicity (usually with rapid IV administration and high doses).
- Example agents: furosemide (Lasix), bumetanide (Bumex), torsemide (Demadex).

c. **Potassium-Sparing Diuretics**
- Some potassium-sparing diuretics (i.e., triamterene) inhibit reabsorption of sodium in exchange for potassium and hydrogen ions through direct effects on the distal tubule. Others (i.e., spironolactone and eplerenone) are renal competitive aldosterone antagonists, inhibiting the effect of aldosterone by competing for the aldosterone-dependent sodium–potassium exchange site in the distal tubule cells. Result is increased secretion of water and sodium, whereas decreasing potassium excretion.
- Therapeutic uses: edema, ascites, heart failure, primary aldosteronism, hypertension.
- Monitor: weight, blood pressure, potassium, BUN, creatinine, gynecomastia (spironolactone).
- Common adverse effects: hyperkalemia, GI upset, gynecomastia (spironolactone).
- Contraindications/cautions: creatinine >2.5 mg per dL (men) or >2 mg per dL (women) and/or potassium >5 mEq per L

(heart failure), patients currently receiving potassium supplementation; avoid large quantities of potassium-rich food.
- Example agents: spironolactone (Aldactone), eplerenone (Inspra), triamterene (Dyrenium), amiloride (Midamor).

2. **β-Adrenergic Blocking Agents**
- Mechanism of action: inhibit interaction of epinephrine, norepinephrine, and sympathomimetic drugs with β-adrenergic receptor sites.
- Therapeutic uses: hypertension (not recommended first line unless there is a compelling indication), angina pectoris, cardiac arrhythmias, MI, heart failure syndrome, pheochromocytoma, migraine, and essential tremor.
- Monitor: blood pressure, heart rate, dizziness, worsening heart failure symptoms.
- Common adverse effects: bradycardia, fatigue, dizziness, dyspnea, sexual dysfunction, worsening heart failure symptoms.
- Contraindications/cautions: sinus bradycardia, second- or third-degree heart block, decompensated cardiac failure, cardiogenic shock; use with caution in diabetes (may mask symptoms of hypoglycemia), airway disease. Do not discontinue medication abruptly.
- Example agents: atenolol (Tenormin), bisoprolol (Zebeta), metoprolol (Lopressor, Toprol XL), nebivolol (Bystolic), nadolol (Corgard), and propranolol (Inderal, Inderal LA).

3. **Calcium-Channel Blocking Agents**
a. **Dihydropyridine Calcium Antagonists**
- Mechanism of action: selectively block the movement of extracellular calcium ions into cardiac muscle and vascular smooth muscle; lowers blood pressure by reducing peripheral vascular resistance by a direct action on vascular smooth muscle.
- Therapeutic uses: angina pectoris, hypertension (preferred over nondihydropyridines), Raynaud phenomenon.
- Monitor: blood pressure, peripheral edema.
- Common adverse effects: headache, peripheral edema, dizziness, flushing, weakness.
- Contraindications/cautions: hepatic dysfunction, hypotension.
- Example agents: amlodipine (Norvasc), felodipine (Plendil), isradipine (Dynacirc), nifedipine (Adalat CC, Procardia XL).

b. **Nondihydropyridine Calcium Antagonists**
- Mechanism of action: exert inotropic and chronotropic effects on the heart.
- Therapeutic uses: hypertension, angina pectoris, atrial fibrillation/flutter, paroxysmal supraventricular tachycardia (PSVT).
- Monitor: blood pressure, heart rate.

- Common adverse effects: GI upset, dizziness, headache, bradycardia, constipation (verapamil).
- Contraindications/cautions: sick sinus syndrome or second- or third-degree AV block except with a functioning pacemaker, hypotension 90 mm Hg systolic, acute MI and pulmonary congestion documented by X-ray on admission, heart failure with reduced ejection fraction (HFrEF), and renal/hepatic dysfunction.
- Example agents: diltiazem (Cardizem), verapamil (Calan SR).

4. **Renin Angiotensin-Aldosterone System Antagonists**
   a. **Angiotensin-Converting Enzyme Inhibitors**
      - Mechanism of action: prevent the conversion of angiotensin I to angiotensin II, a vasoconstrictor agent which decreases vasopressor activity and aldosterone secretion.
      - Therapeutic uses: hypertension, heart failure, MI, kidney disease.
      - Monitor: blood pressure, cough, angioedema, potassium, BUN, creatinine.
      - Common adverse effects: asthenia, cough, dizziness, hyperkalemia; other serious but less common side effects include angioedema, neutropenia, and acute renal failure.
      - Contraindications/cautions: renal artery stenosis, history of angioedema, volume- and/or salt-depletion states; teratogenic.
      - Example agents: captopril (Capoten), benazepril (Lotensin), enalapril (Vasotec), fosinopril (Monopril), ramipril (Altace), lisinopril (Prinivil).
   b. **Angiotensin II Receptor Antagonists**
      - Mechanism of action: selectively block the binding of angiotensin II to the angiotensin II type 1 receptor (AT1) receptors in tissues such as vascular smooth muscle and the adrenal gland.
      - Therapeutic uses: hypertension, heart failure, kidney disease.
      - Monitor: blood pressure, angioedema, potassium, BUN, creatinine.
      - Common adverse effects: headache, dizziness, somnolence, hyperkalemia; serious but less common side effect is acute renal failure and angioedema.
      - Contraindications/cautions: history of angioedema, renal failure; teratogenic.
      - Example agents: valsartan (Diovan), candesartan (Atacand), irbesartan (Avapro), losartan (Cozaar).
   c. **Direct Renin Inhibitors**
      - Mechanism of action: directly inhibit renin, which decreases plasma renin activity (PRA)

and inhibits the conversion of angiotensinogen to angiotensin I.
      - Therapeutic use: hypertension.
      - Monitor: blood pressure, potassium, BUN, creatinine, angioedema (rare).
      - Common adverse effects: dizziness, headache, diarrhea; less common but serious effects include hyperkalemia and angioedema.
      - Contraindications/cautions: concomitant use with an ACEI in patients with diabetes, severe renal impairment, history of angioedema, volume- or salt-depletion states; teratogenic.

5. **α_1-Adrenergic Blockers**
   - Mechanism of action: selectively block α_1-adrenergic receptors and decrease total peripheral resistance and venous return; α_1-blockers produce antihypertensive effects secondary to selective postsynaptic α_1-adrenoceptor blockade. Also inhibit postsynaptic α_1-receptors in prostatic stromal and bladder neck tissues. Reduce the sympathetic tone–induced urethral stricture causing BPH symptoms.
   - Therapeutic uses: hypertension, BPH.
   - Monitor: blood pressure, orthostasis, urinary symptoms.
   - Common adverse effects: hypotension, dizziness, somnolence, headache.
   - Contraindications/cautions: "first-dose" hypotension, priapism.
   - Example agents: prazosin (Minipress), terazosin (Hytrin), doxazosin (Cardura); limited for use with BPH tamsulosin (Flomax) and alfuzosin (Flomax).

6. **α-/β-Adrenergic Blocking Agents**
   - Mechanism of action: selective, competitive postsynaptic α_1-adrenergic blocking and nonselective, competitive β-adrenergic blocking activity.
   - Therapeutic uses: hypertension (not recommended first line unless there is a compelling indication), heart failure.
   - Monitor: blood pressure, heart rate, worsening heart failure.
   - Common adverse effects: hypotension, dizziness, fatigue.
   - Contraindications/cautions: bronchial asthma, decompensated cardiac failure, second- or third-degree heart block, severe bradycardia, cardiogenic shock, abrupt withdrawal, hepatic dysfunction.
   - Example agents: labetalol (Normodyne), carvedilol (Coreg).

7. **Vasodilators**
   - Mechanism of action: direct relaxation of vascular smooth muscle.
   - Therapeutic uses: hypertension, heart failure (hydralazine in combination with isosorbide dinitrate [DN]).
   - Monitor: blood pressure, heart rate, lupus-like syndrome (hydralazine), fluid status, renal function.

- Common adverse effects: blood dyscrasias, rash, palpitations, tachycardia, peripheral neuritis, fluid and electrolyte imbalance, pericardial effusion (minoxidil), hypertrichosis (minoxidil).
- Contraindications/cautions: coronary artery disease (CAD), mitral valvular rheumatic heart disease, pheochromocytoma (minoxidil); use with caution in patients with renal dysfunction and tartrazine sensitivity.
- Example agents: hydralazine (Apresoline), minoxidil (Loniten).

8. **Centrally Acting Neuronal Adrenergic Blockers**
   a. **Clonidine (Catapres), Guanfacine (Tenex)**
      - Mechanism of action: central α_2-adrenergic stimulant that inhibits cardiac workload and vasoconstriction.
      - Therapeutic uses: hypertension, ADHD.
      - Monitor: blood pressure, heart rate, mental status.
      - Common adverse effects: dry mouth, sedation, fatigue.
      - Contraindications/cautions: rebound hypertension—do not discontinue therapy abruptly and do not recommend in patients with compliance issues, ophthalmologic effects.
   b. **Methyldopa (Aldomet)**
      - Mechanism of action: lowers arterial pressure by the stimulation of central inhibitory α_2-adrenergic receptors, false neurotransmission, and/or reduction of PRA.
      - Therapeutic uses: hypertension, hypertensive crises.
      - Monitor: blood pressure, complete blood count (CBC), liver enzymes, Coombs test.
      - Common adverse effects: positive Coombs test/hemolytic anemia, edema, weight gain, bradycardia, hepatic dysfunction, hematologic disorders, sedation, urine discoloration, sulfite sensitivity.
      - Contraindications/cautions: active hepatic disease, coadministration with monoamine oxidase inhibitors (MAOIs).

B. **Heart Failure Syndrome Agents**
   1. **Cardiac Glycosides**
      - Mechanism of action: slow AV conduction, increased contraction.
      - Therapeutic uses: heart failure syndrome, atrial fibrillation.
      - Monitor: heart rate, electrocardiogram (ECG), electrolytes, renal function, digoxin levels.
      - Common adverse effects: nausea, diarrhea, visual disturbances (digoxin toxicity), arrhythmias.
      - Contraindications/cautions: sinus node disease, AV block, renal impairment, elderly, electrolyte abnormalities (hypokalemia, hypercalcemia, hypomagnesemia).
      - Example agent: digoxin (Lanoxin).

2. ACEIs/Angiotensin II Receptor Antagonists (See Antihypertensive Agents)
3. β-Adrenergic Blocking Agents (See Antihypertensive Agents)
4. Diuretics/Aldosterone Antagonists (See Antihypertensive Agents)
5. Vasodilator/Nitrate (See Antihypertensive Agents and Antianginal Agents)
6. **Diuretics**
   a. **Thiazide Diuretics**
      - Mechanism of action: increase the urinary excretion of sodium and chloride in approximately equivalent amounts at distal renal tubule.
      - Therapeutic uses: hypertension, edema.
      - Common adverse effects: hypokalemia, hyponatremia, hypomagnesemia, hypercalcemia, hyperuricemia, muscle cramps, glucose intolerance, dyslipidemia (usually transient and at high doses).
      - Contraindications/cautions: anuria, lupus erythematosus, hypersensitivity to sulfonamides, photosensitivity; use with caution in patients with impaired renal function (increased risk of toxicity or azotemia and decreased diuretic effectiveness).
      - Example agents: hydrochlorothiazide (Esidrix), metolazone (Zaroxolyn), chlorthalidone (Hygroton).
   b. **Loop Diuretics**
      - Mechanism of action: primarily inhibit absorption of sodium and chloride in the renal tubules (ascending loop of Henle, proximal, and distal).
      - Therapeutic uses: hypertension, edema.
      - Common adverse effects: hyperuricemia, hypokalemia, hyponatremia, hypomagnesemia, hypocalcemia, muscle cramps, bladder spasm, loss of appetite.
      - Contraindications/cautions: anuria, liver disease, photosensitivity, ototoxicity.
      - Example agents: furosemide (Lasix), bumetanide (Bumex), torsemide (Demadex).
   c. **Potassium-Sparing Diuretics**
      - Some potassium-sparing diuretics (i.e., triamterene) inhibit reabsorption of sodium in exchange for potassium and hydrogen ions through direct effects on the distal tubule. Others (i.e., spironolactone and eplerenone) are renal competitive aldosterone antagonists inhibiting the effect of aldosterone by competing for the aldosterone-dependent sodium–potassium exchange site in the distal tubule cells. Result is increased secretion of water and sodium, whereas decreasing potassium excretion.

- Therapeutic uses: edema, ascites, heart failure syndrome, primary aldosteronism, hypertension.
- Common adverse effects: hyperkalemia, GI upset, gynecomastia (spironolactone).
- Contraindications/cautions: serum potassium >5.5 mEq per L, patients currently receiving potassium supplementation; avoid large quantities of potassium-rich food.
- Example agents: spironolactone (Aldactone), triamterene (Dyrenium), eplerenone (Inspra).

7. Calcium-Channel Blocking Agents (See Antihypertensive Agents)

C. Antianginal Agents

1. Nitrates
- Mechanism of action: relaxation of vascular smooth muscle through dose-dependent dilation of both arterial and venous beds.
- Therapeutic uses: acute angina, angina prophylaxis.
- Monitor: blood pressure, heart rate, relief of chest pain.
- Contraindications/cautions: severe anemia, closed-angle glaucoma, postural hypotension, early MI, head trauma, or cerebral hemorrhage; tolerance develops to use.
- Common adverse effects: dizziness, headache, hypotension, bradycardia or tachycardia, contact dermatitis (transdermal), burning or tingling sensation of oral cavity (sublingual).
- Example agents: isosorbide mononitrate (Imdur); isosorbide dinitrate (Isordil); nitroglycerin, sublingual (Nitrostat); nitroglycerin, transdermal (Nitro-Dur); nitroglycerin, ointment (Nitro-Bid); nitroglycerin, sublingual spray (NitroMist); nitroglycerin for intravenous injection.

2. β-Blocking Agents (See Antihypertensive Agents)

D. Calcium Channel Agents (See Antihypertensive Agents)

1. Aspirin
- Mechanism of action: potent inhibitor of both prostaglandin synthesis and platelet aggregation.
- Therapeutic uses: unstable angina, patients with previous MI, and reduce the risk of recurrent transient ischemic attacks or stroke in men who have had transient ischemia of the brain due to fibrin platelet emboli.
- Monitor: bleeding, GI.
- Common adverse effects: dyspepsia, nausea, prolongation of bleeding time, hematologic disorders (e.g., iron deficiency anemia, leukopenia, and thrombocytopenia), hematoma.
- Contraindications/cautions: hypersensitivity to salicylates or nonsteroidal anti-inflammatory drugs (NSAIDs), Reye syndrome, caution in patients with chronic renal insufficiency, GI, and hematologic disorders.
- Example agent: aspirin (Ecotrin).

2. Ranolazine (Ranexa)
- Mechanism of action: mechanism is unknown; however, ranolazine can inhibit the inactivating component of the sodium current and inhibits the rapid inward rectifying current, which prolongs the ventricular action potential.
- Therapeutic use: angina pectoris (chronic).
- Monitor: ECG, BUN, creatinine, electrolytes, improvement of symptoms.
- Common adverse effects: constipation, nausea, dizziness, and headache; less common but serious effects include QT prolongation and syncope.
- Contraindications/cautions: hepatic dysfunction, prolonged QT interval, concomitant use with potent CYP3A inhibitors or inducers.

E. Antiarrhythmic Agents

One approach to classifying antiarrhythmic agents is based on their primary electrophysiologic action (see table below), but it is important to note that many agents will possess multiple effects that contribute to their clinical action.

Class	Primary Action
I	Sodium channel blockade
II	β-Blockade
III	Action potential prolongation
IV	Calcium channel blockade

1. Class I

a. Class IA
- Mechanism of action: decrease conduction velocity and prolong repolarization.
- Therapeutic uses: atrial and ventricular arrhythmias.
- Monitor: ECG, electrolytes, renal function, hepatic function, CBC, lupus-like syndrome (procainamide), anticholinergic effects (disopyramide).
- Common adverse effects: torsades de pointes, hypotension, tinnitus, diarrhea, blurred vision, headache, lupus-like syndrome (procainamide), blood dyscrasias.
- Contraindications/cautions: skin eruption or febrile reactions, myasthenia gravis, digitalis intoxication manifested by arrhythmias, conduction disorders, history of long QT syndrome, complete AV block with an AV nodal or AV pacemaker, aberrant ectopic impulses and abnormal rhythms due to escape mechanisms, complete heart block, lupus erythematosus, and torsades de pointes.
- Example agents: quinidine, procainamide, disopyramide.

b. Class IB
- Mechanism of action: decrease conduction velocity and shorten repolarization.
- Therapeutic use: ventricular arrhythmias.
- Monitor: ECG, liver function tests, drug levels.

- Common adverse effects: hypotension, drowsiness, blood dyscrasias (mexiletine), hepatotoxicity (mexiletine), seizure (mexiletine).
- Contraindications/cautions: Stokes–Adams syndrome, Wolff–Parkinson–White syndrome, severe degrees of sinoatrial, AV, or intraventricular block in the absence of an artificial pacemaker.
- Example agents: lidocaine (Xylocaine), mexiletine (Mexitil).

  c. **Class IC**
  - Mechanism of action: decrease conduction velocity.
  - Therapeutic uses: atrial and ventricular arrhythmias.
  - Monitor: ECG, blood pressure, heart rate.
  - Common adverse effects: visual abnormalities, nausea, negative inotrope, dyspnea, headache, metallic taste.
  - Contraindications/cautions: preexisting second- or third-degree AV block, right bundle branch block when associated with a left hemiblock (bifascicular block) unless a pacemaker is present, presence of cardiogenic shock, structural heart disease, conduction disorders in the absence of a pacemaker, bradycardia, marked hypotension, bronchospastic disorders, and electrolyte imbalances.
  - Example agents: flecainide (Tambocor), propafenone (Rythmol).

2. **Class II**
   - Mechanism of action: compete with β-adrenergic agonists to slow ventricular rate.
   - Therapeutic uses: atrial flutter/fibrillation, PSVT, sometimes symptomatic premature ventricular contractions.
   - Monitor: blood pressure, heart rate, dizziness, worsening heart failure symptoms.
   - Common adverse effects: bradycardia, hypotension, fatigue, sexual dysfunction.
   - Contraindications/cautions: sinus bradycardia, greater than first-degree heart block; cardiogenic shock; use with caution in diabetes, asthma, COPD, and PVD.
   - Example agents: propranolol (Inderal), esmolol (Brevibloc), acebutolol (Sectral).

3. **Class III**
   - Mechanism of action: prolong repolarization.
   - Therapeutic uses: atrial and ventricular arrhythmias.
   - Monitor: ECG, electrolytes. Amiodarone has multiple monitoring parameters, including blood pressure, heart rate, pulmonary toxicity assessment, liver function tests, thyroid function, and ophthalmic exam.
   - Common adverse effects: amiodarone (corneal deposits, increased hepatic enzymes, photosensitivity, blue-gray skin discoloration, hypothyroidism/hyperthyroidism, and pulmonary fibrosis), bradycardia, torsades de pointes, and N/V.
   - Contraindications/cautions: severe sinus-node dysfunction causing marked sinus bradycardia, second- and third-degree AV block, cardiogenic shock, electrolyte abnormalities, symptomatic heart failure with recent decompensation requiring hospitalization or New York Heart Association (NYHA) class IV symptoms (dronedarone), and permanent atrial fibrillation (dronedarone).
   - Example agents: amiodarone (Cordarone), sotalol (Betapace), ibutilide (Corvert), dofetilide (Tikosyn), dronedarone (Multaq); amiodarone is known to possess electrophysiologic actions from all four classes of antiarrhythmics.

4. **Class IV**
   - Mechanism of action: decrease heart rate.
   - Therapeutic uses: slow ventricular rate in atrial flutter/fibrillation and PSVT.
   - Monitor: blood pressure, heart rate.
   - Common adverse effects: constipation, dizziness, headache, bradycardia (verapamil), visual disturbances, anorexia, N/V, lethargy (digoxin), chest discomfort, dyspnea, flushing, asystole, headache (adenosine).
   - Contraindications/cautions: sinus node disease or second- or third-degree AV block except with a functioning pacemaker.
   - Example agents: verapamil (Calan SR), diltiazem (Cardizem).

5. **Other Antiarrhythmics: Cardiac Glycosides**
   - Mechanism of action: slow AV conduction, increased contraction.
   - Therapeutic uses: heart failure syndrome, atrial fibrillation.
   - Monitor: heart rate, ECG, electrolytes, renal function, digoxin levels.
   - Common adverse effects: nausea, diarrhea, visual disturbances (digoxin toxicity), arrhythmias.
   - Contraindications/cautions: sinus node disease, AV block, renal impairment, elderly, electrolyte abnormalities (hypokalemia, hypercalcemia, hypomagnesemia).
   - Example agent: digoxin (Lanoxin).

6. **Naturally Occurring Nucleoside**
   - Mechanism of action: slows conduction through the AV node, restoring normal sinus rhythm.
   - Therapeutic use: Treatment of PSVT.
   - Monitor: ECG, heart rate, blood pressure.
   - Common adverse effects: flushing, lightheadedness, chest pressure.
   - Contraindications/cautions: asthma, second- or third-degree AV block.

VI. Anticoagulants

A. Properties
- The coagulation pathway is a complex, multistep process involving thrombin, fibrin, clotting factors, and various other regulatory substances.
- Various conditions can cause the system to function inappropriately. The greatest risks are either clot formation (lack of anticoagulation) or bleeding (excessive anticoagulation).

B. Low-Molecular-Weight Heparins
- Mechanism of action: inhibit factor Xa and thrombin by way of antithrombin III activity.
- Therapeutic uses: thromboembolic complications after surgery or ischemic complications of unstable angina and MI.
- Monitor: CBC; may monitor antifactor Xa in select patients.
- Common adverse effects: hemorrhage, anemia, thrombocytopenia.
- Contraindications/cautions: active bleed, history of heparin-induced thrombocytopenia; use with caution in renal failure, obese, and elderly patients.
- Example agents: enoxaparin (Lovenox), tinzaparin (Innohep), dalteparin (Fragmin).

C. Heparin
- Mechanism of action: inactivates thrombin and factors IX, X, XI, XII, and plasmin. Also inhibits conversion of fibrinogen to fibrin.
- Therapeutic uses: thrombosis, pulmonary embolism, coagulopathies, deep vein thrombosis, clot prevention.
- Monitor: activated partial thromboplastin time (APTT) or activated coagulation time, platelet count, hematocrit, occult blood in stool.
- Common adverse effects: hemorrhage, thrombocytopenia, hypersensitivity reactions, hyperkalemia.
- Contraindications/cautions: severe thrombocytopenia and heparin-induced thrombocytopenia, uncontrolled bleeding.
- Treatment of heparin overdose: protamine sulfate that binds with heparin.

D. Antithrombin Agents
- Mechanism of action: inhibit the formation of thrombin and other activating factors.
- Therapeutic uses: treat thromboembolisms in patients with hereditary antithrombin III deficiency.
- Monitor: antithrombin III levels.
- Common adverse effects: nausea, dizziness, dysgeusia, hemorrhage.
- Example agent: antithrombin III (Thrombate III).

E. Thrombin Inhibitor, Injectable
- Mechanism of action: inhibits human thrombin.
- Therapeutic uses: deep vein thrombosis, pulmonary embolism, atrial fibrillation (prevention of thromboembolism).
- Monitor: APTT, potential for allergic reactions.
- Common adverse effects: hemorrhage, hypersensitivity.
- Contraindications/cautions: active bleeding or irreversible coagulation disorder, hepatic impairment (argatroban).
- Example agents: desirudin (Iprivask), lepirudin (Refludan), argatroban (Argatroban), bivalirudin (Angiomax).

F. Selective Factor Xa Inhibitor, Injectable
- Mechanism of action: inhibition of factor Xa mediated by antithrombin III.
- Therapeutic use: prophylaxis of deep vein thrombosis.
- Monitor: antifactor Xa, if needed.
- Common adverse effect: hemorrhage.
- Contraindications/cautions: active bleeding, uncontrolled arterial hypertension, GI ulceration.
- Example agent: fondaparinux (Arixtra).

G. Warfarin (Coumadin)
- Mechanism of action: inhibits the synthesis of vitamin K–dependent clotting factors (e.g., factors II, VII, IX, and X).
- Therapeutic uses: venous thrombosis, pulmonary embolism, thromboembolic complications of atrial fibrillation/cardiac valve replacement, post-MI.
- Monitor: prothrombin time, international normalized ratio (INR).
- Common adverse effects: hemorrhage, necrosis, thrombocytopenia.
- Contraindications/cautions: protein C deficiency, NSAIDs, high risk for bleeding, numerous food and drug interactions.
- Treatment of excessive warfarin coagulation: oral, SubQ or IV vitamin K_1 or blood product.

H. Dabigatran (Pradaxa)
- An oral anticoagulant used for stroke prevention in patients with nonvalvular atrial fibrillation, postoperative thromboprophylaxis, and treatment/prevention of deep venous thrombosis and pulmonary embolism. Unlike Coumadin, does not require measurement of blood thinning levels and monitor using INR.
- Mechanism of action: direct thrombin inhibitor.
- Monitor: bleeding, CBC, renal function, weight.
- Contraindications: patients with active pathologic bleeding and patients with a known hypersensitivity. Not recommended in patients with body mass index (BMI) >40 or a weight of >120 kg. Mechanical prosthetic heart valve.
- Common adverse effects: bleeding, dyspepsia, abdominal pain, epigastric discomfort, liver enzyme elevation.
- Reversal agent: Idarucizumab (Praxbind).

I. Rivaroxaban (Xarelto)
- An oral anticoagulant used for stroke prevention in patients with nonvalvular atrial fibrillation, treatment of deep vein thrombosis and pulmonary embolism, and deep vein thrombosis prophylaxis. Unlike

Coumadin, does not require measurement of blood thinning levels and monitor using INR.

- Mechanism of action: direct inhibitor of factor Xa.
- Monitor: bleeding, CBC, renal function, weight.
- Contraindications: patients with active pathologic bleeding and patients with a known hypersensitivity. Not recommended in patients with BMI >40 or a weight of >120 kg. Mechanical prosthetic heart valve.
- Common adverse effects: bleeding, abdominal pain, liver enzyme elevation.
- Reversal agent: no specific agent available. May consider prothrombin C concentrate (PCC) or recombinant factor Xa (Andexxa).

J. Apixaban (Eliquis)

- An oral anticoagulant used for stroke prevention in patients with nonvalvular atrial fibrillation, treatment of deep vein thrombosis and pulmonary embolism, and postoperative thromboprophylaxis. Unlike Coumadin, does not require measurement of blood thinning levels and monitor using INR.
- Mechanism of action: direct inhibitor of factor Xa.
- Monitor: bleeding, CBC, renal function, weight.
- Contraindications: patients with active pathologic bleeding, known hypersensitivity, and a CrCl >95 mL per minute (only for atrial fibrillation due to increased rate of ischemic stroke). Not recommended in patients with BMI >40 or a weight of >120 kg. Mechanical prosthetic heart valve.
- Common adverse effects: bleeding, nausea, epistaxis.
- Reversal agent: no specific agent available. May consider PCC or recombinant factor VIIa.

K. Edoxaban (Savaysa)

- An oral anticoagulant used for stroke prevention in patients with nonvalvular atrial fibrillation and treatment of deep vein thrombosis and pulmonary embolism. Unlike Coumadin, does not require measurement of blood thinning levels and monitor using INR.
- Mechanism of action: direct inhibitor of factor Xa.
- Monitor: bleeding, CBC, renal function, weight.
- Contraindications: patients with active pathologic bleeding and known hypersensitivity. Not recommended in patients with BMI >40 or a weight of >120 kg. Mechanical prosthetic heart valve.
- Common adverse effects: bleeding, rash, epistaxis.
- Reversal agent: no specific agent available.

VII. Neurologic Agents

A. Antiepileptics/Anticonvulsants

1. **General Properties**
   - These medications have the ability to depress abnormal neuronal discharges within the CNS, thereby inhibiting seizure activity.
   - Medication initiation and withdrawal should be done only with supervision and caution; avoid abrupt withdrawal of any of the medications.
   - Individual medications have demonstrated varying degrees of efficacy, in part based on the classification type of the seizure.

2. **Hydantoins**
   - Mechanism of action: proposed to stabilize the neurons from hyperexcitability by controlling cellular sodium without causing general depression of the CNS.
   - Therapeutic uses: generalized tonic–clonic and complex partial seizures; treatment and prophylaxis of seizure during and following neurosurgery.
   - Monitor: CBCs, urinalysis, drug level, albumin.
   - Common adverse effects: rash, nystagmus, slurred speech, confusion, dizziness, hematologic complications, gingival hyperplasia.
   - Contraindications/cautions: cardiac conduction abnormalities, significant drug–drug interactions.
   - Example agent: phenytoin (Dilantin).

3. **Succinimides**
   - Mechanism of action: motor cortex depression and elevated stimulatory threshold by reducing low-threshold thalamic Ca^{2+} currents.
   - Therapeutic use: absence seizures.
   - Monitor: CBCs, urinalysis, liver function tests.
   - Common adverse effects: drowsiness, ataxia, dizziness, headache, rash, GI upset.
   - Contraindications/cautions: patients with renal or hepatic failure.
   - Example agents: ethosuximide (Zarontin), methsuximide (Celontin).

4. **Benzodiazepine**
   - Mechanism of action: proposed to potentiate the effects of γ-aminobutyrate (GABA), decrease seizure activity.
   - Therapeutic uses: absence, akinetic, and myoclonic seizures; status epilepticus.
   - Monitor: may lose effectiveness over time, may need to increase dose.
   - Common adverse effects: sedation, ataxia, paradoxical reactions.
   - Contraindications/cautions: multiple seizure types, suicide risk, dependence.
   - Example agents: clonazepam (Klonopin), diazepam (Valium).

5. **Carbamazepine (Tegretol)**
   - Mechanism of action: proposed to reduce response and potentiation of impulses.
   - Therapeutic uses: partial, generalized tonic–clonic, mixed pattern and generalized seizures.
   - Monitor: drug level, CBC, liver function tests, urinalysis, BUN.
   - Common adverse effects: aplastic anemia, agranulocytosis, severe dermatologic reactions.
   - Contraindications/cautions: bone marrow suppression, patients with hypersensitivity to tricyclic antidepressants, MAOIs, potential drug–drug interactions.

- Oxcarbazepine (Trileptal): a metabolite of carbamazepine appears to be as effective as carbamazepine in the treatment of epilepsy; severe adverse effects have occurred less often with oxcarbazepine in some studies.

6. **Valproic Acid**
   - Mechanism of action: varying proposed mechanisms of actions.
   - Therapeutic uses: absence seizures; complex partial epileptic seizure.
   - Monitor: drug level, complete blood cell count, liver function tests, serum ammonia (with lethargy or mental status change), suicidality.
   - Common adverse effects: pancreatitis, thrombocytopenia, hepatotoxicity, GI problems, asthenia.
   - Contraindications/cautions: patients with hepatic dysfunction, urea cycle disorder.
   - Example agents: valproic acid (Depakene), divalproex sodium (Depakote).

7. **Additional Anticonvulsants**
   - A wide variety of additional agents are currently available.
   - Each of the agents has a unique pharmacologic profile and monitoring requirements.
   - Examples: felbamate (Felbatol), gabapentin (Neurontin), lamotrigine (Lamictal), levetiracetam (Keppra), primidone (Mysoline), tiagabine (Gabitril), topiramate (Topamax), pregabalin (Lyrica), lacosamide (Vimpat).

B. **Antiparkinsonian Agents**
1. **General Properties**
   - The biochemical basis is complex with the primary defect appearing to be an imbalance in neurotransmitters.
   - There is not a curative agent.
   - Available medications are aimed at correcting the neurotransmitter defects.

2. **Anticholinergics**
   - Mechanism of action: suppress central cholinergic activity, may prolong activity of dopamine.
   - Therapeutic uses: adjunctive therapy for parkinsonism and drug-induced extrapyramidal symptoms.
   - Monitor: blood pressure, mental status changes.
   - Common adverse effects: mental confusion, disorientation, memory loss, blurred vision, dry mouth, hypotension, appetite changes.
   - Contraindications/cautions: angle-closure glaucoma, prostatic hypertrophy.
   - Example agents: benztropine (Cogentin), diphenhydramine (Benadryl), trihexyphenidyl (Artane).

3. **Amantadine (Symmetrel)**
   - Mechanism of action: may increase dopamine by facilitating dopamine release and block reuptake.
   - Therapeutic uses: parkinsonism, drug-induced extrapyramidal symptoms, influenza A infection.

- Monitor: renal function, CNS, adverse reactions.
- Common adverse effects: dizziness, lightheadedness, insomnia, nausea, orthostatic hypotension, agitation.
- Contraindications/cautions: suicide attempt history, seizure history, untreated angle-closure glaucoma; avoid abrupt withdrawal.

4. **Bromocriptine Mesylate (Parlodel)**
   - Mechanism of action: stimulation of the dopamine receptors in the brain.
   - Therapeutic uses: Parkinson disease, hyperprolactinemia.
   - Monitor: blood pressure.
   - Common adverse effects: hypotension, nausea, headache, dizziness.
   - Contraindications/cautions: ischemic heart or PVD.

5. **Carbidopa (Lodosyn)**
   - Mechanism of action: inhibits decarboxylation of peripheral levodopa, does not cross blood–brain barrier.
   - Therapeutic use: Parkinson disease.
   - Monitor: clinical improvement in parkinsonian symptoms.
   - Common adverse effects: neuroleptic malignant-like syndrome, dyskinesias.
   - Contraindications/cautions: nonselective MAOI; narrow-angle glaucoma, psychotic disorders.

6. **Levodopa**
   - Mechanism of action: a precursor that crosses blood–brain barrier and is converted to dopamine.
   - Therapeutic use: Parkinson disease.
   - Monitor: liver enzymes, CBC, renal function, symptoms of depression.
   - Common adverse effects: "on–off" phenomenon, abnormal body movements, anorexia, N/V.
   - Contraindications/cautions: narrow-angle glaucoma, MAOIs, can activate melanomas, history of MI, tartrazine sensitivity.
   - Example agents: combined use of levodopa plus a peripheral dopa decarboxylase inhibitor enhances efficacy and reduces dose requirements and some adverse effects of levodopa; levodopa is available in combination with carbidopa (Sinemet, Sinemet CR, Rytary).

7. **Entacapone (Comtan)**
   - Mechanism of action: inhibits catechol-*O*-methyltransferase, thereby increasing levodopa concentrations.
   - Therapeutic uses: adjunct to levodopa/carbidopa in treating Parkinson disease.
   - Monitor: blood pressure, liver function tests, clinical improvement.
   - Common adverse effects: hypotension, syncope, diarrhea, nausea, hallucinations, dyskinesia.
   - Contraindications/cautions: MAOIs, hepatic impairment.

8. **Selegiline Hydrochloride**
   - Mechanism of action: increases dopaminergic activity.
   - Therapeutic uses: adjunct to levodopa/carbidopa in treating Parkinson disease.
   - Monitor: blood pressure, clinical improvement, general mood and behavior, potential drug interactions.
   - Common adverse effects: nausea, hallucinations, headache, confusion, cardiac effects.
   - Contraindications/cautions: avoid use with meperidine and use other opioids with caution; avoid concomitant use with MAOIs or dextromethorphan.
   - Example agent: selegiline (Emsam, Eldepryl).
9. **Dopaminergics**
   - Mechanism of action: proposed stimulation of dopamine receptors.
   - Therapeutic uses: Parkinson disease, restless legs syndrome.
   - Monitor: blood pressure, clinical improvement.
   - Common adverse effects: orthostatic hypotension, syncope, hallucinations, dyskinesia.
   - Contraindications/cautions: retinal changes, avoid sudden discontinuation; use with caution with other CNS sedative agents, extensive drug–drug interactions.
   - Example agents: pramipexole (Mirapex), ropinirole (Requip).

VIII. Psychotherapeutic Agents
A. Antidepressants
1. **General Properties**
   - All agents are considered equally effective in treating depression, but their side effect profiles and tolerability vary significantly.
   - Patients should receive a trial of appropriate length before being switched to a second agent; trial duration varies by class of antidepressant.
   - Discontinuation of treatment versus lifelong therapy should be based on the patient's history.
2. **Tricyclic Compounds**
   - Mechanism of action: inhibit reuptake of norepinephrine and serotonin.
   - Therapeutic uses: depression, insomnia, neuropathy.
   - Monitor: CBC, liver function tests, blood glucose, weight, possibly ECG, signs of clinical improvement.
   - Common adverse effects: anticholinergic effects, sedation, weight gain.
   - Contraindications/cautions: avoid use with MAOIs, seizure history, cardiovascular history especially recent MI; use with caution in elderly individuals; avoid abrupt withdrawal.

- Example agents: amitriptyline (Elavil), clomipramine (Anafranil), desipramine (Norpramin), doxepin (Sinequan), imipramine (Tofranil), nortriptyline (Pamelor).
3. **Tetracyclic Compounds**
   - Mechanism of action: enhance central noradrenergic and serotonergic activity.
   - Therapeutic use: depression.
   - Monitor: blood pressure, weight, signs of infection (rare), lipids, signs of clinical improvement.
   - Common adverse effects: sedation, dry mouth, constipation, weight gain, agranulocytosis.
   - Contraindications/cautions: drug–drug interactions, seizure history, avoid use with MAOIs, caution with history of cardiac problems.
   - Example agents: mirtazapine (Remeron, Remeron SolTab).
4. **Trazodone (Desyrel)**
   - Mechanism of action: unknown; has effects on serotonin uptake and serotonin precursor.
   - Therapeutic uses: depression, insomnia; comparative efficacy is generally lower when compared with other classes of antidepressants; thus primary use for trazodone is for the treatment of insomnia.
   - Monitor: signs of clinical improvement.
   - Common adverse effects: priapism, hypotension, sedation, dizziness, blurred vision, syncope, dry mouth.
   - Contraindications/cautions: caution with history of cardiac disease (QT prolongation), drug–drug interactions.
5. **Bupropion Hydrochloride**
   - Mechanism of action: inhibits weakly the neuronal uptake of dopamine and norepinephrine.
   - Therapeutic uses: depression, smoking cessation.
   - Monitor: blood pressure, weight, signs of clinical improvement.
   - Common adverse effects: seizures, agitation, anxiety, restlessness, weight loss, hypertension, headache.
   - Contraindications/cautions: seizure disorder, avoid abrupt withdrawal, bulimia, anorexia nervosa, MAOIs, patients undergoing drug or alcohol detoxification.
   - Example agent: bupropion (Wellbutrin, Zyban—marketed for smoking cessation).
6. **Selective Serotonin–Norepinephrine–Reuptake Inhibitors**
   - Mechanism of action: potentiates the neurotransmitter activity in the CNS; inhibits neuronal serotonin, norepinephrine, and dopamine reuptake (weak).
   - Therapeutic uses: depression, anxiety disorders, diabetic peripheral neuropathic pain (duloxetine).
   - Monitor: blood pressure, weight, electrolytes, liver function tests, signs of clinical improvement.

- Common adverse effects: hypertension, weight loss, anxiety, agitation, dizziness insomnia, hyponatremia.
- Contraindications/cautions: avoid use with MAOIs; use with caution in renal and hepatic impairment, seizure history; avoid abrupt discontinuation.
- Example agent: venlafaxine (Effexor, Effexor XR), duloxetine (Cymbalta).

7. **Selective Serotonin—Reuptake Inhibitors**
   - Mechanism of action: inhibit the CNS reuptake of serotonin.
   - Therapeutic uses: depression, anxiety disorders.
   - Monitor: signs of clinical improvement, weight, electrolytes, ECG (some agents have a high risk of prolonging the QT interval), hyponatremia.
   - Common adverse effects: anxiety, nervousness, insomnia, serotonin syndrome, appetite and weight changes, sexual dysfunction.
   - Contraindications/cautions: MAOIs, drug–drug interactions.
   - Example agents: citalopram (Celexa), escitalopram (Lexapro), fluoxetine (Prozac), paroxetine (Paxil), sertraline (Zoloft), fluvoxamine (Luvox).

8. **Monoamine Oxidase Inhibitors**
   - Mechanism of action: block breakdown of neurotransmitters by inhibiting monoamine oxidase.
   - Therapeutic use: depression (refractory).
   - Monitor: blood pressure, signs of clinical improvement, renal and hepatic function.
   - Common adverse effect: hypertensive crisis.
   - Contraindications/cautions: must avoid tyramine-containing foods.
   - Example agents: phenelzine (Nardil), tranylcypromine (Parnate), isocarboxazid (Marplan).

B. **Antipsychotics**
   1. **General Properties**
      - Antipsychotic medications are used in the treatment of a wide variety of psychiatric disorders and problems.
      - Agents differ significantly in their side effect profiles and tolerability, several agents carry black-box warnings.
      - Agents are typically classified as a typical or atypical antipsychotic based on chemical structure and profile of activity.
      - There are concerns about the development of tardive dyskinesia with long-term use, especially with the typical agents.
      - Patient-specific information may help determine the best agent for a particular patient.
   2. **Phenothiazines**
      - Mechanism of action: related to the inhibition of dopamine receptors.
      - Therapeutic use: psychotic disorders.
      - Monitor: ECG, blood pressure, clinical response.

- Common adverse effects: extrapyramidal symptoms, neuroleptic malignant syndrome, sedation, hypotension, anticholinergic side effects.
- Contraindications/cautions: QT abnormalities, cardiac arrhythmias, BPH, glaucoma.
- Example agents: chlorpromazine (Thorazine), fluphenazine (Prolixin), perphenazine (Trilafon), prochlorperazine (Compazine), trifluoperazine (Stelazine), thioridazine (Mellaril).

3. **Thioxanthenes**
   - Mechanism of action: exact mechanism unknown, effects related to antagonistic actions on receptors.
   - Therapeutic use: schizophrenia.
   - Monitor: abnormal involuntary movement scale, akathisia, CBC, ECG, liver function tests, blood pressure, and heart rate.
   - Common adverse effects: extrapyramidal symptoms, sedation, and orthostatic hypotension.
   - Contraindications/cautions: consider ECG in cardiac patients, caution with elderly patients.
   - Example agents: thiothixene (Navane).

4. **Phenylbutylpiperidines**
   - Mechanism of action: exact mechanism unknown, effects related to antagonistic actions on receptors.
   - Therapeutic use: psychotic disorders.
   - Monitor: abnormal involuntary movement scale, CBC, liver function tests.
   - Common adverse effects: extrapyramidal symptoms, hypotension.
   - Contraindications/cautions: Parkinson disease, anticoagulant use, severe cardiovascular disorders.
   - Example agents: haloperidol (Haldol).

5. **Dihydroindolones**
   - Mechanism of action: exact mechanism unknown, effects related to antagonistic actions on receptors.
   - Therapeutic use: schizophrenia.
   - Monitor: liver function tests, observe for early symptoms of tardive dyskinesia/dystonia.
   - Common adverse effects: extrapyramidal symptoms, sedation.
   - Contraindications/cautions: allergy to sulfites, history of breast cancer, urinary retention, glaucoma, liver impairment.
   - Example agents: molindone (Moban).

6. **Dibenzapines**
   - Mechanism of action: exact mechanism unknown, effects related to antagonistic actions on receptors.
   - Therapeutic use: psychotic disorders.
   - Monitor: weight, blood pressure, blood sugar, lipid profile, clinical response, CBC, liver function test, ECG.
   - Common adverse effects: extrapyramidal symptoms (low risk), increase prolactin levels, hyperglycemia, hyperlipidemia, increased weight, sedation.
   - Contraindications/cautions: diabetes.

- Clozapine risks: agranulocytosis, seizures, myocarditis, special monitoring CBC.
- Example agents: clozapine (Clozaril), loxapine (Loxitane), olanzapine (Zyprexa), quetiapine (Seroquel).

7. **Benzisoxazoles**
   - Mechanism of action: exact mechanism unknown, effects related to antagonistic actions on receptors.
   - Therapeutic use: psychotic disorders.
   - Monitor: CBC, liver function test, ECG, weight, blood pressure.
   - Common adverse effects: extrapyramidal symptoms (higher risk with risperidone), increased prolactin levels, sedation.
   - Contraindications/cautions: QT abnormalities, cardiac arrhythmias, cardiovascular or cerebrovascular problems, Parkinson disease.
   - Example agents: risperidone (Risperdal), ziprasidone (Geodon).

8. **Quinolinones**
   - Mechanism of action: exact mechanism unknown, effects related to antagonistic actions on receptors.
   - Therapeutic use: psychotic disorders.
   - Monitor: blood pressure, heart rate, blood chemistry.
   - Common adverse effects: extrapyramidal symptoms (low risk), agitation, insomnia, dizziness.
   - Contraindications/cautions: dehydration, Parkinson disease, elderly, cardiovascular or cerebrovascular problems.
   - Example agents: aripiprazole (Abilify).

9. **Lithium**
   - Mechanism of action: may be a result of increased norepinephrine reuptake and serotonin receptor sensitivity.
   - Therapeutic use: mania.
   - Monitor: serum creatinine, CBC, urinalysis, sodium, potassium, ECG, thyroid function test, lithium levels, pregnancy test, hydration status (instruct patients to drink 8–12 glasses of water a day).
   - Common adverse effects: hypothyroidism, sodium depletion, electroencephalogram changes, neurologic toxicities, GI problems, headache.
   - Contraindications/cautions: renal failure, elderly, dehydration, pregnancy.
   - Example agents: lithium (Eskalith, Lithobid, Lithonate).

C. **Sedative/Hypnotics/Anxiolytics**
   1. **General Properties**
      - These agents are used both to facilitate sleep and for their sedative effects.
      - Each of the agents has a specific duration of action and approved indications.
   2. **Benzodiazepines**
      - Mechanism of action: potentiate the effects of GABA by binding to the benzodiazepine receptor sites.
      - Therapeutic uses: anxiety disorders, sedation, insomnia, anticonvulsant, skeletal muscle relaxant.
      - Monitor: clinical response, excessive sedation, respiratory function, symptoms of drug abuse or dependence.
      - Common adverse effects: sedation, dizziness, depression, dependency, transient memory impairment, headache.
      - Contraindications/cautions: potential for abuse, dependency, sleep apnea, glaucoma, other CNS depressants, alcohol abuse.
      - Example agents: alprazolam (Xanax), clorazepate (Tranxene), chlordiazepoxide (Librium), clonazepam (Klonopin), diazepam (Valium), lorazepam (Ativan), oxazepam (Serax).
      - **NOTE:** The nonbenzodiazepine hypnotics such as zaleplon (Sonata), eszopiclone (Lunesta), and zolpidem (Ambien) that are indicated for insomnia have similar safety and efficacy profiles within patients with sleep disorders.
   3. **Chloral Hydrate (Aquachloral)**
      - Mechanism of action: unknown; causes mild cerebral depression and deep sleep.
      - Therapeutic use: nocturnal sedation.
      - Monitor: effectiveness, signs of abuse, hangover effect during the day.
      - Common adverse effects: dizziness, drowsiness; potential for abuse, dependency, efficacy may decrease over time.
      - Contraindications/cautions: hepatic or renal impairment, severe cardiac disease, gastritis.

IX. Analgesics

A. **General Overview**
   - A variety of agents are available to treat pain.

B. **Nonsteroidal Anti-inflammatory Drugs**
   - Mechanism of action: inhibition of prostaglandin synthesis by blocking both cyclooxygenase isoenzymes, COX-1 and COX-2 (nonselective) or COX-2 only (selective).
   - Therapeutic uses: analgesia, antipyretic, anti-inflammatory.
   - Monitor: CBC, chemistry profile, occult blood test, liver function test, renal function.
   - Common adverse effects: GI ulcers, bleeding.
   - Contraindications/cautions: active GI bleed, renal insufficiency, concomitant anticoagulant/diuretic/ACEI use, aspirin allergy, liver dysfunction, asthma.
   - Example agents: aspirin (Bayer), diclofenac, etodolac (Lodine), ibuprofen (Motrin), indomethacin (Indocin), ketoprofen (Orudis), ketorolac (Toradol), naproxen (Naprosyn), nabumetone (Relafen),

meloxicam (Mobic), piroxicam (Feldene), celecoxib (Celebrex).
- **NOTE:** Agents such as celecoxib (Celebrex) blocks only COX-2 mainly used as an analgesic; therefore, the agents provide less GI toxicity.

C. Opioids
- Mechanism of action: activity at the opioid receptors in the CNS.
- Therapeutic use: analgesia.
- Monitor: clinical response, signs of abuse, CNS depression, blood pressure/heart rate, liver function.
- Common adverse effects: itching, sedation, dizziness, constipation, N/V, allergic reactions, addiction.
- Contraindications/cautions: severe respiratory disease or depression, including acute asthma (unless patient is mechanically ventilated), potential for abuse, concomitant CNS depressants, alcohol abuse, paralytic ileus, or GI obstruction.
- Example agents: buprenorphine (Buprenex), fentanyl patch (Duragesic), hydromorphone (Dilaudid), methadone (Dolophine), morphine (MS Contin), oxycodone (Roxicodone, OxyContin), hydrocodone (Hysingla ER; Zohydro ER).
- NOTE: Many of the opioids are available commercially in combination products containing aspirin, acetaminophen, or an NSAID.

D. Opioid-like Agents
1. **Tramadol**
   - Binds to μ-opiate receptors in the CNS causing inhibition of ascending pain pathways; also inhibits norepinephrine and serotonin reuptake.
   - Therapeutic use: treatment of moderate-to-severe pain.
   - Common adverse effects: sedation, dizziness, constipation, N/V, somnolence, euphoria/dysphoria.
   - Examples: tramadol (Ultram).
2. **Tapentadol**
   - Binds to μ-opiate receptors in CNS causing inhibition of ascending pain pathways; also inhibits norepinephrine reuptake.
   - Therapeutic use: treatment of moderate-to-severe acute pain.
   - Common adverse effects: nausea, dizziness, hypotension, constipation, sedation.
   - Schedule II drug, same category as morphine.
   - Examples: tapentadol (Nucynta).

X. Pulmonary Agents for Asthma and COPD
A. Quick-Relief Agents
1. **Short-Acting β_2-Agonists**
   - Mechanism of action: relax airway smooth muscle by stimulating β_2-receptors.
   - Therapeutic use: bronchodilation (asthma, COPD, exercise-induced bronchospasm).

- Common adverse effects: palpitations, tachycardia, tremor, nervousness, headache, N/V.
- Contraindications/cautions: cardiac arrhythmias, angina, organic brain damage, narrow-angle glaucoma.
- Example agents: albuterol (Ventolin), levalbuterol (Xopenex), metaproterenol (Alupent).

2. **Anticholinergics**
   - Mechanism of action: inhibit vagally mediated reflexes by antagonizing the effects of ACH resulting in bronchodilation.
   - Therapeutic uses: additive benefits to inhaled β_2-agonists in severe exacerbations or an alternative bronchodilator in patients who do not tolerate inhaled β_2-agonists.
   - Common adverse effects: dry mouth, headache, dyspnea, bronchitis, upper respiratory tract infection.
   - Contraindications/cautions: hypersensitivity to these agents or any of their components.
   - Example agents: ipratropium bromide (Atrovent), tiotropium bromide (Spiriva), umeclidinium (Incruse), aclidinium (Tudorza) are indicated for the maintenance of symptoms in COPD patients.

3. **Systemic Corticosteroids**
   - Mechanism of action: reduce pulmonary inflammation.
   - Therapeutic use: bronchial asthma (including status asthmaticus).
   - Common adverse effects: weight gain, increased appetite, mood swings, weakness, blurred vision, slow healing of cuts and bruises, hyperglycemia, moon face, stomach irritation.
   - Contraindications/cautions: systemic fungal infections, IM use in idiopathic thrombocytopenic purpura, administration of live vaccines in patients receiving immunosuppressive doses, use of caution with prolonged therapy due to adrenal suppression, ocular effects (glaucoma, cataracts), peptic ulcer disease, and osteoporosis and fluid/electrolyte imbalances.
   - Example agents: prednisone (Deltasone), methylprednisolone (Medrol).

B. Long-term Control Agents
1. **Inhaled Corticosteroids**
   - Mechanism of action: reduce pulmonary inflammation.
   - Therapeutic use: asthma.
   - Common adverse effects: cough, sore throat, stomach irritation, upper respiratory tract infections, nasal congestion.
   - Contraindications/cautions: relief of acute bronchospasm, primary treatment of status asthmaticus or other acute episodes of asthma when intensive measures are required; use with caution when withdrawing from oral steroids, monitor

children for reduction in growth velocity; and rare instances of glaucoma, increased intraocular pressure, and cataracts have been reported.
- Example agents: budesonide (Pulmicort), flunisolide (Aerospan), fluticasone (Flovent), mometasone (Asmanex), beclomethasone (Qvar).

2. **Long-Acting β_2-Agonists**
   - Mechanism of action: relax airway smooth muscle by stimulating β_2-receptors.
   - Therapeutic uses: bronchodilation (asthma, COPD, exercise-induced bronchospasm); used in combination with another maintenance therapy, such as an inhaled corticosteroid, by patients with asthma because of increased asthma-related deaths in studies with long-acting β_2-agonist agents as monotherapy.
   - Common adverse effects: palpitations, tachycardia, tremor, nervousness, headache, N/V.
   - Contraindications/cautions: cardiac arrhythmias, angina, organic brain damage, narrow-angle glaucoma; use of a long-acting β_2-agonist without current long-term asthma treatment (such as an inhaled corticosteroid).
   - Example agents: formoterol (Perforomist), salmeterol (Serevent), olodaterol (Striverdi).

3. **Methylxanthines**
   - Mechanism of action: cause bronchodilatation, diuresis, CNS and cardiac stimulation, and gastric acid secretion by blocking phosphodiesterase which promotes stimulation of lipolysis, glycogenolysis, and gluconeogenesis and causes release of epinephrine.
   - Therapeutic uses: asthma, COPD.
   - Common adverse effects: N/V, palpitations, irritability, insomnia, headache.
   - Contraindications/cautions: active peptic ulcer disease, seizure disorders, cardiac arrhythmias.
   - Example agents: theophylline, aminophylline.

4. **Leukotriene Modifiers**
   - Mechanism of action: inhibit inflammation, edema, mucus secretion, bronchoconstriction.
   - Therapeutic uses: asthma, seasonal allergic rhinitis.
   - Common adverse effects: headache, dyspepsia, nausea, liver enzyme elevations, hypersensitivity reactions.
   - Contraindications/cautions: acute liver disease or transaminase elevations greater than or equal to three times the upper limit of normal; patients instructed not to use for acute asthma attacks.
   - Example agents: montelukast (Singulair), zafirlukast (Accolate), zileuton (Zyflo).

5. **Mast Cell Stabilizers**
   - Mechanism of action: reduce bronchial inflammation by inhibiting the release of mediators, histamine, and SRS-A (the slow-reacting substance of anaphylaxis, a leukotriene).
   - Therapeutic uses: asthma, prevention of bronchospasm, allergic rhinitis.

- Common adverse effects: cough, dysgeusia, headache, sneezing, nasal congestion.
- Contraindications/cautions: agents have no role in acute asthma and may cause bronchospasm.
- Example agents: cromolyn sodium (Intal), nedocromil sodium (Alocril).

6. **Monoclonal Antibody Agent**
   - Mechanism of action: inhibits the binding of immunoglobulin E to the surface of mast cells and basophils, and therefore limiting the release of mediators of the allergic response.
   - Therapeutic use: asthma.
   - Common adverse effects: site reactions, viral infections, upper respiratory tract function, sinusitis, headache, pharyngitis.
   - Contraindications/cautions: use has been associated with malignant neoplasms (rare), and patients should be observed after injection for possible anaphylaxis reactions.
   - Example agent: omalizumab (Xolair), reslizumab (Cinqair), mepolizumab (Nucala).

XI. GI Agents
A. Gastrointestinal
1. **Histamine H_2 Antagonists**
   - Mechanism of action: inhibit gastric acid secretion by blocking the histamine-2 receptors in the gastric parietal cells.
   - Therapeutic uses: duodenal ulcers, gastric ulcers, gastroesophageal reflux disease (GERD), erosive esophagitis, pathologic hypersecretory conditions, upper GI bleeding, heartburn.
   - Common adverse effects: drowsiness, confusion, rash, constipation, psychosis, headache.
   - Contraindications/cautions: use with caution in patients with renal/hepatic dysfunction.
   - Example agents: cimetidine, ranitidine (Zantac), nizatidine, famotidine (Pepcid).

2. **Proton Pump Inhibitors**
   - Mechanism of action: suppress gastric acid secretion by specifically inhibiting the hydrogen/potassium (H^+/K^+) ATPase enzyme at the secretory surface of the gastric parietal cell; this inhibition blocks the final step of acid production.
   - Therapeutic uses: duodenal ulcers, gastric ulcers, GERD, pathologic hypersecretory conditions.
   - Common adverse effects: dizziness, rash, headache, nausea, diarrhea, upper respiratory tract infection, long-term use: increased risk for *Clostridium difficile* infection, fractures, hypomagnesemia.
   - Contraindications/cautions: use with caution in patients with hepatic dysfunction.
   - Example agents: omeprazole (Prilosec), esomeprazole (Nexium), lansoprazole (Prevacid), dexlansoprazole (Dexilant), rabeprazole (Aciphex), pantoprazole (Protonix).

B. Antidiarrheals

- Mechanism of action: slow intestinal motility.
- Therapeutic uses: acute diarrhea, chronic diarrhea.
- Common adverse effects: abdominal discomfort, dry skin, dry mouth and mucous membranes, constipation, sedation, rash, tinnitus (bismuth only), blackened tongue (bismuth only).
- Contraindications/cautions: obstructive jaundice, bloody diarrhea, diarrhea associated with pseudomembranous enterocolitis or enterotoxin-producing bacteria, body temperature >101° F; monitor for dehydration.
- Example agents: diphenoxylate with atropine (Lomotil), loperamide (Imodium A-D), bismuth subsalicylate (Pepto-Bismol, Kaopectate).

C. Laxatives

1. Saline Agents

- Mechanism of action: attract/retain water in the intestinal lumen, which increases intraluminal pressure.
- Therapeutic uses: constipation, rectal/bowel examinations.
- Common adverse effects: diarrhea, N/V, perianal irritation, fainting, bloating, flatulence, cramps.
- Contraindications/cautions: signs/symptoms of appendicitis, fecal impaction, intestinal obstruction, undiagnosed abdominal pain. Do not use in patients with megacolon, bowel obstruction, imperforate anus, or CHF.
- Example agents: magnesium hydroxide (milk of magnesia), monobasic sodium phosphate, and dibasic sodium phosphate (Fleet Phospho-soda).

2. Stimulant or Irritant Agents

- Mechanism of action: exhibit direct action on intestinal mucosa or nerve plexus.
- Therapeutic uses: constipation, rectal/bowel examinations.
- Common adverse effects: diarrhea, N/V, perianal irritation, fainting, bloating, flatulence, cramps, urine discoloration.
- Contraindications/cautions: signs/symptoms of appendicitis, fecal impaction, intestinal obstruction, undiagnosed abdominal pain.
- Example agents: sennosides (Ex-Lax, Senokot), bisacodyl (Dulcolax).

3. Bulk-Producing Agents

- Mechanism of action: retain water in the stool to increase bulk-stimulating peristalsis.
- Therapeutic uses: constipation, irritable bowel syndrome, diverticular disease.
- Common adverse effects: diarrhea, N/V, perianal irritation, fainting, bloating, flatulence, cramps.
- Contraindications/cautions: signs/symptoms of appendicitis, fecal impaction, intestinal obstruction, undiagnosed abdominal pain.

- Example agents: psyllium (Metamucil), polycarbophil (FiberCon).

4. Emollient Agents

- Mechanism of action: retard colonic absorption of fecal water and soften the stool.
- Therapeutic uses: constipation, soften stool following surgery/MI, fecal impaction.
- Common adverse effects: diarrhea, N/V, perianal irritation, fainting, bloating, flatulence, cramps, anal seepage, perianal discomfort.
- Contraindications/cautions: signs/symptoms of appendicitis, fecal impaction, intestinal obstruction, undiagnosed abdominal pain, concurrent docusate sodium administration (increase mineral oil absorption).
- Example agent: mineral oil (Fleet Oil).

5. Fecal Softeners/Surfactant Agents

- Mechanism of action: facilitate admixture of fat and water to soften stool.
- Therapeutic uses: constipation, soften stool following surgery/MI.
- Common adverse effects: diarrhea, N/V, perianal irritation, fainting, bloating, flatulence, cramps.
- Contraindications/cautions: signs/symptoms of appendicitis, fecal impaction, intestinal obstruction, undiagnosed abdominal pain, concurrent mineral oil administration (increase mineral oil absorption).
- Example agent: docusate sodium (Colace).

6. Hyperosmotic Agents

- Mechanism of action: retain fluid in the colon, lower the pH and increase the colonic peristalsis.
- Therapeutic use: constipation.
- Common adverse effects: diarrhea, N/V, perianal irritation, fainting, bloating, flatulence, cramps.
- Contraindications/cautions: signs/symptoms of appendicitis, fecal impaction, intestinal obstruction, undiagnosed abdominal pain; use with caution in brittle diabetic patients, and monitor electrolytes in elderly patients on long-term therapy (>6 months).
- Example agents: glycerin, polyethylene glycol, lactulose.

D. Antiemetic Agents

1. Antidopaminergics

- Mechanism of action: block the effect of dopamine in the vomiting center of the brain.
- Therapeutic uses: N/V, motion sickness.
- Common adverse effects: drowsiness, diarrhea, restlessness.
- Contraindications/cautions: comatose or greatly depressed state, blood dyscrasias, bone marrow depression, preexisting liver disease; use with caution in patients with seizure disorder, cardiovascular disease (history of MI, heart failure, ischemic heart disease, conduction abnormalities). Monitor for

any signs/symptoms of tardive dyskinesia or extra-pyramidal symptoms.
   • Example agents: prochlorperazine (Compazine), metoclopramide (Reglan).

   2. **Antihistamines/Anticholinergics**
      • Mechanism of action: act on the brain center that controls N/V and dizziness; act on nerves affecting balance in the inner ear (scopolamine).
      • Therapeutic uses: N/V, motion sickness, vertigo.
      • Common adverse effects: drowsiness, constipation, blurry vision, dry mouth, nose, or throat.
      • Contraindications/cautions: narrow-angle glaucoma, symptomatic prostatic hypertrophy, bladder neck obstruction, MAOI use.
      • Example agents: diphenhydramine (Benadryl), meclizine (Antivert), scopolamine (TransdermScop).

   3. **5-Hydroxytryptamine Antagonists**
      • Mechanism of action: selective blockade of 5-hydroxytryptamine (5-HT3) receptors located in the vagal nerve terminals, GI tract, and centrally in the chemoreceptor trigger zone thus antagonizing nausea and emesis.
      • Therapeutic uses: prevention of N/V associated with cancer chemotherapy, postoperative sequelae, or radiotherapy.
      • Common adverse effects: constipation, fever, headache, diarrhea.
      • Contraindications/cautions: markedly prolonged QTc or AV block II to III (dolasetron), patients receiving class I or III antiarrhythmic agents (dolasetron), monitor for serotonin syndrome and QTc prolongation.
      • Example agents: dolasetron (Anzemet), granisetron (Kytril, Sustol), ondansetron (Zofran), palonosetron (Aloxi).

   4. **Active Cannabinoid**
      • Mechanism of action: activates cannabinoid receptors causing analgesia, appetite enhancement, muscle relaxation, hormonal actions.
      • Therapeutic uses: prevention of N/V associated with cancer chemotherapy, appetite stimulation in AIDS patients.
      • Common adverse effects: dizziness, flushing, tachycardia, abdominal pain.
      • Contraindications/cautions: hypersensitivity to dronabinol, cannabinoids, sesame oil (capsules), alcohol (oral solution); receiving disulfiram- or metronidazole-containing products within 14 days (oral solution).
      • Example agents: dronabinol (Marinol).

E. Benign Prostatic Hyperplasia
   1. **α_1-Adrenergic Blockers**
      • Mechanism of action: block α_1-adrenergic receptors located in the prostate and bladder neck reducing urethral resistance, improving urine flow and BPH symptoms.

   • Therapeutic uses: hypertension, BPH.
   • Common adverse effects: hypotension, dizziness, somnolence, headache.
   • Contraindications/cautions: "first-dose" hypotension, priapism.
   • Example agents: terazosin (Hytrin), doxazosin (Cardura), tamsulosin (Flomax), prazosin (Minipress), silodosin (Rapaflo), alfuzosin (Uroxatral).

   2. **Androgen Hormone Inhibitor**
      • Mechanism of action: inhibits enzyme known as type II 5-α reductase that converts testosterone into dihydrotestosterone; this inhibition decreases the size of the prostate in patients with BPH.
      • Therapeutic uses: BPH, androgenic alopecia.
      • Common adverse effects: erectile dysfunction, decreased libido, breast tenderness and enlargement.
      • Contraindications/cautions: use with caution in patients with hepatic dysfunction and monitor for prostate cancer (e.g., digital rectal examinations).
      • Example agent: finasteride (Proscar), dutasteride (Avodart).

XII. Endocrine Agents
A. Antidiabetic Agents
   1. **Insulin**
      • Mechanism of action: stimulates peripheral glucose uptake and inhibits hepatic glucose production; this mechanism is based on each insulin's individual time to onset and duration of activity.
      • Therapeutic uses: diabetes mellitus (DM; types 1 and 2), hyperkalemia.
      • Common adverse effects: hypoglycemia, injection site reactions, lipodystrophy.
      • Contraindications/cautions: do not use during episodes of hypoglycemia; use with caution when changing insulin and when patients become ill. Inhalation form is contraindicated in patients with chronic lung disease such as asthma or COPD.
      • Example injectable agents: insulin regular (Novolin R, Humulin R), isophane insulin suspension (Novolin N, Humulin N), insulin lispro (Humalog), insulin aspart (Novolog), insulin detemir (Levemir), insulin glargine (Lantus), insulin glulisine (Apidra). Example inhalation agents: insulin regular (Afrezza).

   2. **Sulfonylureas**
      • Mechanism of action: stimulate pancreatic β cells to release insulin.
      • Therapeutic use: DM (type 2).
      • Common adverse effects: hypoglycemia, diarrhea, weakness, nausea, allergic skin reactions.
      • Contraindications/cautions: diabetes complicated by ketoacidosis with or without coma, sole therapy of type 1 DM, diabetes complicated by pregnancy; use with caution in patients with renal/hepatic dysfunction.

- Example agents: glyburide (Diaβeta), glipizide (Glucotrol), glimepiride (Amaryl).

3. **α-Glucosidase Inhibitors**
   - Mechanism of action: delay the absorption of complex carbohydrates, thereby resulting in a smaller rise in blood glucose concentration after meals.
   - Therapeutic use: DM (type 2).
   - Common adverse effects: flatulence, diarrhea, abdominal pain, and elevated serum transaminase levels.
   - Contraindications/cautions: diabetic ketoacidosis or cirrhosis, inflammatory bowel disease, colonic ulceration, partial intestinal obstruction or predisposition to intestinal obstruction, chronic intestinal diseases associated with marked disorders of digestion or absorption or with conditions that may deteriorate as a result of increased gas formation in the intestine. In patients with hypoglycemia taking this drug class with or without other hypoglycemic drugs, use oral glucose (dextrose) instead of sucrose as sucrose hydrolysis is inhibited if taking α-glucosidase inhibitors.
   - Example agents: acarbose (Precose) and miglitol (Glyset).

4. **Biguanides**
   - Mechanism of action: decreases hepatic glucose production and intestinal absorption of glucose and improves insulin sensitivity.
   - Therapeutic use: DM (type 2).
   - Common adverse effects: diarrhea, N/V, flatulence, and abdominal discomfort.
   - Contraindications/cautions: renal disease or dysfunction (estimated GFR < 30 mL/min/1.73 m^2); hepatic disease; acute MI; septicemia; cardiovascular shock; CHF requiring pharmacologic treatment; discontinue use of metformin before undergoing radiologic studies involving administration of iodinated contrast materials, reevaluate renal function 48 hours after procedure before reinstituting metformin; and acute or chronic metabolic acidosis including diabetic ketoacidosis with or without coma. Patients should be informed about the risk of lactic acidosis, its symptoms, and conditions that predispose to its development; monitor renal function closely.
   - Example agent: metformin (Glucophage).

5. **Meglitinides**
   - Mechanism of action: nonsulfonylurea agent that stimulates the release of insulin from the pancreas.
   - Therapeutic use: DM (type 2).
   - Common adverse effects: hypoglycemia, nausea, upper respiratory tract infection, headache.
   - Contraindications/cautions: diabetic ketoacidosis with or without coma; type 1 diabetes; coadministration of gemfibrozil (repaglinide only).
   - Example agents: nateglinide (Starlix), repaglinide (Prandin).

6. **Thiazolidinediones**
   - Mechanism of action: improve sensitivity to insulin in muscle and adipose tissue and inhibit hepatic glucose production.
   - Therapeutic use: DM (type 2).
   - Common adverse effects: edema, weight gain (edema and weight gain can be precursor to rapid development of heart failure), myalgia, fatigue.
   - Contraindications/cautions: not recommended in patients with symptomatic heart failure; is contraindicated in patients with NYHA heart failure class III or IV; use with caution in patients with edema (e.g., CHF); liver enzymes must be monitored.
   - Example agents: pioglitazone (Actos), rosiglitazone (Avandia).

7. **Dipeptidyl Peptidase-4 Inhibitors**
   - Mechanism of action: slow the inactivation of incretin hormones released from the intestine; this inactivation allows incretin to remain active longer, thereby increasing insulin release and decreasing glucagon levels.
   - Therapeutic use: DM (type 2).
   - Common adverse effects: nasopharyngitis, headache, upper respiratory infection, hypoglycemia.
   - Contraindications/cautions: monitor for development of pancreatitis; consider dose adjustment in moderate or severe renal impairment; monitor for development of joint pain; assess for hypersensitivity reactions; assess hepatic function and monitor for hepatotoxicity (alogliptin).
   - Examples: sitagliptin (Januvia), saxagliptin (Onglyza), linagliptin (Tradjenta), alogliptin (Nesina).

8. **Sodium-Glucose Cotransporter 2 Inhibitors**
   - Mechanism of action: reduces reabsorption of filtered glucose at the sodium-glucose cotransporter 2 inhibitors (SGLT2s) site from the tubular lumen; this increases urinary excretion of glucose and reduces plasma glucose concentrations.
   - Therapeutic use: DM (type 2).
   - Common adverse effects: increased serum potassium, urinary tract infection (UTI), polyuria, vaginal infection, balanitis.
   - Contraindications/cautions: severe renal impairment (estimated GFR < 30 mL/min/1.73 m^2); end-stage renal disease; patients on dialysis; monitor for development of hypotension; assess for ketoacidosis development; consider holding drug if acute kidney injury occurs; assess need to withhold drug in patients with fracture risk factors.
   - Examples: canagliflozin (Invokana), dapagliflozin (Farxiga), empagliflozin (Jardiance).

B. **Oral Contraceptives**
   - Mechanism of action: inhibit ovulation by suppressing gonadotropins, follicle-stimulating hormone (FSH), luteinizing hormone; thicken cervical mucus

to inhibit sperm penetration, slow movement of the ovum through the fallopian tubes, and alter the endometrium.
- Therapeutic uses: contraception, emergency contraception, acne vulgaris.
- Common adverse effects: breast tenderness, headache, N/V, breakthrough bleeding, spotting, edema, cramping.
- Contraindications/cautions: thrombophlebitis, thromboembolic disorders, history of deep vein thrombophlebitis, cerebral vascular disease, MI, CAD, known or suspected breast carcinoma or estrogen-dependent neoplasia, carcinoma of endometrium, hepatic adenomas/carcinomas, undiagnosed abnormal genital bleeding, known or suspected pregnancy, acute liver disease, cholestatic jaundice of pregnancy/jaundice with prior pill use; use with caution in patients who smoke and those with gallbladder disease.
- Example agents: ethinyl estradiol/norethindrone (Ortho-Novum), ethinyl estradiol with drospirenone (Yaz, Yasmin), ethinyl estradiol/levonorgestrel (Triphasil), etonogestrel (NuvaRing), norgestrel (Ovrette), levonorgestrel (Plan B).

C. Thyroid Disorders
1. Hypothyroidism Agents
- Mechanism of action: exact mechanism is not known; however, it is believed that the agents listed below restore thyroid hormone that the body may be lacking.
- Therapeutic uses: hypothyroidism, pituitary TSH suppressant, diagnostic use, myxedema coma/precoma (injection only).
- Common adverse effects: palpitations, tachycardia, tremors, headache, weight loss, increased appetite, excessive sweating, muscle weakness.
- Contraindications/cautions: uncorrected adrenal cortical insufficiency, untreated thyrotoxicosis, patients with acute MI, untreated subclinical hypothyroidism; use with caution when switching from one brand to the next.
- Example agents: thyroid desiccated (Armour Thyroid), levothyroxine sodium (Synthroid), liothyronine sodium (Cytomel), levothyroxine/liothyronine (Thyrolar).

2. Hyperthyroidism Agents
- Mechanism of action: inhibit the synthesis of thyroid hormones.
- Therapeutic use: hyperthyroidism.
- Common adverse effects: rash, pruritus, paresthesias, agranulocytosis (see contraindications/cautions).
- Contraindications/cautions: monitor for hepatotoxicity with propylthiouracil; consider propylthiouracil in pregnant patients (especially in the first trimester) as methimazole is associated with fetal abnormalities; monitor patients closely for possible bone marrow suppression—white blood cell count for at the least the first 3 months of therapy, then follow closely for any other signs/symptoms of suppression (e.g., hay fever, sore throat, skin eruptions, fever, headache, or general malaise).
- Example agents: methimazole (Tapazole), propylthiouracil.

D. Hyperlipidemia
1. Bile Acid Sequestrant Agents
- Mechanism of action: bind bile acids in the intestine to form an insoluble complex excreted in the feces. The increased fecal loss of bile acids leads to increased oxidation of cholesterol to bile acids and a decrease in low-density lipoproteins (LDLs) and serum cholesterol levels.
- Therapeutic uses: hyperlipidemia, biliary obstruction.
- Common adverse effects: constipation, abdominal pain, cramping, headache, bloating, flatulence.
- Contraindications/cautions: agents may interfere with normal fat absorption and digestion and may prevent absorption of fat-soluble vitamins such as A, D, E, K, and folic acid.
- Example agents: cholestyramine (Questran), colestipol (Colestid), colesevelam (WelChol).

2. HMG-CoA Reductase Inhibitors
- Mechanism of action: inhibit cholesterol biosynthesis by inhibiting the enzyme HMG-Co-A reductase.
- Therapeutic uses: hyperlipidemia, hypertriglyceridemia, primary prevention of cardiovascular disease in patients with multiple risk factors, secondary prevention of cardiovascular events in patients with clinically evident heart disease.
- Common adverse effects: myalgia, dyspepsia, diarrhea, arthralgia.
- Contraindications/cautions: active liver disease or unexplained persistent elevated liver function tests, pregnancy (all statins are category X), lactation; monitor liver function tests as recommended by each product.
- Example agents: lovastatin (Mevacor), simvastatin (Zocor), pravastatin (Pravachol), fluvastatin (Lescol), atorvastatin (Lipitor), rosuvastatin (Crestor), pitavastatin (Livalo).

3. Fibric Acid Derivatives
- Mechanism of action: inhibit peripheral lipolysis and decrease the hepatic extraction of free fatty acids, thus reducing hepatic triglycerides production.
- Therapeutic uses: hypertriglyceridemia, reduce coronary heart disease risk.

- Common adverse effects: fatigue, dyspepsia, abdominal pain, taste perversion, diarrhea.
- Contraindications/cautions: hepatic or severe renal dysfunction, primary biliary cirrhosis, pre-existing gallbladder disease; monitor for development of pancreatitis; use with caution in patients who are concurrently receiving HMG-CoA reductase inhibitors as skeletal muscle effects may be enhanced.
- Example agents: gemfibrozil (Lopid), fenofibrate (Tricor, Triglide, Trilipix).

4. **Niacin (Nicotinic Acid)**
   - Mechanism of action: decreases serum levels of apolipoprotein B-100, the major component of very low-density lipoprotein (VLDL) and LDL fractions; however, the exact mechanism is not entirely understood.
   - Therapeutic uses: hyperlipidemia, niacin deficiency, pellagra.
   - Common adverse effects: flushing, headache, pruritus, GI distress, activation of peptic ulcer disease, hyperuricemia, hyperglycemia.
   - Contraindications/cautions: hepatic dysfunction, active peptic ulcer, atrial bleeding, frequently monitor liver function tests due to its ability to cause hepatotoxicity; monitor for development of myopathy, especially with concurrent HMG-CoA reductase inhibitors; use with caution when switching from immediate-release to extended-release products, as severe hepatotoxicity may result because of nonequivalency of dosage forms.
   - Example products: extended-release niacin (Niaspan).

5. **Cholesterol Absorption Inhibitor**
   - Mechanism of action: acts at the brush border of the small intestine to inhibit the absorption of cholesterol.
   - Therapeutic uses: hyperlipidemia (often in combination with a HMG-CoA reductase inhibitor).
   - Common adverse effects: diarrhea, abdominal pain, back pain, arthralgia, sinusitis.
   - Contraindications/cautions: same as HMG-CoA reductase inhibitors when used together; use not recommended in moderate/severe hepatic impairment.
   - Example agent: ezetimibe (Zetia).

6. **Proprotein Convertase Subtilisin Kexin Type 9 Inhibitors**
   - Mechanism of action: bind to low-density lipoprotein receptors (LDLR) on hepatocytes surfaces to accelerate LDLR degradation within the liver; this results in increased clearing of circulating LDL.
   - Therapeutic uses: hyperlipidemia as an adjunct to diet and maximal statin therapy.
   - Common adverse effects: diarrhea, injection site reaction, influenza, myalgia.
   - Contraindications/cautions: hypersensitivity reactions.
   - Example agents: alirocumab (Praluent), evolocumab (Repatha).

XIII. Anti-infective Agents
A. General Properties
- Anti-infective agents take advantage of unique features of bacteria and viruses to selectively destroy those organisms while causing minimal toxicity to the host.
- Resistance to anti-infective agents is a major clinical concern.
- Risk of superinfection is a concern (e.g., yeast infections, *C. difficile*–associated diarrhea [CDAD], and pseudomembranous colitis).
- Common adverse effects include allergic reactions and organ-specific toxicity of certain agents.

B. Antibacterial Agents
1. **Cell Wall Synthesis Inhibitors**
   a. **Mechanism of Action**
      - Inhibit synthesis of cell walls, which are unique to bacteria; mammalian cells have membranes, not cell walls.
   b. **Spectrum of Activity**
      - Penicillin G: gram-positive organisms, *Streptococcus*, *Pneumococcus*, *Meningococcus*, anthrax, *Clostridium*, *Bacteroides*, *Neisseria*.
      - Ampicillin and amoxicillin: broad spectrum, including gram-positive and gram-negative organisms including *Escherichia coli*, *Salmonella*, *Haemophilus influenzae*, *Listeria*, and gram-positive organisms susceptible to penicillin G.
      - Nafcillin, oxacillin, dicloxacillin: penicillinase resistant, used in cases of resistance to other penicillins, particularly methicillin-sensitive *Staphylococcus aureus* (MSSA).
      - Ticarcillin and piperacillin: effective against *Pseudomonas aeruginosa*, used in combination with β-lactamase inhibitor to decrease resistance (e.g., ticarcillin + clavulanic acid—Timentin; piperacillin + tazobactam—Zosyn).
      - First-generation cephalosporins (cefazolin [Ancef], cephalexin [Keflex]): primarily useful against gram-positive organisms such as *Staphylococcus* and *Streptococcus*.
      - Second-generation cephalosporins (cefaclor [Ceclor], cefoxitin [Mefoxin]): increased gram-negative activity, including *E. coli*, *Klebsiella*, *Proteus*, and *H. influenzae*.
      - Third-generation cephalosporins (ceftazidime [Fortaz], ceftriaxone [Rocephin]): primarily gram-negative activity, including *P. aeruginosa*, *Enterobacter*, and *Serratia*.
      - Fourth-generation cephalosporins (cefepime [Maxipime]): broad gram-positive and

gram-negative activity; useful in empiric situations such as febrile neutropenia. Fifth-generation cephalosporins (ceftaroline [Teflaro]): effective versus selected *Staphylococcus* species (including MSSA and methicillin-resistant staphylococci [MRSA] in skin infections only), selected *Streptococcus* species, and selected gram-negative organisms (*H. influenzae, Klebsiella, E. coli*).
  - Monobactam (aztreonam [Azactam]): activity against gram-negative rods including *P. aeruginosa, Serratia,* and *Klebsiella.*
  - Carbapenems (imipenem [Primaxin], meropenem [Merrem], ertapenem [Invanz]): broad spectrum including anaerobes, particularly useful in penicillin-resistant pneumococci and *Enterobacter*; imipenem administered with cilastatin to reduce risk of nephrotoxicity.
  - Vancomycin: active against gram-positive organisms, particularly staphylococci, main IV use is against MRSA and given orally only in *C. difficile*-caused diarrhea.
  c. **Common Adverse Effects**
  - Allergic reactions, nephrotoxicity (mainly penicillins and cephalosporins); disulfiram reaction (second- and third-generation cephalosporins); chills, fever, and Redman syndrome (vancomycin); and N/V with rapid infusion, headache (carbapenem).
  d. **Cautions**
  - Resistance with β-lactamase–producing bacteria is common.
2. **Protein Synthesis Inhibitors**
  a. **Mechanism of Action**
  - Bind to ribosomes and prevent protein synthesis, resulting in cell death or decreased replication.
  b. **Spectrum of Activity**
  - Aminoglycosides: active against gram-negative enteric bacteria, in particular *E. coli, Proteus, Mirabilis, Klebsiella, Serratia,* and *Enterobacter*; commonly used in combination with penicillins to provide broad empiric coverage.
  - Tetracyclines: gram-positive and gram-negative coverage, including *Mycoplasma pneumoniae, Chlamydia, Rickettsia,* and Lyme disease.
  - Macrolides: active against gram-positive organisms, useful in Legionnaires disease, *M. pneumoniae, Chlamydia, Helicobacter pylori* (clarithromycin).
  - Chloramphenicol: broad spectrum including *Salmonella,* resistant *H. influenzae* meningitis.
  - Clindamycin: gram-positive anaerobic infections such as *Bacteroides.*
  - Linezolid: *Streptococcus, Staphylococcus, Enterococcus.*

  c. **Common Adverse Effects**
  - Aminoglycosides: nephrotoxicity, ototoxicity, neuromuscular junction blockade (possible drug interaction with anesthetics and paralytics).
  - Tetracyclines: nausea, diarrhea, superinfections, photosensitivity, inhibition of bone growth and teeth discoloration, teratogenic.
  - Macrolides: GI distress, hepatotoxicity, pseudomembranous colitis.
  - Chloramphenicol: bone marrow suppression, gray-baby syndrome.
  - Clindamycin: pseudomembranous colitis.
  - Linezolid: diarrhea, headache, leukopenia, thrombocytopenia, anemia.
  d. **Cautions**
  - Aminoglycosides must be given parenterally, monitoring of plasma levels is required to prevent toxicity; certain macrolides (erythromycin, clarithromycin) are potent inhibitors of cytochrome P450; and macrolides may cause QT prolongation. Linezolid has been reported to cause myelosuppression and optic neuropathy with vision loss (especially with long durations of therapy) and has serotonergic qualities.
  e. **Example Agents**
  - Aminoglycosides: amikacin, gentamicin, tobramycin.
  - Tetracyclines: tetracycline (Achromycin V), minocycline (Minocin), doxycycline (Vibramycin).
  - Macrolides: erythromycin, clarithromycin (Biaxin), azithromycin (Zithromax).
  - Miscellaneous: chloramphenicol; clindamycin (Cleocin); linezolid (Zyvox).
3. **Antimetabolites**
  a. **Mechanism of Action**
  - Block enzymes involved in the synthesis of purine or pyrimidine bases; prevent growth of microorganisms.
  b. **Spectrum of Activity**
  - Sulfonamides: gram positive and gram negative, particularly useful for *E. coli, Salmonella, Shigella,* and *Enterobacter.*
  - Trimethoprim: used in combination with sulfonamides to treat UTIs, *Pneumocystis jiroveci* (formerly *carinii*) pneumonia, *Shigella, Salmonella,* and upper respiratory tract infections.
  c. **Common Adverse Effects**
  - Allergic reactions (Stevens–Johnson syndrome), blood dyscrasias, crystalluria, erythema multiforme, hematuria.
  d. **Cautions**
  - Monitor for development of blood dyscrasias (agranulocytosis, aplastic anemia) and/or skin rash—consider discontinuation of drug if occurs as these may be early signs of severe adverse reactions.

e. **Example Agents**
  * Mainly combination products: Bactrim (sulfa-methoxazole + trimethoprim).

4. **Inhibitors of DNA Gyrase**
  * Mechanism of action: inhibit DNA synthesis in bacteria by way of inhibition of DNA gyrase involved with preventing supercoiling of DNA during replication.
  * Spectrum of activity: quinolones/fluoroquinolones: aerobic gram-negative rods, including *Pseudomonas* and *Neisseria*, active against anthrax.
  * Common adverse effects: nausea; may cause tendinitis and tendon rupture in all ages.
  * Cautions: should not be used during pregnancy, norfloxacin can be used only in UTIs and spontaneous bacterial peritonitis; may exacerbate muscle weakness in patients with myasthenia gravis; avoid concurrent use in this population.
  * Example agents: ciprofloxacin (Cipro), gemifloxacin (Factive), moxifloxacin (Avelox), norfloxacin, ofloxacin, levofloxacin (Levaquin).

C. **Selected Antimycobacterial Agents**
  1. **Isoniazid (INH)**
    * Mechanism of action: inhibits synthesis of mycobacterial cell walls by way of inhibition of mycolic acid synthesis.
    * Spectrum of activity: bactericidal for actively growing *Mycobacterium tuberculosis*.
    * Common adverse effects: allergic reactions, drug-induced lupus, rare (1%) drug-induced hepatitis (mild increases in aminotransferases are common, but usually asymptomatic), neuropathy (high doses).
    * Contraindications/cautions: pyridoxine given in patients at risk for neuropathy, can be used as monotherapy for prevention, but generally used in combination for treatment of active disease.
  2. **Rifampin (Rifadin)**
    * Mechanism of action: inhibits RNA synthesis.
    * Spectrum of activity: bactericidal for tubercle bacilli, many gram-positive and gram-negative organisms are susceptible.
    * Common adverse effects: rash, thrombocytopenia, nephritis.
    * Contraindications/cautions: orange discoloration of urine, sweat, tears; cytochrome P450 inducer so see many drug–drug interactions; generally used in combination for treatment of active disease.
  3. **Miscellaneous Agents Used for TB**
    * Ethambutol (Myambutol).
    * Pyrazinamide.
    * Streptomycin.

D. **Selected Antiviral Agents**
  1. **Nucleoside Reverse Transcriptase Inhibitors**
    * Mechanism of action: inhibit HIV reverse transcriptase.

* Common adverse effects: zidovudine (AZT)—myelosuppression (anemia and neutropenia), GI intolerance, headache, insomnia; didanosine (ddI)—peripheral neuropathy, pancreatitis, diarrhea, hyperuricemia, lactic acidosis, hepatomegaly with steatosis; lamivudine (3TC)—nausea, headache, fatigue, lactic acidosis, hepatomegaly with steatosis; stavudine (d4T)—peripheral neuropathy, oral ulcers lactic acidosis, hepatomegaly with steatosis.
* Contraindications/cautions: resistance is common to monotherapy—use in combination with other retrovirals, drug interactions common.
* Example agents: zidovudine (AZT, Retrovir), didanosine (ddI, Videx), lamivudine (3TC, Epivir), stavudine (d4T, Zerit).

2. **Nonnucleoside Reverse Transcriptase Inhibitors**
  * Mechanism of action: inhibit reverse transcriptase.
  * Common adverse effects: nevirapine and delavirdine—skin reactions, including Stevens–Johnson (nevirapine only), fulminant hepatitis, fever, nausea, headache, fatigue; efavirenz—dizziness, drowsiness/insomnia, headache, confusion, skin rash.
  * Contraindications/cautions: drug interactions common, resistance common with monotherapy.
  * Example agents: etravirine (Intelence), rilpivirine (Edurant), nevirapine (Viramune), delavirdine (Rescriptor), efavirenz (Sustiva).

3. **Protease Inhibitors**
  * Mechanism of action: inhibit production of mature virions, inhibit replication.
  * Common adverse effects: hyperlipidemia, redistribution of fat, truncal obesity and buffalo hump, GI distress, paresthesias (ritonavir), nephrolithiasis, urolithiasis, hyperbilirubinemia (indinavir).
  * Contraindications/cautions: resistance common with monotherapy, drug interactions common.
  * Example agents: darunavir (Prezista), atazanavir (Reyataz), saquinavir (Invirase), ritonavir (Norvir), indinavir (Crixivan), nelfinavir (Viracept), fosamprenavir (Lexiva).

4. **Hepatitis C Virus Direct-Acting Agents**
  * Mechanism of action: affect various stages of the hepatitis C virus (HCV) life cycle that are essential for viral replication, by inhibiting proteases needed for processing of HCV polyproteins, inhibiting RNA-dependent RNA polymerase, or by inhibiting specific proteins.
  * Common adverse effects: chills, headache, insomnia, dizziness, nausea, anemia, arthralgias, weakness, rash.
  * Contraindications/cautions: varies with specific agents; use with caution in advanced or decompensated hepatic insufficiency; monitor for drug interactions (especially CYP3A); assess for immunosuppression or hematologic changes; and monitor for development of severe rashes.

- Example agents: daclatasvir (Daklinza), elbasvir/grazoprevir (Zepatier), ledipasvir/sofosbuvir (Harvoni), ombitasvir/paritaprevir/ritonavir/dasabuvir (Viekira), simeprevir (Olysio), sofosbuvir (Sovaldi), sofosbuvir/velpatasvir (Epclusa).

XIV. Cancer Chemotherapeutic Agents

A. General Principles
- Goal of chemotherapy is to selectively kill cancer cells.
- Generally, chemotherapeutic agents target cancer cells as rapidly dividing cells.
- Common adverse effects include bone marrow suppression, hair loss, and GI distress, all of which are result of lack of specificity of the agents and targeting of rapidly dividing cells.
- Many of these intravenous agents are considered irritants or vesicants, which can cause significant skin damage, local tissue necrosis, and extravasation; take proper precautions upon ordering and administration.
- Resistance to cancer chemotherapeutic agents is a common clinical concern.
- This section provides an overview of major classes of agents; however, therapeutics within oncology is rapidly changing and many experimental agents are used. Therefore, specific protocols are not discussed. Most agents are used in combination in protocols for specific types of cancers.

B. Alkylating Agents
- Mechanism of action: in general, agents transfer an alkyl group to DNA, disrupting DNA replication that can include strand breakage.
- Therapeutic uses: leukemias, lymphomas, myeloma, breast, ovarian, testicular, genitourinary, brain cancers.
- Common adverse reactions: bone marrow suppression, alopecia, N/V, hemorrhagic cystitis (cyclophosphamide), renal dysfunction (cisplatin), local reactions at injection site.
- Example agents: cyclophosphamide (Cytoxan), busulfan (Myleran), carmustine (BCNU), cisplatin (Platinol), carboplatin (Paraplatin), oxaliplatin.

C. Antimetabolite Agents
- Mechanism of action: in general, inhibit enzymes in the replication pathway for cells.
- Therapeutic uses: lymphomas, gastric, breast, colorectal, and skin cancers.
- Common adverse reactions: bone marrow suppression, N/V.
- Example agents: capecitabine (Xeloda), cytarabine (ara-C), gemcitabine (Gemzar), fluorouracil (5FU), mercaptopurine (6-MP), methotrexate (MTX), thioguanine (6-TG).
- Leucovorin is a specific agent that can be given to "rescue" patients from high-dose MTX administration.

D. Inhibitors of Mitosis
- Mechanism of action: in general, agents bind to tubulin and prevent normal mitosis, resulting in disruption of cell division.
- Therapeutic uses: lymphomas, ovarian, breast, and lung cancer.
- Common adverse reactions: alopecia, muscle weakness, bone marrow suppression.
- Cautions: do not administer vinblastine intrathecally as death can result; only give vinblastine intravenously.
- Example agents: vincristine (Oncovin), vinblastine (Velban), paclitaxel (Taxol), docetaxel (Taxotere).

E. Hormone Regulators
- Mechanism of action: block receptors (estrogen receptors for tamoxifen), inhibit cytokine production (glucocorticoids such as prednisone), or mimic the effects of gonadotropin-releasing hormone (leuprolide).
- Therapeutic uses: breast cancer (tamoxifen), prostate cancer (flutamide and leuprolide), used to induce remission in leukemia (prednisone).
- Common adverse effects: related to inhibition of hormone (e.g., hot flashes with tamoxifen).
- Example agents: tamoxifen (Nolvadex), flutamide (Eulexin), prednisone, leuprolide (Lupron).

F. Intercalating Agents
- Mechanism of action: bind to DNA and prevent the synthesis of RNA or DNA.
- Therapeutic uses: leukemias, squamous cell carcinoma (bleomycin), lymphomas, testicular cancer.
- Common adverse effects: GI distress, cardiotoxicity (doxorubicin), alopecia, bone marrow suppression, allergic reaction (bleomycin).
- Cautions: as doxorubicin use can lead to heart failure, monitor lifetime cumulative amount given and do not exceed these limits.
- Example agents: daunorubicin (Cerubidine), doxorubicin (Adriamycin), bleomycin (Blenoxane).

REVIEW QUESTIONS

1. A 42-year-old man has just been prescribed a new drug. After several doses, he notices dry mouth, dry eyes, and a rapid heart rate. This is most likely due to an inhibition of which of the following neurotransmitter:

a) Norepinephrine
b) Serotonin
c) ACH
d) Epinephrine

2. Pindolol and some other β-adrenergic receptor antagonists have an additional property that is referred to as intrinsic sympathomimetic activity (ISA). This additional property indicates these agents are:

a) Full agonists
b) Inverse agonists
c) Partial agonists
d) Noncompetitive antagonists

3. A 53-year-old woman with COPD is using an albuterol inhaler for symptomatic relief of bronchospasm. She does not like using her inhaler because it causes:

a) Her lips to turn black
b) Her heart to beat faster
c) Numbness in her fingers and toes
d) Transient diminished hearing

4. The term "first-pass effect" refers to the:

a) Effect a new drug has on the body after its first administration
b) Time it takes for a drug to be detected in the urine or feces after oral administration
c) Ability of the intestines and liver to reduce the bioavailability of a drug
d) Time it takes for a drug to reach therapeutic concentrations in the target tissue

5. A 28-year-old woman is brought to the emergency department after overdosing on oxycodone, an opiate analgesic. She is unconscious and barely breathing when she arrives at the hospital, but revives and is breathing normally within 2 minutes after receiving an injection of naloxone. After about an hour, she requires another dose of naloxone as the symptoms of opiate overdose begin to redevelop. Naloxone is likely acting as a:

a) Strong stimulant that counteracts the CNS-depressant effects of the opiate
b) Diuretic that increases renal excretion of the opiate
c) Competitive antagonist of opioid receptors
d) Noncompetitive antagonist of opioid receptors

6. Which of the following antihypertensive medications may cause angioedema?

a) HCTZ
b) Lisinopril
c) Valsartan
d) B and C

7. Which of the following antihypertensive medications may cause hyperkalemia?

a) Hydralazine
b) Furosemide
c) Bumetanide
d) Spironolactone

8. All of the following statements regarding dabigatran are correct, EXCEPT:

a) It is an oral direct thrombin inhibitor.
b) It should be avoided in patients weighing >120 kg.
c) An antidote is available.
d) It may be safely used in patients with mechanical heart valves.

9. Which of the following anti-arrhythmic requires monitoring for pulmonary fibrosis?

a) Dofetilide
b) Sotalol
c) Amiodarone
d) Ibutilide

10. Which of the following antidepressants is contraindicated in patients with a history of bulimia?

a) Bupropion
b) Sertraline
c) Venlafaxine
d) Citalopram

11. Which of the following is an appropriate monitoring parameter for patients on opioids?

a) CBC
b) Occult blood test
c) CNS depression
d) Diarrhea

12. Which of the following therapeutic classes is ipratropium categorized as?

a) Short-acting β_2-agonist
b) Anticholinergic
c) Systemic corticosteroid
d) Methylxanthine

13. Which of the following is a common side effect of systemic corticosteroids?

a) Weight gain
b) Dry mouth
c) Headache
d) Sore throat

14. Which of the following medications is an example of a stimulant laxative?

a) Magnesium hydroxide
b) Psyllium
c) Loperamide
d) Bisacodyl

15. Which of the following is NOT a common side effect of α_1-adrenergic blockers?

a) Dizziness
b) Hypertension
c) Somnolence
d) Headache

16. A common side effect seen with sulfonylureas is
    a) Flatulence
    b) Hypoglycemia
    c) Upper respiratory infection
    d) Edema

17. The mechanism of oral contraceptives includes all of the following, EXCEPT:
    a) Inhibit ovulation by suppressing gonadotropins
    b) Thinning of the cervical mucus to inhibit sperm penetration
    c) Slow movement of the ovum through the fallopian tubes
    d) Alter the endometrium

18. A patient presents to your clinic with labs suggestive of hypertriglyceridemia; all other lipids are normal. The best drug choice for him is:
    a) Fenofibrate
    b) Lovastatin
    c) Niacin
    d) Ezetimibe

19. Which of the following is a cell wall inhibitor anti-infective?
    a) Tetracycline
    b) Ciprofloxacin
    c) Linezolid
    d) Vancomycin

20. Common side effects of chemotherapeutic agents include:
    a) Bone marrow suppression
    b) Hair loss
    c) GI distress
    d) All of the above

ANSWERS TO REVIEW QUESTIONS

1. **Answer: C.** These are common anticholinergic side effects. Most commonly, anticholinergics can cause the following side effects, which may be more pronounced in the elderly: drowsiness or sedation, blurred vision, dizziness, urinary retention, confusion or delirium, hallucinations, dry mouth, and constipation. (From Brown JH, Brandl K, Wess, J. Muscarinic receptor agonists and antagonists. In: Brunton LL, Hilal-Dandan R, Knollmann BC, eds. *Goodman and Gilman's: The Pharmacological Basis of Therapeutics.* 13th ed. New York, NY: McGraw-Hill; 2017:chap 9.)

2. **Answer: C.** ISA characterizes a group of β-blockers that are able to stimulate β-adrenergic receptors (agonist effect) and oppose the stimulating effects of catecholamines (antagonist effect) in a competitive way. ISA is defined in the Lexicomp database in the Pindolol drug monograph. (From Westfall TC, Macarthur H, Westfall DP. Adrenergic agonists and antagonists. In: Brunton

LL, Hilal-Dandan R, Knollmann BC, eds. *Goodman and Gilman's: The Pharmacological Basis of Therapeutics.* 13th ed. New York, NY: McGraw-Hill; 2017:chap 12.)

3. **Answer: B.** Tachycardiac listed as a common adverse effect of albuterol in the Lexicomp database in the albuterol drug monograph.

4. **Answer: C.** For some drugs, extensive first-pass metabolism greatly reduces their effectiveness or precludes their use as oral agents (e.g., lidocaine, propranolol, and naloxone). For other agents, the extent of absorption may be very low, thereby reducing bioavailability. (From Buxton ILO. Pharmacokinetics: the dynamics of drug absorption, distribution, metabolism, and elimination. In: Brunton LL, Hilal-Dandan R, Knollmann BC, eds. *Goodman and Gilman's: The Pharmacological Basis of Therapeutics.* 13th ed. New York, NY: McGraw-Hill; 2017:chap 2.)

5. **Answer: C.** The mechanism of action of naloxone as described in Lexicomp: naloxone is a pure opioid antagonist that competes and displaces opioids at opioid receptor sites.

6. **Answer: D.** Angioedema is an adverse effect associated with the ACEI and the angiotensin II receptor blocker classes of medications, described in Lexicomp—lisinopril and valsartan monographs.

7. **Answer: D.** As defined by its mechanism of action: spironolactone is a potassium-sparing diuretic that competes with aldosterone for receptor sites in the distal renal tubules, increasing sodium chloride and water excretion while conserving potassium and hydrogen ions. It may block the effect of aldosterone on arteriolar smooth muscle as well. (From Lexicomp, spironolactone monograph.)

8. **Answer: D.** Dabigatran is contraindicated for use in patients with mechanical prosthetic heart valve(s). (From Lexicomp, dabigatran monograph.)

9. **Answer: C.** Amiodarone has a specific warning that it has several potentially fatal toxicities, the most important of which is pulmonary toxicity (hypersensitivity pneumonitis or interstitial/alveolar pneumonitis) that has resulted in clinically manifest disease at rates as high as 10% to 17% in some series of patients with ventricular arrhythmias given doses of approximately 400 mg per day, and as abnormal diffusion capacity without symptoms in a much higher percentage of patients. Pulmonary toxicity has been fatal approximately 10% of the time. (From Lexicomp, amiodarone monograph.)

10. **Answer: A.** The use of bupropion is contraindicated in patients with a history of anorexia/bulimia. Bupropion is an effective antidepressant; however at higher doses, it may lower the seizure threshold, making it contraindicated in patients with a history of eating disorders and seizure disorders. Selective serotonin reuptake inhibitors (SSRIs) and serotonin-norepinephrine reuptake inhibitors (SNRIs) do not carry these warnings. (From Reference Lexicomp, bupropion monograph.)

11. **Answer: C**. Morphine and related opioids, aside from their effects as analgesics, produce a wide spectrum of effects reflecting the distribution of opiate receptors across organ systems. These effects include respiratory depression, nausea, vomiting, dizziness, mental clouding, dysphoria, pruritus, constipation, increased pressure in the biliary tract, urinary retention, hypotension, and, rarely, delirium. (From Yaksh T, Wallace M. Opioids, analgesia, and pain management. In: Brunton LL, Hilal-Dandan R, Knollmann BC, eds. *Goodman and Gilman's: The Pharmacological Basis of Therapeutics*. 13th ed. New York, NY: McGraw-Hill; 2017:chap 20.)

12. **Answer: B**. Pharmacologic class defined as an anticholinergic agent in Lexicomp, ipratropium monograph.

13. **Answer: A**. Corticosteroids can increase weight because glucocorticoids markedly affect carbohydrate and protein metabolism, which can be viewed as protecting glucose-dependent tissues (e.g., the brain and heart) from starvation. Glucocorticoids stimulate the liver to form glucose from amino acids and glycerol and to store glucose as glycogen. In the periphery, glucocorticoids diminish glucose utilization, increase protein breakdown and the synthesis of glutamine, and activate lipolysis, thereby providing amino acids and glycerol for gluconeogenesis. The net result is to increase blood glucose levels. Through their effects on glucose metabolism, glucocorticoids can worsen glycemic control in patients with overt diabetes and can precipitate the onset of hyperglycemia in susceptible patients. (From Schimmer BP, Funder JW. Adrenocorticotropic hormone, adrenal steroids, and the adrenal cortex. In: Brunton LL, Hilal-Dandan R, Knollmann BC, eds. *Goodman and Gilman's: The Pharmacological Basis of Therapeutics*. 13th ed. New York, NY: McGraw-Hill; 2017:chap 46.)

14. **Answer: D**. Bisacodyl is in the stimulant laxative pharmacologic class. (Listed in Lexicomp, bisacodyl monograph.)

15. **Answer: B**. The α_1A-receptor is the predominant receptor causing vasoconstriction in many vascular beds, including the following arteries: mammary, mesenteric, splenic, hepatic, omental, renal, pulmonary, and epicardial coronary. If the α_1A-receptor is inhibited, vasodilation would be expected. (From Westfall TC, Macarthur H, Westfall DP. Neurotransmission: the autonomic and somatic motor nervous systems (Section: Alpha Adrenergic Receptors). In: Brunton LL, Hilal-Dandan R, Knollmann BC, eds. *Goodman and Gilman's: The Pharmacological Basis of Therapeutics*. 13th ed. New York, NY: McGraw-Hill; 2017:chap 8.)

16. **Answer: B**. A common endocrine and metabolic adverse effect of sulfonylureas is hypoglycemia. (Listed in Lexicomp, glipizide, glimepiride, and glyburide monographs.)

17. **Answer: B**. Mechanism of action of combination oral contraceptives inhibit ovulation via a negative feedback mechanism on the hypothalamus, which alters the normal pattern of gonadotropin secretion of a FSH and luteinizing hormone by the anterior pituitary. The follicular phase FSH and midcycle surge of gonadotropins are inhibited. In addition, combination hormonal contraceptives produce alterations in the genital tract, including changes in the cervical mucus, rendering it unfavorable for sperm penetration even if ovulation occurs. Changes in the endometrium may also occur, producing an unfavorable environment for nidation. Combination hormonal contraceptive drugs may alter the tubal transport of the ova through the fallopian tubes. Progestational agents may also alter sperm fertility. (Listed in Lexicomp, ethinyl estradiol and norethindrone monographs.)

18. **Answer: A**. Fenofibrate is the only drug of the above listed agents indicated for adjunctive therapy to diet for treatment of adult patients with severe hypertriglyceridemia (Fredrickson types IV and V hyperlipidemia). (Listed in Lexicomp, fenofibrate monograph.)

19. **Answer: D**. The mechanism of action of vancomycin is inhibition of bacterial cell wall synthesis by blocking glycopeptide polymerization through binding tightly to D-alanyl-D-alanine portion of cell wall precursor. (Listed in Lexicomp, vancomycin monograph.)

20. **Answer: D**. All of the above are listed as common adverse effects of chemotherapeutic agents. (From Wellstein A, Giaccone G, Atkins MB, Sausville EA. Cytotoxic drugs. In: Brunton LL, Hilal-Dandan R, Knollmann BC, eds. *Goodman and Gilman's: The Pharmacological Basis of Therapeutics*. 13th ed. New York, NY: McGraw-Hill; 2017:chap 66.)

SELECTED REFERENCES

Brown J, Laiken N. Muscarinic receptor agonists and antagonists. In: Brunton LL, Chabner BA, Knollmann BC, eds. *Goodman & Gilman's: The Pharmacological Basis of Therapeutics*. 12th ed. New York, NY: McGraw-Hill; 2011. Also available at: http://accesspharmacy.mhmedical.com/content.aspx?bookid=1613&sectionid=102157962. Accessed June 8, 2017.

Connolly SJ, Ezekowitz MD, Yusuf S, et al; RE-LY Steering Committee and Investigators. Dabigatran versus warfarin in patients with atrial fibrillation. *N Engl J Med*. 2009;361:1139–1151.

Facts and Comparisons. Facts and Comparisons E-answers. online.factsandcomparisons.com. Accessed June 7, 2017.

Giugliano RP, Ruff CT, Braunwald E, et al; ENGAGE AF-TIMI 48 Investigators. Edoxaban versus warfarin in patients with atrial fibrillation. *N Engl J Med*. 2013;369:2093–2104.

Granger CB, Alexander JH, McMurray JJ, et al; ARISTOTLE Committees and Investigators. Apixaban versus warfarin in patients with atrial fibrillation. *N Engl J Med*. 2011;365:981–992.

Jackson CW, Cates ME. Major depressive disorder. In: Chisholm-Burns MA, Schwinghammer TL, Wells BG, et al, eds. *Pharmacotherapy Principles & Practice*. 4th ed. New York, NY: McGraw Hill Medical; 2016:chap 38:583–598.

James PA, Oparil S, Carter BL, et al. Evidence-based guideline for the management of high blood pressure in adults: report from the panel members appointed to the Eighth Joint National Committee (JNC 8). *JAMA*. 2014;311(5):507–520.

Kelly DL, Weiner E, Wehring HJ. Schizophrenia. In: Chisholm-Burns MA, Schwinghammer TL, Wells BG, et al, eds. *Pharmacotherapy Principles & Practice*. 4th ed. New York, NY: McGraw Hill Medical; 2016:chap 37:563–582.

Lexicomp Online. June 7, 2016. Hudson, OH: Lexicomp, Inc. Also available at: online.lexi.com.

McEvoy GK, Miller JL, Snow EK, et al, eds. *AHFS Drug Information*. Bethesda, MD; American Society of Health-System Pharmacists; 2017.

Papadakis MA, McPhee SJ, Rabow MW, eds. *Current Medical Diagnosis & Treatment*. New York, NY: McGraw-Hill; 2017. Also available at: http://accessmedicine.mhmedical.com/content.aspx?bookid=1843&sectionid=135696929. Accessed June 8, 2017.

Parra D, Roman Y, Anastasia E, Straka RJ. Hypertension. In: Chisholm-Burns MA, Schwinghammer TL, Wells BG, et al, eds. *Pharmacotherapy Principles & Practice*. 4th ed. New York, NY: McGraw Hill Medical; 2016:chap 5:45–64.

Patel MR, Mahaffey MD, Garg J, et al; ROCKET AF Investigators. Rivaroxaban versus warfarin in nonvalvular atrial fibrillation. *N Engl J Med*. 2011;365:883–891.

Sampson KJ, Kass RS. Anti-arrhythmic drugs. In: Brunton LL, Chabner BA, Knollmann BC, eds. *Goodman & Gillman's: The Pharmacological Basis of Therapeutics*. 12th ed. New York, NY: McGraw-Hill; 2011. Also available at: http://accesspharmacy.mhmedical.mhmedical.com/content.aspx?bookid=1613&sectionid=102160425. Accessed June 7, 2017.

Smith TR, Wagner ML. Parkinson disease. In: Chisholm-Burns MA, Schwinghammer TL, Wells BG, et al, eds. *Pharmacotherapy Principles & Practice*. 4th ed. New York, NY: McGraw Hill Medical; 2016:chap 33:507–520.

Taylor P. Anticholinesterase agents. In: Brunton LL, Chabner BA, Knollmann BC, eds. *Goodman & Gilman's: The Pharmacological Basis of Therapeutics*. 12th ed. New York, NY: McGraw-Hill; 2011. Also available at: http://accesspharmacy.mhmedical.com/content.aspx?bookid=1613&sectionid=102158067. Accessed June 8, 2017.

Tisdale JE. Arrhythmias. In: Chisholm-Burns MA, Schwinghammer TL, Wells BG, et al, eds. *Pharmacotherapy Principles & Practice*. 4th ed. New York, NY: McGraw Hill Medical; 2016:chap 9:137–162.

Trevor AJ, Katzung BG, Kruidering-Hall M, eds. *Katzung & Trevor's Pharmacology: Examination & Board Review*. 11th ed. New York, NY: McGraw-Hill; 2015:chaps 2–4, 7–10, 43–47, 49, 54. Also available at: http://accesspharmacy.mhmedical.com/content.aspx?bookid=1568&sectionid=95704826. Accessed June 8, 2017.

U.S. Food and Drug Administration. Drugs at FDA. https://www.accessdata.fda.gov/scripts/cder/daf/. Accessed June 7, 2017.

Vardeny O, Ng TM. Heart failure. In: Chisholm-Burns MA, Schwinghammer TL, Wells BG, et al, eds. *Pharmacotherapy Principles & Practice*. 4th ed. New York, NY: McGraw Hill Medical; 2016:chap 6:65–90.

Welty TE, Faught E. Epilepsy. In: Chisholm-Burns MA, Schwinghammer TL, Wells BG, et al, eds. *Pharmacotherapy Principles & Practice*. 4th ed. New York, NY: McGraw Hill Medical; 2016:chap 31:477–496.

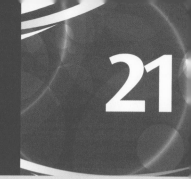

Pediatric Care and Common Disorders

21

Petar Breitinger

I. Evaluation and Care of the Newborn Infant

A. Perinatal Care

- Antenatal evaluation must begin with a thorough history including the current and past medical history of the mother and father, obstetric history, and current pregnancy including the labor and delivery.
- Newborns should have a brief examination at birth consisting of Apgar scores at 1 and 5 minutes; brief examination for congenital anomalies, measurements, vital signs, and skin color; musculoskeletal examination for birth trauma; and examination of the umbilical cord (number of vessels—two arteries and one vein) and the placenta for abnormalities. A complete examination should take place later in the nursery or mother's room within 24 hours of birth.
- Vitamin K should be administered within 4 hours of birth to prevent hemorrhagic disease of the newborn.
- Erythromycin ophthalmic ointment (0.5%) should be administered at the time of delivery for prophylaxis against gonococcal ophthalmia neonatorum.
- Monitoring for hyperbilirubinemia and hypoglycemia.
- Hepatitis B vaccination within 24 hours of delivery.
- Screening for hearing loss, metabolic and genetic disorders, and critical congenital heart disease (CHD).

B. The Newborn Examination

1. **General Survey**
   - **A general inspection of the infant is the first and most important step in the examination and provides much information in a short time.**
   - Determination of sex.
   - Gross deformities or malformations suggesting the presence of a syndrome.
   - Respirations—observe for paradoxical breathing, respiratory distress: nasal flaring, rapid breathing (normal respiratory rate for term neonate is 40–60 breaths per minute), accessory muscle use, and grunting respirations.
   - Activity, cry, tone, and posture. High-pitched cry with or without hypotonia may suggest central nervous system (CNS) disease (hemorrhage, infection, congenital neuromuscular disorder).
   - Edema (may be generalized [hydrops] or localized).

- State of maturity/gestational age. The Dubowitz examination is used to determine a baby's gestational age. It was devised by Lilly Dubowitz, a Hungarian-born British pediatrician, and her husband, the British neurologist Victor Dubowitz. This examination evaluates both physical and neurologic characteristics and in the aggregate, and estimates the baby's gestational age within 1 to 2 weeks of the true gestational age. It assigns a score to various criteria (0–4), the sum of all of which is then extrapolated to the gestational age of the fetus. The physical and neurologic criteria, along with the expected findings, are summarized in Table 21–1.

TABLE 21–1.	**Summary of External Characteristics of the Dubowitz Examination**
Criteria	**Expected Finding**
Edema	No edema
Skin texture	Slight thickening, superficial cracking and peeling, especially hands and feet
Skin color (infant not crying)	Pale, only pink over ears, lips, palms, or soles
Skin opacity (truck)	A few large vessels seen indistinctly over abdomen
Lanugo (over back)	At least half of back devoid of lanugo
Plantar 5 mg/dL creases	Definite deep indentations over more than anterior third
Nipple formation	Areola stippled, edge not raised
Breast size	Breast tissue both sides; one or both >1 cm
Ear form	Ear form incurving whole upper pinna
Ear firmness	Pinna firm, cartilage to edge, instant recoil
Genitalia, male	At least one testis right down
Genitalia, female (with hips half abducted)	Labia majora completely cover labia minora

2. **Vital Signs**
   - **Recorded every 30 to 60 minutes during first 4 to 6 hours of life, and then every 8 to 12 hours thereafter. Normal vital sign values:**
     - Axilla temperature: 36.5° to 37.5° C (97.7°–99.5° F).
     - Respiratory rate: 30 to 60 breaths per minute. Counted for a full minute.
     - Heart rate: 120 to 160 beats per minute.
     - Systolic blood pressure: 50 to 70 mm Hg on day 1 of life. Increases during first week of life.
     - Pulse oximetry: ≥95% in the right hand or foot AND ≤3% difference between the right hand and foot, to be done after 24 hours of life or before hospital discharge.

3. **Skin**
   - Color.
   - Cyanosis.
     - Peripheral cyanosis of the hands and feet, known as acrocyanosis, is normal and will usually disappear after several days of life.
     - Generalized or central cyanosis (tongue and mucous membranes) should prompt evaluation for respiratory, cardiac, or metabolic disorder.
   - Pallor: may represent acute or chronic blood loss.
   - Plethora: seen in polycythemia.
   - Ecchymoses, purpura, or erythema: may represent birth trauma. (Purpura may also represent congenital infection.)
   - Jaundice: always considered pathologic in the first day of life (hemolytic process or congenital hepatitis).
   - Harlequin color change: transient, striking, but normal sign of vasomotor instability and divides the body from head to pubis through the midline, into equal halves of pink and pale color.
   - Lanugo hair: may be present over back and shoulders.
   - Vernix caseosa: a soft creamy substance covering the skin in preterm infants that decreases in amount as fetus approaches term.
   - Meconium staining of skin/umbilical stump.
   - Nevus flammeus (port-wine stain): vascular malformations anywhere on the body; may be benign or associated with other abnormalities (glaucoma) or syndromes (Sturge–Weber or Klippel–Trenaunay syndrome).
   - Common abnormalities.
     - Mongolian spots: dark blue-to-black pigmented macules seen over the lower back and buttocks in 90% of darker pigmented babies.
     - Nevus simplex (salmon patch): pink, macular hemangiomas, usually transient and noted on the back of the neck, eyelids, and forehead.
     - Capillary hemangiomas: benign, raised red lesions.
     - Cavernous hemangiomas: deeper, blue-colored benign masses. **NOTE:** Both capillary and cavernous hemangiomas increase in size after birth, only to resolve between 1 and 4 years of age.
     - Erythema toxicum: benign, erythematous rash characterized by erythematous macules, with central papule or pustule; very common in neonates and usually develops between 24 and 48 hours after birth.
     - Pustular melanosis: more common in infants with darkly pigmented skin; these consist of a small vesicle on a pigmented brown macular base. A scale forms as the vesicle ruptures.
     - Milia: yellow-white epidermal cysts that can be found on the nose.

4. **Head**
   - Head circumference.
   - Shape of the head and molding: resolves 2 to 3 days after birth.
   - Fontanels and suture lines should be palpated. Anterior fontanelle size is 1 to 4 cm in any direction, posterior fontanelle should be <1 cm. Large fontanelles may signify hypothyroidism; trisomy 13, 18, or 21; or bone disease.
   - Craniosynostosis: prematurely fused suture causing abnormal cranial deformity.
   - Craniotabes: slight indentation and recoil of parietal bones elicited by light pressure is normal in newborns.
   - Cephalohematoma: a subperiosteal collection of blood caused by localized trauma that appears as a firm swelling on day 1 and does not cross suture lines. May take weeks to months to resolve.
   - Caput succedaneum: edema of the presenting part of the scalp following a vertex delivery. Edema is soft and crosses the suture lines.
   - Head tilt: congenital torticollis.

5. **Face**
   - Characteristic facies of disease (i.e., Down syndrome, fetal alcohol syndrome, and congenital hypothyroidism).
   - Facial hemiparesis: results from pressure on sacral promontory in utero, or forceps trauma.

6. **Eyes**
   - Lid edema is common.
   - Note symmetry and spacing of eyes. Hypertelorism associated with trisomy 13, where prominent epicanthal folds can suggest trisomy 21.
   - Assess extraocular eye movement.
   - Conjunctival, retinal, and sclera hemorrhage: present during birth trauma.
   - Pupil: papillary reflex should be present.
   - Retina: a red reflex should be present in ophthalmoscopic examination. A white reflex (leukocoria) should be evaluated for glaucoma, cataracts, or retinoblastoma.
   - Chemical conjunctivitis is common in first 24 to 48 hours from erythromycin.

7. **Ears**
   - Low-set ears: may be sign of genetic disorders (i.e., Down syndrome and Turner syndrome).
   - Preauricular skin tags or pits: may be associated with hearing loss or may be familial.
   - Visualize tympanic membranes (TMs): may be opaque in appearance with decreased mobility.
   - Newborn hearing screening test is performed before leaving the hospital.

8. **Nose**
   - Check patency bilaterally: cyanosis that improves with crying is significant for choanal atresia.
   - Check for purulent discharge suggestive of congenital syphilis.

9. **Mouth**
   - Cleft lip.
   - Cleft palate: check for hard and soft palate.
   - Natal teeth: should be removed if mobile.
   - Prominent tongue present with trisomy 21.
   - Epstein pearls: benign, white, beady papules on the hard palate (keratin cysts).

10. **Neck**
    - Mobility.
    - Masses: usually vascular malformations, dermoid cysts, or thyroglossal duct cyst.
    - Torticollis results from sternocleidomastoid muscle trauma by birth injury or intrauterine malposition.
    - Clavicles: the most common fracture resulting from birth trauma is to the clavicle.
    - Redundant skin may represent Turner or Down syndrome.

11. **Chest**
    - Shape and symmetry.
    - Breast hypertrophy: breasts are palpable in mature males and in females.
    - Supernumerary nipples: bilateral and occasionally are associated with renal anomalies.

12. **Lungs**
    - Respiratory rate: typical rate should be 30 to 60 breaths per minute.
    - Character: breathing is abdominal. Expiratory grunting may signify hyaline membrane disease (HMD).
    - Retractions: with tachypnea, may be a sign of respiratory distress syndrome.
    - Auscultation: diminished or absent breath sounds on one side may suggest a pneumothorax or a diaphragmatic hernia.

13. **Heart**
    - Heart rate: typical rate should be 120 to 160 beats per minute. May decrease to 85 to 90 during sleep.
    - Rhythm: initially may be irregular caused by premature atrial contractions. Considered benign and resolves within the first few days of life.
    - Murmurs: transient murmurs heard during the first few hours up to a day are common and benign, but persistent murmurs or murmurs associated with other signs of cardiac disease require further evaluation.
    - Pulses: check both the upper and the lower extremities. Diminished femoral pulses may suggest coarctation of the aorta.

14. **Abdomen**
    - Check for shape and symmetry. Normally slightly protuberant. Distension may indicate intestinal obstruction, ascites, or organomegaly.
    - A scaphoid abdomen with respiratory distress suggests a diaphragmatic hernia.
    - Diastasis recti: a normal finding that represents incomplete closure of the two rectus muscles.
    - Palpation: liver palpated 2 cm below right costal margin. The tip of the spleen may be palpable. Kidneys should be palpated bilaterally.
    - Umbilical cord:
      - Should have three vessels: two arteries and one vein.
      - Erythema of the cord may represent infection (omphalitis).
      - Oozing of blood: provides clue to bleeding disorder.
      - Umbilical or inguinal hernias.
    - Anus: check for patency.

15. **Genitalia**
    - Edema is common.
    - Ambiguous genitalia should be ruled out.
    - Male:
      - Testes: both testes should be descended.
      - Scrotum: scrotal swelling may represent a transient hydrocele.
      - Meatus: check for epispadias, hypospadias, or meatal stenosis.
      - Foreskin: common for newborn to have congenital phimosis; does not forcibly retract foreskin.
    - Female:
      - Imperforate hymen may be visible.
      - A whitish discharge, with or without blood, may be present.

16. **Spine**
    - Midline lumbosacral lesions may represent spinal dysraphism and should have magnetic resonance imaging (MRI) or spinal ultrasound.
      - Myelomeningocele.
      - Lipomas.
      - Dimples.
      - Sinus tracts.
      - Hemangiomas.
      - Hypertrichosis.
    - Scoliosis: check for abnormal curvature of the spine.

17. **Extremities**
    - Symmetry and length.
    - Simian crease: present in Down syndrome.
    - Erb palsy: due to brachial plexus injury during delivery.
    - Deformities: clubfoot, polydactyly, and syndactyly.
    - Hips: examine for signs of developmental dysplasia of the hip.
        - Barlow sign: "clunk" represents dislocatability in posterior–superior direction (Figure 21–1A).
        - Ortolani sign: "clunk" represents relocation into joint (Figure 21–1B).
        - Galeazzi sign: foreshortening of the affected limb (femur will appear shorter with knees flexed) (Figure 21–2).
        - Limited abduction at the hip.
        - Asymmetric subgluteal skin creases (nonspecific sign).

18. **Neurologic**
    - Assess muscle tone and strength.
    - Check for primitive reflexes: Moro, Babinski, palmar grasp, sucking, rooting, stepping, and abdominal reflexes.

C. Care and Discharge of the Normal Newborn
- Following stabilization, the infant's vital signs, voiding, stooling, and feeding patterns should be recorded every 8 hours.
- The normal term neonate passes meconium in the first 24 hours and voids within the first 12 hours. If there is a delay, 48 and 24 hours, respectively, there may be an obstruction.
- Infants should be placed in the supine position to reduce risk of sudden infant death syndrome (SIDS).
- State-mandated newborn metabolic/genetic screening tests are typically performed at 24 to 48 hours of life, and typically include testing for in-born errors of metabolism, congenital hypothyroidism, sickle cell anemia, and cystic fibrosis (CF).
- Prior to discharge, infant has been evaluated for sepsis.
- The decision to circumcise an infant should be made by the parents after consultation with a pediatrician. If circumcised, there should be no evidence of excessive bleeding prior to discharge.
- Neonates and their mothers are typically discharged after 24 to 48 hours. Infants' vital signs should be stable and within normal range for 12 hours prior to discharge.
- Hepatitis B vaccination is typically administered before discharge.
- Parental education on both routine infant care/safety and signs/symptoms of concern to watch for (i.e., fever, jaundice, lethargy, irritability, poor feeding, and vomiting) should be given before discharge.

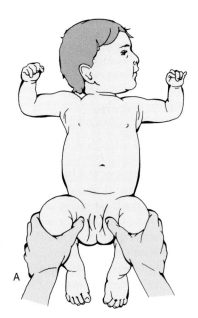
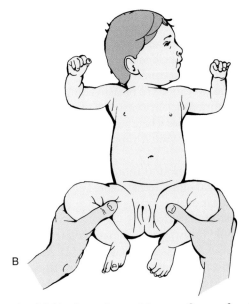

FIGURE 21–1. **Assessing for Barlow and Ortolani signs.** Place the child in the supine position on a firm surface. Be gentle, not forceful. **A:** Barlow test is used to detect hip instability. The located hip is subluxed or dislocated during the maneuver. The examiner's fingers are placed over the child's greater trochanters. Holding the hips and knees at 90° of flexion, a backward pressure is applied while adducting the hips. The femoral head is felt slipping out of the acetabulum posterolaterally when the test is positive. **B:** Ortolani sign is present when the hip is dislocated. The maneuver relocates the femoral head. With the examiner's fingers on the child's greater trochanters, the hips and knees are flexed to 90°. The hips are then abducted while applying upward pressure over the greater trochanter. A positive sign is detected when a "clunk" is felt as the femoral head re-enters the acetabulum. (From Nettina SM. *The Lippincott Manual of Nursing Practice.* 7th ed. Philadelphia, PA: Lippincott Williams & Wilkins; 2001, with permission.)

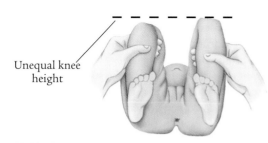

Unequal knee
height

FIGURE 21–2. **Diagnosing developmental dysplasia of the hip (DDH).** Galeazzi sign—when knees are flexed and feet together, the knee on the affected side appears lower. (Asset provided by Anatomical Chart Co.)

D. Feeding the Newborn
1. Breastfeeding
- One of the most important influences on children's health worldwide. The World Health Organization recommends exclusive breastfeeding for the first 6 months of life and continued breastfeeding with age-appropriate supplementation through 2 years of life.
- Advantages of breastfeeding:
  - Numerous immunoactive immunologic factors are present in breast milk and provide protection against gastrointestinal (GI) and upper respiratory infections (URIs), allergic and atopic disease, and some chronic adult diseases.
  - Increased maternal–infant bonding.
  - Decreased cost.
  - Delayed return of maternal fertility.
  - Faster return to prepregnancy weight.
  - Decreased maternal incidence of ovarian and premenopausal breast cancer.
- Absolute contraindications to breastfeeding:
  - Human immunodeficiency virus (HIV) infection in developed countries where suitable formula preparations and safe water supply are available.
  - Active tuberculosis.
  - Use of some medications (lithium, radioactive iodine, antimetabolites, tetracycline, and antithyroid medications).
  - Maternal use of illicit drugs.
- Neonates should breastfeed on demand (typically every 2–3 hours with longer periods at night). After 3 days of life, the infant should feed from 10 to 15 minutes on each side for every feed.
- Failure to pass several stools each day in the early weeks of life suggests inadequate milk intake and supply.
- Common problems:
  - Sore nipples may indicate improper positioning or improper latch on. It may be managed by correcting these, air-drying nipples, and application of lanolin after feeds.

- Breastfeeding jaundice should be managed by increasing the frequency of nursing or temporary formula feeding for 24 to 36 hours.
- Maternal mastitis should be treated with β-lactam antibiotics and analgesics as necessary; breastfeeding should continue. Presence of an abscess requires temporary discontinuation of breastfeeding on the affected side.

2. Formula Feeding
- The standard 20 kcal per oz infant formulas are adequate for use in newborns.
- Soy protein formulas are indicated in infants with lactose intolerance.
- Soy formulas may be substituted when cow's milk protein allergy is suspected; however, infants who are truly allergic to cow's milk protein are frequently allergic to soy protein as well.
- Semielemental formulas are effective in feeding infants who cannot tolerate cow's milk or soy protein and are useful in infants with malabsorptive conditions.

3. Weight Loss
- Term infants can lose up to 10% of their body weight during the first few days despite proper feeding. Typically, the infants will regain body weight by 10 to 14 days.

II. Common Disorders/Diseases of the Newborn
A. Colic
1. Etiology
- The etiology of colic is not well understood; some of the following factors may have a role and have been suggested as causes: GI, behavioral, and parental.

2. Clinical Features
- Characterized by the "Rule of 3s": prolonged bouts of crying for a total of >3 hours a day, for more than 3 days per week, and for longer than 3 weeks in a previously well infant with no apparent underlying cause.
- Crying spells are characterized by clenched fists, posturing with the knees drawn up, and minimal response to attempts to calm the infant.
- Spells typically occur in the late afternoon or evening, but can occur at any time.
- Begins in first few weeks of life and peaks between 2 and 3 months of age. May continue into the fourth and fifth months.

3. Management
- Careful history and physical examination (PE) to search for organic cause of fussiness—that is, URI, otitis media (OM), urinary tract infection (UTI), and GI disease.
- If the evaluation discloses no underlying cause, conservative management is acceptable.

- Supportive, sympathetic instruction to parents regarding colic and its benign nature.
- Regular schedule for feedings and naps to avoid chaotic routines and overfeeding or underfeeding.
- Low-level sound in the infant's sleeping area, such as a radio or vacuum cleaner, may be soothing.
- Gentle movement in a swing, or rides in an automobile.
- A trial of a milk-free diet may help an infant with true cow's milk allergy, but avoid frequent formula changes.
- Rest and assistance for the infant's caretakers is essential to prevent exhaustion.
- Medications are only occasionally useful and include antihistamines, antispasmodics, and antacids.

B. Neonatal Jaundice

1. Epidemiology
- Seen in up to 65% of neonates in the first week of life, with total serum bilirubin (TSB) levels of up to 6 mg per dL.
- Eight to 10% of newborns develop excessive hyperbilirubinemia (TSB > 17 mg per dL), and 1% to 2% have TSB levels above 20 mg.
- Extremely high levels are rare, but potentially dangerous due to risk of kernicterus.

2. Etiology
- Physiologic causes.
- Increased bilirubin production:
  - Antibody-mediated hemolysis (maternal–infant ABO-incompatibility or Rh-isoimmunization). Coombs test positive.
  - Nonimmune hemolysis (hereditary spherocytosis and G6PD deficiency). Coombs test negative.
  - Nonhemolytic increased production (enclosed hemorrhage, i.e., cephalohematoma or excessive bruising from birth trauma, polycythemia, and bowel obstruction).
- Decreased conjugation:
  - Crigler–Najjar syndrome.
  - Gilbert syndrome.
- Unknown factors:
  - Prematurity.
  - Ethnicity (Asians have higher risk than Caucasians or African Americans).
- Breast milk jaundice.
- Congenital infection.

3. Pathophysiology
- Hyperbilirubinemia may be conjugated (always pathologic) or unconjugated (may be physiologic or pathologic).
- Most infants will develop a transient hyperbilirubinemia during the first week of life because of:
  - Increased bilirubin production secondary to increased red blood cell volume, decreased

RBC survival time, and increased enterohepatic circulation.
  - Limited hepatic reuptake of bilirubin.
  - Inadequate conjugation and reduced bilirubin excretion.

4. Clinical Manifestations
- Visible jaundice that progresses in a cephalocaudal direction, and TSB levels may be estimated by the extent of progression of visible jaundice:
  - Involving the face: TSB is approximately 5 mg per dL.
  - Involving the mid-abdomen: TSB is approximately 15 mg per dL.
  - Involving the feet: TSB is approximately 20 mg per dL.
- Estimations should not be relied upon to guide management decisions; the use of transcutaneous bilirubinometry or serum levels is recommended.
- Jaundice will typically appear after 24 hours of life peak at 3 to 5 days of life and resolve by 7 days (term infants) or 14 days (premature infants).
- Breast milk jaundice is seen exclusively in breast-fed infants, and peak levels tend to be higher and last longer.
- Signs of pathologic jaundice include:
  - Clinically evident jaundice in the first 24 hours of life.
  - Indirect unconjugated hyperbilirubinemia lasting longer than 7 days (in a term infant)—suggests hemolysis.
  - Conjugated hyperbilirubinemia (direct fraction exceeds 2 mg per dL or 15% of TSB level).
  - Bilirubin levels increasing at a rate of >0.5 mg/dL/hour.
- Severely elevated levels of bilirubin may result in kernicterus—which is characterized by bilirubin deposition and staining in the basal ganglia and hippocampus. Affected infants show spasticity, muscular incoordination, and variable degrees of cognitive impairment.

5. Diagnostic Studies
- Total bilirubin is increased.
- Indirect bilirubin (increased when unconjugated hyperbilirubinemia is the cause).
- Direct bilirubin (increased when conjugated hyperbilirubinemia is the cause).
- Complete blood count (CBC) with differential and RBC morphology.
- Reticulocyte count (increased with hemolysis).
- Blood type and Rh on mother and infant.
- Direct coombs test on infant (if at risk for ABO or Rh incompatibility).

6. Treatment
- Phototherapy: a commonly used rule of thumb in the Neonate Intensive Care Unit is to start phototherapy when the TSB level is more than five times

the birth weight. For example, in a 1-kg infant, phototherapy is started at a bilirubin level of 5 mg per dL; in a 2-kg infant, phototherapy is started at a bilirubin level of 10 mg per dL.
- Exchange transfusion.
- Treat underlying cause if applicable.

C. Hyaline Membrane Disease
1. **Pathophysiology**
   - Deficiency or inactivation of pulmonary surfactant, leading to a decrease in surface tension in the alveolus.
   - Decreased surface tension results in poor lung compliance and atelectasis.
   - Leads to hypoxemia and ultimately respiratory failure.
2. **Epidemiology**
   - Seen most commonly in preterm infants. Incidence is:
     - Five percent in infants born between 35 and 36 weeks of gestation.
     - Greater than 50% in infants born before 28 weeks.
     - Male gender and white ethnicity associated with increased risk.
   - Other risk factors:
     - Cesarean birth.
     - Birth asphyxia.
     - Infants of diabetic mothers.
     - Siblings with the history of HMD.
3. **Clinical Features**
   - Cyanosis.
   - Grunting with expiration.
   - Tachypnea.
   - Nasal flaring.
   - Intercostal retractions.
   - Progressive dyspnea.
   - Respiratory failure.
4. **Diagnostic Studies**
   - Pulse oximetry: hypoxemia.
   - Chest X-ray (CXR).
     - Bilateral atelectasis with a "ground-glass" appearance.
     - Air bronchograms.
     - Hypoinflation/doming of diaphragms.
5. **Management**
   - Prevention:
     - Administration of steroids to mothers in preterm labor or conditions where preterm labor is likely reduces mortality rate.
     - Administration of artificial surfactant in the delivery room in infants born before 27 weeks.
   - Treatment:
     - Supplemental oxygen.
     - Nasal continuous positive airway pressure (CPAP).
     - Tracheal intubation and administration of artificial surfactant as rescue therapy if oxygen and CPAP ineffective.

D. Meconium Aspiration Syndrome
1. **Etiology/Epidemiology**
   - Passage of meconium before delivery with subsequent aspiration of material.
   - More common in term and post-term infants: up to 20% will pass meconium before delivery. Incidence of meconium aspiration syndrome (MAS) is up to 1.8% in developed countries.
2. **Pathophysiology**
   - Aspiration of the meconium leading to in utero asphyxia.
3. **Clinical Features**
   - Signs of respiratory distress.
     - Tachypnea.
     - Retractions.
     - Nasal flaring.
     - Grunting.
   - Barrel chest.
   - Coarse breath sounds or rales.
4. **Diagnostic Studies**
   - Blood cultures to differentiate pneumonia from MAS.
   - CXR to confirm diagnosis.
     - Hyperinflation with patchy infiltrates.
     - Pneumothorax may be present in 20% to 50% of affected infants.
5. **Management**
   - Amnioinfusion and intrapartum oro/nasopharyngeal suctioning are *not* recommended to prevent MAS.
   - Infants who are covered with thick meconium at delivery should receive adequate tracheal suctioning.
   - Management is otherwise symptomatic:
     - Humidified O_2.
     - Intubation/ventilation.
     - Use of antibiotics is controversial. May begin empirical therapy while awaiting results from blood culture.

E. Perinatal/Congenital Infections (TORCH)
1. **Etiology**
   - "TORCH" represents a group of parasitic, bacterial, and viral pathogens producing congenital and perinatally acquired infections: *Toxoplasmosis, Other, Rubella, Cytomegalovirus* (CMV), and *Herpes simplex virus* (HSV).
   - "Other" represents an increasing number of infections such as syphilis; gonorrhea; TB; HIV; parvovirus; varicella zoster; Zika virus; malaria; *Borrelia burgdorferi*; coxsackievirus; hepatitis B, C, or G; and other viruses.
   - Infections may be acquired in utero, intrapartum, or postnatally.
2. **Clinical Features**
   - Signs and symptoms vary slightly by etiologic agent, but classic presentation includes:
     - Intrauterine growth retardation.
     - Nonimmune hydrops.

- Anemia.
- Thrombocytopenia.
- Jaundice (especially in the first 24 hours of birth).
- Hepatosplenomegaly.
- Chorioretinitis.
- Congenital malformations.
- Seizures.
- Rash.
- Hearing loss.
- Microcephaly.
- Cataract.

3. **Diagnostic Studies**
   - Isolate organism by culture: rubella, HSV, CMV, *Neisseria gonorrhea*, and *Mycobacterium tuberculosis*.
   - Identify antigen: hepatitis B and *Chlamydia trachomatis*.
   - Identify fetal production of antibodies: immunoglobulin M (IgM), or increasing titer of IgG for *Toxoplasma*, syphilis, HIV, and *Borrelia*.

4. **Management**
   - Treat specific pathogen after it is confirmed.

F. Apparent Life-Threatening Events of Infancy
   1. **Episode that is frightening to the observer and involves any combination of apnea, color change, change in muscle tone, choking, or gagging.**
   2. **Epidemiology**
      - Peak incidence between 1 and 2 months of age.
      - Male-to-female ratio is 2:1.
      - Known risk factors include:
        - Prematurity.
        - Respiratory syncytial virus (RSV) infection.
        - Anatomic abnormalities.
        - Known gastroesophageal reflux disease (GERD).
   3. **Etiology**
      - Fifty percent of cases have no identifiable cause and are classified as apnea of infancy.
      - GI (i.e., GERD).
      - Neurologic (i.e., CNS infection, seizure disorder, and central apnea).
      - Respiratory (i.e., bronchiolitis, pneumonia, and upper respiratory tract infection).
      - Cardiovascular (i.e., CHD, dysrhythmias, and cardiomyopathy).
      - Metabolic (i.e., hypoglycemia and electrolyte abnormalities).
      - Infectious (i.e., sepsis).
      - Nonaccidental injury/poisoning (i.e., shaken baby syndrome).
   4. **Clinical Features**
      - Apnea: defined as >20 seconds without breathing, or apneic period of any duration with associated change in color, tone, or heart rate.
        - Central apnea: associated with no chest wall movement.

- Obstructive apnea (i.e., GERD and respiratory secretions): associated with paradoxical chest wall movements.
- Normal periodic breathing of infancy: pauses of several seconds interspersed with normal periods of breathing.
- Color change: usually cyanosis or pallor.
- Change in muscle tone: usually infant will be limp.
- Choking or gagging.

5. **Diagnostic Studies**
   - CBC.
   - Electrolytes.
   - Arterial blood gases (ABGs).
   - O_2 saturation.
   - Blood cultures.
   - CXR.
   - Other studies as guided by history and PE (i.e., lumbar puncture [LP], electroencephalogram [EEG], polysomnography, and esophageal pH).

6. **Treatment**
   - Based on the management of underlying cause (i.e., anti-reflux medications and antibiotics).
   - Caffeine or aminophylline is indicated in certain cases of apnea of infancy.
   - All caregivers should be trained in cardiopulmonary resuscitation (CPR) before discharge from the hospital.
   - Use of home apnea monitors is controversial and has not been shown to reduce the incidence of SIDS.

III. Principles of Health Supervision and Preventive Care of Children

A. General Principles
   - Health supervision visits should focus on the following: disease surveillance, screening, detection and prevention, health promotion, and anticipatory guidance as outlined in the American Academy of Pediatrics (AAP) Bright Futures Guide to Preventive Services.
   - Provide immunizations: the *Red Book*, published by the AAP Committee on Infectious Diseases, is the widely accepted reference for immunizations. It contains guidelines for the many exceptions to the standard childhood schedule. The schedule is also available at https://www.cdc.gov/vaccines/schedules/hcp/imz/child-adolescent.html.
   - Survey developmental progression/milestones: see Figures 21–3 and 21–4.
   - Develop alliance with parent/caregiver through open-ended discussion.
   - Increase caregiver competence in child care through age-appropriate anticipatory guidance.
   - Understand the social determinants of health that may affect children and families.

DIRECTIONS FOR ADMINISTRATION

1. Try to get child to smile by smiling, talking or waving. Do not touch him/her.
2. Child must stare at hand several seconds.
3. Parent may help guide toothbrush and put toothpaste on brush.
4. Child does not have to be able to tie shoes or button/zip in the back.
5. Move yarn slowly in an arc from one side to the other, about 8" above child's face.
6. Pass if child grasps rattle when it is touched to the backs or tips of fingers.
7. Pass if child tries to see where yarn went. Yarn should be dropped quickly from sight from tester's hand without arm movement.
8. Child must transfer cube from hand to hand without help of body, mouth, or table.
9. Pass if child picks up raisin with any part of thumb and finger.
10. Line can vary only 30 degrees or less from tester's line.
11. Make a fist with thumb pointing upward and wiggle only the thumb. Pass if child imitates and does not move any fingers other than the thumb.

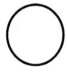

12. Pass any enclosed form. Fail continuous round motions.

13. Which line is longer? (Not bigger.) Turn paper upside down and repeat. (pass 3 of 3 or 5 of 6)

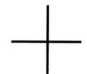

14. Pass any lines crossing near midpoint.

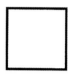

15. Have child copy first. If failed, demonstrate.

When giving items 12, 14, and 15, do not name the forms. Do not demonstrate 12 and 14.

16. When scoring, each pair (2 arms, 2 legs, etc.) counts as one part.
17. Place one cube in cup and shake gently near child's ear, but out of sight. Repeat for other ear.
18. Point to picture and have child name it. (No credit is given for sounds only.)
    If less than 4 pictures are named correctly, have child point to picture as each is named by tester.

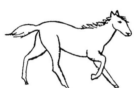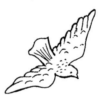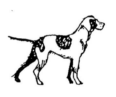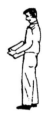

19. Using doll, tell child: Show me the nose, eyes, ears, mouth, hands, feet, tummy, hair. Pass 6 of 8.
20. Using pictures, ask child: Which one flies?...says meow?...talks?...barks?...gallops? Pass 2 of 5, 4 of 5.
21. Ask child: What do you do when you are cold?...tired?...hungry? Pass 2 of 3, 3 of 3.
22. Ask child: What do you do with a cup? What is a chair used for? What is a pencil used for? Action words must be included in answers.
23. Pass if child correctly places <u>and</u> says how many blocks are on paper. (1,5).
24. Tell child: Put block **on** table; **under** table; **in front of** me, **behind** me. Pass 4 of 4. (Do not help child by pointing, moving head or eyes.)
25. Ask child: What is a ball?...lake?...desk?...house?...banana?...curtain?...fence?...ceiling? Pass if defined in terms of use, shape, what it is made of, or general category (such as banana is fruit, not just yellow). Pass 5 of 8, 7 of 8.
26. Ask child: If a horse is big, a mouse is ___? If fire is hot, ice is ___? If the sun shines during the day, the moon shines during the ___? Pass 2 of 3.
27. Child may use wall or rail only, not person. May not crawl.
28. Child must throw ball overhand 3 feet to within arm's reach of tester.
29. Child must perform standing broad jump over width of test sheet (8 1/2 inches).
30. Tell child to walk forward, ⬤⬤⬤⬤⬤➝ heel within 1 inch of toe. Tester may demonstrate. Child must walk 4 consecutive steps.
31. In the second year, half of normal children are non-compliant.

FIGURE 21–3. **Instructions for the Denver development screening test.** Numbers are coded to scoring form (Figure 21–4). "Abnormal" is defined as two or more delays (failure of an item passed by 90% at that age) in two or more categories, or two or more delays in one category with one other category having one delay and an age line that does not intersect one item that is passed. A "suspect" or "questionable" score is given if one category has two or more delays or if one or more categories have one delay and, in the same category, the age line does not pass through one item that is passed. (From Frankenburg WK. *Denver Developmental Screening Test.* 2nd ed. Denver, CO: Denver Developmental Materials, Inc.; 1990, with permission.)

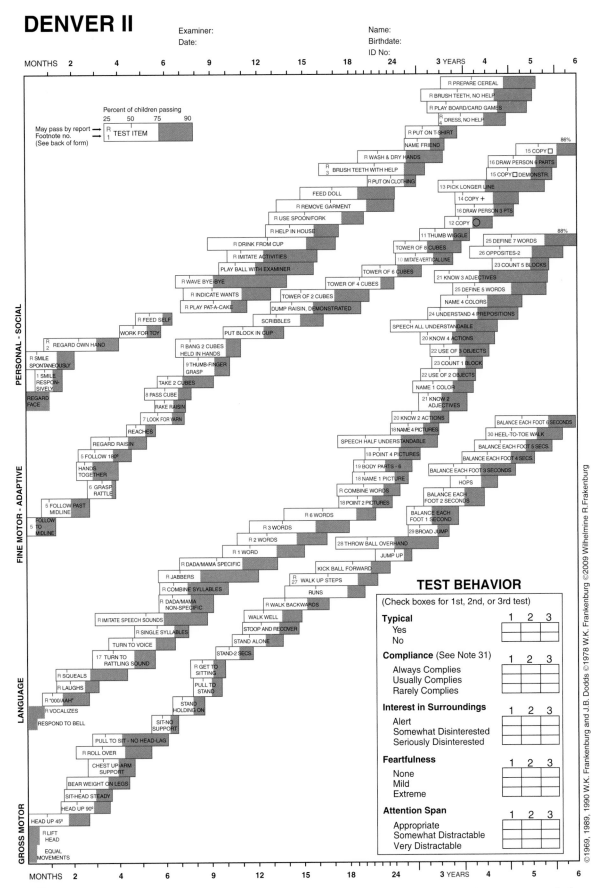

FIGURE 21–4. **Scoring form for the Denver II.** (From Frankenburg WK, Dodds JB. *Denver Developmental Screening Test.* 2nd ed. Denver, CO: Denver Development Materials, Inc.; 1990, with permission.)

- Do history and PE at routine intervals from birth to age 21, including specific attention to height/length, weight, body mass index (BMI) (starting at 2 years), head circumference (up to 2 years), and compare with standardized growth charts.
- Evaluate blood pressure (starting at 3 years), hearing, speech, neurologic findings, deformities, and sexual development.

B. The First 5 Years: Well Care
- Characterized by continuous changes in growth, acquisition of competence in interaction with environment including gross and fine motor skills, language acquisition, and emotional development.
- Continue to monitor growth and development according to standardized charts, and developmental milestones according to the Denver II screening. Autism spectrum disorder (ASD) screening should be done at 18- and 24-month health screening visits.
- Engage in interaction with child to assess expressive and receptive language competence.
- Provide anticipatory guidance for family/social relationships, diet, sleep, toileting, and injury prevention including car seats, gun safety, and bicycle helmets.

C. Middle Childhood: Ages 6 to 12 Years—Well Care
- Characterized by increasing separation from parent/caregiver, development of self-awareness and perception of how others see them, and greater interaction in the social environment beyond immediate family.
- Assess language and development, noting:
  - Acquisition of attention skills.
  - Movement from egocentric to rule-based thinking.
  - Competence in social skills with family, schoolmates, and friends.
- Perform survey of growth according to standardized growth curves, nutrition, hearing, and vision.
  - Growth tends to occur in three to six irregularly spaced spurts each year.
  - Assess for sexual maturity and awareness.
- Provide anticipatory guidance for family/social and school issues, puberty changes, oral health, diet/physical activity, sleep, safety with adults (sexual abuse prevention), bike helmet, seat belt/booster seat, gun safety, water safety, and injury prevention.

D. Adolescence: Ages 13 to 21—Well Care
- Early years (10–13) characterized by progression through puberty.
- Middle years (14–16) characterized by dramatic changes in sexual maturation.
- Late years (17–21) characterized by adult-like characteristics.
- Perform survey of growth according to standardized growth curves, nutrition, hearing, and vision.
- Record sexual maturity rating:
  - Tanner stages (Figures 21–5 to 21–7).
  - Record menses and note cycle length and characteristic of blood flow.
- Explore issues with emotional relationship with parents, family, friends, and school.
  - Perform a "HEADSS" assessment addressing the following issues: *H*ome and Environment, *E*ducation and Employment, *A*ctivities, *D*rugs, *S*exuality, *S*uicidality/Depression.
- Provide anticipatory guidance for risk behaviors, including tobacco/e-cigarettes, drugs and alcohol, driving, counseling regarding sexual behaviors, gender identity, technology usage, pregnancy and contraception, managing conflict nonviolently, and body image.

IV. Genetic Abnormalities
A. Phenylketonuria
1. **Epidemiology**
   - Most common amino acid metabolism disorder.
   - 1:10,000 live births.
2. **Pathology**
   - Autosomal recessive chromosomal disorder.
   - Classic phenylketonuria (PKU) is due to a deficiency in phenylalanine hydroxylase in the liver.
   - Children with PKU are unable to metabolize phenylalanine because of the enzyme deficiency; therefore, with normal dietary intake of phenylalanine, there is a buildup of its toxic metabolites.
3. **Clinical Features**
   - Typically diagnosed through newborn metabolic screen, otherwise symptoms will not manifest until later in childhood.
   - Mental retardation.
   - Hypertonia.
   - Tremors.
   - Behavioral problems.
   - Light complexion/hair.
   - Eczema.
   - Mouse-like odor to urine.
4. **Diagnostic Studies**
   - Neonatal screening demonstrates a hyperphenylalaninemia (20 mg per dL or higher).
   - Diagnosis is confirmed by hyperphenylalaninemia in the presence of a normal or decreased level of plasma tyrosine on a normal diet.
   - Testing should be repeated because elevations may be transient in the perinatal period.
5. **Management**
   - Diet low in phenylalanine (lifelong).
   - Weekly monitoring of phenylalanine levels along with growth and development in the first year of life, twice monthly from 1 to 12 years of age, and monthly after 12 years of age.

Sex Maturity Ratings in Boys

In assigning SMRs in boys, observe each of the three characteristics separately because they may develop at different rates. Record two separate ratings: pubic hair and genital. If the penis and testes differ in their stages, average the two into a single figure for the genital rating.

	Pubic Hair	Genital	
		Penis	*Testes and Scrotum*
Stage 1	Preadolescent—no pubic hair except for the fine body hair (vellus hair) similar to that on the abdomen	Preadolescent—same size and proportions as in childhood	Preadolescent—same size and proportions as in childhood
Stage 2	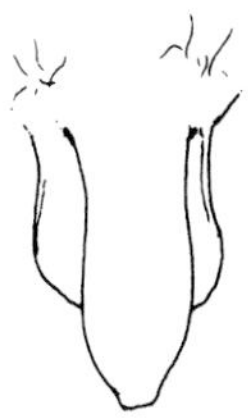 Sparse growth of long, slightly pigmented, downy hair, straight or only slightly curled, chiefly at the base of the penis	Slight or no enlargement	Testes larger; scrotum larger, somewhat reddened, and altered in texture
Stage 3	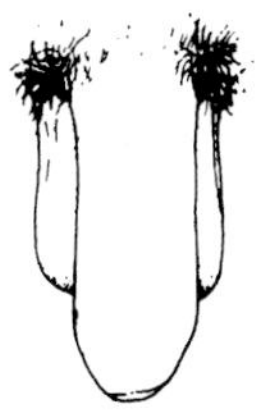 Darker, coarser, curlier hair spreading sparsely over the pubic symphysis	Larger, especially in length	Further enlarged
Stage 4	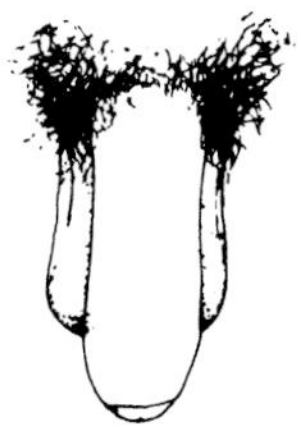 Coarse and curly hair, as in the adult; area covered greater than in stage 3 but not as great as in the adult and not yet including the thighs	Further enlarged in length and breadth, with development of the glans	Further enlarged; scrotal skin darkened
Stage 5	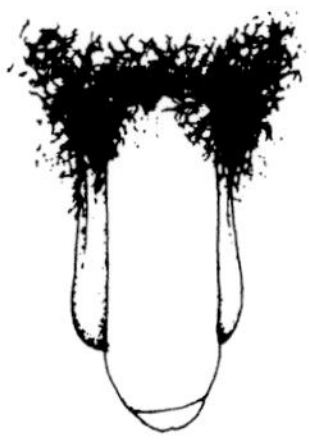 Hair adult in quantity and quality, spread to the medial surfaces of the thighs but not up over the abdomen	Adult in size and shape	Adult in size and shape

FIGURE 21–5. **Sex maturity ratings (SMRs) in boys.** (From Bickley LS, ed. Male genitalia and hernias. In: *Bates' Guide to Physical Examination and History Taking.* 6th ed. Philadelphia, PA: JB Lippincott; 1995:372, with permission.)

Sex Maturity Ratings in Girls: Pubic Hair

Stage 1
Preadolescent—no pubic hair except for the fine body hair (vellus hair) similar to that on the abdomen

Stage 2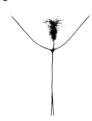

Stage 3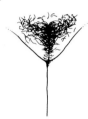

Sparse growth of long, slightly pigmented, downy hair, straight or only slightly curled, chiefly along the labia

Darker, coarser, curlier hair, spreading sparsely over the pubic symphysis

Stage 4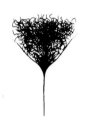

Stage 5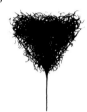

Coarse and curly hair as in adults; area covered greater than in stage 3 but not as great as in the adult and not yet including the thighs

Hair adult in quantity and quality, spread on the medial surfaces of the thighs but not up over the abdomen

FIGURE 21–6. **Sex maturity ratings (SMRs) in girls: pubic hair.** (From Bickley LS, ed. Female genitalia. In: *Bates' Guide to Physical Examination and History Taking*. 6th ed. Philadelphia, PA: JB Lippincott; 1995:388, with permission.)

Sex Maturity Ratings in Girls: Breasts

Stage 1
Preadolescent. Elevation of nipple only

Stage 2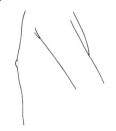

Stage 3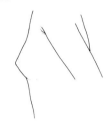

Breast bud stage. Elevation of breast and nipple as a small mound; enlargement of areolar diameter

Further enlargement of elevation of breast and areola, with no separation of their contours

Stage 4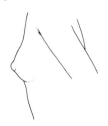

Stage 5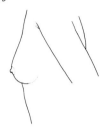

Projection of areola and nipple to form a secondary mound above the level of breast

Mature stage; projection of nipple only. Areola has receded to general contour of the breast (although in some normal individuals the areola continues to form a secondary mound).

FIGURE 21–7. **Sex maturity ratings (SMRs) in girls: breasts.** (From Bickley LS, ed. The breasts and axillae. In: *Guide to Physical Examination and History Taking*. 6th ed. Philadelphia, PA: JB Lippincott; 1995:324, with permission.)

B. Cystic Fibrosis

1. **Epidemiology**
   - Highest in Caucasians (1:3,000 live births).
2. **Pathophysiology**
   - Autosomal recessive inheritance resulting in obstructive lung disease and exocrine gland dysfunction.
3. **Clinical Manifestations**
   - May be diagnosed antenatally by screening or through state newborn screen.
   - Meconium ileus at birth.
   - Failure to thrive (FTT).
   - Productive cough.
   - Wheezing.
   - Recurrent respiratory infections.
   - Steatorrhea.
4. **Diagnostic Testing**
   - Elevated immunoreactive trypsin (IRT) levels at birth.
   - Elevated sweat chloride test associated with typical symptoms or family history.
   - Genotypic analysis.
   - Bronchiectasis on chest imaging.
   - Sputum cultures typically show *Pseudomonas aeruginosa*, *Haemophilus influenzae*, or *Staphylococcus aureus*.
   - Vitamin A, D, E, or K deficiency.
5. **Management**
   - Children with CF should be managed at a facility that is accredited by the CF foundation if possible.
   - Airway clearance therapy.
   - Inhaled mucolytics (recombinant DNAse).
   - Oral and inhaled antibiotics (antipseudomonal).
   - Pancreatic enzyme supplementation.
   - Supplementation of vitamins A, D, E, and K.
6. **Prognosis**
   - Largely determined by progression of lung disease.
   - Median life expectancy is 40 years of age.

C. Down Syndrome (Trisomy 21)

1. **Epidemiology**
   - Most common chromosomal abnormality.
   - Incidence (1:700 newborns).
   - 1:100 mothers age 40.

2. **Etiology**
   - Presence of extra (complete or partial) chromosome. Twenty-one to 95% of these patients have 47 chromosomes with trisomy of 21 (sporadic), 4% translocation, and 1% mosaic.
3. **Clinical Features**
   - Cognitive impairment, IQ is typically between 20 and 80.
   - Characteristic facies:
     - Brachycephaly.
     - Small dysplastic pinnae.
     - Upslanting palpebral fissures.
     - Epicanthal folds.
   - Limb abnormalities.
   - Hypotonia.
   - Associated conditions: hypothyroidism.
   - Cardiovascular defects: septal defects and endocardial cushion defect.
   - GI problems: esophageal/duodenal atresia, celiac disease, feeding problems, and prolonged physiologic jaundice.
   - Leukemia.
   - Alzheimer dementia (average onset 35 years old).
   - Atlantoaxial subluxation.
4. **Diagnostic Studies**
   - Confirmed by chromosomal studies.
5. **Management**
   - Management of specific complications.
   - Goals of treatment are to have child develop to full potential.
   - Educational assistance.
   - Parents are encouraged to use support services.
6. **Prevention**
   - Genetic counseling for at-risk population (advanced maternal age, parents with one child with Down syndrome).
   - Prenatal diagnosis through maternal serum α-feto protein levels, amniocentesis, and chorionic villus sampling.

D. **Trisomy 18 (Edwards Syndrome)**
   1. **Epidemiology**
      - Incidence 1:4,000 births.
      - Male-to-female ratio is 1:3.
   2. **Etiology**
      - Additional copy of chromosome 18.
   3. **Clinical Features**
      - Severe pre- and postnatal growth retardation.
      - Hypertonicity.
      - Dysmorphic facies: prominent occiput, micrognathia, and cleft lip/palate.
      - Cardiac abnormalities: ventricular septal defect (VSD) and patent ductus arteriosus (PDA).
      - Limb abnormalities: rocker bottom feet and overlapping fingers (clinodactyly).
      - Cognitive impairment.
      - Death usually occurs in infancy or early childhood from heart failure or pneumonia.

4. **Diagnostic Studies**
   - Confirmed by chromosomal studies.
5. **Management**
   - General supportive care.
   - Grief counseling.
6. **Prevention**
   - Genetic counseling.
   - Prenatal diagnosis and decision to terminate pregnancy should be discussed with and left up to the parents.

E. **Trisomy 13 (Patau Syndrome)**
   1. **Epidemiology**
      - Incidence 1:12,000 births.
      - Male-to-female ratio is 2:3.
      - Majority die in utero and 90% die within first year of life.
   2. **Etiology**
      - Additional copy of chromosome 13.
   3. **Clinical Features**
      - Usually associated with congenital anomalies incompatible with life; surviving infants usually die of congestive heart failure (CHF) or infection by the second year of life.
      - Characteristic facies: microcephaly, hypotelorism abnormalities of the ears, orbits, nose, and palate.
      - Omphalocele.
      - Polycystic kidneys.
      - Radial bone aplasia.
      - Polydactyly.
      - Skin abnormalities.
   4. **Diagnostic Studies**
      - Confirmed by chromosomal studies.
   5. **Management**
      - General supportive care.
      - Grief counseling.
   6. **Prevention**
      - Genetic counseling.
      - Prenatal diagnosis and decision to terminate pregnancy should be discussed with and left up to the parents.

F. **Turner Syndrome (Gonadal Dysgenesis)**
   1. **Epidemiology**
      - 1:10,000 female live births.
   2. **Etiology**
      - Chromosomal X monosomy.
   3. **Clinical Features**
      - In the newborn: triangular facies, coarctation of the aorta, webbed neck, and edema of the hands and feet.
      - In older children and adolescents: abovementioned symptoms, short stature, shield-shaped chest with widely spaced nipples, primary amenorrhea, absence of secondary sex characteristics, and streak ovaries.
      - Patients with mosaic Turner syndrome: may only have short stature and primary amenorrhea.

4. **Diagnostic Studies**
   - Confirmed by chromosomal studies.
5. **Management**
   - Estrogen replacement therapy.
   - Growth hormone.
   - Fertility management.

G. **Klinefelter Syndrome (XXY)**
   1. **Epidemiology**
      - 1:1,000 live male births.
   2. **Clinical Features**
      - Normal appearance before the onset of puberty.
      - Variable cognitive impairment.
      - In postpubertal boys: microorchidism with otherwise normal external genitalia, gynecomastia, azoospermia, sterility, decreased facial hair, and lack of libido/potency.
   3. **Diagnostic Studies**
      - Confirmed by chromosomal studies.
   4. **Management**
      - Testosterone replacement.
      - Psychosocial and educational counseling as needed.

H. **Fragile X Syndrome**
   1. **Etiology**
      - 1:1,000 in males.
      - Most common cognitive disorder in males.
      - Chromosome mutation of the *FMR1* gene.
   2. **Clinical Features**
      - Variable degrees of intellectual difficulty.
      - Behavioral abnormalities: ranging from social anxiety and shyness to hyperactivity, attention deficit hyperactivity disorder, and autistic characteristics (primarily in males).
      - Characteristic facies with prominent ears and jaw, with oblong face.
      - Macroorchidism.
      - Hyperextensible joints.
      - Mitral valve prolapse.
   3. **Diagnostic Studies**
      - Confirmed by chromosomal studies.
   4. **Management**
      - Management of behavioral and intellectual problems as needed.
      - Multidisciplinary team.
   5. **Prevention**
      - Genetic counseling.

V. Cardiovascular System
A. Tetralogy of Fallot
   1. **Epidemiology**
      - Most common form of cyanotic CHD in infants. Ten percent of all CHD.
      - Associated with 22q11 deletion, DiGeorge syndrome.
   2. **Pathology**
      - Four classic clinical features:
        - A large, unrestricted VSD.

- An aorta overriding the VSD.
- Right ventricular hypertrophy (RVH).
- Right outflow obstruction: infundibular pulmonary stenosis.
   - Anatomic abnormalities that may coexist include right aortic arch (25%), atrial septal defect, absent pulmonary valve, pulmonary atresia, atrioventricular septal defect, and a left superior vena cava to the coronary sinus.

3. **Clinical Features**
   - Symptoms can range from the asymptomatic acyanotic child with a heart murmur ("pink tetralogy") to a severely hypoxic newborn infant.
   - The degree of RV outflow tract obstruction determines whether the infant/child will be cyanotic or acyanotic.
   - Often, at birth, the infant is acyanotic.
   - After the first year of life, the infant is more likely to present with cyanosis.
   - Cyanosis can be exacerbated with exertion in acyanotic patients.
   - Squatting is a common posture in tetralogy of Fallot patients, especially after exercise.
   - Episodes of paroxysmal hypoxemia (tetralogy spells) may be seen.
   - Harsh, systolic ejection murmur along left sternal border possibly radiating to the back.
   - Dyspnea on exertion.
   - Clubbing of the fingers may be present in the older cyanotic child.

4. **Diagnostic Studies**
   - Electrocardiogram (ECG) exhibits RVH and right axis deviation.
   - CXR, as seen in posterior–anterior view, shows a boot-shaped heart (caused by RVH) and a concavity of the upper left heart border (caused by the absence of the main pulmonary artery segment).
   - ECG showing right ventricle wall thickening, overriding aorta, and VSD confirms the diagnosis. In addition, pulmonary valve obstruction can be assessed.
   - Cardiac catheterization will show a right-to-left shunt at the ventricular level. With a large VSD present, the right ventricular pressure will be equal to the left ventricular pressure. A selective right ventriculogram confirms the diagnosis showing the thickened right ventricle, stenotic pulmonary valve, and VSD.

5. **Management**
   - Complete surgical correction involving the closing of the VSD and removing the right ventricular outflow tract obstruction is required if the patient is significantly symptomatic and hypoxemic. Complete repair can be done during the neonatal/infant period.

6. **Prognosis**
   - Surgical mortality rate is <10%.

- The earlier the complete surgical correction, the better the functional capacity as the child ages.
- At risk for sudden death due to ventricular arrhythmias.

B. Ventricular Septal Defect

1. Epidemiology
- The most common cardiac malformation (30% of all CHD).
- More common in males.

2. Pathology
- Range in size from "pinhole" to a virtual absence of septum.
- Membranous defects are more common than muscular defects.
- Most VSDs are small and close spontaneously or do not need repair.

3. Clinical Features
- Patients with small-to-moderate left-to-right shunts (most common) usually have no symptoms.
- Patients with larger shunts usually exhibit diaphoresis with feeding, FTT, frequent URI, and pneumonia in infancy.
- Dyspnea, poor exercise tolerance, fatigue, and CHF in childhood.
- Characteristic loud, harsh, holosystolic, high-pitched murmur heard best along the left sternal border, specifically the third to fifth intercostal spaces.
- A localized thrill may be palpated with moderate left-to-right shunts.

4. Diagnostic Studies
- CXR in small-to-moderate shunts: the findings are usually normal; larger shunts may show cardiomegaly, and the main pulmonary artery segment is dilated with increased pulmonary markings.
- ECG in small-to-moderate shunts: the ECG is normal; larger shunts may show left ventricular hypertrophy.
- Two-dimensional (2-D) ECG: provides visualization of defects 2 mm or larger in about 75% of patients and often can be used to pinpoint the anatomic location. Adding color Doppler can diagnose virtually all defects, including the smallest "pinpoint" lesion. Doppler can estimate the VSD pressure between right and left ventricles.
- Cardiac catheterization is indicated in patient with increased pulmonary vascular resistance.

5. Management
- A significant number of small VSDs (<3 mm), estimated to be 30% to 70%, undergo spontaneous closure usually in the first 2 years of life. Ninety percent may close by age 6 years.
- Small defects that do not close spontaneously require treatment rarely.

- Larger shunts should be surgically repaired before 2 years of age to prevent the possibility of pulmonary hypertension. Primary surgical closure of the defect with a prosthetic patch is used for nearly all isolated symptomatic defects.
- Transcatheter closure of muscular VSDs is indicated on the basis of the size and borders of defect.

6. Prognosis
- Adults with corrected defects have a normal quality of life.
- Functional exercise capacity and O_2 capacity are usually normal.
- Small asymptomatic VSDs that do not close spontaneously require subacute bacterial endocarditis prophylaxis.

C. Patent Ductus Arteriosus

1. Epidemiology
- Females outnumber males, 2:1.
- More common in preterm infants weighing <1,500 g.
- May be seen with VSD and coarctation of the aorta.
- Common in children whose mothers contracted rubella in the first trimester of the pregnancy.

2. Pathology
- PDA is persistence in extrauterine life of the normal fetal vessel that joins the pulmonary artery to the aorta.
- Normally spontaneously closes between 1 and 5 days of life.

3. Clinical Features
- The clinical finding and clinical course depend on the size of the shunt.
- Usually, no symptoms are associated with small patent ductus.
- A moderate-to-large shunt:
  - Bounding pulses and widened pulse pressure due to diastolic runoff.
  - A loud, harsh, continuous murmur or a thrill heard maximally at the second left interspace is often present and may radiate toward the left clavicle and/or down the left sternal border. Has a machine-like quality and is usually unaltered by postural changes.
- May result in CHF.

4. Diagnostic Studies
- CXR in the small patent ductus shunt is normal, whereas the larger shunt may show findings of both the left atrial and the left ventricular hypertrophy, a prominent aorta, and prominent main pulmonary artery segment.
- ECG in the small patent ductus shunt is normal, whereas the larger shunt may show left ventricular or biventricular hypertrophy.
- ECG with a small patent ductus shunt is normal, whereas the larger shunt may show enlargement

of the left atrium or left ventricle or both. Color Doppler and 2-D ECG can show the turbulent blood flow in the pulmonary artery and usually eliminate the need for diagnostic cardiac catheterization.

5. **Management**
   - Surgical correction when the ductus arteriosus is large (except in patients with pulmonary vascular obstruction).
   - Transcatheter closure of small defects with a vascular plug or coil is becoming standard therapy.
   - Although controversial, indomethacin may be used in premature infants to assist closure of the patent ductus.
   - Patients with complex CHD (hypoplastic left heart syndrome/pulmonary atresia) that are ductal dependent require prostaglandin E_2 (PGE_2).

6. **Prognosis**
   - Patients with small-to-moderate PDA shunts do well even without surgery until their third or fourth decade of life. They may then begin to experience easy fatigability and dyspnea on exertion, at which point they require surgical correction.

D. **Kawasaki Disease (Mucocutaneous Lymph Node Syndrome)**

1. **Epidemiology**
   - One of the most common causes of acquired heart disease and inflammatory arthritis.
   - An acute, febrile, multisystem syndrome.
   - Primarily occurs in children <9 years (peak 13–24 months of age).
   - Diagnosis is based entirely on clinical features.
   - Males affected more than females, 1.5:1.

2. **Etiology/Pathology**
   - Unknown.
   - May be related to bacterial toxins.

3. **Clinical Features**
   - The child appears ill.
   - **Diagnostic criteria:**
     - Acute onset of relentless fever (up to 104°–105° F) lasting for at least 5 days.
     - **And at least the presence of four of the following five conditions:**
       - Bilateral, painless, nonpurulent conjunctival injection.
       - Changes of the mucosa of the oropharynx, including pharyngeal injection, dry fissured and cracking lips, and strawberry tongue.
       - Changes of the peripheral extremities, such as edema and erythema of the hands or the feet; desquamation, usually beginning periungually. Desquamation beginning

around the fingers and toes that occurs after the fever has dissipated (about 2 weeks). Rash, primarily truncal; polymorphous but nonvesicular.
       - Unilateral cervical lymphadenopathy ≥1.5 cm.
       - Illness not explained by other known disease process.
   - Associated signs and symptoms:
     - Abdominal pain, vomiting, and diarrhea.
     - Myocarditis and pericarditis.
     - Arthralgia of large joints.

4. **Diagnostic Studies**
   - Elevated white blood cells (WBCs).
   - Elevated ESR.
   - Elevated CRP.
   - Elevated platelets (late finding).
   - Elevated transaminases.
   - UA abnormal with elevated protein and pyuria.
   - **Imaging findings:**
     - ECG abnormalities (peaked T-waves, first-degree heart block, ST-segment elevation or depression, and QT prolongation).
   - Coronary artery aneurysms should be evaluated with ECG.

5. **Complications**
   - Coronary artery aneurysm.
   - Coronary artery thrombosis.
   - Myocardial infarction.
   - Myopericarditis.
   - CHF.
   - Pericardial effusion.
   - Hydrops of gallbladder.
   - Aseptic meningitis.
   - Polyarticular arthritis.
   - Uveitis.
   - Peripheral artery aneurysm.

6. **Management**
   - Intravenous (IV) β-globulin reduces the acute inflammation and also appears to reduce the frequency of coronary artery dilatation and aneurysm.
   - Aspirin at high doses initially to control inflammation, and then low-dose aspirin therapy during the subacute phase (6–8 weeks).
   - Disease is self-limited.

7. **Prognosis**
   - Cardiac damage sustained when the disease was active may be progressive, but it is not proven if they are at an increased risk for atherosclerotic heart disease as adults compared to the normal incidence of atherosclerotic heart disease. Long-term follow-up is required for patients with coronary dilatation or aneurysms.
   - Fatal in 0.1% to 3% of patients.

VI. Pulmonary System

A. Bronchiolitis

1. Epidemiology
- Occurs within first 2 years of life, peak incidence 6 months of age.
- Incidence is highest in the winter and early spring months.
- May occur epidemically or sporadically.
- Frequent cause of hospitalization.
- Infants exposed to secondhand smoke are more likely to develop bronchiolitis than those not exposed.
- Infants who attend daycare centers are more likely to develop bronchiolitis than those who do not.

2. Etiology
- RSV is the most likely pathogen; however, parainfluenza and influenza viruses, adenovirus, *Mycoplasma*, and *Chlamydia* are other causes.

3. Pathology
- Bronchiolitis results from obstruction due to edema and accumulation of mucus and cellular debris and invasion of the small airways by RSV.

4. Clinical Features
- Fever for 1 to 2 days.
- Rhinorrhea.
- Irritability.
- Decreased appetite.
- Cough.
- Wheezing.
- Tachypnea.
- Intercostal retractions.
- Nasal flaring.
- Prolonged expiratory phase.
- May be rales and/or rhonchi.
- The liver and spleen may be palpable because of hyperinflation of the lungs.

5. Diagnostic Studies
- CBC is normal.
- CXR: typical findings are hyperinflation, peribronchial cuffing, and subsegmental atelectasis of the lungs with mild interstitial infiltrates.
- Viral culture or antigen assay from nasopharyngeal secretions may isolate RSV.
- Hypoxemia is common.

6. Complications
- Children with bronchopulmonary dysplasia or certain congenital anomalies (i.e., CHD, neuromuscular disorders, malnutrition, and congenital or acquired abnormalities of immunologic function) have excessive morbidity and mortality.

7. Management
- Most patients are readily managed as outpatients by supportive therapy.
- Patients with respiratory distress and hypoxemia should be hospitalized.
- Treated with humidified O_2 and supportive therapy.
- An antiviral agent, ribavirin, may be of some benefit, especially in patients with respiratory distress or chronic cardiopulmonary disease. Its spectrum includes RSV, influenza, parainfluenza, and adenoviruses.
  - β_2-Agonist bronchodilators can be of some benefit, although controversy exists about their efficacy.
- Prophylaxis:
  - Synagis (palivizumab) is indicated for prevention of serious lower respiratory tract disease caused by RSV in patients at high risk for RSV disease—that is, bronchopulmonary dysplasia and premature infants (<35 weeks' gestational age).
  - The dosage of 15 mg per kg should be administered intramuscularly (IM) on a monthly basis during RSV season.

8. Prognosis
- Overall, the long-term prognosis is good.
- Major concerns include acute effects of bronchiolitis and the development of chronic airway hyper-reactivity (asthma).

B. Epiglottitis

1. Epidemiology
- Most frequently seen in children 3 months to 6 years old, although reported in all age groups.
- Males affected more than females, 2:1.
- Occurs in any season.

2. Etiology
- Usually due to bacteria—*H. influenzae* type B (HiB).

3. Pathology
- An acute infection/inflammation of the epiglottis and edema of the surrounding soft tissue.
- It is an immediate threat to life because complete upper airway obstruction may occur suddenly at any time.

4. Clinical Features
- Sudden with rapid progression.
- Pharyngeal pain.
- Dysphagia.
- Odynophagia (pain on swallowing) is characteristic.
- Fever (~104° F).
- Inspiratory stridor.
- Characteristic posture: TRIPOD-sitting leaning forward, elbows on legs, and drooling.
- Tachypnea: the patient appears anxious.
- Do not examine the mouth or neck if you suspect epiglottitis—it may cause spasm, thereby exacerbating complete upper airway obstruction.

5. Diagnostic Studies
- Obtain a lateral soft-tissue X-ray of the neck.
- Epiglottis will be swollen and displaced posteriorly (thumbprint sign).
- Blood cultures will often be positive.

6. **Management**
- Immediate hospitalization.
- Management of airways, breathing, and circulation is the first priority.
- Consult an anesthesiologist for probable nasotracheal or orotracheal intubation.
- IV antibiotics should be started empirically with cefotaxime (Claforan), ceftriaxone (Rocephin), and Vancomycin.
- Fluids and humidified O_2.

C. Laryngotracheobronchitis (Croup)

1. **Epidemiology**
- Most common in children 6 months to 5 years (but may occur at any age, although uncommon >6 years old).
- Life-threatening airway obstruction more likely to occur in the pediatric population because of the already narrowed airways.
- Males affected more than females, 3:1.
- Increased incidence from October to April.
- One hundred to 1,000 times more common than epiglottitis.

2. **Etiology**
- Almost always caused by viruses (usually parainfluenza types I–III).

3. **Pathology**
- Infection/inflammation of the airway that involves the larynx and subglottic areas.

4. **Clinical Features**
- Slow insidious onset.
- Symptoms may persist up to 14 days (with the worst symptoms lasting 1–2 days).
- Usually, a current or recent URI is noted.
- Hoarseness.
- "Barking," seal-like cough.
- Stridor is common (both inspiratory and expiratory).
- Symptoms usually worse at night or when child is agitated.
- Fever (low-grade), rhinitis, pharyngitis, and wheezing may be present.

5. **Diagnostic Studies**
- Performing diagnostic studies may agitate the patient; therefore, unnecessary invasive studies should be avoided (an ABG may be needed in seriously ill patients).
- An anterior–posterior (AP) or lateral soft-tissue X-ray of the neck showing subglottic narrowing confirms the diagnosis (steeple sign).

6. **Management**
- Always ABCs first.
- Disturb the patient as little as possible.
- Cool air mist is the mainstay of therapy for mild croup, although sitting in a steamed-up bathroom and/or taking the child for a ride with the windows slightly open are simple therapeutic measures.
- Antibiotics are not necessary.

- Observation and adequate hydration.
- Aerosolized racemic epinephrine may be required for severe cases.
- Dexamethasone IM improves symptoms, reduces the duration of hospitalization and frequency of intubations, and permits early discharge from the emergency department.
- Hospitalization is necessary for only the severe cases of croup.

D. Pertussis (Whooping Cough)

1. **Epidemiology**
- Mostly affects children <5 years of age (mortality highest in infants <1 year).
- Females affected more than males.
- Can occur in any season.
- Cases of pertussis have been steadily increasing.

2. **Pathology**
- Predominantly caused by *Bordetella pertussis*, a gram-negative, pleomorphic bacilli.
- Highly contagious; transmission is by droplets released during intense coughing.
- It is postulated that the tracheal cytotoxin, dermonecrotic factor, and adenylate cyclase are responsible for local epithelial damage that produces respiratory symptomology and aids in absorption of pertussis toxin.

3. **Clinical Features**
- Incubation period ranges from 6 to 14 days.
- Illness lasts 6 to 8 weeks and is broken down into three stages:
  - Catarrhal stage (1–2 weeks): prodromal, preparoxysmal:
    - Patients are most contagious during this stage.
    - Rhinorrhea.
    - Conjunctival injection.
    - Lacrimation.
    - Mild cough.
    - Low-grade fever.
    - Pertussis often overlooked during this stage because manifestations resemble those of a simple URI.
  - Paroxysmal stage (2–4 weeks or longer):
    - Episodes of cough increase in severity and frequency.
    - Forceful coughs during expiration are followed by a sudden massive inspiration producing the whoop.
    - Facial petechiae and redness.
    - Cyanosis.
    - Post-tussive vomiting.
    - Recurrent episodes are exhausting; patients appear apathetic.
    - Attacks may be initiated by yawning, sneezing, eating, drinking, and physical exertion.
  - Convalescent stage (1–2 weeks):

- Paroxysmal coughing and vomiting decrease in severity and frequency.
- Chronic cough may persist for several months.

4. **Diagnostic Studies**
   - Isolation of *B. pertussis* during early phase of illness by culture of nasopharyngeal swab on glycerin potato-blood agar medium (Bordet–Gengou), penicillin added to inhibit the growth of other organisms. Polymerase chain reaction (PCR) detection has replaced culture because of improved sensitivity, decreased time of diagnosis, and cost.

5. **Complications**
   - The most frequent complication is pneumonia.
   - OM and sinusitis are also common.

6. **Management**
   - Azithromycin is the drug of choice. Clarithromycin is equally effective.
   - Erythromycin aborts or eliminates pertussis when administered in the catarrhal stage, but does not affect the duration of the paroxysmal stage and is not the preferred treatment.
   - Erythromycin may cause pyloric stenosis if used in infants <1 month.
   - Corticosteroid aerosols may reduce severity.
   - Supportive care includes warm mist O_2, nasopharyngeal suctioning, and parenteral fluids.

7. **Prevention**
   - DTaP vaccine given in multiple doses throughout infancy with an additional booster dose between the ages of 11 and 18 years is recommended.
   - The pertussis vaccine carries with it side effects (seizures and neurologic effects), but a greater chance of mortality exists with pertussis than with the vaccine.

E. Sudden Infant Death Syndrome

1. **Definition**
   - Defined as the sudden death of an infant <1 year, unexpected by history, and unexplained by a thorough postmortem examination, which includes a complete autopsy, investigation of the scene, and review of the medical history.
   - Sudden and unexpected infant death (SUID) is newer terminology being used to further define unexplained versus explained deaths to include deaths caused by infection, arrhythmias, trauma, accidental suffocation, or ingestions.

2. **Epidemiology**
   - The cause of SIDS is unknown.
   - In the United States, SIDS occurs in <1/1,000 live births.
   - Rare before 1 month, peaks at 2 to 4 months, and 95% occur before 6 months of age.
   - Males affected more than females, 3:2.
   - Most common cause of death in the neonatal period (before 1 year of age).
   - Most deaths occur between midnight and 8:00 am, suggesting the common factor is age and sleep.

3. **Pathology**
   - Suggests hypoxia (acute or chronic).
   - Intrathoracic petechiae and mild inflammation and congestion of the respiratory tract may be present.

4. **Risk Factors**
   - Ethnic and racial minorities.
   - Low socioeconomic status.
   - Low birth weight.
   - Maternal drug abuse.
   - Maternal smoking during and after pregnancy.
   - Late or no prenatal care.
   - Sleeping in the prone position.
   - Bed sharing.
   - Family history of SIDS.

5. **Prevention**
   - See Table 21–2 for possible approaches to the prevention of SIDS.

TABLE 21–2.	Possible Approaches to Prevention of Sudden Infant Death Syndrome (SIDS)

Risk reduction

Abandon recommendation of prone sleeping position for all infants (prone sleeping position still recommended for infants with specific clinical indication)

Recommend side-lying or supine sleeping position for healthy infants

Advocate better and more standardized policy concerning death scene investigation

Better educate public about dangers of over-the-counter remedies to young infants

Decrease parental smoking, before and after birth of child

Decrease parental drug use (e.g., crack cocaine smoking), before and after birth of child

Improve access to and use of postnatal medical care

Improve prenatal care (anemia, smoking, nutrition)

Improve recognition of and services for dysfunctional families at risk for intentional injury of infants

Improve services to young mothers living in poor socioeconomic conditions

Improve targeting of very high-risk groups (e.g., Native Americans with very high maternal smoking rates)

Improve understanding of child care practices that may increase SIDS risk

Physiologic component

Improve diagnosis of metabolic disorders leading to SIDS

Increase understanding of possible sources of postnatal vulnerability

Increase understanding of the role of infant sleeping position in increasing SIDS risk

Increase efficacy of home monitoring

Improve compliance with monitor use

Improve monitoring technology

Improve selection of candidates for monitoring

VII. Gastrointestinal System and Nutrition

A. Infectious Gastroenteritis

1. Etiology
- Viruses: rotavirus, Norwalk virus, enterovirus, and astroviruses.
- Bacteria: *Salmonella*, *Shigella*, *Yersinia*, and *Campylobacter* spp.; pathogenic *Escherichia coli*, *Clostridium difficile*, and TB.
- Parasites: *Giardia lamblia*, *Entamoeba histolytica*, and *Cryptosporidium parvum*.

2. Pathology
- Acute inflammation of the intestinal epithelium lining.
- Produces watery and sometimes bloody stool.

3. Clinical Features
- Irritability.
- Vomiting.
- Diarrhea.
- Nausea.
- Abdominal pain.
- May have fever.
- Symptoms and signs of dehydration.

4. Diagnostic Studies
- Stool culture for rotavirus, bacteria, ova and parasites, and *C. difficile* if prolonged or clinically indicated.
- Electrolyte levels should be measured in infants and moderately dehydrated children.
- Imaging studies and GI referral if anatomic abnormalities suspected.

5. Management
- Treatment of diarrhea is directed primarily by the degree of dehydration present and organism identified.
- If mild, use oral rehydrating solution.
- Key to therapy is administering small volumes of glucose–electrolyte solution such as Pedialyte in 5-mL aliquots every 3 to 5 minutes for the first hour, and then advance slowly.
- Wait 15 to 20 minutes after a vomiting episode to give fluid.
- IV solution is necessary to correct electrolyte imbalance or, when vomiting, prolonging BRAT diet (bananas, rice, applesauce, toast) until solids are tolerated.
- Loperamide is not recommended to treat acute diarrhea in children.
- Anticholinergic agents are not recommended in the management of diarrhea in children.
- Bismuth subsalicylate is not recommended because of the possible absorption of salicylate and theoretical concern of Reye syndrome.

B. Intussusception

1. Epidemiology
- One of the most dangerous surgical emergencies in early childhood and the most common cause of intestinal obstruction in the first 2 years of life.
- Most commonly seen in infants 3 months to 1 year of age.
- Male-to-female ratio is 3:1.
- In 85% of the patients, no cause can be found.

2. Pathology
- Characterized by the telescoping of a proximal portion of the intestine into a more distal position. This "telescoping" results in impairment of the blood supply and necrosis of the involved bowel segment.
- In 95% of the patients, the telescoping involves the ileum into the colon (ileocolic).

3. Clinical Features
- Nearly, all affected infants present with an acute onset of episodic colicky pain and drawing up of knees.
- Diarrhea and vomiting.
- Sausage-shaped mass may be palpated in the area of the hepatic flexure.
- Fever.
- Signs of dehydration may be present.
- Currant jelly stools (late finding).

4. Diagnostic Studies
- Abdominal ultrasound 98% to 100% sensitivity diagnosing intussusception and considered study of choice.
- Barium enema discloses the intussusception outlined as an inverted cap, and an obstruction to the progression of the barium is noted.

5. Management
- IV rehydration should be instituted immediately, and a nasogastric (NG) tube is placed.
- Barium and air enema are considered diagnostic and the treatment of choice in a clinically stable child. Seventy-five percent of cases can be reduced successfully using a barium enema under fluoroscopy.
- **Contraindications to hydrostatic (barium) reduction:**
  - Free intraperitoneal air or peritoneal and systemic signs of compromised intestine.
  - These patients should be taken directly to surgery.
  - Surgical reduction or resection and anastomosis should be performed if barium enema reduction is unsuccessful.

6. Prognosis
- Recurrence rate is near 10% and occurs shortly after reduction.

C. Volvulus (Malrotation)

1. **Epidemiology**
   - Accounts for about 10% of neonatal intestinal obstructions.
   - Associated congenital anomalies can occur in 25% of patients. Particularly heterotaxy syndromes with asplenia or polysplenia.

2. **Etiology**
   - Incomplete rotation of the intestine during fetal development.

3. **Pathology**
   - Most common type of malrotation is the failure of the cecum to move into the right lower quadrant. The mesentery, including the superior mesenteric artery, may twist around itself, producing a midgut volvulus.

4. **Clinical Features**
   - Symptoms usually present within the first weeks of life (1–3 weeks).
   - Recurrent bile-stained vomiting.
   - Acute small bowel obstruction (i.e., irritability, distended, rigid abdomen, vomiting, and decreased stooling).
   - Older children may present with abdominal pain (25%–50% may be asymptomatic) and may have an incomplete obstruction.

5. **Diagnostic Studies**
   - Abdominal plain film may demonstrate a "double-bubble" sign.
   - Barium enema shows malposition of the cecum.
   - Upper GI series demonstrates malposition of the ligament of Treitz, confirming the diagnosis of malrotation. This is the procedure of choice in the nonobstructed patient.

6. **Management**
   - A surgical emergency with the Ladd procedure.
   - Bowel necrosis results from occlusion of the superior mesenteric artery, and intestinal resection should be delayed until a second-look operation can be performed 24 to 48 hours later in anticipation that some bowel can be salvaged.

D. Constipation

1. **Etiology**
   - Beyond neonatal period, most common cause is fecal retention and withholding.
   - Prolonged fecal stasis in the colon with reabsorption of fluid.
   - Diet low in fiber.
   - Anal fissures.
   - Hemorrhoids.
   - Structural problems including tumor and inflammatory bowel disease.

2. **Pathology**
   - Subtypes: colonic inertia, obstructed defecation, and generalized slow transit.
   - Rectal wall stretches.
   - Rectum habituates to stimulus of enlarging fecal mass.
   - Urge to defecate subsides.

3. **Clinical Features**
   - Parental concern of change in stool pattern.
   - Fecal soiling in children who are toilet trained.
   - Hard, painful stool.
   - Change in stool size and consistency.
   - Abdominal pain and cramps.
   - Fever, abdominal distension, anorexia, nausea, vomiting, and weight loss or gain may indicate organic disorder.
   - Bloody diarrhea in the infant could be an indicative of enterocolitis complicating Hirschsprung disease.

4. **Diagnostic Studies**
   - Stool for occult blood in all infants.
   - Abdominal radiograph for selected patients.
   - CBC, ESR, thyroid panel, complete metabolic profile, and celiac disease antibodies.
   - Sweat test to rule out CF for all infants and children with FTT.
   - If laboratory values are abnormal, refer to pediatric gastroenterologist.

5. **Management**
   a. **Management for Infants**
      - Rectal disimpaction with glycerin suppositories.
      - Avoid enemas.
      - Give juices that contain sorbitol; for infants <4 months, can add prune juice to formula—several teaspoons to 1 oz of formula or breast milk daily.
      - Avoid mineral oil and stimulant laxatives.
   b. **Management for Children**
      - Disimpaction with medication and/or enemas.
      - Balanced high-fiber diet.
      - Mineral oil and osmotic laxatives.
      - Short-term administration of stimulant laxatives.
      - Polyethylene glycol-electrolyte solution (PEG-ES; MiraLax) given chronically in low dosage for usually 6 months of therapy.
      - Goal of treatment is two soft or runny stools per day.
      - Gradual return to one or two formed stools daily.
      - Psychiatric evaluation may be indicated in children with severe emotional problems or demonstrate resistant symptoms.

E. Pyloric Stenosis

1. **Epidemiology**
   - Incidence 1–8 in 1,000 births and more likely to occur in firstborn infants.
   - More likely to occur in males than in females, 4:1.

2. **Pathology**
   * Marked increase in the circular musculature of the pylorus, causing an obstruction of the lumen.
3. **Clinical Features**
   * Signs and symptoms will likely occur between 2 and 12 weeks of age.
   * Projectile vomiting that occurs within 2 hours of each feeding.
   * Vomitus does not contain bile.
   * Irritability; the child appears hungry.
   * Weight loss and dehydration.
   * Jaundice occurs in 2% to 5% of patients.
   * An olive-shaped mass can be palpated in the right upper quadrant.
   * Mass felt well immediately following vomiting.
4. **Laboratory/Diagnostic Studies**
   * Ultrasonography demonstrates a hypertrophied pyloric muscle.
   * Hypochloremic alkalosis with potassium depletion.
5. **Management**
   * Rehydration and correction of electrolyte imbalance.
   * NG tube insertion.
   * Surgical intervention curative.
6. **Prognosis**
   * Excellent following surgery.
   * Recurrence unlikely.

VIII. Musculoskeletal System

A. Henoch–Schönlein Purpura
1. **Epidemiology**
   * Most common in children 2 to 7 years of age.
   * More likely in boys.
   * Spring and fall has the highest occurrence.
2. **Etiology**
   * Cause unknown.
   * An upper respiratory or other illness or allergy may precede Henoch–Schönlein purpura (HSP).
   * Can affect the skin, GI tract, kidneys, and joints.
3. **Pathology**
   * IgA vasculitis of the small blood vessels in children.
   * An example of nonthrombocytopenic purpura.
4. **Clinical Features**
   * Onset is acute.
   * The hallmark of HSP is circular palpable purpuric lesions 2 to 3 mm in size, found on the legs, buttocks, and elbows.
   * Nonpitting edema about the dorsum of the hands and feet may be present.
   * Colicky abdominal pain.
   * Melena.
   * Ileus.
   * Vomiting.
   * Hematemesis.

* Migratory polyarthritis (most commonly of the knees and ankles, but wrists, elbows, and fingers may be involved).
* Periarticular swelling.
* Joint tenderness.
* Renal disease.

5. **Diagnostic Studies**
   * No specific diagnostic studies for HSP; diagnosis is based on clinical manifestations.
   * Platelets are normal to mildly elevated.
   * Coagulation studies are normal.
   * All other hematologic studies are normal.
   * UA shows hematuria.
   * Antistreptolysin O (ASO) titer may be elevated and throat culture positive for group A β-hemolytic streptococci (GABHS).
   * Stool positive for occult blood.
   * Serum IgA.
6. **Complications**
   * Hypertension.
   * Nephritis.
   * Intussusception.
   * Anemia (secondary to GI bleeding).
7. **Management**
   * Supportive.
   * Most children with HSP have a self-limited course.
   * Most children have a single exacerbation lasting about 4 weeks.
8. **Prognosis**
   * Generally excellent, but depends on the extent of the disease and the age of the child.
   * The younger the child, the better the prognosis.
   * Less than 5% of children progress to end-stage renal disease.

B. Slipped Capital Femoral Epiphysis
1. **Epidemiology**
   * Occurs in adolescence 11 to 16 years.
   * Most common in obese males.
2. **Etiology**
   * Unknown.
   * Hypothesis: perichondrial ring stabilizing the epiphyseal area is weakened by hormonal changes during adolescence such that the overload of excessive body weight can produce a pathologic fracture through the growth plate.
3. **Pathology**
   * Displacement of the proximal femoral epiphysis due to the disruption of the growth plate.
   * Head of the femur is displaced medially and posteriorly relative to the femoral neck.
4. **Clinical Features**
   * In acute instances, it can occur with a fall or direct trauma.

- Most commonly, it is a healthy child who presents with pain and limp.
- Pain can be referred into the thigh or the medial side of the knee.
- On PE, limitation of internal rotation of the hip is found.

5. **Diagnostic Studies**
   - Radiographic findings.
     - AP and frog-leg lateral films.
     - Osteoporosis of the head and neck on AP view early.
     - Indistinct physis widening on AP view.
     - Line along lateral edge of superior femoral neck on AP does not intersect epiphysis.
     - Lateral films make the diagnosis showing posterior displacement and step-off of the epiphysis.

6. **Management**
   - Non–weight bearing on crutches.
   - Immediate referral to an orthopedic surgeon.

7. **Prognosis**
   - Due to the patient's continually being overweight, they have a high incidence of degenerative arthritis, even in those who do not develop avascular necrosis.
   - Development of avascular necrosis almost guarantees a poor prognosis.
   - Thirty percent of patients have bilateral involvement, which may occur as late as 1 or 2 years after the primary episode.

IX. Eyes, Ears, Nose, and Throat

A. Rhinosinusitis

1. **Etiology**
   - Common pathogens include *Streptococcus pneumoniae*, *H. influenzae*, and *Moraxella catarrhalis*.
   - *S. aureus* and anaerobic organisms are recovered more often in chronic sinusitis.

2. **Pathology**
   - Viral infection causes mucosal injury and inflammation, resulting in obstruction and hypersecretion.
   - Inflammation and sinus drainage obstruction most commonly to the maxillary and ethmoid sinuses.
   - Mucus thickening.
   - Symptoms <10 days is a URI, symptoms >10 to 14 days without improvement most likely rhinosinusitis.
   - Acute: <30 days duration.
   - Subacute: 90 days with resolution.
   - Recurrent acute: repeated episodes with resolution in between at least four times a year.
   - Chronic: >90 days with persistent respiratory symptoms such as cough, rhinorrhea, and nasal obstruction.

3. **Clinical Features**
   - Persistent respiratory symptoms.
   - Malodorous breath.
   - Sneezing.
   - Headache and morning painless eye swelling.
   - Sometimes fever.
   - Frequent throat clearing.
   - Hyposmia (diminished smell) in older children.
   - Daytime cough worsening at night.
   - Facial pain when bending forward.
   - Allergic nasal polyps are not common in children and a workup for CF initiated.

4. **Imaging**
   - Should be reserved for patients with complications, those not responsive to medications, or those who may undergo surgical management.
   - Coronal sinus computed tomography (CT) is the most often used study.

5. **Treatment**
   - First-line treatment with Amoxicillin (90 mg/kg/day) for 10 to 14 days or Amoxicillin/clavulanate (80–90 mg/kg/day of amoxicillin with 6.4 mg/kg/d of clavulanate in two divided doses for 14 days) if not improving on amoxicillin alone, daycare exposure, or recent antibiotic use.
   - Alternative therapies include cefdinir, cefuroxime, and cefpodoxime.
   - Highly allergic patients use linezolid, quinolones, or clindamycin for penicillin-resistant *S. pneumoniae*.
   - Failure to improve after 48 to 72 hours of antibiotics may be due to resistant organism or complication, initiate second-line therapies.

6. **Complications**
   - Preseptal cellulitis.
   - Osteitis of the frontal bone (Pott puffy tumor).
   - Orbital or intracranial invasion leading to meningitis and brain abscesses.

B. Otitis Media

1. **Epidemiology**
   - Accounts for 15% to 20% of all ambulatory visits.
   - Classified as acute OM, OM with effusion, chronic OM with effusion, or chronic suppurative.
   - Recurrent OM is >3 episodes in 6 months, or >4 episodes in 1 year (occurs in 20%–30% of pediatric population).

2. **Etiology**
   - Bacterial/viral coinfection: up to 70%.
   - *S. pneumoniae*: 35% to 40%.
   - *H. influenzae*: 30% to 35%.
   - *M. catarrhalis*: 15% to 20%.

3. **Pathology**
   - Antecedent event: URI.
   - Congestion of respiratory mucosa.

- Dysfunction of the Eustachian tube in younger children due to being shorter and horizontal.
- Obstruction of the isthmus portion of the Eustachian tube.
- Increased tube negative pressure.
- Development of effusion.
- Effusion colonization.

4. **Predisposing Factors**
   - Smoke exposure.
   - Daycare attendance.
   - Ages 1 to 3 (greatest risk).
   - Bottle feeding.
   - Immunocompromised.
   - Male gender.
   - Recurrent OM in parents or siblings.
   - Low birth weight or gestational age.
   - Episode of OM before 6 months of age.
   - Prone sleeping position.
   - Pacifier use.
   - Down syndrome.
   - Cleft palate.

5. **Clinical Features**
   - Ear pain.
   - Cold symptoms.
   - Irritability.
   - May or may not have fever.
   - Red TM.
   - Bulging TMs.
   - Decreased TM mobility by pneumatic otoscopy.
   - Perforation with drainage.

6. **Management**
   - Eighty percent of untreated children resolve spontaneously in 7 to 14 days compared with 95% of treated.
   - Treatment prevents progression.
   - Amoxicillin 90 mg/kg/day is considered first-line therapy.
   - Cefdinir in allergic children.
   - For treatment failure, use amoxicillin/clavulanate (80–90 mg/kg/day of the amoxicillin component) and cefuroxime axetil, cefdinir, clindamycin, or ceftriaxone.
   - **Indications for tympanostomy tube placement:**
     - Chronic OM with effusion and associated conductive hearing loss of >15 dB.
     - Failed treatment for recurrent OM.
     - TM retraction with ossicular erosion or cholesteatoma formation.

7. **Complications**
   - Tympanosclerosis.
   - Adhesive otitis.
   - Cholesteatoma.
   - TM perforation.
   - Facial nerve paralysis.

C. **Pharyngitis**
   - Primary goal is to distinguish viral from bacterial etiology.

1. **Etiology**
   a. **Viral (90%)**
      - Rhinovirus, adenovirus, Coxsackie A, enteroviruses, Epstein–Barr virus (EBV), CMV, and HSV.
   b. **Bacterial**
      - Since the use of *H. influenzae* vaccine, incidence is <6 per million annually.
      - GABHS, 20% to 30%.
      - Less than 2 years of age, GABHS is uncommon.
      - GABHS is more common in children >5 years (5–15 years).
      - *Mycoplasma pneumoniae* may be seen in adolescents and adults.

2. **Pathology**
   - Inflammation of the throat.

3. **Clinical Features**
   - Findings suggestive of GABHS:
     - Sudden onset of sore throat.
     - Fever.
     - Pain on swallowing.
     - Marked inflammation and erythema of pharynx and tonsils.
     - Tonsillar hypertrophy.
     - Patchy discrete exudate of tonsils.
     - Tender, enlarged anterior cervical nodes.
     - Scarlatina rash.
     - *Absence* of conjunctivitis, coryza, and cough. If present, suggests a viral etiology.
     - Occurs during winter and early spring.
     - History of exposure to documented case of GABHS.

4. **Diagnostic Studies**
   - Except for the scarlatina rash, *none* of the above clinical findings is specific for GABHS; therefore, the positive predictive value of these findings is low. However, patients with acute pharyngitis whose clinical and epidemiologic findings do not suggest GABHS likely do not have streptococcal disease because the negative predictive value of such findings is high.
   - Therefore, diagnosis can only be confirmed by throat culture or a rapid antigen detection test.
   - **Throat culture versus rapid test**
     - Throat culture is 90% to 95% sensitive (low rate of false negatives) and takes 2 to 3 days for results.
     - Rapid test is more expensive than culture, but results are acquired in 10 minutes. It has excellent specificity (95%), but sensitivity is low (85%–95%). Therefore, one may begin treatment

on the basis of a positive result, but a negative result does not definitively rule out GABHS and must be confirmed by a throat culture.

5. Complications

a. Nonsuppurative Complications

- Acute rheumatic fever: can be prevented by eradication of GABHS from the pharynx.
- Poststreptococcal glomerulonephritis: *cannot* be prevented by antibiotic treatment.

b. Supportive Complications

- Tonsillar and peritonsillar abscess.
- Sinusitis.
- OM.

6. Management

- Supportive and symptomatic care only for viral pharyngitis.
- For GABHS:
  - Penicillin V is the first-line treatment. Cephalexin, clindamycin, and amoxicillin are acceptable.
  - Continue treatment for 10 days.
  - May use IM benzathine penicillin as a one-time dose if compliance is uncertain.
  - If penicillin is allergic, use cephalosporin or macrolide.
  - Recurrent streptococcal tonsillitis, tonsillectomy is indicated.

X. Neurologic System

A. Cerebral Palsy

1. Etiology

- Cerebral injury before birth, during delivery, or in the perinatal period.

2. Types

- Spasticity.
- Ataxia.
- Choreoathetosis.
- Hypotonia without spasticity.

3. Clinical Features

- Motor deficits.
- Seizures.
- Mild-to-severe retardation.
- Disorders of language, speech, vision, hearing, and sensory perception.
- On PE, spasticity, hyper-reflexia, ataxia, and involuntary movements.
- Microcephaly.
- Affected arm and leg may be smaller and shorter than the unaffected limbs.

4. Laboratory/Diagnostic Studies

- MRI.
- Genetic and metabolic testing.

5. Management

- Goal is to attain the maximal physical functioning with physical, occupational, and speech therapy involved.
- Medications to treat seizures.

- Botulinum toxin to treat spasticity.
- Parents and family support through educational programs, counseling, and support groups.

6. Prognosis

- Depends on the child's IQ, cerebral palsy (CP) etiology, severity of the motor deficits, and degree of disability.
- Most common causes of death in severely affected children with CP are aspiration, pneumonia, and other infections.

B. Bacterial Meningitis

1. Epidemiology

- Peak incidence in children <2 months, but can occur at any age.
- Failure to make a prompt diagnosis and institute antibiotic treatment may result in significant illness and possibly death; examiner must have a high suspicion of meningitis.
- Occurs more frequently in the winter and spring, and mostly affects males than females.
- Less commonly, the result of hematogenous dissemination of microorganisms.

2. Etiology

- In children 1 to 3 months old, the usual bacterial organisms that cause meningitis are group B *Streptococcus*, *E. coli*, *Listeria*, *H. influenzae*, *S. pneumoniae*, or *Neisseria meningitidis*.
- In children 3 months to 6 years old, the usual organisms that cause bacterial meningitis are *S. pneumoniae*, *H. influenzae*, *N. meningitidis*, *Salmonella* species, and group A *Streptococcus*.
- In children aged 7 years and older, the usual organisms are *S. pneumoniae*, *N. meningitides*, *Listeria monocytogenes*, and aerobic gram-negative bacilli.

3. Pathology

- An inflammation of the leptomeninges.
- May develop rapidly over several hours with sepsis and brain edema.

4. Clinical Features

- Preceded by several days of upper respiratory tract symptoms.
- Generally appear uncomfortable and look toxic.

a. Infants (<1 Year)

- May be nonspecific.
- Fever.
- Restlessness.
- Irritability (especially increased irritability when being handled).
- Inconsolable crying.
- Poor feeding.
- Emesis.
- Diarrhea.
- Lethargy.
- Decreased tone.

- Respiratory distress.
- Bulging fontanelle (late finding).
- Seizures.
- Neck stiffness, Kernig and Brudzinski signs are not reliable in children <18 months old.

  b. **Children > 18 Months**
- Fever.
- Headache.
- Nausea.
- Vomiting.
- Alterations of consciousness (due to increased intracranial pressure).
- Lethargy.
- Photophobia.
- Nuchal rigidity.
- Seizures.
- Positive Brudzinski sign (involuntary lower extremity flexion elicited with passive neck flexion).
- Positive Kernig sign (pain elicited with passive knee extension).
- Focal neurologic signs.
- Petechial or purpuric lesions most commonly seen with *N. meningitidis*.

5. **Diagnostic Studies**
- Blood cultures × 2, CBC with differential, and complete metabolic profile.
- LP should be performed in every child if bacterial meningitis is suspected.
- CT scan of head before LP if contraindications exist.
- Relative contraindications to LP:
  - Hemodynamic instability (shock or respiratory difficulty).
  - Evidence of mass lesion or increased intracranial pressure, altered pupillary reactions, bradycardia, hypotension, apnea, or posturing.
  - Known bleeding disorder.
  - Infection overlying the LP site (cellulitis).
- If a contraindication exists in a patient with clinical suspicion of meningitis, give antibiotics immediately.
- Cerebrospinal fluid (CSF) examination should include cell count with differential, glucose level, protein level, culture, and gram stain.
  - CSF findings: WBC with increased neutrophils, normal or decreased glucose, increased protein, and positive gram stain.

6. **Management**
- ABCs always first.
- O$_2$ (100% nonrebreather), ECG monitor.
- IV access.
- If truly bacterial meningitis, administer dexamethasone, 0.15 mg per kg IV either before or immediately after the initial antibiotic dose.

- Administer antimicrobial therapy immediately after LP (if CT required first, immediately after blood cultures) based on the child's age and the most likely pathogens.
- Infants <3 months, cefotaxime or ceftriaxone and ampicillin.
- Infants <3 months, ceftriaxone, cefotaxime, or ampicillin plus gentamicin.
- Treat seizures aggressively with anticonvulsants (specifically, lorazepam, phenytoin, and phenobarbital).
- Supportive care.
- Prompt hospitalization, ideally in an intensive care unit.

7. **Prognosis**
- Mortality ranges from 0% to 15%.
- Neurologic sequelae common, including hearing loss, seizures, mental disability, and spasticity/paresis.

C. **Febrile Seizure**

1. **Epidemiology**
- Most common seizure disorder in children under 5 years of age.
- Prevalence: 2% to 5% in the United States.
- Rarely occurs before 3 months or after 5 years (peak onset: 12–18 months of age).
- Spontaneously remits without specific therapy.
- Febrile seizures may represent a serious underlying acute infectious disease (i.e., sepsis and bacterial meningitis).

2. **Etiology**
- Always look for the underlying cause (i.e., URI, OM, and accidental overdose).

3. **Risk Factors for Occurrence of a First Febrile Seizure**
- Two or more of the following, and the patient has a 30% chance of a febrile seizure:
  - First-degree relative with febrile seizures.
  - Second-degree relative with febrile seizures.
  - Slow development as judged by parents.
  - Attendance at day care.

4. **Clinical Features**
- Febrile seizures seem to be associated with a rapidly rising temperature (core temperature to 39° C, or 102.2° F).
- **Febrile seizures characteristics:**
  - Simple:
    - Typically generalized tonic–clonic lasting a few seconds to <15 minutes.
    - Usually benign and require no treatment.
    - Most common.
  - Complex:
    - Typically tonic–clonic lasting >15 minutes.
    - Usually denotes high-risk features (i.e., focal onset, postictal neurologic abnormalities,

prior neurologic or developmental abnormalities, or family history of epilepsy).
- Usually associated with a URI (i.e., viral syndrome, OM, pharyngitis, and adenitis).
- Meningitis must be ruled out.

5. **Diagnostic Studies**
   - Spinal tap (LP) may be considered on children <18 months despite a low positive yield; close observation in the emergency department for older children may negate the necessity to perform a spinal tap on them.
   - EEG for complicated/complex seizures.
   - CBC may help rule in bacteremia.

6. **Management**
   - Always ABCs first.
   - **If active seizure:**
     - IV benzodiazepines (Diazepam/Lorazepam), if no IV access buccal midazolam is effective.
     - O_2.
     - Glucose for children <3 years old, 25% dextrose at 2 mL/kg/dose IV slowly.
     - Three years or older, 50% dextrose at 1 mL/kg/dose IV slowly.
   - **If currently febrile:**
     - Acetaminophen 10 to 15 mg per kg.
     - Ibuprofen 5 to 10 mg per kg.
     - Tepid baths.
     - Sponging.
     - Prophylactic anticonvulsants are not indicated in the uncomplicated febrile seizure patient.
     - Antiepileptics have no effect on febrile seizures.

7. **Prognosis**
   - A uniformly excellent prognosis.
   - Recurrence rate 30% to 35%.
   - Rarely develops into epilepsy.
   - Children presenting with high-risk features (i.e., complex seizures) are at a greater risk for recurrent afebrile seizures or epilepsy.

XI. Genitourinary System

A. Urinary Tract Infection

1. **Epidemiology**
   - Estimated 8% girls/2% boys will have a UTI during childhood.
   - Girls >6 months have UTIs far more commonly than boys.
   - Uncircumcised boys <3 months have more UTIs than girls. Circumcision reduces the risk of UTI in boys. The density of distal urethral and periurethral bacterial colonization with uropathogenic bacteria correlates with the risk of UTI in children.

2. **Pathology**
   - Ascending infections are the most common.

- Adhesions present on the fimbria of uropathogenic bacteria allow colonization of the uroepithelium in the urethra and bladder.
- Uncoordinated relaxation of the urethral sphincter during voiding leads to incomplete emptying of the bladder, increasing the risk of bacterial colonization.

3. **Etiology**
   - Most commonly *E. coli* (>85%).
   - *Klebsiella*.
   - *Proteus*.
   - Less frequently, *Enterococcus* or coagulase-negative staphylococci.

4. **Risk Factors**
   - Constipation.
   - Neurogenic bladder.
   - Poor perineal hygiene.
   - Structural abnormalities of the urinary tract.
   - Catheterization.
   - Instrumentation of the urinary tract.
   - Sexual activity.

5. **Clinical Features**
   - Newborns and infants:
     - Fever, poor feeding, irritability, vomiting, FTT, and sepsis. Suprapubic tenderness, strong, foul-smelling or cloudy urine may be noted.
   - Preschool children:
     - May have abdominal or flank pain, vomiting, fever, urinary frequency, dysuria, urgency, or enuresis.
   - School-aged children:
     - Frequency, dysuria, urgency, fever, vomiting, flank pain, and costovertebral tenderness.

6. **Laboratory/Diagnostic Studies**
   - UA and culture are difficult in children.
   - For toilet-trained, cooperative, older children, a midstream, clean-catch method is satisfactory.
   - For infants and young children, bladder catheterization or suprapubic collection is necessary.
   - Bagged urine specimens are helpful only if negative.
   - Gold standard for diagnosis remains the culture and sensitivity.
   - Blood urea nitrogen (BUN) and serum creatinine concentration should be measured to assess renal function.
   - Routine ultrasound of the kidneys: to detect renal or perirenal abscesses or obstruction of the kidneys.
   - Voiding cystourethrogram: urologic abnormality due to weak stream, dribbling, or perineal abnormalities.

7. **Management**
   - Children <3 months of age, or with dehydration, toxicity, or sepsis should be admitted to the hospital and treated with parenteral antimicrobials.

- Uncomplicated cystitis can be treated preferably with a third-generation cephalosporin for 7 to 10 days instead of amoxicillin, first-generation cephalosporins, or trimethoprim–sulfamethoxazole due to the high *E. coli* resistance.
- Seriously ill children are initially treated parenterally with a third-generation cephalosporin or aminoglycoside.
- Sexually active teenagers use fluoroquinolones such as ciprofloxacin and levofloxacin for 3 days because it is cost-effective.

XII. Dermatologic System

A. Diaper Dermatitis ("Diaper Rash")

1. **Etiology**
   - *Candida albicans* colonization.
   - Due to prolonged contact of the skin with urine and feces.

2. **Pathology**
   - Inability of newborns to control candidal infections is related to relative impairment of specific and nonspecific host–defense mechanisms.
   - Urea and intestinal enzymes from urine and feces acting as an irritant.

3. **Clinical Features**
   - Found in the regions of the body where warmth and moisture lead to maceration of the skin or mucous membranes.
   - Beefy red erythema with elevated margins located in the skin folds.
   - Satellite red lesions.
   - Occasionally, pustules, erythematous papules, and vesicles may be seen.
   - Also seen in the axillary, neck, inguinal, and infra-mammary skin folds in adolescents.

4. **Diagnostic Studies**
   - Potassium hydroxide (KOH) examination: positive for budding yeast hyphae.

5. **Management**
   - Topical therapy using nystatin, miconazole (Monistat), or clotrimazole (Lotrimin) applied four times a day results in complete resolution within 3 to 4 days.
   - Educate the caregivers about proper hygiene (i.e., changing diapers more frequently and letting the patient "air out" between changings).
   - Long-standing dermatitis may benefit from application of zinc oxide and imidazole as a barrier cream with each diaper change.

REVIEW QUESTIONS

1. A mother reports that her infant has been having episodes of crying spells in which he appears to be breathing deeply and rapidly and his lips turn blue. On PE, you note a systolic ejection murmur along the left sternal border that radiates to the back. On CXR, which of the following would you expect to find?
   a) Boot-shaped heart leads to answer.
   b) Course interstitial markings in lungs bilaterally.
   c) Pleural effusion.
   d) Kerley B lines.

2. Which of the following is a LEAST likely clinical manifestation of cystic fibrosis:
   a) Failure to thrive
   b) Steatorrhea
   c) Productive cough
   d) Pernicious anemia

3. Neonatal jaundice is considered pathologic when which of the following is true?
   a) Onset of jaundice is 48 hours after birth.
   b) Jaundice is present in breastfeeding child 6 days after birth.
   c) Hyperbilirubinemia is noted on labs.
   d) Onset of jaundice is 8 hours after birth.

4. On examination of a 25-month-old child, you note leukocoria and mild strabismus. What is the most appropriate next step?
   a) Refer patient to pediatric neurologist for evaluation of cranial nerve deficit immediately.
   b) Monitor patient every 6 months for improvement.
   c) Instruct parent that patient will need glasses prior to grade school entrance.
   d) Refer to ophthalmologist for evaluation immediately.

5. At what age should blood pressure measurements begin in children during routine PEs?
   a) As soon as they are ambulatory
   b) Age 6 or first grade
   c) Age 3
   d) Puberty
   e) Age 10

6. A 5-month-old patient presents to the emergency department with worsening breathing, crying, and a bluish appearance to his lips according to the parents. He has had a "cold" for a few days. The PA suspects possible bronchiolitis from RSV. Which of the following would be indications to hospitalize this patient?
   a) Bluish lips
   b) If the baby was born prematurely
   c) Inconsolable crying
   d) Oxygen saturation < 95%

7. Parents bring in their 25-month-old child to the emergency department because they are worried about his behavior. He does not seem to be interested in playing with other children, avoids eye contact, and gets very emotional when his toys are taken from the places where he likes to keep them. Upon further questioning, you discover he did not start speaking in full single words until a few months ago. Given his presentation, what is your initial recommendation?

   a) Order comprehensive metabolic panel (CMP) and endocrine panel to evaluate growth hormone and thyroid-stimulating hormone (TSH) level.
   b) Send child to pediatric neurologist for EEG.
   c) Order Lyme-specific IgM and IgG tests.
   d) Administer Modified Checklist for Autism in Toddlers (M-CHAT) and refer to psychologist/psychiatrist for evaluation.

ANSWERS TO REVIEW QUESTIONS

1. **Answer: A**. Tetralogy of Fallot presents with a systolic ejection murmur loudest at left sternal border caused by blood flow across a narrowed right ventricular outflow tract, and episodic crying with deep breathing in which the patient may become hypercyanotic (aka Tet spell). The major cardiac deficits are pulmonary stenosis, RVH, an overriding aorta, and VSD. Interstitial markings are seen with pulmonary edema and pneumonitis, as well as with chronic interstitial lung diseases. Pleural effusions can be seen with CHF and pneumonia, and are classified as transudative or exudative. Kerley B lines are a sign of interstitial pulmonary edema associated commonly with CHF.

2. **Answer: D**. FTT, steatorrhea, and productive cough all suggest a diagnosis of CF. Pernicious anemia is not associated with CF, iron deficiency in infants can be a presenting sign.

3. **Answer: D**. Jaundice within the first 24 hours of life is considered pathologic. Jaundice will typically appear 24 hours after birth and peak at days 3 to 5 of life. This is an anticipated pattern in physiologic jaundice. Breast milk jaundice is seen in breastfeeding infants and often causes an exaggerated presentation of physiologic jaundice. Breast milk jaundice usually peaks between days 4 to 16 of life. Hyperbilirubinemia is present in both physiologic and pathologic jaundice.

4. **Answer: D**. Immediate referral is necessary because this child has signs suggesting retinoblastoma. Strabismus can be associated with extraocular muscle deficits (e.g., oculomotor nerve palsy), whereas leukocoria is a finding on retinal examination and is not associated with a cranial nerve deficit. Monitoring is not appropriate; while some strabismus is not uncommon in children (infants up to about 2 months old), any strabismus persisting at 25 months should be assessed by an ophthalmologist. Furthermore, leukocoria is a concerning finding that needs investigation. The recommended answer C is not appropriate without consult from pediatric ophthalmologist.

5. **Answer: C**. According to the American Academy of Family Physicians (AAFP), children should be screened for elevated blood pressure annually beginning at age 3. Under age 13, hypertension is defined as blood pressure in the 95th percentile or higher for age, height, and sex.

6. **Answer: B**. According to AAFP, these are the indications for hospitalization in children with RSV bronchiolitis: age <3 months, gestational age at birth of <34 weeks, cardiopulmonary disease or immunodeficiencies, respiratory rate higher than 70 breaths per minute, lethargic appearance wheezing and respiratory distress associated with oxygen, saturation below 92% on room air, hypercarbia, atelectasis, or consolidation on CXR (see https://www.aafp.org/afp/2004/0115/p325.html).

7. **Answer: D**. This child has symptoms and signs of ASD, including lack of interest in playing and lack of eye contact (social finding), late use of single words (communication finding), and emotional impulsivity when his routine is disturbed. Upon further assessment, this child may also show signs of self-stimulating behavior such as rubbing and scratching (repetitive finding). These are the classic dimensions in which ASD is diagnosed. Given the abovementioned symptoms, the clinician has enough information to illicit further screening/referral to a psychiatrist/psychologist. The M-CHAT is a common and standard screening tool with a clear cutoff range for toddlers with suspected ASD. It is completed by the parents in the setting of a primary care office visit. Growth hormone deficiency in children may have associated behavioral changes; however, the child will also have signs such as short stature and/or poor growth velocity. A CMP would contribute little to the diagnosis suspected in this case. EEG is not an initial test for children with suspected ASD. An EEG and other tests such as MRI are reserved for children with a history of language regression at age 4 years or those suspected of seizure disorder. The clinical presentation of Lyme disease (fever, nausea, vomiting, arthralgia, and erythema migrans) is not present here.

SELECTED REFERENCES

American Academy of Pediatrics Task Force on Sudden Infant Death Syndrome. The changing concept of sudden infant death syndrome: diagnostic coding shifts, controversies regarding the sleeping environment, and new variables to consider in reducing risk. *Pediatrics*. 2005;116:1245.

Garcia-Prats JA. Clinical features and diagnosis of meconium aspiration syndrome. In: Kim MS, ed. *UpToDate*. 2017. https://www.uptodate.com/contents/clinical-features-and-diagnosis-of-meconium-aspiration-syndrome. Accessed May 5, 2018.

Goldenring JM, Rosen DS. Getting into adolescent heads: an essential update. *Contemp Pediatr*. 2004;21:64–90.

Hagan J, Shaw J, Duncan P. *Bright Futures: Guidelines for Health Supervision of Infants, Children, and Adolescents: Pocket Guide*. Itasca, IL: American Academy of Pediatrics; 2017.

Hay W, Levin M, Deterding R, Abzug M. *Current Diagnosis and Treatment Pediatrics*. 23rd ed. New York, NY: McGraw-Hill Education; 2016.

McKee-Garrett TM. Assessment of the newborn infant. In: Kim MS, ed. *UpToDate*. 2018. https://www.uptodate.com/contents/assessment-of-the-newborn-infant. Accessed May 5, 2018.

McKee-Garrett TM. Overview of the routine management of the healthy newborn infant. In: Kim MS, ed. *UpToDate*. 2018. https://www.uptodate.com/contents/overview-of-the-routine-management-of-the-healthy-newborn-infant. Accessed May 5, 2018.

Wessel MA, Cobb JC, Jackson EB, Harris GS Jr, Detwiler AC. Paroxysmal fussing in infancy, sometimes called colic. *Pediatrics*. 1954;14:421–435.

INDEX

Note: Page numbers followed by *f* indicate figures; those followed by *t* indicate tables